Lippincott Q&A Review for

NCLEX-RN®

TWELFTH EDITION

Lippincott Q&A Review for

NCLEX-RN®

TWELFTH EDITION

Diane M. Billings, EdD, RN, FAAN, ANEF
Chancellor's Professor Emeritus
Indiana University School of Nursing
Indianapolis, Indiana

Desiree Hensel, PhD, RN, PCNS-BC, CNE
Associate Professor of Nursing
Indiana University School of Nursing
Bloomington, Indiana

. Wolters Kluwer

Philadelphia • Baltimore • New York • London
Buenos Aires • Hong Kong • Sydney • Tokyo

Acquisitions Editor: Renee A. Gagliardi
Associate Content Strategist: Bernadette Enneg
Production Project Manager: Priscilla Crater
Design Coordinator: Stephen Druding
Art Director: Jennifer Clements
Manufacturing Coordinator: Kathleen Brown
Marketing Manager: Sarah Schuessler
Prepress Vendor: SPi Global

12th edition

9 8 7 6 5 4 3 2 1

Printed in China

Library of Congress Cataloging-in-Publication Data
    Names: Billings, Diane McGovern, author. | Hensel, Desiree, author.
    Title: Lippincott Q & A review for NCLEX-RN / Diane M. Billings, Desiree Hensel.
    Other titles: Lippincott's Q & A review for NCLEX-RN | Lippincott Q and A review for NCLEX-RN | Q & A review for NCLEX-RN
    Description: Twelfth edition. | Philadelphia : Wolters Kluwer, [2017] | Preceded by Lippincott's Q & A review for NCLEX-RN / Diane Billings, Desiree Hensel. 11th ed. c2013. | Includes bibliographical references.
    Identifiers: LCCN 2015040490 | ISBN 9781469886619
    Subjects: | MESH: Nursing Care | Examination Questions Classification: LCC RT55 | NLM WY 18.2 | DDC 610.73076—dc23 LC record available at http://lccn.loc.gov/2015040490

LWW.com

Contributors

Diane M. Billings, EdD, RN, FAAN, ANEF
Chancellor's Professor Emeritus
Indiana University School of Nursing
Indianapolis, Indiana

Ann Butt, MSN, RN
Clinical Assistant Professor
Department of Nursing
Boise State University School of Nursing
Boise, Idaho

Desiree Hensel, PhD, RNC-NIC, CNE
Associate Professor
Indiana University School of Nursing
Bloomington, Indiana

Paula Kelly, RN, MSN
Faculty, School of Nursing
Memorial University of Newfoundland
St. John's, Newfoundland and Labrador, Canada

Cindy Kohtz, RN, EdD, CNE
Professor
Saint Francis Medical Center College of Nursing
Peoria, Illinois

Nicole Lewis-Power, RN, BN, MN
Lecturer
School of Nursing
Memorial University of Newfoundland
St. John's, Newfoundland and Labrador, Canada

Meg Moorman, PhD, RN, WHNP
Clinical Assistant Professor
Indiana University School of Nursing
Indianapolis, Indiana

Cheryl Pollard, PN, RN, BScN, MN, PhD
Assistant Professor
Bachelor of Science in Nursing Program
Faculty of Health and Community Studies
MacEwan University
Edmonton, Alberta, Canada

Julie Poore, RN, MSN, DNP
Clinical Assistant Professor
Family Health Nursing
Indiana University School of Nursing
Indianapolis, Indiana

Wendy Zeiher, MSN, RN, CNOR
Clinical Assistant Professor
Department of Adult Health
Indiana University School of Nursing
Indianapolis, Indiana

Contributors to the Previous Edition

Patricia Allen, MSN, RN
Diane M. Billings, EdD, RN, FAAN
Amy Brauner, RN, MN
Ann Butt, MS, RN
Kelley Connor, RN, MSN, CNE
Debi Drake, MSN, RN
Desiree Hensel, PhD, RNC-NIC, CNE
Margie Hull, MEd, MSN, ACNS-BC, RN, CDE
Patricia Lazare, MSN, RNC
Valerie N. Markley, MSN, PMHCNS-BC
Havoi Patel, MBBS, MS
Julie Poore, RN, MSN
Lee Schwecke, EdD, RN
Evelyn Stephenson, MSN, RNC-NIC, NNP-BC
Sharon Vinten, MSN, WHNP, CNE
Sandra Wood, MSN, RN

Reviewers

OB & PEDS REVIEWERS

Sally Hill Boyster, MS, RNC-OB, CNE
Coordinator/Professor of Nursing Science
Rose State College
Midwest City, Oklahoma

Nancy Fleming, RN, HBScN, MAEd
Professor
Confederation College
Thunder Bay, Ontario, Canada

Krista Kamstra-Cooper, RN, BScN, MN, CRN(C)
Professor of Nursing
Centennial College
Toronto, Ontario, Canada

Rochelle Kuhn, RN, MS, NP
Pediatric Nursing Instructor
Aria Health School of Nursing
Trevose, Pennsylvania

Jeanette Murray, RN, BScN, MA
Educator Emerita
Thompson Rivers University
Kamloops, British Columbia

Linda A. Strong, MSN, RN, CPNP, CNE
Associate Professor
Cuyahoga Community College
Cleveland, Ohio

MED SURG REVIEWERS

Eleanor Benterud, RN, BN, MN
Healthcare Consultant
Calgary, Alberta, Canada

Karen E. Furlong, RN, MN, PhD
Senior Teaching Associate
Department of Nursing and Health Sciences
University of New Brunswick
Saint John, New Brunswick, Canada

Deborah A. Green, MSN, RN, BC
Nursing Education Specialist
Indiana University Health North Hospital
Carmel, Indiana

Verna C. Pangman, RN, MEd, MN
Senior Instructor
College of Nursing, Faculty of Health Sciences
Winnipeg, Manitoba, Canada

Lisa Peden, BSN, MSN
Associate Professor of Nursing
Dalton State College
Dalton, Georgia

Toni Scialdo, RN, MsED, MSN, PhD, CNE
Faculty
Education Affiliates
Port St. Lucie, Florida

Susan K. Tucker, DNP, RN, CNE
Program Director, Nursing Education
Gadsden State Community College
Gadsden, Alabama

Judith Young, DNP, CNE
Clinical Assistant Professor
Department of Community and Health Systems
Indiana University School of Nursing
Indianapolis, Indiana

MENTAL HEALTH REVIEWERS

Edith Claros, PhD, MSN, RN
Assistant Dean and Associate Professor of Nursing
MCPHS University
Boston, Massachusetts

Norma Melanson, BScN, MAEd, MN, PhD
Full Professor
Université de Moncton
Moncton, New Brunswick, Canada

Toni Scialdo, RN, MsED, MSN, PhD, CNE
Faculty
Education Affiliates
Port St. Lucie, Florida

Bernadine Wojtowicz, RN, MSc(N)
NESA BN Programs Co-Chair
University of Lethbridge
Lethbridge, Alberta, Canada

FACULTY MARKET REVIEWERS

Monica Buchanon, RN, BSN, MSN, ED, (PhD ABD)
NLN Ambassador to Education
Director of Nursing
College America
Littleton, Colorado

Mary Burns-Coral, MSN, RN, CNE
Professional Nursing Faculty
Washtenaw Community College
Ann Arbor, Michigan

Rosalie Griffith, RN, MSN, MEd
Nursing Recruitment and Retention Specialist
Chesapeake College
Wye Mills, Maryland

Krista Kamstra-Cooper, RN, BScN, MN, CRN(C)
Professor of Nursing
Centennial College
Toronto, Ontario, Canada

Lenora Marcellus, RN, BSN, MN, PhD
Associate Professor
School of Nursing
University of Victoria
Victoria, British Columbia, Canada

Mary Moseley, EdD, MN, BSN
Professor of Nursing
Nursing Coordinator
Northern Virginia Community College
Springfield, Virginia

Sandra Reed Wilson, MSN, RN, ACNS-BC
Program Coordinator
Crowder College
Neosho, Missouri

STUDENT/RECENT GRADUATE MARKET REVIEWERS

Sierra Emrich
Richmond, Kentucky
Marianne Rowland
Toronto, Ontario, Canada

Sandra Wong, BScN, RN
Toronto, Ontario, Canada

Preface

Introduction to the Q&A Review for NCLEX-RN®

This exam review book and its accompanying study resources available through thePoint have been developed to help you prepare for the National Council Licensing Examination for Registered Nurses (NCLEX-RN®). You will also find this book helpful for review when preparing for course exams, final exams, NCLEX-RN® assessment exams, or other standardized or competency exams.

Features

This edition has been prepared for students who will take the NCLEX-RN® in the United States or in the territories and provinces in Canada. The revision was guided by an editorial board composed of faculty from schools of nursing in both the United States and Canada, with every item written and reviewed by clinical experts in each country.

Features new to this edition include the following:

- Table of definitions of terms used for health providers and healthcare terminology for which meaning and use vary in the United States and Canada.
- List of laboratory values test-takers are expected to know before sitting for the exam.
- Presentation of measurements in test items in both U.S. Standard Units and in metric measurements; presentation of laboratory values in U.S. Standard Units and in International System of Units.
- All test items reviewed for appropriate nursing practice in both the United States and Canada.
- Data-driven item revision, with each item evaluated based on item analysis provided by *Lippincott® PassPoint* data.
- Six comprehensive practice examinations, each of which has been designed to resemble the testing format and content of the NCLEX-RN® test plan; these tests are of varying lengths, including the minimum (75) and maximum (265) possible questions on the licensing exam.
- Table of risk factors for not passing the NCLEX-RN® exam and related study strategies.

- *Content Mastery and Test-Taking Skill Self-Analysis* tear-out sheet to assess exam readiness; this tool is based on current research about effective study skills.
- All questions edited for readability and cultural appropriateness.

Study Resources

This review book includes multiple resources that you can use in any combination to meet your own study and test preparation plans:

- More than 6,000 test questions in the book and accompanying online resource, using all the different formats of question types found on the actual NCLEX (multiple choice, multiple response, hot-spot, fill-in-the-blank, drag-and-drop/ordered response, chart/exhibit, as well as graphic, audio, and video inclusion questions).
- Detailed rationales for correct and incorrect answers to accompany every practice question.
- An online quiz program that provides you with ample opportunity to experience test taking using computer-administered questions and allows you to customize tests for specific review and practice.
- Questions written for all clinical areas of nursing (childbearing family and neonate; nursing care of infants, children, and adolescents; nursing care of adults with medical and surgical health problems; and nursing care of clients with psychiatric disorders and mental health problems).
- Questions organized by major health problems in the United States and Canada to facilitate review for course-specific exams.
- Questions coded by client needs to ensure practice in *all* areas of the NCLEX-RN® test plan.
- Questions coded by cognitive level to guide study and test taking at higher levels of the cognitive domain.
- Questions emphasizing integrative processes (nursing process, caring, communication and documentation, teaching/learning, and culture and spirituality) included on the NCLEX-RN® test plan.

- Questions with teaching feedback and rationales for both correct and incorrect answers.
- Questions written at higher levels of the cognitive domain (application, analysis, synthesis, evaluation, and creation).
- Questions emphasizing clinical decision making, clinical judgment, prioritization, delegation, and management of care.
- Questions to provide practice for calculating drug dosages, intravenous drip rates, intake and output, and other questions requiring calculation and reporting of a numerical response to the question.
- Questions emphasizing pharmacology, medication safety, complementary and alternative modalities, and the nurse's role in administering pharmacotherapeutic agents.
- Questions emphasizing current nursing practice in the areas of client safety, managing care quality, home care, health promotion, care of the older adult, cancer nursing, end-of-life care, perioperative care, community health nursing, and emergency and disaster nursing.
- Questions about managing care quality and safety at the end of each chapter.
- An entire chapter that explains the various test question formats and strategies for answering each type of test item and at each level of the cognitive domain.
- A detailed description of the NCLEX-RN® test plan in effect April 1, 2016.
- A study plan and checklist to guide systematic preparation for the licensing examination.
- A *Content Mastery and Test-Taking Skill Self-Analysis* worksheet to help you identify your own reasons for not answering test items correctly. The "tear-out" worksheet can be copied and used with each test in this book; reviewing all worksheets will help you analyze the reasons for not answering test questions correctly and revise your study plan accordingly.
- Information about developing study skills, taking tests, and managing test anxiety.
- Tips for studying from students who have successfully passed the NCLEX-RN® exam.
- Addresses, telephone numbers, and websites for the National Council of State Boards of Nursing, Inc. and each state board of nursing.
- Bibliography of reference books.

Organization of the Book

The review book is organized in three sections. Each section is designed to build on the previous section.

The first section of the book provides information about the licensing exam and how to prepare for and take high-stakes examinations. A full chapter is devoted to explaining the various types of test question formats and cognitive levels of questions used on the licensing exam; the chapter also provides examples of all types and levels of questions and strategies for answering them.

In the second section of the book, there are four major units—nursing care of the childbearing family and their neonate; nursing care of infants, children, and adolescents; nursing care of adults with medical and surgical health problems; and nursing care of clients with psychiatric disorders and mental health problems. Within each unit, chapter tests are grouped according to health problems and include questions that are matched to the NCLEX-RN® test plan. At the end of each chapter, there is a section of questions about managing client safety and quality care. These questions are essential to test your understanding of important concepts about patient safety and quality. Because the test questions in this section are organized around health problems, this section is ideal for use when preparing for teacher-made or commercially prepared tests that focus on specific content in your curriculum.

The third section of the book contains six comprehensive exams written to simulate the NCLEX-RN® by placing test items in random order of content area. Each test presents a variety of situations commonly encountered in nursing practice and includes test questions from all components of the NCLEX-RN® test plan and all types of questions used on the licensing exam (except video and audio questions, which are found only on thePoint).

thePoint

Additionally, this review package includes access to thePoint, where you will find more than 1,300 practice questions. These questions will allow you to practice with audio and video questions, so be sure to use this feature of this Q&A Review Book.

The questions on thePoint can be used in several ways. For example, you may take a test in the four content areas, arrange a test to present questions in random order, or select questions for particular review and practice. thePoint simulates the actual NCLEX-RN® exam by formatting questions on a computer screen and requiring you to use the keyboard and mouse to enter answers to the questions. It also features a pop-up calculator for use in answering questions that require you to calculate drug doses and drip rates for intravenous infusions.

PassPoint

Lippincott PassPoint NCLEX-RN | Powered by prepU is a separate personalized and comprehensive learning system designed to help students fully prepare for the NCLEX-RN®. *PassPoint* provides students with multiple outlets for individualized review, quizzing, and practice, helping to pinpoint areas requiring additional focus. As students take Practice Quizzes, *PassPoint* quickly determines current knowledge and delivers questions of just the right difficulty. Question data based on actual student usage (e.g., difficulty ratings) from *PassPoint* were collected on the questions in this review book. Usage data helped to ensure items were fairly and appropriately constructed and focused on the most critical topics to master for NCLEX success.

Using This Review Package for Preparing for Nursing Exams

We suggest that you begin your review by using the practice exams in the book to identify areas of strength and areas in which you need further study. Each exam contains specific questions written in the style of the NCLEX-RN®. Answers include rationales for both correct and incorrect answer options to reinforce learning. You may wish to score the results of each practice test and identify areas in which you need further review. To evaluate your results after completing each exam, divide the number of your correct responses by the total number of questions in the test and multiply by 100. For example, if you answered 72 of 90 items correctly, you would divide 72 by 90 and multiply by 100, for a result of 80%. If you answered more than 75% of the items in an area correctly, you are most likely prepared to answer questions in that area on the NCLEX-RN®. If you answered fewer than 75% of the

questions correctly, you need to determine why. Did you answer incorrectly because of lack of content knowledge or because you did not read carefully? As you take each test, use the *Content Mastery and Test-Taking Skill Self-Analysis* worksheet to tally your reasons for not answering the test questions correctly. Understanding the reason for why you are not answering the questions correctly or which content area is most difficult for you is the **most** important aspect of preparing for any exam. Use this information to guide your study.

After reviewing the specific content areas in the practice exams, take the comprehensive exams. These exams more realistically reflect the NCLEX-RN® because each test presents a variety of situations commonly encountered in nursing practice and across all clinical disciplines. Underlying knowledge, skills, and abilities related to the basic sciences, fundamentals of nursing, pharmacology and other therapeutic measures, communicable diseases, legal and ethical considerations, and nutrition are included in items as needed to plan nursing care for individual clients or groups of clients. The comprehensive exams also include test items related to client safety and care quality. These exams are designed with varying numbers of questions so you can time yourself and determine how long it is taking you to complete the minimum and maximum number of possible questions on the licensing exam.

And don't forget to check the online resources available at http://thepoint.lww.com/Billings12e. The study tips and study plan will provide you with a foundation to begin your exam preparation.

Acknowledgments

This book has been developed with the expertise of an Advisory Board of faculty from schools of nursing in the United States and Canada along with a team of internationally recognized test item writers and reviewers. We appreciate the clinical expertise of these faculty and their willingness to develop and review the test questions in this book. We have been most fortunate to have excellent support from Renee Gagliardi, Senior Digital Product Manager, and Bernadette Enneg, Associate Content Strategist, whose wisdom, managerial skills, and editorial eyes have helped us prepare this book. Many future nurses in both the United States and Canada, preparing for NCLEX, will reap the benefits of their dedication to making this the highest quality review book possible. And, not least of all, we thank our husbands, Richard and Tom, for their ongoing support as we worked on this project.

Diane M. Billings, EdD, RN, FAAN, ANEF
Chancellor's Professor Emeritus
Indiana University School of Nursing
Indianapolis, Indiana

Desiree Hensel, PhD, RN, PCNS-BC, CNE
Associate Professor of Nursing
Indiana University School of Nursing
Bloomington, Indiana

About the Authors

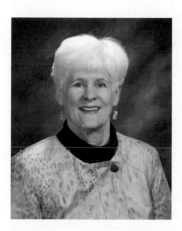

Diane M. Billings, EdD, RN, FAAN, award-winning author and nursing educator, offers more than 40 years' experience teaching nursing from the associate degree through doctoral programs, with a special focus on the NCLEX-RN® examination. Dr. Billings' NCLEX-RN® experience includes developing and teaching NCLEX-RN® review courses, integrating computer-based licensing exam review programs into nursing curricula, and designing NCLEX-RN® test questions. A nationally recognized test-item writer, her NCLEX-RN® preparation books have helped thousands of students pass the NCLEX-RN® exam. Dr. Billings is the recipient of the National League for Nursing's Award for Outstanding Leadership in Nursing Education, the President's Award for Distinguished Teaching at Indiana University, and the Founders Award for Excellence in Teaching from Sigma Theta Tau, International. She is a fellow and Living Legend in the American Academy of Nursing.

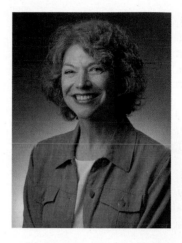

Desiree Hensel, PhD, RN, PCNS-BC, CNE, is an associate professor at Indiana University School of Nursing with more than 10 years of experience teaching pre-licensure students. Her distinct body of research explores the use of innovative teaching strategies to help students acquire the profession's knowledge, skills, and attitudes in both clinical and classroom settings, while more closely examining how nurses define themselves in the 21st century. Dr. Hensel has expertise with mixed-method approaches to evaluate learning outcomes and explore phenomena of interest to the profession of nursing. She has published extensively in top-tier nursing journals and widely disseminated her work in national forums. She has received multiple teaching awards and takes special pride in her work helping students prepare for the NCLEX-RN® exam.

Contents

Part 3 ■ Postreview Tests   865

Appendices   1103

Introduction to the NCLEX-RN® Licensing Examination and Preparation for Test Taking

1 The NCLEX-RN® Licensing Examination

Overview

The National Council Licensure Examination for Registered Nurses (NCLEX-RN®) is administered to graduates of nursing schools in the United States and Canada to test the knowledge, abilities, and skills necessary for entry-level safe and effective nursing practice. The examination is developed by the National Council of State Boards of Nursing, Inc. (NCSBN; ncsbn.org), an organization with representation from all state boards of nursing in the United States and provincial/territorial regulatory bodies in Canada. The same examination is used in all 50 states, the District of Columbia, United States possessions, and Canada. The exam is also administered at international test centers worldwide (National Council of State Boards of Nursing, Inc., 2014). Students who have graduated from pre-licensure programs must pass this examination to meet licensing requirements in the United States and Canada.

The Test Plan

The NCSBN prepares the test plan used to develop the licensing examination. The test plan is based on an analysis of current nursing practice and the skills, abilities, and processes nurses use to provide nursing care.

Practice Analysis: The Foundation of the Test Plan

The NCLEX-RN test plan is based on the results of a practice analysis conducted every 3 years of the entry-level performance of newly licensed registered nurses and on expert judgment provided by members of the National Council's Examination Committee as well as a Job Analysis Panel of Experts. The job analysis asks newly graduated nurses to rank the nursing activities that they perform on a regular basis. The questions used on the test plan, therefore, include those activities that nurses commonly perform. For example, the 2014 RN practice analysis revealed that nursing practice commonly involved activities such as performing procedures necessary to safely admit, transfer, or discharge a client; providing and

receiving reports on assigned clients; and assigning and supervising care provided by others (LPN/VN, unlicensed assistive personnel, other RNs) (National Council of State Boards of Nursing, Inc., 2015).

The NCSBN also used the findings from the practice analysis activity statements to generate knowledge statements, the knowledge needed by newly licensed nurses to provide safe care (National Council of State Boards of Nursing, Inc., 2015). The findings of this second report are used to inform item development for the NCLEX-RN examination.

Test Item Writers

Nurse clinicians and nurse educators volunteer to become item writers. All item writers are approved by the Council of State Boards of Nursing or the provincial/territorial regulatory bodies. Because the item writers come from a variety of geographical areas and practice settings, the test items reflect nursing practice in all parts of the United States and provinces/territories that are using the NCLEX-RN.

Terminology, Measurements, and Laboratory Values Used in This Book

Specific terminology (📖) is used on the licensing exam to be inclusive of the variety of healthcare providers, registered, licensed, and unlicensed assistive personnel (see Table 1.1). Measurements are presented in both U.S. Standard Units and in metric measurements; laboratory values are presented in U.S. Standard Units and in International System of Units (SI units) (see Table 1.1). Students are expected to know a limited list of laboratory values (see Table 1.1). When findings from other laboratory values are included in a test item *in this review book*, information about the value will be provided, for example, if the value is increased or decreased from the normal range (see Table 1.1).

Test Plan Details

Test plans, or test blueprints, are developed to indicate the components and the relative weights of the components that will be tested on an exam. Because

TABLE 1.1
Definitions of Terms, Measurements, and Laboratory Values Used in This Book

Healthcare Personnel

Healthcare Provider (HCP)

- Any person licensed to prescribe medications and treatments. Advanced practice nurses (nurse practitioner, nurse anesthetist), physician assistants, physicians, and surgeons are referred to as healthcare providers.

Licensed Practical/Vocational Nurse (LPN/VN)

- An individual who has completed a state-/province-approved practical or vocational nursing program. This person typically works under the supervision of a registered nurse, advanced practice registered nurse, physician, or other healthcare provider. In the United States, the licensed practical nurse (LPN) must pass the licensing exam offered by the National Council of State Boards of Nursing.

Registered Nurse (RN)

- An individual who has graduated from a state-/province-approved school of nursing and passed the NCLEX-RN examination. This person is licensed by a state/provincial board of nursing to provide client care.

Unlicensed Assistive Personnel (UAP)

- Any unlicensed assistive person, regardless of title, who performs tasks delegated by a nurse. This includes certified nursing aides/assistants (CNAs), patient care assistants (PCAs), patient care technicians (PCTs), state-/province-tested nursing assistants (STNA), nursing assistants-registered (NA/Rs) or certified medication aides/assistants (MA-Cs). Certification of UAPs varies between jurisdictions.

Other Terms

Informed Consent

- Informed consent is a mechanism for communication between a client and a healthcare provider in which the client makes an informed decision about the type of health care, tests, procedures, or treatments he or she is about to receive. There are legal and ethical aspects of informed consent. While each state and province has its own definition of informed consent, in general, the client must be legally able to sign the consent, not be pressured to do so, and must understand the implications of giving the consent. Typically, it is the responsibility of the physician, surgeon, or other healthcare provider who is performing the procedure or treatment to obtain the consent. The nurse's role is to verify that the consent form is signed by the client or designated representative, serve as a witness to the client's signature, document in the nurse's notes that the signature was obtained, and advocate for the client in ensuring the client fully understands the consent.

Medical Record

- The term medical record is used to refer to a "chart," a "health record," "electronic medical record," or an "electronic health record." A medical record is the documentation of health care provided to a client and includes prescriptions, history and physical, laboratory results, miscellaneous reports, imaging results, flow sheets, intake and output records, medication administration record, progress notes, and vital signs.

Rapid Response Team

- A rapid response team is composed of physicians, nurses, hospitalists, and other healthcare providers who are prepared to respond to a situation when a client demonstrates signs of imminent clinical deterioration. The team is called to assess and treat a client with the goal of preventing the need to transfer the client to an intensive care unit or preventing a cardiac arrest. Nurses and healthcare providers may initiate a call to the rapid response team.

Time Out

- A "time out" refers to a protocol for preventing wrong site, wrong procedure, and wrong person surgery. The purpose of a "time out" is to address any discrepancies before the surgery begins or to clarify concerns of any of the surgical team prior to making the incision. This protocol provides an opportunity for nurses and other members of the healthcare team, including the client, to verify the presurgery check list prior to beginning the surgery or invasive procedure.

Measurements

Measurements such as weight, temperature, height, distance, and volume are presented in U.S. Standard Units and metric representation. Examples include the following:
- A client weighs 125 lb (56.7 kg).
- Measurements are rounded to the nearest tenth.
- Blood pressure is presented as mm Hg.

(Continued)

TABLE 1.1

Definitions of Terms, Measurements, and Laboratory Values Used in This Book (*Continued*)

Laboratory Values

Laboratory values are presented in U.S. Standard Units and in the International System of Units (SI units). Examples include the following:

- 140 mEq/L (140 mmol/L)
- A BUN of 26 mg/dL (26 mmol/L)
- Creatinine of 1.2 mg/dL (1.2 μmol/L)

Laboratory Values NCLEX-RN Test Takers Are Expected to Know

Students should know the normal values for these laboratory tests:

- ABGs (pH, PO_2, PCO_2, SaO_2, HCO_3), BUN, cholesterol (total) glucose, hematocrit, hemoglobin, glycosylated hemoglobin ($HgbA_1C$), platelets, potassium, sodium, WBC, creatinine, PT, PTT and APTT, INR.

exams test both content (knowledge) and process (critical thinking, synthesis of information, clinical decision-making), test plans usually have two or three dimensions. The test plan for the NCLEX-RN addresses two components of nursing care: (1) client needs categories and (2) integrated processes, such as the nursing process, caring, communication and documentation, teaching/learning, and culture and spirituality (see Table 1.2). Representative items test knowledge of these components as they relate to specific healthcare situations in all of the four major areas of client needs. The questions developed for the test plan are written to test nursing knowledge and the ability to apply nursing knowledge to client situations.

Client Needs

The health needs of clients are grouped under four broad categories: (1) safe, effective care environment, (2) health promotion and maintenance, (3) psychosocial integrity, and (4) physiologic integrity. Two of these categories include subcategories of related and specified needs (see Table 1.3). The percentage of test items in each subcategory on the NCLEX-RN examination is shown in Figure 1.1. Because candidates receive individualized tests, the percentage of questions any candidate receives from each category varies within a range of ±3%. Understanding the category of client needs is key (🔑) to recognizing the types of questions that are found on the licensing exam and the relative emphasis given to the category based on the percentage of questions from that category on the exam.

Integrated Processes

The NCLEX-RN test plan also is organized according to five integrated processes. These include the nursing process, caring, communication and documentation, teaching/learning, and culture and spirituality (see Table 1.3 and Fig. 1.1).

The Nursing Process

The NCLEX-RN test plan includes questions from all steps of the nursing process. The five phases of the nursing process are (1) assessment, (2) analysis, (3) planning, (4) implementation, and (5) evaluation.

TABLE 1.2

Test Plan Structure

The framework of client needs was selected for the examination because it provides a universal structure for defining nursing actions and competencies and focuses on clients in all settings.

Client Needs

The content of the NCLEX-RN test plan is organized into four major client needs categories. Two of the four categories are divided into subcategories:

A. Safe and Effective Care Environment
   1. Management of care
   2. Safety and infection control
B. Health Promotion and Maintenance
C. Psychosocial Integrity
D. Physiological Integrity
   1. Basic care and comfort
   2. Pharmacological and parenteral therapies
   3. Reduction of risk potential
   4. Physiological adaptation

Integrated Processes

The following processes are fundamental to the practice of nursing and are integrated throughout the client needs categories and subcategories:

- Nursing Process
- Caring
- Communication and Documentation
- Teaching/Learning
- Culture and Spirituality

TABLE 1.3
Overview of Content

All content categories and subcategories reflect client needs across the life span in a variety of settings.

A. Safe, Effective Care Environment
The nurse promotes achievement of client outcomes by providing and directing nursing care that enhances the care delivery setting in order to protect clients and healthcare personnel.

1. *Management of Care*—Providing and directing nursing care that enhances the care delivery setting to protect clients and healthcare personnel. Related content includes but is **not limited** to:
   - Advance Directives/Self-Determination/Life Planning
   - Advocacy
   - Case Management
   - Client Rights
   - Collaboration with Interdisciplinary Team
   - Concepts of Management
   - Confidentiality/Information Security
   - Continuity of Care
   - Assignment, Delegation, and Supervision
   - Establishing Priorities
   - Ethical Practice
   - Informed Consent
   - Information Technology
   - Legal Rights and Responsibilities
   - Organ Donation
   - Performance Improvement (quality improvement)
   - Referrals

2. *Safety and Infection Control*—Protecting clients and healthcare personnel from health and environmental hazards. Related content includes but is **not limited** to:
   - Accident/Error/Injury Prevention
   - Emergency Response Plan
   - Ergonomic Principles
   - Handling Hazardous and Infectious Materials
   - Home Safety
   - Reporting of Incident/Event/Irregular Occurrence/Variance
   - Safe Use of Equipment
   - Security Plan
   - Standard Precautions/Transmission-Based Precautions/Surgical Asepsis
   - Use of Restraints/Safety Devices

B. Health Promotion and Maintenance
The nurse provides and directs nursing care of the client that incorporates the knowledge of expected growth and development principles, prevention and/or early detection of health problems, and strategies to achieve optimal health. Related content includes but is **not limited** to:
   - Aging Process
   - Ante/Intra/Postpartum and Newborn Care
   - Developmental Stages and Transitions
   - Health Promotion/Disease Prevention
   - Health Screening
   - High-Risk Behaviors
   - Lifestyle Choices
   - Self-Care
   - Techniques of Physical Assessment

C. Psychosocial Integrity
The nurse provides and directs nursing care that promotes and supports the emotional, mental, and social well-being of the client experiencing stressful events, as well as clients with acute or chronic mental illness. Related content includes but is **not limited** to:
   - Abuse/Neglect
   - Behavioral Interventions
   - Chemical and Other Dependencies/Substance Use Disorder
   - Coping Mechanisms
   - Crisis Intervention

(Continued)

TABLE 1.3
Overview of Content (*Continued*)

- Cultural Awareness/Cultural Influences on Health
- End-of-Life Care
- Family Dynamics
- Grief and Loss
- Mental Health Concepts
- Religious and Spiritual Influences on Health
- Sensory/Perceptual Alterations
- Stress Management
- Support Systems
- Therapeutic Communication
- Therapeutic Environment

D. Physiological Integrity

The nurse promotes physical health and wellness by providing care and comfort, reducing client risk potential, and managing health alterations.

1. *Basic Care and Comfort*—Providing comfort and assistance in the performance of activities of daily living. Related content includes but is **not limited** to:
   - Assistive Devices
   - Elimination
   - Mobility/Immobility
   - Non-pharmacological Comfort Interventions
   - Nutrition and Oral Hydration
   - Personal Hygiene
   - Rest and Sleep

2. *Pharmacological and Parenteral Therapies*—Providing care related to the administration of medications and parenteral therapies. Related content includes but is **not limited** to:
   - Adverse Effects/Contraindications/Side Effects/Interactions
   - Blood and Blood Products
   - Central Venous Access Devices
   - Dosage Calculation
   - Expected Actions/Outcomes
   - Medication Administration
   - Parenteral/Intravenous Therapies
   - Pharmacological Pain Management
   - Total Parenteral Nutrition

3. *Reduction of Risk Potential*—Reducing the likelihood that clients will develop complications or health problems related to existing conditions, treatments, or procedures. Related content includes but is **not limited** to:
   - Changes/Abnormalities in Vital Signs
   - Diagnostic Tests
   - Laboratory Values
   - Potential for Alterations in Body Systems
   - Potential for Complications of Diagnostic Tests/Treatments/Procedures
   - Potential for Complications from Surgical Procedures and Health Alterations
   - System Specific Assessments
   - Therapeutic Procedures

4. *Physiological Adaptation*—Managing and providing care for clients with acute, chronic, or life-threatening physical health conditions. Related content includes but is **not limited** to:
   - Alterations in Body Systems
   - Fluid and Electrolyte Imbalances
   - Hemodynamics
   - Illness Management
   - Medical Emergencies
   - Pathophysiology
   - Unexpected Response to Therapies

FIGURE 1.1
Distribution of Content

Client Needs Categories

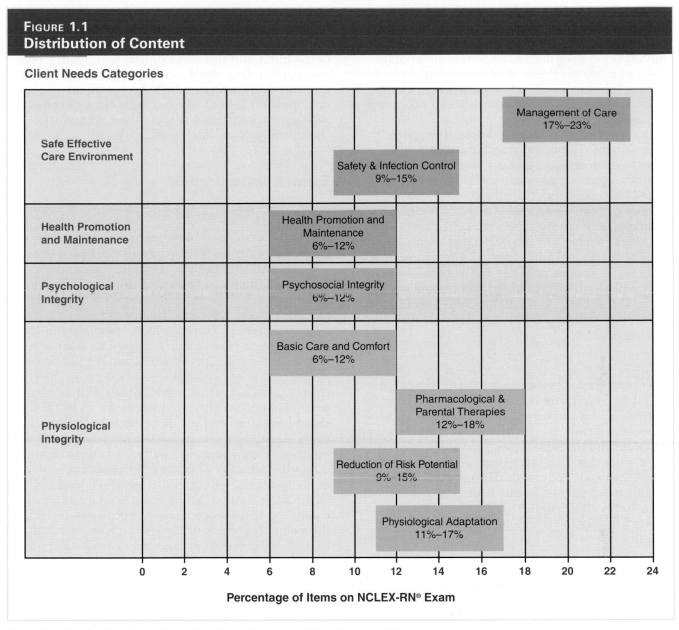

Percentage of Items on NCLEX-RN® Exam

Assessment. Assessment involves establishing a database. The nurse gathers objective and subjective information about the client and then verifies the data and communicates information gained from the assessment.

Analysis. Analysis involves identifying actual or potential healthcare needs or problems based on assessment data. The nurse interprets the data, collects additional data as indicated, and identifies and communicates the client's nursing problem. The nurse also determines the congruency between the client's needs and the ability of the healthcare team members to meet those needs.

Planning. Planning involves setting outcomes and goals for meeting the client's needs and designing strategies to attain them. The nurse determines the goals of care, develops and modifies the plan, collaborates with other health team members for delivery of the client's care, and formulates expected outcomes of nursing interventions.

Implementation. Implementation involves initiating and completing actions necessary to accomplish the defined goals. The nurse organizes and manages the client's care; performs or assists the client in performing activities of daily living;

counsels and teaches the client, significant others, and healthcare team members; and provides care to attain the established client goals. The nurse also provides care to optimize the achievement of the client's healthcare goals; supervises, coordinates, and evaluates delivery of the client's care as provided by nursing staff; and records and exchanges information.

Evaluation. Evaluation determines goal achievement. The nurse compares actual with expected outcomes of therapy, evaluates compliance with prescribed or proscribed therapy, and records and describes the client's response to therapy or care. The nurse also modifies the plan, as indicated, and reorders priorities.

The five phases of the nursing process are equally important. Therefore, each is represented by an equal number of items on the NCLEX-RN test plan, and all phases are integrated throughout the exam. In this book, you will have opportunities to respond to questions involving all five steps of the nursing process.

Caring

The caring process refers to interaction between the nurse, client, and family in a way that conveys mutual respect and trust. The nurse offers encouragement and hope to clients and their families while providing nursing care. Questions about the caring process are threaded throughout the licensing exam to test the candidate's attitudes and values for caring for and about clients. In this book, you will have the opportunity to respond to questions that test your ability to apply the caring process in a variety of situations.

Communication and Documentation

Another element of the licensing exam test plan evaluates the nurse's ability to communicate with clients, families, and health team members. The test also includes questions about documenting nursing care according to standards of nursing practice. In this book, you will be presented with questions that ask you to determine the most effective way to communicate with clients, families, and other health professionals. You will also have the opportunity to respond to questions that require you to select the appropriate information to document or chart.

Teaching/Learning

An important aspect of nursing care is to teach clients and their families about managing their own health status. Nurses also teach other members of the healthcare team. Questions in this book are designed to assist you in answering questions about the teaching and learning process for a variety of clients and healthcare team members.

Culture and Spirituality

Culture and spirituality are integral to person-centered health care and involve the interaction of the nurse and the client (individual, family, or group, including significant others and population) in a way that conveys respect for the client's culture and spiritual beliefs. The nurse assesses the client's self-reported and unique individual preferences and incorporates them into the plan of care.

Exam Administration

Computer Adaptive Testing

The NCLEX-RN is administered using computer adaptive testing (CAT) procedures. CAT uses the memory and speed of the computer to administer a test individualized for each candidate. When the examination begins, the computer randomly selects a relatively easy question. The next question is based on the candidate's response to the previous question. If the question is answered correctly, an item of similar or greater difficulty is generated; if it is answered incorrectly, a less-difficult item is selected. The computer selects items that it thinks the candidate has a 50/50 chance of answering correctly, so test-takers should not be concerned that they are not answering every question correctly. Approximately 50% of the test items every candidate will receive may be too difficult (and will be answered incorrectly), and 50% of the test items will be easily answered based on the candidate's ability. Thus, the test is adapted for each candidate. Once competence has been determined, the exam is completed at a passing level. Since the NCLEX-RN is designed to address specific test plan categories, not content areas, candidates should also not be concerned if it seems they are receiving a large proportion of questions about a specific health problem or client age group.

CAT has several advantages. For example, an exam can be given in less time because candidates potentially have to answer fewer questions. CAT exams also can be administered frequently, allowing a graduate of a nursing program to take the exam following graduation, receive the results quickly, and enter the workforce as a registered nurse in less time than is possible with paper-and-pencil exams. Study results also show that because CAT is self-paced, candidates undergo less stress.

Each NCLEX-RN test is generated from a large pool of questions (a test item bank) based on the NCLEX-RN test plan. The test item bank includes all types of questions, but an individual candidate may or may not receive each type of question, depending on the questions generated from the item bank for each candidate. The exams for all candidates are derived from the same large pool of test items. They contain comparable questions for each component of the test plan. Although the questions are not exactly the same, they test the same knowledge, skills, and abilities from the test plan. All candidates receive comparable percentages of questions from each client need category that aligns with the test plan, and must attain the passing standard from this balanced test plan. Each candidate, therefore, has the same opportunity to demonstrate competence. Although one candidate may answer fewer questions, all candidates have the opportunity to answer a sufficient number of questions to demonstrate competence until the stability of passing or failing is established or the time limit expires.

Each exam includes both "operational" questions (the actual questions used to determine competency) and 15 "pretest" questions (those questions that are being tested for use on subsequent exams). The pretest questions are not included in your final score on the exam. The pretest questions are administered during the early part of the exam, but you will not be able to differentiate pretest items from operational items on the exam. All candidates must answer at least 60 operational test questions. Thus, the minimum number of questions you might receive is 75 (60 operational test questions and 15 pretest questions); the maximum number of possible questions a candidate might receive is 265 (250 operational questions and 15 pretest questions). Most candidates receive about 110 to 130 test questions. Six hours are available to each candidate for completing the test. This time includes an opportunity to review the online candidate tutorial about the test and to take rest breaks. Although some candidates may finish in a shorter time, others will use the entire 6 hours. The amount of time used during testing is not an indication of passing or failing the examination, but rather, reflects the time required to establish competence for each candidate.

Scheduling the Examination

The first step to schedule your NCLEX-RN exam is to apply to the board of nursing/regulatory body (BON/RB), and when you have been declared eligible, you will receive your Authorization to Test (ATT) by email. The next step is to register for the exam with Pearson VUE (pearsonvue.com/nclex). This can be done by a telephone call or online, and confirmation of registration should occur within several days, or immediately if done online. ATT is valid for a specified period of time; check with your state board of nursing for its specific requirements. After receiving the ATT, you can schedule an appointment to take the exam. Check for current information at the NCSBN Web site (www.ncsbn.org) and the Web site of your board of nursing/regulatory body. (See the appendix for State, Provincial, and Territorial Boards of Nursing.) Scheduling to take the examination at an international test

center requires additional steps and fees; consult the Web site of the NCSBN for current information.

Test Center Locations

The Council of State Boards of Nursing contracts with vendors in each state, province, and territory to serve as exam sites. Your school of nursing can inform you of the nearest location. You can also contact your board of nursing/regulatory body for information. (See the appendix for State and Provincial/Territorial Boards of Nursing for the address.) You can also find updated information from the NCSBN at its Web site (www.ncsbn.org).

Computer Use and Screen Design

Test questions are presented on the computer screen (monitor); you select your answer and use the keyboard or a mouse to enter your answer. To practice using computer-generated questions, use the questions on thePoint. To log into thePoint, go to http://thepoint.lww.com. (The code for accessing the site is printed on the inside front cover of the book along with specific instructions for accessing the questions.) At every testing site, written directions are provided at each computer exam station. There are also tutorials and practice questions on the computer that you can complete to be sure you understand how to use the computer before you begin the exam.

The computer used at the testing site has a drop-down clock that indicates elapsed time for taking the exam. This clock can be turned "off" or "on" depending on your preference. Some test takers wish to watch the time as they take the test; others wish to monitor their time periodically. When the exam ends, there will be a message on the screen that indicates, "Examination is ended."

The computer used at the testing site also has a drop-down calculator. The calculator can be used to answer test items requiring calculation. You can use the mouse to drag the calculator to a position on the screen where it is most helpful to you.

Exam Security

Each testing site maintains a high level of security for the exam and for the candidate. The exam is administered on a secured file server and uses password security and host site authentication. All exam sites use test administrators (TA) and video/audio monitoring. Candidates are required to undergo identification verification, which includes showing a valid and recent photo ID (driver's license or passport—passport required at international test centers—provincial/territorial or state identification card, permanent residence card, or military identification card) with signature (the name must match exactly the name on the ATT), and a biometric test such as a palm vein reader. You will also have your photograph taken. Check with your board of nursing/regulatory body and the NCSBN for details about exam security in the jurisdiction in which you are taking the exam, and review information on the testing service Web site (http://www.pearsonvue.com/nclex).

Exam Confidentiality

The NCSBN takes significant steps to protect exam confidentiality. You will not be allowed to bring anything into the exam area, including cellular telephones, watches, handheld electronic devices, paper, or pen/pencil into the exam. While taking the exam, you are not allowed to give or receive test-taking assistance, and you cannot review study materials during a break from the exam; a proctor will be monitoring these areas. Additionally, you will be asked to sign a confidentiality agreement that you will not share information about the test or the test items with others. Social media sites are also monitored to determine if information is shared by way of electronic communication. Students who have posted information through social media about the test will be reported to their state board of nursing or provincial/territorial nursing regulators with a possible consequence of having their license denied.

Special Accommodations

Special accommodations for Americans or Canadians with Disabilities can be made with authorization from the individual boards of nursing/regulatory bodies and the NCSBN. To be eligible for special accommodations, the candidate must have a professionally recognized diagnosis and documentation with recent test results and evaluations. If approved, the accommodations will be noted on the ATT. Candidates approved for testing with accommodations must schedule their testing appointment through the NCLEX Accommodations Coordinator by calling Pearson VUE NCLEX Candidate Services at the telephone number listed on their ATT and asking for the NCLEX Accommodations Coordinator. Check with your board of nursing/regulatory body for additional information.

The Test Center

Although each test center is configured differently, each center will have a small waiting area, a registration area, and a proctored testing area; lockers are provided for valuables. Since the waiting area is small, you should advise your friends and/or family to return to the test center when you have completed the exam.

You should arrive at the test center 30 minutes before you are scheduled to take the test. You should bring your ATT and two forms of identification with you, one of which has photo identification. Leave all unnecessary items in your car or with friends or family. Personal items such as coats, medical devices, and snacks must be placed in provided, lockable storage. If you bring cellular devices to the testing center you will be issued a sealable bag in which to place these devices. If test takers access their phone, or any electronic device, during a break, an incident report will be generated that could result in an exam failure. When you register at the test center, the test center staff will obtain your biometric identification and digital signature. No watches, pencils, or cell phones will be allowed in the test-taking area.

Taking the Exam

Once you have entered the testing area and have settled comfortably at the desk, the test administrator (TA) will turn the computer on. You may request earplugs from the test administrator if the noise of other test takers using the computers in the area is distracting. You may also request an erasable note board with a marking pen, which may be used to make notes or perform math calculations as the test progresses. Before the actual exam begins, there will be an online tutorial that gives you information about the exam and provides an opportunity to practice using the keyboard, mouse, and calculator. Previous computer experience is not necessary to take the NCLEX-RN exam.

You will begin the exam after completing the tutorial. The test questions are presented on the computer screen. You should answer each question; the next question will not appear until you have submitted an answer to the question on the screen. There is no penalty for guessing, but you should make a reasonable attempt to answer the question correctly. Rapid guessing to answer as many questions as possible is not recommended.

As you progress through the test, pace yourself. You should answer the questions at a comfortable speed, not spending too much time on any one question. There is a clock on the computer that can be turned off or on. Some students prefer to turn the clock on periodically rather than watching the time on the clock and feeling rushed. The clock will appear during the last 5 minutes of the test.

You may take a break as needed, but do note that break time counts as test-taking time. Raise your hand, and the test administrator will escort you to the restroom; biometric identification (palm vein reading) will be obtained on your return to the computer desk.

Once you have answered a sufficient number of questions to determine if you have passed or failed the test, or if the allotted time (6 hours) has ended, the exam will end. You will be asked to take a survey about the test experience following the exam, and when you are finished you can raise your hand to indicate to the proctor that you are finished. The proctor then will collect all items at the desk and escort you to the exit.

Results Reporting

Computerized testing allows timely reporting of examination results. The results of the examination are first scored at the testing site and then are verified by Pearson VUE before being forwarded to the board of nursing/regulatory body. The candidate will not receive any results the day of the exam. Results are reported to the candidate up to 6 weeks after taking the exam. Some candidates in the United States can obtain "unofficial" results after 48 business hours through the Quick Results service available on the NCLEX Candidate Web site at www.pearsonvue.com/nclex. The Quick Results service is not available in all states, and there is a minimal fee for this service. The Quick Results service is not available for candidates in Canada.

Exam Failure

If you have failed the exam, you will receive a Candidate Performance Report (CPR), which provides the number of items that you completed and a summary of your relative strengths and weaknesses based on the test plan. You can use this report to guide your study for taking the exam again.

The exam can be retaken as soon as 45 days after the previous test date. Failing the licensing exam can be devastating, but it does not mean that you will never pass the exam or be a good nurse. While you are waiting to retake the exam, you should make a study plan that includes studying a few hours most days of the week, and prepare to take the exam as soon as possible. As a first step, try to determine why you did not pass. Possible reasons include fatigue, stress or illness on the day of the exam, or inadequate preparation. Many students say that the main reason that they do not succeed is test anxiety. Taking practice exams, such as those in Part III, can help you feel more prepared and help reduce your anxiety. Review the information in Chapter 3 about test preparation, and review or complete the

Content Mastery and Test-Taking Skill Self-Analysis (Table 3.2) to identify your particular problems with test taking or your knowledge of the content. Students also find it helpful to form study groups or enroll in an NCLEX-RN test review course.

When to Take the NCLEX-RN®

A study conducted by the National Council of State Boards of Nursing indicates that candidates should take the exam within 6 months of graduating (Wendt, 2009). You should, therefore, plan your own schedule to be prepared to take the NCLEX-RN exam as soon after graduation as possible. Suggestions for developing a study plan are discussed in Chapter 2 of this book.

Additional Information

For further and up-to-date information about the NCLEX-RN, the test plan, test questions, exam format, or testing procedures, visit the NCSBN Web site at www.ncsbn.org. For information about the dates, requirements, and specifics of writing the examination in your state, contact your board of nursing/regulatory body. The addresses and telephone numbers of the NCSBN and board of nursing/regulatory body are provided in the appendix. Information can also be obtained from the vendor who has contracted to provide the testing center for the NCLEX-RN exam. The current vendor is Pearson VUE, and information can be found at their Web site (www.pearsonvue.com/nclex).

References

National Council of State Boards of Nursing, Inc. (2014). NCLEX-RN test plan. Accessed June 16, 2015, from https://www.ncsbn.org

National Council of State Boards of Nursing, Inc. (2015). 2014 practice analysis: Linking the NCLEX-RN examination to practice—U.S. and Canada. Accessed June 16, 2015, from https://www.ncsbn.org

Wendt, A. (2009). 2008 knowledge of newly licensed registered nurses survey. Accessed June 16, 2015, from https://www.ncsbn.org/WEB_08_Newly_Licensed_Nurses_Vol37_small.pdf

2 NCLEX-RN® Test Questions and Strategies for Answering Them

Introduction

The test questions used on the NCLEX-RN exam are written to test the knowledge, skills, and abilities essential to provide safe client care. Understanding the types of questions, the cognitive level of the questions, as well as the thinking processes used to answer the questions is essential for test success. This chapter provides information about the test items used on the NCLEX-RN exam and offers strategies for answering questions for various types of test items and levels of the cognitive domain.

Types of Test Items

The NCLEX-RN examination uses eight types, or formats, of test items (National Council of State Boards of Nursing, Inc., 2015). These include multiple-choice items and seven alternate item formats: multiple-response, fill-in-the-blank (calculation), hot-spot, chart/exhibit, drag-and-drop/ordered-response, graphic options, and audio items. Questions can also be written using video clips as prompts for questions. Although these questions are not currently being used by the National Council of State Boards of Nursing (NCSBN), video questions are included on thePoint as an additional way for you to develop your critical thinking and test taking skills. To log into thePoint, go to http://thepoint.lww.com. (The code for accessing the site is printed on the inside front cover of the book along with specific instructions for accessing the questions.)

Although each type of item tests your understanding of nursing content and is developed using the same test development process, each type of test item requires you to respond in a different way. Because alternate item formats test knowledge, skills, and abilities in a variety of ways, there are increased opportunities for you to demonstrate your competence (Wendt & Kenny, 2009). All test item types are scored as either correct or incorrect; no partial credit is awarded for any question type (National Council of State Boards of Nursing, Inc., 2015).

All eight types of test items and video inclusion test questions are used in this review book and on thePoint to give you the opportunity to learn how to answer each type of question. You can also find examples of these types of questions on the NCSBN Web site (www.ncsbn.org), in the candidate tutorial that precedes each licensing exam at the Pearson VUE Web site (www.pearsonvue.com/nclex), and in the candidates' bulletin that you will receive prior to taking the licensing exam.

Multiple-Choice Item

Multiple-choice items include a scenario/situation, a question, and four answers—only *one* of which is correct (see Fig. 2.1). The scenario provides information about the client or care management situation. The question (stem) poses the problem to solve. The question may be written as a direct question, such as "What should the nurse do **first**?" or as an incomplete sentence, such as "The nurse should:." The answers (options) are possible responses to the stem. Each stem has one correct option and three incorrect options. The options may be written as complete sentences or may complete the sentence stem stated in the question. Multiple-choice items are the most common type of test item used on the licensing exam.

> **FIGURE 2.1**
> **Sample Multiple-Choice Item**
>
> A 7-year-old client with type 1 diabetes is sick with the flu. What is the **most** important information for the nurse to convey regarding diabetes management during illness?
> - ☐ 1. Blood glucose needs to be checked more frequently during illness.
> - ☐ 2. Children require less insulin when they are sick with the flu.
> - ☐ 3. Urine ketones should be checked every other day during illness.
> - ☐ 4. Increase intake of fluids high in carbohydrate to prevent diarrhea.

Strategies for Answering Multiple-Choice Questions

- Read the scenario, and relate the question and answers to the data provided in the scenario. Pay particular attention to information, if included, about the client's age, family status, health status, ethnicity, place of care, or point in the care plan (e.g., early admission vs. preparation for discharge).
- Answer the question before looking at the possible answers.
- Choose the answer that best matches the answer you first thought was correct.
- Recognize that only ONE answer is correct.
- Double-check your answer to be sure you have responded to the question; note particularly key words such as **first, except, not, most, last**; be sure that you are basing your answer on best nursing practice, not experience with one client or in a particular clinical agency.

Multiple-Response Item

Multiple-response items are similar to multiple-choice items, except that they include four to six answers and have two or more correct answers, and the others will be incorrect; there will not be an instance in which the answers are either all correct or all incorrect (see Fig. 2.2). These questions will ask you to identify all of the answers that are correct ("Select all that apply."). Multiple-response questions will be scored as being either correct or incorrect; no partial credit is given for selecting some of the correct responses.

FIGURE 2.2
Sample Multiple-Response Item

The client states to the nurse, "I take citalopram 40 mg every day as my healthcare provider (HCP) prescribed. I have also been taking St. John's wort 750 mg daily for the past 2 weeks." Which findings would indicate that the client is developing serotonin syndrome? Select all that apply.
- ☐ 1. confusion
- ☐ 2. restlessness
- ☐ 3. constipation
- ☐ 4. diaphoresis
- ☐ 5. ataxia

When using the text pages in this book to answer the multiple-response questions, you can make check marks in the boxes located in front of the answers. When taking the actual NCLEX-RN exam, you will place your cursor on the box in front of the

answer you wish to select and click on the box; a check mark will appear indicating that you wish to select that answer. To change an answer, you can use the mouse to remove the check mark from that box.

Strategies for Answering Multiple-Response Questions

- Read the question carefully, and determine what it is you are to select, for example, all possible side effects of a particular drug, all intended outcomes of a particular nursing intervention, all of the elements of a teaching plan for a client with a particular health problem, or all instructions a nurse should give to a client who is being discharged.
- Read each answer, and determine if it is true or false as it pertains to the question.
- Consider how the answers are "clustered" and how the correct answers are related.
- Be sure you have selected ALL of the possible correct answers.
- Double-check your answer by reviewing the answers you did NOT check, and be sure they are incorrect and should not be included in the answer.

Hot-Spot Item

Hot-spot items involve identifying the location of a specific item, such as an appropriate injection site, assessment area, or correct part of a waveform. The question will be phrased, "Identify the location…" or "Select the area…" (see Fig. 2.3).

FIGURE 2.3
Sample Hot-Spot Item

The nurse is preparing the client diagnosed with pleural effusion for a left-sided thoracentesis. The x-ray shows fluid in the pleural cavity. During the preparation for the procedure, the client asks where the healthcare provider (HCP) will "put the needle." Select the appropriate site from the diagram below.

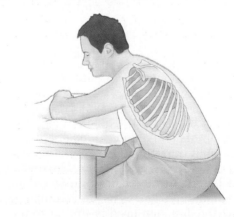

When answering hot-spot questions in the book, you should place an X on the illustration provided to identify the proper area and then refer to the answer section for that chapter to confirm your response. On the actual NCLEX-RN and for the questions on thePoint, you will use the mouse to move your cursor over the area you want to select and then left-click the area. A red "X" will appear over the area you have selected. If you make an error, you can move the cursor to the part of the figure that is the answer you wish to enter.

Strategies for Answering Hot-Spot Questions

- Read the question carefully, and answer the question first by visualizing an answer; then look at the figure to mark your answer.
- Double-check your answer to make sure you have selected the correct "spot" based on evidence for best nursing practice.

Fill-in-the-Blank (Calculation) Item

Fill-in-the-blank items involve calculations, such as determining a drug dose, calculating an IV drip rate, or totaling intake-output records (see Fig. 2.4). These items can be answered with a number. On the NCLEX-RN exam, if you do not enter a number, you will receive an error message that will prompt you to "enter a numeric answer." When an answer includes a measurement amount such as milliliters (mL), grams (g), or inches (in), the measurement unit will be stated in the stem of the question and supplied in the answer box; thus, you will not include the unit of measure as part of your answer. The question will indicate if you are to round your answer and, if so, to how many decimal places.

FIGURE 2.4
Sample Fill-in-the-Blank Item

The healthcare provider (HCP) prescribes an intravenous infusion of 5% dextrose in 0.45 normal saline to be infused at 2 mL/kg/h in an infant who weighs 9 lb (4.1 kg). How many milliliters per hour of the solution should the nurse infuse? Round to one decimal place.

_____ mL/h.

When answering fill-in-the-blank questions on the text pages of this book, you can use paper and pencil, a handheld device with a calculator, or a calculator to determine your answers. However, on the actual NCLEX-RN exam, a drop-down calculator will be available for you to use to calculate your answers. The division sign used is similar to the one used on the Microsoft Calculator (/); be sure to familiarize yourself with the mathematical function keys. To practice calculations required for fill-in-the-blank questions, use the calculator on your computer.

Strategies for Answering Fill-in-the Blank Questions

- Determine what calculation the question is asking you to perform (e.g., add, subtract, or use a formula).
- Write the calculation on the erasable write board provided at the testing center.
- Access the drop-down calculator from the computer to perform the appropriate mathematical function.
- To avoid calculation errors, be sure that you do not enter numbers rapidly when you are using the calculator.
- Round the numbers, as directed, to one or two decimal points; round the number after completing the calculation. If rounded numbers are required to answer the question, the decimal point must be included in the answer.
- Place your answer on the appropriate line.
- Double-check your answer using a logic test—is this answer plausible? Did I perform the correct mathematical function? Is the answer appropriate for the unit of measure required in the question?

Chart/Exhibit Item

Chart/exhibit items present data from a chart, graph, or table. Data from a client's chart will be presented from one or more chart "tabs" such as prescriptions, history and physical, laboratory results, miscellaneous reports, imaging results, flow sheets, intake and output, medication administration record, progress notes, and vital signs (see Fig. 2.5). On the actual NCLEX-RN exam, you will be prompted to "click on the exhibit button below for additional client information." You will then use the data presented in the scenario and on the chart or exhibit to make a nursing decision. For example, you will click on up to three tabs to locate data, and then you will interpret the data, validate if the data are correct or sufficient, and then be asked to respond to a question based on the data.

In this book, chart/exhibit questions show data on 1 or 2 "tabs" and then ask you to use the data to respond to the question. When these types of questions are administered by the computer (as in the NCLEX-RN exam), you may be asked to determine which "tab" to use to locate the information that is required to answer the question. You will click on the tab to open the tab(s), and a "pop-up" window will appear on the computer screen.

Figure 2.5
Sample Chart/Exhibit Item

The nurse is reviewing the history and physical and healthcare provider (HCP) prescriptions on the chart of a newly admitted client.

History and physical tab

Subjective:	19-year-old reports a constant cough for the past "few weeks" with "dark" sputum for the past few days. Has night sweats, 10-lb (4.5-kg) weight loss in the past month, and "always" being tired. He took one Tylenol about an hour prior to arrival.
Objective:	
BP	120/64
HR	84/reg
Resp	26/unlabored/slight wheezing in right lower lobe posteriorly
O² Sat	92%
Temp	99.9°F (37.7°C) oral
Skin	Warm, slightly diaphoretic
Nonproductive cough at this time	
Assessment:	Possible respiratory infection
Physician prescriptions tab	
	Chest x-ray
	Sputum specimen
	Oxygen at 2 L per nasal cannula

The nurse should **first**:
☐ 1. initiate airborne precautions.
☐ 2. apply oxygen at 2 L per nasal cannula.
☐ 3. collect a sputum sample.
☐ 4. reassess vital signs.

🔑 Strategies for Answering Chart/Exhibit Questions

- Read the scenario and question carefully to understand the context for the data to be provided in the chart or exhibit. For example, are you looking for vital signs? Would an elevated pulse or drop in blood pressure be consistent with the context of the question and provide data for making a nursing decision?
- Read the information provided on the chart or exhibit, and identify the information that is essential to answer the question.
- Review the chart or exhibit "pop-up box" as many times as needed.

- If necessary, take notes on the erasable note board provided at the testing center.
- Answer the question only from data provided in the chart or exhibit and from the data presented in the scenario.
- Double-check your answer by being sure you have obtained all of the data necessary to answer the question and that the answer is complete and plausible.

Drag-and-Drop/Ordered-Response Item

Drag-and-drop/ordered-response items require you to place information in a specified order (see Fig. 2.6). For example, the question might ask you to put steps of a procedure in order, or provide information about several clients, and ask you to determine the order of priority in which each client should receive nursing care. Or the question may ask you the order in which to teach a client about a procedure or self-care process. There may be up to six options to arrange in a specific order.

Figure 2.6
Sample Drag-and-Drop/Ordered-Response Item

The nurse's assignment consists of four clients. Prioritize in order from **highest** to **lowest priority** in what order the nurse would assess these clients after receiving report.

1. An 85-year-old client with bacterial pneumonia, temperature of 102.2°F (42°C), and shortness of breath.

2. A 60-year-old client with chest tubes who is 2 days postoperative following a thoracotomy for lung cancer and is requesting something for pain.

3. A 35-year-old client with suspected tuberculosis who has a cough.

4. A 56-year-old client with emphysema who has a scheduled dose of a bronchodilator due to be administered, with no report of acute respiratory distress.

The questions will be scored as correct or incorrect; there is no "partial credit" for having part of the answer in the correct order.

When answering drag-and-drop/ordered-response items in the text of this book, you will write the appropriate step number next to the answer choice. For example, write #1 next to the first step in the process, #2 for the second step in the process, and so on until all answer choices have been used. On the actual licensing exam, you will drag each response from the left-hand column and drop it into the correct order on the right-hand column. You can move the items around until you have them in the correct order and then click "submit" to enter your answer. If you need to change your answer, you can drag the response to another position and reorder the responses. The questions on thePoint function in much the same way, except that you will click on "Next" to proceed to the next question.

Strategies for Answering Drag-and-Drop/ Ordered-Response Questions

- Read the key words in the stem of the question that indicate the order in which you are to place the answers.
- Test the logic of your answer.
- Be sure all items have been placed.
- Double-check your answer by reviewing the correct order for the answers and that you have placed your answers in the order in which you intend to answer the question. One answer out of order will cause the question to be counted as incorrect.

Graphic Option Item

Although graphics can be used as a part of the *question* (see Fig. 2.12), with graphic option items the *answers* to these questions are presented as a graphic (see Fig. 2.7). Graphic option items use graphics (figures, illustrations, photos) in the answers to the questions. You will need to select the correct answer(s) from the graphic options offered as possible answer(s) to the question.

In the text of this book, you can use your pencil to mark the correct answer to a graphic option question. On thePoint and on the actual NCLEX-RN exam, you will click on the circle in front of the graphic that represents your answer. To change your answer, click on another circle.

FIGURE 2.7
Sample Graphic Option Item

Which is the correct knot used to secure a restraint correctly to the bed frame?

☐ 1.

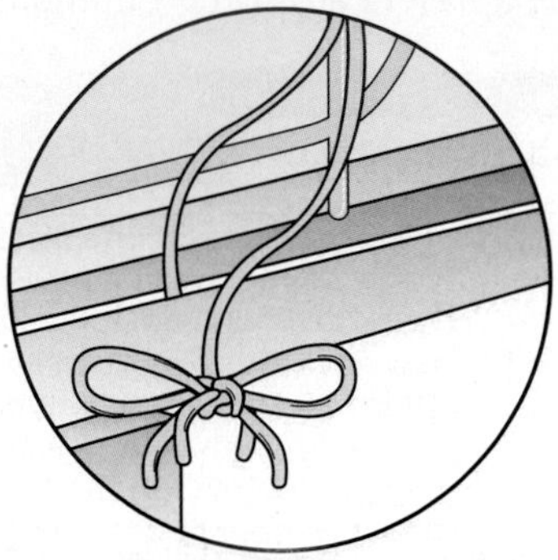

☐ 2.

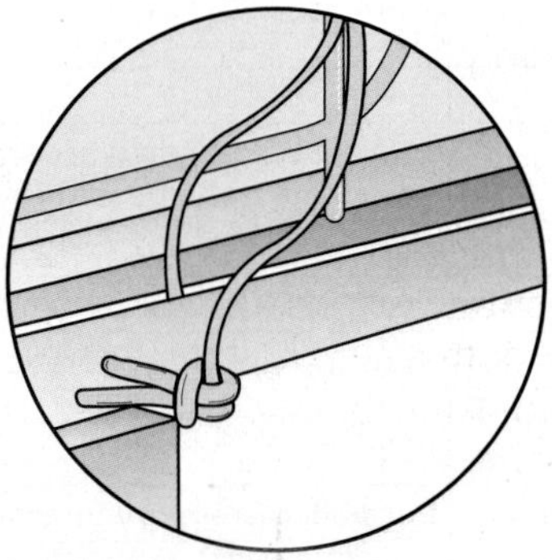

☐ 3.

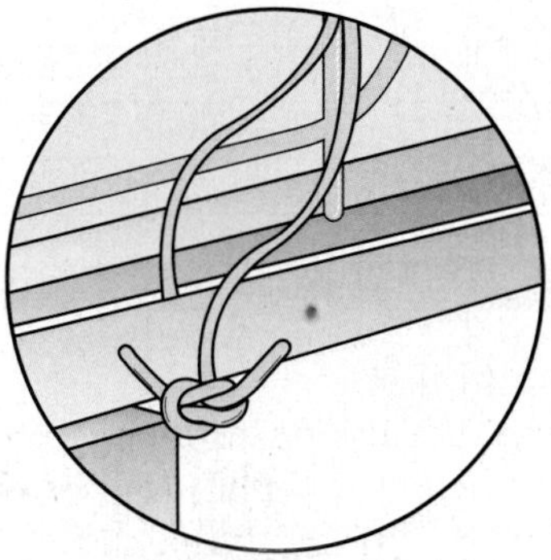

☐ 4.

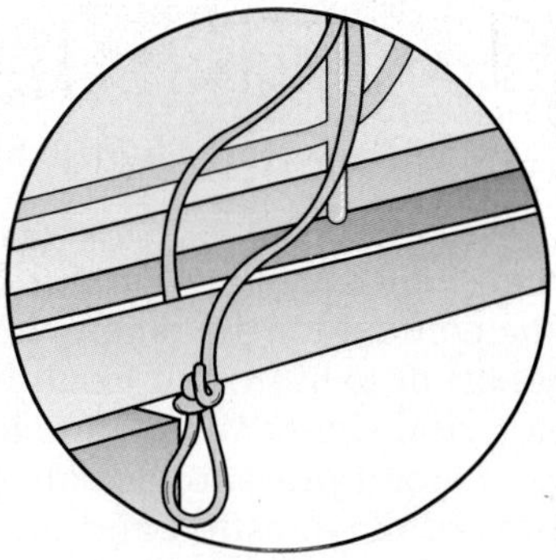

⚿ Strategies for Answering Graphic Option Questions

- Read the question carefully, and visualize the answer before looking at the options presented with the test item.
- Look carefully at each graphic option, and be certain you understand the differences among the options.
- Select the option that best answers the question.
- Double-check your answer by reviewing the question, answering the question based on best nursing practice, and matching the answer to the graphic option.

Audio Item

Audio items include a short audio clip with data that are essential to answer the question. (See Fig. 2.8 for an example of how a question is *written*; go to thePoint to *hear* the actual audio clip or to practice answering other audio questions.) For example, you could be asked to listen to breath sounds, heart sounds, bowel sounds, or verbal interactions. The question will indicate that you should click on the play button to listen to the audio clip. You will be able to play the audio clip as many times as needed to answer the question. The question may ask you to identify the sound on the audio clip, for example, type of breath sound, or you may be asked to make a nursing judgment and/or select a nursing action based on your interpretation of the sound.

In this review book, the audio questions are presented on thePoint. You will be able to listen to the sounds and choose the correct answer. When taking audio test questions on the actual NCLEX-RN exam, you will have headsets to use, and you will be able to adjust the volume.

⚿ Strategies for Answering Audio Questions

- Read the test item carefully to understand the clinical context in which the scenario occurs.
- Listen to the audio clip before answering the question; listen to the audio clip as many times as needed to answer the question.
- Relate the sounds in the audio clip to the scenario in the test item; if the question asks you to make a nursing decision or select a nursing action, base your answer on your interpretation of the sound and best nursing practices.
- Double-check your answer by reviewing the question and answering the question based on best nursing practice.

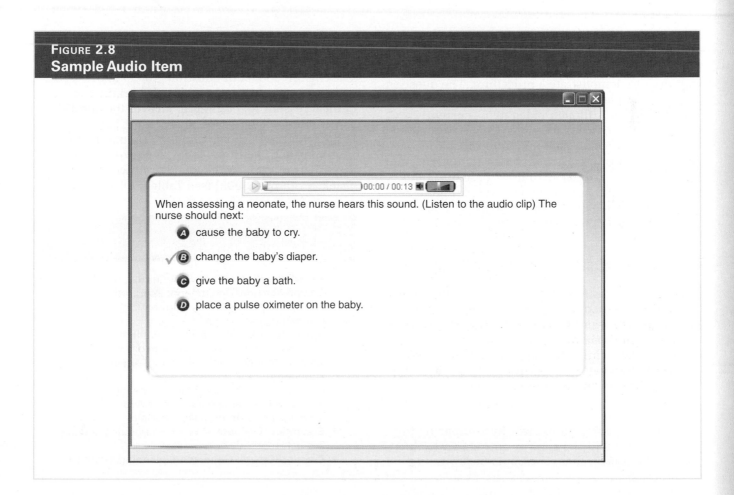

FIGURE 2.8
Sample Audio Item

▷ 〇〇:〇〇 / 〇〇:13

When assessing a neonate, the nurse hears this sound. (Listen to the audio clip) The nurse should next:

- Ⓐ cause the baby to cry.
- ✓Ⓑ change the baby's diaper.
- Ⓒ give the baby a bath.
- Ⓓ place a pulse oximeter on the baby.

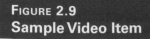

FIGURE 2.9
Sample Video Item

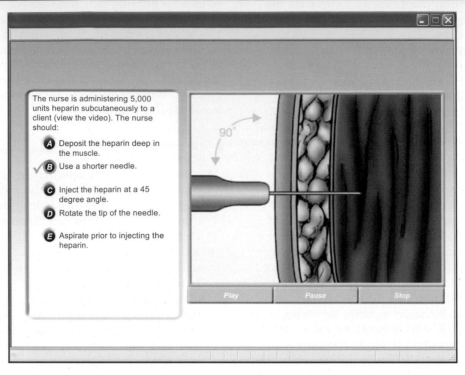

The nurse is administering 5,000 units heparin subcutaneously to a client (view the video). The nurse should:

A. Deposit the heparin deep in the muscle.

✓ B. Use a shorter needle.

C. Inject the heparin at a 45 degree angle.

D. Rotate the tip of the needle.

E. Aspirate prior to injecting the heparin.

Video Item

Video items use video clips to present a clinical situation or to demonstrate a procedure. The question will be based on information you have viewed in the video clip. Although video items currently are not used on the licensing exam, we have included several examples on thePoint. Your faculty may use these questions in classroom testing situations, and you should be familiar with how these questions are designed and how to answer them. (Figure 2.9 shows how video questions are *written*; refer to thePoint for an *actual* example of a video item.)

Strategies for Answering Video Items

- Read the question carefully to understand the clinical context of the question.
- Anticipate what the video clip will show, what you should pay particular attention to when you are watching the clip, and how the question relates to what is being shown in the video clip.
- Play the video clip as often as you need to view the action; look for actions that are correct or not correct.
- Double-check your answer by comparing the video clip and the answer options and selecting the option that represents best nursing practices.

Cognitive Levels of Test Items

The cognitive level of questions refers to the type of mental activity such as critical thinking and clinical reasoning required to answer the question. The cognitive levels used to write test items for the NCLEX-RN are derived from the original Bloom's taxonomy and the Bloom's revised taxonomy of the cognitive domain (Anderson & Krathwohl, 2001; Su, Osiek, & Starnes, 2005) (see Table 2.1). The lowest

TABLE 2.1
Levels of the Cognitive Domain

- **Knowledge/Remember:** Recognizing, recalling
- **Comprehension/Understand:** Interpreting, exemplifying, classifying, summarizing, inferring, comparing, explaining
- **Application/Apply:** Executing, implementing, using knowledge appropriately in new or different situations
- **Analysis/Analyze:** Differentiating, organizing, attributing
- **Synthesis/Synthesize:** Putting parts together to form a whole; using data from several sources to form a conclusion or make a decision
- **Evaluation/Evaluate:** Checking, critiquing, judging against standards or protocols
- **Creation/Create:** Generating, planning, producing

level of the taxonomy is the *knowledge* (or *remember*) level and involves the ability to remember or recall facts. The next level of the cognitive domain, *comprehension* (or *understand*), requires you to interpret, explain, or understand the knowledge. The *application* (or *apply*) level involves using information that you remember and understand and can apply in new situations. *Analysis* (or *analyze*) requires recognizing and differentiating relationships between parts and using clinical reasoning and critical thinking skills. *Synthesis* (or *synthesize*) refers to the ability to take several pieces of information or clinical data and use them to make a nursing care judgment or decision. The next level of the cognitive domain is *evaluation* (or *evaluate*). Here, you must check data, critique information, or judge the outcome of nursing care. The final level of the cognitive domain in Bloom's revised taxonomy is *creation* (or *create*). At this level, you must be able to generate new approaches to nursing care or develop a unique nursing care plan based on available information.

Test items can be written to test at all levels of the cognitive domain, but questions that are written for the NCLEX-RN exam are generally written at application levels and above because nursing requires the ability to apply knowledge to clinical situations, analyze data, think critically, prioritize information, make clinical decisions for client care, evaluate outcomes of nursing interventions or healthcare treatments, and create care plans based on specific client needs. This book and the questions on thePoint present questions at the application level and higher.

Clinical reasoning refers to the higher-order mental activities and critical thinking skills used to solve a problem or make a decision. Nurses use clinical reasoning, critical thinking, critical synthesis, and clinical decision making and make clinical judgments to provide safe client care. Understanding the types of test items written at various levels of the cognitive domain and strategies to answer them is key (🔑) to success on the licensing exam. Examples of questions at higher levels of the cognitive domain are provided here to assist you in further understanding the types of questions used on the licensing exam and the strategies you can use to answer them. A summary of the cognitive levels, with examples of question stems and strategies for answering them, is given in Table 2.2.

Application-Level Item

Application-level items test your ability to apply knowledge to a specific scenario. These questions draw on your ability to know and understand nursing content and to then apply this information to a specific scenario or situation (see Fig. 2.10).

FIGURE 2.10
Sample Application-Level Item

The healthcare provider (HCP) prescribes a serum lithium level tomorrow for a client with bipolar disorder, manic phase, who has been receiving lithium 300 mg PO three times daily for the past 5 days. At what time should the nurse plan to have the blood specimen obtained?

☐ 1. before bedtime
☐ 2. after lunch
☐ 3. before breakfast
☐ 4. during the afternoon

🔑 Strategies for Answering Application-Level Questions

- Read the question, and consider what information you already know and how that information should be used to answer this particular question.
- Consider how information you can recall should be applied to nursing care for the client that is described in the scenario for the question.
- Apply known formulas (divided dose/drip rate calculation), frameworks (e.g., Maslow's hierarchy, developmental stages, stages of moral development), and procedural steps (how to administer a particular medication) to answer the question posed in the new clinical situation (scenario).
- Double-check your answer by recognizing what information you are applying to answer the question.

Analysis-Level Items

Questions at this level ask you to analyze data, clusters of symptoms, and implementation plans and then

---

FIGURE 2.11
Sample Analysis-Level Item

Which statements by the mother of a toddler should lead the nurse to suspect that the child is at risk for iron deficiency anemia? Select all that apply.

☐ 1. "He drinks over 4 glasses of milk per day."
☐ 2. "I cannot keep enough apple juice in the house; he must drink over 10 oz (300 mL) per day."
☐ 3. "He refuses to eat more than two different kinds of vegetables."
☐ 4. "He does not like meat, but he will eat small amounts of it."
☐ 5. "He sleeps 12 hours every night and takes a 2-hour nap."

make clinical decisions. These questions can also ask about what additional information should be obtained to make a clinical decision or plan care (see Fig. 2.11).

🔑 Strategies for Answering Analysis-Level Questions

- Identify the data presented in the scenario that lead you to draw a conclusion.
- Identify how the parts are related and how the nurse should assemble them to make a complete care plan.
- Determine if you have sufficient information to make a decision.
- Review data from all sources possible (client's vital signs, client's responses to medication and treatments, chart information, client assignment list, etc.).
- Double-check your answer by determining that you have understood all of the components of care and have made the correct nursing decision based on those components.

Synthesis-Level Items

Synthesis-level test items ask you to use several pieces of information to make a clinical decision. The focus here is on obtaining sufficient information to make a clinical decision, rather than analyzing data already available. The information may come from the client/family or members of the healthcare team. In synthesis-level items, you must determine accuracy and usefulness of information for the particular situation, sort relevant data from irrelevant data, and use it to plan or give nursing care (see Fig. 2.12).

🔑 Strategies for Answering Synthesis-Level Questions

- Read the question to determine what information is necessary to provide safe client care.
- Determine if you have sufficient and accurate information.
- Interpret all data obtained in context of the question and the client's needs.
- Make a clinical decision about the relevant nursing action.
- Double-check your answer by being sure that the information you have directs you to the correct answer.

Evaluation-Level Items

Evaluation-level items ask you to make judgments about care, determine the effectiveness of nursing care, or evaluate the extent to which an intended outcome has been achieved. Evaluation-level test items can also ask you to determine if the care given by others (client/family, healthcare team, healthcare provider) is appropriate (see Fig. 2.13).

FIGURE 2.13
Sample Evaluation-Level Item

A nurse is reviewing the chart of an adult male with cancer. The healthcare provider (HCP) has prescribed filgrastim 400 µg, subcutaneously once daily. The nurse reviews the laboratory report and determines treatment has been effective when:

Laboratory Results

Test	Result
Hemoglobin	12.0 g/dL (120 g/L)
Platelet count	108,000/mm³ (108 × 10⁹/L)
WBC count	1,600/mm³ (1.6 × 10⁹/L)
ANC	< 1,000/mm³ (1 × 10⁹/L)

☐ 1. hemoglobin is 16 g/dL (160 g/L).
☐ 2. WBC count is 3,500/mm³ (3.5 × 10⁹/L).
☐ 3. platelet count is 200,000/mm³ (200 × 10⁹/L).
☐ 4. RBC count is 4.3 million/mm³ (4.3 × 10¹²/L).

FIGURE 2.12
Sample Synthesis-Level Item

The nurse observes the cardiac rhythm (see below) for a client who is being admitted with a myocardial infarction. What should the nurse do **first**?

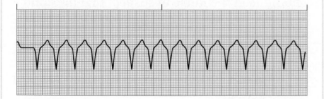

☐ 1. Prepare for immediate cardioversion.
☐ 2. Begin cardiopulmonary resuscitation (CPR).
☐ 3. Check for a pulse.
☐ 4. Prepare for immediate defibrillation.

Strategies for Answering Evaluation-Level Questions

- Review the question to determine what is to be evaluated. Consider if the question is asking you to verify a client's understanding or if the question is asking if a particular outcome has been attained.
- Before looking at possible answers, consider what is the accepted standard of care, ideal level of care, or intended outcome.
- Match the answers with your understanding of the standard of care.
- Double-check your answer with the scenario and expected standard of care in that scenario.

Creation-Level Items

Creation-level test items require you to use information obtained from a client, family, or clinical situation and develop a new, client-centered, or unique approach to solving the clinical problem. For example, the test items may ask you to develop a plan of care, a discharge plan, or an action plan to manage quality improvement (see Fig. 2.14).

FIGURE 2.14
Sample Creation-Level Item

The nurse is caring for a client who is 12 weeks pregnant and speaks Spanish only. Which interventions should the nurse include in the plan of care at the client's initial visit? Select all that apply.

☐ 1. Provide brochures in the client's native language.
☐ 2. Refer the client to a high-risk clinic.
☐ 3. Discuss cultural differences, and emphasize the differences between cultures.
☐ 4. Arrange for an interpreter for her appointments.
☐ 5. Discuss contraception and options.
☐ 6. Review dietary intake and discuss nutrition.

Strategies for Answering Creation-Level Test Questions

- Read the question to determine what is to be developed or created.
- Consider all of the elements necessary to have a complete plan of care, discharge plan, etc.
- Understand what is and is not appropriate to include in the plan being created, and rule out inappropriate aspects of care for the client or situation presented in the scenario.
- Double-check your answer by reviewing the appropriateness of each of the elements in the plan you have developed.

TABLE 2.2
Keys to Answering Test Questions from Various Levels of the Cognitive Domain

Cognitive Level	Descriptions	Examples of Question Stems	Strategies for Answering Questions
Application	Transfer knowledge from classroom to clinical practice.	To assess the breath sounds for a client with heart failure, where should the nurse place the stethoscope?	Use knowledge and understanding of how to auscultate breath sounds to assess a particular client.
	Use a formula or guidelines to perform calculations.	The client is to receive 1,000 mL of fluids in 8 h. The intravenous administration set delivers 15 drops per minute. The nurse should regulate the infusion to provide how many milliliters per minute?	Apply appropriate formula to calculate an intravenous fluid drip rate.
	Apply knowledge and understanding to new situations.	Which nursing intervention is appropriate for this client?	Use knowledge and understanding about nursing interventions, and apply to the client's particular situation.
		The nurse should instruct the client about which side effects that may occur when the client takes this drug? Select all that apply.	Apply knowledge and understanding about drug side effects to instruct a particular client.
		The nurse is teaching a client to use a metered-dose inhaler. In which order (from first to last) should the nurse instruct the client about the steps to take to use the inhaler? All options must be used.	Use knowledge and understanding of correct order of a skill or procedure to teach a particular client.
		The nurse is communicating with an agitated client. Which communication technique is **most** appropriate?	Use knowledge and understanding of communication techniques to apply to this particular client.
Analysis	Organize clinical data into relevant parts in order to identify a client need, form a conclusion, or make a clinical decision.	Based on the clinical assessment, the nurse determines the client has which need?	Review the client's signs and symptoms to determine an appropriate nursing problem.
	Review all data to determine if sufficient data are available to make a decision.	Which (data) indicate(s) the need for nursing action?	Analyze data to determine which nursing action to take next.
	Analyze data to determine priorities.	Which client should the nurse care for **first**?	Organize information about a group of clients, and determine which client requires nursing care first.
	Distinguish relevant from irrelevant data.	Which (data) indicate(s) the nurse should assess the client further?	Analyze data, and determine if additional data are needed.
	Determine what data are needed to plan or implement care.	Based on these findings, the nurse determines the client is in xxx stage of development.	Analyze data/findings, and determine appropriate stage (of development).
		Which client is at risk for xxx?	Analyze data about a group of clients with risk factors and determine the client's risk.
		The client is expressing concerns about xxx and the nurse observes xxx behaviors. The nurse should (do/say/refer):	Analyze clients' verbal and behavioral responses to determine what to say to the client.

Synthesis	Assemble information from several sources to determine the best course of action.	After reviewing (data from the client and the chart), what should the nurse do **first?**	Use information from a variety of appropriate sources such as the client, client responses to medical and nursing interventions, laboratory data, diagnostic tests, and progress notes to determine appropriate nursing action.
		Based on this information (about side effects of medication) and the client's current health status, the nurse should instruct the client to xxx?	
		After assessing the client, the nurse reviews the healthcare provider's prescriptions. The nurse should perform which action **first?**	
		After reviewing the client's rhythm strip, pain medication record, and vital signs chart, what should the nurse do **next?**	
		Which statement indicates the nurse's **best** response to the child's parent?	
Evaluation	Make judgments about the effectiveness of nursing care.	Which statement indicates the client has understood the nurse's teaching?	Determine if the client understands the instructions based on the criteria established in the teaching plan.
	Use standards of care to determine the extent to which the client has met them.	Which finding indicates the intended therapeutic effect has occurred?	Evaluate effectiveness of a nursing intervention, drug, or treatment based on the intended or expected outcome.
	Critique care given by others.	The nurse is observing an unlicensed assistive personnel (UAP) turn a client. Which observation indicates the nurse should intervene?	Evaluate appropriateness of care given by others according to standards of care and knowledge of scope of practice.
		The nurse has administered nitroglycerin to a client with chest pain. In 30 seconds, the client's chest pain should be:	Judge effectiveness of outcome of a nursing action (administering a drug) based on expected therapeutic effect.
Creation	Create or develop a unique or individualized plan, report, or protocol based on client needs.	Which instructions should be included in a discharge plan for the client? Select all that apply.	Develop a discharge plan.
		Which nursing actions best meet this client's needs?	Individualize a standardized care plan for a specific client.
		The nurse is planning care for six clients. The staffing for the team includes one registered nurse (RN) and one unlicensed assistive personnel (UAP). Which clients should be assigned to the UAP? Select all that apply.	Create a care management plan for a group of clients and a team of healthcare professionals.
		The nurse is gathering information for a "hand off" for transferring the client from one nursing unit to another. The nurse should include which information in the report? Select all that apply.	Create a detailed report about the client's health status.

References

Anderson, L. W., & Krathwohl, D., eds. (2001). *A taxonomy for learning, teaching, and assessing: A revision of Bloom's taxonomy of educational objectives*. New York, NY: Longman.

National Council of State Boards of Nursing, Inc. (2015). Accessed June 16, 2015, from https://www.ncsbn.org/nclex.htm

Su, W. M., Osiek, P. J., & Starnes, B. (2005). Using the revised Bloom's Taxonomy in the clinical laboratory. *Nurse Educator, 30*(3), 117–122.

Wendt, A., & Kenny, L. (2009). Alternate item types: Continuing the quest for authentic testing. *The Journal of Nursing Education, 48*(3), 150–156.

3 How to Prepare for and Take the NCLEX-RN® and Other Nursing Exams

Introduction

Studying for the NCLEX-RN or other similar exams requires careful planning and preparation. Evidence from studies about how students prepare for exams indicates that the students who do best on exams have done three things: (1) learned the content in a way that they can apply it to nursing practice (deep learning), (2) learned how to control their anxiety, and (3) fine-tuned their test-taking skills (Thomas & Baker, 2011). This chapter provides information about each of these factors associated with exam success.

You can begin developing your study preparation using a systematic approach to study that includes these five steps to test for success:
- Assess your study needs.
- Develop a study plan.
- Refine your test-taking strategies.
- Rehearse test anxiety management skills.
- Evaluate progress on a regular basis.

Use these five steps as you take your first test in nursing school. Refine your test-taking strategies as you evaluate your progress at each step of the way, so that when you are ready to take the licensing exam, you will be an experienced and successful test taker. Use the Personal Study Plan in Table 3.1 to help develop your own study plan.

Assessing Study Needs

The first step toward test success is to determine your strengths and limitations. Even students who have been successful throughout their academic life, and nurses who are excellent caregivers, have areas in which they need improvement. Be honest with yourself as you assess your own study needs. These steps can help you in your assessment:
- *Review your success in your nursing program.* Review your grades in science courses and the courses in the nursing curriculum. Success on the NCLEX-RN tends to correlate with grades (grade point average) achieved in science and

nursing courses. Subjects in which you received high grades, that you found easy to learn, or in which you have had additional clinical practice or work experience are likely to be areas of strength. On the other hand, subjects you found difficult to learn (or in which you did not achieve high grades) should be areas for concentrated review. Also consider content areas that you have not studied for a while. Recent course work will be the most familiar and, therefore, may require the least amount of study. Candidates should have a strong mastery of materials learned in fundamental skills or assessment courses which are typically offered early in a program. All students, even students who have achieved success in nursing courses, benefit from identifying areas requiring study and spending time practicing test-taking skills. You also can use the practice exams in this book to identify areas needing further study. Begin with the subjects you find most difficult or in which you have the least confidence.

- *Assess your test-taking skills.* Using effective test-taking skills contributes to exam success. What have you done in the past to make you confident about taking a test? How do you feel when you are in the exam situation? What has worked in the past to help you be successful? Review these strategies to build on past successes and work on problem areas. Consider additional strategies suggested in the section "Refining Your Test-Taking Strategies," page 35. You can practice these skills by simulating the testing situation using the practice tests and comprehensive exams in this review book.

- *Assess your ability to take tests that require application, analysis, and evaluation.* Test questions used on the licensing exam are written at higher levels of the cognitive domain. Many candidates' experience with taking tests has come from taking "teacher-made" tests—tests developed by the faculty at your school of nursing. These tests are commonly written to test students' knowledge and understanding of

TABLE 3.1
Personal Study Plan

Assess Study Needs

1. Review your success in nursing school.
☐ I did best in these courses:
_____
_____

☐ I needed to study harder in these courses:
_____
_____

☐ I took these courses near the beginning of the curriculum:
_____
_____

☐ I scored best on these practice exams in this book:
_____
_____

☐ I am not satisfied with my scores on these practice exams in this book:
_____
_____

☐ I need further study in these content areas:
_____
_____

☐ I need further study in these areas of the nursing process:
_____
_____

☐ I need further study in these areas of client needs:
_____
_____

2. Review your test-taking skills.
☐ I can identify the components of a test question.
☐ I read questions carefully before answering.
☐ I can make reasonable guesses if I am not certain of the correct answer.

3. I can recognize patterns of why I miss questions.

4. I can pace myself to complete questions in the allotted time.

5. Review your test-anxiety management skills.
☐ I can do relaxation and deep-breathing exercises.
☐ I can visualize success.
☐ I can give myself positive feedback.
☐ I can concentrate for extended periods of time.

6. Review your computer skills.
☐ I am able to use a computer to read and answer test questions.
☐ I have used thePoint Web site accompanying this book.

Develop a Study Plan
☐ I will study in this location:
_____
_____

☐ I will study at these times and dates:
_____
_____

☐ I have assembled all of the materials I need to study:
_____
_____

☐ I will study with a study group:
_____
_____

Evaluate Progress
☐ I have completed the practice tests in this book.
☐ I have completed the comprehensive tests in this book.
☐ I need to improve my scores in these areas:
_____
_____

☐ I am prepared to take the NCLEX-RN examination.

course content and may not include questions that require application, analysis, or evaluation of course material. Additionally, several of the types of alternate-format questions have recently been added to the exam, and nursing faculty may not yet be designing their own test questions using these formats. Finally, some students are able to "second-guess" the teacher and use this ability to their advantage when taking teacher-made classroom tests. However, it is not as easy to anticipate test questions on standardized and licensing exams, and you will need to develop skills that will help you think critically when presented with an unfamiliar situation. As you prepare to take the licensing exam, spend time on questions where you need to "figure out" the best approach to answering the question. You can use the questions in this book and on thePoint to be sure you understand the difference between questions that require only recall and understanding and those that require you to apply information to provide client care, make clinical judgments, and initiate nursing actions. Use the *Content Mastery and Test-Taking Skill Self-Analysis* table in the back of this book to identify your ability to answer questions in the higher levels of the cognitive domain.

- *Assess your English language skills.* Persons for whom English is an additional language or who do not have well-developed reading and comprehension skills may require additional practice in reading and answering NCLEX-RN-style test questions. If you are one of these persons, plan additional time to practice reading and answering questions, to time yourself when answering questions, and to validate that you understand the question correctly. If necessary, seek assistance. As you study, keep a list of words you do not understand and practice using them.

- *Assess your ability to take timed tests.* Are you always the last one to finish a test? Do you request additional time to complete a test? If so, you will want to practice taking timed tests and doing your best, while completing as many questions as possible. The licensing exam is designed to be completed in 6 hours; only questions completed within that time frame will be scored. As you use the practice questions and tests in this book, time yourself and, if needed, determine ways that you can increase your speed without sacrificing accuracy. The comprehensive tests in this book have been intentionally designed with the minimum and maximum number of operational questions on the licensing exam; time yourself as you take these tests. A typical response time on the exam is under 2 minutes per question. Comprehensive tests in part 3 of this book represent the range of number of questions a candidate might receive offering you an opportunity to time yourself taking exams with the minimum and maximum number of questions.

- *Assess your skills for taking computer-administered exams.* Although previous computer experience is not necessary to take the NCLEX-RN, you should familiarize yourself with the differences between taking a paper-and-pencil exam and taking exams administered by the computer. If you have not used a computer before, find a learning resource center at your college, university, library, or hospital where you can become familiar with basic computer keyboard skills. thePoint, which simulates the computerized NCLEX-RN, offers you the opportunity to practice taking computer-administered test questions. Use these questions to practice reading questions from the computer screen and become acquainted with answering questions in a computerized format. If you are accustomed to underlining key words or making notes in the margins of paper-and-pencil tests, adapt these strategies to reading and answering the questions on the computer screen. Also be sure that you can use a drop-down calculator to answer questions requiring the use of math skills. Use the tutorial offered by the testing company, Pearson VUE at http://www.pearsonvue.com/nclex/, to learn how the test questions will be computer-administered. Note, you cannot move to the next question without answering the question presented on the screen, and you are not able to return to review questions once you have moved to the next question.

- *Assess your reason(s) for not answering the test question accurately.* There are many reasons why students select an incorrect answer. These could include not reading the question carefully (not reading all of the words in the sentence; missing key words), not reading the options carefully, not knowing the answer (lack of knowledge or deep learning), not recognizing the rationale for the correct answer, guessing, not being rested, or dealing with health problems when taking the exam. The most important thing you can do is to assess the *reason* why you are not answering questions correctly. Recent evidence about test taking indicates that understanding the *pattern* of missed questions is essential to changing how you study (Wiles, 2015). For this reason, we have designed the *Content Mastery and Test-Taking Skill Self-Analysis* table (see Table 3.2) so you can identify your specific reason(s) for not answering the questions correctly. Total the check marks in the columns to identify patterns of reasons for not answering the questions correctly. Determine if there is a pattern, and use this information to plan your study. Consider discussing the findings with your faculty member for suggestions for improving your test-taking skills. There is a tear-out copy of the *Content Mastery and Test-Taking Skill Self-Analysis* table (at the back of the book) that you can copy and use for *each* test in this book.

- *Assess your risk for not passing the licensing exam.* Recent evidence indicates that factors associated with not passing the licensing exam can be identified (Breckenridge, Wolf, & Roszkowski, 2012). Table 3.3 lists these factors; having more factors is associated with higher risk. Note that the three top risk factors are poverty, low science GPA prior to the nursing major, and repeating college science courses and, when summed, are predictors of exam failure (Breckenridge et al., 2012). It is important that you identify your risk for not passing the licensing exam and take advantage of all resources available to assist you to lower your risk. Interventions include forming study groups, attending review sessions, establishing effective study habits, practicing test taking on a regular basis, determining reasons for not answering questions correctly (use the *Content Mastery and Test-Taking Skill Self-Analysis* table in this book), and taking action steps to improve knowledge of nursing content and test-taking strategies. The earlier in the academic program that you can identify your risk, use interventions, and monitor your progress, the more likely you are to reverse your risk and improve your chance of passing!

(*text continues on page 36*)

TABLE 3.2
Content Mastery and Test-Taking Skill Self-Analysis

Use the chart below to identify the subject matter and the reason you missed the question. Place a check mark in the columns for questions you did not answer correctly and why, and then total each column. The key (🔑) to effective review is to understand your knowledge deficits and focus additional review on those subjects and reasons for not answering the question.

Review Strategies

Test Number	Subject (care of childbearing family, care of children, care of adults, care of clients with psychiatric disorders and mental health problems)	Score

Total number of questions missed: _____

Use the chart below to identify the subject matter and the reason you missed the question. Use the following codes to note the client need area of the question you missed:

MC, management of care; SI, safety and infection control; HM, health promotion and maintenance; PA, physiological adaptation; PI, psychosocial integrity; PP, pharmacological and parenteral therapies; RR, reduction of risk potential; BC, basic care and comfort.

Question #	Client need	Misread/ Misunderstood the question	Missed key word(s)	Did not read all options	Changed answer	Missed certain type of questions (often multiple-response questions)	Did not understand subject matter	Did not recognize rationale for correct answer	Made an incorrect guess	Did not understand meaning of term in question	Other
1											
2											
3											
4											
5											
5											
6											
7											

Question #	Client need	Misread/ Misunderstood the question	Missed key word(s)	Did not read all options	Changed answer	Missed certain type of questions (often multiple-response questions)	Did not understand subject matter	Did not recognize rationale for correct answer	Made an incorrect guess	Did not understand meaning of term in question	Other
8											
9											
10											
11											
12											
13											
14											
15											
16											
17											
18											
19											
20											
21											
22											
23											
24											
25											
26											
27											
28											
29											
30											
31											
32											
33											
34											
35											
36											
37											

(Continued)

Question #	Client need	Misread/ Misunderstood the question	Missed key word(s)	Did not read all options	Changed answer	Missed certain type of questions (often multiple-response questions)	Did not understand subject matter	Did not recognize rationale for correct answer	Made an incorrect guess	Did not understand meaning of term in question	Other
38											
39											
40											
41											
42											
43											
44											
45											
46											
47											
48											
49											
50											
51											
52											
53											
54											
55											
56											
57											
58											
59											
60											
61											
62											
63											
64											
65											
66											
67											

Question #	Client need	Misread/ Misunderstood the question	Missed key word(s)	Did not read all options	Changed answer	Missed certain type of questions (often multiple-response questions)	Did not understand subject matter	Did not recognize rationale for correct answer	Made an incorrect guess	Did not understand meaning of term in question	Other
68											
69											
70											
71											
72											
73											
74											
75											
76											
77											
78											
79											
80											
81											
82											
83											
84											
85											
86											
87											
88											
89											
90											
91											
92											
93											
94											
95											
96											
97											

(Continued)

Question #	Client need	Misread/ Misunderstood the question	Missed key word(s)	Did not read all options	Changed answer	Missed certain type of questions (often multiple-response questions)	Did not understand subject matter	Did not recognize rationale for correct answer	Made an incorrect guess	Did not understand meaning of term in question	Other
98											
99											
100											
101											
102											
103											
104											
105											
106											
107											
108											
109											
110											
111											
112											
113											
114											
115											
116											
117											
118											
119											
120											
121											
122											
123											
124											
125											
126											
127											

Question #	Client need	Misread/ Misunderstood the question	Missed key word(s)	Did not read all options	Changed answer	Missed certain type of questions (often multiple-response questions)	Did not understand subject matter	Did not recognize rationale for correct answer	Made an incorrect guess	Did not understand meaning of term in question	Other
128											
129											
130											
131											
132											
133											
134											
135											
136											
137											
138											
139											
140											
141											
142											
143											
144											
145											
146											
147											
148											
149											
150											
151											
152											
153											
154											
155											
156											
157											

(Continued)

Question #	Client need	Misread/ Misunderstood the question	Missed key word(s)	Did not read all options	Changed answer	Missed certain type of questions (often multiple-response questions)	Did not understand subject matter	Did not recognize rationale for correct answer	Made an incorrect guess	Did not understand meaning of term in question	Other
158											
159											
160											
161											
162											
163											
164											
165											
166											
167											
168											
169											
170											
171											
172											
173											
174											
175											
176											
177											
178											
179											
180											
181											
182											
183											
184											
185											
186											
187											

Question #	Client need	Misread/ Misunderstood the question	Missed key word(s)	Did not read all options	Changed answer	Missed certain type of questions (often multiple-response questions)	Did not understand subject matter	Did not recognize rationale for correct answer	Made an incorrect guess	Did not understand meaning of term in question	Other
188											
189											
190											

■ How many questions in each area of client needs did you miss?
■ How does this compare with other exam results from this review?

Lower _____ Same _____ Higher _____ NA _____

If you missed questions because you misread questions, missed key words, or changed answers, review *Lippincott Q&A Review for NCLEX-RN* Part I.

If you missed questions because you did not remember or understand the content, review that content in *Lippincott Q&A Review for NCLEX-RN* Part II and your other nursing references.

If you missed questions because you guessed, were you missing because of "rapid guessing" to complete the test on time, or because of "random guessing," making a reasoned attempt to answer the question? Consider how you will approach "guessing" when you do not know the answer.

If you missed questions because you did not pace yourself, practice taking timed test questions and pacing yourself to allow sufficient time for all questions.

What is the pattern of the types of questions you are missing?
What is your action plan for further study?

TABLE 3.3
Factors Associated with Risk of Failure on NCLEX-RN

- Income at or below poverty level
- Science GPA (low grades in science courses—biology, chemistry, microbiology)
- Repeating college science courses
- English is second language
- Low score on standardized admission tests (SAT, ACT)
- Low score on standardized progression tests (ATI, HESI)
- Failure of one or more nursing prerequisite courses (more courses, higher risk)
- Failure of one or more nursing courses (more courses, higher risk)
- GPA (<3.0)
- Working (more hours worked, higher risk)
- Lack of sufficient support to care for children while in school or studying
- First in family to attend college

Developing a Study Plan

Once you have identified areas of strength and areas needing further study, develop a specific plan and begin to study regularly. Students who study a small amount of content over a longer period of time tend to have higher success rates than do students who wait until the last few weeks before the exam and then "cram." Consider these suggestions:

- *Identify a place for study.* The area should be quiet and have room for your books and papers or electronic study materials. Do not study while playing music, responding to text messages, or listening to the television; background noise is distracting and will not be allowed at the actual NCLEX-RN testing site. Your area for study might be in your home, at your nursing school, at your workplace, or in a library. Be sure your friends and family understand the importance of not interrupting you when you are studying.
- *Establish regular study times.* Make appointments with yourself to ensure a commitment to study. Frequent, short study periods (1 or 2 hours) are preferable to sporadic, extended study periods. Test yourself often by taking test questions or generating test questions yourself; using practice test questions is more effective than rereading your textbooks or notes (Shellenbarger, 2011). Plan to finish your studying 1 week before the NCLEX-RN; last-minute cramming tends to increase anxiety.
- *Obtain all necessary resources.* As you begin to study, it is helpful to have easy access to textbooks, electronic resources, notes, and study guides.

- *Make the best use of your time.* Make review cards that you can carry with you to study during free moments throughout the day. Some students record review notes and listen to the tapes or podcasts while driving or exercising. Use electronic devices and smartphones to add test review "apps" to practice test questions on a regular basis.
- *Reduce or eliminate stressful situations.* Students who are juggling multiple responsibilities (such as working, managing a family, taking courses, planning a wedding, or caring for elderly parents) may find it difficult to find time to study or to concentrate when studying. Managing a variety of stressful situations puts students at risk for failing exams. If possible, reduce the number of stressful situations you are involved in during the time you are preparing to take the NCLEX-RN exam.
- *Develop effective study skills.* Study skills enable you to acquire, organize, remember, and use the information you need to take the NCLEX-RN. These skills include outlining, summarizing, applying, synthesizing, reviewing, and practicing test-taking strategies. Some students make concept maps or use reflective journaling to help them learn and remember important content. Use these study skills each time you prepare for an exam.
- *Use study skills with which you are familiar and that have worked well for you in the past.* Recall effective study behaviors that you used in nursing school, such as reviewing highlighted text, outlines, or content/concept maps.
- *Study to learn, not to memorize.* The NCLEX-RN tests application and analysis of knowledge. When reviewing content, continually ask yourself, "How is this information used in client care?" "What clinical decision making will be required of this information?" and "What is the role of the nurse in using this information?" Being able to apply information, rather than just being able to list or recognize information, is one of the most important study skills to master. Study for "deep learning," not surface learning, which emphasizes only comprehension and short-term recall.
- *Identify your learning and study-style preferences.* Each student has a preferred way of learning. For example, some students prefer learning material by listening; they are considered *auditory* learners. If this describes your preference, you will benefit from reviewing recorded notes or class lectures. Some students learn best in a visual mode. They learn by reading, reviewing slide presentations, or looking at illustrations. For these *visual* learners, reading and looking at images is helpful. *Kinesthetic* learners, those who like to touch and manipulate to learn, benefit

from working with models and manikins to reinforce their learning. While you likely have one learning style and study preference, using a variety of styles will enhance the study experience.

■ *Affirm your language skills.* If English is not your first or only language, focus on developing your language skills (Hansen & Beaver, 2012). Make note cards of words that are unfamiliar or keep a list of words from practice tests that you do not know, and review these words. Study with a friend for whom English is the native language, and discuss practice questions to understand meaning of the words and the nursing context. Using concept maps is another useful strategy when studying about particular health problems.

■ *Consider forming a study group.* Some students prefer to study alone, whereas others benefit from study groups; know which approach works best for you, and develop your study plan accordingly. If you participate in a study group, limit the group size to about seven people. The group should develop norms for working together that focus on understanding and applying nursing content, rather than memorizing facts. Talking out loud about the thought processes that go into answering a question is a helpful approach, particularly when students or faculty can provide corrective feedback. In a study group, students can pose questions to each other and discuss rationale or divide the topics for review and practice, but every member must come prepared to contribute. If your school has software that allows you to form online groups of students, set up a study forum. Some students study with a "study buddy." With just two people, it is easy to use Skype or other technology that permits seeing the person with whom you are studying.

■ *Attend faculty-led test review sessions.* Most faculty provide opportunities for group or individual review after each test. Attend these sessions or ask to discuss your exam scores with your faculty. Interaction with faculty and advisors about your test-taking skills is an important element to success on nursing exams and has been shown to improve course grades (Wiles, 2015). Determine the reasons for and patterns of missing particular questions, and plan to use this information in your study plan.

■ *Study the most difficult material before bedtime.* Research indicates that sleeping consolidates information in your memory (Shellenbarger, 2011).

■ *Anticipate questions.* As you study, formulate questions around the content. Practice giving a rationale for your answer to these questions. If you work in a study group, have each member contribute questions that the entire group answers. Frequent testing solidifies learning.

■ *Study common, not unique, nursing care situations.* The NCLEX-RN tests minimum competence for nursing practice; therefore, focus on common health problems and client needs. Review the *RN Practice Analysis*, published by the National Council of State Boards of Nursing, and the current licensing exam test plan to determine common nursing care activities. Both can be found at the NCSBN Web site at ncsbn.org.

■ *Study broad concepts, rather than insignificant details.* Be sure you understand the underlying pathophysiology and nursing implications across the life span for broad concepts such as oxygenation, perfusion, comfort, delegation, and so on. Answers to test questions can be derived from understanding the basic concept and then determining how to implement nursing care for specific client needs.

■ *Simulate test taking.* The comprehensive tests in Part Three of this book are designed to simulate the random order in which questions appear in the NCLEX-RN and the possible number of question you might receive. Make additional copies of answer sheets, and retake the exams on which you had low scores. Use the *Content Mastery and Test-Taking Skill Self-Analysis* table (see Table 3.2 and at the back of the book) to review the *reason* you have missed a question and note *patterns* that may become evident, and use these to guide further study.

Refining Your Test-Taking Strategies

Knowing how to take a test is as important as knowing the content being tested. Strategies for taking tests can be learned and used to improve test scores. Here are some suggestions for building a repertoire of effective test-taking strategies:

■ *Understand the type of test item, the cognitive level, and related thinking processes.* (See Chapter 2 for more information on question types and cognitive levels found on the NCLEX-RN exam.)

■ *Understand which integrated process* (step of the nursing process, caring, communication, documentation, teaching/learning, culture and spirituality) is being tested. For example, as you read the question, determine whether the question is asking you to set priorities (planning) or judge outcomes (evaluation).

■ *Understand client needs.* As you read the question, consider the question in the context of client needs. Be sure to understand if the question is asking you to determine what to do "**first**" or to select the nursing action that is "**best**."

■ *Understand the age of the client, if noted in the test question.* If relevant to answering the question, the age of the client will be specified; consider what information about that age-group will be important to answering the question. If the age of the client is not specified, assume that the client is an adult and base your answers on principles of adult growth and development.

- *Read the question carefully.* This is one of the most important aspects of effective test taking. Read the stem carefully; do not rush. Ask yourself, "What is this question asking?" and "What is the expected response?" If necessary, rephrase the question in your own words, but do not change the meaning of the question when putting the question in your own words, as this is one of the reasons for obtaining an incorrect response.

- *Do not read meaning into a question that is not intended, and do not make a question more difficult than it is.* If you do not understand the question, try to figure it out. If, for example, the question is asking about the fluid balance needs of a client with pheochromocytoma and you do not remember what pheochromocytoma is, then try to answer the question based on your knowledge of the concept of fluid balance.

- *Base your answer to a question on evidence for best nursing practice.* The exam questions reflect national nursing practice standards and are not written to test knowledge of procedures or practices at specific healthcare agencies. Thus, it is important to answer the question from the framework of best nursing practice, not unique practices or procedures that are specific to one clinical agency. For example, "code blue" may be a specific term for a cardiac arrest in one agency, but not in another, or there may be specific steps in the procedure for intravenous line care at each agency. When answering the question, refer to evidence-based practices more than your personal clinical experiences.

- *Determine if the question is asking you to set priorities or place steps of a procedure in a particular order.* Read the stem of the question carefully, and be clear about the priority (first, last) or order (first, last) in which you are to answer the question. Base your answer on commonly used nursing frameworks for setting priorities, such as the nursing process: assess, plan, implement, and evaluate; Maslow's hierarchy of needs: physiological, safety and security; love and belonging, self-esteem; and self-actualization; principles of emergency care: breathing, bleeding, and circulation; principles of triage: resuscitation, emergent, urgent, less urgent, and nonurgent; fire response priorities: rescue, alarm, confine, and extinguish; role of the nurse versus role of the primary care provider versus role of the licensed practical/vocational nurse (LPN/VN) and unlicensed assistive personnel (UAP); or procedures for delegation: scope of practice, workload, ability, and follow-up.

- *Look for key words that provide clues to the correct answer.* For instance, words such as "except," "not," and "but" can change the meaning of a question; words such as "first," "next," and "most" ask you to establish a priority or use an order or sequence of steps; key words such as "most likely" or "least likely" are asking you to determine a probability of a successful outcome. When the question asks you to "select all that apply," be sure you are considering each option as having the possibility of being correct, and have ruled out the ones you have not selected as being incorrect.

- *Be certain you understand the meaning of all words in the question.* If you see a word you do not know, try to figure out its meaning from a familiar base of the word or from the context of the question.

- *Attempt to answer the question before you see the answers, and then look for the answer(s) that is/are similar to the one(s) you generated.* If you do not see the answer you thought was correct, stop and reread the question, be sure you understand what the question is asking, and determine what will help you choose the correct answer.

- *Eliminate answers that you know are not correct.* This will improve your chances of selecting the correct answer. Treat each option in multiple-response questions as "true" or "false"; this will help eliminate incorrect answers.

- *Base answers on nursing knowledge.* Remember that the NCLEX-RN is used to test for safe practice and that you have learned the information needed to answer the question.

- *If you do not know an answer, make a reasonable guess.* Hunches and intuition are often correct. Do not waste time and energy; give yourself permission to not know every question, and move on to the next one. In the computerized adaptive testing format of the NCLEX-RN test, you must answer each question before the next item is administered, and because the level of difficulty will be adjusted as you answer each question, it is likely that you will know the answer to one of the next questions.

- *Learn to pace yourself.* Pacing has been noted to be an important test-taking skill (Thomas & Baker, 2011). Pacing involves spending an appropriate time on each question as well as monitoring the overall amount of time during the test so that you are not rushing at the end. Some students, when they realize they are running out of time, tend to do "rapid guessing," that is, making quick decisions in order to answer more questions. This approach leads to answering with an incorrect response. "Random guessing" on the other hand is a more strategic approach in which you think carefully and make a reasonable guess based on information you can recall to help you answer the question. Pacing also involves recognizing when you need a break. Attention span and concentration levels can start to decline in about 45 minutes, and you should request a break when needed (Wiles, 2015). *Use the comprehensive tests in this book to time yourself and develop an appropriate pace for taking the test.*

Strategies for Managing Test Anxiety

All test takers experience some anxiety. A certain amount of anxiety is motivating; extreme anxiety contributes significantly to poor test performance by causing test takers to change answers, lose concentration, misread or misunderstand questions, or become unable to control the pace of their response to the questions. Be prepared to control unwanted anxiety using the suggestions below.

Anxiety can be managed by both physical and mental activities. Practice anxiety management strategies while you are taking the comprehensive examinations in this book, and use them with *each* exam you take in school or elsewhere. Practicing managing test anxiety when taking "low-stakes" tests, such as practice tests and classroom tests, will make managing test anxiety much easier when you are taking the "high-stakes" tests, such as course or program final exams and, of course, the licensing exam. Commonly used anxiety management strategies include:

- *Mental rehearsal.* Mental rehearsal involves reviewing the events and environment during the examination. Anticipate how you will feel, what the setting will be like, how you will take the exam, what the computer screen will look like, and how you will talk to yourself during the exam. To see an example of a testing center, go to the Pearson VUE Web site, and use the video to take a tour of a typical test center (http://home.pearsonvue.com/test-taker/Pearson-Professional-Center-Tour.aspx). Rehearse what you will do if you have test anxiety.
- *Relaxation exercises.* Relaxation exercises involve tensing and relaxing various muscle groups to relieve the physical effects of anxiety. Practice systematically contracting and relaxing muscle groups from your toes to your neck to release energy for concentration. You can do these exercises during the exam to promote relaxation. Smile! Smiling relaxes tense facial muscles and reminds you to maintain a positive attitude.
- *Deep breathing.* Taking deep breaths by inhaling slowly while counting to 5 and then exhaling slowly while counting to 10 increases oxygen flow to the lungs and brain. Deep breathing also decreases tension and helps manage anxiety by focusing your thoughts on the breathing and away from worries.

- *Positive self-talk.* Talking to yourself in a positive way serves to correct negative thoughts (e.g., "I cannot pass this test" and "I do not know the answers to any of these questions") and reinforces a positive self-concept. Replace negative thoughts with positive ones, for example, tell yourself, "I can do this," "I studied well and am prepared," or "I can figure this out." Visualize yourself as a nurse—you have passed the test!
- *Distraction.* Thinking about something else can clear your mind of negative or unwanted thoughts. Think of something fun, something you enjoy. Plan now what you will think about to distract yourself during the exam.
- *Concentration.* During the exam, be prepared to concentrate. Have tunnel vision. Do not worry if others finish the test before you. Remember that everyone has his or her own speed for taking tests and that each test is individualized. Do not rush; you will have plenty of time. Focus; do not let noises from the keyboard next to you divert your attention. Do not become overwhelmed by the testing environment. Use positive self-talk as you begin the exam. Some students become bored during the exam and then become careless as they answer questions toward the end of the exam. Practice taking tests of at least 265 questions, and discover how long you can focus your attention on the test questions. Practice taking breaks if you begin to lose your concentration. During the actual test, be sure to take breaks when you need them.
- *Seek help.* If you find that you are not able to manage your test anxiety, consult your faculty or resources on your campus. Consider obtaining professional help if needed.

Evaluating Your Progress

The last step of your study plan is to check your progress. Review all of your responses using the tear-out *Content Mastery and Test-Taking Skill Self-Analysis* table (at the back of the book) to identify the number of incorrect responses, the reasons for not answering the question correctly, and how many questions in any one clinical area or categories of client needs you have missed. Note if your scores on the practice and comprehensive tests improve. Do not spend time on content you have mastered, on areas in which you obtained high scores on the practice exam, or on areas with which you feel confident. Use the results of your evaluation to set priorities for study on areas needing additional review. As noted above, evaluate your study skills, your test-taking abilities, and the use of test anxiety management strategies as you take *each* test throughout your academic program. Doing so now will prepare you to test for success.

Tips from Students Who Have Passed the NCLEX-RN®

Students who have successfully passed the NCLEX-RN offer these tips for preparing for, and taking, this exam:

- Study regularly several months before taking the exam. Be sure you are well prepared. Accept responsibility for your study plan—being prepared is up to you!
- Practice taking randomly generated test questions. Most students are accustomed to taking teacher-made exams that cover several topics in the same content area. When taking the NCLEX-RN examination, however, each question will come from a different topic or content area, and you will need to be prepared to shift your focus to a different practice area for each question.
- Use practice questions until you can score at least 75% on the exam. Use practice exams with at least 2,000 questions so you test yourself with a wide range of content and types of questions.
- Use a timer to determine how many questions you can answer in a specified amount of time. Use the timer to be sure you are keeping a steady pace, but not rushing through the test.
- Schedule to take the exam when YOU are ready, but as soon after graduation as is feasible (National Council of State Boards of Nursing, 2007). Candidates who take the exam before they are prepared are not as successful. You are in control of when you take the exam!
- Make sure you know the date, time, and place the exam will be given; how to get to the exam site; how long it takes to drive there; and where you can park. Do locate the exam site, drive to it, and see the room where the exam will be given. Exam sites may be located in small offices in shopping centers and could be difficult to find.
- Visualize yourself in the room taking the test. Use mental rehearsal to practice anxiety-managing strategies.
- Organize the information you will need to bring to the testing center the night before the exam. You will need to present your Authorization to Test. You will also need to provide required identification.
- Make sure you are physically prepared. Get enough rest before the examination; fatigue can impair concentration. If you work, it may be advisable not to work the day before the exam; if you work on a shift that is different from the time of the exam, adjust your work schedule several days ahead of time.
- Avoid planning time-consuming activities (e.g., weddings, vacation trips) immediately before the exam.
- Do not use any drugs you usually do not use (including caffeine and nicotine), and do not use alcohol for 2 days before the exam.
- Eat regular meals before the exam. Remember that high-carbohydrate foods provide energy, but excessive sugar and caffeine can cause hyperactivity. Experts recommend that prior to taking a test, test takers eat high-fiber, high-carbohydrate foods that are slow to digest, such as oatmeal. Eating well-balanced meals the week before the test is also helpful; the diet should include fruits and vegetables; avoid meals high in meat, eggs, and cheese (Shellenbarger, 2011).
- Dress comfortably, in layers that can be added or removed according to your comfort level.

The authors of this review book offer you our best wishes for success on all of the exams you will be taking throughout your academic career. We are confident that your review and preparation have given you a good foundation for a positive testing experience!

References

Breckenridge, D. M., Wolf, Z. R., & Roszkowski, M. J. (2012). Risk assessment profile and strategies for success instrument: Determining prelicensure nursing students' risk for academic success. *The Journal of Nursing Education, 51*(3), 160–166.

Hansen, E., & Beaver, S. (2012). Faculty support for ESL nursing students: Action plan for success. *Nursing Education Perspectives, 33*(4), 246–250.

National Council of State Boards of Nursing. (2007). The NCLEX delay pass rate study. Accessed June 16, 2015, from https://www.ncsbn.org/delay-study2006.pdf

Shellenbarger, S. (2011). Toughest exam question: What is the best way to study? *Wall Street Journal,* October 26, 2011, D1.

Thomas, M. H., & Baker, S. S. (2011). NCLEX-RN success: Evidence-based strategies. *Nursing Educator, 36*(6), 246–249.

Wiles, L. (2015). "Why can't I pass these exams?": Providing individualized feedback for nursing students. *The Journal of Nursing Education, 54*(3 Suppl.), S55–S58.

Practice Tests

1

The Nursing Care of the Childbearing Family

TEST 1

Antepartal Care

- The Preconception Client
- The Pregnant Client Receiving Prenatal Care
- The Pregnant Client in Birth Preparation Classes
- The Pregnant Client with Risk Factors
- Managing Care, Quality, and Safety for Childbearing Clients
- Answers, Rationales, and Test-Taking Strategies

The Preconception Client

1. A client has obtained levonorgestrel as emergency contraception. After unprotected intercourse, the client calls the clinic to ask questions about taking the contraceptives. The nurse realizes the client needs further explanation when she makes which statement?

☒ 1. "I can wait up to 4 days after intercourse to start taking these to prevent pregnancy."

☐ 2. "My boyfriend can buy levonorgestrel from the pharmacy if he is over 18 years old."

☐ 3. "The birth control works by preventing ovulation or fertilization of the egg."

☐ 4. "I may feel nauseated and have breast tenderness or a headache after using the contraceptive."

2. An antenatal G2, T1, P0, A0, L1 client is discussing her postpartum plans for birth control with her health care provider (HCP). In analyzing the available choices, which factor has the **greatest** impact on her birth control options?

☐ 1. satisfaction with prior methods

☐ 2. preference of sexual partner

☒ 3. breast- or bottle-feeding plan

☐ 4. desire for another child in 2 years

3. Which information would be important to include in the teaching plan for the client who wants more information on ovulation and fertility management?

☐ 1. The ovum survives for 96 hours after ovulation, making conception possible during this time.

☐ 2. The basal body temperature falls at least 0.2°F (0.17°C) after ovulation has occurred.

☒ 3. Ovulation usually occurs on day 14, plus or minus 2 days, before the onset of the next menstrual cycle.

☐ 4. Most women can tell they have ovulated because of severe pain and thick, scant cervical mucus.

4. Which instructions about activities during menstruation would the nurse include when counseling an adolescent who has just begun to menstruate?

☒ 1. Take a mild analgesic if needed for menstrual pain.

☐ 2. Avoid cold foods if menstrual pain persists.

☐ 3. Stop exercise while menstruating.

☐ 4. Avoid tampons until you have had your periods for 1 year.

5. After conducting a class for female adolescents about human reproduction, the nurse concludes teaching has been effective when a student makes which statement?

☒ 1. "Under ideal conditions, sperm can reach the ovum in 15 to 30 minutes, resulting in pregnancy."

☐ 2. "I will not become pregnant if I abstain from intercourse during the last 14 days of my menstrual cycle."

☐ 3. "Sperms from a healthy male usually remain viable in the female reproductive tract for 96 hours."

☐ 4. "After an ovum is fertilized by a sperm, the ovum contains 21 pairs of chromosomes."

6. A 20-year-old nulligravid client expresses a desire to learn more about the symptothermal method of family planning. Which information would the nurse include in the teaching plan?

☐ 1. This method has a 50% failure rate during the first year of use.

☐ 2. Couples must abstain from coitus for 5 days after the menses.

☒ 3. Cervical mucus is carefully monitored for changes.

☐ 4. The male partner uses condoms for significant effectiveness.

7. Before advising a 24-year-old client desiring oral contraceptives for family planning, the nurse would assess the client for which signs and symptoms?

☐ 1. anemia

☒ 2. hypertension

☐ 3. dysmenorrhea

☐ 4. acne vulgaris

8. After instructing a 20-year-old nulligravid client about adverse effects of oral contraceptives, the nurse determines that further instruction is needed when the client states which as an adverse effect?

☐ 1. weight gain

☐ 2. nausea

☐ 3. headache

☒ 4. ovarian cancer

9. Which information would the nurse include in the teaching plan for a 32-year-old female client requesting information about using a diaphragm for family planning?

☐ 1. Douching with an acidic solution after intercourse is recommended.

☒ 2. Diaphragms should not be used if the client develops acute cervicitis.

☐ 3. The diaphragm should be washed in a weak solution of bleach and water.

☐ 4. The diaphragm should be left in place for 2 hours after intercourse.

10. After being examined and fitted for a diaphragm, a 24-year-old client receives instructions about its use. Which client statement indicates a need for further teaching?

☐ 1. "I can continue to use the diaphragm for about 2 to 3 years if I keep it protected in the case."

☐ 2. "If I get pregnant, I will have to be refitted for another diaphragm after childbirth."

☐ 3. "Before inserting the diaphragm, I should coat the rim with contraceptive jelly."

☒ 4. "If I gain or lose 20 lb (9 kg), I can still use the same diaphragm."

11. A 22-year-old client tells the nurse that she and her husband are trying to conceive a baby. When teaching the client about reducing the incidence of neural tube defects, the nurse would emphasize the need for increasing the intake of which foods? Select all that apply.

☒ 1. leafy green vegetables

☒ 2. strawberries

☒ 3. beans

☐ 4. milk

☒ 5. sunflower seeds

☒ 6. lentils

12. A couple is inquiring about vasectomy as a permanent method of contraception. Which teaching statement would the nurse include in the teaching plan?

☒ 1. "Another method of contraception is needed until the sperm count is 0."

☐ 2. "Vasectomy is easily reversed if children are desired in the future."

☐ 3. "Vasectomy is contraindicated in males with prior history of cardiac disease."

☐ 4. "Vasectomy requires only a yearly follow-up once the procedure is completed."

13. A 39-year-old multigravid client asks the nurse for information about female sterilization with a tubal ligation. Which client statement indicates effective teaching?

☒ 1. "My fallopian tubes will be tied off through a small abdominal incision."

☐ 2. "Reversal of a tubal ligation is easily done, with a pregnancy success rate of 80%."

☐ 3. "After this procedure, I must abstain from intercourse for at least 3 weeks."

☐ 4. "Both of my ovaries will be removed during the tubal ligation procedure."

14. A 23-year-old nulliparous client visiting the clinic for a routine examination tells the nurse that she desires to use the basal body temperature method for family planning. What instructions should the nurse give the client?

- ☐ 1. Check the cervical mucus to see if it is thick and sparse.
- ☒ 2. Take her temperature at the same time every morning before getting out of bed.
- ☐ 3. Document ovulation when her temperature decreases at least 1°F (0.56°C).
- ☐ 4. Avoid coitus for 10 days after a slight rise in temperature.

15. A couple visiting the infertility clinic for the first time states that they have been trying to conceive for the past 2 years without success. After a history and physical examination of both partners, what would be the **most** appropriate outcome for the couple to accomplish by the end of this visit?

- ☐ 1. Choose an appropriate infertility treatment method.
- ☐ 2. Acknowledge that only 50% of infertile couples achieve a pregnancy.
- ☐ 3. Discuss alternative methods of having a family, such as adoption.
- ☒ 4. Describe each of the potential causes and possible treatment modalities.

16. A client is scheduled to have in vitro fertilization (IVF) as an infertility treatment. Which client statement about IVF indicates that the client understands this procedure?

- ☐ 1. "IVF requires supplemental estrogen to enhance the implantation process."
- ☐ 2. "The pregnancy rate with IVF is higher than that with gamete intrafallopian transfer."
- ☒ 3. "IVF involves bypassing the blocked or absent fallopian tubes."
- ☐ 4. "Both ova and sperm are instilled into the open end of a fallopian tube."

17. A 20-year-old primigravid client tells the nurse that her mother had a friend who died from hemorrhage about 10 years ago during a vaginal birth. Which response would be **most** helpful?

- ☐ 1. "Today's modern technology has resulted in a low maternal mortality rate."
- ☐ 2. "Do not concern yourself with things that happened in the past."
- ☐ 3. "In North America, mothers seldom die in childbirth."
- ☒ 4. "What is it that concerns you about pregnancy, labor, and birth?"

18. A 19-year-old nulligravid client visiting the clinic for a routine examination asks the nurse about cervical mucus changes that occur during the menstrual cycle. Which information would the nurse expect to include in the client's teaching plan?

- ☐ 1. About midway through the menstrual cycle, cervical mucus is thick and sticky.
- ☐ 2. During ovulation, the cervix remains dry without any mucus production.
- ☒ 3. As ovulation approaches, cervical mucus is abundant and clear.
- ☐ 4. Cervical mucus disappears immediately after ovulation, resuming with menses.

19. When instructing a client about the proper use of condoms for pregnancy prevention, the nurse should include which instruction to ensure maximum effectiveness?

- ☒ 1. Place the condom over the erect penis before coitus.
- ☐ 2. Withdraw the condom after coitus when the penis is flaccid.
- ☐ 3. Ensure that the condom is pulled tightly over the tip of the penis before coitus.
- ☐ 4. Obtain a prescription for a condom with nonoxynol 9.

20. A multigravid client will be using medroxyprogesterone acetate as a family planning method. After the nurse instructs the client about this method, which client statement indicates effective teaching?

- ☐ 1. "This method of family planning requires monthly injections."
- ☐ 2. "I should have my first injection during my menstrual cycle."
- ☒ 3. "One possible adverse effect is absence of a menstrual period."
- ☐ 4. "This drug will be given by subcutaneous injections."

21. Which instruction should the nurse include in the teaching plan for a 30-year-old multiparous client who will be using an intrauterine device (IUD) for family planning?

- ☐ 1. Amenorrhea is a common adverse effect of IUDs.
- ☐ 2. The client needs to use additional protection for conception.
- ☐ 3. IUDs are more costly than other forms of contraception.
- ☒ 4. Severe cramping may occur when the IUD is inserted.

22. When developing a teaching plan for an 18-year-old client who asks about treatments for sexually transmitted infections, the nurse should explain that:

☐ 1. acyclovir can be used to cure herpes genitalis.
☐ 2. *Chlamydia trachomatis* infections are usually treated with penicillin.
☒ 3. ceftriaxone may be used to treat *Neisseria gonorrhoeae* infections.
☐ 4. metronidazole is used to treat condylomata acuminata.

23. A couple is visiting the clinic because they have been unable to conceive a baby after 3 years of frequent coitus. The nurse determines that the couple needs further instruction when they identify which factor as a cause of male infertility?

☒ 1. seminal fluid with an alkaline pH
☐ 2. frequent exposure to heat sources
☐ 3. abnormal hormonal stimulation
☐ 4. immunologic factors

24. At a preconception visit, a 24-year-old client is found to have malformation of the uterus. The nurse uses the figure below to explain which type of uterine malformation?

☐ 1. septate uterus
☒ 2. bicornuate uterus
☐ 3. double uterus
☐ 4. uterus didelphys

The Pregnant Client Receiving Prenatal Care

25. A primigravid client at 15 weeks' gestation has had an amniocentesis and has received teaching concerning signs and symptoms to report. Which statement indicates that the client needs further teaching?

☐ 1. "I need to call if I start to leak fluid from my vagina."
☐ 2. "If I start bleeding, I will need to call back."
☒ 3. "If my baby does not move, I need to call my health care provider."
☐ 4. "If I start running a fever, I should let the office know."

26. The nurse is caring for a client who is 12 weeks pregnant and speaks Spanish only. Which interventions should the nurse include in the plan of care at the client's initial visit? Select all that apply.

☒ 1. Provide brochures in the client's native language.
☐ 2. Refer the client to a high-risk clinic.
☐ 3. Discuss cultural differences, and emphasize the differences between cultures.
☒ 4. Arrange for an interpreter for her appointments.
☐ 5. Discuss contraception and options.
☒ 6. Review dietary intake, and discuss nutrition.

27. During a visit to the prenatal clinic, a pregnant client at 32 weeks' gestation has heartburn. The client needs further instruction when she says she must do what?

☐ 1. Avoid highly seasoned foods.
☐ 2. Avoid lying down right after eating.
☐ 3. Eat small, frequent meals.
☒ 4. Consume liquids only between meals.

28. The nurse is teaching a new prenatal client about her iron deficiency anemia during pregnancy. Which statement indicates that the client needs further instruction about her anemia?

☐ 1. "I will need to take iron supplements now."
☒ 2. "I may have anemia because my family is of Asian descent."
☐ 3. "I am considered anemic if my hemoglobin is below 11 g/dL (110 g/L)."
☐ 4. "The anemia increases the workload on my heart."

29. Following a positive pregnancy test, a client begins discussing the changes that will occur in the next several months with the nurse. The nurse should include which information about changes the client can anticipate in the first trimester?

☐ 1. differentiating the self from the fetus
☐ 2. enjoying the role of nurturer
☐ 3. preparing for the reality of parenthood
☒ 4. experiencing ambivalence about pregnancy

30. An antenatal primigravid client has just been informed that she is carrying twins. The plan of care includes educating the client concerning factors that put her at risk for problems during the pregnancy. The nurse realizes the client needs further instruction when she indicates carrying twins puts her at risk for which complication?

☐ 1. preterm labor
☐ 2. twin-to-twin transfusion
☐ 3. anemia
☒ 4. group B streptococcus

31. A 30-year-old multigravid client has missed three periods and now visits the prenatal clinic because she assumes she is pregnant. She is experiencing enlargement of her abdomen, a positive pregnancy test, and changes in the pigmentation on her face and abdomen. These assessment findings reflect this woman is experiencing a cluster of which signs of pregnancy?
- ☐ 1. positive
- ☒ 2. probable
- ☐ 3. presumptive
- ☐ 4. diagnostic

32. When preparing a 20-year-old client for a serum pregnancy test, what information should the nurse tell the client?
- ☒ 1. The test has a high degree of accuracy within 1 week after ovulation.
- ☐ 2. The test is identical in nature to an over-the-counter home pregnancy test.
- ☐ 3. A positive result is considered a presumptive sign of pregnancy.
- ☐ 4. A urine sample is needed to obtain quicker results.

33. After instructing a female client about the radioimmunoassay pregnancy test, the nurse determines that the client understands the instructions when the client states that which hormone is evaluated by this test?
- ☐ 1. prolactin
- ☐ 2. follicle-stimulating hormone
- ☐ 3. luteinizing hormone
- ☒ 4. human chorionic gonadotropin (hCG)

34. Using Nägele's rule for a client whose last normal menstrual period began on May 10, the nurse determines that the client's estimated date of childbirth is what date?
- ☐ 1. January 13
- ☐ 2. January 17
- ☐ 3. February 13
- ☒ 4. February 17

35. After instructing a primigravid client about the functions of the placenta, the nurse determines that the client needs additional teaching when she says that which hormone is produced by the placenta?
- ☐ 1. estrogen
- ☐ 2. progesterone
- ☐ 3. human chorionic gonadotropin (hCG)
- ☒ 4. testosterone

36. The nurse assesses a woman at 24 weeks' gestation and is unable to find the fetal heartbeat. The fetal heartbeat was heard at the client's last visit 4 weeks ago. According to **priority**, the nurse should do the tasks in which order? All options must be used.

1. Call the healthcare provider (HCP).

2. Explain that the fetal heartbeat could not be found at this time.

3. Obtain different equipment and recheck.

4. Ask the client if the baby is or has been moving.

4

3

2

1

37. A primiparous client at 10 weeks' gestation questions the nurse about the need for an ultrasound. She states, "I feel fine, so why should I have the test?" The nurse should incorporate which statements as the underlying reason for performing the ultrasound now? Select all that apply.
- ☒ 1. "The test helps us view the gross anatomy of the fetus."
- ☒ 2. "We need to determine gestational age."
- ☐ 3. "The test will determine if the fetus is viable."
- ☐ 4. "We must determine fetal position."
- ☐ 5. "We must determine that there is a sufficient nutrient supply for the fetus."

38. A 20-year-old married client with a positive pregnancy test states, "Is it really true? I cannot believe I am going to have a baby!" Which response by the nurse would be **most** appropriate at this time?
- ☐ 1. "Would you like some booklets on the pregnancy experience?"
- ☒ 2. "Yes it is true. How does that make you feel?"
- ☐ 3. "You should be delighted that you are pregnant."
- ☐ 4. "What concerns you about this pregnancy?"

39. A newly diagnosed pregnant client tells the nurse, "If I am going to have all of these discomforts, I am not sure I want to be pregnant!" The nurse interprets the client's statement as an indication of which perception?
- ☐ 1. fear of pregnancy outcome
- ☐ 2. rejection of the pregnancy
- ☒ 3. normal ambivalence
- ☐ 4. inability to care for the newborn

40. A client, approximately 11 weeks pregnant, and her husband are seen in the antepartal clinic. The client's husband tells the nurse that he has been experiencing nausea and vomiting and fatigue along with his wife. The nurse interprets these findings as suggesting that the client's husband is experiencing which complication?
- ☐ 1. ptyalism
- ☐ 2. mittelschmerz
- ☒ 3. Couvade syndrome
- ☐ 4. pica

41. A primigravid client asks the nurse if she can continue to have a glass of wine with dinner during her pregnancy. Which statement would be the nurse's **best** response?
- ☐ 1. "The effects of alcohol on a fetus during pregnancy are unknown."
- ☐ 2. "You should limit your consumption to beer and wine."
- ☒ 3. "You should abstain from drinking alcoholic beverages."
- ☐ 4. "You may have 1 drink of 2 oz of alcohol per day."

42. Examination of a primigravid client having increased vaginal secretions since becoming pregnant reveals clear, highly acidic vaginal secretions. The client denies any perineal itching or burning. The nurse interprets these findings as a response related to which factor?
- ☐ 1. a decrease in vaginal glycogen stores
- ☐ 2. development of a sexually transmitted infection
- ☐ 3. prevention of expulsion of the cervical mucus plug
- ☒ 4. control of the growth of pathologic bacteria

43. When measuring the fundal height of a primigravid client at 20 weeks' gestation, the nurse will locate the fundal height at which point?
- ☐ 1. halfway between the client's symphysis pubis and umbilicus
- ☒ 2. at about the level of the client's umbilicus
- ☐ 3. between the client's umbilicus and xiphoid process
- ☐ 4. near the client's xiphoid process and compressing the diaphragm

44. A primigravida at 8 weeks' gestation tells the nurse that she wants an amniocentesis because there is a history of hemophilia A in her family. The nurse informs the client that she will need to wait until she is at 15 weeks' gestation for the amniocentesis. Which is the **most** appropriate rationale for the nurse's statement regarding amniocentesis at 15 weeks' gestation?
- ☐ 1. Fetal development needs to be complete before testing.
- ☒ 2. The volume of amniotic fluid needed for testing will be available by 15 weeks.
- ☐ 3. Cells indicating hemophilia A are not produced until 15 weeks' gestation.
- ☐ 4. Performing an amniocentesis prior to 15 weeks' gestation carries a greater infection rate.

45. After instructing a primigravid client about desired weight gain during pregnancy, the nurse determines that the teaching has been successful when the client makes which statement?
- ☐ 1. "A total weight gain of approximately 20 lb (9 kg) is recommended."
- ☐ 2. "A weight gain of 6.6 lb (3 kg) in the second and third trimesters is considered normal."
- ☐ 3. "A weight gain of about 12 lb (5.5 kg) every trimester is recommended."
- ☒ 4. "Although it varies, a gain of 25 to 35 lb (11.4 to 14.5 kg) is about average."

46. When developing a teaching plan for a client who is 8 weeks pregnant, what foods would the nurse suggest to meet the client's need for increased folic acid? Select all that apply.
- ☒ 1. spinach
- ☐ 2. bananas
- ☐ 3. seafood
- ☐ 4. yogurt
- ☒ 5. beans

47. The nurse instructs a primigravid client about the importance of sufficient vitamin A in her diet. The nurse knows that the instructions have been effective when the client indicates that she should include which foods in her diet?
- ☐ 1. buttermilk and cheese
- ☐ 2. strawberries and broccoli
- ☒ 3. egg yolks and squash
- ☐ 4. oranges and tomatoes

48. The nurse is discussing dietary concerns with pregnant teens. Which of the following choices are convenient for teens yet nutritious for both the mother and fetus? Select all that apply.
- ☒ 1. milkshake or yogurt with fresh fruit or granola bar
- ☐ 2. chicken nuggets with tater tots
- ☒ 3. cheese pizza with spinach and mushroom topping
- ☒ 4. peanut butter with crackers and a juice drink
- ☐ 5. buttery light popcorn with diet cola
- ☐ 6. cheeseburger, pickle, and ketchup

49. An antenatal client is discussing her anemia with the nurse in the prenatal clinic. After a discussion about sources of iron to be incorporated into her daily meals, the nurse knows the client needs further instruction when she responds with which statement?
- ☒ 1. "I can meet two goals when I drink milk: lots of iron and meeting my calcium needs at the same time."
- ☐ 2. "Drinking coffee, tea, and sodas decreases the absorption of iron."
- ☐ 3. "I can increase the absorption of iron by drinking orange juice when I eat."
- ☐ 4. "Cream of wheat and molasses are excellent sources of iron."

50. The nurse instructs a primigravid client to increase her intake of foods high in magnesium because of its role in which process?
- ☐ 1. prevention of demineralization of the mother's bones
- ☒ 2. synthesis of proteins, nucleic acids, and fats
- ☐ 3. amino acid metabolism
- ☐ 4. synthesis of neural pathways in the fetus

51. A client is at 24 weeks' gestation. The nurse is reviewing the report of laboratory tests as noted below.

Laboratory Results

Test	Result
Blood type	A-positive
Blood glucose	90 mg/dL (5 mmol/L)
VDRL	Positive
Rubella titer	Immune

The nurse should report which results to the health care provider (HCP)?
- ☐ 1. blood type
- ☒ 2. VDRL
- ☐ 3. blood glucose
- ☐ 4. rubella titer

52. The nurse is reviewing a pregnant client's immunization record. Which immunizations are contraindicated during pregnancy and are not updated at this time? Select all that apply.
- ☐ 1. tetanus
- ☒ 2. rubella
- ☒ 3. mumps
- ☒ 4. chickenpox
- ☒ 5. live attenuated influenza vaccine (LAIV)
- ☐ 6. hepatitis B

53. A 34-year-old multiparous client at 16 weeks' gestation who received regular prenatal care for all of her previous pregnancies tells the nurse that she has already felt the baby move. How does the nurse interpret this finding?
- ☐ 1. the possibility that the client is carrying twins
- ☐ 2. unusual because most multiparous clients do not experience quickening until 30 weeks' gestation
- ☐ 3. evidence that the client's estimated date of childbirth is probably off by a few weeks
- ☒ 4. normal because multiparous clients can experience quickening between 14 and 20 weeks' gestation

54. A 17-year-old gravid client presents for her regularly scheduled 26-week prenatal visit. She appears disheveled, is wearing ill-fitting clothes, and does not make eye contact with the nurse. Which items should the nurse discuss with the client? Select all that apply.
- ☒ 1. intimate partner violence
- ☒ 2. substance abuse
- ☒ 3. depression
- ☒ 4. blood glucose screening
- ☐ 5. HCG (human chorionic gonadotropin) levels

55. When performing Leopold's maneuvers, which action would the nurse ask the client to perform to ensure optimal comfort and accuracy?
- ☐ 1. breathe deeply for 1 minute
- ☒ 2. empty her bladder
- ☐ 3. drink a full glass of water
- ☐ 4. lie on her left side

56. The nurse performed Leopold's maneuvers and determined that the fetal position is ROA. Identify the area where the nurse would place the Doppler to **most** easily hear fetal heart sounds.

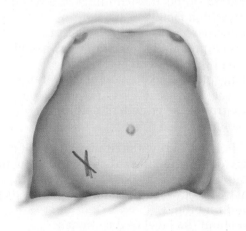

57. The nurse is assessing fetal position for a 32-year-old client in her 8th month of pregnancy. As shown below, the fetus is in which position?

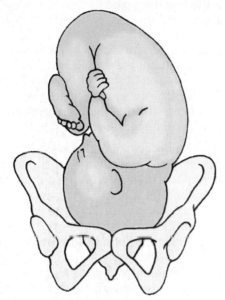

☐ **1.** left occipital transverse
☒ **2.** left occipital anterior
☐ **3.** right occipital transverse
☐ **4.** right occipital anterior

58. Which statement by the nurse would be **most** appropriate when responding to a primigravid client who asks, "What should I do about this brown discoloration across my nose and cheeks?"
☒ **1.** "This usually disappears after childbirth."
☐ **2.** "It is a sign of skin melanoma."
☐ **3.** "The discoloration is due to dilated capillaries."
☐ **4.** "It will fade if you use a prescribed cream."

59. A 36-year-old primigravid client at 22 weeks' gestation without any complications to date is being seen in the clinic for a routine visit. The nurse should assess the client's fundal height to:
☐ **1.** determine the level of uterine activity.
☐ **2.** identify the need for increased weight gain.
☐ **3.** assess the fetal position.
☒ **4.** estimate the fetal growth.

60. After the nurse reviews the primary health care provider's (HCP's) explanation of amniocentesis with a multigravid client, which complication, if stated by the client, indicates that she needs more teaching about the procedure?
☐ **1.** risk of infection
☒ **2.** possible miscarriage
☐ **3.** risk of club foot
☐ **4.** fetal organ malformations

61. A primigravid client at 28 weeks' gestation tells the nurse that she and her husband wish to drive to visit relatives who live several hours away. Which recommendation by the nurse would be **best**?
☐ **1.** "Try to avoid traveling anywhere in the car during your third trimester."
☐ **2.** "Limit the time you spend in the car to a maximum of 4 to 5 hours."
☒ **3.** "Taking the trip is okay if you stop every 1 to 2 hours and walk."
☐ **4.** "Avoid wearing your seat belt in the car to prevent injury to the fetus."

62. The nurse is teaching a woman who is 18 weeks pregnant about seat belt safety. Identify the area that indicates that the client understands where the lap portion of the seat belt should be placed.

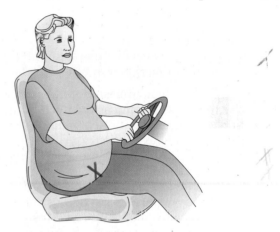

63. Which recommendation would be **most** helpful to suggest to a primigravid client at 37 weeks' gestation who has leg cramps?
☐ **1.** Change positions frequently throughout the day.
☐ **2.** Alternately flex and extend the legs.
☒ **3.** Straighten the knee and flex the toes toward the chin.
☐ **4.** Lie prone in bed with the legs elevated.

64. A nurse eating lunch at a restaurant sees a pregnant woman showing signs of airway obstruction. When the nurse asks the woman if she needs help, the woman nods her head yes. Indicate the area where the nurse's fist should be placed to effectively administer thrusts to clear the foreign body from the airway.

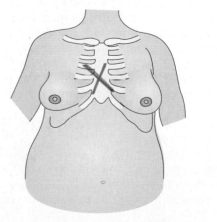

65. When performing Leopold's maneuvers on a primigravid client at 22 weeks' gestation, the nurse performs the first maneuver to accomplish which action?
☐ 1. Locate the fetal back and spine.
☒ 2. Determine what is in the fundus.
☐ 3. Determine whether the fetal head is at the pelvic inlet.
☐ 4. Identify the degree of fetal descent and flexion.

66. A primigravid adolescent client at approximately 15 weeks' gestation is visiting the prenatal clinic to undergo maternal quad screening. What information should the nurse include in the teaching plan for this client?
☐ 1. Ultrasonography usually accompanies maternal quad screen testing.
☐ 2. Results are usually very accurate until 20 weeks' gestation.
☐ 3. A clean-catch midstream urine specimen is needed.
☒ 4. Increased levels of alpha fetoprotein are associated with neural tube defects.

67. Which statement **best** identifies the rationale for why the nurse reinforces the need for continued prenatal care throughout the pregnancy with an adolescent primigravid client?
☒ 1. Pregnant adolescents are at high risk for pregnancy-induced hypertension.
☐ 2. Gestational diabetes during pregnancy commonly develops in adolescents.
☐ 3. Adolescents need additional instruction related to common discomforts.
☐ 4. The father of the baby is rarely involved in the pregnancy.

68. Which information would be included in the teaching plan about pregnancy-related breast changes for a primigravid client?
☐ 1. Growth of the milk ducts is greatest during the first 8 weeks of gestation.
☐ 2. Enlargement of the breasts indicates adequate levels of progesterone.
☒ 3. Colostrum is usually secreted by about the 16th week of gestation.
☐ 4. Darkening of the areola occurs during the last month of pregnancy.

69. A primigravid client at 32 weeks' gestation is enrolled in a breast-feeding class. Which statements indicate that the client understands the breast-feeding education? Select all that apply.
☐ 1. "My milk supply will be adequate since I have increased a whole bra size during pregnancy."
☒ 2. "I can hold my baby several different ways during feedings."
☐ 3. "If my infant latches on properly, I will not develop mastitis."
☒ 4. "If I breast-feed, my uterus will return to prepregnancy size more quickly."
☒ 5. "I need to feed my baby when I see feeding cues and not wait until she is crying."

70. When planning a class for primigravid clients about the common physiologic changes of pregnancy, which information should the nurse include in the teaching plan?
☐ 1. The temperature decreases slightly early in pregnancy.
☒ 2. Cardiac output increases by 25% to 50% during pregnancy.
☐ 3. The circulating fibrinogen level decreases as much as 50% during pregnancy.
☐ 4. The anterior pituitary gland secretes oxytocin late in pregnancy.

71. When teaching a primigravid client at 24 weeks' gestation about the diagnostic tests to determine fetal well-being, which information should the nurse include?
☒ 1. A fetal biophysical profile involves assessments of breathing movements, body movements, tone, amniotic fluid volume, and fetal heart rate reactivity.
☐ 2. A reactive nonstress test is an ominous sign and requires further evaluation with fetal echocardiography.
☐ 3. Contraction stress testing, performed on most pregnant women, can be initiated as early as 16 weeks' gestation.
☐ 4. Percutaneous umbilical blood sampling uses a needle inserted through the vagina to obtain a sample.

72. A client asks why she feels so much variability in fetal activity each day. The nurse explains that fetal movement is affected by which factors? Select all that apply.
☒ 1. fetal sleep
☐ 2. barometric pressure
☒ 3. blood glucose
☒ 4. time of day
☒ 5. cigarette smoking

73. When teaching a primigravid client how to do Kegel exercises, the nurse explains that the expected outcome of these exercises is to:
☐ 1. reduce risk of hemorrhoids.
☐ 2. alleviate lower back discomfort.
☒ 3. strengthen the perineal muscles.
☐ 4. strengthen the abdominal muscles.

74. During a routine clinic visit, a 25-year-old multigravid client who initiated prenatal care at 10 weeks' gestation and is now in her third trimester states, "I've been having strange dreams about the baby. Last week I dreamed he was covered with hair." The nurse should tell the mother:
☐ 1. "Dreams like the ones that you describe are very unusual. Please tell me more about them."
☐ 2. "Commonly when a mother has these dreams, she is trying to cope with becoming a parent."
☐ 3. "Dreams about the baby late in pregnancy usually mean that labor is about to begin soon."
☒ 4. "It is not uncommon to have dreams about the baby, particularly in the third trimester."

75. A primigravid client at 36 weeks' gestation tells the nurse that she has been experiencing insomnia for the past 2 weeks. Which suggestion would be **most** helpful?
- ☒ 1. Practice relaxation techniques before bedtime.
- ☐ 2. Drink a cup of hot chocolate before bedtime.
- ☐ 3. Drink a small glass of wine with dinner.
- ☐ 4. Exercise for 30 minutes just before bedtime.

76. Which client statement indicates a need for additional teaching about self-care during pregnancy?
- ☐ 1. "I should use nonskid pads when I take a shower or bath."
- ☐ 2. "I should avoid using soap on my nipples to prevent drying."
- ☒ 3. "I should sit in a hot tub for 20 minutes to relax after working."
- ☐ 4. "I should avoid douching even if my vaginal secretions increase."

The Pregnant Client in Birth Preparation Classes

77. The nurse is developing a teaching plan for a client entering the third trimester of her pregnancy. The nurse should include which information in the plan? Select all that apply.
- ☐ 1. differentiating the fetus from the self
- ☐ 2. ambivalence concerning pregnancy
- ☒ 3. experimenting with mothering roles
- ☒ 4. realignment of roles and tasks
- ☒ 5. trying various caregiver roles
- ☒ 6. concern about labor and birth

78. A new antenatal G6, T4, P0, A1, L4 client attends her first prenatal visit with her partner. The nurse is assessing this couple's psychological response to the pregnancy. Which finding requires the **most** immediate follow-up?
- ☐ 1. The couple is concerned with financial changes this pregnancy causes.
- ☐ 2. The couple expresses ambivalence about the current pregnancy.
- ☐ 3. The father of the baby states that the pregnancy has changed the mother's focus.
- ☒ 4. The father of the baby is irritated that the mother is not like she was before pregnancy.

79. When preparing a prenatal class about endocrine changes that normally occur during pregnancy, the nurse should include information about which subject?
- ☐ 1. Human placental lactogen maintains the corpus luteum.
- ☐ 2. Progesterone is responsible for hyperpigmentation and vascular skin changes.
- ☐ 3. Estrogen relaxes smooth muscle in the respiratory tract.
- ☒ 4. The thyroid enlarges with an increase in basal metabolic rate.

80. When developing a series of parent classes on fetal development, the nurse should include which feature as being developed by the end of the 3rd month (9 to 12 weeks)?
- ☒ 1. external genitalia
- ☐ 2. myelinization of nerves
- ☐ 3. brown fat stores
- ☐ 4. air ducts and alveoli

81. A primigravid client attending parenthood classes tells the nurse that there is a history of twins in her family. What should the nurse tell the client?
- ☐ 1. Monozygotic twins result from fertilization of one ovum.
- ☒ 2. Monozygotic twins occur by chance regardless of race or heredity.
- ☐ 3. Dizygotic twins are usually of the same sex.
- ☐ 4. Dizygotic twins occur more often in primigravid than in multigravid clients.

82. During a 2-hour birth preparation class focusing on the labor and birth process for primigravid clients, the nurse is describing the maneuvers that the fetus goes through during the labor process when the head is the presenting part. In which order do these maneuvers occur? All options must be used.

1. engagement
2. flexion
3. descent
4. internal rotation

1 ~ engagement
3 ~ descent
2 ~ flexion
4 ~ internal rotation

83. A primigravid client in a preparation for parenting class asks how much blood is lost during an uncomplicated vaginal birth. The nurse should tell the woman:
- ☒ 1. "The maximum blood loss considered within normal limits is 500 mL."
- ☐ 2. "The minimum blood loss considered within normal limits is 1,000 mL."
- ☐ 3. "Blood loss during childbirth is rarely estimated unless there is a hemorrhage."
- ☐ 4. "It would be very unusual if you lost more than 100 mL of blood during childbirth."

84. Which statement by a primigravid client about the amniotic fluid and sac indicates the need for further teaching?

☐ 1. "The amniotic fluid helps to dilate the cervix once labor begins."

☒ 2. "Fetal nutrients are provided by the amniotic fluid."

☐ 3. "Amniotic fluid provides a cushion against impact of the maternal abdomen."

☐ 4. "The fetus is kept at a stable temperature by the amniotic fluid and sac."

85. During a birth preparation class, a primigravid client at 36 weeks' gestation tells the nurse, "My lower back has really been bothering me lately." Which exercise would be **most** helpful?

☒ 1. pelvic rocking

☐ 2. deep breathing

☐ 3. tailor sitting

☐ 4. squatting

86. A client is experiencing pain during the **first** stage of labor. What should the nurse instruct the client to do to manage her pain? Select all that apply.

☒ 1. Walk in the hospital room.

☒ 2. Use slow chest breathing.

☐ 3. Request pain medication on a regular basis.

☒ 4. Lightly massage the abdomen.

☐ 5. Sip ice water.

87. During a preparation for parenting class, one of the participants asks the nurse, "How will I know if I am really in labor?" What should the nurse tell the participant about true labor contractions?

☐ 1. "Walking around helps to decrease true contractions."

☐ 2. "True labor contractions may disappear with ambulation, rest, or sleep."

☐ 3. "The duration and frequency of true labor contractions remain the same."

☒ 4. "True labor contractions are felt first in the lower back, then the abdomen."

88. After instructing participants in a birth education class about methods for coping with discomforts in the first stage of labor, the nurse determines that one of the pregnant clients needs further instruction when she says that she has been practicing which technique?

☐ 1. biofeedback

☐ 2. effleurage

☐ 3. guided imagery

☒ 4. pelvic tilt exercises

89. After a preparation for parenting class session, a pregnant client tells the nurse that she has had some yellow-gray frothy vaginal discharge and local itching. What is the **best** advice for the nurse to give the client?

☐ 1. Use an over-the-counter cream for yeast infections.

☒ 2. Schedule an appointment at the clinic for an examination.

☐ 3. Administer a vinegar douche under low pressure.

☐ 4. Prepare for preterm labor and birth.

90. The topic of physiologic changes that occur during pregnancy is to be included in a parenting class for primigravid clients who are in their first half of pregnancy. Which topic would be important for the nurse to include in the teaching plan?

☐ 1. decreased plasma volume

☒ 2. increased risk for urinary tract infections

☐ 3. increased peripheral vascular resistance

☐ 4. increased hemoglobin levels

The Pregnant Client with Risk Factors

91. A multigravid client at 32 weeks' gestation has experienced hemolytic disease of the newborn in a previous pregnancy. The nurse should prepare the client for frequent antibody titer evaluations obtained from which source?

☐ 1. placental blood

☐ 2. amniotic fluid

☐ 3. fetal blood

☒ 4. maternal blood

92. Which diagnostic test would be the **most** important for a 40-year-old primigravid client to have in the second trimester of her pregnancy?

☐ 1. beta strep screening

☐ 2. chorionic villus sampling

☐ 3. ultrasound testing

☒ 4. quad screen

93. The nurse is caring for a client who has a history of gastric bypass surgery and is now being seen for her first prenatal visit. Which interventions should be included in the plan of care? Select all that apply.

☒ 1. Take a prenatal vitamin with 400 mcg of folic acid.

☒ 2. Refer the client to a registered dietician.

☐ 3. Draw glucose levels at each prenatal visit.

☐ 4. Counsel her that she will most likely gain all of her weight back.

☒ 5. Check urine at each visit for protein and glucose.

☐ 6. Monitor with nonstress tests beginning at 20 weeks.

94. A client with a past medical history of ventricular septal defect repaired in infancy is seen at the prenatal clinic. She has dyspnea with exertion and is very tired. Her vital signs are oxygen saturation 98, pulse 80, respirations 20, blood pressure 116/72 mm Hg. She has +2 pedal edema and clear breath sounds. The nurse determines the client's symptoms indicate which cardiac functional classification?

☐ 1. class I

☒ 2. class II

☐ 3. class III

☐ 4. class IV

95. A primigravid client has completed her first prenatal visit and blood work. Her laboratory test for the hepatitis B surface antigen (HBsAg) is positive. The nurse can advise the client that the plan of care for this newborn will include which interventions? Select all that apply.

1. hepatitis B immune globulin at birth
2. series of three hepatitis B vaccinations per recommended schedule
3. hepatitis B screening when born
4. isolation of infant during hospitalization
5. universal precautions for mother and infant
6. contraindication for breast-feeding

96. A woman with asthma controlled through the consistent use of medication is now pregnant for the first time. Which client statement concerning asthma during pregnancy indicates the need for further instruction?

1. "I need to continue taking my asthma medication as prescribed."
2. "It is my goal to prevent or limit asthma attacks."
3. "During an asthma attack, oxygen needs to continue to be high for mother and fetus."
4. "Bronchodilators should be used only when necessary because of the risk they present to the fetus."

97. A woman at 22 weeks' gestation has right upper quadrant pain radiating to her back. She rates the pain as 9 on a scale of 1 to 10 and says that it has occurred 2 times in the last week for about 4 hours at a time. She does not associate the pain with food. Which nursing measure is the **highest priority** for this client?

1. Educate the client concerning changes occurring in the gallbladder as a result of pregnancy.
2. Refer the client to her health care provider (HCP) for evaluation and treatment of the pain.
3. Discuss nutritional strategies to decrease the possibility of heartburn.
4. Support the client's use of acetaminophen to relieve pain.

98. A client in the triage area who is at 19 weeks' gestation states that she has not felt her baby move in the past week, and no fetal heart tones are found. While evaluating this client, the nurse identifies her as being at the **highest** risk for developing which problem?

1. abruptio placentae
2. HELLP syndrome
3. disseminated intravascular coagulation
4. threatened abortion

99. The nurse performs a routine prenatal assessment on a woman at 35 weeks' gestation and finds vital signs: blood pressure 138/88 mm Hg, pulse 82/min, respirations 18/min, temperature 99.1°F (37.3°C). Which statement is **most** appropriate for the nurse to make at this time?

1. "Your pulse is low. Do you exercise a lot?"
2. "Your blood pressure is slightly high. I will check it again before you leave."
3. "You have a slight temperature. Do you feel hot?"
4. "Your vital signs are all normal. I will document them on your medical record."

100. A 40-year-old client at 8 weeks' gestation has a 3-year-old child with Down syndrome. The nurse is discussing amniocentesis and chorionic villus sampling as genetic screening methods for the expected baby. The nurse is confident that the teaching has been understood when the client makes which statement?

1. "Each test identifies a different part of the infant's genetic makeup."
2. "Chorionic villus sampling can be performed earlier in pregnancy."
3. "The test results take the same length of time to be completed."
4. "Amniocentesis is a more dangerous procedure for the fetus."

101. After conducting a presentation to a group of adolescent parents on the topic of adolescent pregnancy, the nurse determines that one of the parents needs further instruction when the parent says that adolescents are at greater risk for which complication?

1. denial of the pregnancy
2. low-birth-weight infant
3. cephalopelvic disproportion
4. congenital anomalies

102. A dilatation and curettage (D&C) is scheduled for a primigravid client admitted to the hospital at 10 weeks' gestation with abdominal cramping, bright red vaginal spotting, and passage of some of the products of conception. The nurse should assess the client further for the expression of which feeling?

1. ambivalence
2. anxiety
3. fear
4. guilt

103. When providing care to the client who has undergone a dilatation and curettage (D&C) after a spontaneous abortion, the nurse administers hydroxyzine as prescribed. What is an expected outcome?

1. absence of nausea
2. minimized pain
3. decreased uterine cramping
4. improved uterine contractility

104. On entering the room of a client who has undergone a dilatation and curettage (D&C) for a spontaneous abortion, the nurse finds the client crying. Which comment by the nurse would be **most** appropriate?
- [ ] 1. "Are you having a great deal of uterine pain?"
- [ ] 2. "Commonly spontaneous abortion means a defective embryo."
- [x] 3. "I am truly sorry you lost your baby."
- [ ] 4. "It is important that you do not try to get pregnant too soon."

105. Rho (D) immune globulin (RhoGAM) is prescribed for a client before she is discharged after a spontaneous abortion. The nurse instructs the client that this drug is used to prevent which condition?
- [ ] 1. development of a future Rh-positive fetus
- [ ] 2. an antibody response to Rh-negative blood
- [ ] 3. a future pregnancy resulting in abortion
- [x] 4. development of Rh-positive antibodies

106. A multigravid client who stands for long periods while working in a factory visits the prenatal clinic at 35 weeks' gestation, stating, "The varicose veins in my legs have really been bothering me lately." Which instruction would be **most** helpful?
- [ ] 1. Perform slow contraction and relaxation of the feet and ankles twice daily.
- [x] 2. Take frequent rest periods with the legs elevated above the hips.
- [ ] 3. Avoid support hose that reach above the leg varicosities.
- [ ] 4. Take a leave of absence from your job to avoid prolonged standing.

107. A primigravid client at 8 weeks' gestation tells the nurse that since having had sexual relations with a new partner 2 weeks ago, she has noticed flu-like symptoms, enlarged lymph nodes, and clusters of vesicles on her vagina. The nurse refers the client to a primary health care provider (HCP) because the nurse suspects which sexually transmitted infection?
- [ ] 1. gonorrhea
- [ ] 2. *Chlamydia trachomatis* infection
- [ ] 3. syphilis
- [x] 4. herpes genitalis

108. While caring for a 24-year-old primigravid client scheduled for emergency surgery because of a probable ectopic pregnancy, the nurse should:
- [x] 1. prepare to witness an informed consent for surgery.
- [ ] 2. assess the client for massive external bleeding.
- [ ] 3. explain that the fallopian tube can be salvaged.
- [ ] 4. monitor the client for uterine contractions.

Managing Care, Quality, and Safety for Childbearing Clients

109. The nurse is reviewing results for clients who are having antenatal testing. The assessment data from which client warrants prompt notification of the health care provider (HCP) and a further plan of care?
- [ ] 1. primigravida who reports fetal movement 6 times in 2 hours
- [x] 2. multigravida who had a positive oxytocin challenge test
- [ ] 3. primigravida whose infant has a biophysical profile of 9.
- [ ] 4. multigravida whose infant has a reactive non-stress test.

110. A client asks the nurse why taking folic acid is so important before and during pregnancy. The nurse should instruct the client that:
- [x] 1. "Folic acid is important in preventing neural tube defects in newborns and preventing anemia in mothers."
- [ ] 2. "Eating foods with moderate amounts of folic acid helps regulate blood glucose levels."
- [ ] 3. "Folic acid consumption helps with the absorption of iron during pregnancy."
- [ ] 4. "Folic acid is needed to promote blood clotting and collagen formation in the newborn."

111. A nurse is assigned to the obstetrical triage area. When beginning the assignment, the nurse is given a report about four clients waiting to be seen. Place the clients in the order in which the nurse should see them. All options must be used.

1. a primigravid client at 10 weeks' gestation stating she is not feeling well with nausea and vomiting, urinary frequency, and fatigue

2. a multiparous client at 32 weeks' gestation asking for assistance with finding a new primary health care provider (HCP)

3. a single mother at 4 months postpartum fearful of shaking her baby when he cries

4. an antenatal client at 16 weeks' gestation who has occasional sharp pain on her left side radiating from her symphysis to her fundus

3
4
1
2

112. The nurse is working in an ambulatory obstetrics setting. What are emphasized client safety procedures for this setting? Select all that apply.
- ☒ 1. handwashing or antiseptic use when entering and leaving a room
- ☒ 2. use of two client identifiers when initiating contact with a client
- ☒ 3. use same abbreviations as in the hospital setting
- ☒ 4. conduct preprocedure verification asking for client name and procedure to be performed
- ☐ 5. prevent infection by isolating anyone with nausea and vomiting

Answers, Rationales, and Test-Taking Strategies

*The answers and rationales for each question follow below, along with keys (🗝) to the client need (CN) and cognitive level (CL) for each question. In addition, you will also see a glossary icon (📖) high-lighting specific terminology used on the licensing exam. As you check your answers, use the **Content Mastery and Test-Taking Skill Self-Analysis** worksheet (tear-out worksheet in back of book) to identify the reason(s) for not answering the questions correctly. For additional information about test-taking skills and strategies for answering questions, refer to pages 12–23 and pages 35–36 in Part 1 of this book.*

The Preconception Client

1. 1. Levonorgestrel can reduce the chance of pregnancy if taken within 72 hours of unprotected intercourse, and then again 12 hours later. Waiting 4 days to take levonorgestrel reduces effectiveness. Males can purchase this contraceptive as long as they are over 18 years of age. Levonorgestrel works by preventing ovulation or fertilization depending on where a client is in the menstrual cycle. Common side effects include nausea, breast tenderness, vertigo, and stomach pain.

🗝 CN: Physiological adaptation; CL: Evaluate

2. 3. Birth control plans are influenced primarily by whether the mother is breast- or bottle-feeding her infant. The maternal milk supply must be well established prior to the initiation of most hormonal birth control methods. Low-dose oral contraceptives would be the exception. Use of estrogen-/progesterone-based pills and progesterone-only pills are commonly initiated from 4 to 6 weeks postpartum because the milk supply is well established by this time. Prior experiences with birth control methods have an impact on the method chosen as do the preferences of the client's partner; however, they are not the most influential factors. Desire to have another child in 2 years would make some methods, such as an IUD, less attractive but would still be secondary to the choice to breast-feed.

🗝 CN: Pharmacological and parenteral therapies; CL: Analyze

3. 3. For a client with a typical menstrual cycle of 28 days, ovulation usually occurs on day 14, plus or minus 2 days, before the onset of the next menstrual cycle. Stated another way, the menstrual period begins about 2 weeks after ovulation has occurred. Ovulation does not usually occur during the menses component of the cycle when the uterine lining is being shed. In most women, the ovum survives for about 12 to 24 hours after ovulation, during which time conception is possible. The basal body temperature rises 0.5°F to 1.0°F (0.28°C to 0.56°C) when ovulation occurs. Although some women experience some pelvic discomfort during ovulation (mittelschmerz), severe or unusual pain is rare. After ovulation, the cervical mucus is thin and copious.

🗝 CN: Health promotion and maintenance; CL: Create

4. 1. The nurse should instruct the client to take a mild analgesic, such as ibuprofen, if menstrual pain or "cramps" are present. The client should also eat foods rich in iron and should continue moderate exercise during menstruation, which increases abdominal tone. Avoiding cold foods will not decrease dysmenorrhea. Use of pads or tampons is a personal choice. There is no evidence that it is necessary to wait to use tampons.

🗝 CN: Health promotion and maintenance; CL: Apply

5. 1. Under ideal conditions, sperm can reach the ovum in 15 to 30 minutes. This is an important point to make with adolescents who may be sexually active. Many people believe that the time interval is much longer and that they can wait until after intercourse to take steps to prevent conception. Without protection, pregnancy and sexually transmitted diseases can occur. When using the abstinence or calendar method, the couple should abstain from intercourse on the days of the menstrual cycle when the woman is most likely to conceive. Using a 28-day cycle as an example, a couple should abstain from coitus 3 to 4 days before ovulation (days 10 through 14) and 3 to 4 days after ovulation (days 15 through 18). Sperm from a healthy male can remain viable for 24 to 72 hours in the female reproductive tract. If the female client ovulates after coitus, there is a possibility that fertilization can occur. Before fertilization, the ovum and sperm each contain 23 chromosomes. After fertilization, the conceptus contains 46 chromosomes unless there is a chromosomal abnormality.

    📍 CN: Health promotion and maintenance; CL: Evaluate

6. 3. The symptothermal method is a natural method of fertility management that depends on knowing when ovulation has occurred. Because regular menstrual cycles can vary by 1 to 2 days in either direction, the symptothermal method requires daily basal body temperature assessments plus close monitoring of cervical mucus changes. The method relies on abstinence during the period of ovulation, which occurs approximately 14 days before the beginning of the next cycle. Abstinence from coitus for 5 days after menses is unnecessary because it is unlikely that ovulation will occur during this time period (days 1 through 10). Typically, the failure rate for this method is between 10% and 20%. Although a condom may increase the effectiveness of this method, most clients who choose natural methods are not interested in chemical or barrier types of family planning.

    📍 CN: Health promotion and maintenance; CL: Create

7. 2. Before advising a client about oral contraceptives, the nurse needs to assess the client for signs and symptoms of hypertension. Clients who have hypertension, thrombophlebitis, obesity, or a family history of cerebral or cardiovascular accident are poor candidates for oral contraceptives. In addition, women who smoke, are older than 40 years of age, or have a history of pulmonary disease should be advised to use a different method. Iron deficiency anemia, dysmenorrhea, and acne are not contraindications for the use of oral contraceptives. Iron deficiency anemia is a common disorder in young women. Oral contraceptives decrease the amount of menstrual flow and thus decrease the amount of iron lost through menses, thereby providing a beneficial effect when used by clients with anemia. Low-dose oral contraceptives to prevent ovulation may be effective in decreasing the severity of dysmenorrhea (painful menstruation). Dysmenorrhea is thought to be caused by the release of prostaglandins in response to tissue destruction during the ischemic phase of the menstrual cycle. Use of oral contraceptives commonly improves facial acne.

    📍 CN: Reduction of risk potential; CL: Analyze

8. 4. The nurse determines that the client needs further instruction when the client says that one of the adverse effects of oral contraceptive use is

ovarian cancer. Some studies suggest that ovarian and endometrial cancers are reduced in women using oral contraceptives. Other adverse effects of oral contraceptives include weight gain, nausea, headache, breakthrough bleeding, and monilial infections. The most serious adverse effect is thrombophlebitis.

    📍 CN: Pharmacological and parenteral therapies; CL: Evaluate

9. 2. The teaching plan should include a caution that a diaphragm should not be used if the client develops acute cervicitis, possibly aggravated by contact with the rubber of the diaphragm. Some studies have also associated diaphragm use with increased incidence of urinary tract infections. Douching after use of a diaphragm and intercourse is not recommended because pregnancy could occur. The diaphragm should be inspected and washed with mild soap and water after each use. A diaphragm should be left in place for at least 6 hours but no longer than 24 hours after intercourse. More spermicidal jelly or cream should be used if intercourse is repeated during this period.

    📍 CN: Reduction of risk potential; CL: Create

10. 4. The client would need additional instructions when she says that she can still use the same diaphragm if she gains or loses 20 lb (9 kg). Gaining or losing more than 15 lb (6.8 kg) can change the pelvic and vaginal contours to such a degree that the diaphragm will no longer protect the client against pregnancy. The diaphragm can be used for 2 to 3 years if it is cared for and well protected in its case. The client should be refitted for another diaphragm after pregnancy and childbirth because weight changes and physiologic changes of pregnancy can alter the pelvic and vaginal contours, thus affecting the effectiveness of the diaphragm. The client should use a spermicidal jelly or cream before inserting the diaphragm.

    📍 CN: Reduction of risk potential; CL: Evaluate

11. 1,2,3,5,6. The pregnancy requirement for folic acid is 400 to 800 mcg/day. Major sources of folic acid include leafy green vegetables, strawberries and oranges, beans, particularly black and kidney beans, sunflower seeds, and lentils. Milk and fats contain no folic acid.

    📍 CN: Health promotion and maintenance; CL: Apply

12. 1. Another method of contraception is needed until all sperm has been cleared from the body. The number of ejaculates for this to occur varies with the individual, and laboratory analysis is required to determine when that has been accomplished. Vasectomy is considered a permanent sterilization procedure and requires microsurgery for anastomosis of the vas deferens to be completed. Studies have shown that there is no connection between cardiac disease in males and vasectomy. There is no need for follow-up after verification that there is no sperm in the system.

CN: Physiological adaptation; CL: Create

13. 1. Tubal ligation, a female sterilization procedure, involves ligation (tying off) or cauterization of the fallopian tubes through a small abdominal incision (laparotomy). Reversal of a tubal ligation is not easily done, and the pregnancy success rate after reversal is about 30%. After a tubal ligation, the client may engage in intercourse 2 to 3 days after the procedure. The ovaries are not generally removed during a tubal ligation. An oophorectomy involves removal of one or both ovaries.

CN: Health promotion and maintenance; CL: Evaluate

14. 2. The basal body temperature method requires that the client take her temperature each morning before getting out of bed, preferably at the same time each day before eating or any other activity. Just before the day of ovulation, the temperature falls by 0.5°F (0.28°C). At the time of ovulation, the temperature rises 0.4°F to 0.8°F (0.22°C to 0.44°C) because of increased progesterone secretion in response to the luteinizing hormone. The temperature remains higher for the rest of the menstrual cycle. The client should keep a diary of about 6 months of menstrual cycles to calculate "safe" days. There is no mucus for the first 3 or 4 days after menses, and then thick, sticky mucus begins to appear. As estrogen increases, the mucus changes to clear, slippery, and stretchy. This condition, termed spinnbarkeit, is present during ovulation. After ovulation, the mucus decreases in amount and becomes thick and sticky again until menses. Because the ovum typically survives about 24 hours and sperm can survive up to 72 hours, couples must avoid coitus when the cervical mucus is copious and for about 3 to 4 days before and after ovulation to avoid a pregnancy.

CN: Health promotion and maintenance; CL: Apply

15. 4. By the end of the first visit, the couple should be able to identify potential causes and treatment modalities for infertility. If their evaluation shows that a treatment or procedure may help them to conceive, the couple must then decide how to proceed, considering all of the various treatments before selecting one. Treatments can be difficult, painful, or risky. The first visit is not the appropriate time to decide on a treatment plan because the couple needs time to adjust to the diagnosis of

infertility, a crisis for most couples. Although the couple may be in a hurry for definitive therapy, a thorough assessment of both partners is necessary before a treatment plan can be initiated. The success rate for achieving a pregnancy depends on both the cause and the effectiveness of the treatment, and in some cases, it may be only as high as 30%. The couple may desire information about alternatives to treatment, but insufficient data are available to suggest that a specific treatment modality may not be successful. Suggesting that the couple consider adoption at this time may inappropriately imply that the couple has no other choice. If a specific therapy may result in a pregnancy, the couple should have time to consider their options. After a thorough evaluation, adoption may be considered by the couple as an alternative to the costly, time-consuming, and sometimes painful treatments for infertility.

CN: Health promotion and maintenance; CL: Analyze

16. 3. The client's understanding of the procedure is demonstrated by the statement describing IVF as a technique that involves bypassing the blocked or absent fallopian tubes. The primary **health care provider (HCP)** removes the ova by laparoscope- or ultrasound-guided transvaginal retrieval and mixes them with prepared sperm from the woman's partner or a donor. Two days later, up to four embryos are returned to the uterus to increase the likelihood of a successful pregnancy. Supplemental progesterone, not estrogen, is given to enhance the implantation process. Gamete intra-fallopian transfer (GIFT) and tubal embryo transfer have a higher pregnancy rate than does IVF. However, these procedures cannot be used for clients who have blocked or absent fallopian tubes because the fertilized ova are placed into the fallopian tubes, subsequently entering the uterus naturally for implantation. In IVF, fertilization of the ova by the sperm occurs outside the client's body. In GIFT, both ova and sperm are implanted into the fallopian tubes and allowed to fertilize within the woman's body.

CN: Reduction of risk potential; CL: Evaluate

17. 4. The client is verbalizing concerns about death during childbirth, thus providing the nurse with an opportunity to gather additional data. Asking the client about these concerns would be most helpful to determine the client's knowledge base and to provide the nurse with the opportunity to answer any questions and clarify any misconceptions. Although the maternal mortality rate is low in the United States and Canada, maternal deaths do occur, even with modern technology. Leading causes of maternal mortality in the United States and Canada include embolism, pregnancy-induced hypertension, hemorrhage, ectopic pregnancy, and infection. Telling the client not to concern herself about what has happened in the past is not useful. It only serves to discount the client's concerns and block further therapeutic communication. Also, postponing or ignoring the client's need for a discussion about complications of pregnancy may further increase the client's anxiety.

CN: Health promotion and maintenance; **CL:** Apply

18. 3. As ovulation approaches, cervical mucus is abundant and clear, resembling raw egg white. Ovulation generally occurs 14 days (±2 days) before the beginning of menses. During the luteal phase of the cycle, which occurs after ovulation, the cervical mucus is thick and sticky, making it difficult for sperm to pass. Changes in the cervical mucus are related to the influences of estrogen and progesterone. Cervical mucus is always present.

CN: Health promotion and maintenance; **CL:** Create

19. 1. To ensure maximum effectiveness, the condom should always be placed over the erect penis before coitus. Some couples find condom use objectionable because foreplay may have to be interrupted to apply the condom. The penis, covered by the condom, should be withdrawn before the penis becomes flaccid. Otherwise semen may escape from the condom, providing an opportunity for possible fertilization. Rather than having the condom pulled tightly over the penis before coitus, space should be left at the tip of the penis to allow the condom to hold the sperm. The client does not need a prescription for a condom with nonoxynol 9 because these are sold over the counter.

CN: Reduction of risk potential; **CL:** Apply

20. 3. With medroxyprogesterone acetate, irregular menstrual cycles and amenorrhea are common adverse effects. Other adverse effects include weight gain, breakthrough bleeding, headaches, and depression. This method requires deep intramuscular injections every 3 months. The first injection should occur within 5 days after menses.

CN: Reduction of risk potential; **CL:** Evaluate

21. 4. Severe cramping and pain may occur as the device is passed through the internal cervical os. The insertion of the device is generally done when the client is having her menses because it is unlikely that she is pregnant at that time. Common adverse effects of IUDs are heavy menstrual bleeding and subsequent anemia, not amenorrhea.

Uterine infection or ectopic pregnancy may occur. The IUD has an effectiveness rate of 98%. Therefore, additional protection is not necessary to prevent pregnancy. IUDs generally are less costly than other forms of contraception because they do not require additional expense. Only one insertion is necessary, in comparison to daily doses of oral contraceptives or the need for spermicides in conjunction with diaphragm use.

CN: Reduction of risk potential; **CL:** Apply

22. 3. Ceftriaxone may be used to treat *N. gonorrhoeae* infections and is commonly combined with doxycycline. Both the client and her partner should be treated if gonorrhea is present. Acyclovir can be used to treat herpes genitalis; however, the drug does not cure the disease. *C. trachomatis* infections are usually treated with antibiotics such as doxycycline or azithromycin. Metronidazole is used to treat trichomoniasis vaginitis, not condylomata acuminata (genital warts).

CN: Pharmacological and parenteral therapies; **CL:** Create

23. 1. The couple needs further instruction when they identify that one cause of male infertility is decreased sperm count due to seminal fluid that has an alkaline pH. A slightly alkaline pH is necessary to protect the sperm from the acidic secretions of the vagina and is a normal finding. An alkaline pH is not associated with decreased sperm count. However, seminal fluid that is abnormal in amount, consistency, or chemical composition suggests obstruction, inflammation, or infection, which can decrease sperm production. The typical number of sperm produced during ejaculation is 400 million. Frequent exposure to heat sources, such as saunas and hot tubs, can decrease sperm production, as can abnormal hormonal stimulation. Immunologic factors produced by the man against his own sperm (autoantibodies) or by the woman can cause the sperm to clump or be unable to penetrate the ovum, thus contributing to infertility.

CN: Health promotion and maintenance; **CL:** Evaluate

24. 2. A bicornuate uterus has a "Y" shape and appears to be a double uterus but in fact has only one cervix. A septate uterus contains a septum that extends from the fundus to the cervix, thus dividing the uterus into two separate compartments. A double uterus has two uteri, each of which has a cervix. A uterus didelphys occurs when both uteri of a double uterus are fully formed.

CN: Physiological adaptation; **CL:** Apply

The Pregnant Client Receiving Prenatal Care

25. 3. At 15 weeks' gestation, a primipara will not feel the baby moving. Quickening typically occurs between 18 and 20 weeks' gestation for a primipara and between 16 and 18 weeks' gestation for a multipara. Leaking fluid from the vagina should not occur until labor begins and may indicate a rupture of the membranes. Bleeding and a fever are complications that warrant further evaluation and should be reported at any time during the pregnancy.

☠⎯ CN: Health promotion and maintenance; CL: Evaluate

26. 1,4,6. Providing culturally sensitive care includes providing printed material in the client's native language. There is nothing to indicate that this client has a high-risk pregnancy. Discussing cultural differences is not a priority or important at the first visit. Clients need to have an interpreter for each prenatal visit to translate and interpret questions. Contraceptive options are not a priority for the first prenatal visit. Reviewing dietary intake and discussing nutrition are an important component of early prenatal care.

☠⎯ CN: Health promotion and maintenance; CL: Create

27. 4. Consuming most liquids between meals rather than at the same time as eating is an excellent strategy to deter nausea and vomiting in pregnancy but does not relieve heartburn. During the third trimester, progesterone causes relaxation of the sphincter, and the pressure of the fetus against the stomach increases the potential of heartburn. Avoiding highly seasoned foods, remaining in an upright position after eating, and eating small, frequent meals are strategies to prevent heartburn.

☠⎯ CN: Physiological adaptation; CL: Evaluate

28. 2. Iron deficiency anemia is caused by insufficient iron stores in the body, poor iron content in the diet of the pregnant woman, or both. Other thalassemias and sickle cell anemia, rather than iron deficiency anemia, can be associated with ethnicity but occur primarily in clients of African or Mediterranean origin. Because red blood cells increase by about 50% during pregnancy, many clients will need to take supplemental iron to avoid iron deficiency anemia. A pregnant client is considered anemic when the hemoglobin is below 11 mg/dL (110 g/dL). In most types of anemia, the heart must pump more often and harder to deliver oxygen to cells.

☠⎯ CN: Reduction of risk potential; CL: Evaluate

29. 4. Many women in their first trimester feel ambivalent about being pregnant because of the significant life changes that occur for most women who have a child. Ambivalence can be expressed as a list of positive and negative consequences of having a child, consideration of financial and social implications, and possible career changes. During the second trimester, the infant becomes a separate individual to the mother. The mother will begin to enjoy the role of nurturer postpartum. During the third trimester, the mother begins to prepare for parenthood and all of the tasks that parenthood includes.

☠⎯ CN: Health promotion and maintenance; CL: Apply

30. 4. Group B streptococcus is a risk factor for all pregnant women and is not limited to those carrying twins. The multiple gestation client is at risk for preterm labor because uterine distention, a major factor initiating preterm labor, is more likely with a twin gestation. The normal uterus is only able to distend to a certain point, and when that point is reached, labor may be initiated. Twin-to-twin transfusion drains blood from one twin to the second and is a problem that may occur with multiple gestations. The donor twin may become growth restricted and can have oligohydramnios, while the recipient twin may become polycythemic with polyhydramnios and develop heart failure. Anemia is a common problem with multiple gestation clients. The mother is commonly unable to consume enough protein, calcium, and iron to supply her needs and those of the fetuses. A maternal hemoglobin level below 11 mg/dL (110 g/L) is considered anemic.

☠⎯ CN: Physiological adaptation; CL: Evaluate

31. 2. The plan of care should reflect that this woman is experiencing probable signs of pregnancy. She may be pregnant, but the signs and symptoms may have another etiology. An enlarging abdomen and a positive pregnancy test may also be caused by tumors, hydatidiform mole, or other disease processes as well as pregnancy. Changes in the pigmentation of the face may also be caused by oral contraceptive use. Positive signs of pregnancy are considered diagnostic and include evident fetal heartbeat, fetal movement felt by a trained examiner, and visualization of the fetus with ultrasound confirmation. Presumptive signs are subjective and can have another etiology. These signs and symptoms include lack of menses, nausea, vomiting, fatigue, urinary frequency, and breast changes. The word "diagnostic" is not used to describe the condition of pregnancy.

☠⎯ CN: Physiological adaptation; CL: Analyze

32. 1. The serum pregnancy test measures human chorionic gonadotropin (hCG) in blood plasma and is highly accurate within 1 week after ovulation. The test is performed in a laboratory. Over-the-counter or home pregnancy tests are performed on urine and typically require higher levels of hCG to obtain a positive result. A positive pregnancy test is considered a probable sign of pregnancy. Certain conditions other than pregnancy, such as choriocarcinoma, can cause increased hCG levels.

⚷ CN: Reduction of risk potential;
CL: Apply

33. 4. The hormone analyzed in most pregnancy tests is hCG. In the pregnant woman, trace amounts of hCG appear in the serum as early as 24 to 48 hours after implantation owing to the trophoblast production of this hormone. Prolactin, follicle-stimulating hormone, and luteinizing hormone are not used to detect pregnancy. Prolactin is the hormone secreted by the pituitary gland to prepare the breasts for lactation. Follicle-stimulating hormone is involved in follicle maturation during the menstrual cycle. Luteinizing hormone is responsible for stimulating ovulation.

⚷ CN: Reduction of risk potential;
CL: Evaluate

34. 4. When using Nägele's rule to determine the estimated date of birth, the nurse would count back 3 calendar months from the first day of the last menstrual period and add 7 days. This means the client's estimated date is February 17.

⚷ CN: Health promotion and maintenance;
CL: Apply

35. 4. The placenta does not produce testosterone. Human placental lactogen, hCG, estrogen, and progesterone are hormones produced by the placenta during pregnancy. The hormone hCG stimulates the synthesis of estrogen and progesterone early in the pregnancy until the placenta can assume this role. Estrogen results in uterine and breast enlargement. Progesterone aids in maintaining the endometrium, inhibiting uterine contractility, and developing the breasts for lactation. The placenta also produces some nutrients for the embryo and exchanges oxygen, nutrients, and waste products through the chorionic villi.

⚷ CN: Health promotion and maintenance;
CL: Evaluate

36. 4,3,2,1. While initially continuing to attempt to find the fetal heartbeat, the nurse can ask the client if the baby has been moving. This will give a quick idea of status. The next step would be to obtain different equipment and attempt to find the fetal heartbeat again. A simple statement of fact that the nurse cannot find the heartbeat and is taking steps to rule out equipment error is appro-

priate. Calling the **HCP** 📖 would be the last step after it is determined that the baby does not have a heartbeat.

⚷ CN: Reduction of risk potential;
CL: Synthesize

37. 1,2. Although ultrasounds are not considered part of routine care, the ultrasound is able to confirm the pregnancy, identify the major anatomic features of the fetus and possible abnormalities, and determine the gestational age by measuring crown-to-rump length of the embryo during the first trimester. At this time, the ultrasound cannot confirm that the fetus is viable. The ultrasound will provide information about fetal position; however, this information would be more important later in the pregnancy, not during the first trimester. The ultrasound would provide no information about nutrient supply for the fetus.

⚷ CN: Health promotion and maintenance;
CL: Analyze

38. 2. This client is expressing a feeling of surprise about having a baby. Therefore, the nurse's best response would be to confirm the pregnancy, which is something that the client already suspects, and then ascertain how the client is feeling now that the suspicion is confirmed. Studies have shown that a common reaction to pregnancy is summarized as ambivalence or "someday, but not now." Such feelings are normal and are experienced by many women early in pregnancy. Offering a pamphlet on pregnancy does not respond to the client's feelings. Telling the client that she should be delighted ignores, rather than addresses, the client's feelings. Also, doing so imposes the nurse's opinion on the client. Ambivalence is a common reaction to pregnancy. Telling the client that she should be delighted may lead to feelings of guilt. Asking about the client's concerns is premature until the nurse determines the client's overall feelings about the pregnancy.

⚷ CN: Psychosocial integrity;
CL: Synthesize

39. 3. Women normally experience ambivalence when pregnancy is confirmed, even if the pregnancy was planned. Although the client's culture may play a role in openly accepting the pregnancy, most new mothers who have been ambivalent initially accept the reality by the end of the first trimester. Ambivalence also may be expressed throughout the pregnancy; this is believed to be related to the amount of physical discomfort. The nurse should become concerned and perhaps contact a social worker if the client expresses ambivalence in the third trimester. The client's statement reflects ambivalence, not fear. There is no evidence to suggest or imply that the client is rejecting the fetus. The client's statement reflects ambivalence about the pregnancy, not her ability to care for the newborn.

8→ CN: Psychosocial integrity; CL: Analyze

40. 3. Couvade syndrome refers to the situation in which the expectant father experiences some of the discomforts of pregnancy along with the pregnant woman as a means of identifying with the pregnancy. Ptyalism is the term for excessive salivation. Mittelschmerz is the lower abdominal discomfort felt by some women during ovulation. Pica refers to an oral craving for substances such as clay or starch that some pregnant clients experience.

8→ CN: Psychosocial integrity; CL: Analyze

41. 3. Maternal alcohol use may result in fetal alcohol syndrome, marked by mild-to-moderate mental retardation, physical growth retardation, central nervous system disorders, and feeding difficulties. Because there is no definitive answer as to how much alcohol can be safely consumed by a pregnant woman, it is recommended that pregnant clients be taught to abstain from drinking alcohol during pregnancy. Smoking and other medications also may affect the fetus.

8→ CN: Reduction of risk potential; CL: Apply

42. 4. An increase in clear, highly acidic vaginal secretions is a normal finding during pregnancy that aids in controlling the growth of pathologic bacteria. Vaginal secretions increase because of the influence of estrogen secretion and increased vaginal and cervical vascularity. The highly acidic nature of the vaginal secretions is caused by the action of *Lactobacillus acidophilus*, which increases the lactic acid content of the secretions. The increased acidity helps to make the vagina resistant to bacterial growth. During pregnancy, estrogen secretion fosters a glycogen-rich environment. Unfortunately, this glycogen-rich, acidic environment fosters the development of yeast (*Candida albicans*) infections, manifested by itching, burning, and a cheese-like vaginal discharge. If the client had a sexually transmitted infection, most likely she would have additional symptoms, such as lesions in the genital area or changes in color, consistency, or odor of the vaginal secretions. An increase in vaginal secretions does not help prevent expulsion of the mucus plug. The mucus plug is held in place by the cervix until the cervix becomes ripe.

8→ CN: Health promotion and maintenance; CL: Analyze

43. 2. Measurement of the client's fundal height is a gross estimate of fetal gestational age. At 20 weeks' gestation, the fundal height should be at about the level of the client's umbilicus. The fundus typically is over the symphysis pubis

at 12 weeks. A fundal height measurement between these two areas would suggest a fetus with a gestational age between 12 and 20 weeks. The fundal height increases approximately 1 cm/week after 20 weeks' gestation. The fundus typically reaches the xiphoid process at approximately 36 weeks' gestation. A fundal height between the umbilicus and the xiphoid process would suggest a fetus with a gestational age between 20 and 36 weeks. The fundus then commonly returns to about 4 cm below the xiphoid owing to lightening at 40 weeks. Additionally, pressure on the diaphragm occurs late in pregnancy. Therefore, a fundal height measurement near the xiphoid process with diaphragmatic compression suggests a fetus near the gestational age of 36 weeks or older.

8→ CN: Health promotion and maintenance; CL: Apply

44. 2. The volume of fluid needed for amniocentesis is 15 mL, and this is usually available at 15 weeks' gestation. Fetal development continues throughout the prenatal period. Cells necessary for testing for hemophilia A are available during the entire pregnancy but are not accessible by amniocentesis until 12 weeks' gestation. Amniocentesis carries a slight risk of infection regardless of when the procedure is performed.

8→ CN: Reduction of risk potential; CL: Apply

45. 4. The National Academy of Sciences Institute of Medicine and Health Canada recommend that women gain 25 to 35 lb (11.5 to 14.5 kg) during pregnancy. The pattern of weight gain is as important as the total amount of weight gained. Underweight women and women carrying twins should have a greater weight gain. Typically, women should gain 3.5 lb (1.6 kg) during the first trimester and then 1 lb (0.45 kg)/week during the remainder of the pregnancy (24 weeks) for a total of about 27 to 28 lb (12.2 to 12.7 kg). A weight gain of only 6.6 lb (3 kg) in the second and third trimesters is not normal because the client should be gaining about 1 lb (0.45 kg)/week, or 12 lb (5.4 kg) during the second and third trimesters. Gaining 12 lb (5.4 kg) during each trimester would total 36 lb (16.2 kg), which is slightly more than the recommended weight gain. In addition, nausea and vomiting during the first trimester can contribute to a lack of appetite and smaller weight gain during this trimester.

8→ CN: Health promotion and maintenance; CL: Evaluate

46. 1,5. Green, leafy vegetables, such as asparagus, spinach, brussels sprouts, and broccoli, are rich sources of folic acid. Beans, peas, and lentils are also good sources. The pregnant woman needs to eat foods high in folic acid to prevent folic acid deficits, which may result in neural tube defects in the newborn. A well-balanced diet must include whole grains, dairy products, and fresh fruits; however, bananas are rich in potassium, seafood is rich in iodine, and yogurt is rich in calcium, not folic acid.

🔑 CN: Reduction of risk potential;
CL: Apply

47. 3. Egg yolks and squash and other yellow vegetables are rich sources of vitamin A. Buttermilk and cheese are good sources of calcium. Strawberries, broccoli, citrus fruits (such as oranges), and tomatoes are good sources of vitamin C, not vitamin A.

🔑 CN: Basic care and comfort; CL: Evaluate

48. 1,3,4. Dairy products, fresh fruit, vegetables, and foods high in protein (like cheese and peanut butter) are excellent choices. Fried foods, such as chicken nuggets and tater tots, and foods such as cheeseburgers and buttered popcorn are high in fat; carbonated drinks such as diet colas, and foods such as pickles and ketchup contain large amounts of sodium. These foods can lead to an increase in ankle edema and promote weight gain from empty calories.

🔑 CN: Health promotion and maintenance;
CL: Apply

49. 1. Milk contains a large amount of calcium but contains no iron. Coffee, tea, and caffeinated soft drinks inhibit the absorption of iron. The vitamin C found in orange juice enhances the absorption of iron. Cream of wheat (1 cup/10 mg iron) and molasses (1 tbsp/3.0 mg iron) are considered excellent sources of iron as they contain the indicated amounts of iron.

🔑 CN: Physiological adaptation;
CL: Evaluate

50. 2. Magnesium aids in the synthesis of protein, nucleic acids, proteins, and fats. It is important for cell growth and neuromuscular function. Magnesium also activates the enzymes for metabolism of protein and energy. Calcium prevents demineralization of the mother's bones. Vitamin B$_6$ is important for amino acid metabolism. Folic acid assists in the development of neural pathways in the fetus.

🔑 CN: Basic care and comfort; CL: Apply

51. 2. The nurse reports the results of the VDRL to the **HCP** 📖. The pregnant client must be treated for syphilis to prevent perinatal transmission of the disease. The rubella titer and blood sugar values are within normal range. The blood type is not a significant factor in this situation.

🔑 CN Reduction of risk potential;
CL: Analyze

52. 2,3,4,5. During pregnancy, live virus immunizations are not administered because of potential teratogenicity. These immunizations include chickenpox, rubella, mumps, smallpox, and live attenuated influenza vaccine. Vaccines containing killed viruses (tetanus, diphtheria, hepatitis B) may be administered, and in fact are recommended by the CDC if the immunizations are not up-to-date.

🔑 CN: Pharmacologic and parental therapies; CL: Analyze

53. 4. Although most multiparous women experience quickening at about 17½ weeks' gestation, some women may perceive it between 14 and 20 weeks' gestation because they have been pregnant before and know what to expect. Detecting movement early does not suggest a twin pregnancy. If the multiparous client does not experience quickening by 20 weeks' gestation, further investigation is warranted because the fetus may have died, the client has a hydatidiform mole, or the pregnancy dating is incorrect. There is no evidence that the client's expected date of birth is erroneous.

🔑 CN: Health promotion and maintenance;
CL: Analyze

54. 1,2,3,4. Anyone could be a victim of intimate partner violence. Health care workers should routinely assess women for intimate partner violence. Pregnant teens have increased risk for not finishing school, smoking, and substance abuse. It is possible that the client is depressed, and her appearance and lack of eye contact are symptoms of her depression. The nurse expects the blood glucose screening test to be prescribed between 24 and 28 weeks' gestation to screen for gestational diabetes. HCG levels can identify the presence of a pregnancy or give information about an abnormal pregnancy. It would not be done at this time in a normal pregnancy.

🔑 CN: Health promotion and maintenance;
CL: Apply

55. 2. Leopold's maneuvers involve abdominal palpation. The client should empty her bladder before the nurse palpates the abdomen. Doing so increases the client's comfort and makes palpation more accurate. Although breathing deeply may help to relax the client, it has no effect on the accuracy of the results of Leopold's maneuvers. The client does not need to drink a full glass of water before the examination. The client should be lying in a supine position with the head slightly elevated for greater comfort and with the knees drawn up slightly.

🔑 CN: Health promotion and maintenance;
CL: Apply

56. Because the fetus is determined to be in an ROA, a vertex position, the convex portion of the fetus lying closest to the uterine wall would be located in the lower right quadrant of the abdomen. Placing the Doppler ultrasound over that area would produce the loudest fetal heart sounds.

🗝 CN: Management of care; CL: Apply

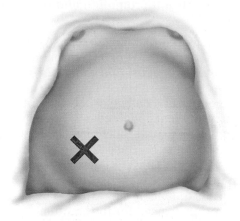

57. 2. In left occipital anterior lie, the occiput faces the left anterior segment of the woman's pelvis. In left occipital transverse lie, the occiput faces the woman's left hip. In right occipital transverse lie, the occiput faces the woman's right hip. In right occipital anterior lie, the occiput faces the right anterior segment of the woman's pelvis.

🗝 CN: Physiological adaptation; CL: Apply

58. 1. Discoloration on the face that commonly appears during pregnancy, called *chloasma* (mask of pregnancy), usually fades postpartum and is of no clinical significance. The client who is bothered by her appearance may be able to decrease its prominence with ordinary makeup. Chloasma is not a sign of skin melanoma. It is not caused by dilated capillaries. Rather, it results from increased secretion of melanocyte-stimulating hormones caused by estrogen and progesterone secretion. No treatment is necessary for this condition.

🗝 CN: Health promotion and maintenance; CL: Apply

59. 4. Assessment of fundal height is a gross estimate of fetal growth. By 20 weeks' gestation, the height of the fundus should be at the level of the umbilicus, after which it should increase 1 cm for each week of gestation until approximately 36 weeks' gestation. Fundal height that is significantly different from that implied by the estimated gestational age warrants further evaluation (e.g., ultrasound examination) because it possibly indicates multiple pregnancy or fetal growth retardation. Fundal height estimation will not determine uterine activity or a need for increased weight gain. Leopold's maneuver will determine fetal position but is not typically done in the second trimester when the fetus is still freely moving.

🗝 CN: Health promotion and maintenance; CL: Apply

60. 2. One of the primary risks of amniocentesis is stimulation of the uterus and possible miscarriage. Other risks include hemorrhage from penetration of the placenta, infection of the amniotic fluid, and puncture of the fetus. Club foot has been associated with amniocentesis especially when it is performed before 15 weeks. There is little risk for fetal organ malformations.

🗝 CN: Reduction of risk potential; CL: Evaluate

61. 3. The client traveling by automobile should be advised to take intermittent breaks of 10 to 15 minutes, including walking, every 1 to 2 hours to stimulate the circulation, which becomes sluggish during long periods of sitting. Automobile travel is not contraindicated during pregnancy unless the client develops complications. There is no set maximum number of hours allowed. The pregnant client should always wear a seat belt when traveling by automobile. The client should be aware of the nearest health care facility in the city to which she is traveling.

🗝 CN: Reduction of risk potential; CL: Apply

62. Seat belt safety is important for pregnant women because proper use reduces maternal mortality in car accidents. Both lap and shoulder belts are to be used. The lap portion of the belt is placed snugly but comfortably to fit under the abdominal bulge. Wearing the lap belt over the abdomen could increase the risk of uterine rupture and fetal complications due to belt tightening as the woman is propelled forward during an automobile accident. The shoulder belt is placed snugly across the shoulder, chest, and upper abdomen.

🗝 CN: Safety and infection control; CL: Apply

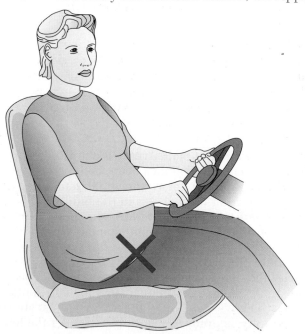

63. 3. Leg cramps are thought to result from excessive amounts of phosphorus absorbed from milk products. Straightening the knee and flexing the toes toward the chin is an effective measure to relieve leg cramps. Also, decreasing milk intake and supplementing with calcium lactate may help to reduce the cramping. Keeping the legs warm and elevating them are good preventive measures. Changing positions frequently aids venous return but is not helpful in relieving leg cramps. Alternately flexing and extending the legs will not help to relieve the leg cramp. Lying prone in the bed is a difficult position for a client at 37 weeks' gestation to achieve and maintain because of the increase in abdominal size and therefore is not considered helpful.

↝ CN: Basic care and comfort; CL: Synthesize

64. The fist is placed against the middle of the woman's sternum, with backward thrusts until the foreign body is expelled. The pressure from the backward thrusts causes compression of the ribs, further adding to the chest and lung pressure, thereby forcing the foreign body to move upward.

↝ CN: Safety and infection control; CL: Apply

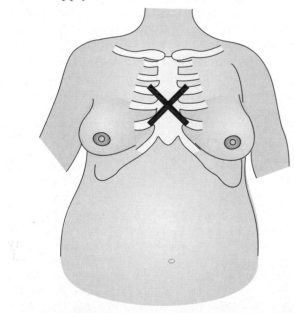

65. 2. In the first maneuver, which is done with the nurse facing the client's head, both hands are used to palpate and determine which fetal body part (e.g., the head or buttocks) is in the fundus. This first maneuver helps to determine the presenting part of the fetus. In the second maneuver, also done with the nurse facing the client's head, the palms of both hands are used to palpate the sides of the uterus and determine the location of the fetal back and spine. In the third maneuver, one hand gently grasps the lower portion of the abdomen just above the symphysis pubis to determine whether the fetal head is at the pelvic inlet. The fourth maneuver, done with the nurse facing the client's feet, determines the degree of fetal descent and flexion into the pelvis.

↝ CN: Health promotion and maintenance; CL: Apply

66. 4. Increased alpha fetoprotein (AFP) is one of the four laboratory values in a maternal quad screen. The labs are *human chorionic gonadotropin, estriol,* and *inhibin-A.* Increased AFP levels are associated with neural tube defects, such as spina bifida, anencephaly, and encephalocele. Ultrasonography is used to confirm a neural tube defect only when AFP levels are increased. Because AFP levels are usually highest at 15 to 18 weeks' gestation, this is the optimum time for testing. Performing the test after this time leads to inaccurate results. The client's blood, not urine, is used for the sample.

↝ CN: Reduction of risk potential; CL: Create

67. 1. Prenatal care is commonly the most critical factor influencing pregnancy outcome. This is especially true for adolescents because the most significant medical complication in pregnant adolescents is pregnancy-induced hypertension. Continued prenatal care helps to allow for early detection and prompt intervention should the complication arise. Other risks for adolescents include low-birth-weight infant, preterm labor, iron deficiency anemia, and cephalopelvic disproportion. Gestational diabetes can occur with any pregnancy regardless of the age of the mother. Generally, all first-time mothers need instruction related to discomforts. Adolescent mothers have better nutrition when they attend group classes and are subject to peer pressure. No evidence demonstrates that most adolescents lack support systems. Fathers may abandon mothers at any time during the pregnancy; other fathers, regardless of age, are supportive throughout the pregnancy.

↝ CN: Health promotion and maintenance; CL: Apply

68. 3. Colostrum is usually secreted by about the 16th week of gestation in preparation for breast-feeding. Growth of the milk ducts is greatest in the last trimester, not in the first 8 weeks of gestation. Enlargement of the breasts is usually caused by estrogen, not progesterone. Darkening of the areola can occur as early as the 6th week of gestation.

↝ CN: Health promotion and maintenance; CL: Create

69. 2,4,5. Understanding of breast-feeding education is demonstrated by statements involving knowledge of the several positions available for comfortable breast-feeding, oxytocin release from the pituitary leading to a let-down reflex and uterine contractions for involution, and feeding cues helpful in successful breast-feeding (because waiting until the infant is hungry and crying is stressful). Breast size does not ensure successful breast-feeding. Mastitis is an infectious process and is not influenced by latching on.

🔑 CN: Basic care and comfort; CL: Evaluate

70. 2. During pregnancy, the circulatory system undergoes tremendous changes. Cardiac output increases by 25% to 50%, and circulatory blood volume increases by about 30%. The client may experience transient hypotension and dizziness with sudden position changes. Early in pregnancy, there is a slight increase in the temperature, and clients may attribute this to a sinus infection or a cold. The client may feel warm, but this sensation is transient. The level of circulating fibrinogen increases as much as 50% during pregnancy, probably because of increased estrogen. Any calf tenderness should be reported because it may indicate a clot. Late in pregnancy, the posterior pituitary gland secretes oxytocin. The client may experience painful Braxton Hicks contractions or early labor symptoms.

🔑 CN: Health promotion and maintenance; CL: Create

71. 1. The fetal biophysical profile includes fetal breathing movements, fetal body movements, tone, amniotic fluid volume, and fetal heart rate reactivity. A reactive nonstress test is a sign of fetal well-being and does not require further evaluation. A nonreactive nonstress test requires further evaluation. A contraction stress test or oxytocin challenge test should be performed only on women who are at risk for fetal distress during labor. The contraction stress test is rarely performed before 28 weeks' gestation because of the possibility of initiating labor. Percutaneous umbilical cord sampling requires the insertion of a needle through the abdomen to obtain a fetal blood sample.

🔑 CN: Reduction of risk potential; CL: Apply

72. 1,3,4,5. The fetus does go through sleep cycles, rendering it less likely to move while it is asleep. Blood glucose does cross the placenta and can affect fetal movement. Cigarette smoking causes carbon monoxide to cross the placenta, which reduces fetal oxygen. Pregnant women are more likely to notice fetal movement while they are sitting or lying down, and time of day often determines this. Most pregnant women notice fetal movement in the evening. Barometric pressure does not affect fetal activity in utero.

🔑 CN: Health promotion and maintenance; CL: Analyze.

73. 3. The purpose of Kegel exercises is to strengthen the perineal muscles in preparation for the labor process. These movements strengthen the pubococcygeal muscle, which surrounds the urinary meatus and vagina. No evidence is available to support the idea that these exercises reduce the risk of hemorrhoids, alleviate lower back discomfort, or strengthen the abdominal muscles.

🔑 CN: Basic care and comfort; CL: Apply

74. 4. During the third trimester, it is not uncommon for clients to have dreams or fantasies about the baby. Sometimes the dreams are about infants who are malformed or, in this example, covered with hair. There is no evidence to suggest that the client is trying to cope with becoming a parent. Having dreams about the baby does not mean that labor will begin soon.

🔑 CN: Psychosocial integrity; CL: Synthesize

75. 1. Insomnia in the later part of pregnancy is not uncommon because the client has difficulty getting into a position of comfort. This is further compounded by frequent nocturia. The best suggestion would be to advise the client to practice relaxation techniques before bedtime. The client should avoid caffeine products such as chocolate and coffee before going to bed because caffeine is a stimulant. Alcohol consumption, regardless of the type or amount, should be avoided. Exercise is advised during the day, but it should be avoided before bedtime because exercise can stimulate the client and decrease the client's ability to fall asleep.

🔑 CN: Basic care and comfort; CL: Apply

76. 3. The client needs further instruction when she says it is permissible to sit in a hot tub for 20 minutes to relax after working. Hot tubs and saunas should be avoided, particularly in the first trimester, because their use can lead to maternal hyperthermia, which is associated with fetal anomalies such as central nervous system defects. The client should use nonskid pads in the shower or bath to avoid slipping because the client's center of gravity has shifted and she may fall. The client should avoid using soap on the nipples to prevent removal of the natural protective oils. Douching is not recommended for pregnant women because it can destroy the normal flora and increase the client's risk of infection.

🔑 CN: Health promotion and maintenance; CL: Evaluate

The Pregnant Client in Birth Preparation Classes

77. 3,4,5,6. During the third trimester of pregnancy, the woman experiments with maternal and caregiver roles and may make plans for changes in employment, managing household tasks, and/or childcare. The woman is also concerned about safety and passage through labor and birth. Other psychological tasks include preparation of the nursery, being tired of the pregnancy, and being introspective. A woman will begin to see herself as someone different from the fetus in the second trimester. Additionally, the mother may fantasize about the infant during the second trimester and be concerned about her changing body image. She may experience ambivalence about pregnancy in the first trimester.

> CN: Psychosocial integrity; CL: Create

78. 4. Pregnancy creates changes in the mother and father. Being considerate, accepting changes, and being supportive of the current situation are considered acceptable responses by the father, rather than feeling irritation about these changes. Expressing concern with the financial changes pregnancy and an expanded family include is normal. The first trimester involves the client and family feeling ambivalent about pregnancy and moving toward acceptance of the changes associated with pregnancy. Maternal acceptance of the pregnancy and a subsequent change in her focus are normal occurrences.

> CN: Health promotion and maintenance; CL: Analyze

79. 4. Thyroid enlargement and increased basal body metabolism are common occurrences during pregnancy. Human placental lactogen enhances milk production. Estrogen is responsible for hyperpigmentation and vascular skin changes. Progesterone relaxes smooth muscle in the respiratory tract.

> CN: Health promotion and maintenance; CL: Create

80. 1. Although sex is not easily discerned at 9 to 12 weeks, external genitalia are developed at this period of fetal development. Myelinization of the nerves begins at about 20 weeks' gestation. Brown fat stores develop at approximately 21 to 24 weeks. Air ducts and alveoli develop later in the gestational period, at approximately 25 to 28 weeks.

> CN: Health promotion and maintenance; CL: Apply

81. 2. Monozygotic twinning is independent of race, age, parity, or heredity. Monozygotic twins result from the fertilization of one ovum that cleaves completely into two embryos. Dizygotic twinning occurs with the fertilization of more than one ovum during conception. Dizygotic twins may be of the same sex or different sexes. Dizygotic twinning is correlated with increased parity, becoming pregnant within 1 month after stopping oral contraception, and infertility treatments. A primigravid client is less likely to conceive dizygotic twins.

> CN: Health promotion and maintenance; CL: Apply

82. 1,3,2,4. Engagement refers to the fetus' entering the true pelvis and occurs before descent in primiparas and concurrently in multiparous women. If the head is the presenting part, the normal maneuvers during labor and birth are (in order) descent, flexion, internal rotation, extension, external rotation, and expulsion. These maneuvers are called the *cardinal movements*. They occur as the fetal head passes through the maternal pelvis during the normal labor process.

> CN: Health promotion and maintenance; CL: Apply

83. 1. In a normal birth and for the first 24 hours postpartum, a total blood loss not exceeding 500 mL is considered normal. Blood loss during childbirth is almost always estimated because it provides a valuable indicator for possible hemorrhage. A blood loss of 1,000 mL is considered hemorrhage.

> CN: Health promotion and maintenance; CL: Apply

84. 2. Although the amniotic fluid promotes normal prenatal development by allowing symmetric development, it does not provide the fetus with nutrients. Rather, nutrients are provided by the placenta. The amniotic fluid does help dilate the cervix once labor begins by pressure and gravity forces. The amniotic fluid helps to protect the fetus from injury by cushioning against impact of the maternal abdomen and allows room and buoyancy for fetal movement. The amniotic fluid and sac keep the fetus at a stable temperature by maintaining a neutral thermal environment.

> CN: Health promotion and maintenance; CL: Evaluate

85. 1. Pelvic rocking helps to relieve backache during pregnancy and early labor by making the spine more flexible. Deep breathing exercises assist with relaxation and pain relief during labor. Tailor sitting and squatting help stretch the perineal muscles in preparation for labor.

> CN: Health promotion and maintenance; CL: Analyze

86. 1,2,4. Pain during the first stage of labor is primarily caused by hypoxia of the uterine and cervical muscle cells during contraction, stretching of the lower uterine segment, dilatation of the cervix and perineum, and pressure on adjacent structures. Ambulating will assist in increasing circulation of blood to the area and relaxing the muscles. Slow chest breathing is appropriate during the first stage of labor to promote increased oxygenation as well as relaxation. The woman or her coach can lightly massage the abdomen (effleurage) while using slow chest breathing. Chest breathing and massaging increase oxygenation and relaxation of uterine muscles. Pain medication is not used during the first stage of labor because most medications will slow labor; anesthesia may be considered during the second stage of labor. Sipping ice water, while helpful for maintaining hydration, will not be useful as a pain management strategy.

🔑 CN: Health promotion and maintenance; CL: Synthesize

87. 4. With true labor, the contractions are felt first in the lower back and then the abdomen. They gradually increase in frequency and duration and do not disappear with ambulation, rest, or sleep. In true labor, the cervix dilates and effaces. Walking tends to increase true contractions. False labor contractions disappear with ambulation, rest, or sleep. False labor contractions commonly remain the same in duration and frequency. Clients who are experiencing false labor may have pain, even though the contractions are not very effective.

🔑 CN: Health promotion and maintenance; CL: Apply

88. 4. Pelvic tilt exercises are useful to alleviate backache during pregnancy and labor but are not useful for the pain from contractions. Biofeedback (a conscious effort to control the response to pain), effleurage (light uterine massage), and guided imagery (focusing on a pleasant scene) are appropriate pain relief techniques to practice before labor begins. Various breathing exercises also can help to alleviate the discomfort from contraction pain.

🔑 CN: Health promotion and maintenance; CL: Evaluate

89. 2. Increased vaginal discharge is normal during pregnancy, but yellow-gray frothy discharge with local itching is associated with infection (e.g., *Trichomonas vaginalis*). The client's symptoms must be further assessed by a health professional because the client needs treatment for this condition. *T. vaginalis* infection is commonly treated with metronidazole; however, this drug is not used in the first trimester. In the first trimester, the typical treatment is topical clotrimazole. Although a yeast infection is associated with vaginal itching, the vaginal discharge is cheese-like. Furthermore, because the client may have a serious vaginal infection, over-the-counter medications are not advised until the client has been evaluated. Douching is not recommended during pregnancy because it would predispose the client to an ascending infection. The client is not exhibiting signs and symptoms of preterm labor, such as contractions or leaking fluid. And although the client's problems are suggestive of a *T. vaginalis* infection, which can lead to preterm labor and premature rupture of the membranes, further evaluation is needed to confirm the cause of the infection.

🔑 CN: Health promotion and maintenance; CL: Synthesize

90. 2. During pregnancy, urinary tract infections are more common because of urinary stasis. Clients need instructions about increasing fluid volume intake. Plasma volume increases during pregnancy. The increase in plasma volume is more pronounced and occurs earlier than does the increase in red blood cell mass, possibly resulting in physiologic anemia. Peripheral vascular resistance decreases during pregnancy, providing a relatively stable blood pressure. Hemoglobin levels decrease during pregnancy even though there is an increase in blood volume.

🔑 CN: Health promotion and maintenance; CL: Apply

The Pregnant Client with Risk Factors

91. 4. For the Rh-negative client who may be pregnant with an Rh-positive fetus, an indirect Coombs test measures antibodies in the maternal blood. Titers should be performed monthly during the first and second trimesters and biweekly during the third trimester and the week before the due date.

🔑 CN: Health promotion and maintenance; CL: Apply

92. 4. A maternal quad screen testing is done to screen for genetic and neural tube abnormalities between the 15th and 18th weeks of gestation. The four tests included are an alpha fetoprotein (AFP), *human chorionic gonadotropin,* estriol, and inhibin-A. Abnormally high levels of AFP found in maternal serum may be indicative of neural tube defects such as anencephaly and spina bifida. Low levels may indicate trisomy 21 (Down syndrome). Beta strep testing is done in the third trimester. Chorionic villus sampling is done as early as 10 weeks' gestation to detect anomalies. Ultrasound testing may be done in the first trimester to determine fetal viability and in the third trimester to determine pelvic adequacy and fetal or placental position.

🔑 CN: Reduction of risk potential; CL: Apply

93. 1,2,5. Prenatal care includes a general supplementation of 400 mcg of folic acid, and clients with a history of gastric bypass should be referred to a dietician to determine adequate nutrient intake. All pregnant clients have their urine routinely checked for protein and sugar. There is no indication for checking glucose levels at each prenatal visit in clients who have undergone gastric bypass. Gastric bypass clients are not at risk of gaining all of their weight back. No evidence supports implementing nonstress tests at 20 weeks.

🔑 CN: Health promotion and maintenance; CL: Create

94. 2. According to both the New York Heart Association and the Canadian Cardiovascular Society, this client would fit under class II because she is symptomatic with increased activity (dyspnea with exertion). Class II clients have cardiac disease and a slight limitation in physical activity. When physical activity occurs, the client may experience angina, difficulty breathing, palpations, and fatigue. All of the client's other symptoms are within normal limits.

 CN: Management of care; CL: Analyze

95. 1,2,5. The test result indicates that the mother has an active hepatitis infection and is a carrier. Hepatitis B immune globulin at birth provides the infant with passive immunity against hepatitis B and serves as a prophylactic treatment. Additionally, the infant will be started on the vaccine series of three injections. The infant should not be screened or isolated because the infant is already hepatitis B positive. As with all clients, universal precautions should be used and are sufficient to prevent transmission of the virus. Women who are positive for hepatitis B surface antigen are able to breast-feed.

 CN: Management of care; CL: Create

96. 4. Asthma medications and bronchodilators should be continued during pregnancy as prescribed before the pregnancy began. The medications do not cause harm to the mother or fetus. Regular use of asthma medication will usually prevent asthma attacks. Prevention and limitation of an asthma attack is the goal of care for a client who is or is not pregnant and is the appropriate care strategy. During an asthma attack, oxygen needs continue as with any pregnant client, but the airways are edematous, decreasing perfusion. Asthma exacerbations during pregnancy may occur as a result of infrequent use of medication rather than as a result of the pregnancy.

 CN: Pharmacological and parenteral therapies; CL: Evaluate

97. 2. The nurse seeing this client should refer her to a **HCP** 📖 for further evaluation of the pain. This referral would allow a more definitive diagnosis and medical interventions that may include surgery. Referral would occur because of her high pain rating as well as the other symptoms, which suggest gallbladder disease. During pregnancy, the gallbladder is under the influence of progesterone, which is a smooth muscle relaxant. Because bile does not move through the system as quickly during pregnancy, bile stasis and gallstone formation can occur. Although education should be a continuous strategy, with pain at this level, a brief explanation is most appropriate. Major emphasis should be placed on determining the cause and treating the pain. It is not appropriate for the nurse to diagnose pain at this

level as heartburn. Discussing nutritional strategies to prevent heartburn are appropriate during pregnancy, but not in this situation. Acetaminophen is an acceptable medication to take during pregnancy but should not be used on a regular basis as it can mask other problems.

 CN: Management of care; CL: Synthesize

98. 3. A fetus that has died and is retained in utero places the mother at risk for disseminated intravascular coagulation (DIC) because the clotting factors within the maternal system are consumed when the nonviable fetus is retained. The longer the fetus is retained in utero, the greater the risk of DIC. This client has no risk factors, history, or signs and symptoms that put her at risk for abruptio placentae such as sharp pain and "woody," firm consistency of the abdomen. HELLP syndrome is a complication of preeclampsia that does not occur before 20 weeks' gestation unless a molar pregnancy is present. There is no evidence that she is threatening to abort as she has no cramping or vaginal bleeding.

 CN: Management of care; CL: Analyze

99. 2. A blood pressure reading of 138/88 mm Hg is nearing hypertension range and could be a sign of developing gestational hypertension. Conversely, the client may be experiencing "white coat" syndrome or could be anxious during the prenatal visit. In order to obtain an accurate blood pressure reading, the nurse should allow the woman to rest for a period of time and recheck the blood pressure in the same arm and while the woman is in the same position. This blood pressure is considered approaching high. All other vitals are within normal range.

 CN: Physiological adaptation; CL: Analyze

100. 2. Chorionic villus sampling (CVS) can be performed from approximately 8 to 12 weeks' gestation, while amniocentesis cannot be performed until between 11 weeks' gestation and the end of the pregnancy. Eleven weeks' gestation is the earliest possible time within the pregnancy to obtain a sufficient amount of amniotic fluid to sample. Because CVS take a piece of membrane surrounding the infant, this procedure can be completed earlier in the pregnancy. Amniocentesis and chorionic villus sampling identify the genetic makeup of the fetus in its entirety, rather than a portion of it. Laboratory analysis of chorionic villus sampling takes less time to complete. Both procedures place the fetus at risk, and postprocedure teaching asks the client to report the same complicating events (bleeding, cramping, fever, and fluid leakage from the vagina).

 CN: Management of care; CL: Evaluate

101. 4. Additional teaching is needed when the parent says that adolescents are at greater risk for congenital anomalies. Although adolescents are at greater risk for denial of the pregnancy, lack of pre-natal care, low-birth-weight infant, cephalopelvic disproportion, anemia, and nutritional deficits and have a higher maternal mortality rate, studies reveal that congenital anomalies are not more common in adolescent pregnancies.

    CN: Health promotion and maintenance; CL: Evaluate

102. 4. With a spontaneous abortion, many clients and their partners feel an acute sense of loss. Their grieving commonly includes feelings of guilt, which may be expressed as wondering whether the woman could have done something to prevent the loss. Anger, sadness, and disappointment are also common emotions after a pregnancy loss. Ambivalence, anxiety, and fear are not common emotions after a spontaneous abortion.

    CN: Psychosocial integrity; CL: Analyze

103. 1. Hydroxyzine has a tranquilizing effect and also decreases nausea and vomiting. It does not decrease fluid retention, reduce pain, decrease uterine cramping, or promote uterine contractility. One of the adverse effects of the medication is sleepiness. Ibuprofen may decrease pain from uterine cramping. Oxytocin may be used to increase uterine contractility.

    CN: Pharmacological and parenteral therapies; CL: Evaluate

104. 3. The death of a fetus at any time during pregnancy is a tragedy for most parents. After a spontaneous abortion, the client and family members can be expected to suffer from grief for several months or longer. When offering support, a simple statement such as "I am truly sorry you lost your baby" is most appropriate. Therapeutic communication techniques help the client and family understand the meaning of the loss, move less stressfully through the grief process, and share feelings. Asking the client whether she is experiencing a great deal of uterine pain is inappropriate because this is a "yes-no" question and doesn't allow the client to express her feelings. Saying that the embryo was defective is inappropriate because this may lead the client to think that she contributed to the fetus's demise. This is not the appropriate time to discuss embryonic or fetal malformations. However, the nurse should explain to the client that this situation was not her fault. Telling the client that she should not get pregnant again too soon is not therapeutic and discounts the feelings of the expectant mother who had already begun to bond with the fetus.

    CN: Psychosocial integrity; CL: Apply

105. 4. Rh sensitization can be prevented by Rho(D) immune globulin, which clears the maternal circulation of Rh-positive cells before sensitization can occur, thereby blocking maternal antibody production to Rh-positive cells. Administration of this drug will not prevent future Rh-positive fetuses, nor will it prevent future abortions. An antibody response will not occur to Rh-negative cells. Rh-negative mothers do not develop sensitivities if the fetus is also Rh negative.

    CN: Pharmacological and parenteral therapies; CL: Apply

106. 2. The client with leg varicosities should take frequent rest periods with the legs elevated above the hips to promote venous circulation. The client should avoid constrictive clothing, but support hose that reach above the varicosities may help alleviate the pain. Contracting and relaxing the feet and ankles twice daily is not helpful because it does not promote circulation. Taking a leave of absence from work may not be possible because of economic reasons. The client should try to rest with her legs elevated or walk around for a few minutes every 2 hours while on the job.

    CN: Reduction of risk potential; CL: Synthesize

107. 4. The client is reporting symptoms typically associated with herpes genitalis. Some women have no symptoms of gonorrhea. Others may experience vaginal itching and a thick, purulent vaginal discharge. *C. trachomatis* infection in women is commonly asymptomatic, but symptoms may include a yellowish discharge and painful urination. The first symptom of syphilis is a painless chancre.

    CN: Physiological adaptation; CL: Apply

108. 1. The client may need surgery to remove a ruptured fallopian tube where the pregnancy has occurred, and the nurse is usually responsible for witnessing the signature on the **informed consent** . Typically, if bleeding is occurring, it is internal, and there is only scant vaginal bleeding with no discoloration. The nurse cannot determine whether the fallopian tube can be salvaged; this can be accomplished only during surgery. If the tube has ruptured, it must be removed. If the tube has not ruptured, a linear salpingostomy may be done to salvage the tube for future pregnancies. With an ectopic pregnancy, although the client is experiencing abdominal pain, she is not having uterine contractions.

    CN: Physiological adaptation; CL: Synthesize

Managing Care, Quality, and Safety for Childbearing Clients

109. 2. Late decelerations during an oxytocin challenge test indicate that the infant is not receiving enough oxygen during contractions and is exhibiting signs of uteroplacental insufficiency. This client would need further medical intervention. Fetal movement 6 times in 2 hours is adequate in a healthy fetus, and a biophysical profile of 9 indicates that the risk of fetal asphyxia is rare. A reactive nonstress test informs the **HCP** 📖 that the fetus has 2 fetal heart rate accelerations of 15 beats per minute above baseline and lasting for 15 seconds within a 20-minute period, which is a normal result and an indication of fetal well-being.

🔑 CN: Management of care; CL: Evaluate

110. 1. Folic acid supplementation is recommended to prevent neural tube defects and anemia in pregnancy. Deficiencies increase the risk of hemorrhage during birth as well as infection. The recommended dose prior to pregnancy is 400 mcg/day; while breast-feeding and during pregnancy, the recommended dosage is 400 to 800 mcg/day. Blood glucose levels are not regulated by the intake of folic acid. Vitamin C potentiates the absorption of iron and is also associated with blood clotting or collagen formation.

🔑 CN: Reduction of risk potential; CL: Apply

111. 3,4,1,2. The first client to be seen should be the postpartum mother who is fearful of shaking her infant. Postpartum depression is a disorder that may occur during the first year postpartum but peaks at 4 weeks postpartum, prior to menses, or upon weaning. As a single mother, this client may not have support, a large factor putting women at risk. Other factors accentuating risk include prior depressive or bipolar illness and self-dissatisfaction. Second, the nurse should see the 16-week antenatal client, who is likely experiencing round ligament syndrome. At this point in the pregnancy, the uterus is stretching into the abdomen causing this type of pain. The pain is on the wrong side to be attributed to appendicitis or gallbladder disease. Nursing interventions to ease the pain include a heating pad or bringing the legs toward the abdomen. The nurse should next see the primigravid client who states she is not feeling well because she is exhibiting signs and symptoms of discomfort experienced by most women in the first trimester. The multiparous client at 32 weeks' gestation is the lowest priority as she is physically well, while the other clients have physical and psychological problems. In most emergency department situations, she may not be seen by medical or nursing staff but would be given the names of **HCPs** 📖 in the reception area.

🔑 CN: Management of care; CL: Synthesize

112. 1,2,3,4. The same safety policies apply to both inpatient and outpatient settings and are adapted to the individual specialty. Handwashing and use of two client identifiers are standard procedures. Abbreviations that are used for inpatient are also used for outpatient as the same mistakes can occur in either setting with confusion in spelling or interpretation of letters and numbers. Preprocedure verification with name and procedure is used in the operating room, inpatient, and in ambulatory settings regardless of the procedure. It is logical to place clients with obvious communicable diseases by themselves, but nausea and vomiting are a "normal" situation in early pregnancy and not contagious.

🔑 CN: Risk reduction; CL: Evaluate

Complications of Pregnancy

The Pregnant Client with Preeclampsia or Eclampsia

1. A laboring client with preeclampsia is prescribed magnesium sulfate 2 g/h IV piggyback. The pharmacy sends the IV to the unit labeled *magnesium sulfate 20 g/500 mL normal saline.* To deliver the correct dose, the nurse should set the pump to deliver how many milliliters per hour? Record your answer using one decimal place.

_____ 50.0 _____ mL.

2. A 32-year-old multigravida returns to the clinic for a routine prenatal visit at 36 weeks' gestation. The assessments during this visit include blood pressure, 140/90 mm Hg; pulse, 80 beats/min; respiratory rate, 16 breaths/min. What further information should the nurse obtain to determine if this client is becoming preeclamptic?
☐ 1. headaches
☐ 2. blood glucose level
☒ 3. proteinuria
☐ 4. peripheral edema

3. The nurse is instructing a preeclamptic client about monitoring the movements of her fetus to determine fetal well-being. Which statement by the client indicates that she needs further instruction

about when to call the healthcare provider (HCP) concerning fetal movement?
☐ 1. "if the fetus is becoming less active than before"
☐ 2. "if it takes longer each day for the fetus to move 10 times"
☐ 3. "if the fetus stops moving for 12 hours"
☒ 4. "if the fetus moves more often than three times an hour"

4. A 29-year-old multigravida at 37 weeks' gestation is being treated for severe preeclampsia and has magnesium sulfate infusing at 3 g/h. To maintain safety for this client, the **priority** intervention is to:
☐ 1. maintain continuous fetal monitoring.
☐ 2. encourage family members to remain at bedside.
☒ 3. assess reflexes, clonus, visual disturbances, and headache.
☐ 4. monitor maternal liver studies every 4 hours.

5. At 32 weeks' gestation, a 15-year-old primigravid client who is 5 feet, 2 inches (151.7 cm) has gained a total of 20 lb (9.1 kg), with a 1-lb (0.45-kg) gain in the last 2 weeks. Urinalysis reveals negative glucose and a trace of protein. The nurse should advise the client that which factor increases her risk for preeclampsia?
☐ 1. total weight gain
☐ 2. short stature
☒ 3. adolescent age group
☐ 4. trace proteinuria

6. After instructing a primigravid client at 38 weeks' gestation about how preeclampsia can affect the client and the growing fetus, the nurse realizes that the client needs additional instruction when she says that preeclampsia can lead to which problem?

☒ 1. hydrocephalic infant
☐ 2. abruptio placentae
☐ 3. intrauterine growth restriction
☐ 4. poor placental perfusion

7. A nurse is completing a prenatal assessment on a woman who is 28 weeks' pregnant with gestational hypertension. Which findings should be reported to the primary care provider? Select all that apply.

☒ 1. dull headache
☐ 2. edematous feet
☒ 3. blurred vision
☒ 4. 1+ urine protein
☐ 5. fundal height of 28 cm

8. When teaching a multigravid client diagnosed with mild preeclampsia about nutritional needs, which type of diet should the nurse discuss?

☐ 1. high-residue diet
☐ 2. low-sodium diet
☒ 3. regular diet
☐ 4. high-protein diet

9. A woman with preeclampsia is receiving magnesium sulfate via infusion pump at 1 g/h. The nurse's assessment includes temperature 36.7°C; pulse 78; respirations 12/minute; B/P 128/82; urinary output 90 mL in last 4 hours via Foley catheter; patellar-tendon reflex absent; ankle clonus absent; fetal heart rate 120 beats/min; cervix 4 cm dilated, 80% effaced, station −1.

Which is the **most** appropriate action for the nurse to take?

☐ 1. Assess the Foley catheter for kinks in the drainage tubing, and obtain a urine sample.
☐ 2. Document findings, and continue to monitor her progress in labor.
☒ 3. Discontinue the magnesium sulfate infusion, and notify the healthcare provider (HCP).
☐ 4. Increase fluid intake intravenously, and measure intake and output.

10. A primigravid client at 38 weeks' gestation diagnosed with mild preeclampsia calls the clinic nurse to say she has had a continuous headache for the past 2 days accompanied by nausea. The client

does not want to take aspirin. The nurse should tell the client:

☐ 1. "Take two acetaminophen tablets. They are not as likely to upset your stomach."
☒ 2. "I think the healthcare provider should see you today. Can you come to the clinic this morning?"
☐ 3. "You need to lie down and rest. Have you tried placing a cool compress over your head?"
☐ 4. "I will ask the healthcare provider to call in a prescription for nausea medications. What is your pharmacy's number?"

11. When preparing the room for admission of a multigravid client at 36 weeks' gestation diagnosed with severe preeclampsia, which item is **most** important for the nurse to obtain?

☐ 1. oxytocin infusion solution
☐ 2. disposable tongue blades
☐ 3. portable ultrasound machine
☒ 4. padding for the side rails

12. A client who is 34 weeks pregnant is admitted to the labor and birth room with the diagnosis of preeclampsia. The client's vital signs are as follows: blood pressure 149/92 mm Hg; pulse, 62 beats/min; respiratory rate, 18 breaths/min; temperature, 98.4°F (36.8°C). What is the **priority** intervention?

☒ 1. Encourage the client to lie in a lateral position.
☐ 2. Administer an antihypertensive agent.
☐ 3. Notify the healthcare provider (HCP) of the client's blood pressure.
☐ 4. Check the cervix.

13. The primary healthcare provider (HCP) prescribes intravenous magnesium sulfate for a primigravid client at 38 weeks' gestation diagnosed with severe preeclampsia. Which medication would be **most** important for the nurse to have readily available?

☐ 1. diazepam
☐ 2. hydralazine
☒ 3. calcium gluconate
☐ 4. phenytoin

14. For the client who is receiving intravenous magnesium sulfate for severe preeclampsia, which assessment finding would alert the nurse to suspect hypermagnesemia?

☒ 1. decreased deep tendon reflexes
☐ 2. cool skin temperature
☐ 3. rapid pulse rate
☐ 4. tingling in the toes

15. A client at 28 weeks' gestation presents to the emergency department with a "splitting headache." What actions are indicated by the nurse at this time? Select all that apply.

☐ 1. Reassure the client that headaches are a normal part of pregnancy.

☒ 2. Assess the client for vision changes or epigastric pain.

☒ 3. Obtain a nonstress test.

☒ 4. Assess the client's reflexes and presence of clonus.

☐ 5. Determine if the client has a documented ultrasound for this pregnancy.

16. Which outcome would the nurse identify as the **priority** to achieve when developing the plan of care for a primigravid client at 38 weeks' gestation who is hospitalized with severe preeclampsia and receiving intravenous magnesium sulfate?

☐ 1. decreased generalized edema within 8 hours

☐ 2. decreased urinary output during the first 24 hours

☐ 3. sedation and decreased reflex excitability within 48 hours

☒ 4. absence of any seizure activity during the first 48 hours

17. The nurse is administering intravenous magnesium sulfate as prescribed for a client at 34 weeks' gestation with severe preeclampsia. What are desired outcomes of this therapy? Select all that apply.

☒ 1. temperature, 98°F (36.7°C); pulse, 72 beats/min; respiratory rate, 14 breaths/min

☐ 2. urinary output less than 30 mL/h

☐ 3. fetal heart rate with late decelerations

☐ 4. blood pressure of less than 140/90 mm Hg

☒ 5. deep tendon reflexes 2+

☒ 6. magnesium level = 5.6 mg/dL (2.8 mmol/L)

18. Soon after admission of a primigravid client at 38 weeks' gestation with severe preeclampsia, the primary healthcare provider (HCP) prescribes a continuous intravenous infusion of 5% dextrose in Ringer's solution and 4 g of magnesium sulfate. While the medication is being administered, which assessment finding should the nurse report **immediately**?

☒ 1. respiratory rate of 12 breaths/min

☐ 2. patellar reflex of +2

☐ 3. blood pressure of 160/88 mm Hg

☐ 4. urinary output exceeding intake

19. As the nurse enters the room of a newly admitted primigravid client diagnosed with severe preeclampsia, the client begins to experience a seizure. Which action should the nurse take **first**?

☐ 1. Insert an airway to improve oxygenation.

☐ 2. Note the time when the seizure begins and ends.

☒ 3. Call for immediate assistance.

☐ 4. Turn the client to her left side.

20. After administering hydralazine 5 mg intravenously as prescribed for a primigravid client with severe preeclampsia at 39 weeks' gestation, the nurse should assess the client for:

☒ 1. tachycardia

☐ 2. bradypnea

☐ 3. polyuria

☐ 4. dysphagia

21. A primigravid client with severe preeclampsia exhibits hyperactive, very brisk patellar reflexes with two beats of ankle clonus present. How does the nurse document the patellar reflexes?

☐ 1. 1+

☐ 2. 2+

☐ 3. 3+

☒ 4. 4+

22. A 16-year-old unmarried primigravid client at 37 weeks' gestation with severe preeclampsia is in early active labor. The client's blood pressure is 164/110 mm Hg. Which finding would alert the nurse that the client may be about to experience a seizure?

☐ 1. decreased contraction intensity

☐ 2. decreased temperature

☒ 3. epigastric pain

☐ 4. hyporeflexia

23. Following an eclamptic seizure, the nurse should assess the client for which complication?

☐ 1. polyuria

☐ 2. facial flushing

☐ 3. hypotension

☒ 4. uterine contractions

24. A client at 36 weeks' gestation begins to exhibit signs of labor after an eclamptic seizure. The nurse should assess the client for:

☒ 1. abruptio placentae.

☐ 2. transverse lie.

☐ 3. placenta accreta.

☐ 4. uterine atony.

25. The nurse is reviewing the medical record of a multigravid client at 39 weeks' gestation with suspected HELLP syndrome. The nurse should notify the healthcare provider (HCP) about which test results?

☐ 1. platelets 200,000 mm³ (200 × 10⁹/L)

☒ 2. lactate dehydrogenase (LDH) > 200 U/L (3.34 μkat/L)

☐ 3. uric acid 3 mg/dL (178.4 μmol/L)

☐ 4. aspartate aminotransferase (AST) 15 U/L (0.25 μkat/L)

hemolysis, elevated liver enzymes, and low platelet count

The Pregnant Client with a Chronic Hypertensive Disorder

26. An obese 36-year-old multigravid client at 12 weeks' gestation has a history of chronic hypertension. She was treated with methyldopa before becoming pregnant. When counseling the client about diet during pregnancy, the nurse realizes that the client needs additional instruction when she makes which statement?

☐ 1. "I need to reduce my caloric intake to 1,200 cal/day."

☐ 2. "A regular diet is recommended during pregnancy."

☐ 3. "I should eat more frequent meals if I get heartburn."

☐ 4. "I need to consume more fluids and fiber each day."

27. After instructing a multigravid client at 10 weeks' gestation diagnosed with chronic hypertension about the need for frequent prenatal visits, the nurse determines that the instructions have been successful when the client makes which statement?

☐ 1. "I may develop hyperthyroidism because of my high blood pressure."

☐ 2. "I need close monitoring because I may have a small-for-gestational-age infant."

☐ 3. "It is possible that I will have excess amniotic fluid and may need a cesarean section."

☐ 4. "I may develop placenta accreta, so I need to keep my clinic appointments."

28. After reinforcing the danger signs to report with a gravida 2 client at 32 weeks' gestation with an elevated blood pressure, which client statements would demonstrate her understanding of when to call the primary healthcare provider's (HCP's) office? Select all that apply.

☐ 1. "if I feel dizzy when I get up quickly"

☐ 2. "if I see any bleeding, even if I have no pain"

☐ 3. "if I have a pounding headache that will not go away"

☐ 4. "if I notice the veins in my legs getting bigger"

☐ 5. "if the leg cramps at night are waking me up"

☐ 6. "if the baby seems to be more active than usual"

The Pregnant Client with Third-Trimester Bleeding

29. A client presents to the OB triage unit with no prenatal care and painless bright red vaginal bleeding. Which interventions are **most** indicated?

☐ 1. applying external fetal monitor and completing a physical assessment

☐ 2. applying external fetal monitor and performing a sterile vaginal exam

☐ 3. obtaining a fundal height physical assessment on the client

☐ 4. obtaining fundal height and a sterile vaginal exam

30. The nurse is caring for a 22-year-old G2, P2 client who has disseminated intravascular coagulation after delivering a dead fetus. Which finding is the **highest priority** to report to the healthcare provider (HCP)?

☐ 1. activated partial thromboplastin time (APTT) of 30 seconds

☐ 2. hemoglobin of 11.5 g/dL (115 g/L)

☐ 3. urinary output of 25 mL in the past hour

☐ 4. platelets at 149,000/mm³ (149 × 10⁹/L)

31. A 24-year-old client, G3, T1, P1, A1, L1 at 32 weeks' gestation, is admitted to the hospital because of vaginal bleeding. After reviewing the client's history, which factor might lead the nurse to suspect abruptio placentae?

☐ 1. several hypotensive episodes

☐ 2. previous low transverse cesarean birth

☐ 3. one induced abortion

☐ 4. history of cocaine use

32. When caring for a multigravid client admitted to the hospital with vaginal bleeding at 38 weeks' gestation, which therapeutic agent would the nurse anticipate administering intravenously if the client develops disseminated intravascular coagulation (DIC)?

☐ 1. Ringer's lactate solution

☐ 2. fresh frozen platelets

☐ 3. 5% dextrose solution

☐ 4. warfarin

33. When assessing a 34-year-old multigravid client at 34 weeks' gestation experiencing moderate vaginal bleeding, which symptom would **most** likely alert the nurse that placenta previa is present?

☐ 1. painless vaginal bleeding

☐ 2. uterine tetany

☐ 3. intermittent pain with spotting

☐ 4. dull lower back pain

34. The primary healthcare provider (HCP) prescribes whole blood replacement for a multigravid client with abruptio placentae. Before administering the intravenous blood product, the nurse should **first:**
- ☒ 1. validate client information and the blood product with another nurse.
- ☐ 2. check the vital signs before transfusing over 5 to 6 hours.
- ☐ 3. ask the client if she has ever had any allergies.
- ☐ 4. administer 100 mL of 5% dextrose solution intravenously.

35. Following a cesarean birth for abruptio placentae, a multigravid client tells the nurse, "I feel like such a failure. None of my other childbirths were like this." Which factor is **most** important for the nurse to consider when responding to the client?
- ☐ 1. The client will most likely have postpartum blues.
- ☐ 2. Maternal-infant bonding is likely to be difficult.
- ☒ 3. The client's feeling of grief is a normal reaction.
- ☐ 4. This type of birth was necessary to save the client's life.

36. A client has received epidural anesthesia to control pain during a vaginal birth. Place an X over the highest point on the body locating the level of anesthesia expected for a vaginal birth.

37. Which action should the nurse take **first** when admitting a multigravid client at 36 weeks' gestation with a probable diagnosis of abruptio placentae?
- ☐ 1. Prepare the client for a vaginal examination.
- ☐ 2. Obtain a brief history from the client.
- ☒ 3. Insert a large-gauge intravenous catheter.
- ☐ 4. Prepare the client for an ultrasound scan.

The Pregnant Client with Preterm Labor

38. The healthcare provider (HCP) has determined that a preterm labor client at 34 weeks' gestation has no fetal fibronectin present. Based on this finding, the nurse would anticipate that within the next week:
- ☐ 1. the client will develop preeclampsia.
- ☐ 2. the fetus will develop mature lungs.
- ☒ 3. the client will not develop preterm labor.
- ☐ 4. the fetus will not develop gestational diabetes.

39. A nurse is discussing preterm labor in a prenatal class. After class, a client asks the nurse to identify again the nursing strategies to prevent preterm labor. The client needs further instruction when she makes which statement?
- ☐ 1. "I need to stay hydrated all the time."
- ☐ 2. "Even dental infections can lead to preterm labor."
- ☐ 3. "I should include frequent rest breaks if I travel."
- ☒ 4. "Cutting back on my smoking will not help my baby."

40. A multigravid client at 34 weeks' gestation is being treated with indomethacin to halt preterm labor. If the client gives birth to a preterm infant, the nurse should notify the nursery personnel about this therapy because of the possibility for which complication?
- ☒ 1. pulmonary hypertension
- ☐ 2. respiratory distress syndrome (RDS)
- ☐ 3. hyperbilirubinemia
- ☐ 4. cardiomyopathy

41. Which statement by the client indicates an understanding of the teaching regarding of the use of corticosteroids during preterm labor?
- ☐ 1. "I will be taking corticosteroids until my baby's due date so that he or she will have the best chance of doing well."
- ☒ 2. "The corticosteroids may help my baby's lungs mature."
- ☐ 3. "The goal of the corticosteroids is to stop contractions and help me get to my due date."
- ☐ 4. "If I take corticosteroids, my baby will not have to spend any time in the neonatal intensive care unit when he or she is born."

42. In which maternal locations would the nurse place the ultrasound transducer of the external electronic fetal heart rate monitor if a fetus at 34 weeks' gestation is in the left occipitoanterior (LOA) position?
- ☐ 1. near the symphysis pubis
- ☐ 2. two inches (5.1 cm) above the umbilicus
- ☒ 3. below the umbilicus on the left side
- ☐ 4. at the level of the umbilicus

43. The primary healthcare provider (HCP) prescribes betamethasone for a 34-year-old multigravid client at 32 weeks' gestation who is experiencing preterm labor. Previously, the client has experienced one infant death due to preterm birth at 28 weeks' gestation. The nurse explains that this drug is given for which reason?
- ☒ 1. to enhance fetal lung maturity
- ☐ 2. to counter the effects of tocolytic therapy
- ☐ 3. to treat chorioamnionitis
- ☐ 4. to decrease neonatal production of surfactant

44. When preparing a multigravid client at 34 weeks' gestation experiencing preterm labor for the shake test performed on amniotic fluid, the nurse would instruct the client that this test is done to evaluate the maturity of which fetal systems?
- ☐ 1. urinary
- ☐ 2. gastrointestinal
- ☐ 3. cardiovascular
- ☒ 4. pulmonary

The Pregnant Client with Premature Rupture of the Membranes

45. The nurse is planning care for a multigravid client hospitalized at 36 weeks' gestation with confirmed rupture of membranes and no evidence of labor. What prescription would the nurse anticipate from the primary healthcare provider (HCP)?
- ☐ 1. frequent assessments of cervical dilation
- ☒ 2. intravenous oxytocin administration
- ☒ 3. vaginal cultures for *Neisseria gonorrhoeae*
- ☐ 4. sonogram for amniotic fluid volume index

46. A multigravid client at 34 weeks' gestation visits the hospital because she suspects that her water has broken. After testing the leaking fluid with nitrazine paper, the nurse confirms that the client's membranes have ruptured when the paper turns which color?
- ☐ 1. yellow
- ☐ 2. white
- ☒ 3. blue
- ☐ 4. red

47. A primigravid client at 30 weeks' gestation has been admitted to the hospital with premature rupture of the membranes without contractions. Her cervix is 2 cm dilated and 50% effaced. The nurse should next assess the client's:
- ☐ 1. red blood cell count.
- ☐ 2. degree of discomfort.
- ☐ 3. urinary output.
- ☒ 4. temperature.

48. A multigravid client at 34 weeks' gestation with premature rupture of the membranes tests positive for group B streptococcus. The client is having contractions every 4 to 6 minutes. Her vital signs are as follows: blood pressure, 120/80 mm Hg; temperature, 100°F (37.8°C); pulse, 100 bpm; respirations, 18 breaths/min. Which medication would the nurse expect the primary healthcare provider (HCP) to prescribe?
- ☒ 1. intravenous penicillin
- ☐ 2. intravenous gentamicin sulfate
- ☐ 3. intramuscular betamethasone
- ☐ 4. intramuscular cefaclor

49. A primigravid client at 36 weeks' gestation with premature rupture of the membranes is to be discharged home on bed rest with follow-up by the nurse. After instruction about care while at home, which client statement indicates effective teaching?
- ☐ 1. "It is permissible to douche if the fluid irritates my vaginal area."
- ☐ 2. "I can take either a tub bath or a shower when I feel like it."
- ☐ 3. "I should limit my fluid intake to less than 1 quart (0.95 L) daily."
- ☒ 4. "I should contact the healthcare provider if my temperature is 100.4°F (38°C) or higher."

50. A primigravid client at 34 weeks' gestation is experiencing contractions every 3 to 4 minutes lasting for 35 seconds. Her cervix is 2 cm dilated and 50% effaced. While the nurse is assessing the client's vital signs, the client says, "I think my bag of water just broke." Which intervention would the nurse do **first?**
- ☒ 1. Check the status of the fetal heart rate.
- ☐ 2. Turn the client to her right side.
- ☐ 3. Test the leaking fluid with nitrazine paper.
- ☐ 4. Perform a sterile vaginal examination.

The Pregnant Client with Diabetes Mellitus

51. The antenatal clinic nurse is educating a client with gestational diabetes soon after diagnosis. Evaluation for this client session will include which outcome? Select all that apply.
- ☒ 1. The client states the need to maintain blood glucose levels between 70 and 110 mg/dL (3.9 to 6.2 mmol/L).
- ☒ 2. The client describes her planned walking program while pregnant.
- ☒ 3. The client will strive to maintain a hemoglobin A1C of less than 6%.
- ☐ 4. The client verbalizes the need to maintain a dietary intake of less than 1,500 cal/day to prevent hyperglycemia.
- ☒ 5. The client will continue taking her prenatal vitamins, iron, and folic acid.

52. A 27-year-old primigravid client with insulin-dependent diabetes at 34 weeks' gestation undergoes a nonstress test, the results of which are documented as reactive. What should the nurse tell the client that the test results indicate?
- ☐ 1. A contraction stress test is necessary.
- ☐ 2. The nonstress test should be repeated.
- ☐ 3. Chorionic villus sampling is necessary.
- ☒ 4. There is evidence of fetal well-being.

53. A primigravid client with insulin-dependent diabetes tells the nurse that the contraction stress test performed earlier in the day was suspicious. The nurse interprets this test result as showing which fetal heart rate pattern?
☐ **1.** frequent late decelerations
☐ **2.** decreased fetal movement
☒ **3.** inconsistent late decelerations
☐ **4.** lack of fetal movement

54. Which statement about a fetal biophysical profile would be incorporated into the teaching plan for a primigravid client with insulin-dependent diabetes?
☐ **1.** It determines fetal lung maturity.
☒ **2.** It is noninvasive using real-time ultrasound.
☐ **3.** It will correlate with the newborn's Apgar score.
☐ **4.** It requires the client to have an empty bladder.

55. A 30-year-old multigravid client at 8 weeks' gestation has a history of insulin-dependent diabetes since age 20. When explaining about the importance of blood glucose control during pregnancy, the nurse should tell the client that which will occur regarding the client's insulin needs during the first trimester?
☐ **1.** They will increase.
☒ **2.** They will decrease.
☐ **3.** They will remain constant.
☐ **4.** They will be unpredictable.

56. The nurse explains the complications of pregnancy that occur with diabetes to a primigravid client at 10 weeks' gestation who has a 5-year history of insulin-dependent diabetes. Which complication, if stated by the client, indicates the need for additional teaching?
☐ **1.** *Candida albicans* infection
☒ **2.** twin-to-twin transfusion
☐ **3.** polyhydramnios
☐ **4.** preeclampsia

57. When developing a teaching plan for a primigravid client with insulin-dependent diabetes about monitoring blood glucose control and insulin dosages at home, what would the nurse expect to include as a desired target range for blood glucose levels?
☐ **1.** 40 to 60 mg/dL (2.2 to 3.3 mmol/L) between 1,400 and 1,600 hours
☒ **2.** 70 to 100 mg/dL (3.3 to 5.6 mmol/L) before meals and bedtime snacks
☐ **3.** 110 to 140 mg/dL (6.2 to 7.8 mmol/L) before meals and bedtime snacks
☐ **4.** 140 to 160 mg/dL (7.8 to 8.9 mmol/L) 1 hour after meals

58. When teaching a primigravid client with diabetes about common causes of hyperglycemia during pregnancy, which information would the nurse include?
☐ **1.** fetal macrosomia
☐ **2.** decreased fetal insulin
☒ **3.** maternal infection
☐ **4.** gestational hypertension

59. After teaching a diabetic primigravida about symptoms of hyperglycemia and hypoglycemia, the nurse determines that the client understands the instruction when she says that hyperglycemia may be manifested by which symptom?
☒ **1.** dehydration
☐ **2.** pallor
☐ **3.** sweating
☐ **4.** nervousness

60. At 38 weeks' gestation, a primigravid client with poorly controlled diabetes and severe preeclampsia is admitted for a cesarean birth. The nurse explains to the client that birth helps to prevent which complication?
☐ **1.** Neonatal hyperbilirubinemia
☐ **2.** Congenital anomalies
☐ **3.** Perinatal asphyxia
☒ **4.** Stillbirth

61. A primigravid client with diabetes at 39 weeks' gestation is seen in the high-risk clinic. The primary healthcare provider (HCP) estimates that the fetus weighs at least 10 lb (4,500 g). The client asks, "What causes the baby to be so large?" The nurse's response is based on the understanding that fetal macrosomia is most related to which factor?
☐ **1.** family history of large infants
☐ **2.** fetal anomalies
☒ **3.** maternal hyperglycemia
☐ **4.** maternal hypertension

62. With plans to breast-feed her neonate, a pregnant client with insulin-dependent diabetes asks the nurse about insulin needs during the postpartum period. Which statement about postpartal insulin requirements for breast-feeding mothers should the nurse include in the explanation?
☒ **1.** They fall significantly in the immediate postpartum period.
☐ **2.** They remain the same as during the labor process.
☐ **3.** They usually increase in the immediate postpartum period.
☐ **4.** They need constant adjustment during the first 24 hours.

The Pregnant Client with Heart Disease

63. After instruction of a primigravid client at 8 weeks' gestation diagnosed with class I heart disease about self-care during pregnancy, which client statement would indicate the need for additional teaching?
☐ 1. "I should avoid being near people who have a cold."
☐ 2. "I may be given antibiotics during my pregnancy."
☒ 3. "I should reduce my intake of protein in my diet."
☐ 4. "I should limit my salt intake at meals."

64. While caring for a primigravid client with class II heart disease at 28 weeks' gestation, the nurse would instruct the client to contact her primary healthcare provider (HCP) immediately if the client experiences which symptom?
☐ 1. mild ankle edema
☐ 2. emotional stress on the job
☐ 3. weight gain of 1 lb (0.45 kg) in 1 week
☒ 4. dyspnea at rest

65. When developing the collaborative plan of care with the healthcare provider (HCP) for a multigravid client at 10 weeks' gestation with a history of cardiac disease who was being treated with digitalis therapy before this pregnancy, the nurse should instruct the client about which modification regarding the client's drug therapy regimen?
☐ 1. need for an increased dosage
☒ 2. continuation of the same dosage
☐ 3. switching to a different medication
☐ 4. addition of a diuretic to the regimen

66. Which anticoagulants would the nurse expect to administer when caring for a primigravid client at 12 weeks' gestation who has class II cardiac disease due to mitral valve stenosis?
☒ 1. heparin
☐ 2. warfarin
☐ 3. enoxaparin
☐ 4. ardeparin

67. A primigravid client with class II heart disease who is visiting the clinic at 8 weeks' gestation tells the nurse that she has been maintaining a low-sodium, 1,800-cal diet. Which instruction should the nurse give the client?
☐ 1. Avoid folic acid supplements to prevent megaloblastic anemia.
☐ 2. Severely restrict sodium intake throughout the pregnancy.
☐ 3. Take iron supplements with milk to enhance absorption.
☒ 4. Increase caloric intake to 2,200 calories daily to promote fetal growth.

The Client with an Ectopic Pregnancy

68. On arrival at the emergency department, a client tells the nurse that she suspects that she may be pregnant but has been having a small amount of bleeding and has severe pain in the lower abdomen. The client's blood pressure is 70/50 mm Hg, and her pulse rate is 120 bpm. The nurse notifies the primary healthcare provider (HCP) immediately because of the possibility of:
☒ 1. ectopic pregnancy.
☐ 2. abruptio placentae.
☐ 3. gestational trophoblastic disease.
☐ 4. complete abortion.

69. The nurse is assessing a multigravid client at 12 weeks' gestation who has been admitted to the emergency department with sharp right-sided abdominal pain and vaginal spotting. Which information should the nurse obtain about the client's history? Select all that apply.
☒ 1. history of sexually transmitted infections
☒ 2. number of sexual partners
☒ 3. last menstrual period
☐ 4. cesarean section
☒ 5. contraceptive use

70. Before surgery to remove an ectopic pregnancy and the fallopian tube, which sign or symptom would alert the nurse to the possibility of tubal rupture?
☐ 1. amount of vaginal bleeding and discharge
☒ 2. profuse sweating
☐ 3. slow, bounding pulse rate of 80 bpm
☐ 4. marked abdominal edema

71. A multigravid client diagnosed with a probable ruptured ectopic pregnancy is scheduled for emergency surgery. In addition to monitoring the client's blood pressure before surgery, which factor is **most** important for the nurse to assess?
☐ 1. uterine cramping
☐ 2. abdominal distention
☐ 3. hemoglobin and hematocrit
☒ 4. pulse rate

72. A 36-year-old multigravid client is admitted to the hospital with possible ruptured ectopic pregnancy. When obtaining the client's history, which finding would be **most** important to identify as a predisposing factor?
☐ 1. urinary tract infection
☐ 2. marijuana use during pregnancy
☒ 3. episodes of pelvic inflammatory disease
☐ 4. use of estrogen-progestin contraceptives

73. A multigravid client is admitted to the hospital with a diagnosis of ectopic pregnancy. The nurse anticipates that, because the client's fallopian

tube has not yet ruptured, which medication may be prescribed?
- ☐ 1. progestin contraceptives
- ☐ 2. medroxyprogesterone
- ☒ 3. methotrexate
- ☐ 4. dyphylline

The Pregnant Client with Hyperemesis Gravidarum

74. After instruction of a primigravid client at 8 weeks' gestation about measures to overcome early morning nausea and vomiting, which client statement indicates the need for additional teaching?
- ☐ 1. "I will eat dry crackers or toast before arising in the morning."
- ☐ 2. "I will drink adequate fluids separate from my meals or snacks."
- ☒ 3. "I will eat two large meals daily with frequent protein snacks."
- ☐ 4. "I will snack on a small amount of carbohydrates throughout the day."

75. A multigravid client thought to be at 14 weeks' gestation reports that she is experiencing such severe morning sickness that she "has not been able to keep anything down for a week." The nurse should assess for signs and symptoms of which condition?
- ☐ 1. hypercalcemia
- ☐ 2. hypobilirubinemia
- ☒ 3. hypokalemia
- ☐ 4. hyperglycemia

76. A multigravid client is admitted at 16 weeks' gestation with a diagnosis of hyperemesis gravidarum. The nurse should explain to the client that hyperemesis gravidarum is thought to be related to high levels of which hormone?
- ☐ 1. progesterone
- ☒ 2. estrogen
- ☐ 3. somatotropin
- ☐ 4. aldosterone

77. The primary healthcare provider (HCP) prescribes 1,000 mL of Ringer's lactate intravenously over an 8-hour period for a 29-year-old primigravid client at 16 weeks' gestation with hyperemesis. The drip factor is 12 gtts/mL. The nurse should administer the IV infusion at how many drops per minute? Record your answer using one decimal place.

_____ 25 _____ gtts/min.

78. In caring for a pregnant client with hyperemesis gravidarum, which is the **priority** nursing intervention?
- ☐ 1. providing adequate sleep for the client
- ☒ 2. correction of fluid-electrolyte imbalance
- ☐ 3. reviewing dietary choices and food intake
- ☐ 4. acetaminophen suppositories

The Client with a Gestational Trophoblastic Disease

79. A client at 15 weeks' gestation presents at the obstetrical triage unit with dark brown vaginal bleeding and continuous nausea and vomiting. Her blood pressure is 142/98 mm Hg and fundal height is 19 cm. Which prescription is **most** important for the nurse to request from the primary care provider?
- ☐ 1. a transfer to the antenatal unit
- ☐ 2. NPO status for 24 hours
- ☐ 3. intravenous magnesium sulfate
- ☒ 4. stat ultrasound

80. A 38-year-old client at about 14 weeks' gestation is admitted to the hospital with a diagnosis of complete hydatidiform mole. Soon after admission, the nurse would assess the client for which signs and symptoms?
- ☒ 1. gestational hypertension
- ☐ 2. gestational diabetes
- ☐ 3. hypothyroidism
- ☐ 4. polycythemia

81. After a dilatation and curettage (D&C) to evacuate a molar pregnancy, assessing the client for which signs and symptoms would be **most** important?
- ☐ 1. urinary tract infection
- ☒ 2. hemorrhage
- ☐ 3. abdominal distention
- ☐ 4. chorioamnionitis

82. When preparing a multigravid client who has undergone evacuation of a hydatidiform mole for discharge, the nurse explains the need for follow-up care. The nurse determines that the client understands the instruction when she says that she is at risk for developing which problem?
- ☐ 1. ectopic pregnancy
- ☒ 2. choriocarcinoma
- ☐ 3. multifetal pregnancies
- ☐ 4. infertility

83. After suction and evacuation of a complete hydatidiform mole, the 28-year-old multigravid client asks the nurse when she can become pregnant again. The nurse would advise the client not to become pregnant again for at least how long?
- ☐ 1. 6 months
- ☒ 2. 12 months
- ☐ 3. 18 months
- ☐ 4. 24 months

84. A woman is diagnosed with complete molar pregnancy. The nurse understands that the woman requires more teaching when she makes which statement?
- ☐ 1. "I need to make follow-up appointments to have my hormone levels checked."
- ☒ 2. "I know the placenta caused problems, and my baby died in my uterus."
- ☐ 3. "I plan to get pregnant again next year."
- ☐ 4. "I understand I may develop a serious type of cancer."

The Pregnant Client with Miscellaneous Complications

85. The nurse is working with four clients on the obstetrical unit. Which client will be the highest **priority** for a cesarean section?
- ☐ 1. client at 40 weeks' gestation whose fetus weighs 8 lb (3,630 g) by ultrasound estimate
- ☐ 2. client at 37 weeks' gestation with fetus in ROP position
- ☐ 3. client at 32 weeks' gestation with fetus in breech position
- ☒ 4. client at 38 weeks' gestation with active herpes lesions

86. The nurse notices that a client who has just given birth is short of breath, is ashen in color, and begins to cough. She becomes limp on the birthing table. At last assessment ½ hour ago, her temperature was 98°F (36.7°C), pulse was 78 beats/min, and respirations were 16 breaths/min. Determine the nursing actions in the order they should occur. All options must be used.

1. Open airway using head tilt-chin lift.
2. Ask staff to activate emergency response system.
3. Establish unresponsiveness.
4. Give two breaths.
5. Begin compressions.

3
2
5
1
4

87. A client in sickle cell crisis has been hospitalized during her pregnancy. After giving discharge instructions, the nurse determines the client needs further teaching when she makes which statement?
- ☐ 1. "I will need more frequent appointments during the remainder of the pregnancy."
- ☐ 2. "Signs of any type of infection must be reported immediately."
- ☐ 3. "At the earliest signs of a crisis, I need to seek treatment."
- ☒ 4. "I will need to take an iron supplement even if my laboratory values are normal."

88. A laboring client at −2 station has a spontaneous rupture of the membranes, and a cord immediately protrudes from the vagina. The nurse should **first:**
- ☒ 1. place gentle pressure upward on the fetal head.
- ☐ 2. place the cord back into the vagina to keep it moist.
- ☐ 3. begin oxygen by face mask at 8 to 10 L/min.
- ☐ 4. turn the client on her left side.

89. A client has just had a cesarean section for a prolapsed cord. In reviewing the client's history, which factors place a client at risk for cord prolapse? Select all that apply.
- ☒ 1. negative 2 station
- ☒ 2. low-birth-weight infant
- ☒ 3. rupture of membranes
- ☒ 4. breech presentation
- ☐ 5. prior abortion
- ☐ 6. low-lying placenta

90. A woman who has given birth to a healthy neonate is being discharged. As part of discharge teaching, the nurse should instruct the client to observe vaginal discharge for postpartum hemorrhage and notify the healthcare provider (HCP) about:
- ☐ 1. bleeding that becomes lighter each day.
- ☐ 2. clots the size of grapes.
- ☒ 3. saturating a pad in an hour.
- ☐ 4. lochia that lasts longer than 1 week.

91. A woman who is Rh negative has given birth to an Rh-positive infant. The nurse explains to the client that she will receive Rho (D) immune globulin (RhoGAM). The nurse determines that the client understands the purpose of RhoGAM when she states:
- ☐ 1. "RhoGAM will protect my next baby if it is Rh negative."
- ☒ 2. "RhoGAM will prevent antibody formation in my blood."
- ☐ 3. "RhoGAM will be given to prevent antigen formation in my baby's blood."
- ☐ 4. "RhoGAM will be used to prevent bleeding in my newborn."

92. A client at 4 weeks postpartum tells the nurse that she cannot cope any longer and is overwhelmed by her newborn. The baby has old formula on her clothes and under her neck. The mother does not remember when she last bathed the baby and states she does not want to care for the infant. The nurse should encourage the client and her husband to call their healthcare provider (HCP) because the mother should be evaluated further for:
- ☐ 1. postpartum blues
- ☒ 2. postpartum depression
- ☐ 3. poor bonding
- ☐ 4. infant abuse

93. The nurse and an unlicensed assistive personnel (UAP) are caring for clients in a birthing center. Which tasks should the nurse delegate to the UAP? Select all that apply.
- [X] 1. removing a Foley catheter from a postpartum client
- [X] 2. assisting an active labor client with breathing and relaxation
- [X] 3. ambulating a postcesarean client to the bathroom
- [ ] 4. calculating hourly IV totals for a preterm labor client
- [ ] 5. intake and output catheterization for culture and sensitivity
- [ ] 6. calling a report of normal findings to the healthcare provider (HCP)

Managing Care, Quality, and Safety for Pregnant Clients

94. Several pregnant clients are waiting to be seen in the triage area of the obstetrical unit. Which client should the nurse see **first**?
- [ ] 1. a client at 13 weeks' gestation who is experiencing nausea and vomiting three times a day with +1 ketones in her urine
- [ ] 2. a client at 37 weeks' gestation who is an insulin-dependent diabetic and experiencing 3 to 4 fetal movements per day
- [X] 3. a client at 32 weeks' gestation who has preeclampsia and +3 proteinuria and who is returning for evaluation of epigastric pain
- [ ] 4. a client at 17 weeks' gestation who is not feeling fetal movement at this point in her pregnancy

95. The nurse is planning care for a group of pregnant clients. Which client should be referred to a healthcare provider (HCP) immediately?
- [ ] 1. a woman who is at 10 weeks' gestation, is having nausea and vomiting, and has +1 ketones in her urine
- [ ] 2. a woman who is at 37 weeks' gestation and has insulin-dependent diabetes experiencing two to three hyperglycemic episodes weekly
- [X] 3. a woman at 32 weeks' gestation who is preeclamptic with +3 proteinuria
- [ ] 4. a woman at 15 weeks' gestation who reports she has not felt fetal movement

96. A client with gestational hypertension is to receive magnesium sulfate to run at 3 g/h with normal saline to maintain the total IV rate at 125 mL/h. The nurse giving the end-of-shift report stated that the client's blood pressures have been elevated during the night. The oncoming nurse checked the client and found magnesium sulfate running at 2 g/h. Identify the nursing actions to be taken from first to last. All options must be used.

1. Notify the primary healthcare provider (HCP) of the incident.
2. Assess the client's current status.
3. Correct the IV rates.
4. Initiate an incident report.

3
2
1
4

97. As the nurse enters the room of a newly admitted primigravid client diagnosed with severe preeclampsia, the client begins to experience a seizure. The nurse should do which in order of **priority** from first to last? All options must be used.

1. Call for immediate assistance.
2. Turn the client to her side.
3. Assess for ruptured membranes.
4. Maintain airway.

1
2
4
3

98. The nurse is receiving shift report on four clients on an antenatal unit. The four clients are (1) a 35-week-gestation mother with severe preeclampsia started on a maintenance dose of magnesium sulfate 1 hour ago, (2) a 30-week-gestation client with preterm labor on an oral tocolytic and having no contractions in 6 hours, (3) a hyperemesis client with emesis four times in the past 12 hours, and (4) a 33-week-gestation client with placenta previa who began to feel pelvic pressure during change of shift report. Which action should the nurse take **first**?

☐ 1. Evaluate the client with preeclampsia for maternal and fetal tolerance of magnesium sulfate and the labor pattern.

☐ 2. Assess the client with preterm labor for tolerance of tocolytics and the labor pattern.

☐ 3. Assess the client with hyperemesis for nausea, further emesis, or dehydration.

☐ 4. Evaluate the client with placenta previa without an exam.

99. Which client findings require the nurse's attention **first**?

☐ 1. a gravida 2, para 1 at 39 weeks' gestation with spontaneous rupture of membranes 1 hour ago but no contractions

☐ 2. a gravida 3, para 2 at 30 weeks' gestation with nausea, vomiting, and epigastric pain

☐ 3. a gravida 5, para 1 at 37 weeks' gestation with pink vaginal discharge and abdominal cramping

☐ 4. a gravida 1, para 0 at 39 weeks' gestation with bruises on the arms and abdomen at various stages of healing

Answers, Rationales, and Test-Taking Strategies

The answers and rationales for each question follow below, along with keys (🔑) to the client need (CN) and cognitive level (CL) for each question. In addition, you will also see a glossary icon (📖) highlighting specific terminology used on the licensing exam. As you check your answers, use the **Content Mastery and Test-Taking Skill Self-Analysis** *worksheet (tear-out worksheet in back of book) to identify the reason(s) for not answering the questions correctly. For additional information about test-taking skills and strategies for answering questions, refer to pages 12–23 and pages 35–36 in Part 1 of this book.*

The Pregnant Client with Preeclampsia or Eclampsia

1. 50 mL

$$\frac{500 \text{ mL}}{20 \text{ g}} \times \frac{2 \text{ g}}{\text{h}} = \frac{\overset{50}{\cancel{1,000}} \text{ g/mL}}{\underset{1}{\cancel{20}} \text{ g/h}} = \frac{500 \text{ mL}}{1 \text{ h}}$$

🔑 CN: Pharmacological and parenteral therapies; CL: Apply

2. 3. The two major defining characteristics of preeclampsia are blood pressure elevation of 140/90 mm Hg or greater and proteinuria. Because the client's blood pressure meets the gestational hypertension criteria, the next nursing responsibility is to determine if she has protein in her urine. If she does not, then she may be having transient hypertension. The peripheral edema is within normal limits for someone at this gestational age, particularly because it is in the lower extremities. While the preeclamptic client may have significant edema in the face and hands, edema can be caused by other factors and is not part of the diagnostic criteria. Headaches are significant in pregnancy-induced hypertension but may have other etiologies. The client's blood glucose level has no bearing on a preeclampsia diagnosis.

🔑 CN: Physiological adaptation; CL: Analyze

3. 4. The fetus is considered well if it moves more often than three times in 1 hour. Daily fetal movement counting is part of all high-risk assessments and is a noninvasive, inexpensive method of monitoring fetal well-being. The **HCP** 📖 should be notified if there is a gradual slowing over time of fetal activity, if each day it takes longer for the fetus to move a minimum of 10 times, or if the fetus stops moving for 12 hours or longer.

🔑 CN: Reduction of risk potential; CL: Evaluate

4. 3. The central nervous system (CNS) functioning and freedom from injury is a priority in maintaining well-being of the maternal-fetal unit. If the mother suffers CNS damage related to hypertension or stroke, oxygenation status is compromised, and the well-being of both mother and infant are at risk. Continuous fetal monitoring is an assessment strategy for the infant only and would be of secondary importance to maternal CNS assessment because maternal oxygenation will dictate fetal oxygenation and well-being. In preeclampsia, frequent assessment of maternal reflexes, clonus, visual disturbances, and headache give clear evidence of the condition of the maternal CNS system. Monitoring the liver studies does give an indication of the status of the maternal system, but the less invasive and highly correlated condition of the maternal CNS system in assessing reflexes, maternal headache, visual disturbances, and clonus is the highest priority. Psychosocial care is a priority and can be accomplished in ways other than having the family remain at the bedside.

🔑 CN: Safety and infection control; CL: Synthesize

5. 3. Clients with increased risk for preeclampsia include primigravid clients younger than 20 years or older than 40 years, clients with 5 or more pregnancies, women of color, women with multifetal pregnancies, women with diabetes or heart disease, and women with hydramnios. A total weight gain of 20 lb (9.1 kg) at 32 weeks' gestation with a 1-lb (0.45-kg) weight gain in the last 2 weeks is within normal limits. Short stature is not associated with the development of preeclampsia. A trace amount of protein in the urine is common during pregnancy. However, protein amounts of 1+ or more may be a symptom of pregnancy-induced hypertension.

CN: Reduction of risk potential; CL: Synthesize

6. 1. Congenital anomalies such as hydrocephalus are not associated with preeclampsia. Conditions such as stillbirth, prematurity, abruptio placentae, intrauterine growth restriction, and poor placental perfusion are associated with preeclampsia. Abruptio placentae occurs because of severe vasoconstriction. Intrauterine growth restriction is possible owing to poor placental perfusion. Poor placental perfusion results from increased vasoconstriction.

CN: Physiological adaptation; CL: Evaluate

7. 1,3,4. The nurse must be alert for any signs and symptoms of superimposed preeclampsia in women with gestational hypertension. Dull headache, blurred vision, and protein in urine are all classic signs of preeclampsia in pregnancy and must be reported to the primary care provider immediately. Edema in lower extremities is not a sign of preeclampsia in pregnancy as it is seen in uncomplicated pregnancy. Fundal height of 28 cm is an expected finding.

CN: Management of care; CL: Analyze

8. 3. For clients with mild preeclampsia, a regular diet with ample protein and calories is recommended. If the client experiences constipation, she should increase the fiber in her diet, such as by eating raw fruits and vegetables, and increase fluid intake. A high-residue diet is not a nutritional need in preeclampsia. Sodium and fluid intake should not be restricted or increased. A high-protein diet is unnecessary.

CN: Basic care and comfort; CL: Apply

9. 3. The nurse must be alert to signs of magnesium sulfate toxicity that include loss of deep tendon reflexes, which is often the first sign (patellar-tendon response is the most common reflex tested); urinary output decreases (should have at least 30 mL/h); respirations decrease (12 respirations/min is low and could be developing respiratory distress). First action would be to stop magnesium sulfate infusion and notify the **IICP** 📖. The Foley catheter tubing maybe kinked; however,

looking at all findings would indicate the woman is experiencing magnesium sulfate toxicity. It is not a priority to obtain a urine sample. Documentation is extremely important to complete; however, the nurse must intervene by stopping the magnesium sulfate and notifying the primary care provider. Increasing fluid intake at this point is not appropriate with a woman who has magnesium sulfate toxicity. Intake and output should be ongoing for a client on intravenous fluids and magnesium sulfate and a diagnosis of preeclampsia.

CN: Pharmacological and parenteral therapies; CL: Apply

10. 2. A client with preeclampsia and a continuous headache for 2 days should be seen by a **healthcare provider (HCP)** 📖 immediately. Continuous headache, drowsiness, and mental confusion indicate poor cerebral perfusion and are symptoms of severe preeclampsia. Immediate care is recommended because these symptoms may lead to eclampsia or seizures if left untreated. Advising the client to take two acetaminophen tablets would be inappropriate and may lead to further complications if the client is not evaluated and treated. Although the application of cool compresses may ease the pain temporarily, this would delay treatment. Treatment for nausea may be indicated but only after the primary care primary provider has seen the client and determined if the preeclampsia requires further treatment.

CN: Reduction of risk potential; CL: Synthesize

11. 4. The client with severe preeclampsia may develop eclampsia, which is characterized by seizures. The client needs a darkened, quiet room and side rails with thick padding. This helps decrease the potential for injury should a seizure occur. Airways, a suction machine, and oxygen also should be available. If the client is to undergo induction of labor, oxytocin infusion solution can be obtained at a later time. Tongue blades are not necessary. However, the emergency cart should be placed nearby in case the client experiences a seizure. The ultrasound machine may be used at a later point to provide information about the fetus. In many hospitals, the client with severe preeclampsia is admitted to the labor area, where she and the fetus can be closely monitored. The safety of the client and her fetus is the priority.

CN: Physiological adaptation; CL: Apply

12. 1. Although the client is being admitted, the first response would be to attempt to lower BP by putting the client in left lateral position. The other interventions may be appropriate later, but left lateral position would be the priority.

CN: Management of care; CL: Analyze

13. 3. The client receiving magnesium sulfate intravenously is at risk for possible toxicity. The antidote for magnesium sulfate toxicity is calcium gluconate, which should be readily available at the client's bedside. Diazepam is used to treat anxiety, and usually it is not given to pregnant women. Hydralazine would be used to treat hypertension, and phenytoin would be used to treat seizures.

    CN: Pharmacological and parenteral therapies; CL: Apply

14. 1. Typical signs of hypermagnesemia include decreased deep tendon reflexes, sweating or a flushing of the skin, oliguria, decreased respirations, and lethargy progressing to coma as the toxicity increases. The nurse should check the client's patellar, biceps, and radial reflexes regularly during magnesium sulfate therapy. Cool skin temperature may result from peripheral vasodilation, but the opposite—flushing and sweating—are usually seen. A rapid pulse rate commonly occurs in hypomagnesemia. Tingling in the toes may suggest hypocalcemia, not hypermagnesemia.

    CN: Physiological adaptation; CL: Analyze

15. 2,3,4. Headaches could be a sign of preeclampsia/eclampsia in pregnancy. The client should be assessed for headache, vision changes, epigastric pain, hyper reflexes, and the presence of clonus. Her fetus should be assessed using a nonstress test. An ultrasound done in this pregnancy does not give information to assess the presence of preeclampsia/eclampsia.

    CN: Management of care; CL: Analyze

16. 4. The highest priority for a client with severe preeclampsia is to prevent seizures, thereby minimizing the possibility of adverse effects on the mother and fetus, and then to facilitate safe birth. Efforts to decrease edema, reduce blood pressure, increase urine output, limit kidney damage, and maintain sedation are desirable but are not as important as preventing seizures. It would take several days or weeks for the edema to be decreased. Sedation and decreased reflex excitability can occur with the administration of intravenous magnesium sulfate, which peaks in 30 minutes, much sooner than 48 hours.

    CN: Physiological adaptation; CL: Create

17. 1,5,6. The use of magnesium sulfate as an anticonvulsant acts to depress the central nervous system by blocking peripheral neuromuscular transmissions and decreasing the amount of acetylcholine liberated. The primary goal of magnesium sulfate therapy is to prevent seizures. While being used, the temperature and pulse of the client should remain within normal limits. The respiratory rate needs to be >12 respirations per minute (rpm). Rates at 12 rpm or lower are associated with respiratory depression and are seen with magnesium toxicity. Renal compromise is identified with

a urinary output of less than 30 mL/h. A fetal heart rate that is maintained within the 112 to 160 range is desired without later or variable decelerations. While extreme elevations of blood pressure must be treated, achieving a normal pressure carries the risk of decreasing perfusion to the fetus. Deep tendon reflexes should not be diminished or exaggerated. The therapeutic magnesium sulfate level of 5 to 8 mg/dL (2.5 to 4 mmol/L) is to be maintained.

    CN: Pharmacological and parenteral therapies; CL: Evaluate

18. 1. A respiratory rate of 12 breaths/min suggests potential respiratory depression, an adverse effect of magnesium sulfate therapy. The medication must be stopped, and the **HCP** should be notified immediately. A patellar reflex of +2 is normal. Absence of a patellar reflex suggests magnesium toxicity. A blood pressure reading of 160/88 mm Hg would be a common finding in a client with severe preeclampsia. Urinary output exceeding intake is not likely in a client receiving intravenous magnesium sulfate. Oliguria is more common.

    CN: Pharmacological and parenteral therapies; CL: Synthesize

19. 3. Principles of emergency management begin with calling for assistance. If a client begins to have a seizure, the first action by the nurse is to remain with the client and call for immediate assistance. The nurse needs to have some assistance in managing this client. After the seizure, the client needs intensive monitoring. An airway can be inserted, if appropriate, after the seizure ends. Noting the time the seizure begins and ends and turning the client to her left side should be done after assistance is obtained.

    CN: Reduction of risk potential; CL: Synthesize

20. 1. One of the most common adverse effects of the drug hydralazine is tachycardia. Therefore, the nurse should assess the client's heart rate and pulse. Hydralazine acts to lower blood pressure by peripheral dilation without interfering with placental circulation. Bradypnea and polyuria are usually not associated with hydralazine use. Dysphagia is not a typical adverse effect of hydralazine.

    CN: Pharmacological and parenteral therapies; CL: Analyze

21. 4. These findings would be documented as 4+. 1+ indicates a diminished response; 2+ indicates a normal response; 3+ indicates a response that is brisker than average but not abnormal. Mild clonus is said to be present when there are two movements.

    CN: Physiological adaptation; CL: Apply

22. 3. Epigastric pain or acute right upper quadrant pain is associated with the development of eclampsia and an impending seizure; this is thought to be related to liver ischemia. Decreased contraction intensity is unrelated to the severity of the preeclampsia. Typically, the client's temperature increases because of increased cerebral pressure. A decrease in temperature is unrelated to an impending seizure. Hyporeflexia is not associated with an impending seizure. Typically, the client would exhibit hyperreflexia.

CN: Physiological adaptation; CL: Analyze

23. 4. After an eclamptic seizure, the client commonly falls into a deep sleep or coma. The nurse must continually monitor the client for signs of impending labor because the client will not be able to verbalize that contractions are occurring. Oliguria is more common than polyuria after an eclamptic seizure. Facial flushing is not common unless it is caused by a reaction to a medication. Typically, the client remains hypertensive unless medications such as magnesium sulfate are administered.

CN: Physiological adaptation; CL: Analyze

24. 1. After an eclamptic seizure, the client is at risk for abruptio placentae due to severe vasoconstriction resulting in hemorrhage into the decidua basalis. Abruptio placentae is manifested by a board-like abdomen and an abnormal fetal heart rate tracing. Transverse lie or shoulder presentation, placenta accreta, and uterine atony are not related to eclampsia. Causes of a transverse lie may include relaxation of the abdominal wall secondary to grand multiparity, preterm fetus, placenta previa, abnormal uterus, contracted pelvis, and excessive amniotic fluid. Placenta accreta, a rare phenomenon, refers to a condition in which the placenta abnormally adheres to the uterine lining. Uterine atony, or relaxed uterus, may occur after childbirth, leading to postpartum hemorrhage.

CN: Physiological adaptation; CL: Analyze

25. 2. The normal value of LDH in a nonpregnant person is 45 to 90 U/L (0.75 to 1.5 μkat/L). LDH elevations indicate tissue destruction that can occur with HELLP syndrome. This platelet range is in the normal range and remains unchanged during pregnancy. Uric acid in a nonpregnant woman is 2 to 6.6 mg/dL (119 to 393 μmol/L). AST normal range is 4 to 20 U/L (0.07 to 0.33 μkat/L).

CN: Reduction of risk potential;
CL: Synthesize

The Pregnant Client with a Chronic Hypertensive Disorder

26. 1. Pregnancy is not the time for clients to begin a diet. Clients with chronic hypertension need to consume adequate calories to support fetal growth and development. They also need an adequate protein intake. Meat and beans are good sources of protein. Most pregnant women report that eating more frequent, smaller meals decreases heartburn resulting from the reflux of acidic secretions into the lower esophagus. Pregnant women need adequate hydration (fluids) and fiber to prevent constipation.

CN: Basic care and comfort; CL: Evaluate

27. 2. Women with chronic hypertension during pregnancy are at risk for complications such as preeclampsia (about 25%), abruptio placentae, and intrauterine growth retardation, resulting in a small-for-gestational-age infant. There is no association between chronic hypertension and hyperthyroidism. Pregnant women with chronic hypertension are not at an increased risk for hydramnios (polyhydramnios), an abnormally large amount of amniotic fluid. Clients with diabetes and multiple gestations are at risk for this condition. Placenta accreta, a rare placental abnormality, refers to a condition in which the placenta abnormally adheres to the uterine lining. It is not associated with chronic hypertension.

CN: Reduction of risk potential;
CL: Evaluate

28. 2,3,6. Vaginal bleeding with or without pain could signify placenta previa or abruptio placentae. Continuous or pounding headache could indicate an elevated blood pressure, and change in the strength or frequency of fetal movements could indicate that the fetus is in distress. Orthostatic hypotension can occur during pregnancy and can be alleviated by rising slowly. Leg veins may increase in size due to additional pressure from the increasing uterine size, while leg cramps may also occur and can commonly be decreased with calcium supplements.

CN: Reduction of risk potential;
CL: Evaluate

The Pregnant Client with Third-Trimester Bleeding

29. 1. Bright red vaginal bleeding without contractions could indicate a placenta previa. A sterile vaginal exam should never be done on a woman with a known or suspected placenta previa. Applying the external fetal monitor will allow the nurse to assess fetal status. A complete physical assessment of the client is indicated. A fundal height is used to monitor fetal growth during pregnancy but does not provide information related to vaginal bleeding.

CN: Reduction of risk potential;
CL: Analyze

30. 3. Urinary output of less than 30 mL/h indicates renal compromise and would be the most important assessment finding to report to the **HCP** 🔲. The APTT is within normal limits, and the hemoglobin is lower than values for an adult female but within normal limits for a pregnant female. Although the platelet level is slightly low and may impact blood clotting, when compared to renal failure, it is less important.

⚷ CN: Management of care; CL: Synthesize

31. 4. Although the exact cause of abruptio placentae is unknown, possible contributing factors include excessive intrauterine pressure caused by hydramnios or multiple pregnancy, cocaine use, cigarette smoking, alcohol ingestion, trauma, increased maternal age and parity, and amniotomy. A history of hypertension is associated with an increased risk of abruptio placentae. A previous low transverse cesarean section and a history of one induced abortion are associated with increased risk of placenta previa, not abruptio placentae.

⚷ CN: Physiological adaptation; CL: Analyze

32. 2. Treatment of DIC includes treating the causative factor, replacing maternal coagulation factors, and supporting physiologic functions. Intravenous infusions of whole blood, fresh frozen plasma, or platelets are used to replace depleted maternal coagulation factors. Although Ringer's lactate solution and 5% dextrose solution may be used as intravenous fluid replacement, the client needs blood component therapy. Therefore, normal saline must be used. Intravenous heparin, not warfarin, may be administered to halt the clotting cascade.

⚷ CN: Physiological adaptation; CL: Analyze

33. 1. The most common assessment finding associated with placenta previa is painless vaginal bleeding. With placenta previa, the placenta is abnormally implanted, covering a portion or all of the cervical os. Uterine tetany, intermittent pain with spotting, and dull lower back pain are not associated with placenta previa. Uterine tetany is associated with oxytocin administration. Intermittent pain with spotting commonly is associated with a spontaneous abortion. Dull lower back pain is commonly associated with poor maternal posture or a urinary tract infection with renal involvement.

⚷ CN: Physiological adaptation; CL: Analyze

34. 1. When administering blood replacement therapy, extreme caution is needed. Before administering any blood product, the nurse should validate the client information and the blood product with another nurse to prevent administration of the wrong blood transfusion. Although baseline vital signs are necessary, she should initiate the infusion of blood slowly for the first 10 to 15 minutes. Then,

if there is no evidence of a reaction, she should adjust the rate of infusion to ensure that the blood product is infused over 2 to 4 hours. The nurse can ask the client if she has ever had a reaction to a blood product, but a general question about allergies may not elicit the most complete response about any reactions to blood product administration. Blood transfusions are typically given with intravenous normal saline solution, not dextrose solutions.

⚷ CN: Pharmacological and parenteral therapies; CL: Apply

35. 3. Feelings of loss, grief, and guilt are normal after a cesarean birth, particularly if it was not planned. The nurse should support the client, listen with empathy, and allow the client time to grieve. The likelihood of the client experiencing postpartum blues is not known, and no evidence is presented. Although maternal-infant bonding may be delayed owing to neonatal complications or maternal pain and subsequent medications, it should not be difficult. Although the nurse is aware that this type of birth was necessary to save the client's life, using this as the basis for the response does not acknowledge the mother's feelings.

⚷ CN: Psychosocial integrity; CL: Apply

36. The level of anesthesia achieved via epidural anesthesia for a vaginal birth is T10 (approximately the level of the umbilicus). Epidural anesthesia for a cesarean birth would be at the level of T4 to T6, approximately the nipple line.

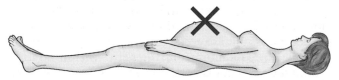

⚷ CN: Pharmacological and parenteral therapies; CL: Apply

37. 3. Abruptio placentae is a medical emergency because the degree of hypovolemic shock may be out of proportion to visible blood loss. On admission, the nurse should plan to first insert a large-gauge intravenous catheter for fluid replacement and oxygen by mask to decrease fetal anoxia. Vaginal examination usually is not performed on pregnant clients who are experiencing third-trimester bleeding due to abruptio placentae because it can result in damage to the placenta and further fetal anoxia. The client's history can be obtained once the client has been admitted and the intravenous line has been started. The goal is birth of the fetus, usually by emergency cesarean section. The nurse should also plan to monitor the client's vital signs and the fetal heart rate. Ultrasound is of limited use in the diagnosis of abruptio placentae.

⚷ CN: Reduction of risk potential; CL: Synthesize

The Pregnant Client with Preterm Labor

38. 3. The absence of fetal fibronectin in a vaginal swab between 22 and 37 weeks' gestation indicates there is less than 1% risk of developing preterm labor in the next week. Fetal fibronectin is an extra cellular protein normally found in fetal membranes and deciduas and has no correlation with preeclampsia, fetal lung maturation, or gestational diabetes.

☌ CN: Reduction of risk potential;
CL: Synthesize

39. 4. Smoking is a major risk factor for preterm labor and decreased fetal weight. Clients struggling to quit should know decreasing cigarette use will help improve outcomes even if they cannot totally quit. Dehydration is a risk factor for preterm labor as is prolonged standing and remaining in one position. Infection anywhere in the body can lead to preterm labor through the inflammation pathway. While taking trips, frequent emptying of the bladder prevents infection and ambulates the woman.

☌ CN: Management of care; CL: Evaluate

40. 1. Indomethacin has been successfully used to halt preterm labor. However, if the client should give birth to a preterm infant, the nurse would notify the nursery personnel about the tocolytic therapy because this drug can lead to premature closure of the fetal ductus arteriosus, resulting in pulmonary hypertension. Prematurity is associated with RDS because of the immaturity of the fetal lungs. RDS is not a result of indomethacin. Hyperbilirubinemia is more common in preterm infants. Use of indomethacin to halt preterm labor is not associated with cardiomyopathy in the infant.

☌ CN: Pharmacological and parenteral therapies; CL: Synthesize

41. 2. Corticosteroids given IM have been shown to increase fetal lung maturity by increasing surfactant and reduce the risk of respiratory distress syndrome in premature infants. It is not a guarantee that a premature newborn would not have problems at birth that would require time in the neonatal intensive care unit. The administration of the corticosteroids is normally completed within 24 to 48 hours.

☌ CN: Pharmacological and parenteral therapies; CL: Evaluate

42. 3. As the uterus contracts, the abdominal wall rises and, when external monitoring is used, presses against the transducer. This movement is transmitted into an electrical current, which is then recorded. With the fetus in the LOA position, the cardiotransducer should be placed below the umbilicus on the side where the fetal back is located and uterine displacement during contractions is greatest. If the fetal back is near the symphysis pubis, the fetus is presenting as a transverse lie. If the fetus is in a breech position, the fetal back may be at or above the umbilicus.

☌ CN: Reduction of risk potential; CL: Apply

43. 1. Betamethasone therapy is indicated when the fetal lungs are immature. The fetus must be between 28 and 34 weeks' gestation, and birth must be delayed for 24 to 48 hours for the drug to achieve a therapeutic effect. Antibiotics would be used to treat chorioamnionitis. Betamethasone is not an antagonist for tocolytic therapy. It increases, not decreases, the production of neonatal surfactant.

☌ CN: Pharmacological and parenteral therapies; CL: Apply

44. 4. The shake test helps determine the maturity of the fetal pulmonary system. The test is based on the fact that surfactant foams when mixed with ethanol. The more stable the foam, the more mature the fetal pulmonary system. A lecithinsphingomyelin ratio is usually determined in conjunction with the shake test. Amniotic fluid volumes are used to evaluate the GI and urinary systems. Ultrasound to evaluate the cardiovascular system.

☌ CN: Reduction of risk potential; CL: Apply

The Pregnant Client with Premature Rupture of the Membranes

45. 3. Because an intrauterine infection may occur when membranes have ruptured, vaginal cultures for *N. gonorrhoeae*, group B streptococcus, and chlamydia are usually taken. Prophylactic antibiotics may be prescribed to reduce the risk of infection in the newborn. Frequent vaginal examinations should be avoided because they can further increase the client's risk for infection. Intravenous oxytocin to initiate labor may be used if an infection occurs. Bed rest can sometimes prolong the pregnancy and prevent a preterm birth. A sonogram may be used to validate rupture of the membranes with an amniotic fluid index. However, it is not needed if the **HCP** □ has confirmed the rupture.

☌ CN: Reduction of risk potential; CL: Apply

46. 3. If the client's membranes have ruptured, the nitrazine paper will turn blue, an alkaline reaction. False positives may occur when the nitrazine paper is exposed to blood or semen. The definitive test for rupture of membranes is fern testing, where amniotic fluid is allowed to dry on a slide and then viewed under a microscope. Dried amniotic fluid will form a fern pattern. No other fluid forms this type of pattern.

⚷ CN: Reduction of risk potential; CL: Analyze

47. 4. Premature rupture of the membranes is commonly associated with chorioamnionitis, or an infection. A priority assessment for the nurse to make is to document the client's temperature every 2 to 4 hours. Temperature elevation may indicate an infection. Lethargy and an elevated white blood cell count also indicate an infection. The red blood cell count would provide information related to anemia, not infection. The client is not in labor. Therefore, assessing the degree of discomfort is not a priority at this time. Urinary output is not a reliable indicator of an infection such as chorioamnionitis.

⚷ CN: Reduction of risk potential; CL: Analyze

48. 1. Because group B streptococcus is a gram-positive bacterium, the **HCP** 📖 probably will prescribe intravenous penicillin to treat the mother's infection and prevent fetal infection. Gentamicin sulfate, which acts on gram-negative bacteria, would be inappropriate. Administering a corticosteroid, such as betamethasone, is inappropriate because the premature rupture of the membranes enhances fetal lung maturity. The lack of amniotic fluid causes early maturation of lung tissue. Cefaclor, which is available only in the oral form, is used for upper and lower respiratory tract infections and urinary tract infections by gram-negative staphylococci.

⚷ CN: Pharmacological and parenteral therapies; CL: Analyze

49. 4. Because of the client's increased risk for infection, successful teaching is indicated when the client states that she will contact the primary care provider if her temperature is 100.4°F (38°C) or greater. The client should be instructed to monitor her temperature twice daily. The client should refrain from coitus, douching, and tub bathing, which can increase the potential for infection. Showering is permitted because water in the shower does not enter the vagina and increase the risk of infection. A fluid intake of at least 2 L daily is recommended to prevent potential urinary tract infection.

⚷ CN: Reduction of risk potential; CL: Evaluate

50. 1. The priority is to determine whether a prolapsed cord has occurred as a result of the spontaneous rupture of membranes. The nurse's first action should be to check the status of the fetal heart rate. Complications of premature rupture of the membranes include a prolapsed cord or increased pressure on the fetal umbilical cord inhibiting fetal nutrient supply. Variable decelerations or fetal bradycardia may be seen on the external fetal monitor. The cord also may be visible. Turning the client to her right side is not necessary. If the cord does prolapse, the client should be placed in a knee-to-chest or Trendelenburg position. Checking the fluid with nitrazine paper and vaginal examination are appropriate once the status of the fetus has been evaluated.

⚷ CN: Reduction of risk potential; CL: Synthesize

The Pregnant Client with Diabetes Mellitus

51. 1,2,3,5. The gestational diabetic needs to maintain blood glucose levels as close to "normal" as the nondiabetic pregnant woman. Walking is an excellent form of exercise for anyone and works well for pregnant diabetics as it burns calories, accelerates the heart rate, and as a result maintains the blood sugar at a lower level. During pregnancy, continuously high blood glucose levels measured by a hemoglobin A1C of >6 mg/dL (60 g/L) carry risks for the dyad. The suggested diet for a gestational diabetic is 1,800 to 2,400 cal/day to avoid the body breaking down maternal fat to maintain blood glucose levels. Continuing prenatal vitamins, iron, and folic acid (800 mcg/day) are general nutritional recommendations for pregnancy.

⚷ CN: Reduction of risk; CL: Evaluate

52. 4. The nonstress test is considered reactive when two or more fetal heart rate accelerations of at least 15 bpm occur (from a baseline fetal heart rate of 120 to 160 bpm), along with fetal movement, during a 10- to 20-minute period. A reactive nonstress test indicates fetal heart rate accelerations and well-being. There is no indication for further evaluation (such as a contraction stress test). However, contraction stress tests are commonly scheduled for pregnant clients with insulin-dependent diabetes in the latter part of pregnancy and are repeated periodically until birth. Chorionic villus sampling is usually performed early in the pregnancy to detect fetal abnormalities.

⚷ CN: Reduction of risk potential; CL: Synthesize

53. 3. A contraction stress test is used to evaluate fetal well-being during a simulated labor. A suspicious contraction stress test indicates inconsistent late deceleration patterns requiring further evaluation. A negative contraction stress test indicates no late decelerations and is the desired outcome. A positive contraction stress test indicates fetal compromise with frequent late decelerations. Fetal movements are one of the parameters of a biophysical profile and are detected with nonstress testing. Decreased or absent fetal movements may indicate central nervous system dysfunction or prematurity. Lack of fetal movement or decreased fetal movement is not associated with contraction stress testing.

CN: Reduction of risk potential; CL: Analyze

54. 2. The fetal biophysical profile, a noninvasive test using real-time ultrasound, assesses five parameters: fetal heart rate reactivity, fetal breathing movements, gross fetal body movements, fetal tone, and amniotic fluid volume. Fetal heart rate reactivity is determined by a nonstress test; the other four parameters are determined by ultrasound scanning. The results are available as soon as the test is completed and interpreted. The lecithin-sphingomyelin ratio is used to determine fetal lung maturity. Although the fetal biophysical profile is useful in predicting which fetuses may be at greater risk for compromise, there is no correlation with the newborn's Apgar score. The biophysical score is sometimes referred to as the fetal Apgar score. A score of 8 to 10 indicates fetal well-being. Use of an ultrasound requires the mother to have a full bladder.

CN: Pharmacological and parenteral therapies; CL: Apply

55. 2. During the first trimester, it is not unusual for insulin needs to decrease, commonly as a result of nausea and vomiting. Progressive insulin resistance is characteristic of pregnancy, particularly in the second half of pregnancy. It is not unusual for insulin needs to increase by as much as four times the nonpregnant dose after about the 24th week of gestation. This resistance is caused by the production of human placental lactogen, also called *human chorionic somatotropin*, by the placenta and by other hormones, such as estrogen and progesterone, which are insulin antagonists.

CN: Pharmacological and parenteral therapies; CL: Apply

56. 2. Clients who are pregnant and have diabetes are not at greater risk for multifetal pregnancy and subsequent twin-to-twin transfusion unless they have undergone fertility treatments. The pregnant diabetic client is at higher risk for complications such as infection, polyhydramnios, ketoacidosis, and preeclampsia, compared with the pregnant nondiabetic client.

CN: Reduction of risk potential; CL: Evaluate

57. 2. The goal is to maintain blood plasma glucose levels at 70 to 100 mg/dL (3.5 to 5.6 mmol/L) before meals and bedtime snacks. Below 60 mg/dL (5.6 mmol/L) indicates hypoglycemia. A range of 110 to 140 mg/dL (6.2 to 7.8 mmol/L) suggests hyperglycemia. The target range 1 hour after meals is 100 to 120 mg/dL (5.6 to 6.7 mmol/L).

CN: Pharmacological and parenteral therapies; CL: Synthesize

58. 3. Maternal infection is the most common cause of maternal hyperglycemia and can lead to ketoacidosis, coma, and death. The client should notify the **healthcare provider (HCP)** immediately if she experiences symptoms of an infection. Fetal macrosomia results from maternal hyperglycemia, but does not cause it. Fetal insulin production increases as maternal glucose crosses the placenta. This helps control glucose in the fetus, but has no bearing on maternal glucose levels. Gestational hypertension does not cause maternal hyperglycemia during pregnancy.

CN: Physiological adaptation; CL: Create

59. 1. Dehydration, polyuria, fatigue, flushed hot skin, dry mouth, and drowsiness are manifestations of hyperglycemia. Hyperglycemia is a medical emergency and requires immediate action to prevent maternal and fetal mortality. Pallor, sweating, and nervousness are early signs of hypoglycemia, not hyperglycemia.

CN: Reduction of risk potential; CL: Evaluate

60. 4. Stillbirths caused by placental insufficiency occur with increased frequency in women with diabetes and severe preeclampsia. Clients with poorly controlled diabetes may experience unanticipated stillbirth as a result of premature aging of the placenta. Therefore, labor is commonly induced in these clients before term. If induction of labor fails, a cesarean section is necessary. Induction and cesarean section do not prevent neonatal hyperbilirubinemia, congenital anomalies, or perinatal asphyxia.

CN: Reduction of risk potential; CL: Apply

61. 3. Maternal hyperglycemia and poor control of the mother's diabetes mellitus have been implicated in fetal macrosomia. When the mother is hyperglycemic, large amounts of amino acids, free fatty acids, and glucose are transferred to the fetus. Although maternal insulin does not cross the placenta, the fetal pancreas responds by hypertrophy of the islet cells of the pancreas. The islet cells produce large amounts of insulin, which acts as a growth hormone. A family history of large infants usually is not the reason for large-for-gestational-age fetuses in diabetic mothers. Maternal hypertension is associated with small-for-gestational-age fetuses because of vasoconstriction of the maternal and placental blood vessels.

 CN: Physiological adaptation; CL: Apply

62. 1. Insulin needs fall significantly for the first 24 hours postpartum because the client has usually been on nothing-by-mouth status for a period of time during labor and the labor process has used maternal glycogen stores. If the client breast-feeds, lower blood glucose levels decrease the insulin requirements. With insulin resistance gone, the client commonly needs little or no insulin during the immediate postpartum period. Although the need for insulin decreases during the intrapartum period, the insulin requirements fall further during the first 24 hours postpartum. After the first 24 hours postpartum, insulin requirements may fluctuate markedly, needing adjustment during the next few days as the mother's body returns to a nonpregnant state.

 CN: Pharmacological and parenteral therapies; CL: Create

The Pregnant Client with Heart Disease

63. 3. The client needs a diet that is adequate in protein and calories to prevent anemia, which can place additional strain on the cardiac system, further compromising the client's cardiac status. The client should avoid contact with people who have infections because of the increased risk for developing endocarditis. The client may need antibiotics during the pregnancy to prevent endocarditis. Limiting sodium intake can help to prevent excessive expansion of blood volume and decrease cardiac workload.

 CN: Reduction of risk potential; CL: Evaluate

64. 4. Clients with class II heart disease have dyspnea upon exertion but not at rest. Dyspnea at rest would indicate a change in condition that must be reported immediately because it may be indicative of increasing congestive heart failure. Mild ankle edema in the third trimester is a common finding. However, generalized or pitting edema, suggesting increasing congestive heart failure, must be reported immediately. Emotional stress on the job increases cardiac demand. However, it needs to be reported only if the client experiences symptoms, such as palpitations or irregular heart rate, indicating heart failure related to the increased stress. Weight gain of 1 lb (0.45 kg) per week is a normal finding during the third trimester.

 CN: Reduction of risk potential; CL: Apply

65. 2. Unless the client has cardiac decompensation during the pregnancy, she will most likely be able to continue taking the same dose of medication. The client may be prescribed prophylactic antibiotics, particularly if she has had rheumatic fever. The medication would be switched only if digitalis toxicity occurs. A diuretic is added only if congestive heart failure is not controlled by sodium and activity restrictions.

 CN: Management of care; CL: Apply

66. 1. Although there is no completely safe anticoagulant therapy during pregnancy, heparin is typically the drug of choice. Warfarin, a pregnancy category D drug, can cause fetal malformations. Enoxaparin is sometimes used, but clients are typically switched to heparin near labor because enoxaparin used along with spinal or epidural anesthesia presents an increased risk of bleeding in the epidural or spinal space. Ardeparin also can cause fetal malformations.

 CN: Pharmacological and parenteral therapies; CL: Apply

67. 4. The client can continue a low-sodium diet but should increase the caloric intake to 2,200 calories daily to provide adequate nutrients to support fetal growth and development. Folic acid supplements, a standard component of care, are used to prevent folic acid deficiency, which is associated with megaloblastic anemia during pregnancy. Severe restriction of sodium intake is not recommended because sodium is necessary to maintain fluid volume. Iron supplements should be taken with acidic foods and fluids (e.g., citrus juices) for maximum absorption. Milk decreases the absorption of iron.

 CN: Reduction of risk potential; CL: Apply

The Client with an Ectopic Pregnancy

68. 1. The client's signs and symptoms indicate a probable ectopic pregnancy, which can be confirmed by ultrasound examination or by culdocentesis. The **HCP** 📖 is notified immediately because hypovolemic shock may develop without external bleeding. Once the fallopian tube ruptures, blood will enter the pelvic cavity, resulting in shock. Abruptio placentae would be manifested by a board-like uterus in the third trimester. Gestational trophoblastic disease would be suspected if the client exhibited no fetal heart rate and symptoms of pregnancy-induced hypertension before 20 weeks' gestation. A client with a complete abortion would exhibit a normal pulse and blood pressure with scant vaginal bleeding.

🔑 CN: Physiological adaptation; CL: Analyze

69. 1,2,3,5. The client may be experiencing an ectopic pregnancy. Contributing factors to an ectopic pregnancy include a prior history of sexually transmitted infection that can scar the fallopian tubes. Multiple sex partners increase the risk of sexually transmitted infections. Knowledge of the client's last menstrual period and contraceptive use may support or rule out the possibility of an ectopic pregnancy. The client's history of cesarean sections would not contribute information valuable to the client's current situation or potential diagnosis of ectopic pregnancy.

🔑 CN: Reduction of risk potential; CL: Analyze

70. 2. Diaphoresis, or profuse sweating, indicates shock, which occurs if the tube ruptures. Other common symptoms of tubal rupture include severe knife-like lower quadrant abdominal pain, referred shoulder pain, and falling blood pressure. The amount of vaginal bleeding that is evident is a poor estimate of actual blood loss. Slight vaginal bleeding, commonly described as *spotting*, is common. A rapid, thready pulse, a symptom of shock, is more common with tubal rupture than a slow, bounding pulse. Abdominal edema is a late sign of a tubal rupture in ectopic pregnancy.

🔑 CN: Reduction of risk potential; CL: Analyze

71. 4. Fallopian tube rupture is an emergency situation because of extensive bleeding into the peritoneal cavity. Shock soon develops if precautionary measures are not taken. The nurse readying a client for surgery should be especially careful to monitor blood pressure and pulse rate for signs of impending shock. The nurse should be prepared to administer fluids, blood, or plasma expanders as necessary through an intravenous line that should already be in place. Because the fertilized ovum has implanted outside the uterus, uterine cramping is unlikely. However, abdominal tenderness or knife-like pain may occur. Abdominal fullness may be present, but abdominal distention is rare unless peritonitis has developed. Although the hemoglobin and hematocrit may be checked routinely before surgery, the laboratory results may not truly reflect the presence or degree of acute hemorrhage.

🔑 CN: Reduction of risk potential; CL: Analyze

72. 3. Anything that causes a narrowing or constriction in the fallopian tubes so that a fertilized ovum cannot be properly transported to the uterus for implantation predisposes an ectopic pregnancy. Pelvic inflammatory disease is the most common cause of constricted or narrow tubes. Developmental defects are other possible causes. Ectopic pregnancy is not related to urinary tract infections. Use of marijuana during pregnancy is not associated with ectopic pregnancy, but its use can result in cognitive reduction if the mother's use during pregnancy is extensive. Progestin-only contraceptives and intra-uterine devices have been associated with ectopic pregnancy.

🔑 CN: Physiological adaptation; CL: Analyze

73. 3. Because the fallopian tube has not yet ruptured, methotrexate may be given, followed by leucovorin. This chemotherapeutic agent attacks the fast-growing zygote and trophoblast cells. RU-486 is also effective. A hysterosalpingogram is usually performed after chemotherapy to determine whether the tube is still patent. Progestin-only contraceptives and medroxyprogesterone are ineffective in clearing the fallopian tube. Dyphylline is a bronchodilator and is not used.

🔑 CN: Pharmacological and parenteral therapies; CL: Analyze

The Pregnant Client with Hyperemesis Gravidarum

74. 3. The client needs further instructions when she says she should eat two meals a day with frequent protein snacks to decrease nausea and vomiting. The client should eat more frequent, smaller meals, with frequent carbohydrate snacks to decrease nausea and vomiting. Eating dry crackers or toast before arising, consuming fluids separately from meals, and avoiding greasy or spicy foods may also help to decrease nausea and vomiting.

🔑 CN: Basic care and comfort; CL: Evaluate

75. 3. Gastrointestinal secretion losses from excessive vomiting, diarrhea, and excessive perspiration can result in hypokalemia, hyponatremia, decreased chloride levels, metabolic alkalosis, and eventual acidosis if precautionary measures are not taken. Ketones may be present in the urine. Dehydration can lead to poor maternal and fetal outcomes. Persistent vomiting can lead to hypocalcemia, not hypercalcemia. Hyperbilirubinemia, not hypobilirubinemia, is typical in clients with hyperemesis. Persistent vomiting may affect liver function and subsequently the excretion of bilirubin from the body. Hypoglycemia, not hyperglycemia, may occur as a result of decreased intake of food and fluids, decreased metabolism of nutrients, and excessive vomiting.

⚷ CN: Reduction of risk potential;
CL: Analyze

76. 2. Although the cause of hyperemesis is still unclear, it is thought to be related to high estrogen and human chorionic gonadotropin levels or to trophoblastic activity or gonadotropin production. Hyperemesis is also associated with infectious conditions, such as hepatitis or encephalitis, intestinal obstruction, peptic ulcer, and hydatidiform mole. Progesterone is a relaxant used during pregnancy and would not stimulate vomiting. Somatotropin is a growth hormone used in children. Aldosterone is a male hormone.

⚷ CN: Physiological adaptation; CL: Apply

77. 25 gtts/min

$$\frac{gtts}{min} = \frac{12\ gtts}{1\ mL} \times \frac{1,000\ mL}{8\ h} \times \frac{1\ h}{60\ min} = 25\ gtts/min$$

⚷ CN: Pharmacological and parenteral therapies; CL: Apply

78. 2. Clients with hyperemesis gravidarum can experience severe vomiting. Some clients will require hospital care to treat dehydration including intravenous fluids, antiemetics, and enteral nutrition. Sleep and dietary choices are important to care but not the priority intervention. Acetaminophen suppositories are not indicated for the care of hyperemesis gravidarum.

⚷ CN: Management of care; CL: Analyze

The Client with a Gestational Trophoblastic Disease

79. 4. The nurse should prepare the client for an ultrasound to determine the cause of the symptoms. Elevated blood pressure at this point in the pregnancy could indicate chronic hypertension as well as hydatidiform mole. The fundal height of 19 cm is higher than is typically found at 15 weeks' gestation and is indicative of a molar pregnancy (hydatidiform mole). The dark brown vaginal bleeding in isolation could indicate an abortion but when placed in context of the other symptoms is likely related to a hydatidiform mole. The continuous nausea and vomiting is abnormal at this point in the pregnancy and can be a result of the high levels of progesterone from a molar pregnancy. There is no fetus involved; the blood pressure elevation and the continuous nausea and vomiting will resolve with evacuation of

the mole, negating the need for magnesium sulfate therapy and placing the client on NPO status. Transferring the client to the antenatal unit is premature before a diagnosis has been made.

⚷ CN: Reduction of risk potential;
CL: Synthesize

80. 1. Hydatidiform mole is suspected when the following are present: gestational hypertension before the 24th week of gestation, brownish or prune-colored vaginal bleeding, anemia, absence of fetal heart tones, passage of hydropic vessels, uterine enlargement greater than expected for gestational age, and increased human chorionic gonadotropin levels. Gestational diabetes is related to an increased risk of preeclampsia and urinary tract infections, but it is not associated with hydatidiform mole. Hyperthyroidism, not hypothyroidism, occurs occasionally with hydatidiform mole. If it does occur, it can be a serious complication, possibly life threatening to the mother and fetus from cardiac problems. Polycythemia is not associated with hydatidiform mole. Rather, anemia from blood loss is associated with molar pregnancies.

⚷ CN: Reduction of risk potential;
CL: Analyze

81. 2. After D&C to evacuate a molar pregnancy, the nurse should assess the client's vital signs and monitor for signs of hemorrhage, because the surgical procedure may have traumatized the uterine lining, leading to hemorrhage. Urinary tract infections, not common after evacuation of a molar pregnancy, are most commonly related to urinary catheterization. Typically, urinary catheters are not used during evacuation of a molar pregnancy. The client should not experience abdominal distention because the contents of the uterus have been removed. Chorioamnionitis is an inflammation of the amniotic fluid membranes. With complete mole, no embryonic or fetal tissue or membranes are present.

⚷ CN: Reduction of risk potential;
CL: Analyze

82. 2. A client who has had a hydatidiform mole removed should have regular checkups to rule out the presence of choriocarcinoma, which may complicate the client's clinical picture. The client's human chorionic gonadotropin (hCG) levels are monitored for 1 year. During this time, she should be advised not to become pregnant because this would be reflected in rising hCG levels. Ectopic or multifetal pregnancy is not associated with hydatidiform mole. Women who have molar pregnancies have fertility rates similar to the general population.

⚷ CN: Reduction of risk potential;
CL: Synthesize

83. **2.** A client who has experienced a molar pregnancy is at risk for development of choriocarcinoma and requires close monitoring of human chorionic gonadotropin (hCG) levels. Pregnancy would interfere with monitoring these levels. High hCG titers are common for up to 7 weeks after the evacuation of the mole, but then, these levels gradually begin to decline. Clients should have a pelvic examination and a blood test for hCG titers every month for 6 months and then every 2 months for 1 year. Gradually declining hCG levels suggest no complications. Increasing levels are indicative of a malignancy and should be treated with methotrexate. If after 1 year the hCG levels are negative, the client is theoretically free of the risk of a malignancy developing and could plan another pregnancy.

⚭ CN: Reduction of risk potential; CL: Apply

84. **2.** Although the woman shows signs and symptoms typical of early pregnancy, in gestational trophoblastic disease, or molar pregnancy, gestational tissue exists but the pregnancy is not viable. The woman must have follow-up human chorionic gonadotropin (hCG) levels for the remaining 12 months to ensure remaining tissue does not turn malignant. Due to the risks of developing malignancy, the woman must avoid pregnancy for at least 1 year following gestational trophoblastic disease. In a complete molar pregnancy, the villi swell and form cysts, and the woman is at risk for choriocarcinoma, which is a rapidly spreading malignancy.

⚭ CN: Health promotion and maintenance; CL: Evaluation

The Pregnant Client with Miscellaneous Complications

85. **4.** Herpes simplex virus can be transmitted to the infant during a vaginal birth. The neonatal effects of herpes are severe enough that a cesarean birth is warranted if active lesions—primary or secondary—are present. A client with a primary infection during pregnancy sheds the virus for up to 3 months after the lesion has healed. The client carrying an infant weighing 8 lb (3,629 g) will be given a trial of labor before a cesarean. The client with a fetus in the right occiput posterior position will have a slow labor with increased back pain but can give birth vaginally. The fetus in a breech position still has many weeks to change positions before being at term. At 7 months' gestation, the breech position is not a concern.

⚭ CN: Physiological adaptation; CL: Evaluate

86. **3,2,5,1,4.** The client's actions indicate distress, and the nurse should initiate emergency procedures. The nurse should first establish unresponsiveness and then ask staff to activate the emergency response system. Next, the nurse should follow CABs of CPR. The nurse should check the pulse and begin CPR. Then after 30 compressions, the nurse should assure the open airway and give two breaths.

⚭ CN: Management of care; CL: Synthesize

87. **4.** Sickle cell disease is an autosomal recessive disorder requiring both parents to have a sickle cell trait to pass the disease to a child. Deoxygenated hemoglobin cells assume a sickle shape and obstruct tissues. Tissue obstruction causes hypoxia to the area (vasoocclusion) and results in pain, called *sickle cell crisis*. This type of anemia is an inherited disorder; it is not caused by lack of iron in the diet. Iron supplementation is needed only if there is laboratory evidence of iron deficiency anemia. Self-monitoring for any type of infections or sickle cell crisis and increased frequency of antenatal care visits are part of the teaching plan of care.

⚭ CN: Physiological adaptation; CL: Evaluate

88. **1.** The nurse should place a hand on the fetal head and provide gentle upward pressure to relieve the compression on the cord. Doing so allows oxygen to continue flowing to the fetus. The cord should never be placed back into the vagina because doing so may further compress it. Administering oxygen is an appropriate measure but will not serve a useful purpose until the pressure is relieved on the cord, enabling perfusion to the infant. Turning the client to her left side facilitates better perfusion to the mother, but until the compression on the cord is relieved, the increased oxygen will not serve its purpose. Placing the client in a Trendelenburg or knee-chest position would be position changes to increase perfusion to the infant by relieving cord compression.

⚭ CN: Management of care; CL: Synthesize

89. **1,2,3,4.** Having the fetus at a negative station places the client at risk for a cord prolapse. With a negative station, there is room between the fetal head and the maternal pelvis for the cord to slip through. A small infant is more mobile within the uterus, and the cord can rest between the fetus and the inside of the uterus or below the fetal head. With a large infant, the head is usually in a vertex presentation and occludes the lower portion of the uterus, preventing the cord from slipping by. When membranes rupture, the cord can be swept through with the amniotic fluid. In a breech presentation, the fetal head is in the fundus, and smaller portions of the fetus settle into the lower portion of the uterus, allowing the cord to lie beside the fetus. Prior abortion and a low-lying placenta have no correlation with cord prolapse.

⚭ CN: Physiological adaptation; CL: Analyze

90. 3. A postpartum client who saturates a pad in an hour or less at any time in the postpartum period is considered to be hemorrhaging. As the normal postpartum client heals, bleeding changes from red to pink to off-white. It also decreases in amount each day. Passing blood clots the size of a fist or larger is a reportable problem. Lochia varies in how long it lasts and is considered normal up to 6 weeks postpartum.

🔑 CN: Health promotion and maintenance; CL: Create

91. 2. RhoGAM is given to new mothers who are Rh negative and not previously sensitized and who have given birth to an Rh-positive infant. RhoGAM must be given within 72 hours of the birth of the infant because antibody formation begins at that time. The vaccine is used only when the mother has borne an Rh-positive infant—not an Rh-negative infant. RhoGAM is not given to a newborn and does not affect antigen formation.

🔑 CN: Pharmacological and parenteral therapies; CL: Evaluate

92. 2. The client is experiencing and verbalizing signs of postpartum depression, which usually appears at about 4 weeks postpartum but can occur at any time within the first year after birth. It is more severe and lasts longer than postpartum blues, also called "baby blues." Baby blues are the mildest form of depression and are seen in the later part of the first week after birth. Symptoms usually disappear shortly. Depression may last several years and is disabling to the woman. Poor bonding may be seen at any time but commonly becomes evident as the mother begins interacting with the infant shortly after birth. Infant abuse may take the form of neglect or injuries to the infant. A depressed mother is at risk for injuring or abusing her infant.

🔑 CN: Reduction of risk potential; CL: Synthesize

93. 1,2,3. The UAP 📖 could assist the client with breathing and relaxation, and ambulate the postcesarean client to the bathroom. UAP can also remove Foley catheters in uncomplicated clients. Calculating the hourly IV totals for a preterm labor client would involve assessments that require nursing expertise. In-and-out catheterization, a sterile procedure, and calling reports to HCPs 📖, which requires gathering and analysis of data, are responsibilities of the nurse.

🔑 CN: Management of care; CL: Evaluate

Managing Care, Quality, and Safety for Pregnant Clients

94. 3. A preeclamptic client with +3 proteinuria and epigastric pain is at risk for seizing, which would jeopardize the mother and the fetus. Thus, this client would be the highest priority. The client at 13 weeks' gestation with nausea and vomiting is a concern because the presence of ketones indicates that her body does not have glucose to break down. However, this situation is a lower priority than the preeclamptic client or the insulin-dependent diabetic. The insulin-dependent diabetic is a high priority; however, fetal movement indicates that the fetus is alive but may be ill. As few as four fetal movements in 12 hours can be considered normal. (The client may need additional testing to further evaluate fetal well-being.) The client who is at 17 weeks' gestation may be too early in her pregnancy to experience fetal movement and would be the last person to be seen.

🔑 CN: Management of care; CL: Evaluate

95. 3. The nurse should refer the preeclamptic client with 3+ proteinuria to an **HCP** 📖. The 3+ urine is significant, indicating there is much protein circulating. The woman who is 37 weeks' gestation with insulin-dependent diabetes who has experienced hypoglycemic episodes in the past week can be managed with food and glucose tablets until the client can obtain an appointment with the care provider. The client at 10 weeks' gestation with nausea and vomiting and +1 ketones should also be seen by an HCP, but at this point, although this client is uncomfortable, her life is not in danger. The 15-week client would not be expected to feel her baby move this soon in the pregnancy, and this would not be considered a problem that requires immediate referral to an HCP.

🔑 CN: Management of care; CL: Evaluate

96. 3,2,1,4. The nurse should first change the IV magnesium sulfate and normal saline infusion rates and then assess the current status of the client. The nurse should then notify the **HCP** 📖 to explain the error and report the action taken. A medication error has occurred, and the nurse will need to initiate an incident report.

🔑 CN: Management of care; CL: Synthesize

97. 1,2,4,3. If a client begins to have a seizure, the first action by the nurse is to remain with the client and call for immediate assistance. Next, the nurse should turn the client to her side and then maintain the airway by keeping the neck hyperextended. When the seizure is over, the nurse should assess the client for ruptured membranes and the fetal status.

🔑 CN: Management of care; CL: Synthesize

98. 4. The first action taken should be to evaluate the placenta previa client who has pelvic pressure. The pelvic pressure may be caused by a fetal head creating pressure in the pelvis indicating a potential birth. This client should be evaluated without a pelvic exam and then consult with the **healthcare provider (HCP)** □. A vaginal exam is contraindicated as it may stimulate bleeding of the placenta. The second action would be to complete an assessment on the client with preeclampsia and her fetus to evaluate for tolerance and effectiveness of the magnesium sulfate. The hyperemesis client needs to be evaluated for hydration status and for medication. The preterm labor client is stable on the oral medication and should be seen last.

    ⚷⟶ CN: Management of care; CL: Apply

99. 2. A woman presenting at 30 weeks with nausea and vomiting and epigastric pain has signs and symptoms of preeclampsia and requires the nurse's attention first. Gravida 2, para 1 with spontaneous rupture of membranes, but no contractions, is not a priority. Gravida 5, para 1 at 37 weeks with pink discharge and abdominal cramping could be in early labor and is not a priority at this time. A gravida 1, para 0 at 39 weeks with bruises at various stages of healing could indicate she is in an abusive relationship, but this is not a priority at this time.

    ⚷⟶ CN: Management of care; CL: Analyze

The Birth Experience

- ■ The Primigravid Client in Labor
- ■ The Multigravid Client in Labor
- ■ The Labor Experience
- ■ The Intrapartal Client with Risk Factors
- ■ Managing Care, Quality, and Safety for Clients Giving Birth
- ■ Answers, Rationales, and Test-Taking Strategies

The Primigravid Client in Labor

1. The nurse is managing care of a primigravida at full term who is in active labor. What should be included in developing the plan of care for this client?
- ☐ **1.** oxygen saturation monitoring every half hour
- ☒ **2.** supine positioning on back, if it is comfortable
- ☒ **3.** anesthesia/pain level assessment every 30 minutes
- ☐ **4.** vaginal bleeding, rupture of membrane assessment every shift

2. The healthcare provider (HCP) prescribes intermittent fetal heart rate monitoring for a 20-year-old obese primigravid client at 40 weeks' gestation in the first stage of labor. The nurse should monitor the client's fetal heart rate pattern at which interval?
- ☐ **1.** every 15 minutes during the latent phase
- ☒ **2.** every 30 minutes during the active phase
- ☐ **3.** every 60 minutes during the pushing phase
- ☐ **4.** every 2 hours during the transition phase

3. The primigravid client is at +1 station and 9 cm dilated. Based on these data, the nurse should **first**:
- ☐ **1.** ask the anesthesiologist to increase epidural infusion rate.
- ☐ **2.** assist the client to push if she feels the need to do so.
- ☒ **3.** encourage the client to breathe through the urge to push.
- ☐ **4.** support family members in providing comfort measures.

4. Assessment of a primigravid client in active labor who has had no analgesia or anesthesia reveals complete cervical effacement, dilation of 8 cm, and the fetus at 0 station. The nurse should expect the client to exhibit which behavior during this phase of labor?
- ☐ **1.** excitement
- ☒ **2.** loss of control
- ☐ **3.** numbness of the legs
- ☐ **4.** feelings of relief

5. The nurse is explaining to a primigravida in labor that her baby is in a breech presentation, with the baby's presenting part in a left, sacrum, posterior (LSP) position. Which illustration should the nurse use to help the client understand how her baby is positioned?

☒ **1.**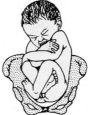

☐ **2.**

☐ **3.**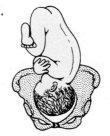

☐ **4.**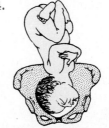

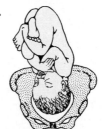

6. The nurse is discussing pain relief methods for a pregnant first-time mother. The discussion should include which labor support methods? Select all that apply.

☒ **1.** effleurage
☐ **2.** positive reinforcement
☒ **3.** guided imagery
☒ **4.** pattern-paced breathing
☐ **5.** self-containment theory
☒ **6.** progressive relaxation

7. A primigravid client at 38 weeks' gestation comes to the labor room because "my water broke." The healthcare provider (HCP) asks the nurse to verify spontaneous rupture of membranes using nitrazine paper. The nurse observes that the nitrazine paper turns bright blue. The nurse's **next** action should be to:

☒ **1.** notify the HCP that the membranes are ruptured.
☐ **2.** perform a sterile vaginal examination to assess the cervix.
☐ **3.** document the findings of the nitrazine test.
☐ **4.** offer the client a sterile sanitary pad after performing perineal care.

8. The healthcare provider (HCP) has prescribed prostaglandin gel to be administered vaginally to a newly admitted primigravid client. Which finding indicates that the client has had a therapeutic response to the medication?

☐ **1.** resting period of 2 minutes between contractions
☐ **2.** normal patellar and elbow reflexes for the past 2 hours
☒ **3.** softening of the cervix and beginning of effacement
☐ **4.** leaking of clear amniotic fluid in small amounts

9. A primigravid client is admitted as an outpatient for an external cephalic version. Which factor would be a contraindication for the procedure?

☒ **1.** multiple gestation
☐ **2.** breech presentation
☐ **3.** maternal Rh-negative blood type
☐ **4.** history of gestational diabetes

10. A primigravida is admitted to the labor area with ruptured membranes and contractions occurring every 2 to 3 minutes, lasting 45 seconds. After 3 hours of labor, the client's contractions are now every 7 to 10 minutes, lasting 30 seconds. The nurse administers oxytocin as prescribed. The expected outcome of this drug is:

☐ **1.** the cervix will begin to dilate 2 cm/h.
☒ **2.** contractions will occur every 2 to 3 minutes, lasting 40 to 60 seconds, moderate intensity, resting tone between contractions.
☐ **3.** the cervix will change from firm to soft, efface to 40% to 50%, and move from a posterior to anterior position.
☐ **4.** contractions will be every 2 minutes, lasting 60 to 90 seconds, with intrauterine pressure of 70 mm Hg.

11. A primigravid client in the second stage of labor feels the urge to push. The client has had no analgesia or anesthesia. Anatomically, what would be the **best** position for the client to assume?

☐ **1.** dorsal recumbent
☐ **2.** lithotomy
☐ **3.** hands and knees
☒ **4.** squatting

12. A 21-year-old primigravid client at 40 weeks' gestation is admitted to the hospital in active labor. The client's cervix is 8 cm and completely effaced at 0 station. During the transition phase of labor, which is a **priority** nursing problem?

☐ **1.** urinary retention
☐ **2.** hyperventilation
☐ **3.** ineffective coping
☒ **4.** pain

13. A 24-year-old primigravid client who gives birth to a viable term neonate is prescribed to receive oxytocin intravenously after delivery of the placenta. Which sign would indicate to the nurse that the placenta is about to be delivered?

☒ **1.** The cord lengthens outside the vagina.
☐ **2.** There is decreased vaginal bleeding.
☐ **3.** The uterus cannot be palpated.
☐ **4.** The uterus changes to discoid shape.

14. A primiparous client, who has just given birth to a healthy term neonate after 12 hours of labor, holds and looks at her neonate and begins to cry. The nurse interprets this behavior as a sign of which response?

☐ **1.** disappointment in the baby's gender
☐ **2.** grief over the ending of the pregnancy
☒ **3.** a normal response to the birth
☐ **4.** indication of postpartum "blues"

15. The cervix of a 15-year-old primigravid client who has been admitted to the labor area is 2 cm dilated and 50% effaced. Her membranes are intact, and contractions are occurring every 5 to 6 minutes. Which intervention should the nurse recommend at this time?

☐ **1.** resting in the right lateral recumbent position
☐ **2.** lying in the left lateral recumbent position
☒ **3.** walking around in the hallway
☐ **4.** sitting in a comfortable chair for a period of time

16. Which technique to promote active relaxation would the nurse include in the teaching plan for a 16-year-old primigravid client in early labor?

☒ **1.** relaxing uninvolved body muscles during uterine contractions
☐ **2.** practicing being in a deep, meditative, sleep-like state
☐ **3.** focusing on an object in the room during the contractions
☐ **4.** breathing rapidly and deeply between contractions

17. The nurse is performing effleurage for a primigravid client in early labor. Which technique should the nurse use?
- ☐ 1. deep kneading of superficial muscles
- ☐ 2. secure grasping of muscular tissues
- ☒ 3. light stroking of the skin surface
- ☐ 4. prolonged pressure on specific sites

18. A 24-year-old primigravid client in active labor requests use of the jet hydrotherapy tub to aid in pain relief. Which condition would the nurse consider to be a contraindication for hydrotherapy?
- ☒ 1. ruptured membranes
- ☐ 2. multifetal gestation
- ☐ 3. diabetes mellitus
- ☐ 4. hypotonic labor patterns

19. The healthcare provider (HCP) prescribes an amniocentesis for a primigravid client at 37 weeks' gestation to determine fetal lung maturity. Which is an indicator of fetal lung maturity?
- ☐ 1. amount of bilirubin present
- ☐ 2. presence of red blood cells
- ☐ 3. Barr body determination
- ☒ 4. lecithin-sphingomyelin (L/S ratio)

20. A 19-year-old primigravid client at 38 weeks' gestation is 7 cm dilated, and the presenting part is at +1 station. The client tells the nurse, "I need to push!" What should the nurse do **next**?
- ☐ 1. Use the McDonald procedure to widen the pelvic opening.
- ☐ 2. Increase the rate of oxygen and intravenous fluids.
- ☒ 3. Instruct the client to use a pant-blow pattern of breathing.
- ☐ 4. Tell the client to push only when absolutely necessary.

21. What would be the **priority** when caring for a primigravid client whose cervix is dilated at 8 cm when the fetus is at 1+ station and the client has had no analgesia or anesthesia?
- ☐ 1. giving frequent sips of water
- ☐ 2. applying extra blankets for warmth
- ☐ 3. providing frequent perineal cleansing
- ☒ 4. offering encouragement and support

22. To determine whether a primigravid client in labor with a fetus in the left occipitoanterior (LOA) position is completely dilated, the nurse performs a vaginal examination. During the examination, the nurse should palpate which cranial sutures?
- ☒ 1. sagittal
- ☐ 2. lambdoidal
- ☐ 3. coronal
- ☐ 4. frontal

23. After a lengthy labor process, a primigravid client gives birth to a healthy newborn boy with a moderate amount of skull molding. What information would the nurse include when explaining to the parents about this condition?
- ☐ 1. It is typically seen with breech births.
- ☒ 2. It usually lasts a day or two before resolving.
- ☐ 3. It is typical when the brow is the presenting part.
- ☐ 4. Surgical intervention may be necessary to alleviate pressure.

24. The healthcare provider (HCP) has informed the labor nurse that he believes the uterus has inverted in a primiparous client who has just given birth. Which findings would help to confirm this diagnosis? Select all that apply.
- ☒ 1. hypotension
- ☒ 2. gush of blood from the vagina
- ☐ 3. intense, severe, tearing type of abdominal pain
- ☐ 4. uterus is hard and in a constant state of contraction
- ☒ 5. inability to palpate the uterus
- ☒ 6. diaphoresis

25. After the birth of a viable neonate, a 20-year-old primiparous client comments to her mother and the nurse about the baby. Which comment would the nurse interpret as a possible sign of potential maternal-infant bonding problems?
- ☐ 1. "He has got my funny-looking ears!"
- ☒ 2. "I think my mother should give him the first feeding."
- ☐ 3. "He is a lot bigger than I expected him to be."
- ☐ 4. "I want to buy him a blue outfit to wear when we get home."

26. The nurse explains to a newly admitted primigravid client in active labor that, according to the gate-control theory of pain, a closed gate means that the client should experience what type of pain?
- ☒ 1. no pain
- ☐ 2. sharp pain
- ☐ 3. light pain
- ☐ 4. moderate pain

27. The cervix of a primigravid client in active labor who received epidural anesthesia 4 hours ago is now completely dilated, and the client is ready to begin pushing. Before the client begins to push, the nurse should assess:
- ☐ 1. fetal heart rate variability
- ☐ 2. cervical dilation again
- ☐ 3. status of membranes
- ☒ 4. bladder status

28. For the past 8 hours, a 20-year-old primigravid client in active labor with intact membranes has been experiencing regular contractions. The fetal heart rate is 136 bpm with good variability. After determining that the client is still in the latent phase of labor, the nurse should observe the client for:
- ☒ **1.** exhaustion
- ☐ **2.** chills and fever
- ☐ **3.** fluid overload
- ☐ **4.** meconium-stained fluid

29. A primigravid client whose cervix is 7 cm dilated with the fetus at 0 station and in a left occipitoposterior (LOP) position has severe back pain. What intervention is **most** indicated?
- ☒ **1.** Provide firm pressure to the client's sacral area.
- ☐ **2.** Prepare the client for a cesarean birth.
- ☐ **3.** Prepare the client for a precipitate birth.
- ☐ **4.** Maintain the client in a left side-lying position.

30. A primigravid client in active labor has had no anesthesia. The client's cervix is 7 cm dilated, and she is starting to feel considerable discomfort during contractions. The nurse should instruct the client to change from slow chest breathing to which breathing technique?
- ☒ **1.** rapid, shallow chest breathing
- ☐ **2.** deep chest breathing
- ☐ **3.** rapid pant-blow breathing
- ☐ **4.** slow abdominal breathing

31. The healthcare provider (HCP) prescribes scalp stimulation of the fetal head for a primigravid client in active labor. When explaining to the client about this procedure, what would the nurse include as the purpose?
- ☐ **1.** assessment of the fetal hematocrit level
- ☐ **2.** increase in the strength of the contractions
- ☒ **3.** increase in the fetal heart rate and variability
- ☐ **4.** assessment of fetal position

32. Assessment of a primigravid client reveals cervical dilation at 8 cm and complete effacement. The client has severe back pain during this phase of labor. The nurse explains that the client's severe back pain is **most** likely caused by the fetal occiput being in which position?
- ☐ **1.** breech
- ☐ **2.** transverse
- ☒ **3.** posterior
- ☐ **4.** anterior

33. The nurse assesses a primiparous client with ruptured membranes in labor for 20 hours. The nurse identifies late decelerations on the monitor and initiates standard procedures for the labor client with this wave pattern. Which interventions should the nurse perform? Select all that apply.
- ☒ **1.** administering oxygen via mask to the client
- ☐ **2.** questioning the client about the effectiveness of pain relief
- ☒ **3.** placing the client on her side
- ☐ **4.** readjusting the monitor to a more comfortable position
- ☒ **5.** applying an internal fetal monitor

34. When performing Leopold's maneuvers on a primigravid client, the nurse is palpating the uterus as shown below. Which maneuver is the nurse performing?

- ☐ **1.** first maneuver
- ☐ **2.** second maneuver
- ☒ **3.** third maneuver
- ☐ **4.** fourth maneuver

35. Before placing the fetal monitoring device on a primigravid client's fundus, the nurse performs Leopold's maneuvers. The nurse explains that third maneuver is done for which reason?
- ☒ **1.** to determine whether the fetal presenting part is engaged
- ☐ **2.** to locate the fetal cephalic prominence
- ☐ **3.** to distinguish between a breech and a cephalic presentation
- ☐ **4.** to locate the position of the fetal arms and legs

The Multigravid Client in Labor

36. The nurse is caring for a G2, T1, P0, A0, L1 client at term. The client is completely effaced, dilated to 2 cm, with contractions every 3 minutes lasting 45 seconds. The client is asking for an epidural to make her more comfortable. Indicate the appropriate response by the nurse.
☐ 1. "We cannot give epidurals until you are 5 to 6 cm dilated. There is IV medication available if you would like it now."
☐ 2. "You cannot have an epidural until your membranes have ruptured."
☐ 3. "Your contraction pattern is slow at this point and will need to accelerate before you can have your epidural."
☒ 4. "It is too early in labor for the epidural, but you can have IV medication to keep you comfortable until you have dilated 1 to 2 cm more."

37. The nurse has just received report on a labor client: a G3, T1, P0, Ab1, L1 who is 80% effaced, 3 cm dilated, 0 station. The nurse anticipates the plan of care for the shift will address what factors? Select all that apply.
☒ 1. This client will give birth before the change of shift in 12 hours.
☒ 2. Pushing the baby out should take 30 minutes or less.
☐ 3. Contractions will remain irregular until transition.
☒ 4. Transition will be shorter for this multiparous client.
☒ 5. This client will withdraw into herself during transition.

38. A multigravida in active labor is 7 cm dilated. The fetal heart rate baseline is 130 bpm with moderate variability. The client begins to have variable decelerations to 100 to 110 bpm. What should the nurse do **next**?
☐ 1. Perform a vaginal examination.
☐ 2. Notify the healthcare provider (HCP) of the decelerations.
☒ 3. Reposition the client, and continue to evaluate fetal heart rate.
☐ 4. Administer oxygen via mask at 2 L/min.

39. A nurse is preparing a change-of-shift report and has been caring for a multigravid client with a normally progressing labor. Which information should be part of this report? Select all that apply.
☒ 1. interpretation of the fetal monitor strip
☒ 2. analgesia or anesthesia being used
☐ 3. previous methods of birth control
☒ 4. support persons with the client
☒ 5. prior birth history

40. A multigravid client is admitted at 4-cm dilation and is requesting pain medication. The nurse gives the client nalbuphine 15 mg. Within 5 minutes, the client tells the nurse she feels like she needs to have a bowel movement. The nurse should **first**:
☐ 1. have naloxone available in the birthing room.
☒ 2. complete a vaginal examination to determine dilation, effacement, and station.
☐ 3. prepare for birth.
☐ 4. document the client's relief due to pain medication.

41. A multigravid laboring client has an extensive documented history of drug addiction. Her last reported usage was 5 hours ago. She is 2 cm dilated with contractions every 3 minutes of moderate intensity. The healthcare provider (HCP) prescribes nalbuphine 15 mg slow IV push for pain relief followed by an epidural when the client is 4 cm dilated. Within 10 minutes of receiving the nalbuphine, the client states she thinks she is going to have her baby now. Of the drugs available at the time of the birth, which should the nurse avoid using with this client in this situation?
☐ 1. lidocaine 1%
☒ 2. naloxone
☐ 3. local anesthetic
☐ 4. pudendal block

42. A 31-year-old multigravid client at 39 weeks' gestation admitted to the hospital in active labor is receiving intravenous lactated Ringer's solution and a continuous epidural anesthetic. During the first hour after administration of the anesthetic, the nurse should monitor the client for:
☒ 1. hypotension.
☐ 2. diaphoresis.
☐ 3. headache.
☐ 4. tremors.

43. A 30-year-old G3, T2, P0, A0, L2 is being monitored internally. She is being induced with IV oxytocin because she is postterm. The nurse notes the pattern below. The client is wedged to her side while lying in bed and is approximately 6 cm dilated and 100% effaced. The nurse should **first**:

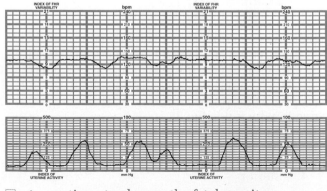

☐ 1. continue to observe the fetal monitor.
☐ 2. anticipate rupture of the membranes.
☒ 3. prepare for fetal oximetry.
☒ 4. discontinue the oxytocin infusion.

44. The nurse, while shopping in a local department store, hears a multiparous woman say loudly, "I think the baby is coming." After asking someone to call 911, the nurse assists the client to give birth to a term neonate. While waiting for the ambulance, the nurse suggests that the mother initiate breast-feeding, primarily for what reason?
- [ ] **1.** to begin the parental-infant bonding process
- [ ] **2.** to prevent neonatal hypothermia
- [ ] **3.** to provide glucose to the neonate
- [x] **4.** to contract the mother's uterus

45. Approximately 15 minutes after birth of a viable term neonate, a multiparous client has chills. What should the nurse do **next**?
- [ ] **1.** Assess the client's pulse rate.
- [ ] **2.** Decrease the rate of intravenous fluids.
- [x] **3.** Provide the client with a warm blanket.
- [ ] **4.** Assess the amount of blood loss.

46. The healthcare provider (HCP) plans to perform an amniotomy on a multiparous client admitted to the labor area at 41 weeks' gestation for labor induction. After the amniotomy, the nurse should **first**:
- [ ] **1.** monitor the client's contraction pattern.
- [x] **2.** assess the fetal heart rate (FHR) for 1 full minute.
- [ ] **3.** assess the client's temperature and pulse.
- [ ] **4.** document the color of the amniotic fluid.

47. A multigravid client who is 10 cm dilated is admitted to the labor and birth unit. In addition to supporting the client, **priority** nursing care includes:
- [x] **1.** turning on the infant warmer.
- [ ] **2.** increasing IV fluids.
- [ ] **3.** determining the client's preferences for pain control.
- [ ] **4.** providing client education regarding care of the newborn.

48. The nurse is assessing fetal presentation in a multiparous client. The illustration below indicates which type of presentation?

- [x] **1.** frank breech
- [ ] **2.** complete breech
- [ ] **3.** footling breech
- [ ] **4.** vertex

49. Two hours ago, a multigravid client was admitted in active labor with her cervix dilated at 5 cm and completely effaced and the fetus at 0 station. Currently, the client is experiencing nausea and vomiting, a slight chill with perspiration beads on her lip, and extreme irritability. The nurse should **first**:
- [ ] **1.** warm the temperature of the room by a few degrees.
- [ ] **2.** increase the rate of intravenous fluid administration.
- [ ] **3.** obtain a prescription for an intramuscular antiemetic medication.
- [x] **4.** assess the client's cervical dilation and station.

50. What interval should the nurse use when assessing the frequency of contractions of a multiparous client in active labor admitted to the birthing area?
- [ ] **1.** acme of one contraction to the beginning of the next contraction
- [ ] **2.** beginning of one contraction to the end of the next contraction
- [ ] **3.** end of one contraction to the end of the next contraction
- [x] **4.** beginning of one contraction to the beginning of the next contraction

51. While a client is being admitted to the birthing unit she states, "My water broke last night, but my labor started 2 hours ago." Which findings are a concern? Select all that apply.
- [ ] **1.** maternal vital signs: T 99.5°F (37.5°C), HR 80, R 24, BP 130/80 mm Hg
- [ ] **2.** blood and mucus on perineal pad
- [x] **3.** baseline fetal heart rate of 140 bpm with a range between 110 and 160 with contractions
- [x] **4.** peripad stained with green fluid
- [x] **5.** client stating, "This baby wants out—he keeps kicking me"

52. While the nurse is caring for a multiparous client in active labor at 36 weeks' gestation, the client tells the nurse, "I think my water just broke." What should the nurse do **first**?
- [ ] **1.** Turn the client to the right side.
- [ ] **2.** Assess the color, amount, and odor of the fluid.
- [x] **3.** Assess the fetal heart rate pattern.
- [ ] **4.** Check the client's cervical dilation.

53. The nurse has obtained a urine specimen from a multiparous client admitted to the labor unit. The woman asks to go to the bathroom and reports that she feels she has to move her bowels. Which actions would be appropriate? Select all that apply.
- [ ] **1.** assisting her to the bathroom
- [ ] **2.** applying an external fetal monitor to obtain fetal heart rate
- [x] **3.** assessing her stage of labor
- [ ] **4.** asking if she had back labor pains like this with any of her other birth experiences
- [ ] **5.** allowing her support person to take her to the bathroom to maintain privacy
- [x] **6.** checking the degree of fetal descent

54. A multigravid client admitted to the labor area is scheduled for a cesarean birth under spinal anesthesia. Which client statement indicates teaching about spinal anesthesia has been understood?
- ☐ 1. "The medication will be administered while I am in prone position."
- ☒ 2. "The anesthetic may cause a severe headache, which is treatable."
- ☐ 3. "My blood pressure may increase if I lie down too soon after the injection."
- ☐ 4. "I can expect immediate anesthesia that can be reversed very easily."

55. The healthcare provider (HCP) determines that the fetus of a multiparous client in active labor is in distress, necessitating a cesarean birth with general anesthesia. Before the cesarean birth, the anesthesiologist prescribes cimetidine 300 mg PO. The nurse explains that the purpose of giving cimetidine is to:
- ☐ 1. incidence of bronchospasm
- ☐ 2. oral and respiratory secretions
- ☒ 3. acid level of the stomach contents
- ☐ 4. incidence of postoperative gastric ulcer

The Labor Experience

56. The nurse is performing a vaginal examination on a client in labor. The nurse finds the fetal presenting part 1 cm above the ischial spines. The nurse should chart the station as:
- ☒ 1. −1 station.
- ☐ 2. +1 station.
- ☐ 3. engaged.
- ☐ 4. floating.

57. The nurse is managing a pregnant client's second stage of labor. The nurse should intervene when observing which action?
- ☒ 1. closed glottis pushing
- ☐ 2. open glottis pushing
- ☐ 3. "rest and descent"
- ☐ 4. squatting while pushing

58. A client in the second stage of labor who planned an unmedicated birth is in severe pain because the fetus is in the ROP position. The nurse should place the client in which position for pain relief?
- ☐ 1. lithotomy
- ☐ 2. right lateral position
- ☒ 3. hands and knees
- ☐ 4. tailor sitting

59. A woman who delivered her last infant by caesarean section is admitted to the hospital at term with contractions every 5 minutes. The healthcare provider (HCP) intends to have her undergo "a trial labor." The nurse explains to the client that:
- ☐ 1. labor will be stimulated with exogenous oxytocin until birth.
- ☐ 2. the HCP needs more information to determine the presence of true labor.
- ☒ 3. labor progress will be evaluated continually to determine appropriate progress for a vaginal birth.
- ☐ 4. labor will be arrested with tocolytic agents after a 2-hour period even if no fetal distress is noted.

60. The nurse prepares a client for lumbar epidural anesthesia. Before anesthesia administration, the nurse instructs the client to assume which position?
- ☐ 1. lithotomy
- ☒ 2. side-lying
- ☐ 3. hands and knees
- ☐ 4. prone

61. A client in labor received an epidural for pain management. Before receiving the epidural, the client's blood pressure was 124/76 mm Hg. Ten minutes after receiving the epidural, the client's blood pressure is 98/56 mm Hg, and the mother is vomiting. Before calling the healthcare provider (HCP), the nurse should:
- ☐ 1. decrease the IV fluid rate.
- ☒ 2. turn the client to her side.
- ☐ 3. catheterize the client.
- ☐ 4. perform a vaginal examination.

62. A nurse is caring for a woman G1 P0 at 40 weeks' gestation in active labor. Assessments include cervix 5 cm dilated; 90% effaced; station 0; cephalic presentation; FHR baseline is 135 bpm and decreases to 125 bpm shortly after onset of five uterine contractions and returns to baseline before the uterine contraction ends.
Based on this assessment, what action should the nurse take **first**?
- ☐ 1. Position the client on her left side, and administer O_2 via face mask.
- ☒ 2. Document findings on the client's chart, and continue to monitor labor progress.
- ☐ 3. Perform vaginal exam to rule out umbilical cord prolapse.
- ☐ 4. Notify the healthcare provider (HCP) immediately, and prepare for emergency caesarean section.

63. The nurse is caring for a full-term, nonmedicated, primiparous client who is in the transition stage of labor. The client is writhing in pain and saying, "Help me, help me!" Her last vaginal exam 1 hour ago showed that she was 8 cm dilated, +1 station, and in what appeared to be a comfortable position. What does the nurse anticipate as the highest **priority** intervention in caring for this client?
☐ 1. Help the client through contractions until a narcotic can be given.
☐ 2. Palpate the bladder to see if it has become distended.
☐ 3. Ask the client for suggestions to make her more comfortable.
☒ 4. Perform a vaginal exam to determine if the client is fully dilated.

64. A client is admitted at 30 weeks' gestation with contractions every 3 minutes. Her cervix is 1 to 2 cm dilated and 75% effaced. Following a 4-g bolus dose, IV magnesium sulfate is infusing at 2 g/h. How will the nurse know the medication is having the intended effect?
☐ 1. Contractions will increase in frequency, leading to birth.
☐ 2. The client will maintain a respiratory rate > 12 breaths/min.
☒ 3. Contractions will decrease in frequency, intensity, and duration.
☐ 4. The client will maintain blood pressure readings of 120/80 mm Hg.

65. A client at 33 weeks' gestation is admitted in preterm labor. She is given betamethasone 12 mg IM every 24 hours × 2. What is the expected outcome of this drug therapy?
☐ 1. The contractions will end within 24 hours.
☐ 2. The client will give birth to a neonate without infection.
☐ 3. The client will give birth to a full-term neonate.
☒ 4. The neonate will be born with mature lungs.

66. A full-term client is admitted for an induction of labor. The healthcare provider (HCP) has assigned a Bishop score of 10. Which drug would the nurse anticipate administering to this client?
☒ 1. oxytocin 30 units in 500 mL D$_5$W
☐ 2. prostaglandin gel 0.5 mg
☐ 3. misoprostol 50 mcg
☐ 4. dinoprostone 10 mg

67. A full-term client is admitted for induction of labor. When admitted, her cervix is effaced 25% but has not dilated. The initial goal is cervical ripening prior to labor induction. Which drug will prepare her cervix for induction?
☐ 1. nalbuphine
☐ 2. oxytocin
☒ 3. dinoprostone
☐ 4. betamethasone

68. The nurse is explaining the medication options available for pain relief during labor. The nurse realizes the client needs further teaching when the client makes which statement?
☐ 1. "Nalbuphine and promethazine will give relief from pain and nausea during early labor."
☒ 2. "I can have an epidural as soon as I start contracting."
☒ 3. "If I have a cesarean, I can have an epidural."
☐ 4. "If I have an emergency cesarean, I may be put to sleep for the birth."

69. The healthcare provider (HCP) has performed an amniotomy on a laboring client. Which details must be included in the documentation of this procedure? Select all that apply.
☐ 1. time of rupture
☐ 2. color and clarity of fluid
☐ 3. fetal heart rate (FHR) and pattern before and after the procedure
☐ 4. size of amnio hook used during the procedure
☐ 5. odor and amount of fluid

70. Following an epidural and placement of internal monitors, a client's labor is augmented. Contractions are lasting greater than 90 seconds and occurring every 1½ minutes. The uterine resting tone is >20 mm Hg with an abnormal fetal heart rate and pattern. Which action should the nurse take **first**?
☐ 1. Notify the healthcare provider (HCP).
☐ 2. Turn off the oxytocin infusion.
☐ 3. Turn the client to her left side.
☐ 4. Increase the maintenance IV fluids.

71. A nurse notices repetitive late decelerations on the fetal heart monitor. The **best** initial actions by the nurse include:
☐ 1. prepare for birth, reposition the client, and begin pushing.
☐ 2. perform sterile vaginal exam, increase IV fluids, and apply oxygen.
☐ 3. notify the provider, explain findings to the client, and begin pushing.
☐ 4. reposition the client, apply oxygen, and increase IV fluids.

72. A client is induced with oxytocin. The fetal heart rate is showing accelerations lasting 15 seconds and exceeding the baseline with fetal movement. What action associated with this finding should the nurse take?
☐ 1. Turn the client to her left side.
☐ 2. Administer oxygen via face mask at 10 to 12 L/min.
☐ 3. Notify the healthcare provider (HCP) of the situation.
☐ 4. Document fetal well-being.

73. As a nurse begins her shift on the obstetrical unit, there are several new admissions. The client with which condition would be a candidate for induction?
☐ 1. preeclampsia
☐ 2. active herpes
☐ 3. face presentation
☐ 4. fetus with late decelerations

74. A nurse and an unlicensed assistive personnel (UAP) are caring for clients in a labor and birth unit. Which task should the registered nurse (RN) assign to the UAP?
☐ 1. Perform a fundal check on a 2-day postpartum client.
☐ 2. Remove a fetal monitor, and assist a client to the bathroom.
☐ 3. Give ibuprofen 800 mg by mouth to a newly postpartum client.
☐ 4. Teach a new mother how to bottle-feed her infant.

75. A laboring client smiles pleasantly at the nurse when asked simple questions. The client speaks only Mandarin, and the interpreter is busy with an emergency situation. At her last vaginal examination, the client was 5 cm dilated, 100% effaced, and at 0 station. While working with this client, which response indicates that the client may be approaching birth?
☐ 1. The fetal monitor strip shows late decelerations.
☐ 2. The client begins to speak to her family in her native language.
☐ 3. The fetal monitor strip shows early decelerations.
☐ 4. The client's facial expressions become animated.

The Intrapartal Client with Risk Factors

76. A client is admitted with a suspected abruptio placentae. The nurse should assess the client for which signs and symptoms? Select all that apply.
☐ 1. bleeding that is concealed or apparent
☐ 2. abdominal rigidity
☐ 3. painful abdomen
☐ 4. painless bleeding
☐ 5. large placenta
☐ 6. bleeding that stops spontaneously

77. A 39-year-old multigravid client at 39 weeks' gestation admitted to the hospital in active labor has been diagnosed with class II heart disease. To ensure cardiac emptying and adequate oxygenation during labor, the nurse plans to encourage the client to:
☐ 1. breathe slowly after each contraction.
☐ 2. avoid the use of analgesics for the labor pain.
☐ 3. remain in a side-lying position with the head elevated.
☐ 4. request local anesthesia for vaginal birth.

78. When developing the plan of care for a multigravid client with class III heart disease, the nurse should expect to assess the client frequently for which problem?
☐ 1. dehydration
☐ 2. nausea and vomiting
☐ 3. iron deficiency anemia
☐ 4. tachycardia

79. A primigravid client at 39 weeks' gestation is admitted to the hospital for induction of labor. The healthcare provider (HCP) has prescribed prostaglandin E2 gel (dinoprostone) for the client. Before administering prostaglandin E2 gel to the client, which action should the nurse do **first**?
☐ 1. Assess the frequency of uterine contractions.
☐ 2. Place the client in a side-lying position.
☐ 3. Determine whether the membranes have ruptured.
☐ 4. Prepare the client for an amniotomy.

80. A primigravida near birth is experiencing a prolonged second stage of labor with a fetus suspected of weighing over 4 kg. Which intervention is **most** important?
☐ 1. preparing for a vacuum-assisted birth
☐ 2. administering an IV fluid bolus
☐ 3. preparing for an emergency cesarean birth
☐ 4. performing the McRoberts maneuver

81. A multigravid client is receiving oxytocin augmentation. When the client's cervix is dilated to 6 cm, her membranes rupture spontaneously with meconium-stained amniotic fluid. Which action should the nurse perform **first**?
☐ 1. Increase the rate of the oxytocin infusion.
☐ 2. Turn the client to a knee-to-chest position.
☐ 3. Assess cervical dilation and effacement.
☐ 4. Assess the fetal heart rate.

82. A multigravid client in active labor at 39 weeks' gestation has a history of smoking one to two packs of cigarettes daily. Which problem is the nurse **most** likely to find during the infant's assessment?
☐ 1. sedation
☐ 2. hyperbilirubinemia
☐ 3. low birth weight
☐ 4. hypocalcemia

83. A primigravid client who has had a prolonged labor but now is completely dilated has received epidural anesthesia. Which statement should the nurse include in the teaching plan about pushing?
☐ 1. The client needs to push for at least 1 to 3 minutes.
☐ 2. Pushing is most effective when the client holds her breath.
☐ 3. The client should be urged to push with an open glottis.
☐ 4. Pushing is limited to times when she feels the urge.

84. The healthcare provider (HCP) determines that outlet forceps are needed to assist in the birth of a primigravid client in active labor with a large-for-gestational-size fetus. The nurse understands that the fetus's skull must be at what point before this procedure can take place?
- ☐ 1. It is engaged past the inlet.
- ☐ 2. It is at +1 station.
- ☐ 3. It is visible at the perineal floor.
- ☐ 4. It has reached the level of the ischial spines.

85. The healthcare provider (HCP) prescribes an amnioinfusion for a primigravid client at term who is diagnosed with oligohydramnios. The nurse explains to the client is the primary purpose of this procedure is to:
- ☐ 1. decreases the frequency and severity of variable decelerations.
- ☐ 2. minimizes the possibility of fetal metabolic alkalosis.
- ☐ 3. increases the fetal heart rate accelerations during a contraction.
- ☐ 4. raises the amniotic fluid index to more than 15 cm.

86. The nurse is admitting a primigravid client at 37 weeks' gestation who has been diagnosed with preeclampsia to the labor and birth area. Which client care room is **most** appropriate for this client?
- ☐ 1. a brightly lit private room at the end of the hall from the nurses' station
- ☐ 2. a semiprivate room midway down the hall from the nurses' station
- ☐ 3. a private room with many windows that is near the operating room
- ☐ 4. a darkened private room as close to the nurses' station as possible

87. A multigravid client is admitted to the labor area from the emergency department. At the time of admission, the fetal head is crowning, and the client yells, "The baby is coming!" To help the client remain calm and cooperative during the imminent birth, which response by the nurse is **most** appropriate?
- ☐ 1. "You are right; the baby is coming, so just relax."
- ☐ 2. "Please do not push because you will tear your cervix."
- ☐ 3. "Your healthcare provider will be here as soon as possible."
- ☐ 4. "I will explain what is happening to guide you as we go along."

88. The nurse is caring for a multigravid client and observes the woman squatting on the bed and the fetal head crowning. After calling for assistance and helping the client lie down, which action should the nurse do **next**?
- ☐ 1. Tell the client to push between contractions.
- ☐ 2. Provide gentle support to the fetal head.
- ☐ 3. Apply gentle upward traction on the neonate's anterior shoulder.
- ☐ 4. Massage the perineum to stretch the perineal tissues.

89. During the first hour after a precipitous birth, the nurse should monitor a multiparous client for signs and symptoms of which complication?
- ☐ 1. postpartum "blues"
- ☐ 2. uterine atony
- ☐ 3. intrauterine infection
- ☐ 4. urinary tract infection

90. A multigravid client in labor at 38 weeks' gestation has been diagnosed with Rh sensitization and probable fetal hydrops and anemia. Which fetal heart rate pattern would the nurse find is **most** concerning?
- ☐ 1. early deceleration pattern
- ☐ 2. sinusoidal pattern
- ☐ 3. variable deceleration pattern
- ☐ 4. late deceleration pattern

91. The nurse in the labor and birth area receives a telephone call from the emergency department announcing that a multigravid client in active labor is being transferred to the labor area. The client has had no prenatal care. When the client arrives by stretcher, she says, "I think the baby is coming … Help!" The fetal skull is crowning. The nurse should obtain which information **first**?
- ☐ 1. estimated date of birth
- ☐ 2. amniotic fluid status
- ☐ 3. gravida and parity
- ☐ 4. prenatal history

92. A multiparous client gives birth to dizygotic twins at 37 weeks' gestation. The twin neonates require additional hospitalization after the client is discharged. What is the **most** appropriate goal to include in the plan of care for the parents while the twins are hospitalized?
- ☐ 1. Discuss how they will cope with twin infants at home.
- ☐ 2. Participate in care of the twins as much as possible.
- ☐ 3. Take turns providing 24-hour observation of the twins.
- ☐ 4. Identify complications that may occur as the twins develop.

93. A primigravid client at 41 weeks' gestation is admitted to the hospital's labor and birth unit in active labor. After 25 hours of labor with membranes ruptured for 24 hours, the client gives birth to a healthy neonate vaginally with a midline episiotomy. Which problem should the nurse identify as the **priority** for the client?
- ☐ **1.** activity intolerance
- ☐ **2.** sleep deprivation
- ☐ **3.** situational low self-esteem
- ☐ **4.** risk for infection

94. The nurse is caring for a primiparous client and her neonate immediately after birth. The neonate was born at 41 weeks' gestation and weighs 9 lb (4,082 g). Assessing for signs and symptoms of which condition should be a **priority** in this neonate?
- ☐ **1.** anemia
- ☐ **2.** hypoglycemia
- ☐ **3.** delayed meconium
- ☐ **4.** elevated bilirubin

95. A multigravid client in active labor at term is diagnosed with polyhydramnios. The healthcare provider (HCP) has instructed the client about possible neonatal complications related to the polyhydramnios. The nurse determines that the client has understood the instructions when the client states that polyhydramnios is associated with which problem in the fetus or neonate?
- ☐ **1.** renal dysfunction
- ☐ **2.** intrauterine growth restriction
- ☐ **3.** pulmonary hypoplasia
- ☐ **4.** gastrointestinal disorders

96. A primigravid client at 39 weeks' gestation is admitted to the hospital in active labor. On admission, the client's cervix is 6 cm dilated. After 2 hours of active labor, the client's cervix is still dilated at 6 cm with 100% effacement at +1 station. Contractions are 3 to 5 minutes apart, lasting 45 seconds, and of moderate intensity. The nurse determines that the client is **most** likely experiencing which problem?
- ☐ **1.** cephalopelvic disproportion
- ☐ **2.** prolonged latent phase
- ☐ **3.** prolonged transitional phase
- ☐ **4.** hypotonic contraction pattern

97. The healthcare provider (HCP) who elects to perform a cesarean birth on a primigravid client for fetal distress has informed the client of possible risks during the procedure. When the nurse asks the client to sign the consent form, the client's husband says, "I will sign it for her. She is too upset by what is happening to make this decision." The nurse should:
- ☐ **1.** ask the client if this is acceptable to her.
- ☐ **2.** have the client and her husband both sign the consent form.
- ☐ **3.** ask the client to sign the consent form.
- ☐ **4.** ask the HCP to witness the consent form.

98. A multigravid client at term is admitted to the hospital for a trial labor and possible vaginal birth. She has a history of previous cesarean birth because of fetal distress. When the client is 4 cm dilated, she receives nalbuphine intravenously. While monitoring the fetal heart rate, the nurse observes minimal variability and a rate of 120 bpm. The nurse should explain to the client that the decreased variability is **most** likely caused by which factor?
- ☐ **1.** maternal fatigue
- ☐ **2.** fetal malposition
- ☐ **3.** small-for-gestational-age fetus
- ☐ **4.** effects of analgesic medication

99. During a scheduled cesarean birth of a primigravid client with a fetus at 39 weeks' gestation in a breech presentation, a neonatologist is present in the operating room. The nurse explains to the client that the neonatologist is present because neonates born by cesarean birth tend to have an increased incidence of which problem?
- ☐ **1.** congenital anomalies
- ☐ **2.** pulmonary hypertension
- ☐ **3.** meconium aspiration syndrome
- ☐ **4.** respiratory distress syndrome

100. A 28-year-old multigravid client at 28 weeks' gestation diagnosed with acute pyelonephritis is receiving intravenous fluids and antibiotics. After teaching the client about the rationale for the aggressive therapy, the nurse determines that the client needs further instruction when she says that acute pyelonephritis can lead to which complication?
- ☐ **1.** preterm labor
- ☐ **2.** maternal sepsis
- ☐ **3.** intrauterine growth restriction
- ☐ **4.** congenital fetal anomalies

101. A primigravid client at 38 weeks' gestation is admitted to the labor suite in active labor. The client's physical assessment reveals a chlamydial infection. The nurse explains that if the infection is left untreated, the neonate may develop which problem?
- ☐ **1.** conjunctivitis
- ☐ **2.** heart disease
- ☐ **3.** harlequin sign
- ☐ **4.** brain damage

102. A 34-year-old primigravid client at 39 weeks' gestation admitted to the hospital in active labor has type B Rh-negative blood. The nurse should instruct the client that if the neonate is Rh positive, the client will receive an Rh immune globulin (RHIG) injection for which reason?
- ☐ **1.** to prevent Rh-positive sensitization with the next pregnancy
- ☐ **2.** to provide active antibody protection for this pregnancy
- ☐ **3.** to decrease the amount of Rh-negative sensitization for the next pregnancy
- ☐ **4.** to destroy fetal Rh-positive cells during the next pregnancy

103. A 16-year-old primigravid client admitted at 38 weeks' gestation with severe preeclampsia is given intravenous magnesium sulfate and lactated Ringer's solution. The nurse should obtain which information?
☐ 1. urinary output every 8 hours
☐ 2. deep tendon reflexes every 4 hours
☐ 3. respiratory rate every hour
☐ 4. blood pressure every 6 hours

104. The nurse has received a telephone call from the emergency department indicating that a multigravid client in early labor and diagnosed with probable placenta previa will be arriving soon. What is the **priority** invention when the client arrives at the unit?
☐ 1. whole blood replacement
☐ 2. continuous blood pressure monitoring
☐ 3. internal fetal heart rate monitoring
☐ 4. an immediate cesarean birth

105. During admission, a multigravida in early active labor acts somewhat euphoric and tells the nurse that she smoked some crack cocaine before coming to the hospital. In addition to fetal heart rate assessment, the nurse should monitor the client for symptoms of which complication?
☐ 1. placenta previa
☐ 2. ruptured uterus
☐ 3. maternal hypotension
☐ 4. abruptio placentae

106. A primigravid client in early labor tells the nurse that she was exposed to rubella at about 14 weeks' gestation. After birth, the nurse should assess the neonate for which complication?
☐ 1. hydrocephaly
☐ 2. cardiac disorders
☐ 3. renal disorders
☐ 4. bulging fontanelles

107. A primigravid client in early labor with abruptio placentae develops disseminated intravascular coagulation (DIC). Which agent should the nurse expect the healthcare provider (HCP) to prescribe?
☐ 1. magnesium sulfate
☐ 2. warfarin sodium
☐ 3. fresh frozen platelets
☐ 4. meperidine hydrochloride

108. A multigravid client diagnosed with chronic hypertension is now in preterm labor at 32 weeks' gestation. The healthcare provider (HCP) has prescribed magnesium sulfate at 3 g/h. Which assessment finding indicates that the intended therapeutic effect has occurred?
☐ 1. decrease in fetal heart rate accelerations
☐ 2. decrease in the frequency and number of contractions
☐ 3. decrease in maternal blood pressure rate
☐ 4. decrease in maternal respiratory rate

109. A primigravid client who was successfully treated for preterm labor at 30 weeks' gestation had a history of mild hyperthyroidism before becoming pregnant. What instructions should the nurse include in the plan of care?
☐ 1. Continue taking low-dose oral propylthiouracil as prescribed.
☐ 2. Discontinue taking the methimazole until after the birth of the neonate.
☐ 3. Consider breast-feeding the neonate after the birth.
☐ 4. Contact the healthcare provider (HCP) if bradycardia occurs.

110. A primigravid client at 37 weeks' gestation has been hospitalized for several days with severe preeclampsia. While caring for the client, the nurse observes that the client is beginning to have a seizure. Which action should the nurse do **first**?
☐ 1. Pad the side rails of the client's bed.
☐ 2. Turn the client to the right side.
☐ 3. Insert a padded tongue blade into the client's mouth.
☐ 4. Call for immediate assistance in the client's room.

111. While assessing a primigravid client admitted at 36 weeks' gestation, the nurse observes multiple bruises on the client's face, neck, and abdomen. When asked about the bruises, the client admits that her boyfriend beats her now and then and says, "I want to leave him because I am afraid he will hurt the baby." Which action is the nurse's **most** appropriate response?
☐ 1. Tell the client to leave the boyfriend immediately.
☐ 2. Ask the client when she last felt the baby move.
☐ 3. Refer the client to a social worker for possible options.
☐ 4. Report the incident to the unit nursing supervisor.

112. A multigravid client in active labor at term suddenly sits up and says, "I cannot breathe! My chest hurts really bad!" The client's skin begins to turn a dusky gray color. After calling for assistance, which action should the nurse take **next**?
☐ 1. Administer oxygen by face mask.
☐ 2. Begin cardiopulmonary resuscitation.
☐ 3. Administer intravenous oxytocin.
☐ 4. Obtain a prescription for intravenous fibrinogen.

Managing Care, Quality, and Safety for Clients Giving Birth

113. A newly postpartum client is asking to go to the bathroom 45 minutes after childbirth. She had an epidural for labor and birth and has an IV infusing, and every 15 minutes assessments are in progress. To provide the safest care for this client, the nurse should:
- ☐ 1. ask her to remain in bed until the 15-minute assessments are complete.
- ☐ 2. assess client's ability to stand and bear weight before going to the bathroom.
- ☐ 3. encourage the client to sit at the side of the bed before ambulating to the bathroom.
- ☐ 4. ask the client to ambulate the first time with a staff member at her side.

114. The charge nurse is preparing for the day shift on the labor and birth unit. Which would be included in the responsibilities for this position? Select all that apply.
- ☐ 1. Review the current status of each labor client with the primary nurse.
- ☐ 2. Admit the new labor client sent from the triage area.
- ☐ 3. Complete the work of the nurse who had to leave 30 minutes early.
- ☐ 4. Follow up with the primary nurse after a birth.
- ☐ 5. Complete report of unit with the oncoming charge nurse.

115. The labor and birth nurse is assigned to triage for the day. There are four clients already in rooms, and reports have been received about each of these clients. To provide the safest care and best manage time, the nurse should plan to see which client **first**?
- ☐ 1. a primipara in active labor at 5 cm asking to be admitted and wanting an epidural
- ☐ 2. a primipara who is 100% effaced, 8 cm dilated, +2 station with nausea
- ☐ 3. a client with no prenatal care, occasional contractions, BP 148/90 mm Hg, and swollen feet
- ☐ 4. a client who is at 42 weeks' gestation with bloody show, no contractions, rupture of membranes 1 hour ago leaking green fluid

116. The triage nurse is giving a telephone report to the receiving nurse in the labor and birth unit. The multigravida client is 8 cm dilated and is being transferred to the labor and birth unit. How should the labor and birth nurse manage the next 10 minutes with the client? Select all that apply.
- ☐ 1. Begin fetal monitoring.
- ☐ 2. Call other staff to set up the birthing table.
- ☐ 3. Assess comfort needs of the client.
- ☐ 4. Determine support systems for the client.
- ☐ 5. Prepare to give an early report to the nurse arriving on the next shift.

117. A client has experienced a postpartum hemorrhage. The healthcare provider (HCP) verbally prescribed carboprost tromethamine 0.25 mg IM stat at the time of the hemorrhage, and this was given by the nurse. The HCP put a prescription into the medical record for 0.25 mg carboprost tromethamine IV stat. When seeing the prescription, how should the nurse administering the carboprost tromethamine respond?
- ☐ 1. Ask the charge nurse to have a discussion with the HCP about the prescription.
- ☐ 2. Initiate an incident report.
- ☐ 3. Call the HCP, discuss the prescription, and request revision if heard correctly.
- ☐ 4. Wait until the HCP returns to the unit, and discuss the situation in person.

118. The nurse is asked to develop an in-service to explain documents guiding professional nursing practice on the obstetrical unit. One of the documents included is the Code of Ethics. The nurse correctly explains that the Code of Ethics asks nurses to demonstrate which behaviors? Select all that apply.
- ☐ 1. Maintain the integrity of practice and shape social policy.
- ☐ 2. Develop, maintain, and improve healthcare environments.
- ☐ 3. Ask the hospital systems for fair compensation for work.
- ☐ 4. Be responsible and accountable for individual practice.
- ☐ 5. Increase professional competence and personal growth.

119. The nurse is preparing to assist the healthcare provider (HCP) with a cervical check for a client whose membranes have ruptured. What equipment should the nurse have ready for the midwife? Select all that apply.
- ☐ 1. sterile speculum
- ☐ 2. sterile gloves
- ☐ 3. sterile lubricant
- ☐ 4. amnio hook
- ☐ 5. cervical dilators

120. Which client is the **best** candidate for a vaginal birth after a caesarean (VBAC)?
- ☐ 1. client who had an emergency caesarean section because of fetal distress during her last delivery and has a classic incision
- ☐ 2. client who had a breech presentation in her last pregnancy, and this pregnancy is a vertex pregnancy
- ☐ 3. client who dilated 6 cm in her last birth and failed to progress beyond this point despite 5 more hours of labor
- ☐ 4. diabetic client whose last infant was over 10 lb (4.5 kg). This infant is larger, as seen on ultrasound.

Answers, Rationales, and Test-Taking Strategies

The answers and rationales for each question follow below, along with keys (🗝) to the client need (CN) and cognitive level (CL) for each question. In addition, you will also see a glossary icon (📖) highlighting specific terminology used on the licensing exam. As you check your answers, use the ***Content Mastery and Test-Taking Skill Self-Analysis*** *worksheet (tear-out worksheet in back of book) to identify the reason(s) for not answering the questions correctly. For additional information about test-taking skills and strategies for answering questions, refer to pages 12–23 and pages 35–36 in Part 1 of this book.*

The Primigravid Client in Labor

1. 3. The nurse should monitor anesthesia/pain levels every 30 minutes during active labor to ascertain that this client is comfortable during the labor process and particularly during active labor when pain often accelerates for the client. When in active labor, oxygen saturation is not monitored unless there is a specific need, such as heart disease. The client should not be on her back but wedged to the right or left side to take the pressure off the vena cava. When lying on the back, the fetus compresses the major blood vessels. Vaginal bleeding in active labor should be monitored every 30 minutes to 1 hour.

🗝 CN: Reduction of risk potential;
CL: Create

2. 2. The first stage of labor is categorized into three phases: latent, active, and transition. During the active stage of labor, intermittent fetal monitoring is performed every 30 minutes to detect changes in fetal heart rate such as bradycardia, tachycardia, or decelerations in a low-risk labor. If complications develop, more frequent or continuous electronic fetal monitoring may be needed. During the latent phase, intermittent monitoring is usually performed every 1 hour because contractions during this time are usually less frequent. During the transition phase, intermittent monitoring is performed every 5 minutes because the client is getting closer to the birth of the baby. Pushing occurs in stage II of labor, and monitoring continues to occur every 5 to 15 minutes.

🗝 CN: Reduction of risk potential;
CL: Analyze

3. 3. The urge to push is often present when the fetus reaches + stations. This client does not have a cervix that is completely dilated, and pushing in this situation may tear the cervix. Encouraging the client to breathe through the urge to push is the most appropriate strategy and allows the cervix to dilate before pushing. Increasing the level of the epidural is inappropriate as nursing would like to have the client be able to push when she is fully dilated. Comfort measures are important for the client at this time but are not the highest priority for the nurse.

🗝 CN: Management of care;
CL: Synthesize

4. 2. Assessment findings indicate that the client is in the transition phase of labor. During this phase, it is not unusual for clients to exhibit a loss of control or irritability. Leg tremors, nausea, vomiting, and an urge to bear down also are common. Excitement is associated with the latent phase of labor. Numbness of the legs may occur when epidural anesthesia has been given; however, it is rare when no anesthesia is given. Feelings of relief generally occur during the second stage, when the client begins bearing-down efforts.

🗝 CN: Health promotion and maintenance;
CL: Analyze

5. 1. This figure shows the client's baby in a breech presentation with the baby facing the pelvis on the left, the sacrum as the presenting part, and the presenting part (sacrum) is posterior in the pelvis. Figure 2 shows a vertex presentation with the baby in a left occipitoanterior (LOA) position. Figure 3 shows a vertex presentation, left occipitoposterior (LOP). Figure 4 shows a face position with the baby in a left mentotransverse (LMT) position.

🗝 CN: Physiological adaptation;
CL: Synthesize

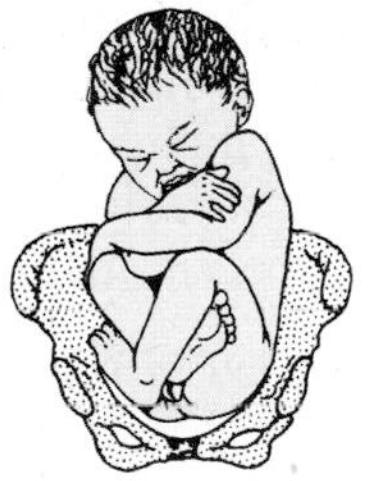

6. 1,3,4,6. Effleurage is a method of light massage that can provide pain relief. Guided imagery is a relaxation technique used in birth preparation, as is pattern-paced breathing. Positive reinforcement is not a labor support method, nor is self-containment theory.

🗝 CN: Basic care and comfort;
CL: Synthesize

7. 1. Nitrazine paper responds to alkaline fluids by changing blue; amniotic fluid is alkaline so the color verifies that the membranes are ruptured. The nurse notifies the provider that membranes are ruptured so that a plan of action can be developed. Rupture of membranes in the absence of labor increases the risk of infection. Vaginal examinations are limited until labor is initiated. Wearing a sanitary pad increases potential for infection. Documentation of the nitrazine test is completed after notifying the provider.

> CN: Reduction of risk potential; CL: Apply

8. 3. Prostaglandin gel may be used for cervical ripening before the induction of labor with oxytocin. It is usually administered by catheter or suppository, or by vaginal insertion. Two to three doses are usually needed to begin the softening process. Common adverse effects include nausea, vomiting, fever, and diarrhea. Continuous fetal heart rate monitoring and close monitoring of maternal vital signs are necessary to detect subtle changes or adverse effects. Prostaglandin gel usually does not initiate contractions; therefore, the rest period between contractions will be > 2 minutes. There is no need to assess reflexes based on prostaglandin use. Leaking of amniotic fluid is not caused by the use of this gel.

> CN: Pharmacological and parenteral therapies; CL: Evaluate

9. 1. External cephalic version is the turning of the fetus from a breech position to the vertex position to prevent the need for a cesarean birth. Gentle pressure is used to rotate the fetus in a forward direction to a cephalic lie. Contraindications to the procedure include multiple gestation because of the potential for fetal injury or uterine injury, severe oligohydramnios (decreased amniotic fluid), contraindications to a vaginal birth (e.g., cephalopelvic disproportion), and unexplained third-trimester bleeding. If the mother has Rh-negative blood type, the procedure can be performed, and Rh immunoglobulin should be administered in case minimal bleeding occurs. A history of gestational diabetes is not a contraindication unless the fetus is large for gestational age and the client has cephalopelvic disproportion.

> CN: Reduction of risk potential; CL: Analyze

10. 2. The goal of oxytocin administration in labor augmentation is to establish an adequate contraction pattern to enhance the forces of labor. The expected outcome is a pattern of contractions occurring every 2 to 3 minutes, lasting 40 to 60 seconds, of moderate intensity with a palpable resting tone between contractions. Other contraction patterns will cause the cervix to dilate too quickly or too slowly. Cervical changes in softening, effacement, and moving to an anterior position are associated with use of cervical ripening agents, such as prostaglandin gel. Cervical dilation of 2 cm/h is too rapid for the induction/augmentation process.

> CN: Pharmacological and parenteral therapies; CL: Evaluate

11. 4. Anatomically, the best position for the client to assume is the squatting position because this enhances pelvic diameters and allows gravity to assist in the expulsion stage of labor. This position also provides for natural pressure anesthesia as the fetal presenting part presses on the stretched perineum. If the client is extremely fatigued from a lengthy labor process, she may prefer the dorsal recumbent position. However, this position is not considered the best position anatomically. The lithotomy position may be ineffective and uncomfortable for a client who is ready to push. The hands and knees position may help to alleviate some back pain. However, this position can cause discomfort to the arms and wrists and is tiring over a long period of time.

> CN: Health promotion and maintenance; CL: Apply

12. 4. During transition, contractions are increasing in frequency, duration, and intensity. The most appropriate nursing problem is pain related to strength and duration of the contractions. Insufficient information is provided in the scenario to support the other listed nursing diagnoses. Urinary retention would be appropriate if the client had a full bladder and was unable to void. Hyperventilation might apply if client was breathing too rapidly, but there is no evidence this is occurring. Ineffective coping might apply if the client said, "I cannot do this" or something similar.

> CN: Health promotion and maintenance; CL: Analyze

13. 1. The most reliable sign that the placenta has detached from the uterine wall is lengthening of the cord outside the vagina. Other signs include a sudden gush of (rather than a decrease in) vaginal blood. Usually, when placenta detachment occurs, the uterus becomes more firm and changes in shape from discoid to globular. This process takes about 5 minutes. If the placenta does not separate, manual removal may be necessary to prevent postpartum hemorrhage.

> CN: Health promotion and maintenance; CL: Analyze

14. 3. Birth is a very emotional experience. An expression of happiness with tears is a normal reaction. Cultural factors, exhaustion, and anxieties over the new role can all affect maternal responses, so the nurse must be sensitive to the client's emotional expressions. There is no evidence to suggest that the mother is disappointed in the baby's gender, grieving over the end of the pregnancy, or a candidate for postpartum "blues." However, approximately 80% of postpartum clients experience transient postpartum blues several days after childbirth.

> CN: Health promotion and maintenance; CL: Analyze

15. 3. Most authorities suggest that a woman in an early stage of labor should be allowed to walk if she wishes as long as no complications are present. Birthing centers and single-room maternity units allow women considerable latitude without much supervision at this stage of labor. Gravity and walking can assist the process of labor in some clients. If the client becomes tired, she can rest in bed in the left lateral recumbent position or sit in a comfortable chair. Resting in the left lateral recumbent position improves circulation to the fetus.

> CN: Health promotion and maintenance;
> CL: Synthesize

16. 1. Birth educators use various techniques and methods to prepare parents for labor and birth. Active relaxation involves relaxing uninvolved muscle groups while contracting a specific group and using chest breathing techniques to lift the diaphragm off the contracting uterus. A deep, meditative, sleep-like state is a form of passive relaxation. Focusing on an object in the room is part of Lamaze technique for distraction. Breathing rapidly and deeply can lead to hyperventilation and is not recommended.

> CN: Health promotion and maintenance;
> CL: Synthesize

17. 3. Light stroking of the skin, or *effleurage*, is commonly used with the Lamaze method of birth preparation. Light abdominal massage with just enough pressure to avoid tickling is thought to displace the pain sensation during a contraction. Deep kneading and secure grasping are typically associated with relaxation massages to relieve stress. Prolonged pressure on specific sites is associated with acupressure.

> CN: Health promotion and maintenance;
> CL: Apply

18. 1. Some **healthcare providers (HCPs)** 📖 do not allow clients with ruptured membranes to use a hot tub or jet hydrotherapy tub during labor for fear of infections. The temperature of the water should be between 98°F and 100°F (36.7°C and 37.8°C) to prevent hyperthermia. Jet hydrotherapy is not contraindicated for clients with multifetal gestation, diabetes mellitus, or hypotonic labor patterns.

> CN: Reduction of risk potential;
> CL: Synthesize

19. 4. To determine fetal lung maturity, the sample of amniotic fluid will be tested for the L/S ratio. When fetal lungs are mature, the ratio should be 2:1. Bilirubin indicates hemolysis and, if present in the fluid, suggests Rh disease. Red blood cells should not appear in the amniotic fluid because their presence suggests fetal bleeding. Barr body determination is a chromosome analysis of the sex chromosomes that is sometimes used when a child is born with ambiguous genitalia.

> CN: Health promotion and maintenance;
> CL: Analyze

20. 3. Pushing during the first stage of labor, when the urge is felt but the cervix is not completely dilated, may produce cervical swelling, making labor more difficult. The client should be encouraged to use a pant-blow (or blow-blow) pattern of breathing to help overcome the urge to push. The McDonald procedure is used for cervical cerclage for an incompetent cervix and is inappropriate here. Increasing the rate of oxygen and intravenous fluids will not alleviate the pressure that the client is feeling. The client should not push even if she feels the urge to do so because this may result in cervical edema at 7-cm dilation.

> CN: Health promotion and maintenance;
> CL: Synthesize

21. 4. The client is in the transition phase of the first stage of labor. During this phase, the client needs encouragement and support because this is a difficult and painful time, when contractions are especially strong. Usually, the client finds it difficult to maintain self-control. Everything else seems secondary to her as she progresses into the second stage of labor. Although ice chips may be given, typically the client does not desire sips of water. Labor is hard work. Generally, the client is perspiring and does not desire additional warmth. Frequent perineal cleansing is not necessary unless there is excessive amniotic fluid leaking.

> CN: Health promotion and maintenance;
> CL: Synthesize

22. 1. The sagittal suture is the most readily felt during a vaginal examination. When the fetus is in the LOA position, the occiput faces the mother's left. The lambdoid suture is on the side of the skull. The coronal suture is a horizontal suture across the front portion of the fetal skull that forms the anterior fontanelle. It may be felt with a brow presentation. The frontal suture may be felt with a brow or face presentation.

> CN: Health promotion and maintenance;
> CL: Apply

23. 2. Molding occurs with vaginal births and is commonly seen in newborns. This is especially true with primigravid clients experiencing a lengthy labor process. Parents need to be reassured that it is not permanent and that it typically lasts a day or two before resolving. Molding rarely is present if the fetus is in a breech or brow presentation. Surgical intervention is not necessary.

> CN: Health promotion and maintenance;
> CL: Create

24. 1,2,5,6. Uterine inversion is indicated by a sudden gush of blood from the vagina leading to decreased blood pressure, and an inability to palpate the uterus since it may be in or protruding from the vagina, and any signs of blood loss such as diaphoresis, paleness, or dizziness could be observed at this time. Intense pain and a hard contracting uterus are not associated with uterine inversion.

⚷ CN: Reduction of risk potential;
CL: Analyze

25. 2. Avoidance, hostility, or low-key (passive) behavior toward the baby may be a cue to potential bonding problems. The nurse should encourage the client to give the baby the first feeding to begin the bonding process. Expressions of disappointment with the baby's gender may also signal problems with maternal-infant bonding. Comparing the baby's features to her own indicates identification of the neonate as belonging to her, suggesting bonding with neonate. Comparing the actual neonate with the "fantasized neonate" is a normal maternal reaction. Wanting to buy a blue outfit indicates an interest in and connection with the neonate and is a sign of bonding.

⚷ CN: Reduction of risk potential;
CL: Analyze

26. 1. According to the gate-control theory of pain, a closed gate means that the client should feel no pain. The gate-control theory of pain refers to the gate-control mechanisms in the substantia gelatinosa that are capable of halting an impulse at the level of the spinal cord so the impulse is never perceived at the brain level as pain (i.e., a process similar to keeping a gate closed).

⚷ CN: Health promotion and maintenance;
CL: Evaluate

27. 4. The bladder status should be monitored throughout the labor process, but especially before the client begins pushing. A full bladder can impede the progress of labor and slow fetal descent. Because she has had an epidural anesthetic, it is most likely that the client is receiving intravenous fluids, contributing to a full bladder. The client also does not feel the urge to void because of the anesthetic. Although it is important to monitor membrane status and fetal heart rate variability throughout labor, this does not affect the client's ability to push. There is no need to recheck cervical dilation because increasing the frequency of examinations can increase the client's risk for infection.

⚷ CN: Reduction of risk potential;
CL: Analyze

28. 1. The normal length of the latent stage of labor in a primigravid client is 6 hours. If the client is having prolonged labor, the nurse should monitor the client for signs of exhaustion as well as dehydration. Hypotonic contractions, which are painful but ineffective, may be occurring. Oxytocin augmentation may be necessary. Chills and fever are manifestations of an infection and are not associated with a prolonged latent phase of labor. Fluid overload can occur from rapid infusion of intravenous fluids administered if the client is experiencing hemorrhage or shock. It is not associated with prolonged latent phase. The client's membranes are intact, so it would be difficult to assess meconium staining of the fluid. Meconium-stained fluid is associated with fetal distress, and this fetus appears to be in a healthy state, as evidenced by a fetal heart rate within normal range and good variability.

⚷ CN: Reduction of risk potential;
CL: Analyze

29. 1. The client who has back pain during labor experiences marked discomfort because the fetus is in an LOP position. This pain is much greater than when the fetus is in the anterior position because the fetal head impinges on the sacrum in the course of rotating to the anterior position. Application of firm pressure to the sacral area can help alleviate the pain. Problems of severe back pain during labor do not typically require a cesarean birth. The **healthcare provider (HCP)** ▢ may elect to do an episiotomy, but it is not necessarily required. It is unlikely that a primigravid client with a fetus in an LOP position will have a precipitous birth; rather, labor is usually more prolonged. A hands-and-knees position or a right side-lying position may help to rotate the fetal head and thus alleviate some of the back pain.

⚷ CN: Health promotion and maintenance;
CL: Synthesize

30. 1. The psychoprophylaxis method of birth suggests using slow chest breathing until it becomes ineffective during labor contractions, then switching to shallow chest breathing (mostly at the sternum) during the peak of a contraction. The rate is 50 to 70 breaths/min. Deep chest breathing is appropriate for the early phase of labor, in which the client exhibits less frequent contractions. When transition nears, a rapid pant-blow pattern of breathing is used. Slow abdominal breathing is very difficult for clients in labor.

⚷ CN: Health promotion and maintenance;
CL: Apply

31. 3. Fetal scalp stimulation is commonly prescribed when there is decreased fetal heart rate variability. Pressure is applied with the fingers to the fetal scalp through the dilated cervix. This should cause a tactile response in the fetus and increase the fetal heart rate and variability. However, if the fetus is in distress and becoming acidotic, fetal heart rate acceleration will not occur. The fetal hematocrit level can be measured by fetal blood sampling. Scalp stimulation does not increase the strength of the contractions. However, it can increase fetal heart rate and variability. Fetal position is assessed by identifying skull landmarks (sutures) during a vaginal examination.

🔑 CN: Reduction of risk potential;
CL: Apply

32. 3. When a client has severe back pain during labor, the fetus is most likely in an occipitoposterior position. This means that the fetal head presses against the client's sacrum, causing marked discomfort during contractions. These sensations may be so intense that the client requests medication for relief of the back pain rather than the contractions. Breech presentation and transverse lie are usually known prior to 8-cm dilation and a cesarean section is performed. Fetal occiput anterior position does not increase the pain felt during labor.

🔑 CN: Health promotion and maintenance;
CL: Apply

33. 1,3,5. Decelerations alert the nurse that the fetus is experiencing decreased blood flow from the placenta. Administering oxygen will increase tissue perfusion. Placing the mother on her side will increase placental perfusion and decrease cord compression. Using an internal fetal monitor would help in identifying the possible underlying cause of the decelerations, such as metabolic acidosis. Assessing for pain relief and readjusting the monitor would have no effect on correcting the late decelerations.

🔑 CN: Reduction of risk potential;
CL: Synthesize

34. 3. The third maneuver involves grasping the lower portion of the abdomen just above the symphysis pubis between the thumb and index finger. This maneuver determines whether the fetal presenting part is engaged. The first maneuver involves facing the woman's head and using the tips of the fingers to palpate the uterine fundus. This maneuver is used to identify the part of the fetus that lies over the inlet to the pelvis. The second maneuver involves placing the palms of each hand on either side of the abdomen to locate the back of the fetus. The fourth maneuver involves placing the fingers on both sides of the uterus and pressing downward and inward in the direction of the birth canal. This maneuver is done to determine fetal attitude and degree of extension and should only be done if the fetus is in the cephalic presentation.

🔑 CN: Physiological adaptation; CL: Apply

35. 1. Leopold's maneuvers are performed to determine the presentation and position of the fetus. The third maneuver determines whether the fetal presenting part is engaged in the maternal pelvis. The first maneuver distinguishes between a breech and a cephalic presentation through palpation of the top of the fundus. The second maneuver locates the fetal back, arms, and legs. The fetal heart rate monitoring device should be placed near the fetal skull and back for optimal fetal heart rate monitoring. The fourth maneuver is done to locate the fetal cephalic prominence if the fetus is in a cephalic position.

🔑 CN: Health promotion and maintenance;
CL: Apply

The Multigravid Client in Labor

36. 4. Epidurals are given when labor is established, usually at 3- to 4-cm dilation. The effect of the epidural should be that labor will continue and not be slowed down by the administration of the epidural. The use of an epidural is not correlated with rupture of membranes. The contraction pattern for this client is adequate, not slow, and considered normal for 2-cm dilation. Epidurals are given at 3- to 4-cm dilation, and if there is medication available, it can be given to make the client comfortable until an epidural can be given.

🔑 CN: Management of care; CL: Apply

37. 1,2,4,5. A multiparous client usually gives birth within 12 hours of the time labor began. The pushing phase statistically takes 30 minutes or less and many multiparous clients go immediately from 10-cm dilation to birth. Contractions become regular and increase in frequency, intensity, and duration as labor progresses for both primiparous and multiparous clients. Transition will be shorter for a multiparous client than it will for a primiparous client, as the entire labor process takes less time for someone who has had a baby before. This client will withdraw into herself during transition, and this is a common characteristic for those in the transition phase.

🔑 CN: Management of care; CL: Create

38. 3. The cause of variable decelerations is cord compression, which may be relieved by moving the client to one side or another. If the client is already on the left side, changing the client to the right side is appropriate. Performing a vaginal examination will let the nurse know how far dilated the client is but will not relieve the cord compression. If the decelerations are not relieved by position changes, oxygen should be initiated, but the rate should be 8 to 10 L/min. Notifying the **HCP** 📖 should occur if turning the client and administering oxygen does not relieve the decelerations.

🔑 CN: Management of care; CL: Synthesize

39. **1,2,4,5.** Knowledge of how the fetus is tolerating contractions as well as the frequency, intensity, and duration of contractions, as indicated on the fetal monitor strip, are extremely important. The type of analgesia or anesthesia being used, the client's response, and her pain rating should be included as well. The amount of vaginal bleeding indicates whether this labor is in the normal range. The support persons with the client are an integral part of the labor process and greatly influence how she manages labor emotionally and, commonly, physically. A complete change-of-shift report would include the client's name, age, gravida and parity, current and prior illnesses that may influence this hospitalization, prior labor and birth history if applicable, last vaginal examination time and findings, vaginal bleeding, support persons with the client, current IVs and other medications being used, and pertinent laboratory test results. Previous use of birth control is not important at this time.

🔑 CN: Physiological adaptation; CL: Create

40. **2.** The feeling of needing to have a bowel movement is commonly caused by pressure on the receptors low in the perineum when the fetal head is creating pressure on them. This feeling usually indicates advances in fetal station and that the client may be close to birth. The nurse should respond initially to the client's signs and symptoms by checking to validate current effacement, dilation, and station. If the fetus is ready to be born, having the room ready for the birth and having naloxone available are important. Naloxone completely or partially reverses the effects of natural and synthetic opioids, including respiratory depression. Documenting pain relief takes time away from the vaginal examination, preparing for birth, and obtaining naloxone. The birth may be occurring rapidly. Being prepared for the birth is a higher priority than documentation for this client.

🔑 CN: Safety and infection control;
CL: Synthesize

41. **2.** Naloxone would not be used in a client who has a history of drug addiction. Naloxone would abruptly withdraw this woman from the drug she is addicted to as well as the nalbuphine. The withdrawal would occur within a few minutes of injection and, if severe enough, could jeopardize the mother and fetus. Lidocaine is a local anesthetic and numbs rather than decreases the effects of nalbuphine. The local anesthetic and the pudendal block are both appropriate for this birth but are used to numb the maternal perineum for birth.

🔑 CN: Pharmacological and parenteral therapies; CL: Synthesize

42. **1.** When a client receives an epidural anesthetic, sympathetic nerves are blocked along with the pain nerves, possibly resulting in vasodilation and hypotension. Other adverse effects include bladder distention, prolonged second stage of labor, nausea and vomiting, pruritus, and delayed respiratory depression for up to 24 hours after administration. Diaphoresis and tremors are not usually associated with the administration of epidural anesthesia. Headache, a common adverse effect of many drugs, also is not associated with administration of epidural anesthesia.

🔑 CN: Pharmacological and parenteral therapies; CL: Analyze

43. **4.** The fetal monitor strip shows late decelerations. The first intervention would be to turn off the oxytocin because the medication is causing the contractions. The stress caused by the contractions demonstrates that the fetus is not being perfused during the entire contraction (as shown by the late decelerations). There is no time to continue to observe in this situation; intervention is a priority. The client is attached to an internal fetal monitor, which would be possible only if her membranes had already ruptured. If the fetus continues to experience stress, fetal oximetry may be initiated.

🔑 CN: Physiological adaptation; CL: Analyze

44. **4.** After an emergency birth, the nurse suggests that the mother begin breast-feeding to contract the uterus. Breast-feeding stimulates the natural production of oxytocin. In a multiparous client, uterine atony is a potential complication because of the stretching of the uterine fibers following each subsequent pregnancy. Although breast-feeding does help to begin the parental-infant bonding process, this is not the primary reason for the nurse to suggest breast-feeding. Prevention of neonatal hypothermia is accomplished by placing blankets on both the neonate and the mother. Although colostrum in breast milk provides the neonate with nutrients and immunoglobulins, the primary reason for breast-feeding is to stimulate the natural production of oxytocin to contract the uterus.

🔑 CN: Reduction of risk potential;
CL: Apply

45. **3.** A chill shortly after birth is a common, normal occurrence. Warm blankets can help provide comfort for the client. It has been suggested that the shivering response is caused by a difference between internal and external body temperatures. A different theory proposes that the woman is reacting to fetal cells that have entered the maternal bloodstream through the placental site. Assessing the client's pulse rate will provide no further information about the chill. Decreasing the IV rate will not influence the length of time the client trembles. Assessing blood loss is a standard of care at this point postpartum but has no correlation with the chill.

🔑 CN: Health promotion and maintenance;
CL: Synthesize

46. 2. After an amniotomy, the nurse should plan to first assess the FHR for 1 full minute. One of the complications of amniotomy is cord compression and/or prolapsed cord, and an FHR of 100 bpm or less should be promptly reported to the **HCP** ⬜. A cord prolapse requires prompt birth by cesarean section. The client's contraction pattern should be monitored once labor has been established. The client's temperature, pulse, and respirations should be assessed every 2 to 4 hours after rupture of the membranes to detect an infection. The nurse should document the color, quantity, and odor of the amniotic fluid, but this can be done after the FHR is assessed and a normal pattern is present.

🔑 CN: Health promotion and maintenance; CL: Synthesize

47. 1. Nursing care for this client includes providing support, preparing for birth, assessing for potential complications, and providing for care of the newborn. Turning on the warmer is the best choice for providing for the care of the newborn. Oxygen and IV fluids may be indicated if variable or late decelerations are noted on the fetal heart monitor, but decelerations are not indicated in the question. It is likely too late for pharmacologic pain relief for a multigravid client. Education regarding care of the newborn is not appropriate at this time.

🔑 CN: Management of care; CL: Apply

48. 1. Breech presentations account for 5% of all births, and the most common is frank breech. In frank breech, there is flexion of the fetal thighs and extension of the knees. The feet rest at the side of the fetal head. In complete breech, there is flexion of the fetal thighs and knees; the fetus appears to be squatting. Footling breech occurs when there is an extension of the fetal knees and one or both feet protrude through the cervix. Vertex presentation occurs in 95% of births with the head engaged in the pelvis.

🔑 CN: Physiological adaptation; CL: Apply

49. 4. The nurse should assess the client's cervical dilation and station because the client's symptoms are indicative of the transition phase of labor. Multiparous clients can proceed 5 to 9 cm/h during the active phase of labor. Warming the temperature of the room is not helpful because the client will soon be ready to begin expulsive pushing. Increasing the intravenous fluid rate is not warranted unless the client is experiencing dehydration. Administration of an antiemetic at this point in labor is not warranted and may result in neonatal depression should a rapid birth occur.

🔑 CN: Health promotion and maintenance; CL: Synthesize

50. 4. To assess the frequency of the client's contractions, the nurse should assess the interval from the beginning of one contraction to the beginning of the next contraction. The duration of a contraction is the interval between the beginning and the end of a contraction. The acme identifies the peak of a contraction.

🔑 CN: Health promotion and maintenance; CL: Analyze

51. 3,4,5. The range of fetal heart rate fluctuating more than 25 beats per minutes could indicate fetal distress. The green peripad fluid indicates meconium, which could be associated with fetal distress. Increased fetal activity during labor may also indicate distress. The maternal vital signs noted and a perineal pad with blood and mucus are normal findings.

🔑 CN: Reduction of risk potential; CL: Analyze

52. 3. After spontaneous rupture of the amniotic fluid, the gushing fluid may carry the umbilical cord out of the birth canal. Sudden deceleration of the fetal heart rate commonly signifies cord compression and/or prolapse of the cord, which would require immediate birth. This client is particularly at risk because the fetus is preterm and the fetal head may not be engaged. Turning the client to the right side is not a priority action. However, changing the client's position would be appropriate if variable decelerations are present. The nurse should assess the color, amount, and odor of the fluid, but this can be done once the fetal heart rate is assessed and no problems are detected. Cervical dilation should be checked but only after the fetal heart rate pattern is assessed.

🔑 CN: Reduction of risk potential; CL: Synthesize

53. 3,6. The pressure from the fetus descending into the birth canal can cause the client to feel she needs to move her bowels and could be near childbirth. Failure to assess the stage of labor and degree of fetal descent before allowing the client to go to the bathroom may lead to progression of labor and could result in a birth in the bathroom. Applying a fetal monitor may reassure the nurse that the fetus is doing well; however, it does not help to determine if the fetus is ready to be born, which is the higher priority in this situation. Regardless of the client's prior experience with back labor pain, the fetal head moving lower into the birth canal causes pressure in the lower back area similar to the feeling of pressure with a bowel movement.

🔑 CN: Safety and infection control; CL: Synthesize

54. 2. Spinal anesthesia is used less commonly today because of preference for epidural block anesthesia. One of the adverse effects of spinal anesthesia is a "spinal headache" caused by leakage of spinal fluid from the needle insertion. This can be treated by applying a cool cloth to the forehead, keeping the client in a flat position, or using a blood patch that can clot and seal off any further leakage of fluid. Spinal anesthesia is administered with the client in a sitting position or side lying. Another adverse effect of spinal anesthesia is hypotension caused by vasodilation. General anesthesia provides immediate anesthesia, whereas the full effects of spinal anesthesia may not be felt for 20 to 30 minutes. General anesthesia can be discontinued quickly when the anesthesiologist administers oxygen instead of nitrous oxide. Epidural anesthesia may take 1 to 2 hours to wear off.

⚷ CN: Pharmacological and parenteral therapies; CL: Evaluate

55. 3. Cimetidine is prescribed by some anesthesiologists who will be giving a general anesthetic to reduce the level of acid in the stomach contents, altering the pH to reduce the risk of complications should aspiration of vomitus occur. Aspiration of vomitus is the fifth most common cause of maternal mortality. Most anesthesiologists insert an endotracheal tube to reduce the incidence of aspiration. Isoproterenol is used to decrease the incidence of bronchospasm. Atropine sulfate is administered to dry oral and nasal secretions. Although cimetidine is useful for gastric ulcer therapy, gastric ulcers are not a common effect associated with operative births.

⚷ CN: Pharmacological and parenteral therapies; CL: Apply

The Labor Experience

56. 1. If presenting part is above the ischial spines 1 cm, the station is −1. If the presenting part is 1 cm below the ischial spines, the station is +1. Engaged and floating are not descriptive of station.

⚷ CN: Reduction of risk potential; CL: Apply

57. 1. Closed glottis pushing, or when a woman is told to hold her breath when she pushes typically while the nurse typically counts to 10, creates the Valsalva maneuver and is associated with decreased perfusion. Open glottis pushing, on the other hand, encourages women to listen to their own body cues for when to breathe and when to bear down. "Rest and descent" and squatting have positive influences on second stage of labor and birth.

⚷ CN: Reduction of risk potential; CL: Analyze

58. 3. Placing the client in the hands and knees position pulls the fetal head away from the sacral promontory (relieving pain) and facilitates rotation of the fetus to the anterior position. Lithotomy is the position preferred by some **healthcare providers (HCP)** ▢ for birth but does not facilitate rotation. The right lateral position will perpetuate the ROP position. Tailor sitting facilitates descent in OA positions.

⚷ CN: Basic care and comfort; CL: Apply

59. 3. A trial labor in this context means that the woman is allowed to go into labor, and her progress is assessed by cervical dilation and effacement as well as fetal descent evaluated to determine whether to allow the labor to progress to birth. If there are indications that labor is not progressing, other means of birth are considered. Labor stimulation is used cautiously and may not be safe. The presence of contractions every 5 minutes indicates true labor. If fetal distress is noted and an emergency cesarean section cannot be done immediately, tocolytic agents may be considered to stop contractions.

⚷ CN: Management of care; CL: Analyze

60. 2. Lumbar epidural anesthesia is usually administered with the client in a sitting or a left side-lying position with shoulders parallel and legs slightly flexed. These positions expose the vertebrae to the anesthesiologist. Paracervical and local anesthetics are usually administered with the client in the lithotomy position. The hands and knees and prone positions are not used for anesthesia administration.

⚷ CN: Pharmacological and parenteral therapies; CL: Apply

61. 2. The nurse should turn the client to the side to reduce pressure on the abdominal aorta. The IV fluid rate would be increased, not decreased. There is no information indicating the client has a full bladder or requires a vaginal examination.

⚷ CN: Management of care; CL Synthesize

62. 2. The nurse would document these findings as "early" decelerations. Early decelerations are thought to be the result of vagal nerve stimulation caused by compression of the fetal head during labor. They are considered normal physiologic response to labor and do not require any intervention. Early decelerations do not require position change or O2 as they are not a sign of fetal distress. Variable decelerations are thought to be due to umbilical cord compression. Early decelerations are not emergent and do not require immediate reporting to the **healthcare provider (HCP)** ▢ or preparing for caesarean section.

⚷ CN: Management of care CL; Synthesize

63. 4. Transition is the most difficult period of the labor process, and often when clients are tired, pain becomes more intensified. Clients during this stage verbalize anger and are outspoken and difficult to comfort. The most logical next step would be to determine if the client has completed transition and is ready to begin pushing. Performing a vaginal exam would provide this answer. The use of narcotic medications is discouraged at this stage as they can lead to respiratory depression in the neonate. Palpating the bladder is an important intervention but not the highest priority as it was done less than an hour ago. Since the nurse has correctly completed the most logical steps, asking for the client's input would certainly be in order but not the highest priority intervention.

CN: Basic care and comfort; CL: Apply

64. 3. The expected outcome of magnesium sulfate administration is suppression of the contractions because the client is in preterm labor. Magnesium sulfate is a smooth muscle relaxant used to slow and stop contractions and is one of the most common tocolytic agents in the United States. Having contractions that lead to birth is not the intended effect of this drug when used for preterm labor. Respirations lower than 12 breaths/min may indicate magnesium sulfate toxicity. Another use of magnesium sulfate is to treat preeclampsia by preventing seizures and, secondarily, lowering maternal blood pressure. However, in this scenario, preterm labor—not preeclampsia—is being treated.

CN: Pharmacological and parenteral therapies; CL: Evaluate

65. 4. Betamethasone is a corticosteroid that induces the production of surfactant. The pulmonary maturation that results causes the fetal lungs to mature more rapidly than normal. Because the lungs are mature, the risk of respiratory distress in the neonate is lowered but not eliminated. Betamethasone also decreases the surface tension within the alveoli. Betamethasone has no influence on contractions or carrying the fetus to full term. It also does not prevent infection.

CN: Pharmacological and parenteral therapies; CL: Evaluate

66. 1. A Bishop score evaluates cervical readiness for labor based on five factors: cervical softness, cervical effacement, dilation, fetal position, and station. A Bishop score of 5 or greater in a multipara or a score of 8 or greater in a primipara indicate that a vaginal birth is likely to result from the induction process. The nurse should expect that labor will be induced using oxytocin because the Bishop score indicates that the client is 60% to 70% effaced, 3 to 4 cm dilated, and in an anterior position. The cervix is soft and the presenting part is at a −1 to 0 position. Prostaglandin gel, misoprostol, and dinoprostone are all cervical ripening agents, and the doses are accurate; however, cervical ripening has already taken place.

CN: Pharmacological and parenteral therapies; CL: Synthesize

67. 3. Cervical ripening, or creating a cervix that is soft, anterior, and dilated to 2 to 3 cm, must occur before the cervix can efface and dilate with oxytocin. Drugs to accomplish this goal include dinoprostone, misoprostol, and prostaglandin E2. Nalbuphine is a narcotic analgesic used in early labor and has no influence on the cervix. Betamethasone is a corticosteroid given to mature fetal lungs.

CN: Pharmacological and parenteral therapies; CL: Apply

68. 2. Typically, a client will be able to have an epidural when she is 3 to 4 cm dilated or the active phase of labor has been established. Waiting until the cervix is dilated to this point ensures that the client is in labor and the epidural is less likely to halt labor contractions. Nalbuphine and promethazine are used to provide relief until the client is about 7 cm dilated. If given after this time, narcotics may cause neonatal respiratory depression in the neonate. The majority of clients have an epidural or spinal for a cesarean section. The only time general anesthesia is used is for an emergency cesarean section.

CN: Pharmacological and parenteral therapies; CL: Evaluate

69. 1,2,3,5. The time of rupture; color, odor, amount, and clarity of amniotic fluid; and FHR and pattern before and after the procedure are all information that must be documented on the client's record. There is only one size for an amnio hook.

CN: Management of care; CL: Create

70. 2. The client is experiencing uterine hyperstimulation from the oxytocin. The first intervention should be to stop the oxytocin infusion, which may be the cause of the long, frequent contractions, elevated resting tone, and abnormal fetal heart patterns. Only after turning off the oxytocin should the nurse turn the client to her left side to better perfuse the mother and fetus. Then, she should increase the maintenance IV fluids to allow available oxygen to be carried to the mother and fetus. When all other interventions are initiated, she should notify the **HCP** 📖.

CN: Management of care; CL: Synthesize

71. 4. Late decelerations on a fetal heart monitor indicate uteroplacental insufficiency. Interventions to improve perfusion include repositioning the client, oxygen, and IV fluids. A sterile vaginal exam is not indicated at this time. Late decelerations are not expected findings and do not indicate an imminent birth.

CN: Management of Care; CL: Analyze

72. 4. Accelerations that are episodic and occur during fetal movement demonstrate fetal well-being. Turning the client to the left side, applying oxygen by face mask, and notifying the **HCP** ☐ are interventions used for late and variable decelerations indicating the fetus is not tolerating the induction process well.

    CN: Physiological adaptation; CL: Synthesize

73. 1. The client with preeclampsia would be a candidate for the induction process because ending the pregnancy is the only way to cure preeclampsia. A client with active herpes would be a candidate for a cesarean section to prevent the fetus from contracting the virus while passing through the birth canal. The woman with a face presentation will not be able to give birth vaginally due to the extended position of the neck. The client whose fetus exhibits late decelerations without oxytocin would be at greater risk for fetal distress with use of this drug. Late decelerations indicate the fetus does not have enough placental reserves to remain oxygenated during the entire contraction. This client may require a cesarean section.

    CN: Management of care; CL: Evaluate

74. 2. Removing a fetal monitor from a client and assisting her to the bathroom are within the realm of practice of a **UAP** ☐. Performing a fundal check is an assessment, which is a responsibility of an **RN** ☐. A UAP is not permitted to administer medication by any route. Education is also part of the professional nursing role. Although a UAP can assist a mother with bottle-feeding, the formal client education must be completed and validated by the nurse.

    CN: Management of care; CL: Evaluate

75. 3. When the fetal head is compressed, early decelerations are seen as a vagal response occurs and the fetal heart rate decelerates and inversely mirrors the contraction. This response commonly occurs when the client is 9 to 10 cm dilated or pushing. If communication cannot be facilitated, early decelerations are one indicator that birth may be approaching. Late decelerations may occur at this time but indicate uteroplacental insufficiency rather than imminent birth. At any time during the labor process, the client may communicate with her family in her native language. The client's facial expressions may change at any point during labor and cannot be used as an indicator of imminent birth.

    CN: Physiological adaptation; CL: Analyze

The Intrapartal Client with Risk Factors

76. 1,2,3. With abruptio placentae, bleeding may occur vaginally, may be obstructed by the fetal head, or it may be hidden behind a portion of the placenta. Abdominal rigidity occurs, particularly with a concealed hemorrhage because the girth and fundal height increase. Abdominal pain is one of the classic symptoms of abruption. The pain may be intermittent, as in labor contractions, or continuous. The placenta with abruption is not larger than a normal placenta, and the bleeding does not end spontaneously.

    CN: Physiological adaptation; CL: Analyze

77. 3. The multigravid client with class II heart disease has a slight limitation of physical activity and may become fatigued with ordinary physical activity. A side-lying or semi-Fowler's position with the head elevated helps to ensure cardiac emptying and adequate oxygenation. In addition, oxygen by mask, analgesics and sedatives, diuretics, prophylactic antibiotics, and digitalis may be warranted. Although breathing slowly during a contraction may assist with oxygenation, it would have no effect on cardiac emptying. It is essential that the laboring woman with cardiac disease be relieved of discomfort and anxiety. Effective intrapartum pain relief with analgesia and epidural anesthesia may reduce cardiac workload as much as 20%. Local anesthetics are effective only during the second stage of labor.

    CN: Reduction of risk potential; CL: Synthesize

78. 4. Assessing for signs and symptoms associated with cardiac decompensation is the priority. Class III heart disease during pregnancy has a 25% to 50% mortality. These clients are markedly compromised, with marked limitation of physical activity. They frequently experience fatigue, palpitations, dyspnea, or anginal pain. A pulse rate >100 bpm or a respiratory rate >25 breaths/min may indicate cardiac decompensation that could result in cardiac arrest. Additional symptoms include dyspnea, peripheral edema, orthopnea, tachypnea, rales, and hemoptysis.

    CN: Reduction of risk potential; CL: Analyze

79. 1. Before administering prostaglandin E2 gel, the nurse would assess the frequency and duration of any uterine contractions first because prostaglandin E2 gel is contraindicated if the client is having contractions. If there are no contractions, the client should be placed in a semi-Fowler's position to allow for vaginal insertion of the gel. Although determining whether the client's membranes have ruptured is part of the assessment of any client in labor, it is not specifically related to the administration of prostaglandin E2 gel. If the membranes remain intact, an amniotomy may be performed once the client begins to dilate and the fetal head is engaged. However, it is not necessary for the nurse to prepare the client for this procedure at this time.

🔑 CN: Pharmacological and parenteral therapies; CL: Synthesize

80. 4. A prolonged second stage of labor with a large fetus could indicate a shoulder dystocia at birth. Immediate nursing actions for a shoulder dystocia include suprapubic pressure and the McRoberts maneuver. If after interventions for vaginal birth with a shoulder dystocia fail, an emergency cesarean birth may be needed but is not indicated at this time. A vacuum-assisted birth would be contraindicated due to increased risk of shoulder dystocia with a macrosomic infant. An IV fluid bolus may be indicated for fetal distress, but there is not enough information to establish that they are needed at this time.

🔑 CN: Physiologic adaptation; CL: Apply

81. 4. Assessing the fetal heart rate is always a priority after spontaneous rupture of membranes has occurred. Also a common sign of fetal distress related to an inadequate transfer of oxygen to the fetus is meconium-stained fluid. Because the fetus has suffered hypoxia, close fetal heart rate monitoring is necessary. In addition, all clients are monitored continuously after rupture of membranes for fetal distress caused by cord prolapse. If there are increasing signs of fetal distress (e.g., late decelerations), the **healthcare provider (HCP)** 📖 should be notified immediately. A cesarean birth may be performed for fetal distress. Increasing the rate of the oxytocin infusion could lead to further fetal distress. Turning the client to the left side, rather than a knee-chest position, improves placental perfusion. The HCP may wish to determine the extent of cervical dilation to make a decision about whether a cesarean birth is warranted, but continuous fetal heart rate monitoring is essential to determine fetal status.

🔑 CN: Reduction of risk potential; CL: Synthesize

82. 3. Neonates born to mothers who smoke tend to have lower-than-average birth weights. Neonates born to mothers who smoke also are at higher risk for stillbirth, sudden infant death syndrome, bronchitis, allergies, delayed growth and development, and polycythemia. Maternal smoking is not related to higher neonatal sedation, hyperbilirubinemia, or hypocalcemia. Smoking may cause irritability, not sedation. Hyperbilirubinemia is associated with Rh or ABO incompatibility or the administration of

intravenous oxytocin during labor. Approximately 50% of neonates born to mothers with insulin-dependent diabetes experience hypocalcemia during the first 3 days of life.

🔑 CN: Health promotion and maintenance; CL: Analyze

83. 3. The client should be urged to push with an open glottis to prevent the Valsalva maneuver. Pushing with a closed glottis increases intrathoracic pressure, preventing venous return. Blood pressure also falls, and cardiac output decreases. Pushing for at least 1 to 3 minutes is too long; prolonged pushing can lead to reduced blood flow and fatigue. Pushing for the duration of the contraction is sufficient. Pushing while holding the breath results in the Valsalva maneuver. Because the client has had an epidural anesthetic, she may not feel the urge to push and may need coaching during the pushing phase.

🔑 CN: Pharmacological and parenteral therapies; CL: Create

84. 3. When the fetal skull is on the perineum with the scalp visible at the perineal floor or vaginal opening, this is considered outlet forceps application. When the head is higher in the pelvis but engaged and its greatest diameter has passed the inlet, the operation is termed midforceps. Midforceps births are not recommended because they are extremely dangerous for the mother and fetus because of the possibility of uterine rupture. If the head is not engaged, at −1 station, this is termed high forceps. High-forceps births also are exceedingly dangerous for both the mother and fetus because of the possibility of uterine rupture and are not recommended. Cesarean birth is preferred in these situations. The fetal head at station +2 or lower is termed low forceps.

🔑 CN: Reduction of risk potential; CL: Apply

85. 1. Oligohydramnios, or a decrease in the volume of amniotic fluid, is associated with variable fetal heart rate decelerations due to cord compression. Maintenance of an adequate amniotic fluid volume during labor provides protective cushioning of the umbilical cord and minimizes cord compression. Cord compression can result in fetal metabolic acidosis, not alkalosis. Amnioinfusion is used to minimize cord compression, not to increase the fetal heart rate accelerations during a contraction. The goal is to maintain the amniotic fluid index at 8 cm. This can be determined by ultrasound.

🔑 CN: Reduction of risk potential; CL: Apply

86. 4. A primigravid client diagnosed with preeclampsia has the potential for developing seizures (eclampsia). This client should be in a room with the least amount of stimulation possible to reduce the risk of seizures and as close to the nurses' station as possible in case the client requires immediate assistance. Bright lighting and sunshine can be a stimulant, possibly increasing the risk of seizures, as can being in a semiprivate room with roommate, visitors, conversation, and noise.

🔑 CN: Management of care; CL: Synthesize

87. 4. The client is experiencing a precipitous birth. The nurse should remain calm during a precipitous birth. Explaining to the client what is happening as the birth progresses and how she can assist is likely to help her remain calm and cooperative. Maintaining eye contact is also beneficial. Telling the client that she is right and to just relax is inappropriate because the client may not be able to relax because of the strong urge to push the fetus out of the birth canal. Telling the client not to push because she may tear the cervix can instill fear, not cooperation. Saying that the **healthcare provider (HCP)** 📖 will be there soon may not be an accurate statement and is not reassuring if the client is concerned about the birth.

🔑 CN: Psychosocial integrity; CL: Apply

88. 2. During a precipitous birth, after calling for assistance and helping the client lie down, the nurse should provide support to the fetal head to prevent too rapid of emergence leading to injury. It is not appropriate to tell the client to push between contractions because this may lead to lacerations. The shoulder should be delivered by applying downward traction until the anterior shoulder appears fully at the introitus, then upward pressure to lift out the other shoulder. Priority should be given to safe birth of the infant over protecting the perineum by massage.

🔑 CN: Reduction of risk potential; CL: Synthesize

89. 2. Because birth occurs so rapidly and the fetus is propelled quickly through the birth canal, the major complication of a precipitous birth is a boggy fundus, or uterine atony. The neonate should be put to the breast, if the mother permits, to allow for the release of natural oxytocin. In a hospital setting, the **healthcare provider (HCP)** 📖 will probably prescribe administration of oxytocin. The nurse should gently massage the fundus to ensure that it is firm. There is no relationship between a precipitous birth and postpartum "blues" or intrauterine infection. Postpartum "blues" usually do not occur until about 3 days postpartum, and symptoms of postpartum infection usually occur after the first 24 hours. There is no relationship between a precipitous birth and urinary tract infection even though the birth has been accomplished under clean rather than sterile technique. Symptoms of urinary tract infection typically begin on the first or second postpartum day.

🔑 CN: Reduction of risk potential; CL: Analyze

90. 2. A sinusoidal pattern is an ominous sign that reflects an absence of autonomic nervous control over the fetal heart rate resulting from severe hypoxia. Sinusoidal patterns, while rare, are associated with Rh sensitization, fetal hydrops, and anemia. This client will most likely require a cesarean birth to improve the fetal outcome. Variable decelerations, associated with cord compression, and late decelerations, associated with poor placental perfusion, are concerning but may correct with appropriate interventions. Early decelerations are associated with head compression and are considered a normal variation.

🔑 CN: Reduction of risk potential; CL: Analyze

91. 1. A priority assessment for the nurse to make is to determine the estimated date of birth or probable gestational age of the fetus. If the gestation is <37 weeks, the neonatal team should be called to begin resuscitative efforts if needed. Amniotic fluid status is not important at this point, because if the fetal skull is crowning, birth is imminent. Determination of gravida and parity is part of the normal nursing history, but the priority is the status of the fetus and safe birth. Prenatal history is part of the nursing assessment, but this information is not especially relevant until the fetus is safely born and has been given immediate care.

🔑 CN: Health promotion and maintenance; CL: Analyze

92. 2. It is important that the parents be allowed to touch, hold, and participate in care of the twins whenever they desire. Ideally, this will be on a daily basis, to promote parent-infant bonding. It is not appropriate to discuss how the couple will cope with twin infants at home until they are ready to take the infants home. They are too overwhelmed at this point and are focused on the well-being of their infants while hospitalized. Having the couple visit the twins to provide care on a 24-hour basis is not warranted. Identifying complications that may occur is not appropriate. If complications arise, the parents should be well informed and given opportunities for discussion related to the care provided.

🔑 CN: Psychosocial integrity; CL: Create

93. 4. Birth trauma and prolonged ruptured membranes make risk for infection the priority problem for this client. Infection can be a serious postpartum complication. Although the client may be fatigued, she should not be experiencing activity intolerance. Clients with heart disease may experience activity intolerance due to excessive cardiac workload. Although the client may be experiencing sleep deprivation, most clients are alert and awake after birth of a neonate. Situational low self-esteem is not a priority. Clients who undergo a cesarean birth commonly feel a sense of failure because of not having a vaginal birth experience, but this is not the case for this client.

⚷ CN: Reduction of risk potential; CL: Analyze

94. 2. Postmature neonates commonly have difficulty maintaining adequate glucose reserves and usually develop hypoglycemia soon after birth. Other common problems include meconium aspiration syndrome, polycythemia, congenital anomalies, seizure activity, and cold stress. These complications result primarily from a combination of advanced gestational age, placental insufficiency, and continued exposure to amniotic fluid. Delayed meconium is not associated with postterm gestation. Hyperbilirubinemia occurs in term neonates as well as postterm neonates, but unless there is an Rh incompatibility, it does not develop until after the first 24 hours of life.

⚷ CN: Reduction of risk potential; CL: Analyze

95. 4. Polyhydramnios is an abnormally large amount of amniotic fluid in the uterus. The client has understood the instructions when the client states that polyhydramnios is associated with gastrointestinal disorders (e.g., tracheoesophageal fistula). Polyhydramnios is also associated with maternal illnesses such as diabetes and anemia. Other fetal/neonatal disorders associated with this condition include congenital anomalies of the central nervous system (e.g., anencephaly), upper gastrointestinal obstruction, and macrosomia. Polyhydramnios can lead to preterm labor, premature rupture of the membranes, and cord prolapse. Renal dysfunction and intrauterine growth restriction are associated with oligohydramnios, not polyhydramnios. Pulmonary hypoplasia (poorly developed lungs) is associated with prolonged oligohydramnios.

⚷ CN: Reduction of risk potential; CL: Evaluate

96. 1. If a client has been in active labor and there is no change in cervical dilation after 2 hours, the nurse should suspect cephalopelvic disproportion. This may be caused by an inadequate pelvis size of the mother or by a large-for-gestational-age fetus. The **healthcare provider (HCP)** ▢ should be notified about the client's lack of progress. If the fetus cannot descend, a cesarean birth is warranted. The client is not experiencing a prolonged latent phase (0- to 3-cm dilation) because her cervix is dilated to 6 cm. She has not reached the transitional phase, characterized by a cervical dilation of 8 to 10 cm. With a hypotonic labor pattern, contractions are painful but far apart and not very intense. This client's contractions are of moderate intensity.

⚷ CN: Reduction of risk potential; CL: Analyze

97. 3. Preparation for cesarean birth is similar to preparation for any abdominal surgery. The client must give **informed consent** ▢. Another person may not sign for the client unless the client is unable to sign the form. If this is the case, only certain designated people can do so legally. The husband does not need to sign the form unless his wife is unable to do so. In a life threatening emergency, surgery may be performed without a written consent. The HCP does not need to witness the consent.

⚷ CN: Management of care; CL: Synthesize

98. 4. Decreased variability may be seen in various conditions. However, it is most commonly caused by analgesic administration. Other factors that can cause decreased variability include anesthesia, deep fetal sleep, anencephaly, prematurity, hypoxia, tachycardia, brain damage, and arrhythmias. Maternal fatigue, fetal malposition, and small-for-gestational-age fetus are not commonly associated with decreased variability.

⚷ CN: Health promotion and maintenance; CL: Apply

99. 4. Respiratory distress syndrome is more common in neonates born by cesarean section than in those born vaginally. During a vaginal birth, pressure is exerted on the fetal chest, which aids in the fetal inhalation and exhalation of air and lung expansion. This pressure is not exerted on the fetus with a cesarean birth. Congenital anomalies are not more common with cesarean birth. Pulmonary hypertension occurs more commonly in infants with meconium aspiration syndrome, congenital diaphragmatic hernia, respiratory distress syndrome, or neonatal sepsis, not with cesarean birth. Meconium aspiration syndrome occurs more commonly with vaginal birth, postterm neonate, and prolonged labor, not with cesarean birth.

⚷ CN: Health promotion and maintenance; CL: Apply

100. 4. Congenital anomalies are not related to maternal urinary tract infections. A multigravid client with acute pyelonephritis is susceptible to preterm labor, premature rupture of the membranes, maternal sepsis, intrauterine growth restriction, and fetal loss. The most common organism responsible for the urinary tract infection is *Escherichia coli*.

⚷ CN: Reduction of risk potential; CL: Evaluate

101. 1. Conjunctivitis is a common complication of neonates who are born to mothers with untreated chlamydial infection. Neonatal pneumonia is another condition associated with chlamydial infection of the mother. Untreated chlamydial infection is not associated with heart disease or brain damage. Exposure to rubella may lead to neonatal heart defects, and brain damage may occur as a result of prolonged shoulder dystocia or difficulty delivering the fetal head during a vaginal breech birth. Occasionally, because of immature circulation, a neonate who has been lying on his or her side appears red on one side of the body. This "harlequin sign" is transient and is of no clinical significance. Presence of a harlequin sign is unrelated to untreated chlamydial infection.

🔑 CN: Reduction of risk potential; CL: Apply

102. 1. The purpose of the RhoGAM is to provide passive antibody immunity and prevent Rh-positive sensitization with the next pregnancy. It should be given within 72 hours after birth of an Rh-positive neonate. Clients who are Rh negative and conceive an Rh-negative fetus do not need antibody protection. Rh-positive cells contribute to sensitization, not Rh-negative cells. The RhoGAM does not cross the placenta and destroy fetal Rh-positive cells.

🔑 CN: Reduction of risk potential; CL: Apply

103. 3. Because magnesium sulfate is a central nervous system depressant, the nurse should plan to assess the client's respiratory rate every hour. If the respiratory rate is <12 breaths/min, the client may be experiencing magnesium sulfate overdose. Urinary output via an indwelling catheter should be assessed hourly and should be at least 30 mL/h. Deep tendon reflexes and blood pressure should also be assessed every hour. At some institutions, continuous electronic blood pressure monitoring will be performed.

🔑 CN: Pharmacological and parenteral therapies; CL: Analyze

104. 2. For a client diagnosed with probable placenta previa, hypovolemic shock is a complication. Continuous blood pressure monitoring with an electronic cuff is the priority assessment after the client's admission. Once the client is admitted, an ultrasound examination will be performed to determine the placement of the placenta. Whole blood replacement is not warranted at this time. However, it may be necessary if the client demonstrates signs and symptoms of hemorrhage or shock. Internal fetal heart rate monitoring is contraindicated because the monitoring device may puncture the placenta and place both the mother and fetus in jeopardy. An immediate cesarean birth is not necessary until there has been an assessment of the amount of bleeding and the location of the placenta previa.

🔑 CN: Reduction of risk potential; CL: Apply

105. 4. Dramatic vasoconstriction occurs as a result of sniffing crack cocaine. This can lead to increased respiratory and cardiac rates and hypertension. It can severely compromise placental circulation, resulting in abruptio placentae and preterm labor and birth. Infants of these women can experience intracranial hemorrhage and withdrawal symptoms of tremulousness, irritability, and rigidity. Placenta previa, ruptured uterus, and maternal hypotension are not associated with cocaine use. Placenta previa may be associated with grand multiparity. Ruptured uterus may be associated with a large-for-gestational-age fetus.

🔑 CN: Reduction of risk potential; CL: Analyze

106. 2. Pregnant women who become infected with the rubella virus early in pregnancy risk having a neonate born with rubella syndrome. The symptoms include thrombocytopenia, cataracts, cardiac disorders, deafness, microcephaly, and motor and cognitive impairment. The most extensive neonatal effects occur when the mother is exposed during the first 2 to 6 weeks and up to 12 weeks' gestation, when critical organs are forming. Bulging fontanelles are associated with increased intracranial pressure and bacterial meningitis. Rubella is not associated with renal defects.

🔑 CN: Reduction of risk potential; CL: Analyze

107. 3. To stop the process of DIC, the underlying insult that began the phenomenon must be halted. Treatment includes fresh frozen platelets or blood administration. The **HCP** 📖 also may prescribe heparin before the administration of blood products to restore the normal clotting mechanism. Immediate birth of the fetus is essential. Magnesium sulfate is given for pregnancy-induced hypertension or preterm labor. Heparin, not warfarin sodium, is used to treat DIC. Meperidine hydrochloride is used for pain relief.

🔑 CN: Pharmacological and parenteral therapies; CL: Apply

108. 2. Magnesium sulfate may be used as an anticonvulsive or a tocolytic agent. The intended effect for this client is to decrease the number and frequency of contractions. Even though this client has chronic hypertension, the first goal is to prevent birth in a 34 weeks' gestation client. If the blood pressure moves into the therapeutic range, that is a benefit for the client, but it is not the major goal. Magnesium sulfate may decrease the accelerations found in this fetus as it decreases the ability of the infant to respond, acting on the infant in the same way it does on the mother. Maternal respiratory rate may also decrease, and a lower respiratory rate to 12 respirations/min indicates that this level of magnesium sulfate is becoming toxic to this client.

🔑 CN: Pharmacological and parenteral therapies; CL: Evaluate

109. 1. Although thioamides such as propylthiouracil and methimazole are considered teratogenic to the fetus and can lead to congenital hyperthyroidism (goiter) in the neonate, they still represent the treatment of choice. The client should be regulated on the lowest possible dose. Hyperthyroidism is associated with preterm labor and a low-birth-weight infant, so the client should contact the **HCP** 📖 if the contractions begin again. The client should not be urged to breast-feed, because medications such as propylthiouracil and methimazole are secreted in breast milk. Tachycardia (not bradycardia) is associated with thyroid storm, a medical emergency, and should be reported to the HCP.

🔑 CN: Pharmacological and parenteral therapies; CL: Apply

110. 4. The first action by the nurse should be to call for immediate assistance in the client's room because this is an emergency. Throughout the seizure, the nurse should note the time and length of the seizure and continue to monitor the status of both client and fetus. The side rails should have been padded at the time of the client's admission to the hospital as part of seizure precautions. The client should be turned to her left side to improve placental perfusion. Inserting a tongue blade is not recommended because it can further obstruct the airway or cause injury to the client's teeth.

🔑 CN: Safety and infection control; CL: Synthesize

111. 3. In an abusive situation, the client's safety is the priority. The nurse should refer the client to a social worker who can provide the client with options such as a safe shelter. Commonly clients who are battered feel powerless and fear that the batterer will kill them. As a result, they remain in the abusive situation. Telling the client to leave the boyfriend immediately is not helpful and reflects the values of the nurse. Although asking about fetal movement is important and is part of a routine assessment, a sonogram can be performed to confirm fetal well-being. The referral is more important at this time. Although it may be part of the unit's policies and procedures to report any incidents such as this one to the unit supervisor, the client's immediate need for safety must be addressed first.

🔑 CN: Management of care; CL: Apply

112. 1. The client's symptoms are indicative of amniotic fluid embolism, which is a medical emergency. After calling for assistance, the first action should be to administer oxygen by face mask or cannula to ensure adequate oxygenation of mother and fetus. If the client needs cardiopulmonary resuscitation, this can be started once oxygen has been administered. If the client survives, disseminated intravascular coagulation will probably develop, and the client will need intravenous fibrinogen and heparin. Oxytocin, a vasoconstrictor, is not warranted for amniotic fluid embolism.

🔑 CN: Physiological adaptation; CL: Synthesize

Managing Care, Quality, and Safety for Clients Giving Birth

113. 2. The nurse will need to assess the client's ability to bear weight before taking her to the bathroom. If she cannot bear weight, she will be unable to ambulate. Asking the client to remain in bed until the assessments are complete sets the client up for increased postpartum bleeding, as the bladder will displace the uterus. Encouraging the client to sit at the bedside is an excellent strategy to prevent orthostatic hypotension, but it will not give the nurse an idea if the client can ambulate. Having a staff member with the client is also correct for the first ambulation of this client, but the ability to bear weight and walk will need to be assessed first.

🔑 CN: Reduction of risk potential; CL: Synthesize

114. 1,4,5. In most settings, the charge nurse coordinates and directs the activities of the unit. Prior to the change of shift, the nurse will review and update the status of each of the laboring clients on the unit to include any difficulties or unusual situations that may be occurring with each of them, including following up with a primary nurse after a birth. A change-of-shift report with the oncoming charge nurse is among the last activities completed before ending the shift. Activities such as admitting a client in labor and completing the nursing responsibilities of the nurse who had to leave 30 minutes early can be delegated to staff members. In an emergency, the charge nurse could assume responsibility for client care.

🔑 CN: Management of care; CL: Create

115. 4. The client at 42 weeks' is the greatest concern, and the nurse should make rounds on this client first based on the length of the pregnancy and the green color of the amniotic fluid. Bloody show is a normal sign of impending labor as the cervix may be beginning to dilate. Not having contractions after rupture of membranes is not unusual within a 1-hour time frame. The green amniotic fluid indicates that fetal distress has recently occurred to the point that the fetus had a bowel movement in utero. Along with the 42-week gestation, this fetus is at greatest risk. The nurse can see the primipara in active labor at 5-cm dilation last; this client is in pain, but nothing about her situation indicates anything, but a normal labor process and as a primipara, her labor process will be slow. The client who is completely effaced, 8 cm dilated, and at +2 station as a primipara usually moves through labor at a slower pace than does a multiparous client. She is experiencing nausea that is an expected situation as a laboring client enters transition. The client with no prenatal care is a cause for concern as the nurse knows nothing about her background. Her blood pressure is elevated, an indicator of mild preeclampsia, but there is no other indications of worsening preeclampsia, such as headache, visual disturbances, or epigastric pain.

CN: Management of care; CL: Synthesize

116. 1,2,3,4. Assuring the safety of this client is the top priority. The nurse should begin either intermittent or continuous fetal and contraction monitor depending on the client's risk status. Since the client is 8 cm dilated and a multigravid client, asking other staff members to set up the birthing table would be in order. This client is not a candidate for medication as this may have an influence on the baby. This client is past the point of offering an epidural as she may have given birth by the time the medication is in effect, but comfort measures such as warm or cool cloths, back rubs, etc., may be helpful. The support system is an important aspect of the birthing process and is an easily settled situation. Preparing to give an early report to the oncoming nurse does not apply in this situation.

CN: Management of care; CL: Create

117. 3. In emergency situations, verbal prescriptions should be entered into the **medical record** 📖 or chart and signed immediately after the emergency. The nurse taking this prescription and giving the medication needs to call the **HCP** 📖, explain the prescription and that the medication was administered per the verbal prescription, and request that the HCP write the correct prescription. If the nurse misunderstood the prescription and gave the medication by the wrong route, an incident report will need to be initiated. The charge nurse would become involved if an error has occurred, an incident report is needed, or there is difficulty between the nurse and HCP that cannot be remediated. Rectifying this prescription is the responsibility of the implementing nurse. Waiting until the HCP comes back to the hospital unit may not occur quickly enough to safely care for the client.

CN: Management of care; CL: Synthesize

118. 1,2,4,5. The Code of Ethics describes those actions by the nurse that guide their practice. It is the responsibility of each nurse to be active in determining policy for health care for all citizens and assuring that the way nursing is practiced is of the highest caliber. Nursing needs to participate in the development of health care of the future, while caring for all members of society. In order to be productive in shaping policy, nurses need to be politically astute while growing personally and professionally to meet the needs of clients. The Code of Ethics does not address compensation for work.

CN: Management of care; CL: Apply

119. 2,3. Intact membranes act as a barrier to prevent infections. Once a client's membranes have ruptured, it is important to take precautions to limit introducing bacteria into the genital tract. Using sterile gloves and sterile lubricant for cervical checks help reduce the risk of infection. A sterile speculum is only needed to diagnose if the membranes have ruptured. An amnio hook would only be indicated if the plan was to artificially rupture the membranes. Cervical dilators are not used for cervical checks in labor.

CN: Management of care; CL: Apply

120. 2. The best candidate for a VBAC is a woman who had a cesarean section in her last birth because of a problem related to the infant that is not repeated in this pregnancy. The woman with the breech presentation in her last birth and a vertex pregnancy in this pregnancy would be the best candidate, especially if she had other vaginal births. The woman who was unable to dilate beyond 6 cm (failure to progress) may try a VBAC but is likely to experience the same problem with this birth. The woman with the very large infant is likely to experience cephalopelvic disproportion with this birth if she experienced cephalopelvic disproportion with her last infant who was large. A classic cesarean section scar is a contraindication for a VBAC because that type of scar may not be strong enough to withstand the stress of hours of uterine contractions and may result in a uterine disruption.

CN: Management of care; CL: Analyze

Postpartal Care

- ■ The Postpartal Client with a Vaginal Birth
- ■ The Postpartal Client Who Breast-feeds
- ■ The Postpartal Client Who Bottle-feeds
- ■ The Postpartal Client with a Cesarean Birth
- ■ The Postpartal Client with Complications
- ■ Managing Care, Quality, and Safety of Postpartal Clients
- ■ Answers, Rationales, and Test-Taking Strategies

The Postpartal Client with a Vaginal Birth

1. The nurse from the nursery is bringing a newborn to a mother's room. The nurse took care of the mother yesterday and knows the mother and baby well. The nurse should implement which action next to ensure the safest transition of the infant to the mother?
- ☐ **1.** Assess whether the mother is able to ambulate to care for the infant.
- ☐ **2.** Ask the mother if there is anything else she needs for the care of her baby.
- ☐ **3.** Check the crib to determine if there are enough diapers and formula.
- ☐ **4.** Complete the hospital identification procedure with mother and infant.

2. A client is in the first hour of her recovery after a vaginal birth. During an assessment, the lochia is moderate, is bright red, and is trickling from the vagina. The nurse locates the fundus at the umbilicus; it is firm and midline with no palpable bladder. The client's vital signs remain at their baseline. Based on this information, the nurse would implement which action?
- ☐ **1.** Increase the IV rate.
- ☐ **2.** Recheck the admission hematocrit and hemoglobin levels.
- ☐ **3.** Report the findings to the healthcare provider (HCP).
- ☐ **4.** Document the findings as normal.

3. The nurse is caring for a multigravida woman who is 1 day postpartum following a vaginal birth. Which finding indicates a need for further assessment?
- ☐ **1.** hemoglobin 12.1 g/dL (121 g/L)
- ☐ **2.** WBC count of 15,000 (15 × 10⁹/L)
- ☐ **3.** pulse of 60 beats/min
- ☐ **4.** temperature of 100.8°F (38.2°C)

4. The nurse is providing follow-up care with clients 10 days after the birth of their neonate. The nurse would anticipate what outcomes from the new mother? Select all that apply.
- ☐ **1.** The client feels tired but is able to care for herself and her new infant.
- ☐ **2.** The family has adequate support from one another and others.
- ☐ **3.** Lochia is changing from red to pink and is smaller in amount.
- ☐ **4.** The client feeds the baby every 6 to 8 hours without difficulty.
- ☐ **5.** The client has positive comments about her new infant.

5. A client gave birth vaginally 2 hours ago and has a third-degree laceration. There is ice in place on her perineum. However, her perineum is slightly edematous, and the client is having pain rated 6 on a scale of 1 to 10. Which nursing intervention would be the **most** appropriate at this time?
- ☐ **1.** Begin sitz baths.
- ☐ **2.** Administer pain medication per prescription.
- ☐ **3.** Replace ice packs to the perineum.
- ☐ **4.** Initiate prescription anesthetic sprays to the perineum.

6. A primigravid client gave birth vaginally 2 hours ago with no complications. As the nurse plans care for this postpartum client, which postpartum goal would have the **highest priority**?
- ☐ **1.** By discharge, the family will bond with the neonate.
- ☐ **2.** The nurse will demonstrate self-care and infant care by the end of the shift.
- ☐ **3.** The nurse will state instructions for discharge during the first postpartum day.
- ☐ **4.** By the end of the shift, the nurse will describe a safe home environment.

7. In response to the nurse's question about how she is feeling, a postpartum client states that she is fine. She then begins talking to the baby, checking the diaper, and asking infant care questions. The nurse determines the client is in which postpartal phase of psychological adaptation?
☐ **1.** taking in
☐ **2.** taking on
☐ **3.** taking hold
☐ **4.** letting go

8. A client has admitted use of cocaine prior to beginning labor. After the infant is born, the nurse should anticipate the need to include which actions in the infant's plan of care?
☐ **1.** urine toxicology screening
☐ **2.** notifying hospital security
☐ **3.** limiting contact with visitors
☐ **4.** contacting local law enforcement

9. The nurse is evaluating the client who gave birth vaginally 2 hours ago and is experiencing postpartum pain rated 8 on scale of 1 to 10. The client is a multigravida breast-feeding mother who would like medication to decrease the pain in her uterus. Which of the medications listed on the prescriptions sheet would be the **most** appropriate for this client?
☐ **1.** aspirin 1,000 mg PO every 4 to 6 hour PRN
☐ **2.** ibuprofen 800 mg PO every 6 to 8 hour PRN
☐ **3.** docusate 100 mg PO twice a day
☐ **4.** acetaminophen and hydrocodone 10 mg 1 tab PO every 4 to 6 hour PRN

10. At which location would the nurse expect to palpate the fundus of a primiparous client immediately after birth of a neonate?
☐ **1.** halfway between the umbilicus and the symphysis pubis
☐ **2.** at the level of the umbilicus
☐ **3.** just below the level of the umbilicus
☐ **4.** above the level of the umbilicus

11. When instilling erythromycin ointment into the eyes of a neonate 1 hour old, the nurse would explain to the parents that the medication is used to prevent which problem?
☐ **1.** chorioretinitis from cytomegalovirus
☐ **2.** blindness secondary to gonorrhea
☐ **3.** cataracts from beta-hemolytic streptococcus
☐ **4.** strabismus resulting from neonatal maturation

12. The healthcare provider (HCP) prescribes an intramuscular injection of vitamin K for a term neonate. The nurse explains to the mother that this medication is used to prevent which problem?
☐ **1.** hypoglycemia
☐ **2.** hyperbilirubinemia
☐ **3.** hemorrhage
☐ **4.** polycythemia

13. The nurse assesses a swollen ecchymosed area to the right of an episiotomy on a primiparous client 6 hours after a vaginal birth. The nurse should **next**:
☐ **1.** apply an ice pack to the perineal area.
☐ **2.** assess the client's temperature.
☐ **3.** have the client take a warm sitz bath.
☐ **4.** contact the healthcare provider (HCP) for prescriptions for an antibiotic.

14. Two hours after the vaginal birth under epidural anesthesia, a client with a midline episiotomy ambulates to the bathroom to void. After voiding, the nurse assesses the client's bladder, finding it distended. The nurse interprets this finding based on the understanding that the client's bladder distention is **most** likely caused by which factor?
☐ **1.** prolonged first stage of labor
☐ **2.** urinary tract infection
☐ **3.** pressure of the uterus on the bladder
☐ **4.** edema in the lower urinary tract area

15. A primiparous client who is bottle-feeding her neonate at 12 hours after birth asks the nurse, "When will my menstrual cycle return?" Which response by the nurse would be **most** appropriate?
☐ **1.** "Your menstrual cycle will return in 3 to 4 weeks."
☐ **2.** "It will probably be 6 to 10 weeks before it starts again."
☐ **3.** "You can expect your menses to start in 12 to 14 weeks."
☐ **4.** "Your menses will return in 16 to 18 weeks."

16. While the nurse is preparing to assist the primiparous client to the bathroom to void 6 hours after a vaginal birth under epidural anesthesia, the client says that she feels dizzy when sitting up on the side of the bed. The nurse explains that this is **most** likely caused by which factor?
☐ **1.** effects of the anesthetic during labor
☐ **2.** hemorrhage during the birth process
☐ **3.** effects of analgesics used during labor
☐ **4.** decreased blood volume in the vascular system

17. The nurse enlists the aid of an interpreter when caring for a primiparous client from Mexico who speaks only Spanish and gave birth to a term neonate 8 hours ago. When developing the postpartum dietary plan of care for the client, the nurse would encourage the client's intake of which foods?
☐ **1.** tomatoes
☐ **2.** potatoes
☐ **3.** corn products
☐ **4.** meat products

18. Three hours postpartum, a primiparous client's fundus is firm and midline. On perineal inspection, the nurse observes a small, constant trickle of blood. Which condition should the nurse assess further?
- [ ] **1.** retained placental tissue
- [ ] **2.** uterine inversion
- [ ] **3.** bladder distention
- [ ] **4.** perineal lacerations

19. At a postpartum checkup 11 days after childbirth, the nurse asks the client about the color of her lochia. Which color is expected?
- [ ] **1.** dark red
- [ ] **2.** pink
- [ ] **3.** brown
- [ ] **4.** white

20. After instructing a primiparous client about episiotomy care, which client statement indicates successful teaching?
- [ ] **1.** "I will use hot, sudsy water to clean the episiotomy area."
- [ ] **2.** "I wipe the area from front to back using a blotting motion."
- [ ] **3.** "Before bedtime, I will use a cold water sitz bath."
- [ ] **4.** "I can use ice packs for 3 to 4 days after birth."

21. A primiparous client, 20 hours after childbirth, asks the nurse about starting postpartum exercises. Which instruction would be **most** appropriate to include in the plan of care?
- [ ] **1.** Start in a sitting position, then lie back, and return to a sitting position, repeating this five times.
- [ ] **2.** Assume a prone position, and then do push-ups by using the arms to lift the upper body.
- [ ] **3.** Flex the knees while supine, and then inhale deeply and exhale while contracting the abdominal muscles.
- [ ] **4.** Flex the knees while supine, and then bring chin to chest while exhaling and reach for the knees by lifting the head and shoulders while inhaling.

22. A multiparous client whose fundus is firm and midline at the umbilicus 8 hours after a vaginal birth tells the nurse that when she ambulated to the bathroom after sleeping for 4 hours, her dark red lochia seemed heavier. Which information would the nurse include when explaining to the client about the increased lochia on ambulation?
- [ ] **1.** Her bleeding needs to be reported to the healthcare provider (HCP) immediately.
- [ ] **2.** The increased lochia occurs from lochia pooling in the vaginal vault.
- [ ] **3.** The increase in lochia may be an early sign of postpartum hemorrhage.
- [ ] **4.** This increase in lochia usually indicates retained placental fragments.

23. A primiparous client who gave birth vaginally 8 hours ago desires to take a shower. The nurse anticipates remaining near the client to assess for which problem?
- [ ] **1.** fatigue
- [ ] **2.** fainting
- [ ] **3.** diuresis
- [ ] **4.** hygiene needs

24. A primiparous client who gave birth 12 hours ago under epidural anesthesia with a midline episiotomy tells the nurse that she is experiencing a great deal of discomfort when she sits in a chair with the baby. Which instructions would be **most** appropriate?
- [ ] **1.** "Ask for some pain medication before you sit down."
- [ ] **2.** "Squeeze your buttock muscles together before sitting down."
- [ ] **3.** "Keep a relaxed posture before sitting down with your full weight."
- [ ] **4.** "Ask the healthcare provider for some analgesic cream or spray."

25. Which information would the nurse include in the primiparous client's discharge teaching plan about measures to provide visual stimulation for the neonate?
- [ ] **1.** Maintain eye contact while talking to the baby.
- [ ] **2.** Paint the baby's room in bright colors accented with teddy bears.
- [ ] **3.** Use brightly colored animals and cartoon figures on the wall.
- [ ] **4.** Move a brightly colored rattle in front of the baby's eyes.

26. A primiparous client has just given birth to a healthy male infant. The client and her husband are Muslim, and the husband begins chanting a song while holding the neonate. How does the nurse interpret the father's actions?
- [ ] **1.** thanking Allah for giving him a male heir
- [ ] **2.** singing to his son from the Koran in praise of Allah
- [ ] **3.** expressing appreciation that his wife and son are healthy
- [ ] **4.** performing a ritual similar to baptism in other religions

27. An adolescent primiparous client 24 hours postpartum asks the nurse how often she can hold her baby without "spoiling" him. Which response would be **most** appropriate?
- [ ] **1.** "Hold him when he is fussy or crying."
- [ ] **2.** "Hold him as much as you want to hold him."
- [ ] **3.** "Try to hold him infrequently to avoid overstimulation."
- [ ] **4.** "You can hold him periodically throughout the day."

28. On the first postpartum day, the primiparous client reports perineal pain of 5 on a scale of 1 to 10 that was unrelieved by ibuprofen 800 mg given 2 hours ago. The nurse should further assess the client for:
☐ 1. puerperal infection.
☐ 2. vaginal lacerations.
☐ 3. history of drug abuse.
☐ 4. perineal hematoma.

29. The nurse assigns an unlicensed assistive personnel (UAP) to care for a client who is 1 day postpartum. Which tasks would be appropriate to delegate to this person? Select all that apply.
☐ 1. changing the perineal pad and reporting the drainage
☐ 2. teaching the mother to latch the infant onto the breast
☐ 3. checking the location of the fundus prior to ambulating the client
☐ 4. reinforcing good hygiene while assisting the client with washing the perineum
☐ 5. discussing postpartum depression with the client who is found crying
☐ 6. assisting the client with ambulation shortly after birth

30. While the nurse is caring for a primiparous client on the first postpartum day, the client asks, "How is that woman doing who lost her baby from prematurity? We were in labor together." Which response by the nurse would be **most** appropriate?
☐ 1. Ignore the client's question and continue with morning care.
☐ 2. Tell the client, "I'm not sure how the other woman is doing today."
☐ 3. Tell the client, "I need to ask the woman's permission before discussing her well-being."
☐ 4. Explain to the client that "Nurses are not allowed to discuss other clients on the unit."

31. A newly postpartum primiparous client asks the nurse, "Can my baby see?" Which statement about neonatal vision should the nurse include in the explanation?
☐ 1. Neonates primarily focus on moving objects.
☐ 2. They can see objects up to 12 inches (30.5 cm) away.
☐ 3. Usually they see clearly by about 2 days after birth.
☐ 4. Neonates primarily distinguish light from dark.

32. While assessing the fundus of a multiparous client 36 hours after birth of a term neonate, the nurse notes a separation of the abdominal muscles. The nurse should tell the client:
☐ 1. that she will have a surgical repair at 6 weeks postpartum.
☐ 2. to remain on bed rest until resolution occurs.
☐ 3. that the separation will resolve on its own with the right posture and diet.
☐ 4. to perform exercises involving head and shoulder raising in a lying position.

33. A postpartum client gave birth 6 hours ago without anesthesia and just voided 100 mL. The nurse palpates the fundus two fingerbreadths above the umbilicus and off to the right side. What should the nurse do **first**?
☐ 1. Administer ibuprofen.
☐ 2. Reassess in 1 hour.
☐ 3. Catheterize the client.
☐ 4. Obtain a prescription for a fluid bolus.

34. While the nurse is assessing the fundus of a multiparous client who gave birth 24 hours ago, the client asks, "What can I do to get rid of these stretch marks?" Which response would be **most** appropriate?
☐ 1. "As long as you do not get pregnant again, the marks will disappear completely."
☐ 2. "They usually fade to a silvery-white color over a period of time."
☐ 3. "You will need to use a specially prescribed cream to help them disappear."
☐ 4. "If you lose the weight you gained during pregnancy, the marks will fade to a pale pink."

35. A primiparous client who gave vaginal birth to a viable term neonate 48 hours ago has a midline episiotomy and repair of a third-degree laceration. When preparing the client for discharge, which assessment would be **most** important?
☐ 1. constipation
☐ 2. diarrhea
☐ 3. excessive bleeding
☐ 4. rectal fistulas

36. In preparation for discharge, the nurse discusses sexual issues with a multiparous client who had a routine vaginal birth with a midline episiotomy. The client asked, "I've heard recommendations about when to resume intercourse have changed since my last baby. What are they saying now?" When should the nurse instruct the client that she can resume sexual intercourse?
☐ 1. in 6 weeks when the episiotomy is completely healed
☐ 2. after a postpartum check by the healthcare provider (HCP)
☐ 3. whenever the client is feeling amorous and desirable
☐ 4. when lochia flow and episiotomy pain have stopped

37. While caring for a multiparous client 4 hours after vaginal birth of a term neonate, the nurse notes that the mother's temperature is 99.8°F (37.2°C), the pulse is 66 beats/min, and the respirations are 18 breaths/min. Her fundus is firm, midline, and at the level of the umbilicus. The nurse should:
☐ 1. continue to monitor the client's vital signs.
☐ 2. assess the client's lochia for large clots.
☐ 3. notify the client's healthcare provider (HCP) about the findings.
☐ 4. offer the mother an ice pack for her forehead.

38. While assessing the episiotomy site of a primiparous client on the first postpartum day, the nurse observes a fairly large hemorrhoid at the client's rectum. After instructing the client about measures to relieve hemorrhoid discomfort, which client statement indicates the need for additional teaching?
- ☐ **1.** "I should ask my healthcare provider about using a stool softener."
- ☐ **2.** "Analgesic sprays and witch hazel pads can relieve the pain."
- ☐ **3.** "I should lie on my back as much as possible to relieve the pain."
- ☐ **4.** "I should drink lots of water and eat foods that have a lot of roughage."

39. A primiparous client is on a regular diet 24 hours postpartum. She is from Guatemala and speaks only Spanish. The client's mother asks the nurse if she can bring her daughter some "special foods from home." The nurse responds based on the understanding about which principle?
- ☐ **1.** Foods from home are generally discouraged on the postpartum unit.
- ☐ **2.** The mother can bring the daughter any foods that she desires.
- ☐ **3.** This is permissible as long as the foods are nutritious and high in iron.
- ☐ **4.** The client's healthcare provider (HCP) needs to give permission for the foods.

40. A primiparous client, 48 hours after a vaginal birth, is to be discharged with a prescription for vitamins with iron because she is anemic. To maximize absorption of the iron, the nurse instructs the client to take the medication with which liquid?
- ☐ **1.** orange juice
- ☐ **2.** herbal tea
- ☐ **3.** milk
- ☐ **4.** grape juice

41. The nurse is caring for a multiparous client after vaginal birth of a set of male twins 2 hours ago. The nurse should encourage the mother and partner to:
- ☐ **1.** bottle-feed the twins to prevent exhaustion and fatigue.
- ☐ **2.** plan for each parent to spend equal amounts of time with each twin.
- ☐ **3.** avoid assistance from other family members until attachment occurs.
- ☐ **4.** relate to each twin individually to enhance the attachment process.

42. Twelve hours after a vaginal birth with epidural anesthesia, the nurse palpates the fundus of a primiparous client and finds it to be firm, above the umbilicus, and deviated to the right. What should the nurse do **next**?
- ☐ **1.** Document this as a normal finding in the client's record.
- ☐ **2.** Contact the healthcare provider (HCP) for a prescription for oxytocin.
- ☐ **3.** Encourage the client to ambulate to the bathroom and void.
- ☐ **4.** Gently massage the fundus to expel the clots.

43. A nurse is discussing discharge instructions with a client. Which statement indicates that the client understands the resources and information available if needed after discharge? Select all that apply.
- ☐ **1.** "My fertility can return as early as 21 days after my baby's birth."
- ☐ **2.** "I have the hospital phone number if I have any questions."
- ☐ **3.** "If I have any breathing problems, chest pain, or pounding fast heart rate, I will seek medical assistance."
- ☐ **4.** "My mother is coming to help for a month, so I will be fine."
- ☐ **5.** "I know if I get fever or chills or change in lochia to call the healthcare provider."
- ☐ **6.** "I will continue my prenatal vitamins until my postpartum checkup or longer."

The Postpartal Client Who Breast-feeds

44. The nurse is reviewing discharge instructions with a postpartum breast-feeding client who is going home. She has chosen depot medroxyprogesterone acetate (DMPA) as birth control. Which statement by the client identifies that she needs further instruction concerning birth control?
- ☐ **1.** "I will wait for my 6-week checkup to get my first DMPA injection."
- ☐ **2.** "DMPA injections last for 90 days."
- ☐ **3.** "My milk supply should be well established before receiving a birth control injection."
- ☐ **4.** "You will give me my first DMPA injection before I leave today."

45. A postpartum primiparous client is having difficulty breast-feeding her infant. The infant latches on to the breast, but the mother's nipples are extremely sore during and after each feeding. The client needs further instruction about breast-feeding when she states:
- ☐ **1.** "The baby needs to have as much of the nipple and areola in the mouth as possible to prevent sore and cracked nipples."
- ☐ **2.** "I can put breast milk on my nipples to heal the sore areas."
- ☐ **3.** "As long as some of my nipple is in the baby's mouth, the baby will receive enough milk."
- ☐ **4.** "Feeding the baby for a half-hour on each side will not make my breasts sore."

46. The nurse is caring for a primipara who gave birth yesterday and has chosen to breast-feed her neonate. Which assessment finding is considered unusual for the client at this point postpartum?
☐ **1.** milk production
☐ **2.** diaphoresis
☐ **3.** constipation
☐ **4.** diuresis

47. The nurse is caring for several mother-baby couplets. In planning the care for each of the couplets, which mother would the nurse expect to have the **most** severe afterbirth pains?
☐ **1.** G4, P1 client who is breast-feeding her infant
☐ **2.** G3, P3 client who is breast-feeding her infant
☐ **3.** G2, P2 cesarean client who is bottle-feeding her infant
☐ **4.** G3, P3 client who is bottle-feeding her infant

48. A breast-feeding client is seen at home by the visiting nurse 10 days after a vaginal birth. The client has a warm, red, painful breast, a temperature of 100°F (37.7°C), and flu-like symptoms. What should the nurse do?
☐ **1.** Encourage the client to breast-feed her infant using the unaffected breast.
☐ **2.** Refer the woman to her healthcare provider (HCP).
☐ **3.** Inform the client that she needs to discontinue breast-feeding.
☐ **4.** Instruct the woman to apply warm compresses to the affected breast.

49. A diabetic postpartum client plans to breast-feed. The nurse determines that the client's understanding of breast-feeding instructions is sufficient when she states:
☐ **1.** "Insulin will be transferred to the baby through breast milk."
☐ **2.** "Breast-feeding is not recommended for diabetic mothers."
☐ **3.** "Breast milk from diabetic mothers contains few antibodies."
☐ **4.** "Breast-feeding will assist in lowering maternal blood glucose."

50. A 1-day-old breast-fed infant has a bilirubin level that is at an intermediate risk for jaundice. Which statement by the infant's mother indicates an understanding of the teaching regarding jaundice?
☐ **1.** "I should breast-feed my baby as often as possible."
☐ **2.** "I should supplement with formula after every feeding."
☐ **3.** "I should discontinue breast-feeding and change to formula feeding."
☐ **4.** "I should place my baby in direct sunlight several times a day."

51. During a home visit, a breast-feeding client asks the nurse what contraception method she and her partner should use until she has her 6-week postpartal examination. Which method would be **most** appropriate for the nurse to suggest?
☐ **1.** condom with spermicide
☐ **2.** oral contraceptives
☐ **3.** rhythm method
☐ **4.** abstinence

52. A primiparous client who is beginning to breast-feed her neonate asks the nurse, "Is it important for my baby to get colostrum?" When instructing the client, the nurse would explain that colostrum provides the neonate with:
☐ **1.** more fat than breast milk.
☐ **2.** vitamin K, which the neonate lacks.
☐ **3.** delayed meconium passage.
☐ **4.** passive immunity from maternal antibodies.

53. Which principle forms the basis for the teaching plan about avoiding nonprescription medication for a primiparous client who is breast-feeding?
☐ **1.** Breast milk quality and richness are decreased.
☐ **2.** The mother's motivation to breast-feed is diminished.
☐ **3.** Medications may be excreted in breast milk to the nursing neonate.
☐ **4.** Medications interfere with the mother's let-down reflex.

54. A breast-feeding primiparous client with a midline episiotomy is prescribed ibuprofen 200 mg orally. The nurse instructs the client to take the medication:
☐ **1.** before going to bed.
☐ **2.** midway between feedings.
☐ **3.** immediately after a feeding.
☐ **4.** when providing supplemental formula.

55. A multiparous client, 28 hours after cesarean birth, who is breast-feeding has severe cramps or afterpains. The nurse explains that these are caused by:
☐ **1.** flatulence accumulation after a cesarean birth.
☐ **2.** healing of the abdominal incision after cesarean birth.
☐ **3.** adverse effects of the medications administered after birth.
☐ **4.** release of oxytocin during the breast-feeding session.

56. After the nurse counsels a primiparous, breast-feeding client about diet and nutritional needs during the lactation period, which client statement indicates a need for additional teaching?
☐ **1.** "I need to increase my intake of vitamin D."
☐ **2.** "I should drink at least five glasses of fluid daily."
☐ **3.** "I need to get an extra 500 cal/day."
☐ **4.** "I need to make sure I have enough calcium in my diet."

57. A breast-feeding primiparous client asks the nurse how breast milk differs from cow's milk. The nurse responds by saying that breast milk is higher in which nutrient?
- ☐ **1.** fat
- ☐ **2.** iron
- ☐ **3.** sodium
- ☐ **4.** calcium

58. While assisting a primiparous client with her first breast-feeding session, which action should the nurse instruct the mother to do to stimulate the neonate to open the mouth and grasp the nipple?
- ☐ **1.** Pull down gently on the neonate's chin, and insert the nipple.
- ☐ **2.** Squeeze both of the neonate's cheeks simultaneously.
- ☐ **3.** Place the nipple into the neonate's mouth on top of the tongue.
- ☐ **4.** Brush the neonate's lips lightly with the nipple.

59. A 25-year-old primiparous client who gave birth 2 hours ago has decided to breast-feed her neonate. Which instructions should the nurse address as the highest **priority** in the teaching plan about preventing nipple soreness?
- ☐ **1.** keeping plastic liners in the brassiere to keep the nipple drier
- ☐ **2.** placing as much of the areola as possible into the baby's mouth
- ☐ **3.** smoothly pulling the nipple out of the mouth after 10 minutes
- ☐ **4.** removing any remaining milk left on the nipple with a soft washcloth

60. Which client statement indicates effective teaching about burping a breast-fed neonate?
- ☐ **1.** "Breast-fed babies who are burped frequently will take more on each breast."
- ☐ **2.** "If I supplement the baby with formula, I will rarely have to burp the baby."
- ☐ **3.** "I will breast-feed my baby every 3 hours so I will not have to burp the baby."
- ☐ **4.** "When I switch to the other breast, I will burp the baby."

61. After the nurse teaches a primiparous client planning to return to work in 6 weeks about storing breast milk, which client statement indicates the need for further teaching?
- ☐ **1.** "I can safely store my milk at room temperature for 8 hours."
- ☐ **2.** "I will be sure to label the milk with the date, time, and amount."
- ☐ **3.** "I must discard any breast milk stored for more than 3 days in the refrigerator."
- ☐ **4.** "I can keep the milk in a deep freeze in clean glass bottles for up to 1 year."

62. During a home visit on the fourth postpartum day, a primiparous client tells the nurse that she is aware of a "letdown sensation" in her breasts and asks what causes it. The nurse explains that the letdown sensation is stimulated by which hormone?
- ☐ **1.** progesterone
- ☐ **2.** estrogen
- ☐ **3.** prolactin
- ☐ **4.** oxytocin

63. During a home visit on the fourth postpartum day, a primiparous client tells the nurse that she has been experiencing breast engorgement. To relieve engorgement, the nurse teaches the client to use which intervention before nursing her baby?
- ☐ **1.** Apply an ice cube to the nipples.
- ☐ **2.** Rub her nipples gently with lanolin cream.
- ☐ **3.** Express a small amount of breast milk.
- ☐ **4.** Offer the neonate a small amount of formula.

64. A breast-feeding primiparous client who gave birth 8 hours ago asks the nurse, "How will I know that my baby is getting enough to eat?" Which guideline should the nurse include in the teaching plan as evidence of adequate intake?
- ☐ **1.** six to eight wet diapers by the 5th day
- ☐ **2.** three to four transitional stools on the 4th day
- ☐ **3.** ability to fall asleep easily after feeding on the first day
- ☐ **4.** regain of lost birth weight by the 3rd day

65. Which information should the nurse include in the teaching plan for a primiparous client who asks about weaning her neonate?
- ☐ **1.** "Wait until you have breast-fed for at least 4 months."
- ☐ **2.** "Eliminate the baby's favorite feeding times first."
- ☐ **3.** "Plan to omit the daytime feedings last."
- ☐ **4.** "Gradually eliminate one feeding at a time."

66. A nurse is caring for a client who is 3 days postpartum and breast-feeding her baby girl. The following assessment is made by the nurse: episiotomy area: red and edematous; breasts: firm and tender on palpation; fundus: firm 2 finger breaths below umbilicus. What nursing actions are indicated? Select all that apply.
- ☐ **1.** Suggest the client apply cool compress to breasts.
- ☐ **2.** Encourage the client to sit on a supportive device.
- ☐ **3.** Ask the client how often the baby feeds.
- ☐ **4.** Suggest the client take cool sitz baths twice a day.
- ☐ **5.** Obtain specimen for culture and sensitivity from episiotomy site.

67. Two weeks after a breast-feeding primiparous client is discharged, she calls the birthing center and says that she is afraid she is "losing my breast milk. The baby had been nursing every 4 hours, but now she is crying to be fed every 2 hours." The nurse interprets the neonate's behavior as **most** likely caused by which factor?
☐ 1. lack of adequate intake to meet maternal nutritional needs
☐ 2. the mother's fears about the baby's weight gain
☐ 3. preventing the neonate from sucking long enough with each feeding
☐ 4. the neonate's temporary growth spurt, which requires more feedings

68. During a home visit to a breast-feeding primiparous client at 1 week postpartum, the client tells the nurse that her nipples have become sore and cracked from the feedings. Which instruction should the nurse give the client?
☐ 1. Wipe off any lanolin creams from the nipple before each feeding.
☐ 2. Position the baby with the entire areola in the baby's mouth.
☐ 3. Feed the baby less often for the next several days.
☐ 4. Use a mild soap while in the shower to prevent an infection.

69. A new father indicates he feels left out of the new family relationship since he is not able to bond the same way as the breast-feeding mother. What is the **most** appropriate response by the nurse?
☐ 1. "This is normal, and these feelings will go away within a few days."
☐ 2. "Holding, talking to, and playing with the infant will facilitate bonding between baby and Dad."
☐ 3. "Bonding occurs later in the first year of life, and Dad can become involved when the infant is better able to recognize him."
☐ 4. "Maternal infant bonding takes priority over paternal infant bonding."

70. The triage nurse in the pediatrician's office returns a call to a mother who is breast-feeding her 4-day-old infant. The mother is concerned about the yellow seedy stool that has developed since discharge home. What is the **best** reply by the nurse?
☐ 1. "This type of stool indicates the infant may have diarrhea and should be seen in the office today."
☐ 2. "The stool will transition into a soft, brown, formed stool within a few days and is appropriate for breast-feeding."
☐ 3. "The stool results from the gassy food eaten by the mother. Refrain from eating these foods while breast-feeding."
☐ 4. "Soft seedy unformed stools with each feeding are normal for this age infant and will continue through breast-feeding."

The Postpartal Client Who Bottle-feeds

71. The nurse is assessing a client at her postpartum checkup 6 weeks after a vaginal birth. The mother is bottle-feeding her baby. Which client finding indicates a problem at this time?
☐ 1. firm fundus at the symphysis
☐ 2. white, thick vaginal discharge
☐ 3. striae that are silver in color
☐ 4. soft breasts without milk

72. A client gave birth 2 days ago and has been given instructions on breast care for bottle-feeding mothers. Which statement indicates that the nurse should reinforce the instructions to the client?
☐ 1. "I will wear a sports bra or a well-fitting bra for several days."
☐ 2. "When showering, I will direct water onto my shoulders."
☐ 3. "I will use only water to clean my nipples."
☐ 4. "I will use a breast pump to remove any milk that may appear."

73. A 24-year-old primipara who has given birth to a healthy neonate plans to bottle-feed her neonate. What information regarding normal weight gain should the nurse include in the teaching plan?
☐ 1. A baby normally loses 15% of weight before beginning to gain weight.
☐ 2. Adding rice cereal to the bottle is a good way to increase calories if weight gain is slow.
☐ 3. Gaining 30 g/day is a normal weight gain pattern.
☐ 4. Babies typically double birth weight by 3 months.

74. A primiparous client with a neonate who is 36 hours old asks the nurse, "Why does my baby spit up a small amount of formula after feeding?" The nurse explains that the regurgitation is thought to result from which factor?
☐ 1. an immature cardiac sphincter
☐ 2. a defect in the gastrointestinal system
☐ 3. burping the infant too frequently
☐ 4. moving the infant during the feeding

75. A primiparous client who will be bottle-feeding her neonate asks, "What is the **best** position for the baby after feeding?" Which position should the nurse recommend?
☐ 1. supine position
☐ 2. on the left side
☐ 3. prone without a pillow
☐ 4. sitting on the caregiver's lap for 20 minutes

76. A primiparous client who is bottle-feeding her neonate asks, "When should I start giving the baby solid foods?" The nurse instructs the client to introduce solid foods no sooner than at which age?
- ☐ **1.** 2 months
- ☐ **2.** 6 months
- ☐ **3.** 8 months
- ☐ **4.** 10 months

77. After instructing a primiparous client who is bottle-feeding about burping, which client statement indicates that the client needs further teaching?
- ☐ **1.** "I will burp him after 15 minutes of feeding him formula."
- ☐ **2.** "After he takes one-half ounce of formula, I will burp him."
- ☐ **3.** "I will burp him while he is in an upright position."
- ☐ **4.** "I will gently pat his back to get him to burp."

78. When teaching a primiparous client about the growth and development of the neonate, the nurse should explain that **most** babies are able to drink independently from a sippy cup at what age?
- ☐ **1.** 5 to 7 months
- ☐ **2.** 8 to 10 months
- ☐ **3.** 12 to 14 months
- ☐ **4.** 15 to 16 months

The Postpartal Client with a Cesarean Birth

79. The nurse is assessing a cesarean section client who gave birth 12 hours ago. Findings include a distended abdomen with faint bowel sounds × 1 quadrant, fundus firm at umbilicus, lochia scant, rubra, and pain rated 2 on a scale of 1 to 10. The IV and Foley catheter have been discontinued, and the client received medication 3 hours ago for pain. The client can have pain medication every 3 to 4 hours. The nurse should **first:**
- ☐ **1.** give the client pain medication.
- ☐ **2.** have the client use the incentive spirometry.
- ☐ **3.** ambulate the client from the bed to the hallway and back.
- ☐ **4.** encourage the client to begin caring for her baby.

80. Carboprost was injected into the uterus of a client to treat uterine atony during a cesarean section. In preparing to care for this client postpartum, the nurse should assess the client for which common adverse effects of the medication?
- ☐ **1.** vertigo and confusion
- ☐ **2.** nausea and diarrhea
- ☐ **3.** restlessness and increased vaginal bleeding
- ☐ **4.** headache and hypertension

81. A multigravida 30-year-old woman has given cesarean birth to a healthy term female neonate due to an abnormal fetal heart rate tracing. At 2 hours postpartum, the nurse assesses the client's Foley catheter and observes that the client's urine is slightly red-tinged. What should the nurse do **next**?
- ☐ **1.** Continue to monitor the client's input and output.
- ☐ **2.** Palpate the client's fundus gently every 15 minutes.
- ☐ **3.** Assess the placement of the Foley catheter.
- ☐ **4.** Contact the client's healthcare provider (HCP) for further instructions.

82. Four hours after cesarean birth of a neonate weighing 8 lb, 13 oz (4,000 g), the primiparous client asks, "If I get pregnant again, will I need to have a cesarean?" When responding to the client, the nurse should base the response to the client about vaginal birth after cesarean (VBAC) on which standard of practice?
- ☐ **1.** VBAC may be possible if the client has not had a classic uterine incision.
- ☐ **2.** A history of rapid labor is a necessary criterion for VBAC.
- ☐ **3.** A low transverse incision contraindicates the possibility for VBAC.
- ☐ **4.** VBAC is not possible because the neonate was large for gestational age.

83. A primiparous client who underwent a cesarean birth 30 minutes ago is to receive Rho (D) immune globulin (RhoGAM). The nurse should administer the medication within which time frame after birth?
- ☐ **1.** 24 hours
- ☐ **2.** 48 hours
- ☐ **3.** 72 hours
- ☐ **4.** 96 hours

84. While the nurse is caring for a primiparous client with cephalopelvic disproportion 4 hours after a cesarean birth, the client requests assistance in breast-feeding. To promote maximum maternal comfort, which position would be **most** appropriate for the nurse to suggest?
- ☐ **1.** football hold
- ☐ **2.** scissors hold
- ☐ **3.** cross-cradle hold
- ☐ **4.** cradle hold

The Postpartal Client with Complications

85. A multigravid client gave birth vaginally 2 hours ago. A family member notifies the nurse that the client is pale and shaky. Which are the **priority** assessments for the nurse to make?
- ☐ **1.** Blood glucose and vital signs
- ☐ **2.** Temperature and level of consciousness
- ☐ **3.** Uterine infection and pain
- ☐ **4.** fundus and lochia

86. A postpartum woman has unrelenting pain in her rectum after vaginal birth despite administration of pain medications. Which action is **most** indicated?
- ☐ **1.** administering additional pain medications
- ☐ **2.** assessing the perineum
- ☐ **3.** reassuring the client that pain is normal after vaginal birth
- ☐ **4.** preparing a warm sitz bath for the client

87. A multiparous client at 24 hours postpartum is found to have a swelling and pain in her right leg. She demonstrates a positive Homans sign with discomfort. The nurse should:
- ☐ **1.** place a cold pack on the client's perineal area.
- ☐ **2.** place the client in semi-Fowler's position.
- ☐ **3.** notify the client's healthcare provider (HCP) immediately.
- ☐ **4.** ask the client to ambulate around the room.

88. Prophylactic heparin therapy is prescribed to treat thrombophlebitis in a multiparous client who gave birth 24 hours ago. After instructing the client about the medication, the nurse determines that the client understands the instructions when she states which as the purpose of the drug?
- ☐ **1.** to thin the blood clots
- ☐ **2.** to increase the lochial flow
- ☐ **3.** to increase the perspiration for diuresis
- ☐ **4.** to prevent further blood clot formation

89. While caring for a the postpartum client who is receiving treatment with bed rest and intravenous heparin therapy for a deep vein thrombosis, the nurse should contact the client's healthcare provider (HCP) immediately if the client exhibited which symptom?
- ☐ **1.** pain in her calf
- ☐ **2.** dyspnea
- ☐ **3.** hypertension
- ☐ **4.** bradycardia

90. A primiparous client 3 days postpartum is to be discharged on heparin therapy. After teaching her about possible adverse effects of heparin therapy, the nurse determines that the client needs further instruction when she states that the adverse effects include which symptom?
- ☐ **1.** epistaxis
- ☐ **2.** bleeding gums
- ☐ **3.** slow pulse
- ☐ **4.** petechiae

91. After being treated with heparin therapy for thrombophlebitis, a multiparous client who gave birth 4 days ago is to be discharged on oral warfarin. After teaching the client about the medication and possible effects, which client statement indicates successful teaching?
- ☐ **1.** "I can take two aspirin if I get uterine cramps."
- ☐ **2.** "Protamine sulfate should be available if I need it."
- ☐ **3.** "I should use a soft toothbrush to brush my teeth."
- ☐ **4.** "I can drink an occasional glass of wine if I desire."

92. A nurse is explaining basic principles of asepsis and infection control to a client who has a respiratory tract infection following birth. The nurse determines the client understands principles of infection control to follow when the client says:
- ☐ **1.** "I must ask visitors to wear a mask."
- ☐ **2.** "I must wear gloves when I handle my baby."
- ☐ **3.** "I must use individual client care equipment."
- ☐ **4.** "I must practice frequent handwashing."

93. The nurse is caring for a woman who gave birth vaginally 4 hours ago. Which factors would likely contribute to the development of endometritis in this woman? Select all that apply.
- ☐ **1.** manual removal of placenta
- ☐ **2.** in-and-out catheterization during labor
- ☐ **3.** epidural use
- ☐ **4.** prolonged labor
- ☐ **5.** placement of fetal scalp electrode

94. A postpartum multiparous client diagnosed with endometritis is to receive intravenous antibiotic therapy with ampicillin. Before administering this drug, the nurse must take which action?
- ☐ **1.** Ask the client if she has any drug allergies.
- ☐ **2.** Assess the client's pulse rate.
- ☐ **3.** Place the client in a side-lying position.
- ☐ **4.** Check the client's perineal pad.

95. Which intervention would be **most** important for the nurse to encourage in a primiparous client diagnosed with endometritis who is receiving intravenous antibiotic therapy?
- ☐ **1.** Ambulate to the bathroom frequently.
- ☐ **2.** Discontinue breast-feeding temporarily.
- ☐ **3.** Maintain bed rest in Fowler's position.
- ☐ **4.** Restrict visitors to prevent contamination.

96. Which measure would the nurse expect to include in the teaching plan for a multiparous client who gave birth 24 hours ago and is receiving intravenous antibiotic therapy for cystitis?
- ☐ **1.** Limiting fluid intake to 1 L daily to prevent overload
- ☐ **2.** Emptying the bladder every 2 to 4 hours while awake
- ☐ **3.** Washing the perineum with povidone-iodine after voiding
- ☐ **4.** Avoiding the intake of acidic fruit juices until the treatment is discontinued

97. A primiparous client diagnosed with cystitis at 48 hours postpartum who is receiving intravenous ampicillin asks the nurse, "Can I still continue to breast-feed my baby?" The nurse should tell the client:
☐ 1. "You can continue to breast-feed as long as you want to do so."
☐ 2. "Alternate your breast-feeding with formula feeding to help you rest."
☐ 3. "You will need to discontinue breast-feeding until the antibiotic therapy is stopped."
☐ 4. "You will need to modify your technique by manually pumping your breasts."

98. Four days after a vaginal birth, a client has excessive lochia rubra with clots. The healthcare provider (HCP) prescribes carboprost 0.25 mg intramuscularly. Which statement by the client reflects the need for more teaching about carboprost?
☐ 1. "This medication may cause nausea and vomiting."
☐ 2. "This medication sometimes causes hypotension that leads to dizziness."
☐ 3. "I will also receive medication to help prevent severe diarrhea."
☐ 4. "I may run a fever after being treated with carboprost."

99. During the first hour postpartum, assessment of a multiparous client who gave cesarean birth to a neonate weighing 10 lb, 2 oz (4,593 g) reveals a soft fundus with excessive lochia rubra. The nurse should include which interventions in the client's plan of care?
☐ 1. administration of intravenous oxytocin
☐ 2. placement of the client in a side-lying position
☐ 3. rigorous fundal massage every 5 minutes
☐ 4. preparation for an emergency hysterectomy

100. A primiparous client who was diagnosed with hydramnios and breech presentation while in early labor is diagnosed with early postpartum hemorrhage at 1 hour after a cesarean birth. The client asks, "Why am I bleeding so much?" The nurse responds based on the understanding that the **most** likely cause of uterine atony in this client is which factor?
☐ 1. trauma during labor and birth
☐ 2. moderate fundal massage after birth
☐ 3. lengthy and prolonged second stage of labor
☐ 4. overdistention of the uterus from hydramnios

101. Thirty-six hours after a vaginal birth, a multiparous client is diagnosed with endometritis. When assessing the client, which symptom would the nurse expect to find?
☐ 1. profuse amounts of lochia
☐ 2. abdominal distention
☐ 3. nausea and vomiting
☐ 4. fever greater than 100.4°F (38.0°C)

102. A multiparous client visits the urgent care center 5 days after a vaginal birth, experiencing persistent lochia rubra in a moderate to heavy amount. The client asks the nurse, "Why am I continuing to bleed like this?" The nurse should instruct the client that this type of postpartum bleeding is **most** likely caused by which problem?
☐ 1. uterine atony
☐ 2. cervical lacerations
☐ 3. vaginal lacerations
☐ 4. retained placental fragments

103. A 26-year-old primiparous client is seen in the urgent care clinic 2 weeks after giving birth to a viable female neonate. The client, who is breast-feeding, is diagnosed with mastitis of the right breast. The client asks the nurse, "Can I continue breast-feeding?" The nurse should tell the client:
☐ 1. "You can continue to breast-feed, feeding your baby more frequently."
☐ 2. "You can continue once your symptoms begin to decrease."
☐ 3. "You must discontinue breast-feeding until antibiotic therapy is completed."
☐ 4. "You must stop breast-feeding because the breast is contaminated."

104. A primiparous client who had a vaginal birth 1 hour ago voices anxiety because she has a nephew with Down syndrome. After teaching the client about Down syndrome, which client statement indicates the need for additional teaching?
☐ 1. "Down syndrome is an abnormality that can result from a missing chromosome."
☐ 2. "Down syndrome usually results in some degree of mental retardation."
☐ 3. "There are several methods available to determine whether my baby has Down syndrome."
☐ 4. "Older mothers are more likely to have a baby with chromosomal abnormalities."

105. A 15-year-old unmarried primiparous client is being cared for in the hospital's birthing center after vaginal birth of a viable neonate. The neonate is being placed for adoption through a social service agency. Four hours postpartum, the client asks if she can feed her baby. Which of the response would be **most** appropriate?
☐ 1. "I will bring the baby to you for feeding."
☐ 2. "I think we should ask your healthcare provider (HCP) if this is a good idea."
☐ 3. "It is not a good idea for you to have any contact with the baby."
☐ 4. "I will check with the social worker to see if the adopting parents will permit this."

106. After teaching a primiparous client about treatment and self-care of mastitis of the right breast, the nurse determines that the client needs further instruction when she makes which statement?
- ☐ 1. "I can apply localized heat to the infected area."
- ☐ 2. "I should increase my fluid intake to 2,000 mL/day."
- ☐ 3. "I will need to take antibiotics for 7 to 10 days before I am cured."
- ☐ 4. "I should begin breast-feeding on the right side to decrease the pain."

107. During a home visit to a primiparous client who gave birth vaginally 14 days ago, the client says, "I have been crying a lot the last few days. I just feel so awful. I am a rotten mother. I just do not have any energy. Plus, my husband just got laid off from his job." The nurse observes that the client's appearance is disheveled. What would be the nurse's **best** response?
- ☐ 1. "These feelings commonly indicate symptoms of postpartum blues and are normal. They will go away in a few days."
- ☐ 2. "I think you are probably overreacting to the labor and birth process. You are doing the best you can as a mother."
- ☐ 3. "It is not unusual for some mothers to feel depressed after the birth of a baby. I think I should contact your healthcare provider."
- ☐ 4. "This may be a symptom of a serious mental illness. I think you should probably go to the hospital."

108. A teen client, who is 1 week postpartum, is concerned about the possibility of postpartum depression because she has a history of depression. Which comment by the client would indicate that she understood the nurse's teaching about the postpartum period and her risks for postpartum depression?
- ☐ 1. "Sleep should not be too much of a problem because the baby will soon start to sleep through the night."
- ☐ 2. "Since I am breast-feeding, I can eat all the food I want and not feel fat. The baby will use all the calories."
- ☐ 3. "If I am feeling guilty or not capable of caring for the baby and am not sleeping or eating well, I need to contact the office."
- ☐ 4. "I am going to give the baby the best care possible without asking anyone for help to show all those people who think I cannot do it."

Managing Care, Quality, and Safety of Postpartal Clients

109. The nurse is catheterizing a client who cannot void after a normal birth 8 hours ago. The nurse begins the catheterization process, and the client states, "I forgot to tell the nurse I get hives to betadine." The nurse should take which steps in order of priority from first to last? All options must be used.

1. Document the incident.

2. Clean povidone-iodine from the client's vaginal area.

3. Notify the healthcare provider (HCP) prescribing catheterization.

4. File an incident report.

110. A nurse is walking down the hall in the main corridor of a hospital when the infant security alert system sounds and a code for an infant abduction is announced. The **first** responsibility of the nurse when this situation occurs is to take which action?
- ☐ 1. Move to the entrance of the hospital, and check each person leaving.
- ☐ 2. Go to the obstetrics unit to determine if they need help with the situation.
- ☐ 3. Call the nursery to ask which baby is missing.
- ☐ 4. Observe individuals in the area for large bags or oversized coats.

111. The nurse on a mother-baby unit who is working on the night shift is revising the planning worksheet for the remaining 2 hours of the shift. The nurse has tasks and prescriptions to complete prior to the change of shift at 0700. Using the work plan below, how should the nurse organize the tasks from first to last so that everything is completed by 0700? All options must be used.

1. Draw blood for the prescribed laboratory tests (complete blood counts [CBCs]) on three postpartum clients with report on medical records by shift change.

2. Start IV of D5 ½ NS at keep vein open (KVO) rate on postpartum client just prior to change of shift.

3. Complete admission assessment of newborn turned over to nurse at 0500.

4. Draw newborn bilirubin level at 0600.

Nurse Worksheet

0500	
0530	
0600	
0630	

112. A nurse is caring for a woman who gave birth to her baby boy 2 hours ago. The nurse notes the woman's perineal pad contains some small clots and a moderate amount of lochia has accumulated under her buttocks. What is the **first** action the nurse should take at this time?
- ☐ 1. Request a prescription to administer oxytocin.
- ☐ 2. Perform an in-and-out catheter immediately.
- ☐ 3. Measure blood loss by measuring perineal pad.
- ☐ 4. Check fundus for position and consistency.

113. The nurse is reviewing the laboratory values on the medical record of a woman who is postpartum day 2. (See Exhibit.)

History	Physical	**Labs**		Prescriptions

Value	Traditional Units	SI Units
WBC	18,000	18 x/L
Hematocrit	40%	0.40%
Hemoglobin	9 g/dL	90 gL
Platelets	400,000	40 x/L

Based on this information, the nurse should:
- ☐ 1. contact the healthcare provider (HCP).
- ☐ 2. obtain a prescription for intravenous antibiotics.
- ☐ 3. assess the woman's vital signs.
- ☐ 4. prepare to administer pain medication.

114. The nurse assesses a client, who delivered vaginally 6 days ago, during a home visit. Which finding should the nurse report immediately to the healthcare provider (HCP)? Select all that apply.
- ☐ 1. foul-smelling lochia
- ☐ 2. engorged breasts bilaterally
- ☐ 3. client who cries easily
- ☐ 4. soaking 1 peripad every 3 to 4 hours
- ☐ 5. temperature of 100.8°F (38.2°C)

115. The night nurse has completed the change of shift report. As the day nurse makes rounds on a postpartum client receiving magnesium sulfate, it is noted the client developed significantly elevated blood pressure during the past shift. Further assessment reveals the magnesium sulfate rate is infusing well below the prescribed rate. In addition to adjusting the infusion rate and notifying the healthcare provider (HCP), what is the **most** important action by the nurse?
- ☐ 1. Complete an incident report.
- ☐ 2. Discuss the matter with the nurse the next time she works.
- ☐ 3. Ask the charge nurse if an incident report is necessary.
- ☐ 4. Evaluate the client's BP for 4 hours before making a decision.

116. The nurse is serving on the Quality Improvement Committee for the maternity unit. Quality improvement projects for this unit impacting safety and quality of care include which projects? Select all that apply.
- ☐ 1. use of recycling bins on the unit
- ☐ 2. infant identification system
- ☐ 3. sibling and family visitation policies
- ☐ 4. postpartum discharge instructions
- ☐ 5. rooming in guidelines

117. A nurse working on the postpartum unit is asked to participate in the unit Client Safety Committee. The nurse wants to know what type of projects would be conducted for the unit. Select all that apply.
☐ **1.** prevention of infant abduction
☐ **2.** safe medication administration
☐ **3.** adequate nourishment on unit
☐ **4.** proper restraints during procedures
☐ **5.** maternal/infant identification system

118. A nurse who works on an obstetrical inpatient unit has been assigned to the client safety committee. What client safety goals are **most** applicable to this setting? Select all that apply.
☐ **1.** effective and timely "hand-off reports" between labor and birth staff and mother-baby staff
☐ **2.** ensuring that preprocedure verifications are completed by healthcare providers (HCP) for any invasive procedure
☐ **3.** involving clients in education to cord infections
☐ **4.** identification of safety risks specific to the unit, such as infant abduction
☐ **5.** car seat instruction allowing infants to ride facing backward in the front seat

119. The nurse is making a postpartum visit at the home of a client who delivered 14 days earlier. After assessing the vital signs (temperature, 99°F (37.2°C); pulse, 88 beats/min; respiration rate, 20 breaths/min; and blood pressure, 112/60 mm Hg), the nurse records other findings as follows:

Breasts	Heart	Lungs	Abdomen
Soft +	Regular	Clear +	Soft +
Firm −	rate, 88		Distended −
Nipples			Bowel sounds +
intact +			Fundus
Cracks −			firm +
Blisters −			Midline +
			4 CM⇓U
			Nontender +
			Bladder empty +

Perineum	Lochia	Extremities
Midline episiotomy	Serosa	Legs: 1+ ankle
redness −	scant	edema
Ecchymosis −		Redness −
Edema −		Tenderness −
Discharge −		Homans −
Approximated +		
Hemorrhoids −		

Which finding indicates delayed involution?
☐ **1.** vital signs
☐ **2.** fundus
☐ **3.** lochia
☐ **4.** edema of the ankles

Answers, Rationales, and Test-Taking Strategies

The answers and rationales for each question follow below, along with keys (🔑) to the client need (CN) and cognitive level (CL) for each question. In addition, you will also see a glossary icon (📖) highlighting specific terminology used on the licensing exam. As you check your answers, use the **Content Mastery and Test-Taking Skill Self-Analysis** *worksheet (tear-out worksheet in back of book) to identify the reason(s) for not answering the questions correctly. For additional information about test-taking skills and strategies for answering questions, refer to pages 12–23 and pages 35–36 in Part 1 of this book.*

The Postpartal Client with a Vaginal Birth

1. 4. The hospital identification procedures for mothers and infants need to be completed each time a newborn is returned to a family's room. It does not matter how well the nurse knows the mother and infant; this validation is a standard of care in an obstetrical setting. Assessing the mother's ability to ambulate, asking the mother if there is anything else she needs to care for the infant, and checking the crib to determine if there are enough supplies are important steps that are part of the process of transferring a baby to the mother, but identification verification is a safety measure that must occur first.

🔑 CN: Safety and infection control; CL: Create

2. 3. At any point in the postpartum period, the lochia should be dark in color, rather than bright red. The volume should not be great enough to trickle or run from the vagina. The information provided states the fundus is firm, midline, and at the umbilicus, which are the expected outcomes at this point postpartum. These findings would indicate to the nurse that the bleeding is not coming from the uterus or from uterine atony. The bladder is not palpable, which indicates that the bleeding is not related to a full bladder, which is further validated by the fundus being at the umbilicus. The most likely etiology is cervical or vaginal lacerations or tears. The nurse is unable to do anything to stop this type of bleeding and must notify the **HCP** 📖. Increasing the IV rate will not decrease the amount or type of vaginal bleeding. Rechecking the hematocrit and hemoglobin will only provide background information for the nurse and identify the beginning levels for this mother, rather than where she is now. It will do nothing to stop the bleeding. The bleeding level and color is not normal, and documenting such findings as normal is incorrect.

🔑 CN: Management of care; CL: Synthesize

3. 4. Within the first 24 hours postpartum, maternal temperature may increase to 100.4°F (38°C), a normal postpartum finding attributed to dehydration. A temperature above 100.4°F (38°C) after the first 24 hours indicates a potential for infection. The hemoglobin is in the normal range. WBC count is normally elevated as a response to the inflammation, pain, and stress of the birthing process. A pulse rate of 60 beats/min is normal at this period and results from an increased cardiac output (mobilization of excess extracellular fluid into the vascular bed, decreased pressure from the uterus on vessels, blood flow back to the heart from the uterus returning to the central circulation) and alteration in stroke volume.

🔑 CN: Physiological adaptation; CL: Analyze

4. 1,2,3,5. Outcome evaluation for a family about 7 days after birth would include a mother who is tired but is able to care for herself and her baby. Having adequate support systems enables the mother to care better for herself and family members, as they can provide the backup for situations that may arise and a resource for new families. The normal progression for lochia is to change from red to pink to off-white while decreasing in amount. This is within the usual time periods for a postpartum mother. The baby should be feeding more frequently than every 6 to 8 hours. It is expected that a 7-day-old infant feeds every 3 to 4 hours if bottle-feeding and every 1½ to 3 hours if breast-feeding. Follow-up questions the nurse would ask to further evaluate this situation include "How many wet diapers does the infant have daily? How alert is the infant? Did the infant gain any weight at the first checkup?" It is expected that the mother has positive comments about the infant, but the nurse will evaluate to determine if there is at least one positive comment.

🔑 CN: Management of care; CL: Evaluate

5. 2. Pain medication is the first strategy to initiate at this pain level. When trauma has occurred to any area, the usual intervention is ice for the first 24 hours and heat after the first 24 hours. Sitz baths are initiated at the conclusion of ice therapy. Ice has already been initiated and will prevent further edema to the rectal sphincter and perineum and continue to reduce some of the pain. Anesthetic sprays can also be utilized for the perineal area when pain is involved but would not lower the pain to a level that the client considers tolerable.

🔑 CN: Physiological adaptation; CL: Synthesize

6. 2. Educating the client about caring for herself and her infant are the two highest priority goals. Following childbirth, all mothers, especially the primigravida, require instructions regarding self-care and infant care. Learning needs should be assessed in order to meet the specific needs of each client. Bonding is significant, but is only one aspect of the needs of this client, and the bonding process would have been implemented immediately postpartum, rather than waiting 2 hours. Planning the discharge occurs after the initial education has taken place for mother and infant and the nurse is aware of any need for referrals. Safety is an aspect of education taught continuously by the nurse and should include maternal as well as newborn safety.

🔑 CN: Management of care; CL: Create

7. 3. The client is in the taking hold phase with a demonstrated focus on the neonate and learning about and fulfilling infant care and needs. The taking in phase is the first period after birth where there is emphasis on reviewing and reliving the labor and birth process, concern with self, and needing to be mothered. Eating and sleep are high priorities during this phase. Taking on is not a phase of postpartum psychological adaptation. Letting go is the process beginning about 6 weeks postpartum when the mother may be preparing to go back to work. During this time, she can have other individuals assume care of the infant and begin the separation process.

🔑 CN: Psychosocial integrity; CL: Analyze

8. 1. A urine toxicology screening will be collected to document that the infant has been exposed to illegal drug use. This documentation will be the basis for legal action for the protection of this infant. If the infant tests positive for cocaine, the legal system will be activated to provide and ensure protective custody for this child. Hospital security would not become involved unless the mother is obtaining or using drugs on hospital premises. The mother and infant have the same privileges as do any hospitalized clients unless the safety of the infant is jeopardized; thus, limiting contact with visitors would not be appropriate. Local law enforcement agencies would be contacted only if the mother initiates use of drugs on hospital premises, and such contact would be made through the hospital security system.

🔑 CN: Physiological adaptation; CL: Synthesize

9. 4. Acetaminophen and hydrocodone would be the drug of choice for this situation because the pain level is so high. Aspirin is not usually used because of the bleeding risk associated with its use. Although ibuprofen would typically be a good choice because it inhibits the prostaglandin synthesis associated with a multiparous client breast-feeding, the pain level is too high for this drug to have an acceptable effect. Docusate is used as a stool softener postpartum but does not provide pain relief.

🔑 CN: Pharmacological and parenteral therapies; CL: Synthesize

10. 1. Immediately after delivery of the placenta, the nurse would expect to palpate the fundus halfway between the umbilicus and the symphysis pubis. Within 2 hours postpartum, the fundus should be palpated at the level of the umbilicus. The fundus remains at this level or may rise slightly above the umbilicus for approximately 12 hours. After the first 12 hours, the fundus should decrease one fingerbreadth (1 cm) per day in size. By the 9th or 10th day, the fundus usually is no longer palpable.

🔑 CN: Health promotion and maintenance; CL: Apply

11. 2. The instillation of erythromycin into the neonate's eyes provides prophylaxis for ophthalmia neonatorum, or neonatal blindness caused by gonorrhea in the mother. Erythromycin is also effective in the prevention of infection and conjunctivitis from *Chlamydia trachomatis*. The medication may result in redness of the neonate's eyes, but this redness will eventually disappear. Erythromycin ointment is not effective in treating neonatal chorioretinitis from cytomegalovirus. No effective treatment is available for a mother with cytomegalovirus. Erythromycin ointment is not effective in preventing cataracts. Additionally, neonatal infection with beta-hemolytic streptococcus results in pneumonia, bacterial meningitis, or death. Cataracts in the neonate may be congenital or may result from maternal exposure to rubella. Erythromycin ointment is also not effective for preventing and treating strabismus (crossed eyes). Infants may exhibit intermittent strabismus until 6 months of age.

🔑 CN: Pharmacological and parenteral therapies; CL: Apply

12. 3. Vitamin K acts as a preventive measure against neonatal hemorrhagic disease. At birth, the neonate does not have the intestinal flora to produce vitamin K, which is necessary for coagulation. Hypoglycemia is prevented and treated by feeding the infant. Hyperbilirubinemia severity can be decreased by early feeding and passage of meconium to excrete the bilirubin. Hyperbilirubinemia is treated with phototherapy. Polycythemia may occur in neonates who are large for gestational age or postterm. Clamping of the umbilical cord before pulsations cease reduces the incidence of polycythemia. Generally, polycythemia is not treated unless it is extremely severe.

🔑 CN: Pharmacological and parenteral therapies; CL: Apply

13. 1. The client has a hematoma. During the first 24 hours postpartum, ice packs can be applied to the perineal area to reduce swelling and discomfort. Ice packs usually are not effective after the first 24 hours. Although vital signs, including temperature, are important assessments, taking the client's temperature is unrelated to the hematoma and would provide no additional information about swelling. After 24 hours, the client may obtain more relief by taking a warm sitz bath. This moist heat is an effective way to increase circulation to the perineum and provide comfort. Usually, hematomas resolve without further treatment within 6 weeks. Additionally, the nurse should measure the hematoma to provide a baseline for subsequent measurements and should notify the **HCP** 📖 of its presence. An antibiotic is not warranted at this point because the client is not exhibiting any signs or symptoms of infection.

🔑 CN: Health promotion and maintenance; CL: Synthesize

14. 4. Urinary retention soon after childbirth is usually caused by edema and trauma of the lower urinary tract; this commonly results in difficulty with initiating voiding. Hyperemia of the bladder mucosa also commonly occurs. The combination of hyperemia and edema predisposes to decreased sensation to void, overdistention of the bladder, and incomplete bladder emptying. A prolonged first stage of labor can contribute to exhaustion and uterine atony, not urinary retention. If the client had a urinary tract infection, she would exhibit symptoms such as dysuria and a burning sensation. After birth, the uterus is contracting, which leads to less pressure on the bladder. Pressure of the uterus on the bladder occurs during labor.

🔑 CN: Health promotion and maintenance; CL: Analyze

15. 2. For clients who are bottle-feeding, the menstrual flow should return in 6 to 10 weeks, after a rise in the production of follicle-stimulating hormone by the pituitary gland. Nonlactating mothers rarely ovulate before 4 to 6 weeks postpartum. Therefore, 3 to 4 weeks is too early for the menstrual cycle to resume. For women who are breast-feeding, the menstrual flow may not return for 3 to 4 months (12 to 16 weeks) or, in some women, for the entire period of lactation, because ovulation is suppressed.

🔑 CN: Health promotion and maintenance; CL: Apply

16. 4. The client's dizziness is most likely caused by orthostatic hypotension secondary to the decreased volume of blood in the vascular system resulting from the physiologic changes occurring in the mother after birth. The client is experiencing dizziness because not enough blood volume is available to perfuse the brain. The nurse should first allow the client to "dangle" on the side of the bed for a few minutes before attempting to ambulate. By 6 hours postpartum, the effects of the anesthesia should be worn off completely. Typically, the effects of epidural anesthesia wear off by 1 to 2 hours postpartum, and the effects of local anesthesia usually disappear by 1 hour. The client scenario provides no information to indicate that the client experienced any postpartum hemorrhage. Normal blood loss during birth should not exceed 500 mL.

⊝🔑 CN: Health promotion and maintenance; CL: Apply

17. 4. Because the diet of immigrants from Mexico and Central America commonly includes beans, corn products, tomatoes, chili peppers, potatoes, milk, cheeses, and eggs, the nurse needs to encourage an intake of meats, dark green leafy vegetables, and other high-protein products that are rich in iron. Doing so helps to compensate for the significant blood loss and subsequent iron loss that occurs during the postpartum period. Additionally, fresh fruits, meats, and green leafy vegetables may be scarce, possibly resulting in deficiencies of vitamin A, vitamin D, and iron. Tomatoes are high in vitamin C, potatoes are good sources of carbohydrates and vitamin C, and corn products are high in thiamine, but these are not rich sources of iron.

⊝🔑 CN: Health promotion and maintenance; CL: Create

18. 4. A small, constant trickle of blood and a firm fundus are usually indicative of a vaginal tear or cervical laceration. If the client had retained placental tissue, the fundus would fail to contract fully (uterine atony), exhibiting as a soft or boggy fundus. Also, vaginal bleeding would be evident. Uterine inversion occurs when the uterus is displaced outside of the vagina and is obvious on inspection. Bladder distention may result in uterine atony because the pressure of the bladder displaces the fundus, preventing it from fully contracting. In this case, the fundus would be soft, possibly boggy, and displaced from midline.

⊝🔑 CN: Reduction of risk potential; CL: Analyze

19. 4. On about the 11th postpartum day, the lochia should be lochia alba, clear or white in color. Lochia rubra, which is dark red to red, may persist for the first 2 to 3 days postpartum. From day 3 to about day 10, lochia serosa, which is pink or brown, is normal.

⊝🔑 CN: Health promotion and maintenance; CL: Evaluate

20. 2. The nurse should instruct the client to cleanse the perineal area with warm water and to wipe from front to back with a blotting motion. Warm water is soothing to the tender tissue, and wiping from front to back reduces the risk of contamination. Hot, sudsy water may increase the client's discomfort and may even burn the client in a very tender area. After the first 24 hours, warm water sitz baths taken three or four times a day for 20 minutes can help increase circulation to the area. Ice packs are helpful for the first 24 hours.

⊝🔑 CN: Health promotion and maintenance; CL: Evaluate

21. 3. After an uncomplicated birth, postpartum exercises may begin on the first postpartum day with exercises to strengthen the abdominal muscles. These are done in the supine position with the knees flexed, inhaling deeply while allowing the abdomen to expand and then exhaling while contracting the abdominal muscles. Exercises such as sit-ups (sitting, then lying back, and returning to a sitting position) and push-ups or exercises involving reaching for the knees are ordinarily too strenuous for the first postpartum day. Sit-ups may be done later in the postpartum period, after approximately 3 to 6 weeks.

⊝🔑 CN: Health promotion and maintenance; CL: Apply

22. 2. Lochia can be expected to increase when the client first ambulates. Lochia tends to pool in the uterus and vagina when the client is recumbent and flows out when the client arises. If the client had reported that her lochia was bright red, the nurse would suspect bleeding. In this situation, the client would be put back in bed and the **HCP** □ would be notified. Early postpartum hemorrhage occurs during the first 24 hours, but typically the fundus is soft or "boggy." The client's fundus here is firm and midline. Late postpartal hemorrhage, occurring after the first 24 hours, is usually caused by retained placental fragments or abnormal involution of the placental site.

⊝🔑 CN: Health promotion and maintenance; CL: Synthesize

23. 2. Clients sometimes feel faint or dizzy when taking a shower for the first time after birth because of the sudden change in blood volume in the body. Primarily for this reason, the nurse remains nearby while the client takes her first shower after birth. If the client becomes dizzy or expresses symptoms of feeling faint, the nurse should get the client back to bed as soon as possible. If the client faints while in the shower, the nurse should cover the client to protect her privacy, stay with the client, and call for assistance. Fatigue postpartum is common and will precede taking a shower. Diuresis is a normal physiologic response during the postpartum period and not associated with showering. Hygiene needs also precede the shower.

🔑 CN: Safety and infection control; CL: Analyze

24. 2. The nurse should instruct the client to squeeze or contract the muscles of the buttocks together before sitting down in the chair; this contracts the pelvic floor muscles, which reduces the tension on the tender perineal area. Then the client should put her full weight slowly down on the chair. Pain medication may only be prescribed for every 3 to 4 hours, so the client may not be able to receive pain medication every time she desires to sit in the chair. The episiotomy pain usually fades by the 5th or 6th postpartum day. Maintaining a relaxed posture before sitting does not contract the pelvic floor muscles. Most **healthcare providers (HCPs)** 📖 prescribe an analgesic cream or spray when a client has an episiotomy, but they provide only temporary relief.

🔑 CN: Health promotion and maintenance; CL: Synthesize

25. 1. Neonates like to look at eyes, and eye-to-eye contact is a highly effective way to provide visual stimulation. The parent's eyes are circular, move from side to side, and become larger and smaller. Neonates have been observed to fix on them. In general, neonates prefer circular objects of darkness against a white background. Sharp black and white images of geometric figures are appropriate. Use of bright colors on the walls and moving a colorful rattle do not provide as much visual stimulation as eye-to-eye contact with talking. Brightly colored animals and cartoon figures are more appropriate at approximately 1 year of age.

🔑 CN: Health promotion and maintenance; CL: Create

26. 2. The father is praying to Allah because of the Muslim belief that the first sounds a child hears should be from the Koran in praise of and supplication to Allah. Although male children are revered in this culture, this practice is performed by Muslims whether the child is male or female. The father's actions are unrelated to his wife and son's being healthy. The nurse should allow the practice because doing so demonstrates cultural sensitivity and builds a trusting relationship with the family. The Muslim faith does not have a baptism rite whereby the child becomes a member of the faith.

🔑 CN: Health promotion and maintenance; CL: Analyze

27. 2. According to Erikson, infants are in the trust versus mistrust stage. Holding, talking to, singing to, and patting neonates helps them develop trust in caregivers. Tactile stimulation is important and should be encouraged. Holding neonates often is unlikely to spoil them because they are totally dependent on other human beings to meet their needs. Being held makes infants feel loved and cared for and should be encouraged. The mother can hold the neonate as often as she wants, not just when the baby is crying or fussy. Overstimulation typically does not result from holding an infant.

🔑 CN: Health promotion and maintenance; CL: Synthesize

28. 4. If the client continues to have perineal pain after an analgesic medication has been given, the nurse should inspect the client's perineum for a hematoma because this is the usual cause of such discomfort. Ibuprofen is a nonsteroidal anti-inflammatory medication used to relieve mild pain. Pain from a perineal hematoma can be moderate to severe, possibly requiring a stronger analgesic, such as acetaminophen with codeine). Ice applied to the perineum during the first 24 hours postpartum may decrease the severity of hematoma formation. Application of warm heat, such as a sitz bath 3 times daily for 20 minutes, also can help to relieve the discomfort when implemented after the first 24 hours. Typically, hematomas resolve themselves within 6 weeks. A puerperal infection would be indicated if the client's temperature were 100.4°F (41°C) or higher. Also, lochia most likely would be foul smelling. A continuous trickle of lochia rubra would suggest a possible vaginal laceration. No evidence is presented to suggest a history of drug abuse.

🔑 CN: Reduction of risk potential; CL: Analyze

29. 1,4,6. Delegating care to **UAP** 📖 requires that the nurse knows which tasks are within that individual's capability. Changing the perineal pad and reporting drainage, reinforcing hygiene with perineal care, and assisting with ambulation are within the individual's capacity. UAP should never be asked to complete any assessments, such as checking fundal location or performing skilled procedures on a client. In addition, it would be beyond the scope of the job of UAP to conduct client teaching such as teaching the mother how to latch or discussing postpartum depression with the client.

🔑 CN: Management of care; CL: Synthesize

30. 4. Legal regulations and ethical decision making require that the nurse maintain confidentiality at all times. The nurse's best response is to explain to the client that nurses are not allowed to discuss other clients on the unit. Ignoring the client's question is inappropriate because doing so would interfere with the development of a trusting nurse-client relationship.

Confidentiality must be maintained at all times. Telling the client that the nurse is not sure may imply that the nurse will find out and then tell the client about the other woman. Asking the other woman's permission to discuss her with another client is inappropriate because confidentiality must be maintained at all times.

🔑 CN: Management of care; CL: Apply

31. 2. The neonate has immature oculomotor coordination, an inability to accommodate for distance, and poorly developed eyes, visual nerves, and brain. However, the normal neonate can see objects clearly within a range of 9 to 12 inches (22.9 to 30.5 cm), whether or not they are moving. Visual acuity at birth is 20/100 to 20/150, but it improves rapidly during infancy and toddlerhood. Newborns can distinguish colors as well as light from dark.

🔑 CN: Health promotion and maintenance; CL: Apply

32. 4. The client is experiencing diastasis recti, a separation of the longitudinal muscles (recti) of the abdomen that is usually palpable on the 3rd postpartum day. An exercise involving raising the head and shoulders about 8 inches (20.3 cm) with the client lying on her back with knees bent and hands crossed over the abdomen is preferred. This exercise helps to pull the abdominal muscles together, and the client gradually works up to performing this exercise 50 times per day. However, until the diastasis has closed, the client should avoid exercises that rotate the trunk, twist the hips, or bend the trunk to one side, because further separation may occur. The condition does not need a surgical repair, and limited activity and bed rest are not necessary. Correct posture and adequate diet assist the body to return to its prepregnancy state more quickly but do not resolve the separation of abdominal muscles.

🔑 CN: Reduction of risk potential; CL: Synthesize

33. 3. A uterine fundus located off to one side and above the level of the umbilicus is commonly the result of a full bladder. Although the client had voided, the client may be experiencing urinary retention with overflow. If anesthesia has been used for birth, the inability to void may be related to the lingering effects of anesthesia; however, that is not the case here. **Healthcare providers (HCP)** 📖 commonly write a one-time prescription for catheterization, after which, typically, enough edema has subsided to make it easier and less painful for the client to void and completely empty her bladder. Administering ibuprofen would have no effect on the uterine fundus. Waiting to reassess in 1 hour could be detrimental since the client's distended bladder is interfering with uterine involution, predisposing

her to possible hemorrhage. Administering a bolus of fluid would be inappropriate because it would only add to the client's full bladder.

🔑 CN: Reduction of risk potential; CL: Synthesize

34. 2. Stretch marks, or *striae gravidarum*, are caused by stretching of the tissues, particularly over the abdomen. After birth, the tissues atrophy, leaving silver scars. These skin pigmentations will not disappear completely. The striae gravidarum may reappear as pink streaks if the client becomes pregnant again. Special creams are not warranted because they are not helpful and may be expensive. Weight loss does not make the marks disappear. Striae gravidarum tend to run in families.

🔑 CN: Health promotion and maintenance; CL: Synthesize

35. 1. The client with a third-degree laceration should be assessed for constipation because a third-degree laceration extends into a portion of the anal sphincter. Constipation, not diarrhea, is more likely because this condition is extremely painful, possibly causing the client to be reluctant to have a bowel movement. The laceration has been sutured and should not be bleeding at 48 hours postpartum. Rectal fistulas may develop at a later time, but not at 48 hours postpartum.

🔑 CN: Reduction of risk potential; CL: Create

36. 4. For most clients, sexual intercourse can be resumed when the lochia has stopped flowing and episiotomy pain has ceased, usually about 3 weeks postpartum. Sexual intercourse may be painful until the episiotomy has healed. The client also needs instructions about the possibility that pregnancy may occur before the return of the client's menstrual flow. The postpartum check by the **HCP** 📖 typically occurs 4 to 6 weeks after birth, and most women have already had intercourse by this time. Typically, new mothers are exhausted and may not feel amorous or desirable for quite a while. In addition, the mother's physiologic responses may be diminished because of low hormonal levels, adjustments to the maternal role, and fatigue due to lack of rest and sleep.

🔑 CN: Health promotion and maintenance; CL: Synthesize

37. 1. The nurse needs to continue to monitor the client's vital signs. During the first 24 hours postpartum, it is normal for the mother to have a slight temperature elevation because of dehydration. A temperature of 100.4°F (38°C) that persists after the first 24 hours may indicate an infection. Bradycardia during the first week postpartum is normal because of decreased blood volume, diuresis, and diaphoresis. The client's respiratory rate is within normal limits. Large clots are indicative of hemorrhage. However, the client's vital signs are within normal limits and her fundus is firm and midline. Therefore, large clots and possible hemorrhage can be ruled out. The **HCP** 📖 does not need to be notified at this time. An ice pack is not necessary because the client's temperature is within normal limits.

🔑 CN: Health promotion and maintenance; CL: Synthesize

38. 3. The client needs more teaching when she states, "I should lie on my back as much as possible to relieve the pain." Instead, the client should lie in the Sims position as much as possible to aid venous return to the rectal area and to reduce discomfort. Stool softeners can decrease pain with defecation, but clients should discuss their use with their provider before taking them. Analgesic sprays and witch hazel pads are helpful in reducing the discomfort of hemorrhoids. Drinking lots of water and eating roughage aid in bowel elimination, minimizing the risk of straining and subsequent hemorrhoidal development or enlargement.

🔑 CN: Basic care and comfort; CL: Evaluate

39. 2. On most postpartum units, clients on regular diets are allowed to eat whatever kinds of food they desire. Generally, foods from home are not discouraged. The nurse does not need to obtain the **HCP's** 📖 permission. Although it is preferred, the foods do not necessarily have to be high in iron. In some cultures, there is a belief in the "hot-cold" theory of disease; certain foods (hot) are preferred during the postpartum period, and other foods (cold) are avoided. Therefore, the nurse should allow the mother to bring her daughter "special foods from home." Doing so demonstrates cultural sensitivity and aids in developing a trusting relationship.

🔑 CN: Basic care and comfort; CL: Synthesize

40. 1. Iron is best absorbed in an acid environment or with vitamin C. For maximum iron absorption, the client should take the medication with orange juice or a vitamin C supplement. Herbal tea has no effect on iron absorption. Milk decreases iron absorption. Grape juice is not acidic and therefore would have no effect on iron absorption.

🔑 CN: Pharmacological and parenteral therapies; CL: Synthesize

41. 4. It is believed that the process of attachment is structured so that the parents become attached to only one infant at a time. Therefore, the nurse should encourage the parents to relate to each twin individually, rather than as a unit, to enhance the attachment process. Mothers of twins are usually able to breast-feed successfully because the milk supply

increases on demand. However, possible fatigue and exhaustion require that the mother rest whenever possible. It would be highly unlikely and unrealistic that each parent would be able to spend equal amounts of time with both twins. Other responsibilities, such as employment, may prevent this. The parents should try to engage assistance from family and friends, because caring for twins or other multiple births (e.g., triplets) can be exhausting for the family.

🔑 CN: Psychosocial integrity; CL: Synthesize

42. 3. At 12 hours postpartum, the fundus normally should be in the midline and at the level of the umbilicus. When the fundus is firm yet above the umbilicus, and deviated to the right rather than in the midline, the client's bladder is most likely distended. The client should be encouraged to ambulate to the bathroom and attempt to void because a full bladder can prevent normal involution. A firm but deviated fundus above the level of the umbilicus is not a normal finding, and if voiding does not return it to midline, it should be reported to the **HCP** 📖. Oxytocin is used to treat uterine atony. This client's fundus is firm, not boggy or soft, which would suggest atony. Gentle massage is not necessary because there is no evidence of atony or clots.

🔑 CN: Reduction of risk potential; CL: Synthesize

43. 1,2,3,5,6. The nurse is responsible for providing discharge instructions that include signs and symptoms that need to be reported to the **health-care provider (HCP)** 📖 as well as resources and follow-up for home care if needed. Phone numbers and health practices to promote healing, such as the use of prenatal vitamins, are also essential pieces of information. Fertility can return in as little as 21 days, especially among women who are not breast-feeding. So it is important to discuss the client's contraception plan. Although the client's mother may be helpful, the client's statement that she will be fine because her mother is coming indicates that she is unaware or ignoring information about valuable information and resources.

🔑 CN: Reduction of risk potential; CL: Evaluate

The Postpartal Client Who Breast-feeds

44. 4. Depot medroxyprogesterone acetate (DMPA) is an injectable progestin contraceptive that can reduce the initial production of breast milk. It is given to a breast-feeding woman when she returns for the 6-week postpartum checkup. By this time, the milk supply is well established and will remain at that level. DMPA is effective as a contraceptive for 90 days. DMPA can be given within 5 days of birth only if a mother is not breast-feeding.

8— CN: Pharmacological and parenteral therapies; CL: Evaluate

45. 3. As much of the mother's nipple and areola as possible need to be in the infant's mouth in order to establish a latch that does not cause nipple cracks or fissures. Having the nipple and the areola deep in the infant's mouth decreases the stress on the end of the nipple, therefore decreasing pain, cracking, and fissures. Breast milk has been found to heal nipples when placed on the nipple at the completion of a feeding. The length of time the baby feeds on each nipple is not a factor as long as the nipple is correctly placed in the infant's mouth.

8— CN: Health promotion and maintenance; CL: Evaluate

46. 1. New mothers usually begin to produce milk at about the 3rd day postpartum and colostrum is produced until that time. For clients who have breast-fed another infant during pregnancy, having milk shortly after birth is not unusual. Diaphoresis and diuresis are considered normal during this time as the body excretes the additional fluids that are no longer needed after the pregnancy. Constipation may continue for several days as a result of progesterone remaining in the system, the consummation of iron, and trauma to the perineum.

8— CN: Physiological adaptation; CL: Analyze

47. 2. The major reasons for afterbirth pains are breast-feeding, high parity, overdistended uterus during pregnancy, and a uterus filled with blood clots. Physiologically, afterbirth pains are caused by intermittent contraction and relaxation of the uterus. These contractions are stronger in multigravidas in order to maintain a contracted uterus. The release of oxytocin when breast-feeding also stimulates uterine contractions. There are no data to suggest any of these clients has had an overdistended uterus or currently has clots within the uterus. The G3, P3 client who is breast-feeding has the highest parity of the clients listed, which—in addition to breast-feeding—places her most at risk for afterbirth pains. The G2, P2 postcesarean client may have cramping, but it should be less than the G3, P3 client. The G3, P3 client who is bottle-feeding would be at risk for afterbirth pains because she has given birth to several children, but her choice to bottle-feed reduces her risk of pain.

8— CN: Physiological adaptation; CL: Evaluate

48. 2. The client is exhibiting signs and symptoms of a breast infection (mastitis). The nurse should instruct her to contact her **HCP** 🖥, who will likely prescribe a prescription for antibiotics. She should continue to breast-feed the infant from both breasts. Frequent breast-feeding is encouraged rather than discontinuing the process for anyone having a breast infection. Applying warm compresses may relieve pain. However, the underlying infection indicated by the elevated temperature indicates that additional treatment with antibiotics will be needed.

8— CN: Management of care; CL: Synthesize

49. 4. Breast-feeding consumes maternal calories and requires energy that increases the maternal basal metabolic rate and assists in lowering the maternal blood glucose level. Insulin is not transferred to the infant through breast milk. Breast-feeding is recommended for diabetic mothers because it does lower blood glucose levels. The number of antibodies in breast milk is not altered by maternal diabetes.

8— CN: Physiological adaptation; CL: Evaluate

50. 1. Jaundice in a breast-feeding infant is common and is not pathological. Mothers should be taught to breast-feed as often as possible, at least every 2 to 3 hours and until the infant is satiated. Breast-fed babies rarely need to be supplemented with formula. Mothers should be encouraged to continue breast-feeding their infants due to the numerous benefits it provides. Infants should never be placed in direct sunlight.

8— CN: Health promotion and maintenance; CL: Evaluate

51. 1. If not contraindicated for moral, cultural, or religious reasons, a condom with spermicide is commonly recommended for contraception after birth until the client's 6-week postpartal examination. This method has no effect on the neonate who is breast-feeding. Oral contraceptives containing estrogen are not advised for women who are breast-feeding because the hormones decrease the production of breast milk. Women who are not breast-feeding may use oral contraceptive agents. The rhythm method is not effective because the client is unlikely to be able to determine when ovulation has occurred until her menstrual cycle returns. Although breast-feeding is not considered an effective form of contraception, breast-feeding usually delays the return of both ovulation and menstruation. The length of the delay varies with the duration of lactation and the frequency of breast-feeding. While abstinence is one form of birth control and safe while breast-feeding, it may not be acceptable to this couple who is asking about a method that will allow them to resume sexual relations.

> CN: Health promotion and maintenance; CL: Synthesize

52. 4. Colostrum is a thin, watery, yellow fluid composed of protein, sugar, fat, water, minerals, vitamins, and maternal antibodies (e.g., immunoglobulin A). It is important for the neonate to receive colostrum for passive immunity. Colostrum is lower in fat and lactose than mature breast milk. Colostrum does not contain vitamin K. The neonate will produce vitamin K once a feeding pattern is established. Colostrum may speed, rather than delay, the passage of meconium.

> CN: Health promotion and maintenance; CL: Apply

53. 3. Various medications can be excreted in the breast milk and affect the nursing neonate. The client should avoid all nonprescribed medications (such as acetaminophen) unless approved by the **healthcare provider (HCP)** 📖. Medications typically do not affect the quality of the mother's breast milk. Medications usually do not interfere with or diminish the mother's motivation to breast-feed, nor do they interfere with the mother's letdown reflex.

> CN: Health promotion and maintenance; CL: Apply

54. 3. Taking ibuprofen 200 mg orally immediately after breast-feeding helps minimize the neonate's exposure to the drug because drugs are most highly concentrated in the body soon after they are taken. Most mothers breast-feed on demand or every 2 to 3 hours, so the effects of the ibuprofen should be decreased by the next breast-feeding session. Taking the medication before going to bed is inappropriate because, although the mother may go to bed at a certain time, the neonate may wish to breast-feed soon after the mother goes to bed. If the mother takes the medication midway between feedings, then its peak action may occur midway between feedings. Breast milk is sufficient for the neonate's nutritional needs. Most breast-feeding mothers should not be encouraged to provide supplemental feedings to the infant because this may result in nipple confusion.

> CN: Pharmacological and parenteral therapies; CL: Apply

55. 4. Breast-feeding stimulates oxytocin secretion, which causes the uterine muscles to contract. These contractions account for the discomfort associated with afterpains. Flatulence may occur after a cesarean birth. However, the mother typically would have abdominal distention

and a bloating feeling, not a "cramp-like" feeling. Stretching of the tissues or healing may cause slight tenderness or itching, not cramping feelings of discomfort. Medications such as mild analgesics or stool softeners, commonly administered postpartum, typically do not cause cramping.

> CN: Health promotion and maintenance; CL: Apply

56. 2. For the breast-feeding client, drinking at least 8 to 10 glasses of fluid a day is recommended. Breast-feeding women need an increased intake of vitamin D for calcium absorption. A breast-feeding woman requires an extra 500 cal/day above the recommended nonpregnancy intake to produce quality breast milk. Breast-feeding women need adequate calcium for blood clotting and strong bones and teeth.

> CN: Basic care and comfort; CL: Evaluate

57. 1. Breast milk has a higher fat content than cow's milk. Thirty to fifty-five percent of the calories in breast milk are from fat. Breast milk contains less iron than cow's milk does. However, the iron absorption from breast milk is greater in the neonate than with cow's milk. Breast milk contains less sodium and calcium than does cow's milk.

> CN: Basic care and comfort; CL: Apply

58. 4. Lightly brushing the neonate's lips with the nipple causes the neonate to open the mouth and begin sucking. The neonate should be taught to open the mouth and grasp the nipple on his or her own. The neonate should not be forced to nurse.

> CN: Health promotion and maintenance; CL: Apply

59. 2. Several methods can be used to prevent nipple soreness. Placing as much of the areola as possible into the neonate's mouth is one method. This action prevents compression of the nipple between the neonate's gums, which can cause nipple soreness. Other methods include changing position with each feeding, avoiding breast engorgement, nursing more frequently, and feeding on demand. Plastic liners are not helpful because they prevent air circulation, thus promoting nipple soreness. Instead, air drying is recommended. Pulling the baby's mouth out smoothly after only 10 minutes may prevent the baby from getting the entire feeding and increases nipple soreness. Any breast milk remaining on the nipples should not be wiped off because the milk has healing properties.

> CN: Health promotion and maintenance; CL: Synthesize

60. 4. Breast-fed neonates do not swallow as much air as bottle-fed neonates, but they still need to be burped. Good times to burp the neonate are when the mother switches from one breast to the other and at the end of the breast-feeding session. Neonates do not eat more if they are burped frequently. Breast-feeding mothers are advised not to supplement the feedings with formula because this may cause nipple confusion and decrease milk production. If supplements are given, the baby still needs to be burped. Neonates who are fed every 3 hours still need to be burped.

CN: Health promotion and maintenance; CL: Evaluate

61. 3. While there is some variation in recommendations, stored breast milk can be safely kept in the refrigerator for 5 to 7 days or in a deep freeze at 0°F (−18°C) for 12 months. Breast milk should be stored in glass containers because immunoglobulin tends to stick to plastic bottles. Breast milk can remain without refrigeration or loss of nutrients for up to 8 to 10 hours. The containers should be labeled with date, time, and amount to prevent inadvertent administration of spoiled milk. Frozen breast milk should be thawed in the refrigerator for a few hours, placed under warm tap water, and then shaken.

CN: Health promotion and maintenance; CL: Evaluate

62. 4. Oxytocin stimulates the letdown reflex when milk is carried to the nipples. A lactating mother can experience the letdown reflex suddenly when she hears her baby cry or when she anticipates a feeding. Some mothers have reported feeling the letdown reflex just by thinking about the baby. Progesterone plays an important role in pregnancy, but levels drop after giving birth. This hormone if taken for contraception too soon after birth may decrease milk supply. Estrogen influences development of female secondary sex characteristics and controls menstruation. Prolactin stimulates milk production.

CN: Health promotion and maintenance; CL: Apply

63. 3. Expressing a little milk before nursing, massaging the breasts gently, or taking a warm shower before feeding also may help to improve milk flow. Although various measures such as ice, heat, and massage may be tried to relieve breast engorgement, prevention of breast engorgement by frequent feedings is the method of choice. Applying ice to the nipples does not relieve breast engorgement. However, it may temporarily relieve the discomfort associated with breast engorgement. Using lanolin on the nipples does not relieve breast engorgement and is unnecessary. Use of lanolin may cause sensitivity and irritation. Having frequent breast-feeding sessions, rather than offering the neonate a small amount of formula, is the method of choice for preventing and relieving breast

engorgement. In addition, offering the neonate small amounts of formula may result in nipple confusion.

CN: Health promotion and maintenance; CL: Apply

64. 1. The nurse should instruct the client that the baby is getting enough to eat when there are six to eight wet diapers by the 5th day of age. Other signs include good suckling sounds during feeding, dripping breast milk at the mouth, and quiet rest or sleep after the feeding. By the 4th day of age, the infant should have soft yellow stools, not transitional (greenish) stools. Falling asleep easily after feeding on the first day is not a good indicator because most infants are sleepy during the first 24 hours. Most infants regain their lost birth weight in 7 to 10 days after birth. An infant who has gained weight during the first well-baby checkup (usually at 2 weeks) is getting sufficient breast milk at feedings.

CN: Health promotion and maintenance; CL: Apply

65. 4. The client should wean the infant gradually, eliminating one feeding at a time. The baby can be weaned to a bottle (formula) anytime the mother desires; she does not have to breast-feed for 4 months. Most infants (and mothers) develop a "favorite feeding time," so this feeding session should be eliminated last. The client may wish to begin weaning with daytime feedings when the infant is busy.

CN: Health promotion and maintenance; CL: Create

66. 1,3. The client is experiencing symptoms of engorgement. Cool compresses between feedings can help decrease swelling. Determining when the baby last fed is critical as frequent feedings can help relieve symptoms. The nurse must also assess how long baby feeds, if it has a correct latch, and if baby empties breast during feeds. Sitting on supportive devices is not necessary as the epitiostomy is healing. Cool sitz baths do not promote circulation to the area; instead they cause vasoconstriction and decrease blood flow to the area, therefore prolonging healing and increasing discomfort. Swab for a culture and sensitivity is not warranted at this time. If edema and redness continue for more than two days then further assessment is required to rule out infection.

CN: Basic care and comfort; CL: Synthesize

67. 4. Neonates normally increase breast-feeding during periods of rapid growth (growth spurts). These can be expected at age 10 to 14 days, 5 to 6 weeks, 2.5 to 3 months, and 4.5 to 6 months.

Each growth spurt is usually followed by a regular feeding pattern. Lack of adequate intake to meet maternal nutritional needs is not associated with the neonate's desire for more frequent breast-feeding sessions. However, an intake of adequate calories is necessary to produce quality breast milk. The mother's fears about weight gain and preventing the neonate from sucking long enough are not associated with the desire for more frequent breast-feeding sessions.

🗝 CN: Health promotion and maintenance; CL: Analyze

68. 2. Even if the nipples are sore and cracked, the mother should position the baby with the entire areola in the baby's mouth so that the nipple is not compressed between the baby's gums during feeding. The best method is to prevent cracked nipples before they occur. This can be done by feeding frequently and using proper positioning. Warm, moist tea bags can soothe cracked nipples because of tannic acid in the tea. Creams on the nipples should be avoided; wiping off any lanolin creams from the nipple before each feeding can cause further soreness. Feeding the baby less often for the next few days will cause engorgement (and possible neonatal weight loss), leading to additional problems. Soap use while in the shower should be avoided to prevent drying and removal of protective oils.

🗝 CN: Reduction of risk potential; CL: Synthesize

69. 2. Time for bonding with their newborns is a frequent concern for fathers of breast-fed babies. It is common for fathers to express concern about having less intimate contact time. These feelings are normal, but they do not go away in a few days. The father of the baby has to dedicate time to spend with the infant where he can talk to, hold, cuddle, and/or play with the infant. These strategies provide the infant with the contact and stimulation to establish a close bond between them. Bonding occurs from the moment of birth and continues in various ways between mother, father, and infant. Infants recognize and respond to touch, light, and voice immediately after birth. Bonding between both parents is equally important, and one does not take priority over the other.

🗝 CN: Psychosocial integrity; CL: Apply

70. 4. A soft seedy unformed stool is the norm for a 4-day-old infant. It may surprise the mother as it is a change from the meconium the infant had since birth. This stool is not diarrhea even though it has no form. There is no need for the infant to be seen for this. As long as the infant is breast-feeding, the stools will remain of this color and consistency.

Brown and formed stool is common for an infant who is bottle-fed or after the breast-feeding infant has begun eating food.

🗝 CN: Physiologic adaptation; CL: Apply

The Postpartal Client Who Bottle-feeds

71. 1. By 4 to 6 weeks postpartum, the fundus should be deep in the pelvis and the size of a nonpregnant uterus. Subinvolution, caused by infection or retained placental fragments, is a problem associated with a uterus that is larger than expected at this time. Normal expectations include a white, thick vaginal discharge, striae that are beginning to fade to silver, and breasts that are soft without evidence of milk production (in a bottle-feeding mother).

🗝 CN: Physiological adaptation; CL: Analyze

72. 4. The use of a breast pump to remove milk is contraindicated in bottle-feeding mothers. Nipple and breast stimulation and emptying of the breasts produce milk, rather than eliminate milk production. The bottle-feeding client is discouraged from stimulating the breasts in any way. A sports bra that is well fitting provides support and decreases stimulation. (Binders are not suggested.) Having the water in a shower land on the shoulders of the mother rather than the breasts also decreases stimulation. Only water is necessary to clean nipples when breast or bottle-feeding.

🗝 CN: Basic care and comfort; CL: Evaluate

73. 3. Gaining 1 oz (30 g) a day is normal for a neonate. Initial weight loss that exceeds 10% of birth weight is abnormal. Adding rice cereal to a bottle without a medical indication increases the risk of aspiration and may promote obesity. Doubling the birth weight is typical at 5 months.

🗝 CN: Basic care and comfort; CL: Apply

74. 1. Initial regurgitation in the neonate during the first 12 to 24 hours may be caused by excessive mucus and gastric irritation from foreign substances in the stomach. After the first 24 hours, regurgitation is thought to be caused by the neonate's immature cardiac sphincter. It represents an overflow of stomach contents and is probably a result of feeding the neonate too fast or too much. A defect in the gastrointestinal system usually results in more severe symptoms. A small amount of regurgitation is normal, but vomiting or forceful fluid expulsion is not. Burping the infant often during a feeding can decrease the amount of air in the stomach from swallowing. However, burping too often can lead the neonate to become tired or fussy. Moving the infant usually does not result in regurgitation.

⚷ CN: Health promotion and maintenance; CL: Apply

75. 1. The neonate should be placed in a supine position. Placing infants on their side or prone in a crib after a feeding is no longer recommended due to the increased risk of sudden infant death syndrome (SIDS). Although the mother may desire to hold the infant in her lap after feeding, this is not necessary for the neonate's digestion unless the infant has reflux.

⚷ CN: Health promotion and maintenance; CL: Apply

76. 2. Pediatricians recommend that infants be given either breast milk or formula until at least 6 months of age because of the neonate's difficulty digesting solid foods. Giving solid foods too early can lead to food allergies. Because chewing movements do not begin until 7 to 9 months of age, foods requiring chewing should be delayed until this time.

⚷ CN: Health promotion and maintenance; CL: Apply

77. 1. The client needs further instruction when she says burping should be done after 15 minutes of formula feeding. The entire feeding should take only 15 to 20 minutes, and the neonate should be burped before the feeding is complete. During initial feedings, the burping should be done after each half-ounce of formula with the neonate in an upright position, patting the neonate gently on the back.

⚷ CN: Health promotion and maintenance; CL: Evaluate

78. 2. Most babies are developmentally ready to drink independently from a cup by the age of 8 to 10 months. If the child has not mastered drinking from a cup by this time, there may be a problem with motor development that requires further investigation.

⚷ CN: Health promotion and maintenance; CL: Apply

The Postpartal Client with a Cesarean Birth

79. 3. The client should have more active bowel sounds by this time postpartum. Ambulation will encourage passing flatus and begin peristaltic action in the gastrointestinal track. Medicating the client should be evaluated prior to ambulating, but it is probably too soon because the last dose was 3

hours ago and her pain assessment rating is fairly low. Pain medications should not have codeine as a component as it decreases peristaltic activity. Incentive spirometry or asking the client to turn, cough, and deep breathe is appropriate to encourage good oxygen exchange in the lungs prior to ambulation, and walking can be used concurrently with these interventions. Participating in infant care is another way to encourage the mother to move about, but the primary goal would be to have her walk on the unit, a more purposeful activity.

⚷ CN: Physiological adaptation; CL: Synthesize

80. 2. Carboprost is an oxytocic prostaglandin that causes uterine contraction in women who are bleeding heavily. Nausea, vomiting, diarrhea, and fever are common adverse effects of prostaglandin administration. Vertigo and confusion are not associated with this drug. Carboprost may not control all cases of hemorrhage, but it does not cause bleeding. Restlessness typically is a sign of shock, not a reaction to carboprost. If too large a dose is given, the client may experience headache and hypertension because carboprost contracts smooth muscles.

⚷ CN: Pharmacological and parenteral therapies; CL: Evaluate

81. 4. Slightly red-tinged urine may indicate that the bladder was accidentally cut during the cesarean birth. The nurse should notify the **HCP** 📖 as soon as possible about the urine color. Continuing to monitor the client's input and output should be done after the HCP is contacted. Palpating the fundus every 15 minutes is not necessary unless the client's fundus becomes soft or "boggy." Assessment of the Foley catheter is a normal part of the elimination assessment by the nurse, but displacement is not the cause of the red-tinged urine.

⚷ CN: Reduction of risk potential; CL: Synthesize

82. 1. VBAC can be attempted if the client has not had a classic uterine incision. This type of incision carries a danger of uterine rupture. A **healthcare provider (HCP)** 📖 must be available, and a cesarean birth must be possible within 30 minutes. A history of rapid labor is not a criterion for VBAC. A low transverse incision is not a contraindication for VBAC. A classic (vertical) incision is a contraindication because the client has a greater possibility for uterine rupture. Estimated fetal weight greater than 4,000 g by itself is not a contraindication if the mother is not diabetic.

⚷ CN: Health promotion and maintenance; CL: Apply

83. 3. For maximum effectiveness, RhoGAM should be administered within 72 hours postpartum. Most Rh-negative clients also receive RhoGAM during the prenatal period at 28 weeks' gestation and then again after birth. The drug is given to Rh-negative mothers who have a negative Coombs test and give birth to Rh-positive neonates. If there is doubt about the fetus's blood type after pregnancy is terminated, the mother should receive the medication.

CN: Pharmacological and parenteral therapies; CL: Apply

84. 1. After a cesarean birth, most mothers have the greatest comfort when the neonate is positioned in the football hold with the mother in semi-Fowler's position, supporting the neonate's head in her hand and resting the neonate's body on pillows alongside her hip. This position prevents pressure on the uterine incision yet allows the neonate easy access to the mother's breast. The scissors hold, where the mother places her hand well back on the breast to prevent touching the areola and interfering with the neonate's mouth placement, is used by the mother to hold the breast and support it during breast-feeding. The cross-cradle hold is done when the mother holds the neonate's head in the hand opposite from the breast on which the neonate will feed and the mother's arm supports the neonate's body across her lap. This position can be uncomfortable because of the pressure placed on the client's incision line. For the cradle hold, the mother cradles the infant alongside the arm at the breast on which the neonate will feed. This position also can be uncomfortable because of the pressure placed on the incision line.

CN: Basic care and comfort; CL: Synthesize

The Postpartal Client with Complications

85. 4. A client who is pale and shaking could be experiencing hypovolemic shock likely caused by blood loss. A primary cause of blood loss after the birth of an infant is uterine atony. Therefore, the priority assessments should be the fundus of the uterus for firmness and location. In addition, the amount of vaginal bleeding (lochia) should also be assessed. An immediate intervention for uterine atony is fundal massage that will help the uterus to contract and therefore stop additional bleeding. Assessing the client's level of consciousness does not require additional time and can be done by the nurse while the fundus and lochia are assessed. Obtaining vital signs, blood glucose, and temperature are important but either should be done

after the fundus has been assessed and massaged or should be obtained by a second responder. Assessing for uterine infection and pain should be done after treatment for hypovolemic shock has been initiated.

CN: Reduction of risk potential; CL: Analyze

86. 2. Pain after childbirth is generally well managed with pain control medications; since they did not help this woman, further assessment is necessary. The first nursing action would be to assess the source of the pain; the woman may have sustained a laceration or a hematoma as a result of childbirth. Assessing the perineum may help the nurse to determine the source of the pain and may require follow-up by the **healthcare provider (HCP)** 📖. Subsequent nursing interventions may include pain medication, sitz bath, or education regarding the healing process.

CN: Basic care and comfort; CL: Analyze

87. 3. A pain and swelling may be indicative of thrombophlebitis. Redness at the site and may be more reliable as an indicator of thrombophlebitis. The nurse should notify the **HCP** 📖 immediately and ask the client to remain in bed to minimize the risk for pulmonary embolus, a serious consequence of thrombophlebitis should a clot dislodge. Placing an ice pack on the perineal area is inappropriate. However, ice to the perineum would be useful for episiotomy pain and swelling. The client does not need to be positioned in semi-Fowler's position but should remain on bed rest to prevent dislodgement of a potential clot.

CN: Reduction of risk potential; CL: Synthesize

88. 4. Heparin therapy is prescribed to prevent further clot formation by inhibiting further thrombus and clot formation. Heparin, an anticoagulant, does not make blood clots thinner. An adverse effect of heparin therapy during the puerperium is increased lochia flow, so the nurse must be observant for symptoms of hemorrhage, such as heavy lochial flow. Heparin does not increase diaphoresis, which is normal for the postpartum client.

CN: Pharmacological and parenteral therapies; CL: Evaluate

89. 2. A major complication of deep vein thrombosis is pulmonary embolism. Signs and symptoms, which may occur suddenly and require immediate treatment, include dyspnea, severe chest pain, apprehension, cough (possibly accompanied by hemoptysis), tachycardia, fever, hypotension, diaphoresis, pallor, shortness of breath, and friction rub. Pain in the calf is common with a diagnosis of deep vein thrombosis. Hypotension, not hypertension, would suggest a possible pulmonary embolism. It also could suggest possible hemorrhage secondary to intravenous heparin therapy. Bradycardia for the first 7 days in the postpartum period is normal.

CN: Reduction of risk potential; CL: Synthesize

90. 3. A slow pulse (bradycardia) is normal for the first 7 days postpartum as the body begins to adjust to the decrease in blood volume and return to the prepregnant state. Adverse effects of heparin therapy suggesting prolonged bleeding include hematuria, epistaxis, increased lochial flow, and bleeding gums. Typically, tachycardia, not bradycardia, would be associated with hemorrhage. Petechiae indicate bleeding under the skin or in subcutaneous tissue.

CN: Reduction of risk potential; CL: Evaluate

91. 3. Successful teaching is demonstrated when the client says, "I should use a soft toothbrush to brush my teeth." Heparin therapy can cause the gums to bleed, so a soft toothbrush should be used to minimize this adverse effect. Use of aspirin and other nonsteroidal anti-inflammatory medications should be avoided because of the increased risk for possible hemorrhage. Protamine sulfate is the antidote for heparin therapy. Vitamin K is the antidote for warfarin excess. Alcohol can inhibit the metabolism of oral anticoagulants and should be avoided.

CN: Pharmacological and parenteral therapies; CL: Evaluate

92. 4. Frequent handwashing is the most important aspect of infection control. The nurse can emphasize, monitor, and ensure this strategy for all who come in contact with this client. The use of gloves is not needed for clients caring for their own infants. The best practice is to restrict visitation if the client has a respiratory illness. If visitation is necessary, it is better if the client with the known infection wears the mask. Individual client care equipment is not needed in this situation.

CN: Reduction of risk potential; CL: Evaluate

93. 1,4,5. Endometritis is an ascending infection where organisms from the lower reproductive tract contaminate the normally sterile uterine lining. When the amniotic membranes rupture, bacteria from the cervix, vagina, perineum, and bowel can ascend into the uterus and infect the lining. Manual removal of placenta, prolonged labors, and the use of fetal scalp electrodes all increase the risk of developing endometritis postpartum. The use of in-and-out catheters during labor is not a risk factor

for developing endometritis. Epidural use for pain relief in labor is not a risk factor for developing endometritis postpartum.

CN: Reduction of risk potential; CL: Analyze

94. 1. Before administering ampicillin intravenously, the nurse must ask the client if she has any drug allergies, especially to penicillin. Antibiotic therapy can cause adverse effects, such as rash or even anaphylaxis. If the client is allergic to penicillin, the **healthcare provider (HCP)** □ should be notified, and ampicillin should not be given. Checking the client's pulse rate or placing her in a side-lying position is not necessary. Assessing the amount of lochia by checking the perineal pad is important for all postpartum clients but is not necessary before antibiotic therapy.

CN: Pharmacological and parenteral therapies; CL: Apply

95. 3. The nurse should encourage the client to maintain Fowler's position, which promotes comfort and facilitates drainage. Endometritis can make the client feel extremely uncomfortable and fatigued, so ambulation during intravenous therapy is not as important at this time. The client does not need to discontinue breast-feeding, although she may become quite fatigued and need assistance in caring for the neonate. Typically, breast-feeding would be discontinued only if the mother lacks the necessary energy. The institution's policy regarding visitors is to be followed. However, visitors do not need to be restricted to prevent contamination because the client is not considered to be contagious. The nurse should maintain the client's need for privacy and rest and should respect the client's wishes related to visitors.

CN: Reduction of risk potential; CL: Synthesize

96. 2. The client diagnosed with cystitis needs to void every 2 to 4 hours while awake to keep her bladder empty. In addition, she should maintain adequate fluid intake; 3,000 mL/day is recommended. Intake of acidic fruit juices (e.g., cranberry, apricot) is recommended because of their association with reducing the risk for infection. The client should wear cotton underwear and avoid tight-fitting slacks. She does not need to wash with povidone-iodine after voiding. Plain warm water is sufficient to keep the perineal area clean.

CN: Basic care and comfort; CL: Create

97. 1. The client can continue to breast-feed as often as she desires. Continuation of breast-feeding is limited only by the client's discomfort or malaise. Antibiotics for treatment are chosen carefully so that they avoid affecting the neonate through breast milk. Drugs such as sulfonamides, nitrofurantoin, and cephalosporins usually are not prescribed for breast-feeding mothers. Manual pumping of the breasts is not necessary.

⚷ CN: Health promotion and maintenance; CL: Apply

98. 1. Carboprost tromethamine may cause hypertension, not hypotension. More commonly carboprost tromethamine, a synthetic prostaglandin, causes nausea, vomiting, diarrhea, and fever. Gastrointestinal symptoms are so common that antiemetic and antidiarrheal medications are often given as a pretreatment or immediately following carboprost.

⚷ CN: Pharmacological and parenteral therapies; CL: Analyze

99. 1. The client is exhibiting signs of early postpartal hemorrhage, defined as blood loss greater than 500 mL in the first 24 hours postpartum. Rapid intravenous oxytocin infusion of 30 units in 500 mL of normal saline, oxygen therapy, and gentle fundal massage to contract the uterus are usually effective. If bleeding persists, the nurse should inspect the cervix and vagina for lacerations. Other pharmacologic interventions may be needed. Severe uncontrolled hemorrhage may require bimanual uterine compression, a dilation and curettage to remove any retained placental tissue, or a hysterectomy to prevent maternal death from hemorrhage. The client should be placed in the supine position to allow evaluation of the fundus. The side-lying position is not helpful in controlling postpartum hemorrhage. Vigorous fundal massage every 5 minutes is unnecessary. In addition, it can be very painful for the mother. Rather, gentle massage along with oxytocin administration is used to stimulate the uterus to contract. A hysterectomy is used to remove fibroid tumors. With massive hemorrhage, a hysterectomy (removal of the uterus) may be necessary to control the bleeding.

⚷ CN: Health promotion and maintenance; CL: Create

100. 4. The most likely cause of this client's uterine atony is overdistention of the uterus caused by the hydramnios. As a result, the stretched uterine musculature contracts less vigorously. Besides hydramnios, a large infant, bleeding from abruptio placentae or placenta previa, and rapid labor and birth can also contribute to uterine atony during the postpartum period. Trauma during labor and birth is not a likely cause. In addition, no evidence of excessive trauma was described in the scenario. Moderate fundal massage helps to contract the uterus, not contribute to uterine atony. Although a

lengthy or prolonged labor can contribute to uterine atony, this client had a cesarean birth for breech presentation. Therefore, it is unlikely that she had a long labor.

⚷ CN: Physiological adaptation; CL: Apply

101. 4. The classic symptoms of endometritis are fever and foul-smelling lochia. Odorless, heavy bleeding is associated with retained placental fragments. Abdominal distention is associated with parametritis as the pelvic cellulitis advances and spreads, causing severe pain and distention. Nausea and vomiting are associated with parametritis, resulting from an abscess and advancing pelvic cellulitis.

⚷ CN: Reduction of risk potential; CL: Analyze

102. 4. The most likely cause of delayed postpartum hemorrhage is retained placental fragments. The client may be scheduled for a dilatation and curettage to remove remaining placental fragments. Uterine atony, cervical lacerations, and vaginal lacerations are commonly associated with early, not late, postpartum hemorrhage.

⚷ CN: Health promotion and maintenance; CL: Apply

103. 1. The client being treated for mastitis should continue to breast-feed often, or at least every 2 to 3 hours. Treatment also includes bed rest, increased fluid intake, local heat application, analgesics, and antibiotic therapy. Continually emptying the breasts decreases the risk of engorgement or breast abscess. The client should not discontinue breast-feeding unless she chooses to do so. The client may continue breast-feeding while receiving antibiotic therapy. Generally, the breast milk is not contaminated by the offending organism and is safe for the neonate.

⚷ CN: Physiological adaptation; CL: Synthesize

104. 1. Down syndrome is a genetic abnormality that is caused by an extra chromosome that results in mental retardation. The degree of mental retardation is difficult to predict in a neonate, although most children born with Down syndrome have some degree of mental retardation. Various methods can be used to determine whether a neonate has Down syndrome, which is commonly manifested by hypotonia, poor Moro reflex, flat facial profile, up-slanting palpebral fissures, epicanthal folds, and hyperflexible joints. Genetic studies can be indicative of this disorder. Mothers older than 35 years of age are at a higher risk for having a child with Down syndrome. However, chromosomal abnormalities can occur regardless of the mother's age.

⚷ CN: Reduction of risk potential; CL: Evaluate

105. **1.** After birth, the client should make the decision about how much she would like to participate in the neonate's care. Seeing and caring for the neonate commonly facilitates the grief process. The nurse should be nonjudgmental and should allow the client any opportunity to see, hold, and care for the neonate. The **healthcare provider (HCP)** 📖 does not need to be contacted about the client's desire to see the baby, which is a normal reaction. The social worker and the adoptive parents do not need to give the client permission to feed the baby.

🔑 CN: Health promotion and maintenance; CL: Synthesize

106. **4.** The client needs further instruction when she says that she should begin feeding on the right (painful) breast to decrease the pain. Starting the feeding on the unaffected (left) breast can stimulate the milk ejection reflex in the right breast and thereby decrease the pain. Frequent nursing or pumping is recommended to empty the breast. For some mothers, mastitis is so painful that they choose to discontinue breast-feeding, so these mothers need a great deal of support. Applying heat to the infected area before starting to feed is appropriate because heat stimulates circulation and promotes comfort. Increasing fluid intake is advised to ensure adequate hydration. Antibiotics need to be taken until all medication has been used, usually 7 to 10 days to ensure eradication of the infection.

🔑 CN: Reduction of risk potential; CL: Evaluate

107. **3.** The client is probably experiencing postpartum depression, and the **healthcare provider (HCP)** 📖 should be contacted. Postpartum depression is usually treated with psychotherapy, social support groups, and antidepressant medications. Contributing factors include hormonal fluctuations, a history of depression, and environmental factors (e.g., job loss). An estimated 50% to 70% of women experience some degree of postpartum "blues," but these feelings of sadness disappear within 1 to 2 weeks after birth. However, the client is voicing more than just sadness. Telling her that she is overreacting is not helpful and may make her feel even less worthy. She is not exhibiting symptoms of a serious mental illness (loss of contact with reality) and does not need hospitalization.

🔑 CN: Health promotion and maintenance; CL: Synthesize

108. **3.** Feelings of guilt combined with a lack of self-care (not eating or sleeping enough) can predispose a new mother to postpartum depression, especially one who has had previous episodes of depression. Sleep is essential to both the mother and baby, but sleeping through the night does not usually occur in the first few weeks after birth. While breast-feeding mothers do need good nutrition, eating as much as you want after birth may inhibit the return to a normal weight and could create depression in a new mother, especially a vulnerable one. Attempting to care for an infant with no help from others is likely to cause stress that could lead to depression, especially in an adolescent.

🔑 CN: Psychosocial integrity; CL: Evaluate

Managing Care, Quality, and Safety of Postpartal Clients

109. **2,3,1,4.** The nurse should then clean the solution from the client, notify the **healthcare provider (HCP)** 📖 of the incident, and ask for a prescription for medication if needed to counteract the povidone-iodine. The nurse will need to document the incident on the client's **medical record** 📖 as soon as the client has physically been taken care of. The nurse also will need to file an incident report.

🔑 CN: Management of care; CL: Synthesize

110. **4.** The process for infant abduction in a hospital system focuses on utilizing all healthcare workers to observe for anyone who may possibly be concealing an infant in a large bag or under an oversized coat and is attempting to leave the building. Moving to the entrances and exits and checking each individual would be a responsibility of the doorman or security staff within the hospital system. Going to the obstetrics unit to determine if they need help would not be advised as the doors to the unit will be locked and access will not be available. Calling the nursery to ask about a missing baby wastes time, and the nursery staff should not reveal such information.

🔑 CN: Safety and infection control; CL: Synthesize

111.

0500	3
0530	1
0600	4
0630	2

Drawing the bilirubin levels at 0600 must occur at a specific time. The admission assessment should be completed as soon after admission as possible; 0500 is available to complete this task. The IV should be started at 0630 and completed as close to change of shift as possible. The nurse should then draw the blood at 0530, right after the newborn assessment.

🔑 CN: Management of care; CL: Create

112. 4. While the greatest risk of postpartum hemorrhage is within the first hour following birth, a woman can develop an early postpartum hemorrhage anytime within the first 24 hours postbirth. As soon as the nurse notices an increased amount of lochia and clots, the fundus must be assessed for firmness and position. Normally, it should be firm, midline, and either just above or below the umbilicus. Massaging the fundus if it is not firm will assist with a uterine contraction to help decrease blood loss postpartum. Administering oxytocin would not be the first action for the nurse to take. Performing an in-and-out catheterization at this time is not appropriate. The nurse should assist the woman to the washroom to void on her own first. The nurse can measure the blood loss by measuring the perineal pad; however, this would be done after the nurse has first assessed the fundus.

🔑 CN: Management of care; CL: Synthesize

113. 1. Hemoglobin (hgb) values following birth remains close to that during pregnancy. This value would indicate low hgb value and requires further follow-up by notifying **HCP** 📖 and documentation. WBC of 18,000 × 10⁹/L is considered normal during postpartum period. This is normal value for hematocrit. 9 mmol/L for serum iron is within normal range. WBC is within normal range for postpartum period and will not require parenteral antibiotics. Vital signs can be assessed following contacting the HCP. Pain medication is not indicated at this time based on these lab values.

🔑 CN: Management of care; CL: Synthesize

114. 1,5. Foul-smelling lochia and an elevated temperature greater than 100.8°F (38.2°C) are signs of a postpartum infection and should be reported to the **HCP** 📖. Bilateral engorgement is not an unusual finding and typically responds to nursing interventions such as use of ice packs. Postpartum blues can cause the client to cry easily for up to 2 weeks after birth. Soaking a peripad every 3 to 4 hours is a normal amount of lochia for a postpartum client within a week of birth.

🔑 CN: Management of care; CL: Synthesize

115. 1. Safety is the highest priority, and a nursing error has occurred. If the day nurse decides to tell the night nurse, the timing of the notification will be up to the nurse initiating the incident report. The nurse should confer with the charge nurse concerning the incident, but completion of the report is required. Waiting for several hours to initiate the report based on changes in client data and assessment is not an ethical or professional decision and should not be considered; again, safety is the highest priority.

🔑 CN: Reduction of risk; CL: Analyze

116. 2,3,4,5. The use of recycling bins on the unit does not impact safety or contribute to the quality of care. The infant identification system is a safety practice. Nursing influences the type of system used and how monitoring and identification occur, which improves the quality of care. The sibling and family visitation policy can be an excellent project. Sibling policies regarding visitation can influence safety (safety of mother and infant by keeping children with colds/flus, infections away from the obstetrics unit). Nursing influences development of the policy utilized and implemented on a daily basis. Postpartum instructions represent an area where the skill level, quality, and quantity of instruction represent nursing contributions to care. The ability for a family to remain together during a hospital stay is important to families. The quality of the obstetrical experience can be enhanced or determined to be negative by this particular policy, one that is often looked at by these committees.

🔑 CN: Management of care; CL: Apply

117. 1,2,4,5. The safety of clients on an obstetrical unit does include prevention of infant abduction. Safe medication administration guidelines apply in obstetrics as well as all units in the hospital system. Adequate nourishment on the unit is essential for promotion of breast-feeding and for those clients who want to eat shortly after birth but is not a safety concern. Adequate restraints as used during procedures, such as circumcisions, are a safety concern. An infant always needs proper identification when admitted, discharged, and taken to or away from parents, and this is also a great safety issue.

🔑 CN: Reduction of risk; CL: Apply

118. 1,2,3,4. Specific safety concerns on an obstetrical unit include a very specific "hand-off report" after birth and recovery has been completed and the couplet is transitioned to mother-baby care. In any invasive procedure including tubal ligations and circumcisions, preprocedure verification is a standard procedure. Client education concerning the potential for infection in obstetrics is essential for any incision areas. Infant abduction is an ever-present concern for those working in a mother-baby unit. Car seat instructions for new parents involve the infant being in the back seat of a car facing backward—**not** in the front seat. Education for the family includes this important area.

🔑 CN: Reduction of risk potential; CL: Evaluate

119. 2. The fundus descends at the rate of 1 to 2 cm/day and by 2 weeks is no longer a pelvic organ. The vital signs, breasts, heart, lungs, abdomen (with exception of fundus), lochia, perineum, and extremities are within normal limits.

🔑 CN Reduction of risk potential; CL: Analyze

The Neonatal Client

- **Neonatal Care**
- **Physical Assessment of the Neonatal Client**
- **The Preterm Neonate**
- **The Postterm Neonate**
- **The Neonate with Risk Factors**
- **Managing Care, Quality, and Safety of Neonatal Clients**
- **Answers, Rationales, and Test-Taking Strategies**

Neonatal Care

1. A primiparous woman has recently given birth to a term infant. Priority teaching for the client includes information on:
- ☐ **1.** sudden infant death syndrome (SIDS).
- ☐ **2.** breast-feeding.
- ☐ **3.** infant bathing.
- ☐ **4.** infant sleep-wake cycles.

2. A newborn who is 20 hours old has a respiratory rate of 66, is grunting when exhaling, and has occasional nasal flaring. The newborn's temperature is 98°F (36.6°C); he is breathing room air and is pink with acrocyanosis. The mother had membranes that were ruptured 26 hours before birth. What nursing actions are **most** indicated?
- ☐ **1.** Continue recording vital signs, voiding, stooling, and eating patterns every 4 hours.
- ☐ **2.** Place a pulse oximeter, and contact the healthcare provider (HCP) for a prescription to draw blood cultures.
- ☐ **3.** Arrange a transfer to the neonatal intensive care unit with diagnosis of possible sepsis.
- ☐ **4.** Draw a complete blood count (CBC) with differential and feed the infant.

3. A neonate is born by cesarean section at 36 weeks' gestation. The temperature in the birthing room is 70°F (21.1°C). To prevent heat loss from convection, which action should the nurse take?
- ☐ **1.** Dry the neonate quickly after birth.
- ☐ **2.** Keep the neonate away from air conditioning vents.
- ☐ **3.** Place the neonate away from outside windows.
- ☐ **4.** Prewarm the bed.

4. The healthcare provider (HCP) prescribes ampicillin 100 mg/kg/dose for a newly admitted neonate. The neonate weighs 1,350 g. How many milligrams should the nurse administer? Record your answer using one decimal place.
_____ mg.

5. A neonate born at 30 weeks' gestation and weighing 2,000 g is admitted to the neonatal intensive care unit. What nursing measure will decrease insensible water loss in a neonate?
- ☐ **1.** bathing the baby as soon after birth as possible
- ☐ **2.** use of eye patches with phototherapy
- ☐ **3.** use of humidity in the incubator
- ☐ **4.** use of a radiant warmer

6. A septic preterm neonate's IV was removed due to infiltration. The nurse prioritizes restarting the IV to help which complication?
- ☐ **1.** fever
- ☐ **2.** hyperkalemia
- ☐ **3.** hypoglycemia
- ☐ **4.** tachycardia

7. The nurse makes a home visit to a 3-day-old full-term neonate who weighed 3,912 g (8 lb, 10 oz) at birth. Today the neonate, who is being bottle-fed, weighs 3,572 g (7 lb, 14 oz). Which instructions should the nurse give to the mother?
- ☐ **1.** Continue feeding every 3 to 4 hours since the weight loss is normal.
- ☐ **2.** Contact the healthcare provider (HCP).
- ☐ **3.** Switch to a soy-based formula because the current one seems inadequate.
- ☐ **4.** Change to a higher-caloric formula to prevent further weight loss.

8. Commercial formulas contain 20 calories per 30 mL. A 1-day-old infant was fed 45 mL at 0200, 0530, 0800, 1,100, 1,400, 1,630, 2,000, and 2,230. What is the total amount of calories the infant received today? Record your answer using one decimal place.
_____ calories.

9. A healthy neonate was just born in stable condition. In addition to drying the infant, what is the preferred method to prevent heat loss?
- ☐ **1.** placing the infant under a radiant warmer
- ☐ **2.** wrapping the infant in warm blankets
- ☐ **3.** applying a knit hat
- ☐ **4.** placing the infant skin-to-skin on the mother

10. The nurse is preparing to administer a vitamin K injection to a male neonate shortly after birth. What statement by the mother indicates that she understands the purpose of the injection?
☐ 1. "My baby does not have the normal bacteria in his intestines to produce this vitamin."
☐ 2. "My baby is at a high risk for a problem involving his blood's ability to clot."
☐ 3. "The red blood cells my baby formed during pregnancy are destroying the vitamin K."
☐ 4. "My baby's liver is not able to produce enough of this vitamin so soon after birth."

11. The nurse is teaching the mother of a newborn to develop her baby's sensory system. To further improve the infant's most developed sense, the nurse should instruct the mother to:
☐ 1. speak in a high-pitched voice to get the newborn's attention.
☐ 2. place the newborn about 12 inches from maternal face for best sight.
☐ 3. stroke the newborn's cheek with her nipple to direct the baby's mouth to nipple.
☐ 4. give infant formula with a sweetened taste to stimulate feeding.

12. The nurse has completed discharge teaching with new parents who will be bottle-feeding their normal term newborn. Which statement by the parents reflects the need for more teaching?
☐ 1. "Our baby will require feedings through the night for several weeks or months after birth."
☐ 2. "The baby should burp during and after each feeding with no projective vomiting."
☐ 3. "Our baby should have one to three soft, formed stools a day."
☐ 4. "We should weigh our baby daily to make sure he is gaining weight."

13. The nurse knows the mother of a neonate has understood her car seat safety instructions when she comments:
☐ 1. "I did not realize that even children between 1 to 2 years old are safer in rear-facing car seats."
☐ 2. "I should put my car seat in the front so I can watch my baby when I drive."
☐ 3. "I plan to use the car seat I saved from my last baby 10 years ago."
☐ 4. "The front-facing car seats do a better job supporting the head and neck of my baby."

14. While making a home visit to a primiparous client and her 3-day-old son, the nurse observes the mother changing the baby's disposable diaper. Before putting the clean diaper on the neonate, the mother begins to apply baby powder to the neonate's buttocks. Which information about baby powder should the nurse relate to the mother?
☐ 1. It may cause pneumonia to develop.
☐ 2. It helps prevent diaper rash.
☐ 3. It keeps the diaper from adhering to the skin.
☐ 4. It can result in allergies later in life.

15. After teaching a new mother about the care of her neonate after circumcision with a Gomco clamp, which statement by the mother indicates to the nurse that the mother needs additional instructions?
☐ 1. "The petroleum gauze may fall off into the diaper."
☐ 2. "A few drops of blood oozing from the site is normal."
☐ 3. "I will leave the gauze in place for 24 hours."
☐ 4. "I will remove any yellowish crusting gently with water."

16. After completing discharge instructions for a primiparous client who is bottle-feeding her term neonate, the nurse determines that the mother understands the instructions when the mother says that she should contact the healthcare provider (HCP) if the neonate exhibits which sign or symptom?
☐ 1. ability to fall asleep easily after each feeding
☐ 2. spitting up of a tablespoon of formula after feeding
☐ 3. passage of a liquid stool with a watery ring
☐ 4. production of one to two light brown stools daily

17. The nurse instructs a primiparous client about bottle-feeding her neonate. Which action demonstrates that the mother has understood the nurse's instructions?
☐ 1. placing the neonate on his back after the feeding
☐ 2. bubbling the baby after 1 oz (30 mL) of formula
☐ 3. putting three-fourths of the bottle nipple into the baby's mouth
☐ 4. pointing the nipple toward the neonate's palate

18. The nurse is to draw a blood sample for glucose testing from a term neonate during the first hour after birth. The nurse should obtain the blood sample from the neonate's foot near which area?

☐ **1.**

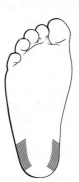

☐ **2.**

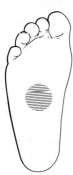

☐ **3.**

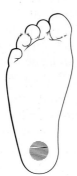

☐ **4.**

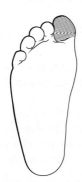

19. After circumcision with a Plastibell, the nurse should instruct the neonate's mother to cleanse the circumcision site using which agent?
☐ **1.** antibacterial soap
☐ **2.** warm water
☐ **3.** povidone-iodine solution
☐ **4.** diluted hydrogen peroxide

20. Based on the understanding of periods of reactivity, the nurse should encourage the mother of a term neonate to do which approximately 90 minutes after birth?
☐ **1.** Feed the neonate.
☐ **2.** Allow the neonate to sleep.
☐ **3.** Get to know the neonate.
☐ **4.** Change the neonate's diaper.

Physical Assessment of the Neonatal Client

21. The nurse is to assess a newborn for incurving of the trunk. Which illustration indicates the position in which the nurse should place the newborn?

☐ **1.**

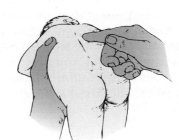

☐ **2.**

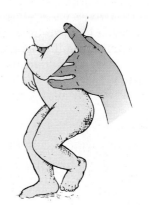

☐ **3.**

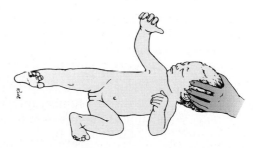

☐ **4.**

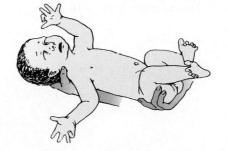

22. A full-term neonate is admitted to the normal newborn nursery. When lifting the baby out of the crib, the nurse notes the baby's arms move sideways with the palms up and the thumbs flexed. What should the nurse do **next**?
☐ **1.** Call a code.
☐ **2.** Identify this reflex as a normal finding.
☐ **3.** Place the neonate on seizure precautions.
☐ **4.** Start supplemental oxygen.

23. After the birth of a neonate, a quick assessment is completed. The neonate is found to be apneic. After quickly drying and positioning the neonate, what should the nurse do **next**?
☐ **1.** Assign the first Apgar score.
☐ **2.** Start positive pressure ventilation.
☐ **3.** Administer oxygen.
☐ **4.** Start cardiac compressions.

24. A 6-lb, 8-oz (2,948 g) neonate was born vaginally at 38 weeks' gestation. At 5 minutes of life, the neonate has the following signs: heart rate 110, intermittent grunting with respiratory rate of 70, flaccid tone, no response to stimulus, and overall pale white in color. The Apgar score is:
☐ **1.** 2
☐ **2.** 3
☐ **3.** 4
☐ **4.** 6

25. A neonate has a large amount of secretions. After vigorously suctioning the neonate, the nurse should assess for what possible result?
☐ **1.** bradycardia
☐ **2.** rapid eye movement
☐ **3.** seizures
☐ **4.** tachypnea

26. When reviewing the prenatal history for a newly born neonate, the nurse notes that the mother has neurofibromatosis. The nurse should further assess the neonate for:
☐ **1.** acrocyanosis.
☐ **2.** café au lait spots.
☐ **3.** port-wine nevus.
☐ **4.** strawberry hemangiomas.

27. A 24-hour-old, full-term neonate is showing signs of possible sepsis. The nurse is assisting the healthcare provider (HCP) with a lumbar puncture on this neonate. What should the nurse do to assist in this procedure? Select all that apply.
☐ **1.** Administer the IV antibiotic.
☐ **2.** Hold the neonate steady in the correct position.
☐ **3.** Ensure a patent airway.
☐ **4.** Maintain a sterile field.
☐ **5.** Obtain a serum glucose level.

28. After vaginal birth of a term neonate, the nurse observes that the neonate has one artery and one vein in the umbilical cord. The nurse notifies the healthcare provider (HCP) based on the analysis that this may be indicative of which anomalies?
☐ **1.** respiratory anomalies
☐ **2.** musculoskeletal anomalies
☐ **3.** cardiovascular anomalies
☐ **4.** facial anomalies

29. While changing the neonate's diaper, the client asks the nurse about some red-tinged drainage from the neonate's vagina. Which response would be **most** appropriate?
☐ **1.** "It is of no concern because it is such a small amount."
☐ **2.** "The cause is usually related to swallowing blood during the birth."
☐ **3.** "Sometimes baby girls have this from hormones received from the mother."
☐ **4.** "This vaginal spotting is caused by hemorrhagic disease of the newborn."

30. Which finding would the nurse expect as common for a multiparous client giving birth to a viable neonate at 41 weeks' gestation with the aid of a vacuum extractor?
☐ **1.** caput succedaneum
☐ **2.** cephalohematoma
☐ **3.** maternal lacerations
☐ **4.** neonatal intracranial hemorrhage

31. After explaining to a primiparous client about the causes of her neonate's cranial molding, which statement by the mother indicates the need for further instruction?
☐ **1.** "The molding was caused by an overlapping of the baby's cranial bones during my labor."
☐ **2.** "The amount of molding is related to the amount and length of pressure on the head."
☐ **3.** "The molding will usually disappear in a couple of days."
☐ **4.** "Brain damage may occur if the molding does not resolve quickly."

32. Which observation is expected when the nurse is assessing the gestational age of a neonate born at term?
☐ **1.** ear lying flat against the head
☐ **2.** absence of rugae in the scrotum
☐ **3.** sole creases covering the entire foot
☐ **4.** square window sign angle of 90 degrees

33. While performing a complete assessment of a term neonate, which finding would alert the nurse to notify the healthcare provider (HCP)?
☐ **1.** red reflex in the eyes
☐ **2.** expiratory grunt
☐ **3.** respiratory rate of 45 breaths/min
☐ **4.** prominent xiphoid process

34. After instructing a mother about normal reflexes of term neonates, the nurse determines that the mother understands the instructions when she describes the tonic neck reflex as occurring when the neonate displays which behavior?
- [ ] 1. steps briskly when held upright near a firm, hard surface
- [ ] 2. pulls both arms and does not move the chin beyond the point of the elbows
- [ ] 3. turns head to the left, extends left extremities, and flexes right extremities
- [ ] 4. extends and abducts the arms and legs with the toes fanning open

35. A primiparous client expresses concern, asking the nurse why her neonate's eyes are crossed. Which information would the nurse include when teaching the mother about neonatal strabismus?
- [ ] 1. The neonate's eyes are unable to focus on light at this time.
- [ ] 2. Neonates commonly lack eye muscle coordination.
- [ ] 3. Congenital cataracts may be present.
- [ ] 4. The neonate is able to fixate on distant objects immediately.

36. While performing a physical assessment on a term neonate shortly after birth, which finding would cause the nurse to notify the healthcare provider (HCP)?
- [ ] 1. deep creases across the soles of the feet
- [ ] 2. frequent sneezing during the assessment
- [ ] 3. single crease on each of the palms
- [ ] 4. absence of lanugo on the skin

37. Metabolic screening of an infant revealed a high phenylketonuria (PKU) level. Which statement by the infant's mother indicates understanding of the disease and its management? Select all that apply.
- [ ] 1. "My baby cannot have milk-based formulas."
- [ ] 2. "My baby will grow out of this by the age of 2."
- [ ] 3. "This is a hereditary disease, so any future children will have it, too."
- [ ] 4. "My baby will eventually become mentally challenged because of this disease."
- [ ] 5. "We have to follow a strict low-phenylalanine diet."
- [ ] 6. "A dietitian can help me plan a diet that keeps a safe phenylalanine level but lets my baby grow."

38. Assessment of a term neonate at 2 hours after birth reveals a heart rate of less than 100 bpm, periods of apnea approximately 25 to 30 seconds in length, and mild cyanosis around the mouth. The nurse notifies the healthcare provider (HCP) based on the interpretation that these findings may lead to which condition?
- [ ] 1. respiratory arrest
- [ ] 2. bronchial pneumonia
- [ ] 3. intraventricular hemorrhage
- [ ] 4. epiglottitis

39. A new mother asks, "When will the soft spot near the front of my baby's head close?" The nurse should tell the mother the soft spot will close in about:
- [ ] 1. 2 to 3 months
- [ ] 2. 6 to 8 months
- [ ] 3. 9 to 10 months
- [ ] 4. 12 to 18 months

40. Which assessment finding in a term neonate would cause the nurse to notify the healthcare provider (HCP)?
- [ ] 1. absence of tears
- [ ] 2. unequally sized corneas
- [ ] 3. pupillary constriction to bright light
- [ ] 4. red circle on pupils seen with a penlight

41. At 24 hours of age, assessment of the neonate reveals the following: eyes closed, skin pink, no sign of eye movements, heart rate of 120 bpm, and respiratory rate of 35 breaths/min. What is this neonate **most** likely experiencing?
- [ ] 1. drug withdrawal
- [ ] 2. first period of reactivity
- [ ] 3. a state of deep sleep
- [ ] 4. respiratory distress

42. While assessing a male neonate whose mother desires him to be circumcised, the nurse observes that the neonate's urinary meatus appears to be located on the ventral surface of the penis. The healthcare provider (HCP) is notified because the nurse suspects which complication?
- [ ] 1. phimosis
- [ ] 2. hydrocele
- [ ] 3. epispadias
- [ ] 4. hypospadias

The Preterm Neonate

43. The nurse is discussing kangaroo care with the parents of a premature neonate. The nurse should tell the parents that the advantages of kangaroo care include which benefits? Select all that apply.
- [ ] 1. enhanced bonding
- [ ] 2. increased IQ
- [ ] 3. improved physiologic stability
- [ ] 4. decreased length of stay in the neonatal intensive care unit
- [ ] 5. improved breast-feeding

44. After a vaginal birth, a preterm neonate is to receive oxygen via mask. While administering the oxygen, the nurse would place the neonate in which position?
- [ ] 1. left side, with the neck slightly flexed
- [ ] 2. back, with the head turned to the left side
- [ ] 3. abdomen, with the head down
- [ ] 4. back, with the neck slightly extended

45. Which action should the nurse take when performing external chest compressions on a neonate born at 28 weeks' gestation?
☐ 1. Maintain a compression-to-ventilation ratio of 3:1.
☐ 2. Compress the sternum with the palm of the hand.
☐ 3. Compress the chest 70 to 80 times/min.
☐ 4. Displace the chest wall half the depth of the anterior-posterior diameter of the chest.

46. A preterm neonate who has been stabilized is placed in a radiant warmer and is receiving oxygen via an oxygen hood. Which action should the nurse take while administering oxygen in this manner?
☐ 1. Humidify the air being delivered.
☐ 2. Cover the neonate's scalp with a warm cap.
☐ 3. Record the neonate's temperature every 3 to 4 minutes.
☐ 4. Assess the neonate's blood glucose level.

47. Two hours ago, a neonate at 38 weeks' gestation and weighing 3,175 g (7 lb) was born to a primiparous client who tested positive for beta-hemolytic Streptococcus. Which finding would alert the nurse to notify the healthcare provider (HCP)?
☐ 1. alkalosis
☐ 2. increased muscle tone
☐ 3. temperature instability
☐ 4. positive Babinski's reflex

48. Assessment of a 2-day-old neonate born at 34 weeks' gestation reveals absent apical pulse left of the midclavicular line, cyanosis, grunting, and diminished breath sounds. After beginning oxygen, the **priority** intervention is to:
☐ 1. obtain a prescription for a stat chest x-ray.
☐ 2. reposition the neonate and then assess if the grunting and cyanosis resolve.
☐ 3. obtain a prescription for an echocardiogram.
☐ 4. obtain a complete blood count to determine infection.

49. Twenty-four hours after cesarean birth, a neonate at 30 weeks' gestation is diagnosed with respiratory distress syndrome (RDS). When explaining to the parents about the cause of this syndrome, the nurse should include a discussion about an alteration in the body's secretion of which substance?
☐ 1. somatotropin
☐ 2. surfactant
☐ 3. testosterone
☐ 4. progesterone

50. A viable male neonate born to a 28-year-old multiparous client by cesarean section because of placenta previa is diagnosed with respiratory distress syndrome (RDS). Which factor would the nurse explain as the factor placing the neonate at the **greatest** risk for this syndrome?
☐ 1. mother's development of placenta previa
☐ 2. neonate born preterm
☐ 3. mother receiving analgesia 4 hours before birth
☐ 4. neonate with sluggish respiratory efforts after birth

51. While the nurse is caring for a neonate at 32 weeks' gestation in an isolette with continuous oxygen administration, the neonate's mother asks why the neonate's oxygen is humidified. The nurse should tell the mother:
☐ 1. "The humidity promotes expansion of the neonate's immature lungs."
☐ 2. "The humidity helps to prevent viral or bacterial pneumonia."
☐ 3. "Oxygen is drying to the mucous membranes unless it is humidified."
☐ 4. "Circulation to the baby's heart is improved with humidified oxygen."

52. A preterm neonate admitted to the neonatal intensive care unit at about 30 weeks' gestation is placed in an oxygenated isolette. The neonate's mother tells the nurse that she was planning to breast-feed the neonate. Which instructions about breast-feeding would be **most** appropriate?
☐ 1. Breast-feeding is not recommended because the neonate needs increased fat in the diet.
☐ 2. Once the neonate no longer needs oxygen and continuous monitoring, breast-feeding can be done.
☐ 3. Breast-feeding is contraindicated because the neonate needs a high-calorie formula every 2 hours.
☐ 4. Gavage feedings using breast milk can be given until the neonate can coordinate sucking and swallowing.

53. What is the best reason for assessing a neonate weighing 1,500 g at 32 weeks' gestation for retinopathy of prematurity (ROP)?
☐ 1. The neonate is at risk because of multiple factors.
☐ 2. Oxygen is being administered at a level of 21%.
☐ 3. The neonate was alkalotic immediately after birth.
☐ 4. Phototherapy is likely to be prescribed by the healthcare provider (HCP).

54. Which subject should the nurse include when teaching the mother of a neonate diagnosed with retinopathy of prematurity (ROP) about possible treatment for complications?
☐ 1. laser therapy
☐ 2. anti-inflammatory eye drops
☐ 3. frequent testing for glaucoma
☐ 4. corneal transplants

55. Three days after admission of a neonate born at 30 weeks' gestation, the neonatologist plans to assess the neonate for intraventricular hemorrhage (IVH). The nurse should plan to assist the neonatologist by preparing the neonate for which test?
☐ 1. cranial ultrasonography
☐ 2. arterial blood specimen collection
☐ 3. radiographs of the skull
☐ 4. complete blood count specimen collection

56. Which finding would the nurse **most** expect to find in a neonate born at 28 weeks' gestation who is diagnosed with intraventricular hemorrhage (IVH)?
☐ 1. increased muscle tone
☐ 2. hyperbilirubinemia
☐ 3. bulging fontanelles
☐ 4. hyperactivity

57. An infant born premature at 34 weeks is receiving gavage feedings. The client holding her infant asks why the nurse places a pacifier in the infant's mouth during these feedings. The nurse replies that the pacifier helps in what ways? Select all that apply.
☐ 1. teaches the infant to coordinate the swallow
☐ 2. provides oral stimulation
☐ 3. keeps oral mucous membranes moist while the tube is in place
☐ 4. reminds the infant how to suck
☐ 5. stimulates secretions that help gastric emptying

58. While caring for a neonate born at 32 weeks' gestation, which finding would **most** suggest the infant is developing necrotizing enterocolitis (NEC)?
☐ 1. the presence of 1 mL of gastric residual before a gavage feeding
☐ 2. jaundice appearing on the face and chest
☐ 3. an increase in bowel peristalsis
☐ 4. abdominal distention

59. Which statement by the mother of a neonate diagnosed with bronchopulmonary dysplasia (BPD) indicates effective teaching?
☐ 1. "BPD is an acute disease that can be treated with antibiotics."
☐ 2. "My baby may require long-term respiratory support."
☐ 3. "Bronchodilators can cure my baby's condition."
☐ 4. "My baby may have seizures later on in life because of this condition."

60. A preterm infant born 2 hours ago at 34 weeks' gestation is experiencing rapid respirations, grunting, no breath sounds on one side, and a shift in location of heart sounds. The nurse should prepare to assist with which procedure?
☐ 1. placement of the neonate on a ventilator
☐ 2. administration of bronchodilators through the nares
☐ 3. suctioning of the neonate's nares with wall suction
☐ 4. insertion of a chest tube into the neonate

61. Which finding would lead the nurse to suspect that a neonate born at 34 weeks' gestation receiving intravenous fluids has developed overhydration?
☐ 1. hypernatremia
☐ 2. polycythemia
☐ 3. hypoproteinemia
☐ 4. increased urine specific gravity

62. A newborn weighing 6½ lb (2,950 g) is to be given naloxone due to respiratory depression as a result of a narcotic given to the mother shortly before birth. The drug is to be given 0.01 mg/kg into the umbilical vein. The vial is marked 0.4 mg/mL. How many milligrams would the newborn receive? Record your answer using two decimal places.

_____ mg.

The Postterm Neonate

63. A neonate born by cesarean at 42 weeks' gestation, weighing 4.1 kg (9 lb), with Apgar scores of 8 at 1 minute and 9 at 5 minutes after birth, develops an increased respiratory rate and tremors of the hands and feet 2 hours postpartum. What is the **priority** problem for this neonate?
☐ 1. ineffective airway clearance
☐ 2. hyperthermia
☐ 3. decreased cardiac output
☐ 4. hypoglycemia

64. At a home visit, the nurse assesses a neonate born vaginally at 41 weeks' gestation 5 days ago. Which of these findings warrants further assessment?
☐ 1. Frequent hiccups
☐ 2. Loose, watery stool in diaper
☐ 3. Pink papular vesicles on the face
☐ 4. Dry, peeling skin

65. When performing an initial assessment of a postterm male neonate weighing 4,000 g (8 lb, 13 oz) who was admitted to the observation nursery after a vaginal birth with low forceps, the nurse detects Ortolani's sign. Which action should the nurse take **next**?
- ☐ 1. Determine the length of the mother's labor.
- ☐ 2. Notify the healthcare provider (HCP) immediately.
- ☐ 3. Keep the neonate under the radiant warmer for 2 hours.
- ☐ 4. Obtain a blood sample to check for hypoglycemia.

66. A neonate is admitted to the neonatal intensive care unit for observation with a diagnosis of probable meconium aspiration syndrome (MAS). The neonate weighs 10 lb, 4 oz (4,650 g) and is at 41 weeks' gestation. What would be the **priority** problem for this neonate?
- ☐ 1. impaired skin integrity
- ☐ 2. hyperglycemia
- ☐ 3. risk for impaired parent-infant-child attachment
- ☐ 4. impaired gas exchange

67. The neonate in the nurse's care has a pneumothorax. The nurse knows the signs of early decompensation and to observe carefully for changes in which assessments? Select all that apply.
- ☐ 1. blood pressure
- ☐ 2. temperature
- ☐ 3. urinary output
- ☐ 4. color
- ☐ 5. heart rate

The Neonate with Risk Factors

68. A nurse is attempting to resuscitate a neonate. Thirty seconds of chest compressions have been completed. The neonate's heart rate remains less than 60 bpm. Epinephrine is given. What is the expected outcome for a neonate who has received epinephrine during resuscitation?
- ☐ 1. increased urine output
- ☐ 2. a normal heart rate
- ☐ 3. pain relief
- ☐ 4. sedation

69. A mother is visiting her neonate in the neonatal intensive care unit. Her baby is fussy, and the mother wants to know what to do. In order to quiet a sick neonate, what can the nurse teach the mother to do?
- ☐ 1. Bring in toys for distraction.
- ☐ 2. Place a musical mobile over the crib.
- ☐ 3. Stroke the neonate's back.
- ☐ 4. Use constant, gentle touch.

70. A neonate born at 40 weeks' gestation admitted to the nursery is found to be hypoglycemic. At 4 hours of age, the neonate appears pale and his pulse oximeter is reading 75% on room air. The nurse should:
- ☐ 1. increase the IV rate.
- ☐ 2. provide supplemental oxygen.
- ☐ 3. record the finding on the medical record and repeat the reading in 30 minutes.
- ☐ 4. wrap the neonate to increase body temperature.

71. A neonate with heart failure is being discharged home. In teaching the parents about the neonate's nutritional needs, the nurse should explain that:
- ☐ 1. fluids must be restricted.
- ☐ 2. decreased activity level should reduce the need for additional calories.
- ☐ 3. the formula should be low in sodium.
- ☐ 4. the neonate may need a more calorie-dense formula.

72. During an assessment of a neonate born at 33 weeks' gestation, a nurse finds and reports a heart murmur. An echocardiogram reveals patent ductus arteriosus, for which the neonate received indomethacin. An expected outcome after the administration of indomethacin to a neonate with patent ductus arteriosus is:
- ☐ 1. closure of a patent ductus arteriosus.
- ☐ 2. decreased bleeding time.
- ☐ 3. increased gastrointestinal function.
- ☐ 4. increased renal output.

73. A nurse is reviewing a client's maternal prenatal record and notes that the mother used narcotics during her pregnancy. A primary nursing intervention when caring for a drug-exposed neonate is to:
- ☐ 1. assess vital signs including blood pressure every hour.
- ☐ 2. minimize environmental stimuli.
- ☐ 3. place the infant in a well-lighted area.
- ☐ 4. increase eye contact with caregiver.

74. The nurse is receiving over the telephone a laboratory results report of a neonate's blood glucose level. The nurse should:
- ☐ 1. write down the results, read back the results to the caller from the laboratory, and receive confirmation from the caller that the nurse understands the results.
- ☐ 2. repeat the results to the caller from the laboratory, write the results on scrap paper first, and then transfer the results to the medical record.
- ☐ 3. indicate to the caller that the nurse cannot receive verbal results from laboratory tests for neonates, and ask the laboratory to bring the written results to the nursery.
- ☐ 4. request that the laboratory send the results by e-mail to transfer to the client's medical record.

75. A multiparous client who has a neonate diagnosed with hemolytic disease of the newborn asks the nurse why the neonate has developed this problem. Which response by the nurse would be **most** appropriate?
- ☐ 1. "You are Rh positive, and the baby is Rh negative."
- ☐ 2. "You and the baby are both Rh negative."
- ☐ 3. "You are Rh negative, and the baby is Rh positive."
- ☐ 4. "The baby and you are both Rh positive."

76. After teaching the multiparous mother about hemolytic disease of the newborn and Rh sensitization, the nurse determines that the client understands why she was not sensitized during her other pregnancy when she makes which statement?
- ☐ 1. "My other baby had a different father."
- ☐ 2. "Like most women, I have immunity against the Rh factor."
- ☐ 3. "Antibodies are not usually formed until after exposure to an antigen."
- ☐ 4. "My blood could not neutralize antibodies formed from my first pregnancy."

77. After teaching a multiparous client about the effects of hemolysis due to Rh sensitization on the neonate at birth, the nurse determines that the client needs further instruction when the mother reports that the neonate may have which complication?
- ☐ 1. cardiac decompensation
- ☐ 2. polycythemia
- ☐ 3. anemia
- ☐ 4. splenic enlargement

78. After birth, a direct Coombs test is performed on the umbilical cord blood of a neonate with Rh-positive blood born to a mother with Rh-negative blood. The nurse explains to the client that this test is done to detect which information?
- ☐ 1. degree of anemia in the neonate
- ☐ 2. initial bilirubin level
- ☐ 3. antibodies coating the neonate's red blood cells
- ☐ 4. antigens coating the neonate's red blood cells

79. The nurse recognizes that teaching about the need for an exchange transfusion in a neonate with erythroblastosis fetalis has been effective if the parents describe the purpose of the transfusion is:
- ☐ 1. to replenish the neonate's leukocytes.
- ☐ 2. to restore the fluid and electrolyte balance.
- ☐ 3. to correct the neonate's anemia.
- ☐ 4. to replace Rh-negative blood with Rh-positive blood.

80. The nurse explains to the mother of a neonate diagnosed with erythroblastosis fetalis that the exchange transfusion is necessary to prevent damage primarily to which organ in the neonate?
- ☐ 1. kidneys
- ☐ 2. brain
- ☐ 3. lungs
- ☐ 4. liver

81. The nurse determines that a newborn is experiencing hypoglycemia based on which findings? Select all that apply.
- ☐ 1. a blood glucose reading of less than 30 mg/dL (1.7 mmol/L) at 1 hour
- ☐ 2. family history of insulin-dependent diabetes
- ☐ 3. internal fetal monitor tracing
- ☐ 4. irregular respirations, tremors, and hypothermia
- ☐ 5. large for gestational age

82. The nurse is caring for a newborn of a primiparous woman with insulin-dependent diabetes. When the mother visits the neonate at 1 hour after birth, the nurse explains to the mother that the neonate is being closely monitored for symptoms of hypoglycemia because of which reason?
- ☐ 1. increased use of glucose stores during a difficult labor and birth process
- ☐ 2. interrupted supply of maternal glucose and continued high neonatal insulin production
- ☐ 3. a normal response that occurs during transition from intrauterine to extrauterine life
- ☐ 4. increased pancreatic enzyme production caused by decreased glucose stores

83. When caring for a neonate weighing 4,564 g (10 lb, 1 oz) born vaginally to a mother with diabetes, the nurse should assess the neonate for fracture of the:
- ☐ 1. clavicle
- ☐ 2. skull
- ☐ 3. wrist
- ☐ 4. rib cage

84. While caring for a neonate of a woman with diabetes soon after birth, the nurse has fed the newborn formula to prevent hypoglycemia. The nurse checks the neonate's blood glucose level, and it is 60 mg/dL (3.3 mmol/L), but the neonate continues to exhibit jitteriness and tremors. The nurse should **first:**
- ☐ 1. request a prescription for a blood calcium level.
- ☐ 2. administer glucose intravenously based on infant glucose level.
- ☐ 3. take the neonate's temperature and place him in the radiant warmer.
- ☐ 4. refeed the infant to continue to increase the blood glucose level.

85. The nurse is caring for a neonate weighing 4,536 g (10 lb) who was born via cesarean section 1 hour ago to a mother with insulin-dependent diabetes. She asks the nurse, "Why is my baby in the neonatal intensive care unit?" The nurse bases a response on the understanding that neonates of mothers with diabetes commonly develop which condition?
- ☐ 1. anemia
- ☐ 2. persistent pulmonary hypertension
- ☐ 3. hemolytic disease
- ☐ 4. hypoglycemia

86. While assessing a neonate weighing 3,175 g (7 lb) who was born at 39 weeks' gestation to a primiparous client who admits to opiate use during pregnancy, which finding would alert the nurse to possible opiate withdrawal?
- ☐ 1. bradycardia
- ☐ 2. high-pitched cry
- ☐ 3. sluggishness
- ☐ 4. hypocalcemia

87. The nurse recognizes that parent teaching about complications of neonatal opioid exposure has been effective when the parents state that the baby may exhibit which gastrointestinal problem?
- ☐ 1. hypotonia
- ☐ 2. constipation
- ☐ 3. vomiting
- ☐ 4. abdominal distention

88. When teaching a primiparous client who used cocaine during pregnancy how to comfort her fussy neonate, the nurse can advise the mother to:
- ☐ 1. tightly swaddle the neonate.
- ☐ 2. feed the neonate extra, high-calorie formula.
- ☐ 3. keep the neonate in a brightly lit environment.
- ☐ 4. touch the baby only when he or she is crying.

89. A neonate born at 38 weeks' gestation is admitted to the neonatal nursery for observation. The neonate's mother, who is positive for human immunodeficiency virus (HIV) infection, has received no prenatal care. The mother asks the nurse if her neonate is positive for HIV. The nurse can tell the mother which information?
- ☐ 1. "More than 50% of neonates born to mothers who are positive for HIV will be positive at 18 months of age."
- ☐ 2. "An enlarged liver at birth generally means the neonate is HIV positive."
- ☐ 3. "A complete blood count analysis is the primary method for determining whether the neonate is HIV positive."
- ☐ 4. "We will test your baby now, but testing will need to be repeated for an accurate diagnosis."

90. When caring for a multiparous client who is human immunodeficiency virus (HIV) positive and asking to breast-feed her neonate as soon as possible, which instructions about breast milk should the nurse include in the teaching plan?
- ☐ 1. It may help prevent the spread of the HIV virus.
- ☐ 2. It contains antibodies that can protect the neonate from HIV.
- ☐ 3. It can be beneficial for the bonding process.
- ☐ 4. It has been found to contain the retrovirus HIV.

91. While caring for the neonate of a human immunodeficiency virus–positive mother, the nurse prepares to administer a prescribed vitamin K intramuscular injection at 1 hour after birth. Which action should the nurse do **first**?
- ☐ 1. Bathe the neonate.
- ☐ 2. Place the neonate under a radiant warmer.
- ☐ 3. Wash the injection site with povidone-iodine solution.
- ☐ 4. Wait until the first dose of antiretroviral medication is given.

92. A 6-hour-old neonate born at 38 weeks' gestation by cesarean section after prolonged rupture of the membranes and a maternal oral temperature of 102°F (38.8°C) is being observed for signs and symptoms of infection. Which sign would alert the nurse to notify the healthcare provider (HCP)?
- ☐ 1. leukocytosis
- ☐ 2. apical heart rate of 132 bpm
- ☐ 3. behavioral changes
- ☐ 4. warm, moist skin

93. The nurse is caring for a neonate diagnosed with early-onset sepsis and is being treated with intravenous antibiotics. Which instruction will the nurse include in the parents' teaching plan?
- ☐ 1. Wear protective gear near the isolation incubator.
- ☐ 2. Visit but do not touch the neonate.
- ☐ 3. Wash hands thoroughly before touching the neonate.
- ☐ 4. Wear a mask when holding the neonate.

94. A female neonate born vaginally at term with a cleft lip and cleft palate is admitted to the regular nursery. Which action should the nurse take the first time that the parents visit the neonate in the nursery?
- ☐ 1. Explain the surgical interventions that will be performed.
- ☐ 2. Stress that this defect is not life-threatening.
- ☐ 3. Emphasize the neonate's normal characteristics.
- ☐ 4. Reassure the parents about the success rate of the surgery.

95. After teaching the parents of a neonate born with a cleft lip and cleft palate about appropriate feeding techniques, the nurse determines that the mother needs further instruction when the mother makes which statement?
- ☐ 1. "I should clean her mouth each feeding."
- ☐ 2. "I should feed her in an upright position."
- ☐ 3. "I need to remember to burp her often."
- ☐ 4. "I may need to use a special nipple for feeding."

96. A male neonate born at 36 weeks' gestation is admitted to the neonatal intensive care nursery with a diagnosis of probable fetal alcohol syndrome (FAS). The mother visits the nursery soon after the neonate is admitted. Which instructions should the nurse expect to include when developing the teaching plan for the mother about FAS?
- [ ] 1. Withdrawal symptoms usually do not occur until 7 days postpartum.
- [ ] 2. Large-for-gestational-age size is common with this condition.
- [ ] 3. Facial deformities associated with FAS can be corrected by plastic surgery.
- [ ] 4. Symptoms of withdrawal include tremors, sleeplessness, and seizures.

97. Which characteristic should the nurse teach the mother about her neonate diagnosed with fetal alcohol syndrome (FAS)?
- [ ] 1. Neonates are commonly listless and lethargic.
- [ ] 2. The IQ scores are usually average.
- [ ] 3. Hyperactivity and speech disorders are common.
- [ ] 4. The mortality rate is 70% unless treated.

98. A newborn is diagnosed with fetal alcohol syndrome. The nurse is teaching this mother what to expect when she goes home with her baby. The nurse determines the mother needs further instruction when she makes which statement?
- [ ] 1. "The way my baby's face looks now will stay that way."
- [ ] 2. "My baby may be irritable as a newborn."
- [ ] 3. "I may need some help coping with my newborn."
- [ ] 4. "My baby will be fine soon after we are home."

99. The father of a neonate diagnosed with gastroschisis tells the nurse that his wife had planned on breast-feeding the neonate. Which information should the nurse include in the preoperative teaching plan about feeding the neonate?
- [ ] 1. The neonate will remain on nothing-by-mouth (NPO) status until after surgery.
- [ ] 2. An iron-fortified formula will be given before surgery.
- [ ] 3. The neonate will need total parenteral nutrition for nourishment.
- [ ] 4. The mother may breast-feed the neonate before surgery.

100. The nurse is developing a plan of care for a neonate who is to undergo gastroschisis surgery. What should be included? Select all that apply.
- [ ] 1. prevention of hypothermia
- [ ] 2. maintenance of fluid and electrolyte balance
- [ ] 3. controlling preoperative pain
- [ ] 4. prevention of infection
- [ ] 5. providing developmental care

101. While caring for a male neonate diagnosed with gastroschisis, the nurse observes that the parents seem hesitant to touch the neonate because of his appearance. The nurse determines that the parents are **most** likely experiencing which stage of grief?
- [ ] 1. denial
- [ ] 2. shock
- [ ] 3. bargaining
- [ ] 4. anger

102. Which instructions should the nurse give to the parents of a neonate diagnosed with hyperbilirubinemia who is receiving phototherapy?
- [ ] 1. Keep the neonate's eyes completely covered.
- [ ] 2. Use a regular diaper on the neonate.
- [ ] 3. Offer feedings every 4 hours.
- [ ] 4. Check the rectal temperature every 8 hours.

103. While caring for a term neonate who has been receiving phototherapy for 8 hours, the nurse should notify the healthcare provider (HCP) if which finding is noted?
- [ ] 1. bronze-colored skin
- [ ] 2. maculopapular chest rash
- [ ] 3. urine specific gravity of 1.018
- [ ] 4. absent Moro reflex

104. The nurse is caring for a neonate at 38 weeks' gestation when the nurse observes marked peristaltic waves on the neonate's abdomen. After this observation, the neonate exhibits projectile vomiting. The nurse notifies the healthcare provider (HCP) because these signs are indicative of which problem?
- [ ] 1. esophageal atresia
- [ ] 2. pyloric stenosis
- [ ] 3. diaphragmatic hernia
- [ ] 4. hiatal hernia

105. The nurse is caring for a term neonate who is diagnosed with patent ductus arteriosus. While performing a physical assessment of the neonate, the nurse anticipates that the neonate will exhibit which signs?
- [ ] 1. decreased cardiac output with faint peripheral pulses
- [ ] 2. profound cyanosis over most of the body
- [ ] 3. loud cardiac murmur through systole and diastole
- [ ] 4. harsh systolic murmur with a palpable thrill

106. Assessment of a term neonate at 8 hours after birth reveals tachypnea, diminished femoral pulses, and poor lower body perfusion. The nurse notifies the healthcare provider (HCP) based on the interpretation that these symptoms are associated with which complication?
- [ ] 1. coarctation of the aorta
- [ ] 2. atrioventricular septal defect
- [ ] 3. pulmonary atresia
- [ ] 4. transposition of the great arteries

107. The nurse is caring for a 2-day-old neonate in the postanesthesia care unit 30 minutes after surgical correction for the cardiac defect, transposition of the great vessels. Which finding would alert the nurse to notify the healthcare provider (HCP)?
- ☐ **1.** oxygen saturation of 90%
- ☐ **2.** pale pink extremities
- ☐ **3.** warm, dry skin
- ☐ **4.** femoral pulse of 90 bpm

108. Assessing a neonate at 8 hours of age, the nurse records findings on the medical record below:

Nurses Progress Notes

Time	1100
Respiration	92, no nasal flaring, retractions, grunting
Heart rate	128, no murmur noted
Temperature	98.9°F (32.3°C)

At 1130, the nurse notices the neonate has central cyanosis, and the respiratory rate is now 102; no nasal flaring, no retractions, or grunting was noted, and breath sounds were clear. The nurse should:
- ☐ **1.** change the neonate's position.
- ☐ **2.** encourage the baby to cry.
- ☐ **3.** notify the healthcare provider.
- ☐ **4.** suction the nose and mouth.

109. The nurse is performing an admission assessment on a neonate and finds the femoral pulses to be weaker than the brachial and radial pulses. The **next** nursing action should be to:
- ☐ **1.** call for a cardiac consult.
- ☐ **2.** note and tell the healthcare provider (HCP) when rounds are made.
- ☐ **3.** place the neonate in reverse Trendelenburg position.
- ☐ **4.** take the neonate's blood pressure in all four extremities.

110. A neonate is 4 hours of age. The nursing assessment reveals a heart murmur. The nurse should:
- ☐ **1.** call the healthcare provider immediately.
- ☐ **2.** continue routine care.
- ☐ **3.** feed the neonate.
- ☐ **4.** further assess for signs of distress.

111. During change of shift report, it was reported that a neonate was experiencing subcostal retractions. Identify where you would expect to see the retractions.

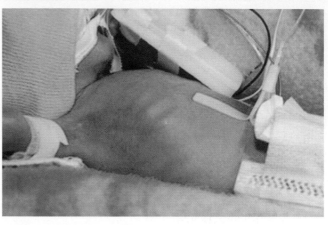

112. A woman has just given birth to a stillborn baby at 39 weeks' gestation. What is the **most** appropriate response for the nurse to make at this time?
- ☐ **1.** "I understand how you must feel."
- ☐ **2.** "I am sorry for your loss."
- ☐ **3.** "Time heals all wounds."
- ☐ **4.** "You can have another baby."

Managing Care, Quality, and Safety of Neonatal Clients

113. The nurse is making clinical rounds on a group of clients in a newborn nursery. Which infant is at **greatest** risk of developing respiratory distress syndrome (RDS)?
- ☐ **1.** a neonate born at 36 weeks' gestation
- ☐ **2.** a neonate born by cesarean section
- ☐ **3.** a neonate experiencing apneic episodes
- ☐ **4.** a neonate who is 42 weeks' gestation

114. The nurse has received a shift report on a group of newborns. The nurse should make rounds on which client **first**?
- ☐ **1.** a newborn who is large for gestational age (LGA) who needs a repeat blood glucose prior to the next feeding in 15 minutes
- ☐ **2.** a neonate born at 36 weeks' gestation weighing 5 lb (2,270 g) who is due to breast-feed for the first time in 15 minutes
- ☐ **3.** a neonate who was born 24 hours ago by cesarean section and had a respiratory rate of 62, 30 minutes ago
- ☐ **4.** a newborn who had a borderline low temperature and was double-wrapped with a hat half an hour ago to bring up the temperature

115. The nurse is caring for a 2-hour-old, full-term, breast-feeding newborn. The nurse notes the following assessments: apical pulse, 122 bpm; axilla temperature, 96.6°F (35.9°C); jitteriness. Based on this assessment, the nurse should **first**:
- ☐ 1. assist the newborn to breast-feed.
- ☐ 2. notify the healthcare provider (HCP).
- ☐ 3. obtain a blood glucose sample.
- ☐ 4. place the newborn under a radiant heater.

116. The nurse is assigned to care for four mothers and their term newborns. Which mother and newborn couplet requires the nurse's attention **first**?
- ☐ 1. Mother: fundus firm 2 cm below umbilicus, minimal lochia rubra. Infant: color is pink on room air, respirations 67 breaths/min; bilateral crackles on auscultation.
- ☐ 2. Mother: fundus firm 3 cm above umbilicus and to the right, moderate rubra lochia. Infant: color pink when active, currently dusky while quiet, respirations 70 breaths/min.
- ☐ 3. Mother: fundus firm 1 cm above umbilicus, small amount lochia rubra. Infant: color pink with acrocyanosis, respirations 68 breaths/min and intermittent expiratory grunting.
- ☐ 4. Mother: fundus firm at umbilicus, small amount lochia rubra. Infant: pale pink, quiet alert; respirations 65 breaths/min; periodic breathing noted.

117. The nurse in a postpartum couplet room is making rounds prior to ending the shift. Which findings indicate that the safety needs of the clients have been met? Select all that apply.
- ☐ 1. infant lying on abdomen
- ☐ 2. security tags in place
- ☐ 3. identification system on mother and infant
- ☐ 4. bulb syringe within sight
- ☐ 5. someone in room able to care for infant
- ☐ 6. infant in the mother's arms, both asleep

118. After receiving change of shift report in the normal newborn nursery, which neonate should the nurse see **first**?
- ☐ 1. neonate A, ½ hour of age with occasional respiratory grunting
- ☐ 2. neonate B, 4 hours of age with a blood glucose of 25 (1.38 mmol/L)
- ☐ 3. neonate C, 12 hours of age with a temperature of 97.4°F (36.4°C)
- ☐ 4. neonate D, 24 hours of age with no urine output for past 12 hours

119. The newborn nurse has just received shift report about a group of newborns and is to receive another admission in 30 minutes. In order to provide the safest care and plan for the new admission, the nurse should do which tasks in order of first to last? All options must be used.

1. Move quickly from room to room, and assess all clients.

2. Check the room to which the new client will be admitted to be sure all supplies and equipment are available.

3. Log on to the clinical information system, and determine if there are new prescriptions.

4. Review notes from shift report, and prioritize all clients; make rounds on the most critical first.

120. The charge nurse in the newborn nursery has an unlicensed assistive personnel (UAP) with her for the shift. Under their care are eight babies rooming in with their mothers, and one infant in the nursery for the night on tube feedings. There is a new client whose infant will be brought to the nursery in 15 minutes. Which tasks would the nurse assign to the UAP? Select all that apply.
- ☐ 1. newborn admission
- ☐ 2. vital signs on all stable infants
- ☐ 3. tube feeding
- ☐ 4. document feedings of infants
- ☐ 5. record voids/stools
- ☐ 6. bath and initial feeding for new admission

Answers, Rationales, and Test-Taking Strategies

The answers and rationales for each question follow below, along with keys (🔑) to the client need (CN) and cognitive level (CL) for each question. In addition, you will also see a glossary icon (📖) highlighting specific terminology used on the licensing exam. As you check your answers, use the **Content Mastery and Test-Taking Skill Self-Analysis** *worksheet (tear-out worksheet in back of book) to identify the reason(s) for not answering the questions correctly. For additional information about test-taking skills and strategies for answering questions, refer to pages 12–23 and pages 35–36 in Part 1 of this book.*

Neonatal Care

1. 2. Breast-fed infants should eat within the first hour of life and approximately every 2 to 3 hours. Successful breast-feeding will likely require sustained support, encouragement, and instruction from the nurse. Information on SIDS, infant bathing, and sleep-wake cycles are also important topics for the new parent, but can be done at any time prior to discharge.

🔑 CN: Health promotion and maintenance; CL: Analyze

2. 2. The concern with this infant is sepsis based on prolonged rupture of membranes before birth. Blood cultures would provide an accurate diagnosis of sepsis but will take 48 hours from the time drawn. Frequent monitoring of infant vital signs, looking for changes, and maintaining contact with the parents is also part of care management while awaiting culture results. Continuing with vital signs, voiding, stooling, and eating every 4 hours is the standard of care for a normal newborn, but a respiratory rate greater than 60, grunting, and occasional flaring are not normal. Although not normal, the need for the intensive care unit is not warranted as newborns with sepsis can be treated with antibiotics at the maternal bedside. The CBC does not establish the diagnosis of sepsis, but the changes in the WBC levels can identify an infant at risk. Many experts suggest that waiting until an infant is 6 to 12 hours old to draw a CBC will give the most accurate results.

🔑 CN: Reduction of risk potential; CL: Synthesize

3. 2. The neonate should be kept away from drafts, such as from air conditioning vents, which may cause heat loss by convection. Evaporation is one of the most common mechanisms by which the neonate will lose heat, such as when the moisture on the newly born neonate's body is converted to vapor. Drying the infant prevents heat loss by evaporation, Keeping infants away from outside windows helps prevent heat loss by radiation defined as heat loss between solid objects that are not in contact with one another such as walls and windows. Conduction is when heat is transferred between solid objects in contact with one another, such as when a neonate comes in contact with a cold mattress or scale. Placing the infant in a radiant warmer or skin-to-skin reduces heat loss from conduction.

🔑 CN: Reduction of risk potential; CL: Synthesize

4. 135 mg
The recommended dose of ampicillin for a neonate is 100 mg/kg/dose. First, determine the neonate's weight in kilograms, and then multiply the kilograms by 100 mg. The nurse should use this formula:

$$1,000 \text{ g} = 1 \text{ kg}$$
$$1,350 \text{ g} = 1.35 \text{ kg}$$
$$100 \text{ mg} \times 1.35 \text{ kg} = 135 \text{ mg/kg}$$

🔑 CN: Pharmacological and parenteral therapies; CL: Apply

5. 3. Adding humidity to the incubator adds moisture to the ambient air, which helps to decrease the insensible water loss. Bathing and the use of eye patches has no impact on insensible water loss. The use of a radiant warmer will increase the insensible water loss by drawing moisture out of the skin.

🔑 CN: Reduction of risk potential; CL: Synthesize

6. 3. Neonates that are septic use glucose at an increased rate. During the time the IV is not infusing, the neonate is using the limited glucose stores available to a preterm neonate and may deplete them. Hypoglycemia is too little glucose in the blood; without the constant infusion of IV glucose, hypoglycemia will result. Fevers and hyperkalemia are not related to glucose levels. Tachycardia is the result of untreated hypoglycemia.

🔑 CN: Reduction of risk potential; CL: Analyze

7. 1. This 3-day-old neonate's weight loss falls within a normal range, and therefore no action is needed at this time. Full-term neonates tend to lose 5% to 10% of their birth weight during the first few days after birth, most likely because of minimal nutritional intake. With bottle-feeding, the neonate's intake varies from one feeding to another. Typically, neonates regain any weight loss by 7 to 10 days of life. If the weight loss continues after that time, the **HCP** 📖 should be called.

🔑 CN: Health promotion and maintenance; CL: Synthesize

8. 240 calories

Eight feedings × 45 mL per feeding equals 360 mL. 360 mL × 20 cal/30 mL = 240 calories.

🔑 CN: Basic care and comfort; CL: Apply

9. 4. Placing an infant on a mother's bare chest or abdomen facilitates transition to extrauterine life and is the preferred method of thermoregulation for stable infants. A radiant warmer should be used if an infant is unstable and needs medical intervention. Blankets may be placed over a newborn and mom's chest. A hat may be added to prevent heat loss from the head, but these methods are supplemental to skin-to-skin care.

🔑 CN: Health promotion and maintenance; CL: Apply

10. 1. For vitamin K synthesis in the intestines to begin, food and normal intestinal flora are needed. However, at birth, the neonate's intestines are sterile. Therefore, vitamin K is administered via injection to prevent a vitamin K deficiency that may result in a bleeding tendency. When administered, vitamin K promotes formation in the liver of clotting factors II, VII, IX, and X. Neonates are not normally susceptible to clotting disorders, unless they are diagnosed with hemophilia or demonstrate a deficiency of or a problem with clotting factors. Hemolysis of fetal red blood cells does not destroy vitamin K. Hemolysis may be caused by Rh or ABO incompatibility, which leads to anemia and necessitates an exchange transfusion. Vitamin K synthesis occurs in the intestines, not the liver.

🔑 CN: Pharmacological and parenteral therapies; CL: Evaluate

11. 3. Currently, touch is believed to be the most highly developed sense at birth. It is probably why neonates respond well to touch. Auditory sense typically is relatively immature in the neonate, as evidenced by the neonate's selective response to the human voice. By 4 months, the neonate should turn his eyes and head toward a sound coming from behind. Visual sense tends to be relatively immature. At birth, visual acuity is estimated at 20/100 to 20/150, but it improves rapidly during infancy and toddlerhood. Taste is well developed, with a preference toward glucose; however, touch is more developed at birth.

🔑 CN: Health promotion and maintenance; CL: Synthesize

12. 4. Healthy infants are weighed during their visits to their **healthcare provider (HCP)** 📖, so it is not necessary to monitor weights at home. Infants may require one to three feedings during the night initially. By 3 months, 90% of babies sleep through the night. Projective vomiting may indicate pyloric stenosis and should not be seen in a normal newborn. Bottle-fed infants may stool one to three times daily.

🔑 CN: Health promotion and maintenance; CL: Evaluate

13. 1. The head and neck are best supported in a rear-facing seat in infants and toddlers, and infants should remain rear facing for as long possible until they outgrow their car seat. In the United States, the American Academy of Pediatrics recommends a rear-facing car seat for children younger than 2 years. The middle of the back seat is safest for a car seat. Because plastic can become brittle over time, car seats have an expiration date that must be checked before use. Ten years would generally be outside of most car seats' expiration dates.

🔑 CN: Health promotion and maintenance; CL: Evaluate

14. 1. The nurse should inform the mother that baby powder can enter the neonate's lungs and result in pneumonia secondary to aspiration of the particles. The best prevention for diaper rash is frequent diaper changing and keeping the neonate's skin dry. The disposable diapers have moisture-collecting materials and generally do not adhere to the skin unless the diaper becomes saturated. Typically, allergies are not associated with the use of baby powder in neonates.

🔑 CN: Reduction of risk potential; CL: Synthesize

15. 4. The mother needs further instruction when she says that a yellowish crust should be removed with water. The yellowish crust is normal and indicates scar formation at the site. It should not be removed because to do so might cause increased bleeding. The petroleum gauze prevents the diaper from sticking to the circumcision site, and it may fall off in the diaper. If this occurs, the mother should not attempt to replace it but should simply apply plain petroleum jelly to the site. The gauze should be left in place for 24 hours, and the mother should continue to apply petroleum jelly with each diaper change for 48 hours after the procedure. A few drops of oozing blood is normal, but if the amount is greater than a few drops, the mother should apply pressure and contact the **healthcare provider (HCP)** 📖. Any bleeding after the first day should be reported.

🔑 CN: Reduction of risk potential; CL: Evaluate

16. 3. The mother demonstrates understanding of the discharge instructions when she says that she should contact the **HCP** 🔲 if the baby has a liquid stool with a watery ring, because this indicates diarrhea. Infants can become dehydrated very quickly, and frequent diarrhea can result in dehydration. Normally, babies fall asleep easily after a feeding because they are satisfied and content. Spitting up a tablespoon of formula is normal. However, projectile or forceful vomiting in larger amounts should be reported. Bottle-fed infants typically pass one to two light brown stools each day.

⚷ CN: Reduction of risk potential;
CL: Evaluate

17. 1. Placing the neonate on his back after the feeding is recommended to minimize the risk for sudden infant death syndrome (SIDS). Placing the neonate on the abdomen after feeding has been associated with SIDS. The mother should bubble or burp the baby more than once during a feeding including at least after ½ oz (15 mL) of formula has been taken and then again when the baby is finished. Waiting until the baby has eaten 1 oz (30 mL) of formula can lead to regurgitation. The entire nipple should be placed on top of the baby's tongue and into the mouth to prevent excessive air from being swallowed. The nipple is pointed directly into the mouth, not toward the neonate's palate, to provide adequate sucking.

⚷ CN: Reduction of risk potential;
CL: Evaluate

18. 1. In a neonate, the lateral aspect of the heel is the most appropriate site for obtaining a blood specimen. Using this area prevents damage to the calcaneus bone, which is located in the middle of the heel. The middle of the heel is to be avoided because of the increased risk for damaging the calcaneus bone located there. The middle of the foot contains the medial plantar nerve and the medial plantar artery, which could be injured if this site is selected. Using the base of the big toe as the site for specimen collection would cause a great deal of discomfort for the neonate; therefore, it is not the preferred site.

⚷ CN: Reduction of risk potential;
CL: Apply

19. 2. After circumcision with a Plastibell, the most commonly recommended procedure is to clean the circumcision site with warm water with each diaper change. Other treatments are necessary only if complications, such as an infection, develop. Antibacterial soap or diluted hydrogen peroxide may cause pain and is not recommended. Povidone-iodine solution may cause stinging and burning, and therefore its use is not recommended.

⚷ CN: Health promotion and maintenance;
CL: Apply

20. 2. As part of the neonate's physiologic adaptation to birth at 90 minutes after birth the neonate typically is in the rest or sleep phase. During this time, the heart and respiratory rates slow and the neonate sleeps, unresponsive to stimuli. At this time, the mother should rest and allow the neonate to sleep. Feedings should be given during the first period of reactivity, considered the first 30 minutes after birth. During this period, the neonate's respirations and heart rate are elevated. Getting to know the neonate typically occurs within the first hour after birth and then when the neonate is awake and during feedings. Changing the neonate's diaper can occur at any time, but at 90 minutes after birth, the neonate is usually in a deep sleep, unresponsive, and probably has not passed any meconium.

⚷ CN: Health promotion and maintenance;
CL: Apply

Physical Assessment of the Neonatal Client

21. 1. When assessing the incurving of the trunk tests for automatic reflexes in the newborn, the nurse places the infant horizontally and in a prone position with one hand, and strokes the side of the newborn's trunk from the shoulder to the buttocks using the other hand. If the reflex is present, the newborn's trunk curves toward the stimulated side. Answer 2 shows a figure for testing for a stepping response. Answer 3 shows a figure for testing for a tonic neck reflex. Answer 4 shows a figure for testing for the Moro (startle) reflex.

⚷ CN: Physiological adaptation;
CL: Apply

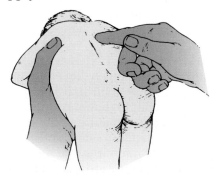

22. 2. The baby is displaying a normal Moro reflex that occurs with a sudden loss of support and requires no intervention. Calling a code, placing the neonate on seizure precautions, and starting supplemental oxygen are not necessary for a normally occurring reflex.

⚷ CN: Basic care and comfort;
CL: Synthesize

23. 2. If an infant is not breathing after the initial steps of resuscitation, the next thing the nurse must do is begin positive pressure ventilation. Apgar scores are an evaluation of the neonate's status at 1 and 5 minutes of life. Waiting to restore respirations until after assigning an Apgar score would be a waste of valuable time. Oxygen alone does little good if the infant is not breathing. Chest compressions must be accompanied by adequate oxygenation.

⚷ CN: Physiological adaptation; CL: Synthesize

24. 3. The neonate has a heart rate greater than 100, which earns him 2 points. His respiratory rate of 70 is equivalent to a 2 on the scale. His flaccid muscle tone is equal to 0 on the scale. The lack of response to stimulus also equals 0, as does his overall pale white color. Thus, the total score equals 4.

⚷ CN: Basic care and comfort; CL: Apply

25. 1. After performing vigorous suctioning, the nurse must watch for bradycardia due to potential vagus nerve stimulation. Rapid eye movement is not associated with vagus nerve stimulation. Vagal stimulation will not cause seizures or tachypnea.

⚷ CN: Reduction of risk potential; CL: Analyze

26. 2. There is a correlation between café au lait spots and the development of neurofibromatosis. Acrocyanosis is a normal finding of bluish hands and feet as a result of poor capillary perfusion. Port-wine nevus and strawberry hemangiomas are a collection of dilated capillaries and are not associated with any other disease process.

⚷ CN: Reduction of risk potential; CL: Analyze

27. 2,3,4. Holding the neonate steady and in the proper position will help ensure a safe and accurate lumbar puncture. The neonate is usually held in a "C" position to open the spaces between the vertebral column. This position puts the neonate at risk for airway obstruction. Thus, ensuring the patency of the airway is the first priority, and the nurse should observe the neonate for adequate ventilation. Maintaining a sterile field is important to avoid infection in the neonate. It is not necessary to administer antibiotics or obtain a serum glucose level during the procedure.

⚷ CN: Safety and infection control; CL: Synthesize

28. 3. Normally, the umbilical cord has two umbilical arteries and one vein. When a neonate is born with only one artery and one vein, the nurse should notify the **HCP** 📖 for further evaluation of cardiac anomalies. Other common congenital problems associated with a missing artery include renal anomalies, central nervous system lesions, tracheoesophageal fistulas, trisomy 13, and trisomy 18. Respiratory anomalies are associated with dyspnea and respiratory distress; musculoskeletal anomalies include fractures or dislocated hip; and facial anomalies are associated with fetal alcohol syndrome or Down syndrome, not a missing umbilical artery.

⚷ CN: Reduction of risk potential; CL: Analyze

29. 3. The most appropriate response would be to explain that the vaginal spotting in female neonates is associated with hormones received from the mother. Estrogen is believed to cause slight vaginal bleeding or spotting in the female neonate. The condition disappears spontaneously, so there is no need for concern. Telling the mother that it is of no concern does not allay the mother's worry. The vaginal spotting is related to hormones received from the mother, not to swallowing blood during the birth or hemorrhagic disease of the neonate. Anemia is associated with hemorrhagic disease.

⚷ CN: Health promotion and maintenance; CL: Synthesize

30. 1. Caput succedaneum is common after the use of a vacuum extractor to assist the client's expulsion efforts. This edema may persist up to 7 days. Vacuum extraction is not associated with cephalohematoma. Maternal lacerations may occur, but they are more common when forceps are used. Neonatal intracranial hemorrhage is a risk with both vacuum extraction and forceps births, but it is not a common finding.

⚷ CN: Health promotion and maintenance; CL: Analyze

31. 4. The mother needs further instruction if she says the molding can result in brain damage. Brain damage is highly unlikely. Molding occurs during vaginal birth when the cranial bones tend to override or overlap as the head accommodates to the size of the mother's birth canal. The amount and duration of pressure on the head influence the degree of molding. Molding usually disappears in a few days without any special attention.

⚷ CN: Health promotion and maintenance; CL: Evaluate

32. 3. Sole creases covering the entire foot are indicative of a term neonate. If the neonate's ear is lying flat against the head, the neonate is most likely preterm. An absence of rugae in the scrotum typically suggests a preterm neonate. A square window sign angle of 0 degrees occurs in neonates of 40 to 42 weeks' gestation. A 90-degree square window angle suggests an immature neonate of approximately 28 to 30 weeks' gestation.

> CN: Health promotion and maintenance;
> CL: Apply

33. 2. An expiratory grunt is significant and should be reported promptly because it may indicate respiratory distress and the need for further intervention such as oxygen or resuscitation efforts. The presence of a red reflex in the eyes is normal. An absent red reflex may indicate congenital cataracts. A respiratory rate of 45 breaths/min and a prominent xiphoid process are normal findings in a term neonate.

> CN: Reduction of risk potential;
> CL: Synthesize

34. 3. The tonic neck reflex, also called the fencing position, is present when the neonate turns the head to the left side, extends the left extremities, and flexes the right extremities. This reflex disappears in a matter of months as the neonatal nervous system matures. The stepping reflex is demonstrated when the infant is held upright near a hard, firm surface. The prone crawl reflex is demonstrated when the infant pulls both arms but does not move the chin beyond the elbows. When the infant extends and abducts the arms and legs with the toes fanning open, this is a normal Babinski's reflex.

> CN: Health promotion and maintenance;
> CL: Apply

35. 2. Convergent strabismus is common during infancy until about age 6 months because of poor oculomotor coordination. The neonate has peripheral vision and can fixate on close objects for short periods. The neonate can also perceive colors, shapes, and faces. Neonates can focus on light and should blink or close their eyes in response to light. However, this is not associated with strabismus. An absent red reflex or white areas over the pupils, not strabismus, may indicate congenital cataracts. Most neonates cannot focus well or accommodate for distance immediately after birth.

> CN: Health promotion and maintenance;
> CL: Apply

36. 3. A single crease across the palm (simian crease) is most commonly associated with chromosomal abnormalities, notably Down syndrome. Deep creases across the soles of the feet is a normal finding in a term neonate. Frequent sneezing in a term neonate is normal. This occurs because the neonate is a nose breather and sneezing helps to clear the nares. An absence of lanugo on the skin of a term neonate is a normal finding.

> CN: Reduction of risk potential;
> CL: Synthesize

37. 1,5,6. Phenylketonuria, an inherited autosomal recessive disorder, involves the body's inability to metabolize the amino acid phenylalanine. A diet low in phenylalanine must be followed. Such foods as meats, eggs, and milk are high in phenylalanine. Assistance from a dietitian is commonly necessary to keep phenylalanine levels low and to provide the essential amino acids necessary for cell function and tissue growth. With autosomal recessive disorders, future children will have a 25% chance of having the disease, a 50% chance of carrying the disease, and a 25% chance of being free of the disease. If a diet low in phenylalanine is followed until brain growth is complete (sometime in adolescence), the child should achieve normal intelligence.

> CN: Health promotion and maintenance;
> CL: Evaluate

38. 1. Periods of apnea lasting longer than 20 seconds, mild cyanosis, and a heart rate of <100 bpm (bradycardia) are associated with a potentially life-threatening event and subsequent respiratory arrest. The neonate needs further evaluation by the **HCP** ▢. Pneumonia is associated with tachycardia, anorexia, malaise, cyanosis, diminished breath sounds, and crackles. Intraventricular hemorrhage is associated with prematurity. Assessment findings include bulging fontanelles and seizures. Epiglottitis is a bacterial form of croup. Assessment findings include inspiratory stridor, cough, and irritability. It occurs most commonly in children age 3 to 7 years.

> CN: Reduction of risk potential;
> CL: Analyze

39. 4. Normally, the anterior fontanelle closes between ages 12 and 18 months. Premature closure (craniostenosis or premature synostosis) prevents proper growth and expansion of the brain, resulting in an intellectual disability. The posterior fontanel typically closes by ages 2 to 3 months.

> CN: Health promotion and maintenance;
> CL: Apply

40. 2. Corneas of unequal size should be reported because this may indicate congenital glaucoma. An absence of tears is common because the neonate's lacrimal glands are not yet functioning. The neonate's pupils normally constrict when a bright light is focused on them. The finding implies that light perception and visual acuity are present, as they should be after birth. A red circle on the pupils is seen when a penlight or ophthalmoscope's light shines onto the retina and is a normal finding. Called the red reflex, this indicates that the light is shining onto the retina.

> CN: Reduction of risk potential;
> CL: Synthesize

41. 3. At 24 hours of age, the neonate is probably in a state of deep sleep, as evidenced by the closed eyes, lack of eye movements, normal skin color, and normal heart rate and respiratory rate. Jitteriness, a high-pitched cry, and tremors are associated with drug withdrawal. The first period of reactivity occurs in the first 30 minutes after birth, evidenced by alertness, sucking sounds, and rapid heart rate and respiratory rate. There is no evidence to suggest respiratory distress because the neonate's respiratory rate of 35 breaths/min is normal.

CN: Health promotion and maintenance; CL: Analyze

42. 4. The condition in which the urinary meatus is located on the ventral surface of the penis, termed hypospadias, occurs in 1 of every 500 male infants. Circumcision is delayed until the condition is corrected surgically, usually between 6 and 12 months of age. Phimosis is an inability to retract the prepuce at an age when it should be retractable or by age 3 years. Phimosis may necessitate circumcision or surgical intervention. Hydrocele is a painless swelling of the scrotum that is common in neonates. It is not a contraindication for circumcision. Epispadias occurs when the urinary meatus is located on the dorsal surface of the penis. It is extremely rare and is commonly associated with bladder exstrophy.

CN: Reduction of risk potential; CL: Analyze

The Preterm Neonate

43. 1,3,4,5. Kangaroo care is skin-to-skin holding of a neonate by one of the parents. Research has shown increased bonding, physiologic stability, decreased length of stay, and improved breast-feeding for neonates who experience this method of holding. Research has not shown an increase in IQ as a developmental outcome. The experience is usually limited to 1 to 2 hours, two to three times per day.

CN: Health promotion and maintenance; CL: Apply

44. 4. When receiving oxygen by mask, the neonate is placed on the back with the neck slightly extended, in the "sniffing" or neutral position. This position optimizes lung expansion and places the upper respiratory tract in the best position for receiving oxygen. Placing a small rolled towel under the neonate's shoulders helps to extend the neck properly without overextending it. Once stabilized and transferred to an isolette in the intensive care unit, the neonate can be positioned in the prone position, which allows for lung expansion in the oxygenated environment. Placing the neonate on

the left side does not allow for maximum lung expansion. Also, slightly flexing the neck interferes with opening the airway. Placing the neonate on the back with the head turned to the left side does not allow for lung expansion. Placing the neonate on the abdomen interferes with proper positioning of the oxygen mask.

CN: Pharmacological and parenteral therapies; CL: Synthesize

45. 1. Chest compressions should be alternated with ventilation to ensure breathing and circulation. Two fingers or two thumbs encircling hands, not the palm of the hand, are used to compress a neonate's sternum. The chest is compressed 100 to 120 times/min. The proper technique recommended by the Neonatal Resuscitation Program is to use enough pressure to depress the sternum to a depth of approximately one-third of the anterior-posterior diameter of the chest.

CN: Physiological adaptation; CL: Apply

46. 1. Whenever oxygen is administered, it should be humidified to prevent drying of the nasal passages and mucous membranes. Because the neonate is under a radiant warmer, a stocking cap is not necessary. Temperature, continuously monitored by a skin probe attached to the radiant warmer, is recorded every 30 to 60 minutes initially. Although the oxygen concentration in the hood requires close monitoring and measurement of blood gases, checking the blood glucose level is not necessary.

CN: Pharmacological and parenteral therapies; CL: Apply

47. 3. The neonate is at high risk for sepsis due to exposure to the mother's infection. Temperature instability in a neonate at 38 weeks' gestation is an early sign of sepsis. Other signs include tachycardia, decreased muscle tone, acidosis, apnea, respiratory distress, hypotension, poor feeding behaviors, vomiting, and diarrhea. Late signs of infection include jaundice, seizures, enlarged liver and spleen, respiratory failure, and shock. Alkalosis is not typically seen in neonates who develop sepsis. Acidosis and respiratory distress may develop unless treatment such as antibiotics is started. A positive Babinski's reflex is a normal finding and does not need to be reported.

CN: Reduction of risk potential; CL: Analyze

48. 1. With an absent apical pulse left of the midclavicular line accompanied by cyanosis, grunting, and diminished breath sounds, the neonate is most likely experiencing pneumothorax. Pneumothorax occurs when alveoli are overdistended and subsequently the lung collapses, compressing the heart and lung and compromising the venous return to the right side of the heart. This condition can be confirmed by x-ray. An echocardiogram would be indicated if the chest x-ray did not reveal a respiratory cause for the problem or suggested a cardiac problem. Repositioning the infant may open the airway, and obtaining blood studies for infection will rule that out, but until pneumothorax is resolved, the other symptoms will continue.

⚷— CN: Physiological adaptation;
CL: Synthesize

49. 2. RDS, previously called hyaline membrane disease, is a developmental condition involving a decrease in lung surfactant leading to improper expansion of the lung alveoli. Surfactant contains a group of surface-active phospholipids, of which one component—lecithin—is the most critical for alveolar stability. Surfactant production peaks at about 35 weeks' gestation. This syndrome primarily attacks preterm neonates, although it can also affect term and postterm neonates. Altered somatotropin secretion is associated with growth disorders such as gigantism or dwarfism. Altered testosterone secretion is associated with masculinization. Altered progesterone secretion is associated with spontaneous abortion during pregnancy.

⚷— CN: Physiological adaptation; CL: Apply

50. 2. RDS is a developmental condition that primarily affects preterm infants before 35 weeks' gestation because of inadequate lung development from deficient surfactant production. The development of placenta previa has little correlation with the development of RDS. Although excessive analgesia can depress the neonate's respiratory condition if it is given shortly before birth, the scenario presents no information that this has occurred. The neonate's sluggish respiratory activity postpartum is not the likely cause of RDS but may be a sign that the neonate has the condition.

⚷— CN: Reduction of risk potential;
CL: Synthesize

51. 3. Oxygen should be humidified before administration to help prevent drying of the mucous membranes in the respiratory tract. Drying impedes the normal functioning of cilia in the respiratory tract and predisposes to mucous membrane irritation. Humidification of oxygen does not promote expansion of the immature lungs. Expansion is promoted by placing the infant in a prone position or providing the preterm infant with surfactant medication. Humidified oxygen does not prevent viral or bacterial pneumonia. In fact, in some nurseries, *Staphylococcus aureus* has been detected in moist environments and on the hands and nails of staff members, predisposing the neonate

to pneumonia. Humidified oxygen does not improve blood circulation in the cardiac system.

⚷— CN: Pharmacological and parenteral therapies; CL: Apply

52. 4. Many intensive care units that care for high-risk neonates recommend that the mother pump her breasts, store the milk, and bring it to the unit so the neonate can be fed with it, even if the neonate is being fed by gavage. As soon as the neonate has developed a coordinated suck-and-swallow reflex, breast-feeding can begin. Secretory immunoglobulin A, found in breast milk, is an important immunoglobulin that can provide immunity to the mucosal surfaces of the gastrointestinal tract. It can protect the neonate from enteric infections, such as those caused by Escherichia coli and Shigella species. Some studies have also shown that breast-fed preterm neonates maintain transcutaneous oxygen pressure and body temperature better than bottle-fed neonates. There is some evidence that breast milk can decrease the incidence of necrotizing enterocolitis. The preterm neonate does not need additional fat in the diet. However, some neonates may need an increased caloric intake. In such cases, breast milk can be fortified with an additive to provide additional calories. Neonates who are receiving oxygen can breast-feed. During feedings, supplemental oxygen can be delivered by nasal cannula.

⚷— CN: Health promotion and maintenance;
CL: Apply

53. 1. ROP, previously called retrolental fibroplasia, is associated with multiple risk factors, including high arterial blood oxygen levels, prematurity, and very low birth weight (less than 1,500 g). In the early acute stages of ROP, the neonate's immature retinal vessels constrict. If vasoconstriction is sustained, vascular closure follows, and irreversible capillary endothelial damage occurs. Normal room air is at 21%. Acidosis, not alkalosis, is commonly seen in preterm neonates, but this is not related to the development of ROP. Phototherapy is not related to the development of ROP. However, during phototherapy, the neonate's eyes should be constantly covered to prevent damage from the lights.

⚷— CN: Reduction of risk potential;
CL: Apply

54. 1. Because the retina may become detached with ROP, laser therapy has been used successfully in some medical centers to treat ROP. Anti-inflammatory eye drops may be used to treat seasonal allergies. ROP is not associated with glaucoma, so frequent testing is not necessary.

Because the vessels of the eye are affected and not the corneas, corneal transplantation is not used.

🔑 CN: Physiological adaptation; CL: Apply

55. 1. Neonates who weigh less than 1,500 g or are born at less than 34 weeks' gestation are susceptible to IVH. Cranial ultrasound scanning can confirm the diagnosis. The spinal fluid will show an increased number of red blood cells. Arterial blood gas specimen collection is done to evaluate the neonate's oxygen saturation level. Skull radiographs are not commonly used because of the danger of radiation. Additionally, computed tomography scans have replaced the use of skull x-ray films because they can provide more definitive results. Complete blood count specimen collection is usually performed to determine the hemoglobin, hematocrit, and white blood cell count. The results are not specific for IVH.

🔑 CN: Reduction of risk potential; CL: Apply

56. 3. A common finding of IVH is a bulging fontanelle. The most common site of hemorrhage is the periventricular subependymal germinal matrix, where there is a rich blood supply and where the capillary walls are thin and fragile. Rapid volume expansion, hypercarbia, and hypoglycemia contribute to the development of IVH. Other common manifestations include neurologic signs such as hypotonia, lethargy, temperature instability, nystagmus, apnea, bradycardia, decreased hematocrit, and increasing hypoxia. Seizures also may occur. Hyperbilirubinemia refers to an increase in bilirubin in the blood and may be seen if bleeding was severe.

🔑 CN: Physiological adaptation; CL: Analyze

57. 2,4,5. Nonnutritive sucking has been seen in infants as early as 28 weeks, and ultrasound examinations have shown thumb sucking in utero even earlier. Nonnutritive sucking provides oral stimulation and allows the baby to maintain the sucking reflex needed for breast- or bottle-feedings later. It does not teach the infant how to suck and swallow. Sucking is thought to help with gastric emptying by stimulating secretions of GI peptides. Moisture of the mucous membranes is an indication of adequate hydration, and nonnutritive sucking will not have an effect.

🔑 CN: Basic care and comfort; CL: Apply

58. 4. Indications of NEC include abdominal distention with gastric retention and vomiting. Other signs may include lethargy, irritability, positive blood culture in stool, absent or diminished bowel sounds, apnea, diarrhea, metabolic acidosis, and unstable temperature. A gastric residual of 1 mL is not significant. Jaundice of the face and chest is associated with the neonate's immature liver function and increased bilirubin, not NEC. Typically with NEC, the neonate would exhibit absent or diminished bowel sounds, not increased peristalsis.

🔑 CN: Physiological adaptation; CL: Analyze

59. 2. BPD is a chronic illness that may require prolonged hospitalization and permanent assisted ventilation. The disease typically occurs in compromised very-low-birth-weight neonates who require oxygen therapy and assisted ventilation for treatment of respiratory distress syndrome. The cause is multifactorial, and the disease has four stages. The neonate's activities may be limited by the disease. Antibiotics may be prescribed and bronchodilators may be used, but these medications will not cure the chronic disease state. Seizure activity is associated with periventricular-intraventricular hemorrhage, not BPD.

🔑 CN: Physiological adaptation; CL: Evaluate

60. 4. The client data support the diagnosis of pneumothorax, which would be confirmed with a chest x-ray. Pneumothorax is an accumulation of air in the thoracic cavity between the parietal and visceral pleurae and requires immediate removal of the accumulated air. Resolution is initiated with insertion of a chest tube connected to continuous negative pressure. The neonate does not need to be placed on a ventilator unless there is evidence of severe respiratory distress. The goal of treatment is to reinflate the collapsed lung. Administering bronchodilators through the nares or suctioning the neonate's nares would do nothing to aid in lung reinflation.

🔑 CN: Physiological adaptation; CL: Synthesize

61. 3. Decreased protein or hypoproteinemia is a sign of overhydration, which can lead to patent ductus arteriosus or congestive heart failure. Bulging fontanelles, decreased serum sodium, decreased urine specific gravity, and decreased hematocrit are other signs of overhydration. Hypernatremia (increased serum sodium concentration) or increased urine specific gravity would suggest dehydration, not overhydration. Polycythemia evidenced by an elevated hematocrit would suggest hypoxia or congenital heart disorder.

🔑 CN: Reduction of risk potential; CL: Analyze

62. 0.03 mg

2,950 g = 2.95 kg

2.95 kg × 0.01 mg = 0.029 mg, rounded to 0.03 mg

🔑 CN: Pharmacological and parenteral therapies; CL: Apply

The Postterm Neonate

63. 4. Increased respiratory rate and tremors are indicative of hypoglycemia, which commonly affects the postterm neonate because of depleted glycogen stores. There is no indication that the neonate has ineffective airway clearance, which would be evidenced by excessive amounts of mucus or visualization of meconium on the vocal cords. Lethargy, not tremors, would suggest infection or hyperthermia. Furthermore, the postterm neonate typically has difficulty maintaining temperature, resulting in hypothermia, not hyperthermia. Decreased cardiac output is not indicated, particularly because the neonate was born by cesarean section, which is not considered a difficult birth.

🔑 CN: Health promotion and maintenance; CL: Analyze

64. 2. A loose, watery stool in the diaper is indicative of diarrhea and needs immediate attention. The infant may become severely dehydrated quickly because of the higher percentage of water content per body weight in the neonate, compared with the adult. Frequent hiccups are considered normal in a neonate and do not warrant additional investigation. Pink papular vesicles (erythema toxicum) on the face are considered normal in a neonate and disappear without treatment. Dry, peeling skin is normal in a postterm neonate.

🔑 CN: Health promotion and maintenance; CL: Analyze

65. 2. Ortolani's maneuver involves flexing the neonate's knees and hips at right angles and bringing the sides of the knees down to the surface of the examining table. A characteristic click or "clunk," felt or heard, represents a positive Ortolani's sign, suggesting a possible hip dislocation. The nurse should notify the **HCP** 📖 promptly because treatment is needed, while maintaining the dislocated hip in a position of flexion and abduction. It should be noted that many institutions now limit performing the Ortolani's maneuver to APNs or HCPs. Determining the length of the mother's labor provides no useful information related to the nurse's finding. Keeping the infant under the radiant warmer is necessary only if the neonate's temperature is low or unstable. Checking for hypoglycemia is not indicated at this time, unless the neonate is exhibiting jitteriness.

🔑 CN: Reduction of risk potential; CL: Synthesize

66. 4. The priority problem for the neonate with probable MAS is impaired gas exchange related to the effects of respiratory distress. Obstruction of the airways may be complete or partial. Meconium aspiration may lead to pneumonia or pneumothorax. Establishing adequate respirations is the primary goal. Impaired skin integrity is a concern, but establishing and maintaining an airway and gas exchange is always the priority. Hypoglycemia tends to be a problem for large-for-gestational-age babies, not hyperglycemia. If the parents do not express interest or concern for the neonate, then risk for impaired parent-infant-child attachment may be appropriate once the airway is established.

🔑 CN: Physiological adaptation; CL: Analyze

67. 1,4,5. The pneumothorax may affect cardiac output, thus affecting perfusion causing a decrease in blood pressure and changes in color from pallor to cyanosis. As the neonate attempts to compensate, bradycardia or tachycardia may be exhibited. A change in temperature and urinary output are very late signs of decompensation.

🔑 CN: Physiologi al adaptation; CL: Analyze

The Neonate with Risk Factors

68. 2. Epinephrine is given for severe bradycardia and hypotension. An expected outcome would be an increased heart rate to a normal range. Epinephrine decreases renal blood flow, so a decrease in urine output would be expected. Epinephrine also stimulates alpha- and beta-adrenergic receptors, which do not offer pain relief or sedation.

🔑 CN: Pharmacological and parenteral therapies; CL: Evaluate

69. 4. Neonates that are sick do not have the physical resources or energy to respond to all elements of the environment. The use of a constant touch provides comfort and only requires one response to a stimulus. To comfort a sick neonate, the care provider applies gentle, constant physical support or touch. Toys for distraction are not developmentally appropriate for a neonate. Sick neonates react to any stimulus; in responding, the sick neonate may have increased energy demands and increased oxygen requirements. A musical mobile may be too much audio stimulation and thus increases energy and oxygen demands. Repetitive touching with a hand going off and on the neonate, as with stroking or patting, requires the neonate to respond to every touch, thus increasing energy and oxygen demands.

🔑 CN: Basic care and comfort; CL: Synthesize

70. 2. Recommended pulse oximetry reading in a full-term neonate is 95% to 100%. The saturation reading of only 75% is an indication that the neonate is not adequately oxygenating in room air. Providing supplemental oxygen will increase the neonate's oxygen saturation. Increasing the IV rate will not improve the oxygen saturation. Documenting the finding and taking no action is not appropriate with a saturation of 75%. Wrapping and increasing the body temperature of the neonate may increase the saturation reading only if it is inaccurate due to cold extremities. Caution must be used because overheating a neonate can be harmful.

CN: Reduction of risk potential; CL: Synthesize

71. 4. Neonates with heart failure may need calorie-dense formula to provide extra calories for growth. Fluids should not be restricted because the nutritional requirements are based on calories per ounce of formula. Decreasing fluid intake will decrease calories needed for growth. These neonates may have limited energy due to their heart condition but have a high caloric need to stimulate proper growth and development. The sodium level should be at a normal level to ensure adequate fluid and electrolyte balance unless prescribed by the **healthcare provider (HCP)** 📖.

CN: Health promotion and maintenance; CL: Create

72. 1. The indication for the use of indomethacin is to close a patent ductus arteriosus. Adverse effects include decreased renal blood flow, platelet dysfunction with coagulation defects, decreased GI motility, and an increase in necrotizing enterocolitis. Thus, increased bleeding time, decreased gastrointestinal function, and decreased renal output would be expected outcomes after the administration of indomethacin.

CN: Pharmacological and parenteral therapies; CL: Evaluate

73. 2. A quiet environment with decreased stimulation is the best treatment for a drug-exposed neonate. The drug-exposed neonate has limited ability to deal with stress and cope with stimuli. Assessing vital signs with blood pressure every hour will disturb the neonate's rest periods and cause increased physical and psychological demands. Placement in a well-lighted environment and increasing eye contact can be overwhelming for the neonate and will increase the neonate's stress level.

CN: Physiological adaptation; CL: Apply

74. 1. To ensure client safety, the nurse should first write the results on the **medical record** 📖, then read them back to the caller, and wait for the caller to confirm that the nurse has understood the results. Using scrap paper increases the risk of losing the results as well as transcription errors. The nurse may receive results by telephone, and while electronic transfer to the client's medical record is appropriate, the nurse can also accept the telephone results if the laboratory has called the results to the nursery. Sending client information via e-mail is unacceptable due to potential security and privacy issues.

CN: Safety and infection control; CL: Apply

75. 3. Hemolytic disease of the newborn is associated with Rh problems. Hemolytic disease of the newborn occurs most commonly when the mother is Rh negative and the infant is Rh positive. About 13% of Caucasians, 7% to 8% of people of African descent, and 1% of people of Asian descent are Rh negative. Rh-positive cells enter the mother's Rh-negative bloodstream, and antibodies to the Rh-positive cells are produced. In a subsequent pregnancy, the antibodies cross the placenta to the Rh-positive fetus and begin the destruction of Rh-positive cells through hemolysis. This results in severe fetal anemia.

CN: Physiological adaptation; CL: Apply

76. 3. The problem of Rh sensitivity arises when the mother's blood develops antibodies after fetal red blood cells enter the maternal circulation. In cases of Rh sensitivity, this usually does not occur until after the first pregnancy. Hence, hemolytic disease of the newborn is rare in a primiparous client. A mismatched blood transfusion in the past or an unrecognized spontaneous abortion could also result in hemolytic disease because the transfusion or abortion would have the same effects on the client. The statement about the other baby having a different father may be true. However, if both fathers were Rh positive, then sensitization could occur. Most women do not have immunity against the antibodies formed when Rh-positive cells enter the mother's bloodstream. Antibodies are not neutralized by the mother's system.

CN: Reduction of risk potential; CL: Evaluate

77. 2. The Rh-sensitized neonate generally does not have problems related to polycythemia. Therefore, the client needs additional teaching. In general, moderate-to-severe Rh sensitization can cause anemia, enlarged spleen, and cardiac decompensation. Cardiac decompensation (as in heart failure) occurs because of severe anemia. Anemia is caused by the destruction of red blood cells by antibodies as the severity of hemolytic disease of the neonate increases. Splenic enlargement is caused by the excessive destruction of fetal red blood cells.

CN: Physiological adaptation; CL: Evaluate

78. 3. A direct Coombs test is done on umbilical cord blood to detect antibodies coating the neonate's red blood cells. Hematocrit is used to detect anemia. A direct Coombs does not measure bilirubin but may help explain the underlying cause of increased bilirubin levels. Antigens on the neonate's red blood cells are proteins that help determine the neonate's blood type.

🔑 CN: Reduction of risk potential; CL: Apply

79. 3. An exchange transfusion is done to reduce the blood concentration of bilirubin and correct the anemia. The exchange transfusion does not replenish the white blood cells or restore the fluid and electrolyte balance. The neonate's Rh-positive blood is replaced by Rh-negative blood.

🔑 CN: Reduction of risk potential; CL: Apply

80. 2. The organ most susceptible to damage from uncontrolled hemolytic disease is the brain. Bilirubin levels increase as the red blood cells are destroyed. Bilirubin crosses the blood-brain barrier and damages the cells of the central nervous system. This condition, called kernicterus, is potentially fatal. Although the kidneys, lungs, and liver may be affected by increased bilirubin levels, the brain will sustain the most life-threatening injury.

🔑 CN: Reduction of risk potential; CL: Apply

81. 1,4. A blood glucose reading at or below 30 mg/dL (1.7 mmol/L) within 2 hours of birth and irregular respirations, tremors, and hypothermia are indicative of hypoglycemia. Blood glucose should be 45 mg/dL (2.5 mmol/L) by 24 hours of age. Internal fetal monitors detect the strength of contractions and the fetal heart rate. An infant of an insulin-dependent mother and a large-for-gestational-age infant are at greater risk of developing hypoglycemia and need to be observed carefully, but these findings are not definitive for the diagnosis of hypoglycemia.

🔑 CN: Physiological adaptation; CL: Analyze

82. 2. Glucose crosses the placenta, but insulin does not. Hence, a high maternal blood glucose level causes a high fetal blood glucose level. This causes the fetal pancreas to secrete more insulin. At birth, the neonate loses the maternal glucose source but continues to produce much insulin, which commonly causes a drop in blood glucose levels (hypoglycemia), usually at 30 to 60 minutes postpartum. Most neonates do not develop hypoglycemia if their mothers are not insulin dependent unless they are preterm. Therefore, hypoglycemia is not a normal response as the neonate transitions to extrauterine life.

🔑 CN: Reduction of risk potential; CL: Analyze

83. 1. Infants born to mothers with diabetes tend to be larger than average, and this neonate weighs 10 lb, 1 oz (4,564 g). The most common fractures are those of the clavicle and long bones, such as the femur. In a neonate, the skull bones are not fused and move to allow for vaginal birth, so skull fracture is rarely seen. Wrist and rib cages are rarely fractured.

🔑 CN: Reduction of risk potential; CL: Apply

84. 1. This neonate has a mother with diabetes who tends to have higher calcium levels, which can cause secondary hypoparathyroidism in their neonates. This lack of calcium may be the cause of the tremors and jitteriness of this neonate, and a serum calcium level should be obtained. Other factors contributing to hypocalcemia in neonates include hypophosphatemia from tissue metabolism, vitamin D antagonism from increased cortisol levels, and decreased serum magnesium levels. Beginning a glucose IV based on a normal infant glucose level would have no benefit. Rechecking the neonate's temperature is a precaution that can be taken to assure that it is within normal limits but is not the action to take first. Refeeding the infant who has a normal newborn blood glucose level is not appropriate.

🔑 CN: Management of care; CL: Synthesize

85. 4. Hypoglycemia is caused by the rapid depletion of glucose stores. In addition, neonates born to class women with insulin-dependent diabetes are about seven times more likely to suffer from respiratory distress syndrome than neonates born to nondiabetic women. This neonate should be closely monitored for symptoms of hypoglycemia and respiratory distress. Neonates of diabetic mothers commonly have polycythemia, not anemia. Anemia and hemolytic disease are associated with erythroblastosis fetalis. Persistent pulmonary hypertension is associated with meconium aspiration syndrome.

🔑 CN: Reduction of risk potential; CL: Apply

86. 2. Manifestations of opiate withdrawal in the neonate include an increased central nervous system irritability, such as a shrill, high-pitched cry, gastrointestinal symptoms, and metabolic, vasomotor, and respiratory disturbances. These signs usually appear within 72 hours and persist for several days. These neonates are difficult to console, have poor feeding behaviors, and have diarrhea. Bradycardia is associated with preterm neonates. Sluggishness and lethargy are associated with neonates whose mothers received analgesia shortly before birth. Hypocalcemia occurs most commonly in infants of mothers with diabetes, premature infants, and low-birth weight infants.

🔑 CN: Reduction of risk potential; CL: Analyze

87. 3. Neonates experiencing opiate withdrawal have gastrointestinal problems similar to those of adults withdrawing from opiates. The neonates exhibit poor sucking, vomiting, drooling, diarrhea, regurgitation, and anorexia. In addition, they are difficult to console and difficult to feed. Because of these problems, the neonate withdrawing from opiates needs to be monitored carefully to prevent dehydration. Neonates with opiate exposure experience hypertonia, not hypotonia, due to increased central nervous system irritability. Diarrhea, not constipation, is seen in these neonates. Abdominal distention is associated with necrotizing enterocolitis, not opiate withdrawal.

☛ CN: Reduction of risk potential; CL: Evaluate

88. 1. A neonate undergoing cocaine withdrawal is irritable, often restless, difficult to console, and often in need of increased activity. It is commonly helpful to swaddle the neonate tightly with a blanket, offer a pacifier, and cuddle and rock the neonate. Offering extra nourishment is not advised because overfeeding tends to increase gastrointestinal problems such as vomiting, regurgitation, and diarrhea. Environmental stimuli such as bright lights and loud noises should be kept to a minimum to decrease agitation. Minimizing touching of the neonate to only when he or she is crying will not aid the bonding process between mother and neonate. Frequent holding and touching are permissible.

☛ CN: Reduction of risk potential; CL: Synthesize

89. 4. New recommendations state that virologic diagnostic testing at birth should be considered for infants at high risk of HIV infection, but it may take several months before an accurate diagnosis can be made. New guidelines suggest that infants should be tested at 2 to 3 weeks, 1 to 2 months, and again 4 to 6 months. It is estimated that 15% to 30% of all HIV-positive mothers without treatment will give birth to HIV-positive infants. With appropriate drug intervention to the mother during pregnancy, 95% of these neonates can be born unaffected. An enlarged liver at birth is associated with erythroblastosis fetalis, not HIV infection. Virologic testing, such as deoxyribonucleic acid polymerase chain reaction, viral culture, or ribonucleic acid plasma assay, can diagnose HIV infection by 6 months of age and commonly in the first month.

☛ CN: Reduction of risk potential; CL: Apply

90. 4. Breast milk has been found to contain the retrovirus HIV. In general, mothers are discouraged from breast-feeding if they are HIV positive because of the risk of possible transmission of the virus if the neonate is HIV negative. Breast milk does contain some immunoglobulins, but it does not protect the neonate from HIV infection.

☛ CN: Health promotion and maintenance; CL: Create

91. 1. Newborns are typically bathed 2 to 4 hours after birth when their temperatures have had time to stabilize, but early/immediate bathing is recommended for the infants of HIV-positive mothers to decrease blood exposure. Placing the neonate under the radiant warmer for the vitamin K injection is not necessary unless the neonate's temperature is subnormal. Washing the injection site with povidone-iodine is not recommended and may increase the risk for possible allergy to iodine preparations. The first dose of zidovudine is given when the newborn is 6 to 12 hours old, but vitamin K is recommended to be given within an hour of birth to be most effective. Therefore, the vitamin K should not be delayed.

☛ CN: Safety and infection control; CL: Synthesize

92. 3. Symptoms of infection in a neonate include subtle behavioral changes, such as lethargy and irritability, and color changes such as pallor or cyanosis. Other symptoms include temperature instability, poor feeding, gastrointestinal disorders, hyperbilirubinemia, and apnea. Leukocytosis, an elevated white blood cell count possibly as high as 30,000 cells/mm3 (30 × 109/L) or more, may be normal during the first 24 hours. An apical heart rate of 132 bpm is normal. Warm, moist skin is not a typical sign of infection in neonates. Typically, temperature instability is common. The neonate's temperature is low, and the skin is cool and dry.

☛ CN: Health promotion and maintenance; CL: Analyze

93. 3. The parents of a neonate with an infection should be allowed to participate in daily care as long as they use good handwashing technique. This includes touching and holding the neonate. It is not necessary for parents to wearing protective gear new the isolette. Restricting parental visits has not been shown to have any effect on the infection rate and may have detrimental effects on the neonate's psychological development. Normally, the neonate does not need to be isolated. The baby will not spread sepsis via respiratory droplets to parents so is not necessary for the parents to wear a mask.

☛ CN: Safety and infection control; CL: Apply

94. 3. On the initial visit, the parents may be shocked, fearful, and anxious. Nursing care should include spending time with the parents to allow them to express their emotions. The nurse should initially emphasize the neonate's normal characteristics. After the parents have had sufficient time to adjust to the neonate's special needs, surgical interventions can be discussed. Telling the parents that this is not a life-threatening defect or that everything will be all right after the surgery is not helpful. Doing so discounts their feelings. Reassuring the parents about the success rate of the surgery can be done once the parents have had time to adjust to the neonate and express their emotions.

⚿ CN: Psychosocial integrity;
CL: Synthesize

95. 1. It is not necessary to clean the mouth of an infant with an unrepaired cleft palate after each feeding. The neonate needs to be fed in an upright position to prevent aspiration. The neonate with a cleft lip and palate commonly swallows large amounts of air during feeding. Therefore, the neonate needs to be burped frequently to help eliminate the air and decrease the risk for regurgitation. The neonate with a cleft lip and palate should be fed with a special soft nipple that fills the cleft and facilitates sucking.

⚿ CN: Reduction of risk potential;
CL: Evaluate

96. 4. The long-term prognosis for neonates with FAS is poor. Symptoms of withdrawal include tremors, sleeplessness, seizures, abdominal distention, hyperactivity, and inconsolable crying. Symptoms of withdrawal commonly occur within 6 to 12 hours or, at the latest, within the first 3 days of life. The neonate with FAS is usually growth deficient at birth. Most neonates with FAS are mildly to severely mentally handicapped. The facial deformities, such as short palpebral fissures, epicanthal folds, broad nasal bridge, flattened midface, and short, upturned nose, are not easily corrected with plastic surgery.

⚿ CN: Reduction of risk potential;
CL: Create

97. 3. Central nervous system disorders are common in neonates with FAS. Speech and language disorders and hyperactivity are common manifestations of central nervous system dysfunction. Mild-to-severe mental retardation and feeding problems also are common. Delayed growth and development is expected. These neonates feed poorly and commonly have persistent vomiting until age 6 to 7 months. These neonates do not have a 70% mortality rate, and there is no treatment for FAS.

⚿ CN: Reduction of risk potential;
CL: Apply

98. 4. Changes seen in the facial features of newborns with fetal alcohol syndrome remain that way. These include epicanthal folds, whorls, irregular hair, cleft lip or palate, small teeth, and lack of philtrum. Newborns with fetal alcohol syndrome are usually difficult to calm and frequently cry for long periods of time. Parents do need assistance with caring for themselves and their infants, particularly with continued alcohol use. A supportive family or support systems are essential. The problems seen with this newborn do not go away and remain with the infant throughout life and are compounded when the child begins to develop mentally.

⚿ CN: Health promotion and maintenance;
CL: Evaluate

99. 1. The parents need to know that the neonate will be kept on NPO status and will receive intravenous therapy before surgery. After surgery, feeding will depend on the neonate's condition. Total parenteral nutrition may be prescribed after surgery, but not before. Breast-feeding may be started after surgery if the neonate's condition is stable. The mother can pump the breasts until that time.

⚿ CN: Reduction of risk potential;
CL: Apply

100. 1,2,4. The major goals for the neonate include preventing hypothermia, maintaining fluid and electrolyte balance, and preventing infection. Pain medication will be needed after surgery but is not typically needed before the procedure. In many cases, surgery is done very soon after birth. So while developmental care is important, it should be addressed after the closure of the abdominal wall defect.

⚿ CN: Reduction of risk potential;
CL: Create

101. 2. The physical appearance of the anomaly and the life-threatening nature of the disorder may result in shock to the parents. The parents may hesitate to form a bond with the neonate because of the guarded prognosis. Denial would be evidenced if the parents acted as if nothing were wrong. Bargaining would be evidenced by parental statements involving "if-then" phrasing, such as, "If the surgery is successful, I will go to church every Sunday." Anger would be evidenced if the parents attempted to blame someone, such as healthcare personnel, for the neonate's condition.

⚿ CN: Psychosocial integrity; CL: Analyze

102. 1. To prevent eye damage from phototherapy, the eyes must remain covered at all times while under the lights. The eye patches can be removed when the neonate is held out of the lights by the parents for feeding. Instead of a regular diaper, a "string" diaper or disposable face mask may be used to help contain loose stools, while allowing maximum skin exposure. Feeding formula or breast milk every 2 to 3 hours is recommended to prevent hypoglycemia and to encourage gastrointestinal motility. Because the phototherapy lights can overheat the neonate, the temperature should be checked by the axillary route every 2 to 4 hours.

    CN: Reduction of risk potential;
CL: Apply

103. 4. An absent Moro reflex, lethargy, opisthotonos, and seizures are symptoms of bilirubin encephalopathy, which, although rare, can be life-threatening. Bronze discoloration of the skin and maculopapular chest rash are normal and are caused by the phototherapy. They will disappear once the phototherapy is discontinued. A urine specific gravity of 1.001 to 1.020 is normal in term neonates.

    CN: Reduction of risk potential;
CL: Analyze

104. 2. Marked visible peristaltic waves in the abdomen and projectile vomiting are signs of pyloric stenosis. If the condition progresses without surgical intervention, the neonate will become dehydrated and develop metabolic alkalosis. Signs of esophageal atresia include coughing and regurgitation with feedings. Diaphragmatic hernia, a life-threatening event in which the abdominal contents herniate into the thoracic cavity, may be evidenced by breath sounds being heard over the abdomen and significant respiratory distress with cyanosis. Signs of hiatal hernia include vomiting, failure to thrive, and short periods of apnea.

    CN: Reduction of risk potential;
CL: Analyze

105. 3. With a patent ductus arteriosus, a cardiac defect marked by a failure of the patent ductus arteriosus to close completely at birth, blood from the aorta flows into the pulmonary arteries to be reoxygenated in the lungs and returned to the left atrium and ventricle. The effect of this altered circulation includes increased workload on the left side of the heart and increased pulmonary vascular congestion. Term infants are commonly asymptomatic, but a loud, machinery-like murmur may be heard throughout systole and diastole. This murmur may be accompanied by a suprasternal thrill, and the heart may be enlarged. Decreased cardiac output with faint peripheral pulses, poor peripheral perfusion, feeding difficulties, and severe congestive heart failure are symptoms associated with severe aortic stenosis. With this defect, the aortic valve is thickened and rigid, leading to decreased cardiac output and reduced myocardial

blood flow. Profound cyanosis over most of the body, fatigue on exertion, feeding difficulties, and chronic hypoxemia are associated with tetralogy of Fallot. With this defect, malalignment of the ventricular system results in nonrestricted ventral septal defects, pulmonic stenosis, overriding of the aorta, and hypertrophy of the left ventricle. The heart appears boot shaped. A harsh systolic murmur with a palpable thrill is associated with truncus arteriosus. It is marked by incomplete division of the great vessel. This is caused by a ventral septal defect. Bounding pulses and a widening pulse pressure may also be present.

    CN: Reduction of risk potential;
CL: Analyze

106. 1. Coarctation of the aorta accounts for 5% to 7% of congenital heart disease. There is localized constriction of the aorta, at or near the insertion site of the ductus arteriosus, that increases afterload and decreases cardiac output. The infant with coarctation of the aorta presents with symptoms of poor lower body perfusion, weak lower extremity pulses, and congestive heart failure, including respiratory distress. The child with a partial atrioventricular septal defect may be asymptomatic at birth. The symptoms in a child with a complete defect depend on the pulmonary artery pressure. The child with pulmonary atresia has profound (complete) cyanosis. Transposition of the great arteries is associated with complete cyanosis during the first few hours of life.

    CN: Reduction of risk potential;
CL: Analyze

107. 4. The normal pulse rate in a neonate is 120 to 160 bpm. Therefore, a femoral pulse rate of 90 bpm is too low. Diminished peripheral pulses, coolness and mottling of the extremities, delayed capillary refill, hypotension, and decreased urine output are indicative of low cardiac output and poor perfusion. The neonate may be experiencing a complication of the surgery, such as blood loss or leaking of fluid into the interstitial space. The surgeon should be notified immediately to correct the diminished pulse, through either medications or transfusions. An oxygen saturation between 85% and 100% is considered normal. The surgeon does not need to be notified unless the oxygen saturation falls below 85%. Pale pink extremities are considered a normal finding. If mottling or cyanosis develops, the surgeon should be notified immediately. Warm, dry skin is also a normal finding. If the skin becomes cool or appears cyanotic, the surgeon should be notified.

    CN: Reduction of risk potential;
CL: Synthesize

108. 3. The neonate is experiencing quiet tachypnea with central cyanosis, which is a sign of possible congenital heart disease, so notifying the **HCP** 📖 is the correct answer. The baby is showing no signs of increased work of breathing, except increased respiratory rate. Breath sounds are clear; therefore, suctioning is not necessary and may cause further distress due to trauma to the nasal passage. Changing the neonate's position would have no impact on the cyanosis. Encouraging the baby to cry would increase the distress by decreasing oxygen consumption.

🔑 CN: Physiological adaptation; CL: Analyze

109. 4. The next nursing action in this situation would be to assess the blood pressure in all four extremities and compare the findings. A difference of 15 mm Hg in the systolic blood pressure between the arms and legs is an indication of a narrowed aorta. This could be an emergency, and the **HCP** 📖 needs to be notified as soon as the blood pressure data have been collected. Generally, prescribing an HCP consult is not a nursing function. Placing the neonate in reverse Trendelenburg will only decrease the perfusion to the lower extremities.

🔑 CN: Physiological adaptation; CL: Analyze

110. 4. Further assessment for signs of distress is necessary. At 4 hours of age, a transient murmur may be heard as the fetal shunts are closing. This is a normal finding. If no other distress is noted, the **HCP** 📖 does not need to be called. Result can be noted on the **medical record** 📖. Further assessment is needed to know if continuing routine care and feeding are appropriate and safe for the neonate.

🔑 CN: Physiological adaptation; CL: Analyze

111.

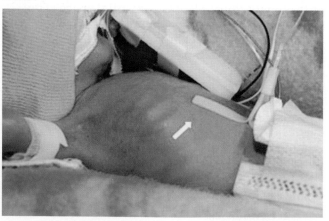

Subcostal retractions are noted under the rib cage. Intercostal retractions are noted between the ribs. Suprasternal retractions are found above the sternum, and the substernal retractions are found below the sternum.

🔑 CN: Physiological adaptation; CL: Apply

112. 2. Parents who have experienced perinatal loss have described statements such as "I am sorry for your loss" as helpful. All other statements are not helpful. A nurse can empathize, but may not know what clients are feeling unless they have been given an opportunity to express their emotions. Stating that time heals is a cliché. Suggesting the client can have another child makes a false assumption that one child can replace another. Also the client may not have the ability to have another child.

🔑 CN: Psychosocial integrity; CL: Apply

Managing Care, Quality, and Safety of Neonatal Clients

113. 1. The preterm infant is at greatest risk for developing RDS as the lungs are immature and unable to produce adequate surfactant to reduce the surface tension in the lungs and promote the stability of the alveoli. The neonate born at 42 weeks' gestation is at greater risk of having meconium-stained amniotic fluid and developing meconium aspiration syndrome. The neonate born by cesarean section is at greater risk of fluid retention in the lungs as the lungs are not compressed during the birth process as they are in a vaginal birth. Generally, these infants are able to overcome this situation with adequate crying. Apneic episodes in infants may be related to several conditions, including hypothermia, sepsis, and hypoglycemia, or a result of a rapid increase in the infant's temperature.

🔑 CN: Management of care; CL: Analyze

114. 3. The nurse should make rounds and first assess the neonate with the respiratory rate of 62. The respiratory rate is out of the normal range and needs reevaluation. The nurse should next assess the newborn with a borderline low temperature to determine if his body temperature is increasing. The newborn who is LGA still has 15 minutes before being due for the feeding, and much can be accomplished by the nurse in that time. A 36-week newborn weighing 5 lb (2,270 g) will need to be fed on time to maintain the blood glucose level.

🔑 CN: Management of care; CL: Synthesize

115. 3. A temperatur... jitteriness are signs of... newborn. The nurse m... blood sample for blood... preferably skin-to-skin... immediately following... treat the suspected hy... be notified once the bl... and the baby is succes... newborn temperature... 99.1°F (37.3°C). A tem... low, another sign of hy... feeding takes preceder... Also, breast-feeding vi... been found as the mos... newborn's temperature...

CN: Manage...

116. 2. The mother d... bladder and vaginal bl... with bladder emptying... assess the origination... requires further assess... when quiet and respira... indicate the beginning... and requires prompt in... are recovering normall... in a newborn could in... pink color indicates th... oxygenation. Normal respiration is ... to ... breaths/ min. While a respiratory rate of 67 is slightly elevated, the baby is not demonstrating any other signs of respiratory distress. The newborn with acrocyanosis (bluish hands and feet) is a normal newborn finding and shows the ability to maintain oxygenation. Respirations of 70 breaths/min and intermittent expiratory grunt would indicate close observation but does not require immediate intervention if the infant is pink. The last newborn is maintaining oxygenation, with respirations just slightly above normal. Periodic breathing, featuring pauses in breathing of less than 15 seconds, is a normal newborn finding.

CN: Management of care; CL: Synthesize

117. 2,3,4,5. A hospital-specific security system is the standard of care to prevent neonatal abduction. The bulb syringe should be visible and easily accessible to both the mother and the nurse in case of choking. Someone should remain in the room who is able to safely care for the infant. This may

be the mother or a family member if the mother is physically not able to care for the infant. The infant should be lying on the back or side, rather than the abdomen to prevent sudden infant death syndrome ("back to sleep"). Infant falls from a mother's bed are a serious safety problem. The infant should be in the mother's arms or in the crib rather than lying on a bed, even with the side rails up, as an infant can slip through the rails. A sleeping mother is not aware of the status of the infant who can easily fall out of her arms; the infant can be in the mother's arms only if she is awake.

CN: Safety and infection control; CL: Evaluate

118. 2. The blood glucose of 25 (1.38 mmol/L) is the most critical. Glucose is the only fuel that the brain can use. It is important to protect the central nervous system, and levels less than 30 (1.7 mmol/L) in the first 6 hours of life of a neonate indicate hypoglycemia. Occasional grunting at ½ hour of age may be normal transitioning to extrauterine life. A temperature of 97.4°F (36.4°C) is only slightly low for a neonate at this age. Ninety-five percent of all neonates will void at least once in the first 24 hours. This is not unusual at this age.

CN: Management of care; CL: Analyze

119. 4,1,3,2. Based on the report given by the preceding nurse, the nurse should plan to prioritize all clients and first make rounds on the client needing the highest level of nursing care. The nurse can then make rounds on all other clients. The nurse can then check for new prescriptions and, finally, inspect the room in which the next client will be admitted to be sure all of the equipment is available.

CN: Management of care; CL: Synthesize

120. 2,4,5. The role of the UAP 📖 allows this member of the healthcare team to take vital signs on clients, record feedings, and voids and stools of infants according to hospital guidelines. The newborn assessment is completed by a licensed care provider as is the tube feeding. Bathing of the newborn is within the scope of practice for the UAP, but the initial assessment of patency of the gastrointestinal tract, which is initiated by the first feeding, is within the scope of licensed care providers. If there is a trachea esophageal fistula, this is the time when it may become evident.

CN: Management of care; CL: Apply

the mother-fucking NCLEX aint got shit on you!

2

The Nursing
of Children

Health Promotion of the Infant and Family

1. After reading the vaccine information sheets, the parent of a 2-month-old infant is hesitant to consent to the recommended vaccinations. The nurse should **first** ask the parent:
- ☐ **1.** "Did you know that vaccinations are required by law for school entry?"
- ☐ **2.** "What concerns do you have about vaccinations?"
- ☐ **3.** "Would you prefer that fewer vaccines are given at a time?"
- ☐ **4.** "Can you please sign this vaccine waiver form?"

2. Which is appropriate language development for an 8-month-old? The child should be:
- ☐ **1.** saying "dada" and "mama" specifically ("dada" to father and "mama" to mother).
- ☐ **2.** saying three other words besides "mama" and "dada."
- ☐ **3.** saying "dada" and "mama" nonspecifically.
- ☐ **4.** saying "ball" when parents point to a ball.

3. The nurse should refer the parents of an 8-month-old child to a healthcare provider (HCP) if the child is unable to:
- ☐ **1.** stand momentarily without holding onto furniture.
- ☐ **2.** stand unsupported well for long periods of time.
- ☐ **3.** stoop to recover an object.
- ☐ **4.** sit without support for long periods of time.

4. The nurse is teaching the parents of an 8-month-old about what the child should eat. The nurse should include which information points in the teaching plan?
- ☐ **1.** Vegetables should be introduced before fruits.
- ☐ **2.** Solid foods should not be introduced until the infant is 10 months old.
- ☐ **3.** Iron-fortified cereals should not be introduced until the infant is 8 months old.
- ☐ **4.** The infant's diet can be changed from formula to whole milk when the infant is 12 months old.

2

The Nursing Care of Children

Health Promotion

- Health Promotion of the Infant and Family
- Health Promotion of the Toddler and Family
- Health Promotion of the Preschooler and Family
- Health Promotion of the School-Age Child and Family
- Health Promotion of the Adolescent and Family
- Common Childhood and Adolescent Health Problems
- Managing Care, Quality, and Safety of Children
- Answers, Rationales, and Test-Taking Strategies

Health Promotion of the Infant and Family

1. After reading the vaccine information sheets, the parent of a 2-month-old infant is hesitant to consent to the recommended vaccinations. The nurse should **first** ask the parent:
- ☐ **1.** "Did you know that vaccinations are required by law for school entry?"
- ☐ **2.** "What concerns do you have about vaccinations?"
- ☐ **3.** "Would you prefer that fewer vaccines are given at a time?"
- ☐ **4.** "Can you please sign this vaccine waiver form?"

2. Which is appropriate language development for an 8-month-old? The child should be:
- ☐ **1.** saying "dada" and "mama" specifically ("dada" to father and "mama" to mother).
- ☐ **2.** saying three other words besides "mama" and "dada."
- ☐ **3.** saying "dada" and "mama" nonspecifically.
- ☐ **4.** saying "ball" when parents point to a ball.

3. The nurse should refer the parents of an 8-month-old child to a healthcare provider (HCP) if the child is unable to:
- ☐ **1.** stand momentarily without holding onto furniture.
- ☐ **2.** stand unsupported well for long periods of time.
- ☐ **3.** stoop to recover an object.
- ☐ **4.** sit without support for long periods of time.

4. The nurse is teaching the parents of an 8-month-old about what the child should eat. The nurse should include which information points in the teaching plan?
- ☐ **1.** Vegetables should be introduced before fruits.
- ☐ **2.** Solid foods should not be introduced until the infant is 10 months old.
- ☐ **3.** Iron-fortified cereals should not be introduced until the infant is 8 months old.
- ☐ **4.** The infant's diet can be changed from formula to whole milk when the infant is 12 months old.

115. 3. A temperature of 96.6°F (35.9°C) and jitteriness are signs of hypoglycemia in the newborn. The nurse must first obtain a heel stick blood sample for blood glucose. Breast-feeding, preferably skin-to-skin, should be initiated immediately following the heel stick puncture to treat the suspected hypoglycemia. The **HCP** 📖 can be notified once the blood glucose value is known and the baby is successfully breast-feeding. Normal newborn temperature ranges from 97.7°F (36.5°C) to 99.1°F (37.3°C). A temperature of 96.6°F (35.9°C) is low, another sign of hypoglycemia; however, breast-feeding takes precedence over the radiant heater. Also, breast-feeding via skin-to-skin contact has been found as the most effective way to maintain a newborn's temperature.

🗝️ CN: Management of care; CL: Synthesize

116. 2. The mother demonstrates signs of full bladder and vaginal bleeding and requires assistance with bladder emptying and uterine massage to assess the origination of the bleeding. The newborn requires further assessment because turning dusky when quiet and respiration rate of 70 breaths/min indicate the beginning signs of respiratory distress and requires prompt intervention. All other mothers are recovering normally. While bilateral crackles in a newborn could indicate excessive fluid, a pink color indicates the infant is maintaining oxygenation. Normal respiration is 30 to 60 breaths/min. While a respiratory rate of 67 is slightly elevated, the baby is not demonstrating any other signs of respiratory distress. The newborn with acrocyanosis (bluish hands and feet) is a normal newborn finding and shows the ability to maintain oxygenation. Respirations of 70 breaths/min and intermittent expiratory grunt would indicate close observation but does not require immediate intervention if the infant is pink. The last newborn is maintaining oxygenation, with respirations just slightly above normal. Periodic breathing, featuring pauses in breathing of less than 15 seconds, is a normal newborn finding.

🗝️ CN: Management of care; CL: Synthesize

117. 2,3,4,5. A hospital-specific security system is the standard of care to prevent neonatal abduction. The bulb syringe should be visible and easily accessible to both the mother and the nurse in case of choking. Someone should remain in the room who is able to safely care for the infant. This may be the mother or a family member if the mother is physically not able to care for the infant. The infant should be lying on the back or side, rather than the abdomen to prevent sudden infant death syndrome ("back to sleep"). Infant falls from a mother's bed are a serious safety problem. The infant should be in the mother's arms or in the crib rather than lying on a bed, even with the side rails up, as an infant can slip through the rails. A sleeping mother is not aware of the status of the infant who can easily fall out of her arms; the infant can be in the mother's arms only if she is awake.

🗝️ CN: Safety and infection control; CL: Evaluate

118. 2. The blood glucose of 25 (1.38 mmol/L) is the most critical. Glucose is the only fuel that the brain can use. It is important to protect the central nervous system, and levels less than 30 (1.7 mmol/L) in the first 6 hours of life of a neonate indicate hypoglycemia. Occasional grunting at ½ hour of age may be normal transitioning to extrauterine life. A temperature of 97.4°F (36.4°C) is only slightly low for a neonate at this age. Ninety-five percent of all neonates will void at least once in the first 24 hours. This is not unusual at this age.

🗝️ CN: Management of care; CL: Analyze

119. 4,1,3,2. Based on the report given by the preceding nurse, the nurse should plan to prioritize all clients and first make rounds on the client needing the highest level of nursing care. The nurse can then make rounds on all other clients. The nurse can then check for new prescriptions and, finally, inspect the room in which the next client will be admitted to be sure all of the equipment is available.

🗝️ CN: Management of care; CL: Synthesize

120. 2,4,5. The role of the **UAP** 📖 allows this member of the healthcare team to take vital signs on clients, record feedings, and voids and stools of infants according to hospital guidelines. The newborn assessment is completed by a licensed care provider as is the tube feeding. Bathing of the newborn is within the scope of practice for the UAP, but the initial assessment of patency of the gastrointestinal tract, which is initiated by the first feeding, is within the scope of licensed care providers. If there is a trachea esophageal fistula, this is the time when it may become evident.

🗝️ CN: Management of care; CL: Apply

5. A 10-month-old looks for objects that have been removed from his view. The nurse should instruct the parents that:

☐ **1.** neuromuscular development enables the child to reach out and grasp objects.

☐ **2.** the child's curiosity has increased.

☐ **3.** the child understands the permanence of objects even though the child cannot see them.

☐ **4.** the child is now able to transfer objects from hand to hand.

6. Which structure should be closed by the time the child is 2 months old?

☐ **1.** A
☐ **2.** B
☐ **3.** C
☐ **4.** D

7. Which statement by a parent reflects the need for further teaching regarding car seat safety?

☐ **1.** "My baby should stay in a rear-facing car seat until he is 1 year old."

☐ **2.** "I should check my old car seat's expiration date before using it for this baby."

☐ **3.** "My older child will need to stay in a booster seat until he is 4 feet 9 inches (144.8 cm)."

☐ **4.** "My children should ride in the back seat until they are 13 years old."

8. The parents of a 3-week-old healthy newborn ask the nurse why their child is intermittently cross-eyed. The nurse's **best** response is:

☐ **1.** "An eye patch may be necessary for 6 weeks to correct your child's vision."

☐ **2.** "Your child will likely need an ophthalmology consult."

☐ **3.** "It is normal to have eye-crossing in the newborn period."

☐ **4.** "Surgery may be necessary to correct your child's vision."

9. A parent brings a 4-month-old to the clinic for a regular well visit and expresses concern that the infant is not developing appropriately. Which finding in the infant would indicate the need for further developmental screening?

☐ **1.** has no interest in peekaboo games
☐ **2.** does not turn front to back
☐ **3.** does not babble
☐ **4.** sits unsupported

10. The nurse assesses a 6-month-old for vaccination readiness. Which finding would **most** likely indicate the need to delay administering the diphtheria, tetanus, and acellular pertussis (DTaP) vaccine?

☐ **1.** a family history of sudden infant death syndrome (SIDS)

☐ **2.** a fever of 38.5°C (101.3°F) following the 4-month vaccinations

☐ **3.** an acute bilateral ear infection

☐ **4.** living with a family member who is immunosuppressed

11. The parents of a 9-month-old bring the infant to the clinic for a regular checkup. The infant has received no immunizations. Which vaccine if prescribed would the nurse question?

☐ **1.** diphtheria, tetanus, and acellular pertussis (DTaP)

☐ **2.** Haemophilus influenzae type B (Hib)

☐ **3.** measles, mumps, and rubella (MMR)

☐ **4.** inactivated influenza (Flu)

12. To assess the development of a 1-month-old, the nurse asks the parent if the infant is able to:

☐ **1.** smile and laugh out loud.
☐ **2.** roll from back to side.
☐ **3.** hold a rattle briefly.
☐ **4.** lift head from prone position.

13. The parent of a 6-month-old reports starting 2% milk. The nurse should **first** ask the parent:

☐ **1.** "Do you think your baby will be fine with this milk?"

☐ **2.** "Is it possible for you to switch your baby to whole milk?"

☐ **3.** "Can you tell me more about the reason you switched your baby to 2% milk?"

☐ **4.** "You cannot switch to 2% milk right now. Did your pediatrician tell you to do this?"

14. The nurse notes that an infant stares at an object placed in his hand and takes it to his mouth, coos and gurgles when talked to, and sustains part of his own weight when held in a standing position. The nurse correctly interprets these findings as characteristic of an infant at which age?

☐ **1.** 2 months
☐ **2.** 4 months
☐ **3.** 7 months
☐ **4.** 9 months

15. An 8-month-old infant is seen in the well-child clinic for a routine checkup. The nurse should expect the infant to be able to do which tasks? Select all that apply.
- ☐ **1.** say "mama" and "dada" with specific meaning
- ☐ **2.** feed self with a spoon
- ☐ **3.** play peekaboo
- ☐ **4.** walk independently
- ☐ **5.** stack two blocks
- ☐ **6.** transfer object from hand to hand

16. The parent of a 9-month-old infant is concerned that the infant's front soft spot is still open. The nurse should tell the parent:
- ☐ **1.** "I will measure your baby's head to see if it is a normal size."
- ☐ **2.** "Your infant will need to be referred for more testing."
- ☐ **3.** "You should contact your healthcare provider immediately."
- ☐ **4.** "This is normal because this soft spot usually closes between 12 and 18 months."

17. The parent of a 9-month-old expressed concern that the baby "is developing slowly." The nurse is concerned about a developmental delay when finding the baby is unable to accomplish which skill?
- ☐ **1.** vocalizing single syllables
- ☐ **2.** standing alone
- ☐ **3.** building a tower of two cubes
- ☐ **4.** drinking from a cup with little spilling

18. Which infant **most** needs a developmental referral for a gross motor delay?
- ☐ **1.** the 2-month-old who does not roll over
- ☐ **2.** the 4-month-old who does not sit without support
- ☐ **3.** the 6-month-old who does not crawl
- ☐ **4.** the 9-month-old who does not stand holding on

19. Which intervention should the nurse employ to reduce trauma caused by vaccine administration to an infant?
- ☐ **1.** Use a 5/8-inch (1.6-cm) needle.
- ☐ **2.** Simultaneously administer vaccines at separate sites with a second nurse.
- ☐ **3.** Aspirate to verify needle placement.
- ☐ **4.** Breast-feed right before administering the vaccines.

Health Promotion of the Toddler and Family

20. An uncle is shopping for a toy to give his niece. He has no children of his own and asks his neighbor, a nurse, what would be the **most** appropriate toy to give a 15-month-old child. Which toy should the nurse recommend to facilitate learning and development?
- ☐ **1.** a stuffed animal
- ☐ **2.** a music box
- ☐ **3.** a push-pull toy
- ☐ **4.** a nursery mobile

21. A 2-year-old tells his parent he is afraid to go to sleep because "the monsters will get him." The nurse should tell his parent to:
- ☐ **1.** allow him to sleep with his parents in their bed whenever he is afraid.
- ☐ **2.** increase his activity before he goes to bed so he eventually falls asleep from being tired.
- ☐ **3.** read a story to him before bedtime, and allow him to have a cuddly animal or a blanket.
- ☐ **4.** allow him to stay up an hour later with the family until he falls asleep.

22. A 2-year-old always puts his teddy bear at the head of his bed before he goes to sleep. The parents ask the nurse if this behavior is normal. The nurse should explain to the parents that toddlers use ritualistic patterns to:
- ☐ **1.** establish a sense of identity.
- ☐ **2.** establish control over adults in their environment.
- ☐ **3.** establish sequenced patterns of learning behavior.
- ☐ **4.** establish a sense of security.

23. Which development is necessary for toilet training readiness for a 2-year-old? Select all that apply.
- ☐ **1.** adequate neuromuscular development for sphincter control
- ☐ **2.** appropriate chronological age
- ☐ **3.** ability to communicate the need to use the toilet
- ☐ **4.** desire to please the parents
- ☐ **5.** ability to play with other 2-year-olds

24. A parent of a toilet-trained 3-year-old expresses concern over her child's bed-wetting while hospitalized. The nurse should tell the parent:
- ☐ **1.** "Your child was too immature to be toilet trained. In a few months your child should be old enough."
- ☐ **2.** "Children are afraid in the hospital and frequently wet their bed."
- ☐ **3.** "It is very common for children to regress when they are in the hospital."
- ☐ **4.** "This is normal. Your child probably received too much fluid the night before."

25. The nurse is to obtain a urine specimen from a toddler hospitalized with a urinary tract infection. In what order should the nurse perform the following steps? Place in order from first to last. All options must be used.

| 1. Cleanse the genital area. |
| 2. Apply gloves. |
| 3. Offer fluids. |
| 4. Apply collection bag. |

| |
| |
| |
| |

26. A parent brings in an 18-month-old to the clinic because the child "eats ashes, crayons, and paper." Which information about the toddler should the nurse assess **first**?
- ☐ **1.** evidence of eruption of large teeth
- ☐ **2.** amount of attention from the parent
- ☐ **3** any changes in the home environment
- ☐ **4.** intake of a soft, low-roughage diet

27. When assessing a 2-year-old child at the clinic for a routine checkup, which skill should the nurse expect the child to be able to perform?
- ☐ **1.** ride a tricycle
- ☐ **2.** tie his or her shoelaces
- ☐ **3.** kick a ball forward
- ☐ **4.** use blunt scissors

28. A 2-year-old child brought to the clinic by her parents is uncooperative when the nurse tries to look in her ears. What should the nurse try **first**?
- ☐ **1.** Ask another nurse to assist.
- ☐ **2.** Allow a parent to assist.
- ☐ **3.** Wait until the child calms down.
- ☐ **4.** Restrain the child's arms.

29. When observing the parent instilling prescribed ear drops prescribed twice a day for a 2-year-old, the nurse decides that the teaching about positioning of the pinna for instillation of the drops is effective when the parent pulls the toddler's pinna in which direction?
- ☐ **1.** up and forward
- ☐ **2.** up and backward
- ☐ **3.** down and forward
- ☐ **4.** down and backward

30. The mother asks the nurse for advice about discipline for her 18-month-old. Which discipline strategy should the nurse suggest that the mother use?
- ☐ **1.** reprimand
- ☐ **2.** spanking
- ☐ **3.** reasoning
- ☐ **4.** time-out

31. When assessing for pain in a toddler, which method should be the **most** appropriate?
- ☐ **1.** Ask the child about the pain.
- ☐ **2.** Observe the child for restlessness.
- ☐ **3.** Use a numeric rating pain scale.
- ☐ **4.** Assess for changes in vital signs.

32. Which amount of daily milk intake should the nurse include in the plan of care for a 15-month-old?
- ☐ **1.** ½ to 1 cup (125 to 250 mL)
- ☐ **2.** 2 to 3 cups (500 to 750 mL)
- ☐ **3.** 3 to 4 cups (750 to 1,000 mL)
- ☐ **4.** 4 to 5 cups (1,000 to 1,250 mL)

Health Promotion of the Preschooler and Family

33. The nurse teaches the parents of a 4-year-old diagnosed with iron deficiency anemia about potential side effects of taking an iron supplement. The nurse knows more teaching is required when the parents state a side effect of taking an iron supplement is:
- ☐ **1.** teeth staining.
- ☐ **2.** black stools.
- ☐ **3.** anorexia.
- ☐ **4.** dark urine.

34. The parent of a 4-year-old expresses concern that the child may be hyperactive. The parent describes the child as always in motion, constantly dropping and spilling things. Which action would be appropriate at this time?
- ☐ **1.** Determine whether there have been any changes at home.
- ☐ **2.** Explain that this is not unusual behavior.
- ☐ **3.** Explore the possibility that the child is being abused.
- ☐ **4.** Suggest that the child be seen by a pediatric neurologist.

35. The parent of a preschooler reports that the child creates a scene every night at bedtime. What is the **best** course of action?
- ☐ **1.** Allow the child to stay up later one or two nights a week.
- ☐ **2.** Establish a set bedtime and follow a routine.
- ☐ **3.** Encourage active play before bedtime.
- ☐ **4.** Give the child a cookie if bedtime is pleasant.

36. The parents of a preschooler ask the nurse how to handle their child's temper tantrums. Which technique should the nurse include in the teaching plan? Select all that apply.
- ☐ 1. putting the child in "time-out"
- ☐ 2. ignoring the child
- ☐ 3. putting the child to bed
- ☐ 4. spanking the child
- ☐ 5. trying to reason with the child

37. After teaching a group of parents of preschoolers attending a well-child clinic about oral hygiene and tooth brushing, the nurse determines that the teaching has been successful when the parents state that children can begin to brush their teeth without help at which age?
- ☐ 1. 3 years
- ☐ 2. 5 years
- ☐ 3. 7 years
- ☐ 4. 9 years

38. After having a blood sample drawn, a 5-year-old child insists that the site be covered with a bandage. When the parent tries to remove the bandage before leaving the office, the child screams that all the blood will come out. The nurse encourages the parent to leave the bandage in place and tells the parent that the child:
- ☐ 1. fears another procedure.
- ☐ 2. does not understand body integrity.
- ☐ 3. is expressing pain.
- ☐ 4. is attempting to regain control.

39. The family of a 5-year-old, only child has just moved to a rural setting. At the well-child visit, the father expresses concern that his child seems prone to minor accidents such as skinning his elbow and knees or falling off his scooter. The nurse tells the father:
- ☐ 1. "Only children use accidents as a way to seek parental attention."
- ☐ 2. "Children who live in the suburbs typically have more accidents."
- ☐ 3. "Children frequently have more accidents when families experience change."
- ☐ 4. "We see a relationship between accidents and parental education."

40. When developing the teaching plan about illness for the parent of a preschooler, which information should the nurse include about how a preschooler perceives illness?
- ☐ 1. a necessary part of life
- ☐ 2. a test of self-worth
- ☐ 3. a punishment for wrongdoing
- ☐ 4. the will of God

Health Promotion of the School-Age Child and Family

41. To interpret the results of blood pressure screenings in children over 3 years of age, the nurse compares the results to percentiles for systolic and diastolic blood pressure based on what factors? Select all that apply.
- ☐ 1. age
- ☐ 2. body mass index (BMI)
- ☐ 3. gender
- ☐ 4. height
- ☐ 5. occipital frontal circumference (OFC)
- ☐ 6. weight

42. A nurse is assessing the growth and development of a 10-year-old. What is the expected behavior of this child?
- ☐ 1. enjoys physical demonstrations of affection
- ☐ 2. is selfish and insensitive to the welfare of others
- ☐ 3. is uncooperative in play and school
- ☐ 4. has a strong sense of justice and fair play

43. To assess a 9-year-old's social development, the nurse asks the parent if the child:
- ☐ 1. thinks independently.
- ☐ 2. is able to organize and plan.
- ☐ 3. has a best friend.
- ☐ 4. enjoys active play.

44. A 10-year-old child proudly tells the nurse that brushing and flossing her teeth is her responsibility. How does the nurse interpret the statement?
- ☐ 1. She is too young to be given this responsibility.
- ☐ 2. She is most likely capable of this responsibility.
- ☐ 3. She should have assumed this responsibility much sooner.
- ☐ 4. She is probably just exaggerating the responsibility.

45. The parent tells the nurse that an 8-year-old child is continually telling jokes and riddles to the point of driving the other family members crazy. The nurse should explain this behavior is a sign of:
- ☐ 1. inadequate parental attention.
- ☐ 2. mastery of language ambiguities.
- ☐ 3. inappropriate peer influence.
- ☐ 4. excessive television watching.

46. The parent asks the nurse about a 9-year-old child's apparent need for between-meal snacks, especially after school. When developing a sound nutritional plan for the child with the mother, the nurse should advise the parent that:
- ☐ **1.** the child does not need to eat between-meal snacks.
- ☐ **2.** the child should eat the snacks the mother thinks are appropriate.
- ☐ **3.** the child should help with preparing his or her own snacks.
- ☐ **4.** the child will instinctively select nutritional snacks.

47. A nurse compares a child's height and weight with standard growth charts and finds the child to be in the 50th percentile for height and in the 25th percentile for weight. The nurse interprets these findings as indicating that the child is:
- ☐ **1.** typical height and weight.
- ☐ **2.** overweight for height.
- ☐ **3.** underweight for height.
- ☐ **4.** abnormal in height.

Health Promotion of the Adolescent and Family

48. The nurse is assessing an 11-year-old female, using the Tanner staging of puberty. Which finding indicates preadolescent development of the breasts?

☐ **1.**

☐ **2.**

☐ **3.**

☐ **4.**

49. The parents of a 12-year-old girl ask why their daughter, who is not sexually active, should receive the human papillomavirus (HPV) vaccine. The nurse should tell the parents:
- ☐ **1.** "The vaccine is most effective against cervical cancer if given before becoming sexually active."
- ☐ **2.** "Parents are never sure when their child might become sexually active."
- ☐ **3.** "HPV is most common is teens and women in their late 20s."
- ☐ **4.** "If your daughter is sexually assaulted, she may be exposed to HPV."

50. The nurse is teaching an adolescent with asthma how to use an inhaler. In which order should the nurse instruct the client to follow the steps from first to last? All options must be used.

1. Put the inhaler in your mouth.

2. Breathe out.

3. Depress the top of the inhaler.

4. Begin to slowly breath in.

5. Hold the breath 5 to 10 seconds.

6. Shake the inhaler.

51. A 16-year-old client and who has been confined to a wheelchair since early childhood has lately been acting rebellious and rude. Her parents ask the nurse, "Are all adolescents like this?" The nurse should respond with which statement?
- ☐ **1.** "Yes, although your daughter's behaviors are more like those of an adolescent boy."
- ☐ **2.** "No. Your daughter must need some help in dealing with her feelings."
- ☐ **3.** "Your daughter's behavior seems to be typical adolescent behavior. Let us talk more about it."
- ☐ **4.** "Your daughter's behavior results from feelings about her disability; ignore them."

52. The parents of an adolescent boy are concerned their son seems to need 9 hours of sleep a night. The nurse should advise the parents:
☐ **1.** "As long as he seems otherwise well, this sounds like a typical teenager."
☐ **2.** "Adolescents need only 8 hours of sleep a night; anything over this is excessive."
☐ **3.** "Your son is probably engaged in too many activities and is wearing himself out."
☐ **4.** "The side effect of many drugs is sleepiness."

53. An adolescent tells the nurse that she would like to use tampons during her period. The nurse should **first**:
☐ **1.** assess her usual menstrual flow pattern.
☐ **2.** determine whether she is sexually active.
☐ **3.** provide information about preventing toxic shock syndrome.
☐ **4.** refer her to a specialist in adolescent gynecology.

54. Several high-school seniors are referred to the nurse because of suspected alcohol misuse. When the nurse assesses the situation, what would be **most** important to determine?
☐ **1.** what they know about the legal implications of drinking
☐ **2.** the type of alcohol they usually drink
☐ **3.** the reasons they choose to use alcohol
☐ **4.** when and with whom they use alcohol

Common Childhood and Adolescent Health Problems

55. Which action initiated by the parents of an 8-month-old indicates they need further teaching about preventing childhood accidents?
☐ **1.** placing a fire screen in front of the fireplace
☐ **2.** placing a car seat in a front-seat, front-facing position
☐ **3.** inspecting toys for loose parts
☐ **4.** placing toxic substances out of reach or in a locked cabinet

56. A nurse is assessing the growth and development of a 14-year-old boy. He reports that his 13-year-old sister is 2 inches (5 cm) taller than he is. The nurse should advise the boy that the growth spurt in adolescent boys, compared with the growth spurt of adolescent girls:
☐ **1.** occurs about at the same time.
☐ **2.** occurs about 2 years earlier.
☐ **3.** occurs about 2 years later.
☐ **4.** occurs about 1 year earlier.

57. Parents of a 15-year-old state that their child is moody and rude. The nurse should advise the parents to:
☐ **1.** restrict their child's activities.
☐ **2.** discuss their feelings with their child.
☐ **3.** obtain family counseling.
☐ **4.** talk to other parents of adolescents.

58. Which statement by a parent whose child was just diagnosed with pediculosis capitis (head lice) demonstrates an understanding of the safety and efficacy of the common medications used to treat the infection?
☐ **1.** "I am going to request a prescription for lindane since it works the best."
☐ **2.** "After I shampoo, I will use the special comb to get the nits out."
☐ **3.** "Most OTC lice treatments are 100% effective at killing all the eggs."
☐ **4.** "I like the OTC lice treatments because you can give a second treatment the next day if any lice remain."

59. A parent asks, "Can I get head lice too?" The nurse indicates that adults can also be infested with head lice but that pediculosis is more common among school-age children, primarily for what reason?
☐ **1.** An immunity to pediculosis usually is established by adulthood.
☐ **2.** School-age children tend to be more neglectful of frequent handwashing.
☐ **3.** Pediculosis usually is spread by close contact with infested children.
☐ **4.** The skin of adults is more capable of resisting the invasion of lice.

60. After teaching the parents about the cause of ringworm of the scalp (tinea capitis), which statement by the parent indicates successful teaching?
☐ **1.** "It results from overexposure to the sun."
☐ **2.** "It is caused by infestation with a mite."
☐ **3.** "It is a fungal infection of the scalp."
☐ **4.** "It is an allergic reaction."

61. Griseofulvin was prescribed to treat a child's ringworm of the scalp. The nurse instructs the parents to use the medication for several weeks for which reason?
☐ **1.** A sensitivity to the drug is less likely if it is used over a period of time.
☐ **2.** Fewer side effects occur as the body slowly adjusts to a new substance over time.
☐ **3.** Fewer allergic reactions occur if the drug is maintained at the same level long-term.
☐ **4.** The growth of the causative organism into new cells is prevented with long-term use.

62. A parent asks the nurse, "How did my children get pinworms?" The nurse explains that pinworms are **most** commonly spread by which route?
- ☐ **1.** food
- ☐ **2.** hands
- ☐ **3.** animals
- ☐ **4.** toilet seats

63. A parent asks the nurse how to care for a child with chickenpox. What should the nurse include in the plan of care? Select all that apply.
- ☐ **1.** Use OTC aspirin for fever.
- ☐ **2.** Encourage oatmeal baths.
- ☐ **3.** Keep fingernails short.
- ☐ **4.** Avoid overheating.
- ☐ **5.** Do not return to school until all lesions have crusted over.

64. A mother states that a healthcare provider (HCP) described her daughter as having 20/60 vision, and she asks the nurse what this means. The nurse responds based on the interpretation that the child is experiencing which condition?
- ☐ **1.** a loss of approximately one-third of her visual acuity
- ☐ **2.** ability to see at 60 feet what she should see at 20 feet
- ☐ **3.** ability to see at 20 feet what she should see at 60 feet
- ☐ **4.** visual acuity three times better than average

65. The nurse discusses the eating habits of school-age children with their parents, explaining that these habits are **most** influenced by:
- ☐ **1.** food preferences of their peers.
- ☐ **2.** smell and appearance of foods offered.
- ☐ **3.** examples provided by parents at mealtimes.
- ☐ **4.** parental encouragement to eat nutritious foods.

66. When discussing the onset of adolescence with parents, the nurse explains that it occurs at what time?
- ☐ **1.** same age for both boys and girls
- ☐ **2.** 1 to 2 years earlier in boys than in girls
- ☐ **3.** 1 to 2 years earlier in girls than in boys
- ☐ **4.** 3 to 4 years later in boys than in girls

67. A mother has heard that several children have been diagnosed with mononucleosis. She asks the nurse what precautions should be taken to prevent this from occurring in her child. The nurse should instruct the mother to:
- ☐ **1.** take no particular precautionary measures.
- ☐ **2.** sterilize the child's eating utensils before they are reused.
- ☐ **3.** wash the child's linens separately in hot, soapy water.
- ☐ **4.** have the child vaccinated.

68. A father asks the nurse how he would know if his child had developed mononucleosis. The nurse explains that in addition to fatigue, which symptom would be **most** common?
- ☐ **1.** liver tenderness
- ☐ **2.** enlarged lymph glands
- ☐ **3.** persistent nonproductive cough
- ☐ **4.** a blush-like generalized skin rash

Managing Care, Quality, and Safety of Children

69. A 17-year-old high school senior calls the clinic because she thinks she might have gonorrhea. She wants to be seen but wants assurances that no one will know. Which is the **most** appropriate response by the nurse?
- ☐ **1.** "Because you are underage, we will need your parent's consent to treat you."
- ☐ **2.** "We can treat you without your parents' consent, but they have the right to review your medical record."
- ☐ **3.** "We can see you without your parents' consent but have to report any positive results to the public health department."
- ☐ **4.** "We can see you and will not share your results with anyone."

70. A parent brings a 5-year-old child to a weekend vaccination clinic to prepare for school entry. The nurse notes that the child has not had any vaccinations since 4 months of age. What is the **best** way for the nurse to determine how to catch up the child's vaccinations?
- ☐ **1.** Ask the child's healthcare provider (HCP).
- ☐ **2.** Check nationally published immunization guidelines.
- ☐ **3.** Read each vaccine's manufacturer's insert.
- ☐ **4.** Contact the pharmacist.

71. A 13-month-old has a febrile seizure 3 weeks after the administration of the chickenpox vaccine. The nurse should:
- ☐ **1.** recognize that the events are unrelated.
- ☐ **2.** report the event through an immunization surveillance system.
- ☐ **3.** explain to the parents that this is a rare but acceptable risk.
- ☐ **4.** refer the child to a neurologist.

72. The nurse is invited to attend a meeting with several parents who express frustration with the amount of time their adolescents spend in front of the mirror and the length of time it takes them to get dressed. The nurse explains that this behavior indicates:
☐ 1. an abnormal narcissism.
☐ 2. a method of procrastination.
☐ 3. a way of testing the parents' limit-setting.
☐ 4. a result of developing self-concept.

73. A child who is 18 months of age is brought to the emergency department by her babysitter. The babysitter states, "She fell from the sofa an hour ago and has not been herself since." On questioning, the babysitter appears to be unsure of time and other facts about the incident. Which question below would be **most** effective in obtaining more information about the child's injuries?
☐ 1. "Why did you leave the child alone on the couch?"
☐ 2. "Have you taken a course in safe babysitting?"
☐ 3. "Tell me what was happening before she fell."
☐ 4. "Where are her parents? Do they know this happened?"

Answers, Rationales, and Test-Taking Strategies

The answers and rationales for each question follow below, along with keys (🔑) to the client need (CN) and cognitive level (CL) for each question. In addition, you will also see a glossary icon (📖) highlighting specific terminology used on the licensing exam. As you check your answers, use the **Content Mastery and Test-Taking Skill Self-Analysis** *worksheet (tear-out worksheet in back of book) to identify the reason(s) for not answering the questions correctly. For additional information about test-taking skills and strategies for answering questions, refer to pages 12–23 and pages 35–36 in Part 1 of this book.*

Health Promotion of the Infant and Family

1. 2. By trying to determine the source of parents' concerns, the nurse is able to acknowledge their feelings and provide the most appropriate information. This approach increases the likelihood parents will listen to the **healthcare provider's (HCP's)** 📖 views. Exemptions for vaccines vary by state, province, or territory, and many parents feel legal requirements for vaccinations take away parental rights. The number of vaccinations given at one time may not be the issue. Waivers are used only if clients refuse vaccination after a discussion of risks and benefits.

🔑 CN: Health promotion and maintenance; CL: Synthesize

2. 3. It is important for the nurse to assist parents in assessing speech development in their child so that developmental delays can be identified early. According to the Denver Developmental Screening Examination, at 8 months of age, the child should say "mama" and "dada" nonspecifically and imitate speech sounds. Children cannot say "dada" or "mama" specifically or use more than three words until they are about 12 months of age. A child cannot respond to specific commands or point to objects when requested until about 17 months of age.

🔑 CN: Health promotion and maintenance; CL: Apply

3. 4. According to the Denver Developmental Screening Examination, a child of 8 months should sit without support for long periods of time. An 8-month-old child does not have the ability to stand without hanging onto a stationary object for support. His or her muscles are not developed enough to support all his weight without assistance. His or her balance has not developed to the point that he or she can stand and stoop over to reach an object.

🔑 CN: Health promotion and maintenance; CL: Synthesize

4. 4. Infants should be kept on formula or breast milk until 1 year of age. The protein in cow's milk is harder to digest than is that found in formula. It does not matter in what order fruits and vegetables are introduced as long as the foods are introduced slowly. Solids are introduced into the infant's diet around 4 to 6 months, after the extrusion reflex has diminished and when the child will accept new textures. Iron deficiency develops in term infants between 4 to 6 months when the prenatal iron stores are depleted. Fortified cereals can be added to the infant's diet at 4 to 6 months to prevent iron deficiency anemia.

🔑 CN: Health promotion and maintenance; CL: Create

5. 3. Understanding object permanence means that the child is aware of the existence of objects that are covered or displaced. Neuromuscular development, curiosity, and the ability to transfer objects are not associated with the principle of object permanence. Although, at 10 months, neuromuscular development is sufficient to grasp objects and a child's curiosity has increased, neither are related to the thought process involved in object permanence.

🔑 CN: Health promotion and maintenance; CL: Apply

6. **3.** The posterior fontanelle should be closed by age 2 months. The anterior fontanelle and sagittal and frontal sutures should be closed by age 18 months.

   ⚷ CN Health promotion and maintenance; CL: Apply

7. **1.** New guidelines recommend that parents keep their toddlers in a rear-facing car seat until 2 years of age or they reach maximum height and weight for the seat. Car seats are marked with an expiration date because the integrity of the plastic may deteriorate with age. Booster seats are recommended for older children until they are 4 feet 9 inches (144.8 cm). This typically occurs between the ages 8 and 12 years. Children should ride in the back seat until they are 13 years of age to minimize injury should airbags be deployed.

   ⚷ CN: Health promotion and maintenance; CL: Evaluate

8. **3.** During the first few months of life, an infant's eyes may wander and appear to be crossing. As the eye muscles mature, between 2 and 3 months of age, both eyes will focus on the same thing. No intervention is necessary, as crossing of the eyes is normal in the first few months of life.

   ⚷ CN: Health promotion and maintenance; CL: Apply

9. **3.** By the end of 3 months, infants should babble. Lack of babbling suggests a language delay and warrants further investigation. Infants typically would begin playing peekaboo around 7 months. The ability to roll front to back typically occurs at 5 months. Sitting unsupported is expected at 6 months.

   ⚷ CN: Health promotion and maintenance; CL: Analyze

10. **3.** Vaccination in the presence of a moderate-to-severe infection, with or without fever, increases the risk of injury and decreases the chance of mounting good immunity. There is currently no evidence to suggest vaccines raise the risk of SIDS. A mild temperature may be expected with the DTaP. A fever of >40.5°C (105°F) within 48 hours of vaccination would warrant caution. The DTaP is not a live vaccine. No special precautions are needed regarding immunosuppressed family members.

   ⚷ CN: Reduction of risk potential; CL: Synthesize

11. **3.** The MMR is a live vaccine. Neither the American Academy of Pediatrics nor the Public Health Agency of Canada recommends routine vaccination with the MMR (either alone or combined with the varicella vaccine) to children younger than 12 months. The DTaP, Hib, and influenza are all indicated.

   ⚷ CN: Health promotion and maintenance; CL: Synthesize

12. **4.** A 1-month-old infant is usually able to lift the head from a prone position. The full-term infant with no complications has probably been able to do this since birth. Smiling and laughing is expected behavior at 2 to 3 months. Rolling from back to side and holding a rattle are characteristics of a 4-month-old.

   ⚷ CN: Health promotion and maintenance; CL: Analyze

13. **3.** The American Academy of Pediatrics and Canadian Pediatric Society recommend that infants remain on iron-fortified formula or breast milk until 1 year of age. The nurse needs to first assess if the parent switched the baby prematurely to due to lack of information or lack of resources. Then appropriate teaching or referrals may be determined. At 1 year of age, the infant may be switched to whole milk, which has a higher fat content than 2%. The higher fat content is needed for brain growth. Demanding clients change behaviors without addressing the cause is unlikely to produce desired results.

   ⚷ CN: Health promotion and maintenance; CL: Analyze

14. **2.** Holding the head erect when sitting, staring at an object placed in the hand, taking the object to the mouth, cooing and gurgling, and sustaining part of his body weight when in a standing position are behaviors characteristic of a 4-month-old infant. A 2-month-old typically vocalizes, follows objects to the midline, and smiles. A 7-month-old typically is able to sit without support, turns toward the voice, and transfers objects from hand to hand. Usually, a 9-month-old can crawl, stand while holding on, and initiate speech sounds.

   ⚷ CN: Health promotion and maintenance; CL: Analyze

15. **3,6.** Typical abilities demonstrated by 8-month-old infants include playing peekaboo and transferring objects from one hand to another. The ability to say "dada" and "mama" is more typical of 10-month-old infants. Infants usually are at least 12 months old when they achieve the ability to walk independently. Infants who are 15 months old commonly can feed themselves with a spoon and stack two blocks.

   ⚷ CN: Health promotion and maintenance; CL: Analyze

16. 4. The anterior fontanelle, commonly known as the soft spot, closes between 12 to 18 months in most infants. The nurse normally measures an infant's occipital frontal circumference at each well-child visit. This action alone does not relieve the parent's concerns. Referrals would be indicated for premature or delayed closures of the fontanelle especially if there were other abnormal findings. Closure of the anterior fontanelle by 12 months can only be expected to occur in approximately a third of all infants.

CN: Health promotion and maintenance; CL: Synthesize

17. 1. Typically, a 9-month-old infant should have been voicing single syllables since 6 months of age. Absence of this finding would be a cause for concern. An infant usually is able to stand alone at about 10 months of age. An infant usually is able to build a tower of two cubes at about 15 months of age. An infant usually is able to drink from a cup with little spilling at about 15 months of age.

CN: Health promotion and maintenance; CL: Analyze

18. 4. More than 90% of 9-month-olds are able to stand holding onto objects. Rolling over is expected at 4 to 6 months, and sitting without support is expected at 6 months. Crawling is expected at 9 months.

CN: Health promotion and maintenance; CL: Analyze

19. 2. Simultaneous injection reduces the anxiety from anticipation of the next injection. Needle length must be long enough to deposit the vaccine into the muscle. A 5/8-inch (1.6-cm) needle is appropriate for newborns but is not long enough for infants older than 1 month or other children. Aspirating for blood return does not confirm needle placement. Breast-feeding during vaccinations, not before, has been found to reduce pain.

CN: Basic care and comfort; CL: Apply

Health Promotion of the Toddler and Family

20. 3. A push-pull toy will aid in development of gross motor skills and muscle development. A stuffed animal is age appropriate for a toddler but is not the toy to promote development. A music box and nursery mobile are most appropriate to stimulate development for an infant.

CN: Health promotion and maintenance; CL: Apply

21. 3. Behavior problems related to sleep and rest are common in young children. Consistent rituals around bedtime help to create an easier transition from waking to sleep. Allowing a child to sleep with his parents commonly creates more problems for the family and child and does not alleviate the problem or foster autonomy. Increasing activity before bedtime does not alleviate the separation anxiety in the toddler and causes further anxiety. Allowing him to stay up later than his normal time for bed will increase his anxiety, make it more difficult for him to fall asleep, and do nothing to lessen his fear.

CN: Psychosocial integrity; CL: Synthesize

22. 4. Toddlers establish ritualistic patterns to feel secure, despite inconsistencies in their environment. Establishing a sense of identity is the developmental task of the adolescent. The toddler's developmental task is to use rituals and routines to help in making autonomy easier to accomplish. Ritualistic patterns do involve patterns of behavior, but they are not utilized to develop learning behaviors.

CN: Psychosocial integrity; CL: Apply

23. 1,3,4. Readiness for toilet training is based on neurological, psychological, and physical developmental readiness. The nurse can introduce concepts of readiness for toilet training and encourage parents to look for adaptive and psychomotor signs such as the ability to walk well, balance, climb, sit in a chair, dress oneself, please the parent, and communicate awareness of the need to urinate or defecate. Chronological age is not an indicator for toilet training. Two-year-olds engage in parallel play, which is not an indicator of readiness for toilet training.

CN: Health promotion and maintenance; CL: Apply

24. 3. A child will regress to a behavior used in an earlier stage of development in order to cope with a perceived threatening situation. Readiness for toilet training should be based on neurological, physical, and psychological development, not the age of the child. Children are afraid of hospitalization, but the bed-wetting is a compensatory mechanism done to regress to a previous stage of development that is more comfortable and secure for the child. Telling the mother that bed-wetting is related to fluid intake does not provide an adequate explanation for the underlying regression to an earlier stage of development.

CN: Psychosocial integrity; CL: Synthesize

25. **3,2,1,4.** When obtaining a urine specimen from an infant, the nurse assists the client to drink fluids 30 to 60 minutes prior to specimen collection so the client voids as soon as possible after the collection bag is applied. Next, the nurse applies gloves and then cleanses the genital area with sterile water to prevent contamination of the urine. Finally, the nurse applies the collection bag and then removes the bag when the specimen is obtained.

CN: Safety and infection control; CL: apply

26. **3.** A craving to eat nonfood substances is known as pica. Toddlers use oral gratification as a means to cope with anxiety. Therefore, the nurse should first assess whether the child is experiencing any change in the home environment that could cause anxiety. Teething or the eruption of large teeth and the amount of attention from the mother are unlikely causes of pica. Nutritional deficiencies, especially iron deficiency, were once thought to cause pica, but research has not substantiated this theory. A soft, low-roughage diet is an unlikely cause.

CN: Physiological adaptation; CL: Analyze

27. **3.** A 2-year-old child usually can kick a ball forward. Riding a tricycle is characteristic of a 3-year-old child. Tying shoelaces is a behavior to be expected of a 5-year-old child. Using blunt scissors is characteristic of a 3-year-old child.

CN: Health promotion and maintenance; CL: Analyze

28. **2.** Parents can be asked to assist when their child becomes uncooperative during a procedure. Most commonly, the child's difficulty in cooperating is caused by fear. In most situations, the child will feel more secure with a parent present. Other methods, such as asking another nurse to assist or waiting until the child calms down, may be necessary, but obtaining a parent's assistance is the recommended first action. Restraints should be used only as a last resort, after all other attempts have been made to encourage cooperation.

CN: Health promotion and maintenance; CL: Synthesize

29. **4.** In a child younger than 3 years of age, the pinna is pulled back and down because the auditory canals are almost straight in children. In children over 3 through adulthood, the pinna is pulled up and backward because the auditory canals are directed inward, forward, and down.

CN: Pharmacological and parenteral therapies; CL: Evaluate

30. **4.** Time-out is the most appropriate discipline for toddlers. It helps to remove them from the situation and allows them to regain control. Structuring interactions with 3-year-olds helps minimize unacceptable behavior. This approach involves setting clear and reasonable rules and calling attention to unacceptable behavior as soon as it occurs. Reprimanding a young child can reinforce undesirable behavior over time because it provides attention. Physical punishment, such as spanking, has limited effectiveness and serious negative effects. Reasoning is more appropriate for older children, such as preschoolers and those older, especially when moral issues are involved. Unfortunately, reasoning combined with scolding often takes the form of shame or criticism, and children take such remarks seriously, believing that they are "bad."

CN: Health promotion and maintenance; CL: Synthesize

31. **2.** Toddlers usually express pain through such behaviors as restlessness, facial grimaces, irritability, and crying. It is not particularly helpful to ask toddlers about pain. In most instances, they would be unable to understand or describe the nature and location of their pain because of their lack of verbal and cognitive skills. However, preschool and older children have the verbal and cognitive skills to be able to respond appropriately. While the FACES pain scale can be used in young children, numeric rating pain scales are more appropriate for children who are of school age or older. Changes in vital signs do occur as a result of pain, but behavioral changes usually are noticed first.

CN: Physiological adaptation; CL: Analyze

32. **2.** Toddlers around the age of 15 months need 2 to 3 cups (500 to 750 mL) of milk per day to supply necessary nutrients such as calcium. A daily intake of more than 3 cups (750 mL) of milk may interfere with the ingestion of other necessary nutrients.

CN: Health promotion and maintenance; CL: Apply

Health Promotion of the Preschooler and Family

33. **4.** Dark urine is not a potential side effect of taking an iron supplement. Families need education about the possible side effects, including placing liquid iron behind the teeth to avoid teeth staining. Stools may become dark in color, even turn black, and some clients may experience anorexia.

CN: Pharmacological and parenteral therapies; CL: Evaluate

34. 2. Preschool-age children have been described as powerhouses of gross motor activity who seem to have endless energy. A limitation of their motor ability is that in moving as quickly as they do, they are not always able to judge distances, nor are they able to estimate the amount of strength and balance needed for activities. As a result, they have frequent mishaps. This level of activity typically is not associated with changes at home. However, if the behavior intensifies, a referral to a pediatric neurologist would be appropriate. Children who have been abused usually demonstrate withdrawn behaviors, not endless energy.

CN: Health promotion and maintenance; CL: Synthesize

35. 2. Bedtime is often a problem with preschoolers. Recommendations for reducing conflicts at bedtime include establishing a set bedtime, having a dependable routine, such as story reading, and conveying the expectation that the child will comply. Allowing the child to stay up late one or two nights interferes with establishing the needed bedtime rituals. Excitement, such as active play, just before bedtime should be avoided because it stimulates the child, making it difficult for the child to calm down and prepare for sleep. Using food such as a cookie as a reward if bedtime is pleasant should be avoided because it places too much importance on food. Other rewards, such as stickers, could be used as an alternative.

CN: Health promotion and maintenance; CL: Synthesize

36. 1,2. Some parents find that putting the child in time-out until control is regained is very effective. Others find that ignoring the behaviors works just as well with their child. Both suggestions are appropriate to include in the teaching plan. Spanking the child is never an option. Attempting to reason with a child having a temper tantrum does not work because the child is out of control. A more appropriate time to discuss it with the child is when the child regains control.

CN: Health promotion and maintenance; CL: Create

37. 3. Children younger than 7 years of age do not have the manual dexterity needed for tooth brushing. Therefore, parents need to help with this task until that time.

CN: Health promotion and maintenance; CL: Evaluate

38. 2. The preschool-age child does not have an accurate concept of skin integrity and can view medical and surgical treatments as hostile invasions that can destroy or damage the body. The child does not understand that exsanguinations will not occur from the injection site. Here, the child is verbalizing a fear consistent with the developmental age. The child would most likely verbalize concerns of not wanting another procedure or exhibit other symptoms associated with pain if those were the underlying issues. If control was the main issue, the child would try to control more than just the bandage removal.

CN: Psychosocial integrity; CL: Analyze

39. 3. Family changes and stresses (e.g., moving, having company, taking a vacation, adding a new member) can distract parents and contribute to accidents. Only children typically receive more attention than those with siblings. Thus, the risk would be less. Families who live in the suburbs frequently are more affluent and, therefore, better able to maintain a home less conducive to accidents. A parent's formal education is unrelated to accidents.

CN: Health promotion and maintenance; CL: Synthesize

40. 3. Preschool-age children may view illness as punishment for their fantasies. At this age, children do not have the cognitive ability to separate fantasies from reality and may expect to be punished for their "evil thoughts." Viewing illness as a necessary part of life requires a higher level of cognition than preschoolers possess. This view is seen in children of middle school age and older. Perceiving illness as a test of self-worth or as the will of God is more characteristic of adults.

CN: Health promotion and maintenance; CL: Apply

Health Promotion of the School-Age Child and Family

41. 1,3,4. Blood pressures percentiles for children are referenced by the age, sex, and height. Measurements at or above the 95th percentile are considered indicative of hypertension. Weight and elevated BMI contribute to hypertension but are not used to define it. The OFC is not routinely measured in children over 2 years of age and is not used to reference blood pressure readings.

CN: Health promotion and maintenance; CL: Analyze

42. 4. School-age children are concerned about justice and fair play. They become upset when they think someone is not playing fair. Physical affection makes them embarrassed and uncomfortable. They are concerned about others and are cooperative in play and school.

CN: Health promotion and maintenance; CL: Analyze

43. 3. During the school-age years, children learn to socialize with children of the same age. The "best friend" stage, which occurs around 9 or 10 years of age, is important in providing a foundation for self-esteem and later relationships. Thinking independently, organizing, and planning are cognitive skills. Active play relates to motor skills.

◕⚷ CN: Health promotion and maintenance; CL: Analyze

44. 2. Children are capable of mastering the skills required for flossing when they reach 9 years of age. At this age, many children are able to assume responsibility for personal hygiene. She is not too young to assume this responsibility, and she should not have been expected to assume this responsibility much earlier. It is not likely that she is exaggerating; this is an expected behavior at this age.

◕⚷ CN: Health promotion and maintenance; CL: Analyze

45. 2. School-age children delight in riddles and jokes. Mastery of the ambiguities of language and of sentence structure allows the school-age child to manipulate words, and telling riddles and jokes is a way of practicing this skill. Children who suffer from inadequate attention from parents tend to demonstrate abnormal behavior. Peer influence is less important to school-age children, and while the child may learn the joke from a friend, he or she is telling the joke to master language. Watching television does not influence the extent of joke telling.

◕⚷ CN: Health promotion and maintenance; CL: Analyze

46. 3. Snacks are necessary for school-age children because of their high energy level. School-age children are in a stage of cognitive development in which they can learn to categorize or classify and can also learn cause and effect. By preparing their own snacks, children can learn the basics of nutrition (such as what carbohydrates are and what happens when they are eaten). The mother and child should make the decision about appropriate foods together. School-age children learn to make decisions based on information, not instinct. Some knowledge of nutrition is needed to make appropriate choices.

◕⚷ CN: Health promotion and maintenance; CL: Synthesize

47. 1. The values of height and weight percentiles are usually similar for an individual child. Measurements between the 5th and 95th percentiles are considered normal. Marked discrepancies identify overweight or underweight children.

◕⚷ CN: Health promotion and maintenance; CL: Analyze

Health Promotion of the Adolescent and Family

48. 3. This figure indicates elevation of the papilla, without breast buds, considered stage 1 and typical of a preadolescent. Figure 1 shows stage 2, breast bud enlargement; there is elevation of the breast and the diameter of the areola has increased. Figure 2 shows stage 3, enlargement of the breast and areola. Figure 4 shows stage 4, in which there is projection of areola and papilla to form a secondary mound above the level of the breast.

◕⚷ CN: Physiological adaptation; CL: Analyze

49. 1. Vaccines are preventative in nature and ideally given before exposure. Focusing on the benefits of cancer prevention is most appropriate, as opposed to discussing with parents the potential that their child may become sexually active without their knowledge. It is true HPV is most common in adolescents and women in their late twenties, but parents still may not perceive that their child is at risk. Discussing the possibility of exposure through assault raises fears and does not focus on prevention.

◕⚷ CN: Health promotion and maintenance; CL: Apply

50. 6,2,1,4,3,5. When dispensing medication from an inhaler, the client should first shake the inhaler and then breathe out through the mouth before putting the inhaler in the mouth. Next, the client inhales slowly and then presses the canister to dispense the medication while continuing to inhale. The client should hold the breath for 5 to 10 seconds before exhaling.

◕⚷ CN: Pharmacological and parenteral therapies; CL: Apply

51. 3. It is normal behavior for adolescents to assert independence and begin to separate from their parents; the behavior is not changed by their daughter's disability, nor is it unique to a girl. The nurse offers reassurance to the parents and then opens the conversation for additional discussion.

◕⚷ CN: Health promotion; CL: Analyze

52. 1. Many teenagers feel fatigued from a combination of fast-food diets, many activities, and a rapid growth spurt; this is normal behavior, and the nurse should explain possible reasons for the sleep pattern. Adolescents typically need 8.5 to 9.5 hours of sleep. There are no data to suggest that activities are tiring this teenager. It is not appropriate to suggest the child is taking drugs based on the question the parents are asking the nurse.

◕⚷ CN: Health Promotion; CL: Analyze

53. 3. The nurse should provide the adolescent with information about toxic shock syndrome because of the identified relationship between tampon use and the syndrome's development. Additionally, about 95% of cases of toxic shock syndrome occur during menses. Most adolescent females can use tampons safely if they change them frequently. Using tampons is not related to menstrual flow or sexual activity. There is no need to refer the girl to a gynecologist; a nurse can provide health teaching about tampon use.

⚿ CN: Reduction of risk potential;
CL: Synthesize

54. 3. Information about why adolescents choose to use alcohol or other drugs can be used to determine whether they are becoming responsible users or problem users. The senior students likely know the legal implications of drinking, and the nurse will establish a more effective relationship with the students by understanding motivations for use. The type of alcohol and when and with whom they are using it are not the first data to obtain when assessing the situation.

⚿ CN: Health promotion and maintenance;
CL: Analyze

Common Childhood and Adolescent Health Problems

55. 2. It is recommended that children up to 2 years of age ride in a rear-facing car seat. The middle of the back seat is considered the safest area of the car. Burns are a major cause of childhood accidents, and using fire screens in front of fireplaces can help prevent children from getting too close to a fire in a fireplace. Toys that contain loose parts or plastic eyes that can be swallowed or aspirated by small children should be avoided. Parents should inspect all toys for these parts before giving one to a child. Poisonings are most commonly caused by improper storage of a toxic substance. Keeping toxic substances in a childproof container in a locked cabinet and continually observing the child's activities can prevent most poisonings.

⚿ CN: Safety and infection control;
CL: Evaluate

56. 3. Adolescent boys lag about 2 years behind adolescent girls in growth. Most girls are 1 to 2 inches (3 to 5 cm) taller than boys at the beginning of adolescence but tend to stop growing approximately 2 to 3 years after menarche with the closure of the epiphyseal lines of the long bones.

⚿ CN: Health promotion and maintenance;
CL: Apply

57. 2. Parents need to discuss with their adolescent how they perceive his or her behavior and how they feel about it. Moodiness is characteristic of adolescents. The adolescent may have a reason for or not be aware of his behavior. Restricting the adolescent's activities will not change his or her mood or the way he or she responds to others. It may increase his or her unacceptable responses. Counseling may not be needed at this time if the parents are open to communicating and listening to the adolescent. Talking to other parents may be of some help, but what is helpful to others may not be helpful to their child.

⚿ CN: Health promotion and maintenance;
CL: Synthesize

58. 2. The makers of many of the pediculicides recommend manual removal of the nits following treatment with an extra–fine-tooth comb. None of the pediculicides are 100% effective in killing all the eggs. The FDA has issued a warning regarding the use of lindane because of the potential for neurotoxicity. Clients are treated with lindane only when the benefits outweigh the risks. Lice treatments may be repeated in 7 to 10 days; the next day is too soon.

⚿ CN: Health promotion; CL: synthesize

59. 3. Lice are spread by close personal contact and by contact with infested clothing, bed and bathroom linens, and combs and brushes. Lice are more common in school-age children than in adults because of the close contact in school or at sleepovers and the common practice of sharing possessions. Lice are not commonly spread by hand contact. There is no immunity conferred by having head lice. Adults can have head lice, particularly if they come in close contact with their children's infested clothing or linens.

⚿ CN: Physiological adaptation; CL: Apply

60. 3. Ringworm of the scalp is caused by a fungus of the dermatophyte group of the species. Overexposure to the sun would result in sunburn. Mites, such as chiggers or ticks, produce bites on the skin, resulting in inflammation. An allergic reaction commonly is manifested by hives, rash, or anaphylaxis.

⚿ CN: Physiological adaptation;
CL: Evaluate

61. 4. Griseofulvin is an antifungal agent that acts by binding to the keratin that is deposited in the skin, hair, and nails as they grow. This keratin is then resistant to the fungus. But as the keratin is normally shed, the fungus enters new, uninfected cells unless drug therapy continues. Long-term administration of griseofulvin does not prevent sensitivity or allergic reactions. As the body adjusts to a new substance over time, side effects are variable and do not necessarily decrease.

🔑 CN: Pharmacological and parenteral therapies; CL: Apply

62. 2. The adult pinworm emerges from the rectum and colon at night onto the perianal area to lay its eggs. Itching and scratching introduces the eggs to the hands, from where they can easily reinfect the child or infect others. Nightclothes and bed linens can be sources of infection. The eggs can also be transmitted by dust in the home. Although transmission through contaminated food and water supplies is possible, it is rare. Contaminated animals can spread histoplasmosis and salmonella. The spread of infections by toilet seats has not been supported by research.

🔑 CN: Physiological adaptation; CL: Apply

63. 2,3,4,5. The care of a child with chickenpox focuses keeping the child comfortable and preventing infection in the lesions. Oatmeal baths may ease severe itching. Keeping fingernails short reduces trauma from scratching and helps prevent skin infections. Overheating can make itching worse. Children may return to school once all lesions have crusted over. The use of aspirin in children with chickenpox is contraindicated because it has been linked to Reye syndrome.

🔑 CN: Basic care and comfort; CL: Synthesize

64. 3. A child with 20/60 vision sees at 20 feet what those with 20/20 vision see at 60 feet. A visual acuity of 20/200 is considered to be the boundary of legal blindness.

🔑 CN: Physiological adaptation; CL: Analyze

65. 3. Although children may be influenced by their peers and smell and appearance of foods may be important, children are most likely to be influenced by the example and atmosphere provided by their parents. Coaxing and badgering a child to eat most likely will aggravate poor eating habits.

🔑 CN: Health promotion and maintenance; CL: Apply

66. 3. Girls experience the onset of adolescence about 1 to 2 years earlier than do boys. The reason for this is not understood.

🔑 CN: Health promotion and maintenance; CL: Apply

67. 1. The cause of infectious mononucleosis is thought to be the Epstein-Barr virus. The virus is believed to be spread only by direct intimate contact. No precautionary measures for the general public are recommended to prevent mononucleosis. However, it is recommended that sharing food items

and kissing be avoided with persons known to have mononucleosis. There currently is no vaccine for the disease.

🔑 CN: Physiological adaptation; CL: Synthesize

68. 2. Mononucleosis usually has an insidious onset, with fatigue and the inability to maintain usual activity levels as the most common symptoms. The lymph nodes are typically enlarged, and the spleen also may be enlarged. Fever and a sore throat often accompany mononucleosis. A persistent nonproductive cough can follow an upper respiratory tract infection. A blush-like generalized skin rash is more characteristic of rubella.

🔑 CN: Physiological adaptation; CL: Analyze

Managing Care, Quality, and Safety of Children

69. 3. While some areas may specify a minimum age for treatment (usually 12 to 14 years), generally adolescents have the right to seek treatment for sexually transmitted infections without their parents' permission. These **medical records** 📖 are not shared with parents without the client's permission. However, adolescents must be made aware that certain infections, including gonorrhea, must be reported by law to public health agencies. Partner notification will also take place, but methods vary.

🔑 CN: Management of care; CL: Apply

70. 2. National advisory committees on immunization practices review vaccination evidence and update recommendations yearly. Current vaccination catch-up schedules are readily available on their Web sites. The lack of vaccinations is a strong indicator that the child probably does not have an **HCP** 📖. Even if the client had a provider, however, that person might be difficult to reach on a weekend during the time frame of a vaccination clinic. If consulted, the pharmacist would most likely have to review the latest guidelines that are equally available to the nurse. Reading each of manufacturer's inserts for multiple vaccines would be time consuming, and synthesis of the information could possibly lead to errors.

🔑 CN: Management of care; CL: Apply

71. 2. Any unusual event that occurs after the administration of a vaccination should be reported through an immunization surveillance system, especially if it happens with 1 month of the vaccine administration. In the United States, it is the Vaccine Adverse Event Reporting System (VAERS). In Canada, it is Canadian Adverse Events Following Immunization Surveillance System

(CAEFISS). A high fever, with or without a seizure, that occurs within 6 weeks of vaccination may have been caused by the vaccine. A febrile seizure is considered a moderate reaction that warrants caution with future chickenpox vaccination. A single febrile seizure does not require referral to a neurologist.

⊶ CN: Safety and infection control;
CL: Synthesize

72. 4. An adolescent's body is undergoing rapid changes. Adolescence is a time of integrating these rapidly occurring physical changes into the self-concept to achieve the developmental task of a positive self-identity. Thus, most adolescents spend much time worrying about their personal appearance. This behavior is not abnormal narcissism, a method of procrastination, or a way of testing the parents' limits.

⊶ CN: Health promotion and maintenance;
CL: Analyze

73. 3. An open-ended question is apt to supply more information when a person is under stress and easily susceptible to being influenced by the question. The other questions are direct and only require an answer with limited information.

⊶ CN Management of care; CL: Analyze

The Child with Respiratory Health Problems

- The Client with Tonsillitis
- The Client with Otitis Media
- The Client with Foreign Body Aspiration
- The Client with Asthma
- The Client with Cystic Fibrosis and Bronchopneumonia
- The Client with Sudden Infant Death Syndrome
- The Client Who Requires Immediate Care and Cardiopulmonary Resuscitation
- The Client with Croup
- The Client with Bronchiolitis or Pharyngitis
- Managing Care, Quality, and Safety of Children with Respiratory Health Problems
- Answers, Rationales, and Test-Taking Strategies

The Client with Tonsillitis

1. The nurse is inspecting the child's throat (see figure). The nurse should:

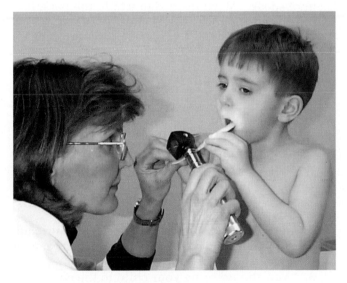

- ☐ **1.** remove the tongue blade from the child's hands after he has experienced what it feels like in his mouth.
- ☐ **2.** ask the child to hold the tongue blade with both hands in his lap while the nurse uses another tongue blade.
- ☐ **3.** have the parent hold the child with arms restrained.
- ☐ **4.** guide the tongue blade while the child is holding it to depress the tongue to visualize the throat.

2. The nurse has identified a problem of anxiety for a 4-year-old preparing for a tonsillectomy. The nurse should tell the child:
- ☐ **1.** "You will not have so many sore throats after your tonsils are removed."
- ☐ **2.** "The doctor will put you to sleep so you do not feel anything."
- ☐ **3.** "Show me how to give the doll an IV."
- ☐ **4.** "When it is done, you will get to see your mommy and get an ice pop."

3. After a tonsillectomy and adenoidectomy, which finding should alert the nurse to suspect early hemorrhage in a 5-year-old child?
- ☐ **1.** drooling of bright red secretions
- ☐ **2.** pulse rate of 95 bpm
- ☐ **3.** vomiting of 25 mL of dark brown emesis
- ☐ **4.** blood pressure of 95/56 mm Hg

4. The nurse is offering nutritional instruction to the parents of a preschooler who has undergone a tonsillectomy and adenoidectomy. What food choice by the parents would indicate successful teaching?
- ☐ **1.** meat loaf and uncooked carrots
- ☐ **2.** pork and noodle casserole
- ☐ **3.** cream of chicken soup and orange sherbet
- ☐ **4.** hot dog and potato chips

5. A nurse is teaching the parents of a preschooler about the possibility of postoperative hemorrhage after a tonsillectomy and adenoidectomy. When should the nurse explain that the risk of bleeding is the **greatest**?
☐ 1. 1 to 3 days after surgery
☐ 2. 4 to 6 days after surgery
☐ 3. 7 to 10 days after surgery
☐ 4. 11 to 14 days after surgery

The Client with Otitis Media

6. An adolescent female is prescribed amoxicillin for an ear infection. The nurse should teach the adolescent about the risks associated with her concurrent use of:
☐ 1. OTC antihistamines.
☐ 2. oral contraceptives.
☐ 3. multiple vitamins.
☐ 4. ibuprofen.

7. A toddler is scheduled to have tympanostomy tubes inserted. When approaching the toddler for the first time, which should the nurse do?
☐ 1. Talk to the mother first so that the toddler can get used to the new person.
☐ 2. Hold the toddler so that the toddler becomes more comfortable.
☐ 3. Walk over and pick the toddler up right away so that the mother can relax.
☐ 4. Pick up the toddler and take the child to the play area so that the mother can rest.

8. After insertion of bilateral tympanostomy tubes in a toddler, which instructions should the nurse include in the child's discharge plan for the parents?
☐ 1. Insert ear plugs into the canals when the child bathes.
☐ 2. Gently clean the ear canal with cotton swabs.
☐ 3. Administer the prescribed antibiotic while the tubes are in place.
☐ 4. Disregard any drainage from the ear after 1 week.

9. The nurse caring for a 3-year-old with otitis media notes that the client has an allergy to amoxicillin that causes wheezing. Which prescription should the nurse question?
☐ 1. azithromycin
☐ 2. cephalexin
☐ 3. trimethoprim-sulfamethoxazole
☐ 4. cefdinir

The Client with Foreign Body Aspiration

10. After teaching the parents of a toddler about commonly aspirated foods, which food, if identified by the parents as easily aspirated, would indicate the need for additional teaching?
☐ 1. popcorn
☐ 2. raw vegetables
☐ 3. round candy
☐ 4. crackers

11. A toddler who has been treated for a foreign body aspiration begins to fuss and cry when the parents attempt to leave the hospital for an hour. As the nurse tries to take the child out of the crib, the child pushes the nurse away. The nurse interprets this behavior as indicating which stage of separation anxiety?
☐ 1. protest
☐ 2. despair
☐ 3. regression
☐ 4. detachment

12. The nurse teaches the three cardinal signs of choking to the parents of a toddler who was treated for a foreign body obstruction. When asked to repeat the signs, the parents identify "turn blue" and "cannot speak." What third sign would the parents identify if teaching was successful?
☐ 1. vomits
☐ 2. gasps
☐ 3. gags
☐ 4. collapses

13. The father of a 2-year-old phones the emergency department on a Sunday evening and informs the nurse that his son put a bead in his nose. What is the **most** appropriate recommendation made by the nurse?
☐ 1. "Try to remove the bead at home as soon as possible; you might try using a pair of tweezers."
☐ 2. "Be sure to take your child to the pediatrician in the morning so the pediatrician can remove the bead in the office."
☐ 3. "You should bring your child to the emergency department tonight so the bead can be removed as soon as possible."
☐ 4. "Ask your child to blow his nose several times; this should dislodge the bead."

The Client with Asthma

14. An 11-year-old is admitted for treatment of an asthma attack. Which finding indicates immediate intervention is needed?
- ☐ **1.** thin, copious mucous secretions
- ☐ **2.** productive cough
- ☐ **3.** intercostal retractions
- ☐ **4.** respiratory rate of 20 breaths/min

15. A 12-year-old with asthma wants to exercise. Which activity should the nurse suggest to improve breathing?
- ☐ **1.** soccer
- ☐ **2.** swimming
- ☐ **3.** track
- ☐ **4.** gymnastics

16. When preparing the teaching plan for the mother of a child with asthma, what information should the nurse include as a sign to alert the mother that her child is having an asthma attack?
- ☐ **1.** secretion of thin, copious mucus
- ☐ **2.** tight, productive cough
- ☐ **3.** wheezing on expiration
- ☐ **4.** temperature of 99.4°F (37.4°C)

17. Which assessment findings should lead the nurse to suspect that a toddler is experiencing respiratory distress? Select all that apply.
- ☐ **1.** coughing
- ☐ **2.** respiratory rate of 35 breaths/min
- ☐ **3.** heart rate of 95 beats/min
- ☐ **4.** restlessness
- ☐ **5.** malaise
- ☐ **6.** diaphoresis

18. A child, who uses an inhaled bronchodilator only when needed for asthma, has a best peak expiratory flow rate of 270 L/min. The child's current peak flow reading is 180 L/min. How does the nurse interpret this reading?
- ☐ **1.** The child's asthma is under good control, so the routine treatment plan should continue.
- ☐ **2.** The child needs to use short-acting, inhaled beta$_2$-agonist medication.
- ☐ **3.** This is a medical emergency requiring a trip to the emergency department for treatment.
- ☐ **4.** The child needs to use inhaled cromolyn sodium.

19. An adolescent with chest pain goes to the nurse. The nurse determines that the teenager has a history of asthma but has had no problems for years. What should the nurse do **next**?
- ☐ **1.** Call the adolescent's parent.
- ☐ **2.** Have the adolescent lie down for 30 minutes.
- ☐ **3.** Obtain a peak flow reading.
- ☐ **4** Have the teen take two puffs of his or her short-acting bronchodilator.

20. A 7-year-old child with a history of asthma controlled without medications is referred to the school nurse by the teacher because of persistent coughing. What should the nurse do **first**?
- ☐ **1.** Obtain the child's heart rate.
- ☐ **2.** Give the child a nebulizer treatment.
- ☐ **3.** Call a parent to obtain more information.
- ☐ **4.** Have a parent come and pick up the child.

21. When developing a teaching plan for the parent of an asthmatic child concerning measures to reduce allergic triggers, which suggestion should the nurse include?
- ☐ **1.** Keep the humidity in the home between 50% and 60%.
- ☐ **2.** Have the child sleep in the bottom bunk bed.
- ☐ **3.** Use a scented room deodorizer to keep the room fresh.
- ☐ **4.** Vacuum the carpet once or twice a week.

22. After discussing asthma as a chronic condition, which statement by the parent of a child with asthma **best** reflects the family's positive adjustment to this aspect of the child's disease?
- ☐ **1.** "We try to keep him happy at all costs; otherwise, he has an asthma attack."
- ☐ **2.** "We keep our child away from other children to help cut down on infections."
- ☐ **3.** "Although our child's disease is serious, we try not to let it be the focus of our family."
- ☐ **4.** "I'm afraid that when my child gets older, he will not be able to care for himself like I do."

23. A child with asthma states, "I want to play some sports like my friends. What can I do?" The nurse responds to the child based on the understanding of which information?
- ☐ **1.** Physical activities are inappropriate for children with asthma.
- ☐ **2.** Children with asthma must be excluded from team sports.
- ☐ **3.** Vigorous physical exercise frequently precipitates an asthmatic episode.
- ☐ **4.** Most children with asthma can participate in sports if the asthma is controlled.

The Client with Cystic Fibrosis and Bronchopneumonia

24. A child with cystic fibrosis does not like taking a pancreatic enzyme supplement with meals and snacks. The parent does not like to force the child to take the supplement. The **most** important reason for the child to take the pancreatic enzyme supplement with meals and snacks is:
- ☐ 1. the child will become dehydrated if the supplement is not taken with meals and snacks.
- ☐ 2. the child needs these pancreatic enzymes to help the digestive system absorb fats, carbohydrates, and proteins.
- ☐ 3. the child needs the pancreatic enzymes to aid in liquefying mucus to keep the lungs clear.
- ☐ 4. the child will experience severe diarrhea if the supplement is not taken as prescribed.

25. An adolescent with cystic fibrosis has been hospitalized several times. On the latest admission, the client has labored respirations, fatigue, malnutrition, and failure to thrive. Which initial nursing actions are **most** important?
- ☐ 1. placing the client on bed rest and obtaining a prescription for a blood gas analysis
- ☐ 2. implementing a high-calorie, high-protein, low-fat, vitamin-enriched diet and pancreatic granules
- ☐ 3. applying an oximeter and initiating respiratory therapy
- ☐ 4. inserting an IV line and initiating antibiotic therapy

26. A child with cystic fibrosis is receiving gentamicin. Which nursing action is **most** important?
- ☐ 1. monitoring intake and output
- ☐ 2. obtaining daily weights
- ☐ 3. monitoring the client for indications of constipation
- ☐ 4. obtaining stool samples for hemoccult testing

27. When developing the plan of care for a child with cystic fibrosis (CF) who is scheduled to receive postural drainage, the nurse should anticipate performing postural drainage at which times?
- ☐ 1. after meals
- ☐ 2. before meals
- ☐ 3. after rest periods
- ☐ 4. before inhalation treatments

28. What type of diet should the nurse teach the parents to give an older infant with cystic fibrosis (CF)?
- ☐ 1. low-protein diet
- ☐ 2. high-fat diet
- ☐ 3. low-carbohydrate diet
- ☐ 4. high-calorie diet

29. At a follow-up appointment after being hospitalized, an adolescent with a history of cystic fibrosis (CF) describes his stools to the nurse. Which description should the nurse interpret as indicative of continued problems with malabsorption?
- ☐ 1. soft with little odor
- ☐ 2. large and foul-smelling
- ☐ 3. loose with bits of food
- ☐ 4. hard with streaks of blood

30. What toy should the nurse include as part of a recreational therapy plan of care for a 3-year-old child hospitalized with pneumonia and cystic fibrosis?
- ☐ 1. 100-piece jigsaw puzzle
- ☐ 2. child's favorite doll
- ☐ 3. fuzzy stuffed animal
- ☐ 4. scissors, paper, and paste

31. Which factor, if described by the parents of a child with cystic fibrosis (CF), indicates understanding the underlying problem of the disease?
- ☐ 1. an abnormality in the body's mucus-secreting glands
- ☐ 2. formation of fibrous cysts in various body organs
- ☐ 3. failure of the pancreatic ducts to develop properly
- ☐ 4. reaction to the formation of antibodies against streptococcus

32. Which outcome criterion would the nurse develop for a child with cystic fibrosis who has ineffective airway clearance related to increased pulmonary secretions and inability to expectorate?
- ☐ 1. respiratory rate and rhythm within expected range
- ☐ 2. absence of chills and fever
- ☐ 3. ability to engage in age-related activities
- ☐ 4. ability to tolerate usual diet without vomiting

33. A school-age child with cystic fibrosis asks the nurse what sports she can become involved in as she becomes older. Which activity would be appropriate for the nurse to suggest?
- ☐ 1. swimming
- ☐ 2. track
- ☐ 3. baseball
- ☐ 4. soccer

The Client with Sudden Infant Death Syndrome

34. When explaining to parents how to reduce the risk of sudden infant death syndrome (SIDS), the nurse should teach about which measures? Select all that apply.
- ☐ 1. Maintain a smoke-free environment.
- ☐ 2. Use a wedge for side-lying positions.
- ☐ 3. Breast-feed the baby.
- ☐ 4. Place the baby on his or her back to sleep.
- ☐ 5. Use bumper pads over the bed rails.
- ☐ 6. Have the baby sleep in the parent's bed.

35. Which child is **most** at risk for sudden infant death syndrome (SIDS)?
- ☐ **1.** infant who is 3 months old
- ☐ **2.** 2-year-old who has apnea lasting up to 5 seconds
- ☐ **3.** firstborn child whose parents are in their early forties
- ☐ **4.** 6-month-old who has had two bouts of pneumonia

36. Parents bring their infant to the emergency department because the child has stopped breathing. A nurse obtains a brief history of events occurring before and after the parents found the infant not breathing. Which question should the nurse ask the parents **first?**
- ☐ **1.** "Was the infant sleeping while wrapped in a blanket?"
- ☐ **2.** "Was the infant lying on his stomach?"
- ☐ **3.** "What did the infant look like when you found him?"
- ☐ **4.** "When had you last checked on the infant?"

37. When planning a visit to the parents of an infant who died of sudden infant death syndrome (SIDS) at home, the nurse should visit the parents at which time?
- ☐ **1.** a few days after the funeral
- ☐ **2.** 2 weeks after the funeral
- ☐ **3.** as soon as the parents are ready to talk
- ☐ **4.** as soon after the infant's death as possible

The Client Who Requires Immediate Care and Cardiopulmonary Resuscitation

38. A child has just ingested about 10 adult-strength acetaminophen tablets an hour ago. The mother brings the child to the emergency department. What should the nurse do? Place the interventions in the order of priority from first to last. All options must be used.

1. Administer activated charcoal.

2. Assess the airway.

3. Check serum acetaminophen levels.

4. Administer acetylcysteine.

39. On finding a child who is not breathing, the nurse has someone activate the emergency medical system and then does what **first?**
- ☐ **1.** Clear the airway.
- ☐ **2.** Begin mouth-to-mouth resuscitation.
- ☐ **3.** Initiate oxygen therapy.
- ☐ **4.** Start chest compressions.

40. Which breathing rates should the nurse use when performing rescue breathing during cardiopulmonary resuscitation for a 5-year-old?
- ☐ **1.** 10 breaths/min
- ☐ **2.** 12 breaths/min
- ☐ **3.** 15 breaths/min
- ☐ **4.** 20 breaths/min

41. The nurse begins CPR on a 5-year-old unresponsive client. When the emergency response team arrives, the child continues to have no respiratory effort but has a heart rate of 50 with cyanotic legs. What should the team do **next?**
- ☐ **1.** Discontinue compressions, but continue administering breaths with a bag-mask device.
- ☐ **2.** Establish an intravenous line with a large bore needle while preparing the defibrillator.
- ☐ **3.** Begin 2-person CPR at a ratio of 2 breaths to 15 compressions.
- ☐ **4.** Begin 2-person CPR at a ratio of 2 breaths to 30 compressions.

42. As part of a health education program, the nurse teaches a group of parents CPR. The nurse determines that the teaching had been effective when a parent states:
- ☐ **1.** "If I am by myself, I should call for help before starting CPR."
- ☐ **2.** "I should compress a child's chest using 2 to 3 fingers."
- ☐ **3.** "I should deliver chest compression at a rate of 100 per minute."
- ☐ **4.** "If I cannot get the breaths to make the chest rise, I should administer abdominal thrusts."

43. When performing cardiopulmonary resuscitation (CPR), which finding indicates that external chest compressions are effective?
- ☐ **1.** mottling of the skin
- ☐ **2.** pupillary dilation
- ☐ **3.** palpable pulse
- ☐ **4.** cool, dry skin

44. A nurse walks into the room just as a 10-month-old infant places an object in his mouth and starts to choke. After opening the infant's mouth, which should the nurse do **next** to clear the airway?
- ☐ **1.** Use blind finger sweeps.
- ☐ **2.** Deliver back slaps and chest thrusts.
- ☐ **3.** Apply four subdiaphragmatic abdominal thrusts.
- ☐ **4.** Attempt to visualize the object.

45. A young child has had a cardiac arrest, and the rapid response team has been paged. The nurse arrives in the client's room and observes a licensed practical/vocational nurse (LPN/VN) administering CPR to an infant (see figure). To assist the LPN/VN with CPR, the nurse should:

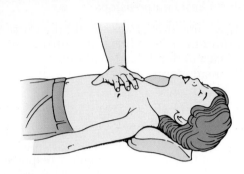

☐ **1.** take over rescue breaths with a rate of 1 breath per 5 compressions using a bag-mask device while the LPN/VN continues compressions.

☐ **2.** take over compressions using one hand while the LPN/VN uses a mask device to administer rescue breaths.

☐ **3.** take over rescue breaths using a rate of 2 breaths per 15 compressions using a bag-mask device while the LPN/VN delivers compressions.

☐ **4.** take over compressions at 80 compressions a minute while the LPN/VN uses a bag-mask device to administer rescue breaths.

46. When teaching the parents of an infant how to perform back slaps to dislodge a foreign body, what should the nurse tell the parents to use to deliver the blows?

☐ **1.** palm of the hand
☐ **2.** heel of the hand
☐ **3.** fingertips
☐ **4.** entire hand

47. While the nurse is delivering abdominal thrusts to a 6-year-old who is choking on a foreign body, the child begins to cry. What should the nurse do **next**?

☐ **1.** Tap or gently shake the shoulders.
☐ **2.** Deliver back slaps.
☐ **3.** Perform a blind finger sweep of the mouth.
☐ **4.** Observe the child closely.

The Client with Croup

48. A 3-year-old is brought into the emergency department in her parent's arms. The child's mouth is open, and she is drooling and lethargic. The parent states that the child became ill suddenly within the past 2 hours. What should the nurse do **first**?

☐ **1.** Draw blood cultures for complete blood count.
☐ **2.** Start an intravenous line.
☐ **3.** Inspect the child's throat with a tongue blade.
☐ **4.** Maintain the child in an undisturbed, upright position.

49. The parent of a 16-month-old child calls the clinic because the child has a low-grade fever, cold symptoms, and a hoarse cough. What should the nurse suggest that the parent do?

☐ **1.** Offer extra fluids frequently.
☐ **2.** Bring the child to the clinic immediately.
☐ **3.** Count the child's respiratory rate.
☐ **4.** Use a hot air vaporizer.

50. A 21-month-old child admitted with the diagnosis of croup now has a respiratory rate of 48 breaths/min, a heart rate of 120 bpm, and a temperature of 100.8°F (38.2°C) rectally. The nurse is having difficulty calming the child. What should the nurse do **next**?

☐ **1.** Administer acetaminophen.
☐ **2.** Notify the healthcare provider (HCP) immediately.
☐ **3.** Allow the toddler to continue to cry.
☐ **4.** Offer clear fluids every few minutes.

The Client with Bronchiolitis or Pharyngitis

51. A child has viral pharyngitis. What should the nurse advise the parents to do? Select all that apply.

☐ **1.** Use a cool mist vaporizer.
☐ **2.** Offer a soft-to-liquid diet.
☐ **3.** Administer amoxicillin.
☐ **4.** Administer acetaminophen.
☐ **5.** Place the child on secretion precautions.

52. A parent brings a 3-month-old infant to the clinic, reporting that the infant has a cold, is having trouble breathing, and "just does not seem to be acting right." Which action should the nurse take **first**?

☐ **1.** Check the infant's heart rate.
☐ **2.** Weigh the infant.
☐ **3.** Assess the infant's oxygen saturation.
☐ **4.** Obtain more information from the parent.

53. A nurse's assessment of a 6-month-old infant reveals a respiratory rate of 52 breaths/min, retractions, and wheezing. The mother states that her infant was doing fine until yesterday. Which action would be **most** appropriate?
☐ **1.** Administer a nebulizer treatment.
☐ **2.** Send the infant for a chest radiograph.
☐ **3.** Refer the infant to the emergency department.
☐ **4.** Provide teaching about cold care to the mother.

54. An infant is being treated at home for bronchiolitis. What should the nurse teach the parent about home care? Select all that apply.
☐ **1.** offering small amounts of fluids frequently
☐ **2.** allowing the infant to sleep prone
☐ **3.** calling the clinic if the infant vomits
☐ **4.** writing down how much the infant drinks
☐ **5.** performing chest physiotherapy every 4 hours
☐ **6.** watching for difficulty breathing

55. In preparation for discharge, the nurse teaches the mother of an infant diagnosed with bronchiolitis about the condition and its treatment. Which statement by the mother indicates successful teaching?
☐ **1.** "I need to be sure to take my child's temperature every day."
☐ **2.** "I hope I do not get a cold from my child."
☐ **3.** "Next time my child gets a cold I need to listen to the chest."
☐ **4.** "I need to wash my hands more often."

56. The nurse observes an 18-month-old who has been admitted with a respiratory tract infection who is drooling (see figure). The nurse should **first**:

☐ **1.** position the child supine.
☐ **2.** call the rapid response team.
☐ **3.** suction the airway.
☐ **4.** administer oxygen.

57. A teaching care plan to prevent the transmission of respiratory syncytial virus (RSV) should include what information? Select all that apply.
☐ **1.** The virus can be spread by direct contact.
☐ **2.** The virus can be spread by indirect contact.
☐ **3.** Palivizumab is recommended to prevent RSV for all toddlers in day care.
☐ **4.** The virus is typically contagious for 3 weeks.
☐ **5.** Older children seldom spread RSV.
☐ **6.** Frequent handwashing helps reduce the spread of RSV.

Managing Care, Quality, and Safety of Children with Respiratory Health Problems

58. A charge nurse is making assignments for a group of children on a pediatric unit. The nurse should **most** avoid assigning the same nurse to care for a 2-year-old with respiratory syncytial virus (RSV) and:
☐ **1.** an 18-month-old with RSV.
☐ **2.** a 9-year-old 8 hours postappendectomy.
☐ **3.** a 1-year-old with a heart defect.
☐ **4.** a 6-year-old with sickle cell crisis.

59. The nurse is preparing to administer the last dose of ceftriaxone before discharge to a 1-year-old but finds the IV has occluded. The nurse should:
☐ **1.** restart the IV.
☐ **2.** administer the medication intramuscularly.
☐ **3.** document that the last dose was withheld.
☐ **4.** contact the prescriber to request a prescription change.

60. A nurse administers cefazolin instead of ceftriaxone to an 8-year-old with pneumonia. The client has suffered no adverse effects. The nurse tells the charge nurse of the incident but fears disciplinary action from reporting the error. The charge nurse should tell the nurse:
☐ **1.** "If you do not report the error, I will have to."
☐ **2.** "Reporting the error helps to identify system problems to improve client safety."
☐ **3.** "Notify the client's healthcare provider to see if she wants this reported."
☐ **4.** "This is not a serious mistake, so reporting it will not affect your position."

61. A 12-year-old with cystic fibrosis is being treated in the hospital for pneumonia. The healthcare provider (HCP) is calling in a telephone prescription for ampicillin. The nurse should take which actions? Select all that apply.

☐ 1. Ask the unit clerk to listen on the speakerphone with the nurse and write down the prescription.

☐ 2. Ask the HCP to come to the hospital and write the prescription on the medical record.

☐ 3. Repeat the prescription to the HCP.

☐ 4. Ask the HCP to confirm that the prescription is correct as understood by the nurse.

☐ 5. Ask the nursing supervisor to cosign the telephone prescription as transcribed by the nurse.

62. The triage nurse in the emergency department must prioritize the children waiting to be seen. Which child is in the **greatest** need of emergency medical treatment?

☐ 1. a 6-year-old with a fever of 104°F (40°C), a muffled voice, no spontaneous cough, and drooling

☐ 2. a 3-year-old with a fever of 100°F (37.8°C), a barky cough, and mild intercostal retractions

☐ 3. a 4-year-old with a fever of 101°F (38.3°C), a hoarse cough, inspiratory stridor, and restlessness

☐ 4. a 13-year-old with a fever of 104°F (40°C), chills, and a cough with thick yellow secretions

63. A 6-month-old on the pediatric floor has a respiratory rate of 68, mild intercostal retractions, and oxygen saturation of 89%. The infant has not been feeding well for the last 24 hours and is restless. Using the situation, background, assessment, and recommendation (SBAR) technique for communication, the nurse calls the healthcare provider (HCP) with the recommendation for:

☐ 1. starting oxygen.

☐ 2. providing sedation.

☐ 3. transferring to pediatric intensive care.

☐ 4. prescribing a chest CT scan.

64. A child with cystic fibrosis has been admitted to the pediatric unit. What type of diet should the nurse request for the client?

☐ 1. high-fat, high-carbohydrate

☐ 2. high-calorie, high-protein

☐ 3. high-calorie, high-carbohydrate

☐ 4. high-carbohydrate, high-protein

Answers, Rationales, and Test-Taking Strategies

The answers and rationales for each question follow below, along with keys (✦➞) to the client need (CN) and cognitive level (CL) for each question. In addition, you will also see a glossary icon (📖) highlighting specific terminology used on the licensing exam. As you check your answers, use the **Content Mastery and Test-Taking Skill Self-Analysis** *worksheet (tear-out worksheet in back of book) to identify the reason(s) for not answering the questions correctly. For additional information about test-taking skills and strategies for answering questions, refer to pages 12–23 and pages 35–36 in Part 1 of this book.*

The Client with Tonsillitis

1. 4. If the child does not stick out his tongue so the nurse can visualize the throat, it is appropriate to use a tongue blade. Having the child participate by holding the tongue blade while the nurse guides it to facilitate visualization of the throat is appropriate technique. It is not useful to remove the tongue blade or have the child hold it because the nurse will need to use the tongue blade to depress the tongue. It is preferable to engage the child's cooperation before asking the parent to restrain the child.

✦➞ CN: Health promotion and maintenance; CL: Apply

2. 4. When preparing a child for a procedure the nurse should use neutral words, focus on sensory experiences, and emphasize the positive aspects at the end. Being reunited with parents and having an ice pop would be considered pleasurable events. Children this age fear bodily harm. To reduce anxiety, the nurse should use the word "fixed" instead of "removed" to describe what is being done to the tonsils. Using the terms "put to sleep" and "IV" may be threatening. Additionally, directing a play experience to focus on IV insertion may be counterproductive as the child may have little recollection of this aspect of the procedure.

✦➞ CN: Psychosocial integrity; CL: Synthesize

3. 1. After a tonsillectomy and adenoidectomy, drooling bright red blood is considered an early sign of hemorrhage. Often, because of discomfort in the throat, children tend to avoid swallowing; instead, they drool. Frequent swallowing would also be an indication of hemorrhage because the child attempts to clear the airway of blood by swallowing.

Secretions may be slightly blood-tinged because of a small amount of oozing after surgery. However, bright red secretions indicate bleeding. A pulse rate of 95 bpm is within the normal range for a 5-year-old child, as is a blood pressure of 95/56 mm Hg. A small amount of blood that is partially digested, and therefore dark brown, is often present in postoperative emesis.

CN: Reduction of risk potential; CL: Analyze

4. 3. For the first few days after a tonsillectomy and adenoidectomy, liquids and soft foods are best tolerated by the child while the throat is sore. Children typically do not chew their food thoroughly, and solid foods are to be avoided because they are difficult to swallow. Although meat loaf would be considered a soft food, uncooked carrots would not be. Pork is frequently difficult to chew. Foods that have sharp edges, such as potato chips, are contraindicated because they are hard to chew and may cause more throat discomfort.

CN: Basic care and comfort; CL: Evaluate

5. 3. The risk of hemorrhage from a tonsillectomy is greatest when the tissue begins sloughing and the scabs fall off. This typically happens 7 to 10 days after a tonsillectomy.

CN: Safety and infection control; CL: Apply

The Client with Otitis Media

6. 2. When a person is taking amoxicillin as well as an oral contraceptive, it renders the contraceptive less effective. Because pregnancy can occur in such a situation, the nurse should advise the client to use additional means of birth control during the time she is taking the antibiotic. There are no risks associated with the concurrent use of amoxicillin and OTC antihistamines, vitamins, or ibuprofen.

CN: Psychosocial integrity; CL: Apply

7. 1. Toddlers should be approached slowly because they are wary of strangers and need time to get used to someone they do not know. The best approach is to ignore them initially and to focus on talking to the parents. The child will likely resist being held by a stranger, so the nurse should not pick up or hold the child until the child indicates a readiness to be approached or the mother indicates that it is okay.

CN: Health promotion and maintenance; CL: Synthesize

8. 1. Placing ear plugs in the ears will prevent contaminated bathwater from entering the middle ear through the tympanostomy tube and causing an infection. Inserting cotton swabs into the ear canal is not recommended. It is not necessary to administer antibiotics continuously to a child with a tympanostomy tube. Antibiotics are appropriate only when an ear infection is present. Drainage from the ear may be a sign of middle ear infection and should be reported to the **healthcare provider (HCP)** .

CN: Reduction of risk potential; CL: Create

9. 2. Cephalexin is a first-generation cephalosporin. Because clients with a history of anaphylaxis to penicillin, or related antibiotics, have an increased risk of having a cross-reaction to first-generation cephalosporin, the nurse should question a prescription for cephalexin. Azithromycin is not usually considered to be a first-line antibiotic for ear infections in pediatric clients but is effective in pediatric clients with an allergy to amoxicillin. Trimethoprim-sulfamethoxazole is effective against middle ear infections and can be used effectively in pediatric clients with an allergy to amoxicillin. Second- and third-generation cephalosporins, like cefdinir, do not have the same rates of cross-sensitivities to penicillins as first-generation cephalosporin and may be prescribed for pediatric clients with an allergy to amoxicillin.

CN: Management of care; CL: Synthesize

The Client with Foreign Body Aspiration

10. 4. Crackers, because they crumble and easily dissolve, are not commonly aspirated. Because children commonly eat popcorn hulls or pieces that have not popped, popcorn can be easily aspirated. Toddlers frequently do not chew their food well, making raw vegetables a commonly aspirated food. Round candy is often difficult to chew and comes in large pieces, making it easily aspirated.

CN: Health promotion and maintenance; CL: Evaluate

11. 1. Young children have specific reactions to separation and hospitalization. In the protest stage, the toddler physically and verbally attacks anyone who attempts to provide care. Here, the child is fussing and crying and visibly pushes the nurse away. In the despair stage, the toddler becomes withdrawn and obviously depressed (e.g., not engaging in play activities and sleeping more than usual). Regression is a return to a developmentally earlier phase because of stress or crisis (e.g., a toddler who could feed himself before this event is not doing so now). Denial or detachment occurs if the toddler's stay in the hospital without the parent is prolonged because the toddler settles in to the hospital life and denies the parents' existence (e.g., not reacting when the parents come to visit).

⚷ CN: Psychosocial integrity; CL: Analyze

12. 4. The three cardinal signs indicating that a child is truly choking and requires immediate life-saving interventions include inability to speak, blue color (cyanosis), and collapse. Vomiting does not occur while a child is unable to breathe. Once the object is dislodged, however, vomiting may occur. Gasping, a sudden intake of air, indicates that the child is still able to inhale. When a child is choking, air is not being exchanged, so gagging will not occur.

⚷ CN: Reduction of risk potential;
CL: Evaluate

13. 3. The bead should be removed by a health-care professional as soon as possible to prevent the risk of aspiration and tissue necrosis. Unskilled individuals should not attempt to remove an object from the nose as they may push the object further increasing the risk for aspiration. Two-year-old children are not skilled at blowing their nose and may breathe in, further increasing the risk of aspiration.

⚷ CN: Management of care; CL: Analyze

The Client with Asthma

14. 3. Intercostal retractions indicate an increase in respiratory effort, which is a sign of respiratory distress. During an asthma attack, secretions are thick, the cough is tight, and respiration is difficult (and shortness of breath may occur). If mucous secretions are copious but thin, the client can expectorate them, which indicates an improvement in the condition. If the cough is productive, it means the bronchospasms and the inflammation have been resolved to the extent that the mucus can be expectorated. A respiratory rate of 20 breaths/min would be considered normal and no intervention would be needed.

⚷ CN: Physiological adaptation; CL: Analyze

15. 2. Swimming is appropriate for this child because it requires controlled breathing, assists in maintaining cardiac health, enhances skeletal muscle strength, and promotes ventilation and perfusion. Stop-and-start activities, such as soccer, track, and gymnastics, commonly trigger symptoms in asthmatic clients.

⚷ CN: Health promotion and maintenance;
CL: Synthesize

16. 3. The child who is experiencing an asthma attack typically demonstrates wheezing on expiration initially. This results from air moving through narrowed airways secondary to bronchoconstriction. The child's expiratory phase is normally longer than the inspiratory phase. Expiration is passive as the diaphragm relaxes. During an asthma attack, secretions are thick and are not usually expelled until the bronchioles are more relaxed. At the beginning of an asthma attack, the cough will be tight but not productive. Fever is not always present unless there is an infection that may have triggered the attack.

⚷ CN: Physiological adaptation; CL: Analyze

17. 1,2,4,6. Coughing, especially at night and in the absence of an infection, is a common symptom of asthma. Early signs of respiratory distress include restlessness, tachypnea, tachycardia, and diaphoresis. Other signs also include hypertension, nasal flaring, grunting, wheezing, and intercostal retractions. A heart rate of 95 bpm is normal for a toddler. Malaise typically does not indicate respiratory distress.

⚷ CN: Physiological adaptation; CL: Analyze

18. 2. The peak flow of 180 L/min is in the yellow zone, or 50% to 80% of the child's personal best. This means that the child's asthma is not well controlled, thereby necessitating the use of a short-acting beta$_2$-agonist medication to relieve the bronchospasm. A peak flow reading greater than 80% of the child's personal best (in this case, 220 L/min or better) would indicate that the child's asthma is in the green zone or under good control. A peak flow reading in the red zone, or less than 50% of the child's personal best (135 L/min or less), would require notification of the **healthcare provider (HCP)** 📖 or a trip to the emergency department. Cromolyn sodium is not used for short-term treatment of acute bronchospasm. It is used as part of a long-term therapy regimen to help desensitize mast cells and thereby help to prevent symptoms.

⚷ CN: Reduction of risk potential;
CL: Evaluate

19. 3. Problems of chest pain in children and adolescents are rarely cardiac. With a history of asthma, the most likely cause of the chest pain is related to the asthma. Therefore, the nurse should check the adolescent's peak flow reading to evaluate the status of the airflow. Calling the adolescent's parent would be appropriate, but this would be done after the nurse obtains the peak flow reading and additional assessment data. Having the adolescent lie down may be an option, but more data need to be collected to help establish a possible cause. Because the adolescent has not experienced any asthma problems for a long time, it would be inappropriate for the nurse to administer a short-acting bronchodilator at this time.

⚷ CN: Reduction of risk potential;
CL: Synthesize

20. 3. Because persistent coughing may indicate an asthma attack and a 7-year-old child would be able to provide only minimal history information, it would be important to obtain information from the parent. Although determining the child's heart rate is an important part of the assessment, it would be done after the history is obtained. More information needs to be obtained before giving the child a nebulizer treatment. Although it may be necessary for the parent to come and pick up the child, a thorough assessment including history information should be obtained first.

⚷ CN: Reduction of risk potential;
CL: Synthesize

21. 1. To help reduce allergic triggers in the home, the nurse should recommend that the humidity level be kept between 50% and 60%. Doing so keeps the air moist and comfortable for breathing. When air is dry, the risk for respiratory infections increases. Too high a level of humidity increases the risk for mold growth. Typically, the child with asthma should sleep in the top bunk bed to minimize the risk of exposure to dust mites. The risk of exposure to dust mites increases when the child sleeps in the bottom bunk bed because dust mites fall from the top bed, settling in the bottom bed. Scented sprays should be avoided because they may trigger an asthmatic episode. Ideally, carpeting should be avoided in the home if the child has asthma. However, if it is present, carpeting in the child's room should be vacuumed often, possibly daily, to remove dust mites and dust particles.

⚷ CN: Reduction of risk potential; CL: Create

22. 3. Positive adjustment to a chronic condition requires placing the child's illness in its proper perspective. Children with asthma need to be treated as normally as possible within the scope of the limitations imposed by the illness. They also need to learn how to manage exacerbations and then resume as normal a life as possible. Trying to keep the child happy at all costs is inappropriate and can lead to the child's never learning how to accept responsibility for behavior and get along with others. Although minimizing the child's risk for exposure to infections is important, the child needs to be with his or her peers to ensure appropriate growth and development. Children with a chronic illness need to be involved in their care so that they can learn to manage it. Some parents tend to overprotect their child with a chronic illness. This overprotectiveness may cause a child to have an exaggerated feeling of importance or later, as an adolescent, to rebel against the overprotectiveness and the parents.

⚷ CN: Psychosocial integrity; CL: Evaluate

23. 4. Physical activities are beneficial to asthmatic children, physically and psychosocially. Most children with asthma can engage in school and sports activities that are geared to the child's condition and within the limits imposed by the disease. The coach and other team members need to be aware of the child's condition and know what to do in case an attack occurs. Those children who have exercise-induced asthma usually use a short-acting bronchodilator before exercising.

⚷ CN: Health promotion and maintenance;
CL: Apply

The Client with Cystic Fibrosis and Bronchopneumonia

24. 2. The child must take the pancreatic enzyme supplement with meals and snacks to help absorb nutrients so he can grow and develop normally. In cystic fibrosis, the normally liquid mucus is tenacious and blocks three digestive enzymes from entering the duodenum and digesting essential nutrients. Without the supplemental pancreatic enzyme, the child will have voluminous, foul, fatty stools due to the undigested nutrients and may experience developmental delays due to malnutrition. Dehydration is not a problem related to cystic fibrosis. The pancreatic enzymes have no effect on the viscosity of the tenacious mucus. Diarrhea is not caused by failing to take the pancreatic enzyme supplement.

⚷ CN: Pharmacological and parenteral therapies; CL: Apply

25. 3. Clients with cystic fibrosis commonly die from respiratory problems. The mucus in the lungs is tenacious and difficult to expel, leading to lung infections and interference with oxygen and carbon dioxide exchange. The client will likely need supplemental oxygen and respiratory treatments to maintain adequate gas exchange, as identified by the oximeter reading. The child will be on bed rest due to respiratory distress. However, although blood gases will probably be prescribed, the oximeter readings will be used to determine oxygen deficit and are, therefore, more of a priority. A diet high in calories, proteins, and vitamins with pancreatic granules added to all foods ingested will increase nutrient absorption and help the malnutrition; however, this intervention is not the priority at this time. Inserting an IV to administer antibiotics is important and can be done after ensuring adequate respiratory function.

⚷ CN: Physiological adaptation;
CL: Synthesize

26. 1. Monitoring intake and output is the most important nursing action when administering an aminoglycoside, such as gentamicin, because a decrease in output is an early sign of renal damage. Daily weight monitoring is not indicated when the client is receiving an aminoglycoside. Constipation and bleeding are not adverse effects of aminoglycosides.

🔑 CN: Pharmacological and parenteral therapies; CL: Synthesize

27. 2. Postural drainage, which aids in mobilizing the thick, tenacious secretions commonly associated with CF, is usually performed before meals to avoid the possibility of vomiting or regurgitating food. Although the child with CF needs frequent rest periods, this is not an important factor in scheduling postural drainage. However, the nurse would not want to interrupt the child's rest period to perform the treatment. Inhalation treatments are usually given before postural drainage to help loosen secretions.

🔑 CN: Reduction of risk potential; CL: Apply

28. 4. CF affects the exocrine glands. Mucus is thick and tenacious, sticking to the walls of the pancreatic and bile ducts and eventually causing obstruction. Because of the difficulty with digestion and absorption, a high-calorie, high-protein, high-carbohydrate, moderate-fat diet is indicated.

🔑 CN: Physiological adaptation; CL: Apply

29. 2. In children with CF, poor digestion and absorption of foods, especially fats, results in frequent bowel movements that are bulky, large, and foul-smelling. The stools also contain abnormally large quantities of fat, which is called *steatorrhea*. An adolescent experiencing good control of the disease would describe soft stools with little odor. Stool described as loose with bits of food indicates diarrhea. Stool described as hard with streaks of blood may indicate constipation.

🔑 CN: Physiological adaptation; CL: Analyze

30. 2. The child's favorite doll would be a good choice of toys. The doll provides support and is familiar to the child. Although a 3-year-old may enjoy puzzles, a 100-piece jigsaw puzzle is too complicated for an ill 3-year-old child. In view of the child's lung pathology, a fuzzy stuffed animal would not be advised because of its potential as a reservoir for dust and bacteria, possibly predisposing the child to additional respiratory problems. Scissors, paper, and paste are not appropriate for a 3-year-old unless the child is supervised closely.

🔑 CN: Health promotion and maintenance; CL: Create

31. 1. CF is characterized by a dysfunction in the body's mucus-producing exocrine glands. The mucus secretions are thick and sticky rather than thin and slippery. The mucus obstructs the bronchi, bronchioles, and pancreatic ducts. Mucus plugs in the pancreatic ducts can prevent pancreatic digestive enzymes from reaching the small intestine, resulting in poor digestion and poor absorption of various food nutrients. Fibrous cysts do not form in various organs. Cystic fibrosis is an autosomal recessive inherited disorder and does not involve any reaction to the formation of antibodies against streptococcus.

🔑 CN: Physiological adaptation; CL: Evaluate

32. 1. After treatment, the client outcome would be that respiratory status would be within normal limits, as evidenced by a respiratory rate and rhythm within expected range. Absence of chills and fever, although related to an underlying problem causing the respiratory problem (e.g., the infection), does not specifically relate to the respiratory problem of ineffective airway clearance. The child's ability to engage in age-related activities may provide some evidence of improved respiratory status. However, this outcome criterion is more directly related to activity intolerance. Although the child's ability to tolerate his or her usual diet may indirectly relate to respiratory function, this outcome is more specifically related to an imbalanced nutrition that may or may not be related to the child's respiratory status.

🔑 CN: Physiological adaptation; CL: Evaluate

33. 1. Swimming would be the most appropriate suggestion because it coordinates breathing and movement of all muscle groups and can be done on an individual basis or as a team sport. Because track events, baseball, and soccer throwing usually are performed outdoors, the child would be breathing in large amounts of dust and dirt, which would be irritating to her mucous membranes and pulmonary system. The strenuous activity and increased energy expenditure associated with track events, in conjunction with the dust and possible heat, would play a role in placing the child at risk for an upper respiratory tract infection and compromising her respiratory function.

🔑 CN: Health promotion and maintenance; CL: Synthesize

The Client with Sudden Infant Death Syndrome

34. 1,3,4. Exposure to environmental tobacco increases the risk for SIDS. Sleeping on the back and breast-feeding both decrease the risk of SIDS. The side-lying position is not recommended for sleep. It is recommended that babies be dressed in sleepers and that cribs are free of blankets, pillows, bumper pads, and stuffed animals. Cobedding with parents is not recommended as parents may roll on the child.

🔑 CN: Safety and infection control;
CL: Create

35. 1. The highest incidence of SIDS occurs in infants between ages 2 and 4 months. About 90% of SIDS occurs before the age of 6 months. Apnea lasting longer than 20 seconds has also been associated with a higher incidence of SIDS. SIDS occurs with higher frequency in families where a child in the family has already died of SIDS, but the age of the parents has not been shown to contribute to SIDS. A respiratory infection such as pneumonia has not been shown to cause a higher incidence of SIDS.

🔑 CN: Health promotion and maintenance;
CL: Analyze

36. 3. Because this is an especially disturbing and upsetting time for the parents, they must be approached in a sensitive manner. Asking what the infant looked like when found allows the parents to verbalize what they saw and felt, thereby helping to minimize their feelings of guilt without implying any blame, neglect, wrongdoing, or abuse. Asking if the child was wrapped in a blanket or lying on his stomach, or when the parents last checked on the infant, implies that the parents did something wrong or failed in their care of the infant, thus blaming them for the event.

🔑 CN: Physiological adaptation; CL: Analyze

37. 4. The community health nurse should visit as soon after the death as possible because the parents may need help to deal with the sudden, unexpected death of their infant. Parents often have a great deal of guilt in these situations and need to express their feelings to someone who can provide counseling.

🔑 CN: Psychosocial integrity; CL: Synthesize

The Client Who Requires Immediate Care and Cardiopulmonary Resuscitation

38. 2,1,3,4. Care of children with an acetaminophen overdose is based on time of ingestion. Immediate care of the child is to ensure airway, breathing, and circulation. If it has been less than 4 hours since ingestion, activated charcoal should be given. Acetaminophen levels should be drawn at 4 hours post ingestion. Depending on the findings, acetylcysteine may also be used as an antidote.

🔑 CN: Safety and infection control;
CL: Synthesize

39. 4. The current CPR guidelines call for a CAB approach. When breathlessness is determined, the priority nursing action is checking a pulse and beginning compressions. After 30 compressions, the nurse opens the airway and gives 2 breaths. Oxygen therapy would not be initiated at this time because the child is not breathing. Also, administering oxygen therapy would interfere with providing mouth-to-mouth resuscitation.

🔑 CN: Physiological adaptation;
CL: Synthesize

40. 1. Rescue breaths should be delivered slowly at a volume that makes the chest rise and fall. For a 5-year-old child, the rate is 10 breaths per minute. If the nurse is also administering chest compressions, the rate is 2 breaths for every 30 compressions.

🔑 CN: Physiological adaptation; CL: Apply

41. 3. CPR is done on children for heart rate of less than 60 with signs of poor perfusion. Rescuers should use a 15:2 compression to ventilation ratio for 2-rescuer CPR for a child. Breaths without compressions are indicated only for respiratory arrests where the heart rate remains above 60. The AED/defibrillator should be used as soon as it is ready, but rescuers should not discontinue compressions until the device is ready for use. The ratio for 2-person CPR in adults is 30:2.

🔑 CN: Physiological adaptation;
CL: Synthesize

42. 3. To maintain the best perfusion, it is recommended that compressions be given at a rate of 100 per minute in a ratio of 30 compressions to 2 breaths for 1-rescuer CPR. Children still are more likely to have had a respiratory arrest than a cardiac arrest and are more likely to respond to opening the airway and rescue breaths. Therefore, it is recommended that unless the collapse was witnessed, a sole rescuer should attempt 5 cycles of CPR before leaving to call for help. Using 2 to 3 fingers for chest compressions is recommended for infant CPR only. Abdominal thrusts are no longer recommended for unconscious victims.

🔑 CN: Physiological adaptation; CL: Evaluate

43. 3. With CPR, effectiveness of external chest compressions is indicated by palpable peripheral pulses, the disappearance of mottling and cyanosis, the return of pupils to normal size, and warm, dry skin. To determine whether the victim of cardiopulmonary arrest has resumed spontaneous breathing and circulation, chest compressions must be stopped for 5 seconds at the end of the first minute and every few minutes thereafter.

🔑 CN: Physiological adaptation; CL: Evaluate

44. **2.** The nurse should use mechanical force—back slaps and chest thrusts—in an attempt to dislodge the object. Blind finger sweeps are not appropriate in infants and children because the foreign body may be pushed back into the airway. Subdiaphragmatic abdominal thrusts are not used for infants aged 1 year or younger because of the risk of injury to abdominal organs. If the object is not visible when opening the mouth, time is wasted in looking for it. Action is required to dislodge the object as quickly as possible.

CN: Reduction of risk potential; CL: Apply

45. **3.** The nurse should first obtain a bag-mask device and assist with CPR by giving breaths at 2 breaths/15 compressions. The **LPN/VN** is using correct technique by using one hand on the chest to administer chest compressions. The heel of both hands is used for older children and adolescents. The compression rate is at least 100/min.

CN: Management of care; CL: Apply

46. **2.** Back slaps are delivered rapidly and forcefully with the heel of the hand between the infant's shoulder blades. Slowly delivered back slaps are less likely to dislodge the object. Using the heel of the hand allows more force to be applied than when using the palm or the whole hand, increasing the likelihood of loosening the object. The fingertips would be used to deliver chest compressions to an infant younger than 1 year of age.

CN: Physiological adaptation; CL: Apply

47. **4.** Crying indicates that the airway obstruction has been relieved. No additional thrusts are needed. However, the child needs to be observed closely for complications, including respiratory distress. Tapping or shaking the shoulders is used initially to determine unresponsiveness in someone who appears unconscious. Delivering chest or back slaps could jeopardize the child's now-patent airway. Because the obstruction has been relieved, there is no need to sweep the child's mouth. Additionally, blind finger sweeps are contraindicated because the object may be pushed further back, possibly causing a complete airway obstruction.

CN: Physiological adaptation;
CL: Synthesize

The Client with Croup

48. **4.** This child is in severe respiratory distress with the potential for complete airway obstruction. The nurse should refrain from disturbing the child at this time to avoid irritating the epiglottis and causing it to completely obstruct the child's airway. The child may be intubated or undergo a tracheotomy. However, initially, the child should be kept as calm as possible with as little disruption as possible. Any attempt to restrain the child, draw blood, insert an IV, or examine her throat could result in total airway obstruction.

CN: Physiological adaptation;
CL: Synthesize

49. **1.** The toddler is exhibiting cold symptoms. A hoarse cough may be part of the upper respiratory tract infection. The best suggestion is to have the father offer the child additional fluids at frequent intervals to help keep secretions loose and membranes moist. There is no evidence presented to suggest that the child needs to be brought to the clinic immediately. Although having the father count the child's respiratory rate may provide some additional information, it may lead the father to suspect that something is seriously wrong, possibly leading to undue anxiety. A hot air vaporizer is not recommended. However, a cool mist vaporizer would cause vasoconstriction of the respiratory passages, making it easier for the child to breathe and loosening secretions.

CN: Physiological adaptation;
CL: Synthesize

50. **2.** The nurse may be having difficulty calming the child because the child is experiencing increasing respiratory distress. The normal respiratory rate for a 21-month-old is 25 to 30 breaths/min. The child's respiratory rate is 48 breaths/min. Therefore, the **HCP** needs to be notified immediately. Typically, acetaminophen is not given to a child unless the temperature is 101°F (38.6°C) or higher. Letting the toddler cry is inappropriate with croup because crying increases respiratory distress. Offering fluids every few minutes to a toddler experiencing increasing respiratory distress would do little, if anything, to calm the child. Also, the child would have difficulty coordinating breathing and swallowing, possibly increasing the risk of aspiration.

CN: Physiological adaptation;
CL: Synthesize

The Client with Bronchiolitis or Pharyngitis

51. **1,2,4.** Viral pharyngitis is treated with symptomatic, supportive therapy. Treatment includes use of a cool mist vaporizer, feeding a soft or liquid diet, and administration of acetaminophen for comfort. Viral infections do not respond to antibiotic administration. The child does not need to be on secretion precautions because viral pharyngitis is not contagious.

    CN: Psychosocial integrity; CL: Synthesize

52. **3.** In an infant with these symptoms, the first action by the nurse would be to obtain an oxygen saturation reading to determine how well the infant is oxygenating. Because the parent probably can provide no other information, checking the heart rate would be the second action done by the nurse. Then the nurse would obtain the infant's weight.

    CN: Reduction of risk potential;
CL: Synthesize

53. **3.** Based on the assessment findings of increased respiratory rate, retractions, and wheezing, this infant needs further evaluation, which could be obtained in an emergency department. Without a definitive diagnosis, administering a nebulizer treatment would be outside the nurse's scope of practice unless there was a prescription for such a treatment. Sending the infant for a radiograph may not be in the nurse's scope of practice. The findings need to be reported to an **HCP** ⬜ who can then determine whether or not a chest radiograph is warranted. The infant is exhibiting signs and symptoms of respiratory distress and is too ill to send out with just instructions on cold care for the mother.

    CN: Physiological adaptation;
CL: Synthesize

54. **1,6.** An infant with bronchiolitis will have increased respirations and will tire more quickly, so it is best and easiest for the infant to take fluids more often in smaller amounts. The parents also would be instructed to watch for signs of increased difficulty breathing, which signal possible complications. Healthy infants and even those with bronchiolitis should sleep in the supine position. Calling the clinic for an episode of vomiting would not be necessary. However, the parents would be instructed to call if the infant cannot keep down any fluids for a period of more than 4 hours. Parents would not need to record how much the infant drinks. Chest physiotherapy is not indicated because it does not help and further irritates the infant.

    CN: Basic care and comfort; CL: Create

55. **4.** Handwashing is the best way to prevent respiratory illnesses and the spread of disease. Bronchiolitis, a viral infection primarily affecting the bronchioles, causes swelling and mucus accumulation of the lumina and subsequent hyperinflation of the lung with air trapping. It is transmitted primarily by direct contact with respiratory secretions as a result of eye-to-hand or nose-to-hand contact or from contaminated fomites. Therefore, handwashing minimizes the risk for transmission. Taking the child's temperature is not appropriate in most cases. As long as the child is getting better, taking the temperature will not be helpful. The mother's statement that she hopes she does not get a cold from her child does not indicate understanding of what to do after discharge. For most parents, listening to the child's chest would not be helpful because the parents would not know what they were listening for. Rather, watching for an increased respiratory rate, fever, or evidence of poor eating or drinking would be more helpful in alerting the parent to potential illness.

    CN: Physiological adaptation; CL: Evaluate

56. **2.** The nurse should suspect epiglottitis in any young child with a respiratory infection who sits leaning forward with an open mouth and protruding tongue and is drooling. Epiglottitis is a medical emergency. The **rapid response team** ⬜ should be notified to secure the airway. While waiting for the team, the child should remain sitting upright to facilitate breathing; complete obstruction may occur if the child is placed prone or becomes agitated. Therefore, it is important to avoid any procedures that upset the child such as suctioning or applying oxygen.

    CN: Reduction of risk potential;
CL: Synthesize

57. **1,2,6.** RSV can be spread through direct contact such as kissing the face of an infected person, and it can be spread through indirect contact by touching surfaces covered with infected secretions. Handwashing is one of the best ways to reduce the risk of disease transmission. Palivizumab can prevent severe RSV infections but is only recommended for the most at-risk infants and children. RSV is typically contagious for 3 to 8 days. RSV frequently manifests in older children as cold-like symptoms. Infected school-age children frequently spread the virus to other family members.

    CN: Safety and infection control;
CL: Create

Managing Care, Quality, and Safety of Children with Respiratory Health Problems

58. 3. RSV may be spread through both direct and indirect contact. While contact and standard precautions should be employed, a measure to further decrease the risk of nosocomial infections is to avoid assigning the same nurse caring for an RSV client to a client at risk for infection. A private room is preferred, but if this is not an option, the nurse should understand that children 2 years of age and younger are most at risk for RSV, especially if they have other chronic problems such as a heart defect. From an infection control perspective, pairing two clients with RSV is ideal. RSV infections are less likely to pose a serious problem in older children.

⚲ CN: Safety and infection control;
CL: Synthesize

59. 4. Restarting an IV for one dose of a medication may not be in the infant's best interest when the medication can be given in an alternate form. The prescriber should be contacted to determine IM or PO options. Ceftriaxone may be given IM, but changing the route of a medication administration requires a prescription. While reasons for giving a medication late would be indicated, the failing to complete an entire course of antibiotics contributes to the emergence of antibiotic resistance, and withholding the medicine would rarely be the best option.

⚲ CN: Management of care; CL: Synthesize

60. 2. Client safety is enhanced when the emphasis on medication errors is to determine the root cause. All errors should be reported so systems can identify patterns that contribute to errors. Here, the similar names probably contributed to the error. The nurse who commits the error knows all the relevant information and is in the best position to report it. While the **healthcare provider (HCP)** 🗔 should be notified, it is a nursing responsibility to report errors, not an HCP's choice. Relating mistakes to a nurse's position focuses on personal blame.

⚲ CN: Safety and infection control;
CL: Synthesize

61. 3,4. To ensure client safety in obtaining telephone prescriptions, the prescription must be received by a **registered nurse (RN)** 🗔. The nurse should write the prescription, read the prescription back to the **HCP** 🗔, and receive confirmation from the HCP that the prescription is correct. It is not necessary to ask the unit clerk to listen to the prescription, to require the HCP to come to the hospital to write the prescription on the **medical record** 🗔, or to have the nursing supervisor cosign the telephone prescription.

⚲ CN: Safety and infection control;
CL: Synthesize

62. 1. This child is exhibiting signs and symptoms of epiglottitis, which is a medical emergency due to the risk of complete airway obstruction. The 3- and 4-year-olds are exhibiting signs and symptoms of croup. Symptoms often diminish after the child has been taken out in the cool night air. If symptoms do not improve, the child may need a single dose of dexamethasone. Fever should also be treated with antipyretics. The 13-year-old is exhibiting signs and symptoms of bronchitis. Treatment includes rest, antipyretics, and hydration.

⚲ CN: Management of care; CL: Analyze

63. 1. The infant is experiencing signs and symptoms of respiratory distress indicating the need for oxygen therapy. Sedation will not improve the infant's respiratory distress and would likely cause further respiratory depression. If the infant's respiratory status continues to decline, she may need to be transferred to the pediatric intensive care. Oxygen should be the priority as it may improve the infant's respiratory status. A chest CT is not indicated. However, a CXR would be another appropriate recommendation for this infant.

⚲ CN: Safety and infection control;
CL: Apply

64. 2. A high-calorie, high-protein diet is necessary to ensure adequate growth. Some children require up to two times the recommended daily allowance of calories (increased calorie diet includes foods high in fat and balanced carbohydrates). Pancreatic enzyme activity is lost, and malabsorption of fats, proteins, and carbohydrates occurs.

⚲ CN: Management of care; CL: Apply

The Child with Cardiovascular and Hematologic Health Problems

- The Client Undergoing a Cardiac Catheterization
- The Client with a Congenital Heart Defect
- The Client with Rheumatic Fever
- The Client with Kawasaki Disease
- The Client with Sickle Cell Anemia
- The Client with Iron Deficiency Anemia
- The Client with Hemophilia
- The Client with Leukemia
- Managing Care, Quality, and Safety of Children with Cardiovascular and Hematologic Health Problems
- Answers, Rationales, and Test-Taking Strategies

The Client Undergoing a Cardiac Catheterization

1. The nurse caring for a 7-year-old child who has undergone a cardiac catheterization 2 hours ago finds the dressing and bed saturated with blood. The nurse should **first**:
☐ 1. assess the vital signs.
☐ 2. reinforce the dressing.
☐ 3. apply pressure just above the catheter insertion site.
☐ 4. notify the healthcare provider (HCP).

2. A 4-year-old has been scheduled for a cardiac catheterization. To help prepare the family, the nurse should:
☐ 1. advise the family to bring the child to the hospital for a tour a week in advance.
☐ 2. explain that the child will need a large bandage after the procedure.
☐ 3. discourage bringing favorite toys that might become associated with pain.
☐ 4. explain that the child may get up as soon as the vital signs are stable.

3. When teaching the parents of a child with a ventricular septal defect who is scheduled for a cardiac catheterization, the nurse explains that this procedure involves the use of which technique?
☐ 1. ultra-high-frequency sound waves
☐ 2. catheter placed in the right femoral vein
☐ 3. cutdown procedure to place a catheter
☐ 4. general anesthesia

4. When developing the discharge teaching plan for the parents of a child who has undergone a cardiac catheterization for ventricular septal defect, which information should the nurse expect to include?
☐ 1. restriction of the child's activities for the next 3 weeks
☐ 2. use of sponge baths until the stitches are removed
☐ 3. use of prophylactic antibiotics before receiving any dental work
☐ 4. maintenance of a pressure dressing until a return visit with the healthcare provider (HCP)

The Client with a Congenital Heart Defect

5. Discharge teaching for a 3-month-old infant with a cardiac defect who is to receive digoxin should include which information? Select all that apply.
☐ 1. Give the medication at regular intervals.
☐ 2. Mix the medication with a small volume of breast milk or formula.
☐ 3. Repeat the dose one time if the child vomits immediately after administration.
☐ 4. Notify the healthcare provider (HCP) of poor feeding or vomiting.
☐ 5. Make up any missed doses as soon as realized.
☐ 6. Notify the HCP if more than two consecutive doses are missed.

6. An 18-month-old with a congenital heart defect is to receive digoxin twice a day. Which instructions should the nurse give the parents?
☐ 1. Digoxin enables the heart to pump more effectively with a slower and more regular rhythm.
☐ 2. Signs of toxicity include increased pulse and visual disturbances.
☐ 3. Digoxin is absorbed better if taken with meals.
☐ 4. If the child vomits within 15 minutes of administration, the dosage should be repeated.

7. Which signs and symptoms would lead the nurse to suspect a child has tetralogy of Fallot (TOF)? Select all that apply.
☐ 1. murmur
☐ 2. history of squatting
☐ 3. bounding pulses
☐ 4. cyanosis
☐ 5. faint pulse
☐ 6. tachypnea

8. The nurse is caring for a newborn with a large ventricular septal defect. The client has undergone pulmonary artery banding. Which assessment findings indicate that the pulmonary artery band is functioning effectively?
☐ 1. Capillary refill is less than 3 seconds.
☐ 2. Urine output is greater than 1 mL/kg/h.
☐ 3. Breath sounds are clear and equal bilaterally.
☐ 4. Radial pulses are bounding.

9. A child diagnosed with tetralogy of Fallot becomes upset, cries, and thrashes around when a blood specimen is obtained. The child becomes cyanotic, and the respiratory rate increases to 44 breaths/min. Which action should the nurse do **first**?
☐ 1. Obtain a prescription for sedation for the child.
☐ 2. Assess for an irregular heart rate and rhythm.
☐ 3. Explain to the child that it will only hurt for a short time.
☐ 4. Place the child in a knee-to-chest position.

10. When teaching a preschool-age child how to perform coughing and deep-breathing exercises before corrective surgery for tetralogy of Fallot, which teaching and learning principles should the nurse address **first**?
☐ 1. organizing information to be taught in a logical sequence
☐ 2. arranging to use actual equipment for demonstrations
☐ 3. building the teaching on the child's current level of knowledge
☐ 4. presenting the information in order from simplest to most complex

11. When assessing a child after heart surgery to correct tetralogy of Fallot, which finding should alert the nurse to suspect a low cardiac output?
☐ 1. bounding pulses and mottled skin
☐ 2. altered level of consciousness and thready pulse
☐ 3. capillary refill of 2 seconds and blood pressure of 96/67 mm Hg
☐ 4. extremities warm to the touch and pale skin

12. Which intervention is the **greatest priority** for the therapeutic management of a child with congestive heart failure (CHF) caused by pulmonary stenosis?
☐ 1. educating the family about the signs and symptoms of infection
☐ 2. administering enoxaparin to improve left ventricular contractility
☐ 3. assessing heart rate and blood pressure every 2 hours
☐ 4. administrating furosemide to decrease systemic venous congestion

13. An infant weighing 9 kg is in the pediatric intensive care unit following arterial switch surgery. In the past hour, the infant has had 16 mL of urine output. Which action should the nurse take?
☐ 1. Notify the healthcare provider (HCP) immediately.
☐ 2. Record the urine output in the medical record.
☐ 3. Administer a fluid bolus immediately.
☐ 4. Assess for other signs of hypervolemia.

14. A child has had open heart surgery to repair a tetralogy of Fallot with a patch. The nurse should instruct the parents to:
☐ 1. notify all healthcare providers (HCPs) before invasive procedures for the next 6 months.
☐ 2. maintain adequate hydration of at least 10 glasses of water a day.
☐ 3. provide for frequent rest periods and naps during the first 4 weeks.
☐ 4. restrict the ingestion of bananas and citrus fruit.

15. As part of the preoperative teaching for the family of a child undergoing a tetralogy of Fallot repair, the nurse tells the family upon returning to the pediatric floor that the child may:
☐ 1. be placed on a reduced sodium diet.
☐ 2. have an activity restriction for several days.
☐ 3. be assigned to an isolation room.
☐ 4. have visits limited to a select few.

16. After surgery to correct a tetralogy of Fallot, the child's parents express concern to the nurse that their 4-year-old child wants to be held more frequently than usual. The nurse recommends:
☐ 1. introducing a new skill.
☐ 2. play therapy.
☐ 3. encouraging the behavior.
☐ 4. having the volunteer hold the child.

17. The parent of a child hospitalized with tetralogy of Fallot tells the nurse that the child's 3-year-old sibling has become quiet and shy and demonstrates more than a usual amount of genital curiosity since this child's hospitalization. The nurse should tell the parent:
- ☐ 1. "This behavior is very typical for a 3-year-old."
- ☐ 2. "This may be how your child expresses feeling a need for attention."
- ☐ 3. "This may be an indication that your child may have been sexually abused."
- ☐ 4. "This may be a sign of depression in your child."

The Client with Rheumatic Fever

18. A 13-year-old has been admitted with a diagnosis of rheumatic fever and is on bed rest. He has a sore throat. His joints are painful and swollen. He has a red rash on his trunk and is experiencing aimless movements of his extremities. Use the chart below to determine what the nurse should do **first**.
- ☐ 1. Report the heart rate to the healthcare provider (HCP).
- ☐ 2. Apply lotion to the rash.
- ☐ 3. Splint the joints to relieve the pain.
- ☐ 4. Request a prescription for medication to treat the elevated temperature.

Vital Signs

Time		0800	1200
Temperature	40°C 39°C 38°C 37°C 36°C 35°C 34°C	X (38°C)	X (37°C)
Respirations	30 25 20 15 10 5	X (22)	X (24)
Apical heart rate	160 150 140 130 120 110 100 90	X (110)	X (150)
Blood pressure	150 140 130 120 110 100 90 80	X (110) X (80)	X (120) X (85)

19. A nurse is planning care for a 12-year-old with rheumatic fever. The nurse should teach the parents to:
- ☐ 1. observe the child closely.
- ☐ 2. allow the child to participate in activities that will not tire him.
- ☐ 3. provide for adequate periods of rest between activities.
- ☐ 4. encourage someone in the family to be with the child 24 hours a day.

20. A 12-year-old with rheumatic fever has a history of long-term aspirin use. Which client statement **most** indicates that the client is experiencing a serious adverse reaction to aspirin?
- ☐ 1. "I hear ringing in my ears."
- ☐ 2. "I put lotion on my itchy skin."
- ☐ 3. "My stomach hurts after I take that medicine."
- ☐ 4. "These pills make me cough."

21. Which outcome indicates that the activity restriction necessary for a 7-year-old child with rheumatic fever during the acute phase has been effective?
- ☐ 1. Joints demonstrate absence of permanent injury.
- ☐ 2. The resting heart rate is between 60 and 100 bpm.
- ☐ 3. The child exhibits a decrease in chorea movements.
- ☐ 4. The subcutaneous nodules over the joints are no longer palpable.

22. Which initial physical finding indicates the development of carditis in a child with rheumatic fever?
- ☐ 1. heart murmur
- ☐ 2. low blood pressure
- ☐ 3. irregular pulse
- ☐ 4. anterior chest wall pain

23. The healthcare provider (HCP) prescribes pulse assessments through the night for a 12-year-old child with rheumatic fever who has a daytime heart rate of 120 bpm. The nurse explains to the mother that this is to evaluate if the elevated heart rate is caused by:
- ☐ 1. the morning digitalis.
- ☐ 2. normal activity during waking hours.
- ☐ 3. a warmer daytime environment.
- ☐ 4. normal variations in day and evening hours.

24. Which action should the nurse perform to help alleviate a child's joint pain associated with rheumatic fever?
- ☐ 1. Maintain the joints in an extended position.
- ☐ 2. Apply gentle traction to the child's affected joints.
- ☐ 3. Support proper alignment with rolled pillows.
- ☐ 4. Use a bed cradle to avoid the weight of bed linens on joints.

The Client with Kawasaki Disease

25. When developing the plan of care for a newly admitted 2-year-old child with the diagnosis of Kawasaki disease (KD), which intervention should be the **priority**?
☐ 1. taking vital signs every 6 hours
☐ 2. monitoring intake and output every hour
☐ 3. minimizing skin discomfort
☐ 4. providing passive range-of-motion exercises

26. A child with Kawasaki disease is receiving low-dose aspirin. The mother calls the clinic and states that the child has been exposed to influenza. Which recommendations should the nurse make? Select all that apply.
☐ 1. Increase fluid intake.
☐ 2. Stop the aspirin.
☐ 3. Keep the child home from school.
☐ 4. Watch for fever.
☐ 5. Weigh the child daily.

27. A 16-month-old child diagnosed with Kawasaki disease (KD) is very irritable, refuses to eat, and exhibits peeling skin on the hands and feet. What should the nurse do **first**?
☐ 1. Apply lotion to the hands and feet.
☐ 2. Offer foods the toddler likes.
☐ 3. Place the toddler in a quiet environment.
☐ 4. Encourage the parents to get some rest.

28. Which information should the nurse include when completing discharge instructions for the parents of a 12-month-old child diagnosed with Kawasaki disease (KD) and being discharged home?
☐ 1. Offer the child extra fluids every 2 hours for 2 weeks.
☐ 2. Take the child's temperature daily for several days.
☐ 3. Check the child's blood pressure daily until the follow-up appointment.
☐ 4. Call the healthcare provider (HCP) if the irritability lasts for 2 more weeks.

The Client with Sickle Cell Anemia

29. The nurse is teaching the parents of a child with sickle cell disease. To instruct them on how to prevent sickle cell crisis, the nurse should include which instructions?
☐ 1. Exercise in cool temperatures.
☐ 2. Drink at least 2 quarts of fluids per day.
☐ 3. Avoid contact sports.
☐ 4. Take anti-inflammatory medications before exercising.

30. The nurse explains to the parents of a 1-year-old child admitted to the hospital in sickle cell crisis that the local tissue damage the child has on admission is caused by which factor?
☐ 1. autoimmune reaction complicated by hypoxia
☐ 2. lack of oxygen in the red blood cells
☐ 3. obstruction to circulation
☐ 4. elevated serum bilirubin concentration

31. The parents of a child with sickle cell disease ask the nurse why their child's hemoglobin was normal at birth but now the child has S hemoglobin. Which response by the nurse is appropriate?
☐ 1. "The placenta bars passage of the hemoglobin S from the mother to the fetus."
☐ 2. "The red bone marrow does not begin to produce hemoglobin S until several months after birth."
☐ 3. "Antibodies transmitted from you to the fetus provide the newborn with temporary immunity."
☐ 4. "The newborn has a high concentration of fetal hemoglobin in the blood for some time after birth."

The Client with Iron Deficiency Anemia

32. Which action indicates that the parents of a 12-month-old with iron deficiency anemia understand how to administer iron supplements? Select all that apply.
☐ 1. They administer iron supplements in combination with fruit juice.
☐ 2. They administer iron supplements with meals.
☐ 3. They report dark stools.
☐ 4. They brush the child's teeth after administering the iron supplements.
☐ 5. They decrease dietary intake of foods fortified with iron.

33. A parent asks the nurse if a child's iron deficiency anemia is related to the child's frequent infections. The nurse responds based on an understanding of which principle?
☐ 1. Little is known about iron deficiency anemia and its relationship to infection in children.
☐ 2. Children with iron deficiency anemia are more susceptible to infection than are other children.
☐ 3. Children with iron deficiency anemia are less susceptible to infection than are other children.
☐ 4. Children with iron deficiency anemia are equally as susceptible to infection as are other children.

34. Which statements by the mother of a toddler should lead the nurse to suspect that the child is at risk for iron deficiency anemia? Select all that apply.
- ☐ 1. "He drinks over four glasses of milk per day."
- ☐ 2. "I cannot keep enough apple juice in the house; he must drink over 10 oz (300 mL) per day."
- ☐ 3. "He refuses to eat more than two different kinds of vegetables."
- ☐ 4. "He does not like meat, but he will eat small amounts of it."
- ☐ 5. "He sleeps 12 hours every night and takes a 2-hour nap."

35. Which foods should the nurse encourage a parent to offer to a child with iron deficiency anemia?
- ☐ 1. rice cereal, whole milk, and yellow vegetables
- ☐ 2. potato, peas, and chicken
- ☐ 3. macaroni, cheese, and ham
- ☐ 4. pudding, green vegetables, and rice

The Client with Hemophilia

36. What is the **most** appropriate method to use when drawing blood from a child with hemophilia?
- ☐ 1. Use finger punctures for lab draws.
- ☐ 2. Prepare to administer platelets.
- ☐ 3. Apply heat to the extremity before venipunctures.
- ☐ 4. Schedule all labs to be drawn at one time.

37. A diagnosis of hemophilia A is confirmed in an infant. Which instruction should the nurse provide the parents as the infant becomes more mobile and starts to crawl?
- ☐ 1. Administer one-half of a children's aspirin for a temperature higher than 101°F (38.3°C).
- ☐ 2. Sew thick padding into the elbows and knees of the child's clothing.
- ☐ 3. Check the color of the child's urine every day.
- ☐ 4. Expect the eruption of the primary teeth to produce moderate to severe bleeding.

38. A child with hemophilia presents with a burning sensation in the knee and reluctance to move the body part. The nurse collaborates with the care team to provide factor replacement and:
- ☐ 1. administer an aspirin-containing compound.
- ☐ 2. institute rest, ice, compression, and elevation (RICE).
- ☐ 3. begin physical therapy with active range of motion.
- ☐ 4. initiate skin traction.

39. Because of the risks associated with administration of antihemophilic factor (recombinant), the nurse should teach the child's family to recognize and immediately report which problem?
- ☐ 1. yellowing of the skin
- ☐ 2. constipation
- ☐ 3. abdominal distention
- ☐ 4. hives

40. The mother tells the nurse she will be afraid to allow her child with hemophilia to participate in sports because of the danger of injury and bleeding. After explaining that physical fitness is important for children with hemophilia, which activity should the nurse suggest as ideal?
- ☐ 1. snow skiing
- ☐ 2. swimming
- ☐ 3. basketball
- ☐ 4. gymnastics

The Client with Leukemia

41. A 15-year-old has been admitted to the hospital with the diagnosis of acute lymphocytic leukemia. Which signs and symptoms require the most immediate nursing intervention?
- ☐ 1. fatigue and anorexia
- ☐ 2. fever and petechiae
- ☐ 3. swollen neck lymph glands and lethargy
- ☐ 4. enlarged liver and spleen

42. A 12-year-old with leukemia is receiving cyclophosphamide. The nurse should assess for the adverse effect of:
- ☐ 1. photosensitivity
- ☐ 2. ataxia
- ☐ 3. cystitis
- ☐ 4. cardiac arrhythmias

43. After teaching the parents of a child newly diagnosed with leukemia about the disease, which description if given by the parent **best** indicates understanding the nature of leukemia?
- ☐ 1. "The disease is an infection resulting in increased white blood cell production."
- ☐ 2. "The disease is a type of cancer characterized by an increase in immature white blood cells."
- ☐ 3. "The disease is an inflammation associated with enlargement of the lymph nodes."
- ☐ 4. "The disease is an allergic disorder involving increased circulating antibodies in the blood."

44. Which problem is the highest risk for a child with leukemia whose lab values are as follows: WBC 6,500 mm³ (6.5×10^9/L), platelet count 40,000 µL (40×10^9/L), and HCT 41.2% (0.412)?
- ☐ 1. activity intolerance
- ☐ 2. bleeding
- ☐ 3. impaired tissue perfusion
- ☐ 4. infection

45. Which statement should the nurse use to describe to the parents why their child with leukemia is at risk for infections?
- ☐ 1. "Abnormal platelets lead to bruising and bleeding."
- ☐ 2. "There are an insufficient number of circulating white blood cells."
- ☐ 3. "The number of red blood cells is inadequate for carrying oxygen."
- ☐ 4. "Immature white blood cells are incapable of handling an infectious process."

46. Which beverage should the nurse plan to give a child with leukemia to relieve nausea?
- ☐ 1. orange juice
- ☐ 2. weak tea
- ☐ 3. plain water
- ☐ 4. a carbonated beverage

47. Which medication prescription to help relieve pain in a child with leukemia should the nurse question?
- ☐ 1. hydromorphone
- ☐ 2. acetaminophen with codeine
- ☐ 3. ibuprofen
- ☐ 4. acetaminophen with hydrocodone

48. After teaching a child with leukemia about a scheduled bone marrow aspiration, the nurse determines that the teaching has been successful when the child identifies which place as the site for the aspiration?
- ☐ 1. right lateral side of the right wrist
- ☐ 2. middle of the chest
- ☐ 3. distal end of the thigh
- ☐ 4. back of the hipbone

49. The nurse and parents are planning for the discharge of a child with leukemia who is receiving dactinomycin and vincristine. The nurse should teach the parents to:
- ☐ 1. encourage increased fluid intake.
- ☐ 2. keep the child out of the sun.
- ☐ 3. monitor the child's heart rate.
- ☐ 4. observe the child for memory loss.

50. After doing well for a period of time, a child with leukemia develops an overwhelming infection. The child's death is imminent. Which statement offers the nurse the **best** guide in making plans to assist the parents in dealing with their child's imminent death?
- ☐ 1. Knowing that the prognosis is poor helps prepare relatives for the death of children.
- ☐ 2. Relatives are especially grieved when a child does well at first but then declines rapidly.
- ☐ 3. Trust in healthcare personnel is most often destroyed by a death that is considered untimely.
- ☐ 4. It is more difficult for relatives to accept the death of an older child than that of a toddler.

51. A 12-year-old with leukemia will be taking vincristine. The nurse should encourage the child to eat what kind of diet?
- ☐ 1. high-residue
- ☐ 2. low-residue
- ☐ 3. low-fat
- ☐ 4. high-calorie

52. A 10-year-old with leukemia is taking immunosuppressive drugs. To maintain health, the nurse should instruct the child and parents to:
- ☐ 1. continue with immunizations.
- ☐ 2. not receive any live attenuated vaccines.
- ☐ 3. receive vitamin and mineral supplements.
- ☐ 4. stay away from peers.

53. A nurse is teaching the family of an 8-year-old with acute lymphocytic leukemia about appropriate activities. Which recommendation should the nurse make?
- ☐ 1. home schooling
- ☐ 2. restriction from participating in athletic activities
- ☐ 3. avoiding trips to the shopping mall
- ☐ 4. being treated as "normal" as much as possible

54. Which signs and symptoms of leukemia would lead the nurse to suspect the client has thrombocytopenia? Select all that apply.
- ☐ 1. fever
- ☐ 2. petechiae
- ☐ 3. epistaxis
- ☐ 4. anorexia
- ☐ 5. bone pain
- ☐ 6. shortness of breath

Managing Care, Quality, and Safety of Children with Cardiovascular and Hematologic Health Problems

55. A transfusion of packed red blood cells has been prescribed for a 1-year-old with a sickle cell anemia. The infant has a 25-gauge IV infusing dextrose with sodium and potassium. Using the situation, background, assessment, and recommendation (SBAR) method of communication, the nurse contacts the healthcare provider (HCP) and recommends:
- ☐ 1. starting a second IV with a 22-gauge catheter to infuse normal saline with the blood.
- ☐ 2. using the existing IV, but changing the fluids to normal saline for the transfusion.
- ☐ 3. replacing the IV with a 22-gauge catheter to infuse the prescribed fluids.
- ☐ 4. starting a second IV with a 25-gauge catheter to infuse normal saline with the transfusion.

56. An infant has been transferred from the ICU to the pediatric floor after undergoing surgery to correct a heart defect. Which tasks can the nurse delegate to the licensed practical/vocational nurse (LPN/VN)? Select all that apply.
- ☐ 1. administering oral medications
- ☐ 2. administering IV morphine
- ☐ 3. obtaining vital signs
- ☐ 4. morning hygiene
- ☐ 5. circulation checks
- ☐ 6. discharge teaching

57. The nurse is assisting with conscious sedation for a 6-year-old undergoing a bone marrow biopsy. The nurse's **most** important responsibility during the procedure is to:
- ☐ 1. administer the topical anesthetic.
- ☐ 2. keep the parents informed.
- ☐ 3. monitor the client.
- ☐ 4. record the procedure.

58. The nurse is transferring a child who has had open heart surgery from the intensive care unit to the pediatric unit. The child's blood pressure has been fluctuating but has been stable during the last 2 hours. The nurse from the pediatric intensive care unit should include which information in the report to the nurse on the pediatric unit? Select all that apply.
- ☐ 1. medications being used
- ☐ 2. current vital signs
- ☐ 3. potential for blood pressure to drop
- ☐ 4. drip rate for the intravenous infusion
- ☐ 5. time of the most recent dose of pain medication
- ☐ 6. medications given during surgery

59. The nurse is preparing to administer furosemide to a 3-year-old with a heart defect. The nurse verifies the child's identity by checking the arm band and:
- ☐ 1. asking the child to state her name.
- ☐ 2. checking the room number.
- ☐ 3. asking the child to tell her birth date.
- ☐ 4. asking the parent the child's name.

60. A 7-year-old with hemophilia A has fallen and badly bruised his knee. Which intervention should be done **first** when managing the client's hemarthrosis?
- ☐ 1. Use active range of motion to prevent immobility.
- ☐ 2. Apply cold packs to promote vasoconstriction.
- ☐ 3. Apply pressure and immobilize the joint.
- ☐ 4. Notify the healthcare provider (HCP) of the injury.

61. An 8-week-old infant with congenital heart disease is being discharged. What is the **most** important information for the nurse to convey regarding feeding?
- ☐ 1. Allow the infant 1 hour to complete each feeding.
- ☐ 2. Position the infant in an upright position after each feeding.
- ☐ 3. Give feedings per nasogastric tube to conserve energy.
- ☐ 4. Provide a higher calorie formula or fortified breast milk.

Answers, Rationales, and Test-Taking Strategies

*The answers and rationales for each question follow below, along with keys (🔑) to the client need (CN) and cognitive level (CL) for each question. In addition, you will also see a glossary icon (📖) highlighting specific terminology used on the licensing exam. As you check your answers, use the **Content Mastery and Test-Taking Skill Self-Analysis** worksheet (tear-out worksheet in back of book) to identify the reason(s) for not answering the questions correctly. For additional information about test-taking skills and strategies for answering questions, refer to pages 12–23 and pages 35–36 in Part 1 of this book.*

The Client Undergoing a Cardiac Catheterization

1. 3. Direct pressure is the first measure that should be used to control bleeding. Taking the vital signs will not control the bleeding. This should be done while another person is being sent to notify the **HCP** 📖. The dressing can be reinforced after the bleeding has been contained.

🔑 CN: Reduction of risk potential; CL: Synthesize

2. 2. The catheter insertion site will be covered with a bandage. This is important for preschool children to know as they are very concerned about bodily harm. The best time to prepare a preschool child for an invasive procedure is the night before. Bringing a favorite toy to the hospital will help decrease the child's anxiety. To prevent bleeding, the child will be expected to keep the extremity straight for 4 to 6 hours after the procedure, either in bed or on the parent's lap.

🔑 CN: Psychosocial integrity; CL: Synthesize

3. 2. In children, cardiac catheterization usually involves a right-sided approach because septal defects permit entry into the left side of the heart. The catheter is usually inserted into the femoral vein through a percutaneous puncture. A cutdown procedure is rarely used. Echocardiography involves the use of ultra-high-frequency sound waves. The catheterization is usually performed under local, not general, anesthesia with sedation.

⚷ CN: Reduction of risk potential; CL: Apply

4. 3. Prophylactic antibiotics are suggested for children with heart defects before dental work is done to reduce the risk of bacterial infection. Typically, activities are not restricted after a cardiac catheterization. A percutaneous approach is used to insert the catheter, so stitches are not necessary. Showering or bathing is allowed as usual. The pressure dressing will be removed before the child is discharged.

⚷ CN: Reduction of risk potential; CL: Create

The Client with a Congenital Heart Defect

5. 1,4,6. To achieve optimal therapeutic levels, digoxin should be given at regular intervals without variation, usually every 12 hours. Vomiting and poor feeding are signs of toxicity. If more than two consecutive doses are missed, interventions may be needed to assure therapeutic drug levels. The medication should not be mixed with any other fluid as refusal may result in inaccurate intake of the medication. Taking makeup doses, or taking the medication at times other than scheduled, may adversely affect serum levels.

⚷ CN: Pharmacological and parenteral therapies; CL: Create

6. 1. Digoxin's effect is to slow the rate of the electrical conduction through the heart and increase the strength of the heart's contraction. Signs of toxicity include anorexia and decreased heart rate, not visual changes or increases in heart rate. Digoxin should be taken 1 hour before meals or 2 hours after meals in order to obtain better absorption of the drug. If the child vomits within 15 minutes of administration, the dose should not be repeated because it is not known how much of the medication has been absorbed.

⚷ CN: Pharmacological and parenteral therapies; CL: Apply

7. 1,2,4,6. TOF is a heart condition with four defects: pulmonic stenosis, right ventricular hypertrophy, ventricular septal defect, and an overriding aorta. A systolic murmur, cyanosis, and tachypnea are all symptoms of TOF. Toddlers with uncorrected defects instinctively squat (knee-chest position) to decrease the return of systemic venous blood to the heart. Coarctation of the aorta is a narrowing in the descending aorta, obstructing the systemic blood outflow. Infants with severe constriction may present with faint pulse in lower extremities and bounding pulses in upper extremities.

⚷ CN: Physiological adaptation; CL: Analyze

8. 3. Pulmonary artery banding is a palliative treatment used in pediatric clients with congenital cardiac defects with increased pulmonary blood flow. The pulmonary artery band reduces excessive pulmonary blood flow and protects the lungs from irreversible damage. When the pulmonary artery band is functioning properly, the lungs should no longer be receiving an increased amount of blood flow, which would be reflected in clear and equal breath sounds. A capillary refill of less than 3 seconds and a urine output greater than 1 mL/kg/h reflect adequate peripheral perfusion. Bounding radial pulses suggest increased pulmonary blood flow.

⚷ CN: Physiological adaptation; CL: Evaluate

9. 4. The child is experiencing tet or hypoxic episode. Therefore, the nurse should place the child in a knee-to-chest position. Flexing the legs reduces venous flow of blood from the lower extremities and reduces the volume of blood being shunted through the interventricular septal defect and the overriding aorta in the child with tetralogy of Fallot. As a result, the blood then entering the systemic circulation has higher oxygen content, and dyspnea is reduced. Flexing the legs also increases vascular resistance and pressure in the left ventricle. An infant often assumes a knee-to-chest position in the crib, or the mother learns to put the infant over her shoulder while holding the child in a knee-to-chest position to relieve dyspnea. If this position is ineffective, then the child may need a sedative. Once the child is in the position, the nurse may assess for an irregular heart rate and rhythm. Explaining to the child that it will only hurt for a short time does nothing to alleviate the hypoxia.

⚷ CN: Physiological adaptation; CL: Synthesize

10. 3. Before developing any teaching program for a child, the nurse's first step is to assess the child to determine what is already known. Most older preschool children have some understanding of a condition present since birth. However, the child's interest will soon be lost if familiar material is repeated too often. The nurse can then organize the information in a sequence because there are several steps to be demonstrated. These exercises do not require the use of equipment. The nurse should judge the amount and complexity of the information to be provided, based on the child's current knowledge and response to teaching.

CN: Psychosocial integrity;
CL: Synthesize

11. 2. With a low cardiac output and subsequent poor tissue perfusion, signs and symptoms would include pale, cool extremities; cyanosis; weak, thready pulses; delayed capillary refill; and decrease in level of consciousness.

CN: Physiological adaptation;
CL: Analyze

12. 4. Pulmonary stenosis can cause right-sided CHF, resulting in venous congestion. Removing accumulated fluid is a primary goal of treatment in right-sided CHF. Furosemide is used to reduce venous congestion. It is important to educate the family about signs and symptoms of CHF, but treating the client's CHF is the priority. Enoxaparin is an anticoagulant and will not help improve left ventricular contractility. It is important to assess vital signs frequently in the child with CHF, but assessments do not treat the problem.

CN: Physiological adaptation;
CL: Apply

13. 2. Urine output for an infant weighing 9 kg should be 1 mL/kg/h. Sixteen milliliters of urine output is more than adequate for 1 hour, so the nurse should record the output in the **medical record** 📖. There is no reason to notify the **HCP** 📖 regarding adequate urine output. The infant has adequate output, so there is no need for a fluid bolus. A fluid bolus could also cause the infant to become fluid overloaded, increasing the workload on the heart. There is no information in the question indicating that the child is hypervolemic.

CN: Physiological adaptation;
CL: Analyze

14. 1. Children who have undergone open heart surgery with a patch are at risk for infection, especially subacute bacterial endocarditis (SBE), for the first 6 months following surgery. The newest evidence-based guidelines suggest that once the patch has epithelialized, these precautions are no longer necessary. Therefore, parents are instructed about SBE precautions including the need to notify providers before invasive procedures so antibiotics can be prescribed for that time period. Having the child drink a very large amount of water may lead to fluid overload. Children gear their rest schedule to their activities making it unnecessary to schedule frequent rest periods. Bananas and citrus fruit are high in potassium, but there is no evidence provided that the child has an elevated serum potassium requiring restriction.

CN: Physiological adaptation;
CL: Synthesize

15. 1. Because of the hemodynamic changes that occur with open heart surgery repair, particularly with septal defects, transient congestive heart failure may develop. Therefore, the child's sodium intake typically is restricted to 2 to 3 g/day. Activity restrictions are inappropriate. Typically, the child is encouraged to walk the halls and unit. Risk for infection after the repair is the same as any postoperative client; therefore, isolation is not necessary. The child may be placed in a room with other children who are not contagious. Visitors are not restricted unless the pediatric unit has restrictive visiting policies.

CN: Physiological adaptation;
CL: Synthesize

16. 2. The child is exhibiting regression. During periods of stress, children frequently revert to behaviors that were comforting in earlier developmental stages; play therapy is one way to help the child cope with the stress. Teaching a new skill most likely would add more stress. Parents should be instructed to praise positive behaviors and ignore regressive behaviors rather than calling attention to them through encouragement or discouragement. Having someone else hold the child does not encourage coping with the stress or promoting appropriate development.

CN: Psychosocial integrity;
CL: Synthesize

17. 2. According to Erikson, the central psychosocial task of a preschooler is to develop a sense of initiative versus guilt. Any environmental situation may affect the child. In this situation, the sibling is probably feeling less attention from the mother and trying to resolve the conflict in an inappropriate way. Three-year-olds are usually active and outgoing. These behaviors represent a change. Data are not sufficient to suggest the child has been exposed to a sexual experience. Symptoms of depression would include withdrawal and fatigue.

CN: Psychosocial integrity;
CL: Synthesize

The Client with Rheumatic Fever

18. 1. The child's heart rate of 150 bpm is significantly above its rate at the time of his admission. The nurse must notify the **HCP** 📖. The increase in heart rate may indicate carditis, a possible complication of rheumatic fever that can cause serious and lifelong effects on the heart. The HCP will intervene with medication and cardiac monitoring. While lotion may provide comfort, the most important action for the nurse is to notify the HCP of the increased heart rate. Splinting will not help the inflammation that is causing the painful joints. The joint pain will migrate and subside with time. The temperature is not elevated at this time and does not require intervention.

🔑 CN: Physiological adaptation;
CL: Synthesize

19. 3. The nurse should teach the parents to provide for sufficient periods of rest to decrease the client's cardiac workload. The client's condition does not warrant close observation unless cardiac complications develop. The child's activity level will be based on the results of the sedimentation rate, c-reactive protein, heart rate, and cardiac function. The family does not need to be with the client 24 hours a day unless carditis develops and his condition deteriorates.

🔑 CN: Basic care and comfort;
CL: Synthesize

20. 1. Tinnitus is an adverse effect of prolonged aspirin therapy, and the child should be examined by a **healthcare provider (HCP)** 📖 for hearing loss. Itchy skin commonly accompanies the rash associated with rheumatic fever, and the nurse can encourage lotion use. The nurse teaches clients to take aspirin with food or milk to avoid abdominal discomfort. The nurse can also address the fact that coughing after ingesting aspirin can be caused by inadequate fluid intake during administration.

🔑 CN: Pharmacological and parenteral therapies; CL: Analyze

21. 2. During the acute phase of rheumatic fever, the heart is inflamed and every effort is made to reduce the work of the heart. Bed rest with limited activity is necessary to prevent heart failure. Therefore, the most reliable indicator that activity restriction has been effective is a resting heart rate between 60 and 100 bpm, normal for a 7-year-old child. No permanent damage to the joints occurs with rheumatic fever. The chorea movements associated with rheumatic fever are self-limited and usually disappear in 1 to 3 months. They are unrelated to activity restrictions. Subcutaneous nodules that occur over joint surfaces also resolve over time with no treatment. Therefore, they are not appropriate for evaluating the effectiveness of activity restrictions.

🔑 CN: Physiological adaptation;
CL: Evaluate

22. 1. In rheumatic fever, the connective tissue of the heart becomes inflamed, leading to carditis. The most common signs of carditis are heart murmurs, tachycardia during rest, cardiac enlargement, and changes in the electrical conductivity of the heart. Heart murmurs are present in about 75% of all clients during the first week of carditis and in 85% of clients by the third week. Signs of carditis do not include hypotension or chest pain. The client may have a rapid pulse, but it is usually not irregular.

🔑 CN: Physiological adaptation;
CL: Analyze

23. 2. An above-average pulse rate that is out of proportion to the degree of activity is an early sign of heart failure in a client with rheumatic fever. The sleeping pulse is used to determine whether the mild tachycardia persists during sleep (inactivity) or whether it is a result of daytime activities. The environmental temperature would need to be quite warmer before it could influence the heart rate. Digitalis lowers the heart rate, so the rate would be decreased during the daytime.

🔑 CN: Reduction of risk potential;
CL: Analyze

24. 4. For a child with arthritis associated with rheumatic fever, the joints are usually so tender that even the weight of bed linens can cause pain. Use of a bed cradle is recommended to help remove the weight of the linens on painful joints. Joints need to be maintained in good alignment, not positioned in extension, to ensure that they remain functional. Applying gentle traction to the joints is not recommended because traction is usually used to relieve muscle spasms, not typically associated with rheumatic fever. Supporting the body in good alignment and changing the client's position are recommended, but these measures are not likely to relieve pain.

🔑 CN: Basic care and comfort;
CL: Synthesize

The Client with Kawasaki Disease

25. 2. Cardiac status must be monitored carefully in the initial phase of KD because the child is at high risk for congestive heart failure (CHF). Therefore, the nurse needs to assess the child frequently for signs of CHF, which would include respiratory distress and decreased urine output. Vital signs would be obtained more often than every 6 hours because of the risk of CHF. Although minimizing skin discomfort would be important, it does not take priority over monitoring the child's hourly intake and output. Passive range-of-motion exercises would be done if the child develops arthritis.

⚷ CN: Physiological adaptation; CL: Create

26. **2,4.** Aspirin needs to be stopped because of its possible link to Reye syndrome. Additionally, the parents need to watch for signs and symptoms of influenza. Children with influenza frequently present with fever, cold symptoms, and gastrointestinal symptoms. Increasing the child's fluid intake and weighing the child daily are not needed at this time because the child is not displaying signs of influenza. Keeping the child home from school is not necessary because the child is not symptomatic and has already been exposed.

⚷ CN: Reduction of risk potential; CL: Synthesize

27. **3.** One of the characteristics of children with KD is irritability. They are often inconsolable. Placing the child in a quiet environment may help quiet the child and reduce the workload of the heart. Although peeling of the skin occurs with KD, the child's irritability takes priority over applying lotion to the hands and feet. Children with KD usually are not hungry and do not eat well regardless of what is served. There is no indication that the parents need rest. Additionally, in this situation, the child takes priority over the parents.

⚷ CN: Physiological adaptation; CL: Synthesize

28. **2.** The child's temperature should be taken daily for several days after discharge because recurrent fever may develop. Offering the child fluids every 2 hours is not necessary. Doing so increases the child's risk for CHF. Checking the child's blood pressure at home usually is not included as part of the discharge instructions because by the time of discharge the child is considered stable and the risk for cardiac problems is minimal. Most children with KD recover fully. Irritability may last for 2 months after discharge.

⚷ CN: Physiological adaptation; CL: Create

The Client with Sickle Cell Anemia

29. **2.** Increasing fluid intake and being well hydrated will help prevent cell stasis in the small vessels. Restricting fluids causes stasis of red blood cells and promotes obstruction and increases the chance of sickling with hypoxia and pain to the part that is involved. Clients with sickle cell disease should avoid exercising in cool temperatures or

swimming in cold water. While contact sports are not recommended because of bleeding risks, they do not cause sickle crisis. Taking an anti-inflammatory medication before exercising does not prevent sickle cell crisis.

⚷ CN: Health promotion and maintenance; CL: Synthesize

30. **3.** Characteristic sickle cells tend to cause "log jams" in capillaries. This results in poor circulation to local tissues, leading to ischemia and necrosis. The basic defect in sickle cell disease is an abnormality in the structure of the red blood cells. The erythrocytes are sickle shaped, rough in texture, and rigid. Sickle cell disease is an inherited disease, not an autoimmune reaction. Elevated serum bilirubin concentrations are associated with jaundice, not sickle cell disease.

⚷ CN: Physiological adaptation; CL: Apply

31. **4.** Sickle cell disease is an inherited disease that is present at birth. However, 60% to 80% of a newborn's hemoglobin is fetal hemoglobin, which has a structure different from that of hemoglobin S or hemoglobin A. Sickle cell symptoms usually occur about 4 months after birth, when hemoglobin S begins to replace the fetal hemoglobin. The gene for sickle cell disease is transmitted at the time of conception, not passed through the placenta. Some hemoglobin S is produced by the fetus near term. The fetus produces all its own hemoglobin from the earliest production in the first trimester. Passive immunity conferred by maternal antibodies is not related to sickle cell disease, but this transmission of antibodies is important to protect the infant from various infections during early infancy.

⚷ CN: Physiological adaptation; CL: Apply

The Client with Iron Deficiency Anemia

32. **1,4.** Parent teaching concerning a child with iron deficiency anemia should include directions about giving iron combined with fruit juice, in divided doses, between meals, and with a dropper for a 12-month-old or through a straw for older toddlers. Iron stains teeth, so brushing the teeth and administering liquid iron through a dropper or straw are necessary to prevent staining the teeth. Iron should not be given with milk, antacids, or tea and should be administered on an empty stomach. Iron will cause the stool to become black or green, which is normal and does not need to be reported. However, light-colored stools indicate the iron is not being absorbed and should be reported.

CN: Pharmacological and parenteral therapies; CL: Evaluate

33. 2. Children with iron deficiency anemia are more susceptible to infection because of marked decreases in bone marrow functioning with microcytosis.

CN: Physiological adaptation; CL: Apply

34. 1,2. Toddlers should have between two and three servings of milk per day and no more than 6 oz (180 mL) of juice per day. If they have more than that, then they are probably not eating enough other foods, including iron-rich foods that have the needed nutrients. Food preferences vary among children. It is acceptable for the child to refuse foods as long as the diet is balanced and contains adequate calories. The child is obtaining a normal amount of sleep.

CN: Basic care and comfort; CL: Evaluate

35. 2. Potatoes, peas, chicken, green vegetables, and fortified cereal contain significant amounts of iron and therefore would be recommended. Milk and yellow vegetables are not good iron sources. Rice by itself also is not a good source of iron. Macaroni, cheese, and ham are not high in iron. While pudding (made with fortified milk) and green vegetables contain some iron, the better diet has protein and iron from the chicken and potato.

CN: Basic care and comfort; CL: Apply

The Client with Hemophilia

36. 4. Coordinating labs to minimize sticks reduces trauma and the risk of bleeding. Fingersticks in general are more painful and associated with more bleeding than are venipunctures. In hemophilia, platelets are typically normal. Heat would increase vasodilatation and increase bleeding.

CN: Reduction of risk potential; CL: Apply

37. 2. As the hemophilic infant begins to acquire motor skills, falls and bumps increase that risk of bleeding. Such injuries can be minimized by padding vulnerable joints. Aspirin is contraindicated because of its antiplatelet properties, which increase the infant's risk for bleeding. Because genitourinary bleeding is not a typical problem in children with hemophilia, urine testing is not indicated. Although some bleeding may occur with tooth eruption, it does not normally cause moderate to severe bleeding episodes in children with hemophilia.

CN: Safety and infection control; CL: Synthesize

38. 2. The child is displaying symptoms of bleeding in the joint and factor replacement is indicated. The RICE method is used additionally as a supportive measure to help control the bleeding. Aspirin-containing compounds contribute to bleeding and should never be used to control pain. Physical therapy is instituted after the acute bleeding to prevent further damage. Orthopedic traction is considered in some rare cases during the rehabilitation phase, but not the acute phase.

CN: Physiological adaptation; CL: Synthesize

39. 4. Administration of antihemolytic factor (recombinant) is a biosynthetic preparation of factor VIII that carries the risk of severe allergic reaction. Signs include hives, difficulty breathing, tachycardia, chills, and fever. Originally, factor VIII preparations were derived from large pools of human plasma and carried the risk of hepatitis, but recombinant preparations do not. Antihemolytic factor (recombinant) is not associated with constipation or abdominal distention.

CN: Pharmacological and parenteral therapies; CL: Synthesize

40. 2. Swimming is an ideal activity for a child with hemophilia because it is a noncontact sport. Many noncontact sports and physical activities that do not place excessive strain on joints are also appropriate. Such activities strengthen the muscles surrounding joints and help control bleeding in these areas. Noncontact sports also enhance general mental and physical well-being. Falls and subsequent injury to the child may occur with snow skiing. Basketball is a contact sport and therefore increases the child's risk for injury. Gymnastics is a very strenuous sport. Gymnasts frequently have muscle and joint injuries that result in bleeding episodes.

CN: Health promotion and maintenance; CL: Apply

The Client with Leukemia

41. 2. Fever and petechiae associated with acute lymphocytic leukemia indicate a suppression of normal white blood cells and thrombocytes by the bone marrow and put the client at risk for other infections and bleeding. The nurse should initiate infection control and safety precautions to reduce these risks. Fatigue is a common symptom of leukemia due to red blood cell suppression. Although the client should be told about the need for rest and meal planning, such teaching is not the priority intervention. Swollen glands and lethargy may be uncomfortable, but they do not require immediate intervention. An enlarged liver and spleen do require safety precautions that prevent injury to the abdomen; however, these precautions are not the priority.

🔑 CN: Reduction of risk potential; CL: Analyze

42. 3. Cystitis is a potential adverse effect of cyclophosphamide. The client should be monitored for pain on urination. Photosensitivity, ataxia, and cardiac arrhythmias are not adverse effects associated with cyclophosphamide.

🔑 CN: Pharmacological and parenteral therapies; CL: Analyze

43. 2. Leukemia is a neoplastic, or cancerous, disorder of blood-forming tissues that is characterized by a proliferation of immature white blood cells. Leukemia is not an infection, inflammation, or allergic disorder.

🔑 CN: Physiological adaptation; CL: Evaluate

44. 2. A normal platelet count is 150,000 to 400,000 μL (150 to 400 × 10^9/L). A platelet count of 40,000 μL (40 × 10^9/L) is low and puts the child at risk for injury, bruising, and bleeding. Hematocrit of 41.2% (0.41) is normal; therefore, the child will have adequate oxygenation and tissue perfusion. The white blood cell count of 6,500 mm^3 (6.5 × 10^9/L) is normal; therefore, the child has no increase in risk for infection.

🔑 CN: Reduction of risk potential; CL: Analyze

45. 4. In leukemia, although there is an increased number of immature white blood cells, they are unable to combat infection. Lack of mature white blood cells puts a child with leukemia at risk for infection. The major morbidity and mortality factor associated with leukemia is infection resulting from the presence of granulocytopenia. Decreased red blood cells are not directly caused by infection. While platelets play a role in the body's response to infection, bleeding does not directly cause infections.

🔑 CN: Reduction of risk potential; CL: Apply

46. 4. Carbonated beverages ordinarily are best tolerated when a child feels nauseated. Many children find cola drinks especially easy to tolerate, but noncola beverages are also recommended. Orange juice usually is not tolerated well because of its high acid content. Tea may also be too acidic, and many children do not like tea. Water does not relieve nausea.

🔑 CN: Basic care and comfort; CL: Apply

47. 3. Ibuprofen prolongs bleeding time and is contraindicated in clients with leukemia. Nonnarcotic drugs other than ibuprofen or aspirin, such as acetaminophen, may be prescribed to control pain and may be used in combination with codeine or hydrocodone if pain is more severe. Hydromorphone may also be used for severe pain.

🔑 CN: Pharmacological and parenteral therapies; CL: Synthesize

48. 4. Although bone marrow specimens may be obtained from various sites, the most commonly used site in children is the posterior iliac crest, the back of the hipbone. This area is close to the body's surface but removed from vital organs. The area is large, so specimens can easily be obtained. For infants, the proximal tibia and the posterior iliac crest are used. The middle of the chest or sternum is the usual site for bone marrow aspiration in an adult. The wrist, chest, and thigh are not sites from which to obtain bone marrow specimens.

🔑 CN: Reduction of risk potential; CL: Evaluate

49. 1. Dactinomycin and vincristine both cause nausea and vomiting. Oral fluids are encouraged, and antiemetics are given to prevent dehydration. Avoiding sun exposure is not necessary because photosensitivity is not associated with these drugs. Heart rate changes and memory issues also are not associated with either of these two drugs.

🔑 CN: Pharmacological and parenteral therapies; CL: Synthesize

50. 2. It has been found that parents are more grieved when optimism is followed by defeat. The nurse should recognize this when planning various ways to help the parents of a dying child. It is not necessarily true that knowing about a poor prognosis for years helps prepare parents for a child's death. Death is still a shock when it occurs. Trust in healthcare personnel is not necessarily destroyed when a death is untimely if the family views the personnel as having done all that was possible. It is not more difficult for parents to accept the death of an older child than that of a younger child.

🔑 CN: Psychosocial integrity; CL: Synthesize

51. 1. Vincristine may cause constipation, so the client should be encouraged to eat a high-residue (fiber) diet. The other diets do not help with constipation that can occur while receiving vincristine.

🔑 CN: Pharmacological and parenteral therapies; CL: Apply

52. 2. Children who are immunosuppressed should not receive any live attenuated vaccines. Clients who are immunosuppressed and are given live attenuated vaccines such as measles, mumps, rubella, and oral polio vaccine can develop severe forms of the diseases for which they are being immunized, which can result in death. Inactivated vaccines may be given if necessary, but the client is not able to adequately produce needed antibodies, and it is recommended that immunizations be delayed for 3 months after the immunosuppressive drugs have been discontinued. Vitamin and mineral supplements are not normally given in conjunction with immunosuppressive drugs. When the client is immunosuppressed, the client should avoid only persons who have an infection.

CN: Health promotion and maintenance; CL: Synthesize

53. 4. Any child with a chronic illness should be treated as normally as possible. Unless the child has severe bone marrow depression, he or she should be allowed to go to school with others and can go to the mall. If the child is in remission, athletic activities are allowed.

CN: Health promotion and maintenance; CL: Synthesize

54. 2,3. Children with acute lymphocytic leukemia have a reduced platelet count (thrombocytopenia), reduced red blood cell count (anemia), and reduced white blood cell count (neutropenia) because of unrestricted proliferation of immature white blood cell. Chemotherapy is used to treat leukemia and contributes to thrombocytopenia, neutropenia, and anemia. Clients with thrombocytopenia are at risk for bleeding. Petechiae (small red or purple spots on the skin) and epistaxis (nose bleeds) are both signs of bleeding. A fever is a result of a decreased white blood cell count. Anorexia and shortness of breath are a result of a decreased red blood cell count. Bone pain is a result of stress on the bone related to the unrestricted proliferation of the leukemic blast cells.

CN: Physiological adaptation; CL: Analyze

Managing Care, Quality, and Safety of Children with Cardiovascular and Hematologic Health Problems

55. 2. The best evidence indicates that a catheter as small as 27 gauge may safely be used for transfusion in children, but blood must be infused with normal saline, not dextrose. A 1-year-old should be able to maintain his or her blood glucose for the 2-hour duration of the infusion without the need for a second IV.

CN: Management of care; CL: Synthesize

56. 1,3,4. The RN's scope of practice includes assessment, planning, implementing, and evaluation. Only aspects of care implementation

may be delegated to the **LPN/VN** , and the exact skills that may be delegated vary by state and institution. In general, LPN/VNs have been trained to perform the tasks of administering oral medications, performing hygiene, and recording the intake and output. LPN/VNs may also take vital signs to gather data, but the nurse must interpret the data. Administering IV morphine requires assessment of the client's respiratory status before, during, and after the procedure. Circulation checks are assessments the RN should complete.

CN: Management of care; CL: Synthesize

57. 3. During conscious sedation, the client may lose protective reflexes, and adequate respiratory and cardiac function may be impaired. At every procedure, there must be one healthcare professional whose sole responsibility is to monitor the client. Topical agents must be given in advance of the procedure to be effective. During the procedure, the nurse would not leave the child to speak with parents. While the procedure would be documented according to the facility's protocols, proper monitoring of the client is the intervention most associated with reducing risks.

CN: Reduction of risk potential; CL: Apply

58. 1,2,3,4,5. The report made when nurses are "handing off" a client from one nursing unit to another must include information about the condition of the client, potential for changes in the client's condition, current medications, and care and services received. It is not necessary to know what medications were given in surgery to provide safe care at this point.

CN: Safety and infection control; CL: Synthesize

59. 4. Safety standards require the use of two identifiers prior to medication administration. A parent can be used as the second identifier. Many young children will only answer to a nickname that does not coincide with the medical identification band or may answer to any name. It is common for children on a pediatric floor to go into each other's rooms. Small children may not know their birth date.

CN: Safety and infection control; CL: Synthesize

60. 3. Application of pressure and immobilization of the affected limb are the first priority. Pressure is required to stop the bleeding, and immobilization aids in reducing swelling and pain. Active range of motion is recommended after the bleeding is controlled. The application of cold packs can be helpful in diminishing swelling and pain. Cold packs will also promote vasoconstriction, which can help reduce the bleeding. The **healthcare provider (HCP)** 📖 should be informed of the bleeding episode after initial measures to control the bleeding are implemented.

🗝️ CN: Management of care; CL: Synthesize

61. 4. Infants with congenital heart disease often have difficulty feeding and gaining weight. They will tire quickly during the feeding. Most will do well with smaller, more frequent feedings. The infant with a congenital heart defect should not be given more than 20 minutes per feeding. Fortified breast milk or a high-calorie formula will help the infant gain weight and conserve energy. Prolonging the feeding to an hour will merely tire the infant. Positioning the infant in an upright position is recommended for infants with gastrointestinal reflux. Some infants with a congenital heart defect may not consume adequate amounts of calories through breast- or bottle-feeding and may require supplemental feeding through a nasogastric tube; however, nasogastric tube feedings are not necessary for all infants with congenital heart defects.

🗝️ CN: Management of care; CL: Synthesize

The Child with Health Problems of the Gastrointestinal Tract

The Client with Cleft Lip and Palate

1. When developing the plan of care for an infant with a cleft lip before corrective surgery is performed, what should be a **priority**?
- ☐ 1. maintaining skin integrity in the oral cavity
- ☐ 2. using techniques to minimize crying
- ☐ 3. altering the usual method of feeding
- ☐ 4. preventing the infant from putting fingers in the mouth

2. Which measure would be **most** effective in helping the infant with a cleft lip and palate to retain oral feedings?
- ☐ 1. Burp the infant at frequent intervals.
- ☐ 2. Feed the infant small amounts at one time.
- ☐ 3. Place the end of the nipple far to the back of the infant's tongue.
- ☐ 4. Maintain the infant in a supine position while feeding.

3. After teaching the parent of an infant who has had a surgical repair for a cleft lip about the use of elbow restraints at home, the nurse determines that the teaching has been successful when the parent makes which statement?
- ☐ 1. "We will keep the restraints on continuously except when checking the skin under them for redness."
- ☐ 2. "We will keep the restraints on during the day while he is awake, but take them off when we put him to bed at night."
- ☐ 3. "After we get home, we will not have to use the restraints because our child does not suck on his hands or fingers."
- ☐ 4. "We will be sure to keep the restraints on all the time until we come to see the care provider for a follow-up visit."

4. The mother of an infant with a cleft lip asks when the repair will be scheduled. What is the nurse's **best** response?
- ☐ 1. at birth
- ☐ 2. during the first 6 months of life
- ☐ 3. after 6 months of age
- ☐ 4. at 1 year of age

5. On the 2nd postoperative day after repair of a cleft palate, what should the nurse use to feed a toddler?
- ☐ 1. cup
- ☐ 2. straw
- ☐ 3. rubber-tipped syringe
- ☐ 4. large-holed nipple

The Client with Tracheoesophageal Fistula

6. The parents report that their 1-day-old is drooling and having choking episodes with excessive amounts of mucus and color changes, especially during feedings. The nurse should contact the healthcare provider (HCP) to further assess the baby and request a prescription for:
☐ **1.** a lactation consultation.
☐ **2.** a blood gas.
☐ **3.** an x-ray with orogastric catheter placement.
☐ **4.** a serum blood glucose.

7. The parents of a child with a tracheoesophageal fistula express feelings of guilt about their baby's anomaly. Which approach by the nurse would **best** support the parents?
☐ **1.** helping the parents accept their feelings as a normal reaction
☐ **2.** explaining that the parents did nothing to cause the newborn's defect
☐ **3.** encouraging the parents to concentrate on planning their baby's care
☐ **4.** urging the parents to visit their newborn as often as possible

8. After teaching the parents of a neonate diagnosed with a tracheoesophageal fistula (TEF) about this anomaly, the nurse determines that the teaching was successful when the parent describes the condition in which way?
☐ **1.** "The muscle below the stomach is too tight, causing the baby to vomit forcefully."
☐ **2.** "There is a blind upper pouch and an opening from the esophagus into the airway."
☐ **3.** "The lower bowel is lacking certain nerves to allow normal function."
☐ **4.** "A part of the bowel is on the outside without anything covering it."

9. Which finding would indicate that an infant with a tracheoesophageal fistula (TEF) needs suctioning?
☐ **1.** barking cough
☐ **2.** substernal retractions
☐ **3.** decreased activity level
☐ **4.** increased respiratory rate

10. The nurse is administering bolus gastrostomy feedings to an infant after surgery to correct a tracheoesophageal fistula (TEF). To prevent air from entering the stomach once the syringe barrel is attached to the gastrostomy, tube the nurse should:
☐ **1.** unclamp the tube after pouring the complete amount of formula to be administered into the syringe barrel.
☐ **2.** pour all of the formula to be administered into the syringe barrel after opening the clamp.
☐ **3.** maintain a continuous flow of formula down the side of the syringe barrel once the clamp is opened.
☐ **4.** allow a small amount of formula to enter the stomach before pouring more formula into the syringe barrel.

11. After surgery to repair a tracheoesophageal fistula, an infant receives gastrostomy tube feedings. The nurse continues holding the infant for about 15 minutes after the feeding primarily to help accomplish what need?
☐ **1.** Promote intestinal peristalsis.
☐ **2.** Prevent regurgitation of formula.
☐ **3.** Relieve pressure on the surgical site.
☐ **4.** Associate eating with a pleasurable experience.

12. A newborn who had a surgical repair of a tracheoesophageal fistula (TEF) is started on oral feedings. What should the nurse include in the teaching plan for the parent about oral feedings?
☐ **1.** They are better tolerated when larger but less frequent feedings are offered.
☐ **2.** They should be offered on a feeding schedule to help the infant accept the feedings more readily.
☐ **3.** They are best accepted by the infant when offered by the same nurse or by the infant's parent.
☐ **4.** They are best planned in conjunction with observations of the infant's behavior.

The Client with an Anorectal Anomaly

13. After completing diagnostic testing, the surgeon has scheduled a newborn with the diagnosis of an imperforate anus for surgery the next day. The infant's parents are Catholic and do not want the surgery to take place unless the infant has first been baptized. The nurse asks the parents:
☐ **1.** "Are you worried your baby might die?"
☐ **2.** "Do you want me to help arrange the baptism?"
☐ **3.** "Do you want to speak with the social worker?"
☐ **4.** "Would you prefer to wait for the surgery?"

14. What should the nurse assess in a newborn diagnosed with an anorectal malformation? Select all that apply.
- ☐ **1.** abdominal distention
- ☐ **2.** loose stools
- ☐ **3.** vomiting
- ☐ **4.** meconium in the urine
- ☐ **5.** meconium stools

15. When performing discharge teaching with the parents of a neonate who has successfully undergone surgery to repair a low anorectal anomaly, which parent statement about the child's prognosis indicates teaching has been successful?
- ☐ **1.** "My child will need to wear protective pads until puberty."
- ☐ **2.** "My child will need extra fluids to prevent constipation."
- ☐ **3.** "My child will probably always need a high-fiber diet."
- ☐ **4.** "My child has a good chance of being potty trained."

16. When the infant returns to the unit after imperforate anus repair, the nurse should place the infant in which position?
- ☐ **1.** on the abdomen, with legs pulled up under the body
- ☐ **2.** on the back, with legs extended straight out
- ☐ **3.** lying on the side with the hips elevated
- ☐ **4.** lying on the back in a position of comfort

17. The father of a neonate scheduled for gastrointestinal surgery asks the nurse how newborns respond to painful stimuli. What is the nurse's **best** response?
- ☐ **1.** "Newborns cry and cannot be distracted to stop crying."
- ☐ **2.** "When faced with a pain, newborns try to roll away from it."
- ☐ **3.** "Newborns typically move their whole body in response to pain."
- ☐ **4.** "Pain causes the newborn to withdraw the affected part."

18. When developing the plan of care for a neonate who was diagnosed with an anorectal malformation and who subsequently underwent surgery, what intervention would be **most** helpful in facilitating parent-infant bonding?
- ☐ **1.** explaining to the parents that they can visit at any time
- ☐ **2.** encouraging the parents to hold their infant
- ☐ **3.** asking the parents to help monitor the infant's intake and output
- ☐ **4.** helping the parents plan for their infant's discharge

The Client with Pyloric Stenosis

19. A 4-week-old infant admitted with the diagnosis of hypertrophic pyloric stenosis presents with a history of vomiting. The nurse should anticipate that the infant's vomitus would contain gastric contents and which other body substances?
- ☐ **1.** bile and streaks of blood
- ☐ **2.** mucus and bile
- ☐ **3.** mucus and streaks of blood
- ☐ **4.** stool and bile

20. When an infant with pyloric stenosis is admitted to the hospital, which aspect of the plan of care should the nurse implement **first**?
- ☐ **1.** Weigh the infant.
- ☐ **2.** Begin an intravenous infusion.
- ☐ **3.** Switch the infant to an oral electrolyte solution.
- ☐ **4.** Orient the mother to the hospital unit.

21. After teaching the parent of an infant with pyloric stenosis about the condition, which cause, if stated by the parent, indicates effective teaching?
- ☐ **1.** "An enlarged muscle below the stomach sphincter."
- ☐ **2.** "A telescoping of the large bowel into the smaller bowel."
- ☐ **3.** "A result of giving the baby more formula than is necessary."
- ☐ **4.** "A result of my baby taking the formula too quickly."

22. A newborn admitted with pyloric stenosis is lethargic and has poor skin turgor. The healthcare provider (HCP) has prescribed IV fluids of dextrose water with sodium and potassium. The baby's admission potassium level is 3.4 mEq/L (3.4 mmol/L). What should the nurse do **first**?
- ☐ **1.** Notify the HCP.
- ☐ **2.** Administer the prescribed fluids.
- ☐ **3.** Verify that the infant has urinated.
- ☐ **4.** Have the potassium level redrawn.

23. After undergoing surgical correction of pyloric stenosis, an infant is returned to the room in stable condition. While standing by the crib, the mother says, "Perhaps if I had brought my baby to the hospital sooner, the surgery could have been avoided." What should be the nurse's **best** response?
- ☐ **1.** "Surgery is the most effective treatment for pyloric stenosis."
- ☐ **2.** "Try not to worry; your baby will be fine."
- ☐ **3.** "Do you feel that this problem indicates that you are not a good mother?"
- ☐ **4.** "Do you think that earlier hospitalization could have avoided surgery?"

24. After surgery to correct pyloric stenosis, the nurse instructs the parents about the postoperative feeding schedule for their infant. The parents exhibit understanding of these instructions when they state that they can start feeding the child within which time frame?
☐ **1.** 6 hours
☐ **2.** 8 hours
☐ **3.** 10 hours
☐ **4.** 12 hours

25. Immediately after the first oral feeding after corrective surgery for pyloric stenosis, a 4-week-old infant is fussy and restless. Which action would be **most** appropriate at this time?
☐ **1.** Encourage the parents to hold the infant.
☐ **2.** Hang a mobile over the infant's crib.
☐ **3.** Give the infant more to eat.
☐ **4.** Give the infant a pacifier to suck on.

26. Which behavior exhibited by the parent of an infant with pyloric stenosis should the nurse correctly interpret as a positive indication of parental coping?
☐ **1.** telling the nurse that they have to get away for a while
☐ **2.** discussing the infant's care realistically
☐ **3.** repeatedly asking if their child is normal
☐ **4.** exhibiting fear that they will disturb the infant

27. A 6-month-old has had a pyloromyotomy to correct a pyloric stenosis. Three days after surgery, the parents have placed their infant in his own infant seat (see figure). What should the nurse do?

☐ **1.** Reposition the infant to the left side.
☐ **2.** Ask the parents to put the infant back in his crib.
☐ **3.** Remind the parents that the infant cannot use a pacifier now.
☐ **4.** Tell the parents they have positioned their infant correctly.

The Client with Intussusception

28. When assessing a 4-month-old infant diagnosed with possible intussusception, the nurse should expect the parent to relate which information about the infant's crying and episodes of pain?
☐ **1.** constant accompanied by leg extension
☐ **2.** intermittent with knees drawn to the chest
☐ **3.** shrill during ingestion of solids
☐ **4.** intermittent while being held in the mother's arms

29. When obtaining the nursing history from the mother of an infant with suspected intussusception, which question would be **most** helpful?
☐ **1.** "What do the stools look like?"
☐ **2.** "When was the last time your child urinated?"
☐ **3.** "Is your child eating normally?"
☐ **4.** "Has your child had any episodes of vomiting?"

30. A nasogastric tube inserted during surgical correction of infant's intussusception is no longer freely removing gastric secretions. What should the nurse do **next**?
☐ **1.** Aspirate the tube with a syringe.
☐ **2.** Irrigate the tube with distilled water.
☐ **3.** Increase the level of suction.
☐ **4.** Rotate the tube.

31. Which assessment should be the **priority** for an infant who has had surgery to correct an intussusception and is now at risk for development of a paralytic ileus postoperatively?
☐ **1.** measurement of urine specific gravity
☐ **2.** auscultation of bowel sounds
☐ **3.** inspection of the first stool passed
☐ **4.** measurement of gastric output

32. An infant is to be discharged after surgery for intussusception. In developing the discharge teaching plan, the nurse should tell the parent:
☐ **1.** the infant will experience a change in the normal home routine.
☐ **2.** the infant can return to the prehospital routine immediately.
☐ **3.** the infant needs to ingest more calories at home than what was consumed in the hospital.
☐ **4.** the infant will continue to experience abdominal cramping for a few days.

The Client with Inguinal Hernia

33. When assessing an infant with suspected inguinal hernia, which finding would be **most** significant?
- [ ] 1. The inguinal swelling is reddened, and the abdomen is distended.
- [ ] 2. The infant is irritable, and a thickened spermatic cord is palpable.
- [ ] 3. The inguinal swelling can be reduced, and the infant has a stool in the diaper.
- [ ] 4. The infant's diaper is wet with urine, and the abdomen is nontender.

34. The healthcare provider (HCP) is able to reduce an infant's hernia and schedules the infant for a herniorrhaphy in 2 days. The parent asks the nurse why the surgery is not being performed now. Which response about delaying the surgery is **most** appropriate?
- [ ] 1. "Delaying the surgery ensures that your infant will receive the proper preoperative preparation."
- [ ] 2. "We need to make sure that your infant receives nothing by mouth for at least 24 hours before the surgery."
- [ ] 3. "Waiting these 2 days helps to allow any edema and inflammation in the area to subside."
- [ ] 4. "Your infant needs to wear a truss for at least 24 hours before any surgery can be attempted."

35. Preoperatively, the nurse develops a plan to prepare a 7-month-old infant psychologically for a scheduled herniorrhaphy the next day. Which intervention should the nurse expect to implement to accomplish this goal?
- [ ] 1. explaining the preoperative and postoperative procedures to the mother
- [ ] 2. having the mother stay with the infant
- [ ] 3. making sure the infant's favorite toy is available
- [ ] 4. allowing the infant to play with surgical equipment

36. Which instruction should the nurse expect to include in the discharge teaching plan for the parent of an infant who has had an inguinal herniorrhaphy?
- [ ] 1. Change diapers as soon as they become soiled.
- [ ] 2. Apply an abdominal binder.
- [ ] 3. Keep the incision covered with a sterile dressing.
- [ ] 4. Restrain the infant's hands.

37. A parent asks, "How should I bathe my baby now that he has had surgery for his inguinal hernia?" Which instruction should the nurse give the parent?
- [ ] 1. "Clean his face and diaper area for 2 weeks."
- [ ] 2. "Use sterile sponges to cleanse the inguinal incision."
- [ ] 3. "Give him a sponge bath daily for 1 week."
- [ ] 4. "Give the infant full tub baths every day."

The Client with Hirschsprung's Disease

38. During physical assessment of a 4-month-old infant with Hirschsprung's disease, the nurse should **most** likely note which finding?
- [ ] 1. scaphoid-shaped abdomen
- [ ] 2. weight less than expected for height and age
- [ ] 3. cyanosis of the fingers and toes
- [ ] 4. hyperactive deep tendon reflexes

39. An infant diagnosed with Hirschsprung's disease is scheduled to receive a temporary colostomy. When initially discussing the diagnosis and treatment with the parents, which action would be **most** appropriate?
- [ ] 1. assessing the adequacy of their coping skills
- [ ] 2. reassuring them that their child will be fine
- [ ] 3. encouraging them to ask questions
- [ ] 4. giving them printed material on the procedure

40. After teaching the parents of an infant diagnosed with Hirschsprung's disease, the nurse determines that the parents understand the diagnosis when the parent makes which statement?
- [ ] 1. "There is no rectal opening for stool to pass."
- [ ] 2. "There is a tube between the trachea and esophagus."
- [ ] 3. "The nerves at the end of the large colon are missing."
- [ ] 4. "The muscle below the stomach is too tight."

41. When developing the preoperative plan of care for an infant with Hirschsprung's disease, which intervention should the nurse include?
- [ ] 1. administering a tap water enema
- [ ] 2. inserting a gastrostomy tube
- [ ] 3. restricting oral intake to clear liquids
- [ ] 4. using povidone-iodine solution to prepare the perineum

42. The nurse is showing the parent of a child with Hirschsprung's disease where the aganglionic area is located. Identify the area the nurse should point out as being aganglionic.

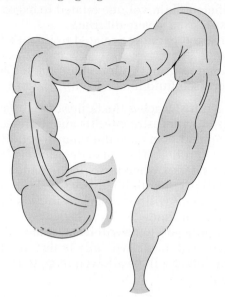

43. An infant diagnosed with Hirschsprung's disease undergoes surgery with the creation of a temporary colostomy. Which statement by the parent regarding the colostomy indicates the need for further teaching?
- ☐ **1.** "The colostomy is only temporary."
- ☐ **2.** "The colostomy will give time for the nerves to return to normal."
- ☐ **3.** "The colostomy may include two separate abdominal openings."
- ☐ **4.** "Right after the procedure, the stoma may appear purple."

44. When teaching the mother of an infant who has received a temporary colostomy for treatment of Hirschsprung's disease about how the stoma should normally appear, which description about the stoma's appearance should the nurse include in the teaching?
- ☐ **1.** becoming dark brown in 2 months
- ☐ **2.** staying deep red in color
- ☐ **3.** changing to several shades of pink
- ☐ **4.** turning almost purple in color

45. When teaching the parent of an infant with Hirschsprung's disease who received a temporary colostomy about the types of foods the infant will be able to eat, which diet would the nurse recommend?
- ☐ **1.** high-fiber diet
- ☐ **2.** low-fat diet
- ☐ **3.** high-residue diet
- ☐ **4.** regular diet

46. A child with Hirschsprung's disease is to be discharged 1 or 2 days after a colostomy takedown surgery. After teaching the infant's parents about the overall effects of their infant's surgery, the nurse determines that the teaching has been effective when the parents make which statement?
- ☐ **1.** "His abdomen will be large for a while."
- ☐ **2.** "Toilet training may be difficult."
- ☐ **3.** "We need to limit his intake of dairy products."
- ☐ **4.** "We will give him vitamin supplements until he is an adolescent."

47. A parent of a 7-year-old child with Hirschsprung's disease and chronic constipation asks about increasing dietary fiber in the child's diet. Which food could the nurse recommend?
- ☐ **1.** fruit juice
- ☐ **2.** white bread
- ☐ **3.** popcorn
- ☐ **4.** pancakes

The Client with Diarrhea, Gastroenteritis, or Dehydration

48. A nurse is caring for a 10-month-old, weighing 8 kg, who was admitted for dehydration. The infant has vomited five times in the last 3 hours and has had no wet diapers in the last 8 hours. The nurse informs the healthcare provider (HCP). Which prescription should the nurse question?
- ☐ **1.** Begin an intravenous line of D5W 0.45% normal saline at 40 mL/h.
- ☐ **2.** NPO while vomiting persists.
- ☐ **3.** Begin an intravenous line, and administer a fluid bolus of dextrose 25%.
- ☐ **4.** Strict intake and output, weighing all diapers.

49. Which signs or symptoms suggest that an infant with diarrhea is dehydrated? Select all that apply.
- ☐ **1.** tacky mucous membranes
- ☐ **2.** sunken anterior fontanelle
- ☐ **3.** salty saliva
- ☐ **4.** restlessness
- ☐ **5.** increased urine output

50. A child is admitted with a tentative diagnosis of shigella. The nurse performs which interventions? Select all that apply.
- ☐ **1.** Assess the child for nausea and vomiting.
- ☐ **2.** Collect a stool specimen for white blood cells (WBCs).
- ☐ **3.** Place the child on airborne precautions.
- ☐ **4.** Monitor the child for signs and symptoms of dehydration.
- ☐ **5.** Initiate an intake and output record.

51. Which finding would **most** likely alert the nurse to the possibility that a preschooler is experiencing moderate dehydration?
☐ 1. deep, rapid respirations
☐ 2. diaphoresis
☐ 3. absence of tear formation
☐ 4. decreased urine specific gravity

52. Which finding would be **most** important in an 8-month-old infant admitted with severe diarrhea?
☐ 1. bowel sounds every 5 seconds
☐ 2. pale yellow urine
☐ 3. normal skin elasticity
☐ 4. depressed anterior fontanelle

53. Which assessment would be the **most** important for the nurse to include in the plan of care for an infant experiencing severe diarrhea?
☐ 1. monitoring the total 8-hour formula intake
☐ 2. weighing the infant each day
☐ 3. checking the anterior fontanelle every shift
☐ 4. monitoring abdominal skin turgor every shift

54. The healthcare provider (HCP) prescribes an intravenous infusion of 5% dextrose in 0.45 normal saline to be infused at 2 mL/kg/h in an infant who weighs 9 lb (4.1 kg). How many milliliters per hour of the solution should the nurse infuse? Round to one decimal place.

_____ mL/h.

55. A 3-year-old with dehydration has vomited three times in the last hour and continues to have frequent diarrhea stools. The child was admitted 2 days ago with gastroenteritis caused by rotavirus. The child weighs 22 kg, has a normal saline lock in his right hand, and has had 30 mL of urine output in the last 4 hours. Using the situation-background-assessment-recommendation (SBAR) technique for communication, the nurse calls the healthcare provider (HCP) with the recommendation for:
☐ 1. giving a dose of loperamide.
☐ 2. starting a fluid bolus of normal saline.
☐ 3. beginning an IV antibiotic.
☐ 4. establishing a Foley catheter.

56. Which intervention would be **most** appropriate for the nurse to teach the mother of a 6-month-old infant hospitalized with severe diarrhea to help her comfort her infant who is fussy?
☐ 1. offering a pacifier
☐ 2. placing a mobile above the crib
☐ 3. sitting at crib side talking to the infant
☐ 4. turning the television on to cartoons

57. What would the nurse identify as a **priority** nursing problem for an infant just admitted to the hospital with a diagnosis of gastroenteritis?
☐ 1. pain related to repeated episodes of vomiting
☐ 2. deficient fluid volume related to excessive losses from severe diarrhea
☐ 3. impaired parenting related to infant's loss of fluid
☐ 4. impaired urinary elimination related to increased fluid intake feeding pattern

58. The nurse teaches the father of an infant hospitalized with gastroenteritis about the next step of the treatment plan once the infant's condition has been controlled. The nurse determines that the father understands when he explains which intervention will occur with his infant?
☐ 1. The infant will receive clear liquids for a period of time.
☐ 2. Formula and juice will be offered.
☐ 3. Blood will be drawn daily to test for anemia.
☐ 4. The infant will be allowed to go to the playroom.

59. The mother of a toddler who has just been admitted with severe dehydration secondary to gastroenteritis says that she cannot stay with her child because she has to take care of her other children at home. Which of the responses by the nurse would be **most** appropriate?
☐ 1. "You really should not leave right now. Your child is very sick."
☐ 2. "I understand, but feel free to visit or call anytime to see how your child is doing."
☐ 3. "It really is not necessary to stay with your child. We will take very good care of him."
☐ 4. "Can you find someone to stay with your children? Your child needs you here."

60. A 9-month-old is admitted because of dehydration. How should the nurse go about accurately monitoring fluid intake and output? Select all that apply.
☐ 1. weighing and recording all wet diapers
☐ 2. changing breast-feedings to bottle-feedings
☐ 3. obtaining an accurate daily weight
☐ 4. restricting fluids prior to weighing the child
☐ 5. obtaining an accurate stool count

61. The healthcare provider (HCP) prescribes intravenous fluid replacement therapy with potassium chloride to be added for a child with severe gastroenteritis. Before hanging the IV fluids with potassium chloride, which assessments would be **most** important?
☐ 1. ability to void
☐ 2. passage of stool today
☐ 3. baseline electrocardiogram
☐ 4. serum calcium level

62. Which finding would alert the nurse to suspect that a child with severe gastroenteritis who has been receiving intravenous therapy for the past several hours may be developing circulatory overload?
- [ ] 1. a drop in blood pressure
- [ ] 2. change to slow, deep respirations
- [ ] 3. auscultation of moist crackles
- [ ] 4. marked increase in urine output

63. The stool culture of a child with profuse diarrhea reveals *Salmonella* bacilli. After teaching the parent about the course of *Salmonella enteritidis*, which statement by the parent indicates effective teaching?
- [ ] 1. "Some people become carriers and stay infectious for a long time."
- [ ] 2. "After the acute stage passes, the organism is usually not present in the stool."
- [ ] 3. "Although the organism may be alive indefinitely, in time it will be of no danger to anyone."
- [ ] 4. "If my child continues to have the organism in the stool, an antitoxin can help destroy the organism."

64. A child undergoes rehydration therapy after having diarrhea and dehydration. A nurse is teaching the child's parents about dietary management after rehydration. The nurse understands that the teaching plan has been successful when the parents tell the nurse that they will follow which type of diet?
- [ ] 1. regular
- [ ] 2. clear liquid
- [ ] 3. full liquid
- [ ] 4. soft

65. When obtaining a history from the parents of a child diagnosed with diarrhea due to *Salmonella*, the nurse should ask the parents if the child has been exposed to which possible sources of infection?
- [ ] 1. nonrefrigerated custard
- [ ] 2. a pet canary
- [ ] 3. undercooked eggs
- [ ] 4. unwashed fruit

66. On a home visit following discharge from the hospital after treatment for severe gastroenteritis, the parent tells the nurse that a toddler answers "No!" and is difficult to manage. After discussing this further with the parent, the nurse explains that the child's behavior is **most** likely the result of which factor?
- [ ] 1. beginning leadership skills
- [ ] 2. inherited personality trait
- [ ] 3. expression of individuality
- [ ] 4. usual lack of interest in everything

67. The parent of a toddler hospitalized for episodes of diarrhea reports that when the toddler cannot have things the way she wants, she throws her legs and arms around, screams, and cries. The mother says, "I do not know what to do!" After teaching the parent about ways to manage this behavior, which statement indicates that the nurse's teaching was successful?
- [ ] 1. "Next time she screams and throws her legs, I will ignore the behavior."
- [ ] 2. "I will allow her to have what she wants once in a while."
- [ ] 3. "I will explain why she cannot have what she wants."
- [ ] 4. "When she behaves like this, I will tell her that she is being a bad girl."

68. The mother of a toilet-trained toddler who was admitted to the hospital for severe gastroenteritis and subsequent dehydration and is now at home asks the nurse why the child still wets the bed. What would be the nurse's **best** response?
- [ ] 1. "Hospitalization is a traumatic experience for children. Regression is common, and it takes time for them to return to their former behavior."
- [ ] 2. "The stress of hospitalization is hard for many children, but usually they have no problems when they return home."
- [ ] 3. "After returning home from being hospitalized, children still feel they should be the center of attention."
- [ ] 4. "Children do not feel comfortable in their home surroundings once they return home from being hospitalized."

The Client with Appendicitis

69. An adolescent is being seen in the clinic for abdominal pain with a fever. In what order should the nurse assess the abdomen? All options must be used.

1. auscultate

2. inspect

3. palpate

4. percuss

70. A child is admitted with a diagnosis of possible appendicitis. The child is in acute pain. Which nursing interventions would be appropriate prior to surgery to decrease pain? Select all that apply.
- [ ] 1. Offer an ice pack.
- [ ] 2. Apply a heating pad.
- [ ] 3. Encourage the child to assume a position of comfort.
- [ ] 4. Limit the child's activity.
- [ ] 5. Request a prescription for a cathartic.

71. A 10-year-old male is 24 hours postappendectomy. He is awake, alert, and oriented. He tells the nurse that he is experiencing pain. He has a prescription for morphine 1 to 2 mg PRN for pain. What is the **priority** nursing action in managing the child's pain?
- [ ] 1. Change the child's position in bed.
- [ ] 2. Obtain vital signs with a pain score.
- [ ] 3. Administer 1 mg morphine as prescribed.
- [ ] 4. Perform a head-to-toe assessment.

72. A typically developing preschool child is experiencing pain after an appendectomy. Which data collection tool is the **most** appropriate for the nurse to use to assess the pain?
- [ ] 1. visual analog scale
- [ ] 2. FLACC scale
- [ ] 3. numerical pain scale
- [ ] 4. FACES pain rating scale

73. A 7-year-old has had an appendectomy on November 12. He has had pain for the last 24 hours. There is a prescription to administer acetaminophen with codeine every 3 to 4 hours as needed. The nurse is beginning the shift, and the child is requesting pain medication. The nurse reviews the chart below for pain history. Based on the information in the medical record, what should the nurse do **next**?
- [ ] 1. Administer the acetaminophen with codeine.
- [ ] 2. Distract the child by giving him breakfast.
- [ ] 3. Instruct the child to take deep breaths and blow his pain away.
- [ ] 4. Assess the child again in 1 hour.

74. When obtaining the initial health history from a 10-year-old child with abdominal pain and suspected appendicitis, which question would be **most** helpful in eliciting data to help support the diagnosis?
- [ ] 1. "Where did the pain start?"
- [ ] 2. "What did you do for the pain?"
- [ ] 3. "How often do you have a bowel movement?"
- [ ] 4. "Is the pain continuous, or does it let up?"

75. When developing the plan of care for a school-age child with a suspected diagnosis of appendicitis who has severe abdominal pain, which measure should the nurse expect to include in the child's plan of care?
- [ ] 1. application of a heating pad
- [ ] 2. insertion of a rectal tube
- [ ] 3. application of an ice bag
- [ ] 4. administration of an intravenous narcotic

76. Which assessment finding should alert the nurse to suspect appendicitis in a male adolescent with severe abdominal pain?
- [ ] 1. Abdomen appears slightly rounded.
- [ ] 2. Bowel sounds are heard twice in 2 minutes.
- [ ] 3. All four abdominal quadrants reveal tympany.
- [ ] 4. The client demonstrates a cremasteric reflex.

77. An adolescent client scheduled for an emergency appendectomy is to be transferred directly from the emergency department to the operating room. Which statement by the client should the nurse interpret as **most** significant?
- [ ] 1. "All of a sudden, it does not hurt at all."
- [ ] 2. "The pain is centered around my navel."
- [ ] 3. "I feel like I am going to throw up."
- [ ] 4. "It hurts when you press on my stomach."

78. A nurse admits a pediatric client weighing 11.6 kg at the time of surgery for appendicitis. The nurse reviews the unit's standing prescription for IV fluids rates (see exhibit). At what hourly rate would the nurse set the IV pump?

Nurses Progress Notes

Date	Time	Progress Notes
11/12	1500	Tylenol with Codeine given PO. FACES pain scale changed from 5 to 2 within 15 minutes
11/12	1800	Tylenol with Codeine given PO. FACES pain scale changed from 5 to 2
11/12	2130	Tylenol with Codeine given PO. FACES pain scale changed from 5 to 2
11/13	0100	Tylenol with Codeine given PO. FACES pain scale changed from 4 to 1
11/13	0700	Client rates pain on FACES pain scale as 4

History	Physical	**Prescriptions**	Diagnostics

1. Start an IV of lactated Ringers.
2. Run infusion at: (100 mL for each of the first 10 kg) + (50 mL for each kg 11-20) + (20 mL for each additional kg beyond 20)/24 hours.

79. What should be the **priority** assessment for an adolescent on return to the nursing unit after an appendectomy?
- [ ] 1. the dressings on the surgical sites
- [ ] 2. intravenous fluid infusion site
- [ ] 3. nasogastric (NG) tube function
- [ ] 4. amount of pain

80. An adolescent who has had an appendectomy and developed peritonitis has nausea. Which intervention should the nurse do **first**?
- [ ] 1. Administer an antiemetic.
- [ ] 2. Irrigate the nasogastric (NG) tube.
- [ ] 3. Notify the surgeon.
- [ ] 4. Take the blood pressure.

81. When developing the postoperative plan of care for an adolescent who has undergone an appendectomy for a ruptured appendix, in which position should the nurse expect to place the client during the early postoperative period?
- [ ] 1. semi-Fowler's position
- [ ] 2. supine
- [ ] 3. lithotomy position
- [ ] 4. prone

82. What would the nurse expect as a normal response from an adolescent who has just returned to her room after an open appendectomy?
- [ ] 1. "I will need plastic surgery for this scar."
- [ ] 2. "I am worried about the size of my scar."
- [ ] 3. "I do not want to have any pain."
- [ ] 4. "What will my boyfriend say about the scar?"

83. Which client action would the nurse judge to be a healthy coping behavior for a male adolescent after an appendectomy?
- [ ] 1. insisting on wearing a T-shirt and gym shorts rather than pajamas
- [ ] 2. avoiding interactions with other adolescents on the nursing unit
- [ ] 3. refusing to fill out the menu, and allowing the nurse to do so
- [ ] 4. not taking telephone calls from friends so he can rest

84. The nurse prepares to teach an adolescent scheduled for an appendectomy about what to expect. The adolescent says, "I would rather look this up on the Internet." The nurse should:
- [ ] 1. explain that completing a teaching checklist is required by the hospital.
- [ ] 2. help the client find information on the Internet.
- [ ] 3. provide the client with written information instead.
- [ ] 4. explain that information found on the Internet cannot be trusted.

Managing Care, Quality, and Safety of Children with Health Problems of the Gastrointestinal Tract

85. The healthcare team has noticed an increase in IV infiltrations on the pediatric floor. As part of a Plan, Do, Study, Act quality improvement plan the team should perform the actions in which order? All options must be used.

1. Analyze the data.

2. Decide to monitor IV gauges.

3. Perform chart audits.

4. Write a new IV insertion policy.

86. The healthcare team wishes to establish a policy regarding sleep positions for infants with gastroesophageal reflux. The **first** step should be to search for:
- [ ] 1. policies from other hospitals.
- [ ] 2. data from retrospective studies.
- [ ] 3. published national standards.
- [ ] 4. expert opinions.

87. The nurse is assisting another member of the healthcare team who is placing a peripherally inserted catheter in a 10-year-old with peritonitis from a ruptured appendix. The family is present in the treatment room to support the child. The nurse observes that the other team member has contaminated a sterile glove. The nurse should:
- [ ] 1. discuss the incident with the team member after the event.
- [ ] 2. report the incident to the nursing unit manager.
- [ ] 3. tell the team member the glove is contaminated.
- [ ] 4. ask the family to leave before confronting the team member.

88. The hospital is responding to a mass casualty disaster with adult and pediatric victims. After reallocating staff, the charge nurse on the pediatric floor should:
☐ 1. ask parents to leave to free up the parent sleep areas for incoming victims.
☐ 2. review the census for clients that are candidates for early discharge.
☐ 3. initiate paper charting backup.
☐ 4. change taking all vital signs to every 8 hours.

89. Eight hours ago, an infant with Hirschsprung's disease had surgery to create a colostomy. Which finding should alert the nurse to notify the healthcare provider (HCP) immediately?
☐ 1. a 3-cm increase in abdominal circumference
☐ 2. periods of occasional fussiness
☐ 3. absence of bowel sounds since surgery
☐ 4. appearance of a bright red stoma

Answers, Rationales, and Test-Taking Strategies

The answers and rationales for each question follow below, along with keys (🔑*) to the client need (CN) and cognitive level (CL) for each question. In addition, you will also see a glossary icon (*📖*) highlighting specific terminology used on the licensing exam. As you check your answers, use the **Content Mastery and Test-Taking Skill Self-Analysis** worksheet (tear-out worksheet in back of book) to identify the reason(s) for not answering the questions correctly. For additional information about test-taking skills and strategies for answering questions, refer to pages 12–23 and pages 35–36 in Part 1 of this book.*

The Client with Cleft Lip and Palate

1. 3. Before corrective surgery for a cleft lip, the infant needs to consume formula or breast milk. Methods for feeding may need to be adjusted to fit the infant's needs because the infant with a cleft lip experiences a decreased ability to suck, which interferes with the infant's ability to compress the nipple. A special feeder may be used to feed the infant to ensure adequate caloric intake. Problems with infection and skin integrity in the mouth are uncommon because the areas of the defect are not open areas. Although crying may cause the infant to swallow more air because of the defect, crying poses no harm to the infant. There is no need to keep the infant's fingers out of the mouth preoperatively. The fingers will not harm the defect or cause an infection.

🔑 CN: Reduction of risk potential; CL: Synthesize

2. 1. An infant with a cleft lip and palate typically swallows large amounts of air while being fed and therefore should be burped frequently. The soft palate defect allows air to be drawn into the pharynx with each swallow of formula. The stomach becomes distended with air, and regurgitation, possibly with aspiration, is likely if the infant is not burped frequently. Feeding frequently, even in small amounts, would not prevent swallowing of large amounts of air. A nipple placed in the back of the mouth is likely to cause the infant to gag and aspirate. Holding the infant in a supine position during feedings can also lead to regurgitation and aspiration of formula. The infant should be fed in an upright position.

🔑 CN: Basic care and comfort; CL: Synthesize

3. 1. To keep the infant from disturbing the suture line by placing fingers or other objects in the mouth, either intentionally or accidentally, the restraints should be in place at all times. They should be removed for a short period, however, so that the underlying skin can be checked for any redness or breakdown. While the restraints are removed, the parents should be instructed to manually restrain the hands and arms.

🔑 CN: Safety and infection control; CL: Evaluate

4. 2. Cleft lips are typically repaired during the first 6 months of life. This allows the child to form a better seal around the nipple of a bottle for feeding and strengthens muscles needed for speech. If the surgery is delayed until after 6 months, the child may have possible dental issues and problems with sucking. The repair is not done at birth because the infant must first gain weight to safely undergo surgery. The palate should be closed by 18 months to protect the formation of tooth buds and allow the infant to develop more normal speech patterns.

🔑 CN: Management of care; CL: Analyze

5. 1. A cup is the preferred drinking or eating utensil after repair of a cleft palate. At the age when repair is done, the child is ordinarily able to drink from a cup. Use of a cup avoids having to place a utensil in the mouth, which would increase the potential for injury to the suture lines.

🔑 CN: Physiological adaptation; CL: Synthesize

The Client with Tracheoesophageal Fistula

6. 3. The drooling and excessive mucus production is highly suggestive of a tracheoesophageal fistula (TEF). The initial diagnosis is made when an orogastric catheter cannot be passed to the stomach. A lactation consult would be warranted only after determining feedings were safe to continue. While cyanosis can be a sign of sepsis and hypoglycemia, the cyanosis is most likely related to the excessive secretions and airway patency. A blood gas may be needed, but only after ruling out a TEF.

✺━ CN: Management of care; CL: Synthesize

7. 1. The parents of children born with defects often have feelings of guilt and ask what they might have done to cause the condition or how they might have avoided it. It is important to allow parents to express their feelings and to accept these feelings as normal reactions. Explaining that the parents are not at fault would not be appropriate until they have dealt with their feelings of guilt. Encouraging long-term planning generally is of little benefit to parents who are emotionally distraught. Additionally, the parents may interpret this as ignoring their feelings and confirming that they played a role in causing their child's anomaly. Urging the parents to visit their infant as often as possible would generally be of little help and could appear to the parents as though they are being "talked out" of their feelings.

✺━ CN: Psychosocial integrity;
CL: Synthesize

8. 2. Although a TEF can include several different structural anomalies, the most common type involves a blind upper pouch and a fistula from the esophagus into the trachea. Other types include a blind pouch at the end of the esophagus with no connection to the trachea and a normal trachea and esophagus with an opening that connects them. A tightened muscle below the stomach and projectile vomiting of normal amounts of formula are characteristic of pyloric stenosis. Aganglionic megacolon is a lack of autonomic parasympathetic ganglion cells in a portion of the lower intestine. Gastroschisis occurs when the bowel herniates through a defect in the abdominal wall and no membrane covers the exposed bowel.

✺━ CN: Physiological adaptation;
CL: Evaluate

9. 2. With a TEF, overflow of secretions into the larynx leads to laryngospasm. This obstruction to inspiration stimulates the strong contraction of accessory muscles of the thorax to assist the diaphragm in breathing. This produces substernal retractions. The laryngospasm that occurs with a TEF resolves quickly when secretions are removed from the oropharynx area. A barking cough is related to a relatively constant laryngeal narrowing, usually caused by edema seen with croup. It is not an indication of the need to suction. A decreased activity level and an increased respiratory rate in an infant with a TEF are usually the result of hypoxia, a relatively long-term and constant phenomenon in infants with a TEF.

✺━ CN: Physiological adaptation;
CL: Analyze

10. 1. The best way to prevent air from entering the stomach when performing a bolus feeding on an infant through a gastrostomy tube is to open the clamp after all the formula has been placed in the syringe barrel. Doing so prevents air from mixing with the formula and thus being introduced into the stomach. Pouring all the formula into the barrel after opening the clamp, maintaining a continuous flow of formula down the side of the barrel after unclamping the tube, and allowing a small amount of formula to enter the stomach before adding more formula to the barrel permit air to enter the stomach.

✺━ CN: Reduction of risk potential;
CL: Apply

11. 4. The nurse can help meet the psychological needs of an infant being fed through a gastrostomy tube by rocking the infant after a feeding. The infant soon learns to associate eating with a pleasurable experience and learns to trust the caregiver. Rocking the infant will not promote peristalsis or prevent regurgitation. Holding the baby will not relieve pressure on the surgical site. However, holding the child right after feeding promotes comfort and pleasure.

✺━ CN: Psychosocial integrity; CL: Apply

12. 4. When initiating oral feedings after surgical repair of a TEF, it is best to follow a plan of care in conjunction with observation of the infant's needs and behavior known as cue-based feedings. When sticking to a strict feeding schedule that overlooks the infant's readiness, plans are likely to be unsatisfactory and are more likely to meet the nurse's needs rather than the infant's needs. After a surgical procedure, infants initially tolerate small amounts of fluids offered more frequently better than larger amounts offered less often. Smaller amounts cause less bloating as the infant becomes used to feeding again. Although infants accept feedings more readily from their mother or from someone who feeds the infant repeatedly, the priority is to meet the infant's nutritional needs based on the infant's behavior.

✺━ CN: Basic care and comfort; CL: Create

The Client with an Anorectal Anomaly

13. 2. The nurse should honor the parent's belief system and help arrange to have the infant baptized. This may be done through the hospital's chaplaincy department or by the family's clergy. The parents may indeed be worried that the infant may die during surgery. Having the infant baptized would help address the family's spiritual needs. At this time, there is an immediate need for chaplaincy, not social service. While surgery may be postponed briefly, the infant cannot begin feeding until an outlet for stool as been established. Therefore, it is not advisable to postpone the surgery for a prolonged period of time.

　　CN: Psychosocial integrity; CL: Analyze

14. 1,3,4. Anorectal malformations present with lack of stool or evidence of meconium in the urine through a fistula. Meconium is not found in the stool. Because stool does not pass, abdominal distention and vomiting occur.

　　CN: Physiological adaptation; CL: Analyze

15. 4. Children who undergo surgical correction for low anorectal anomalies as infants usually are continent. Fecal continence can be expected after successful correction of anal membrane atresia. Therefore, this child probably has a good chance of being potty trained and will not need to wear protective pads. Extra fluids and a high-fiber diet are not required to prevent constipation. Children with high anorectal anomalies may or may not achieve continence.

　　CN: Physiological adaptation; CL: Evaluate

16. 3. After surgical repair for an imperforate anus, the infant should be positioned either supine with the legs suspended at a 90-degree angle or on either side with the hips elevated to prevent pressure on the perineum. A neonate who is placed on the abdomen pulls the legs up under the body, which puts tension on the perineum, as does positioning the neonate on the back with the legs extended straight out.

　　CN: Basic care and comfort; CL: Synthesize

17. 3. The neonate responds to pain with total body movement and brief, loud crying that ceases with distraction. After the age of 6 months, an infant reacts to pain with intense physical resistance and tries to escape by rolling away. A toddler reacts to pain by withdrawing the affected part.

　　CN: Basic care and comfort; CL: Apply

18. 2. Encouraging the parents to hold their neonate promotes parent-infant attachment. Parent-infant bonding is based on a relationship that begins when the parent first touches the infant. Both the parents and the infant have predictable steps that they go through in this process. Explaining that the parents can visit at any time promotes bonding only if they do visit with, talk to, and hold the newborn. Asking the parents to help monitor intake and output at this time may be too anxiety producing, thus interfering with bonding. Helping the parents plan for the infant's discharge involves them in the newborn's care and is important. However, it is not the first step in the development of bonding.

　　CN: Psychosocial integrity; CL: Synthesize

The Client with Pyloric Stenosis

19. 3. The vomitus of an infant with hypertrophic pyloric stenosis contains gastric contents, mucus, and streaks of blood. The vomitus does not contain bile or stool because the pyloric constriction is proximal to the ampulla of Vater.

　　CN: Physiological adaptation; CL: Analyze

20. 1. Unless the infant is in hypovolemic shock, obtaining a baseline weight is an important first action because the weight is used to calculate the child's fluid and electrolyte needs. The intravenous fluid rate and the amounts of electrolytes to be added to the fluid are based on the infant's weight. The weight also helps determine the infant's degree of dehydration. The intravenous infusion is initiated once the weight has been obtained. The child with pyloric stenosis typically experiences vomiting and is at risk for fluid volume deficit and metabolic acidosis. As a result, oral food and fluids are withheld, and the infant is allowed nothing by mouth. Fluid replacement is given intravenously. Orientation can wait until treatment is under way.

　　CN: Physiological adaptation; CL: Synthesize

21. 1. Pyloric stenosis involves hypertrophy of the pylorus muscle distal to the stomach and obstruction of the gastric outlet resulting in vomiting, metabolic acidosis, and dehydration. Telescoping of the bowel is called intussusception. Overfeeding, feeding too quickly, or underfeeding is not associated with pyloric stenosis.

　　CN: Physiological adaptation; CL: Evaluate

22. **3.** Normal serum potassium levels are 3.5 to 4.5 mEq/L (3.5 to 4.5 mmol/L). Elevated potassium levels can cause life-threatening cardiac arrhythmias. The nurse must verify that the client has the ability to clear potassium through urination before administering the drug. Infants with pyloric stenosis frequently have low potassium levels due to vomiting. A level of 3.4 mEq/L (3.4 mmol/L) is not unexpected and should be corrected with the prescribed fluids. The lab value does not need to be redrawn as the findings are consistent with the infant's condition.

🔑 CN: Pharmacological and parenteral therapies; CL: Synthesize

23. **4.** Restating or rephrasing a mother's response provides the opportunity for clarification and validation. It also helps to focus on what the mother is saying and address her concerns and feelings. Although surgery is the most effective treatment for pyloric stenosis, stating this ignores the mother's feelings and does not give her an opportunity to express them. Telling the mother not to worry also ignores the mother's feelings. Additionally, this type of statement gives the mother premature reassurance, which may turn out to be false. Asking the mother if she thinks the problem indicates that she is not a good mother implies such an idea. It does not allow her to express her concerns and feelings and therefore is not a therapeutic response.

🔑 CN: Psychosocial integrity; CL: Synthesize

24. **1.** Clear liquids containing glucose and electrolytes are usually prescribed 4 to 6 hours after surgery. If significant vomiting does not occur, formula or breast milk then can be gradually substituted for clear liquids until the infant is taking normal feedings.

🔑 CN: Physiological adaptation; CL: Evaluate

25. **4.** Giving the infant a pacifier would help meet nonnutritive sucking needs and ensure oral gratification. Additionally, sucking aids in calming the infant. Holding the infant to decrease fussiness and restlessness is more effective in an older infant. Also, the reason for the infant's fussiness needs to be explored. Hanging a mobile over the crib frequently does not decrease fussiness. After surgery to correct pyloric stenosis, feeding the infant more formula would lead to vomiting, putting additional stress on the operative site.

🔑 CN: Reduction of risk potential; CL: Synthesize

26. **2.** The parents' ability to verbalize the infant's care realistically indicates that they are working through their fears and concerns. This behavior demonstrates an understanding of the infant's condition and needs. Without further data, the fact that the parents have to get away could be interpreted as ineffective coping, possibly suggesting that they are unable to handle the situation. Continuing to ask about the child's general condition even after answers have been given does not suggest effective coping. The parents are demonstrating that they are unsure of themselves as parents or are hoping for positive information. Exhibiting fear that they will disturb the infant does not suggest effective coping. This behavior indicates that they are uncertain or lack knowledge about infants.

🔑 CN: Psychosocial integrity; CL: Analyze

27. **4.** Following pyloromyotomy, the infant should be positioned with the head elevated and slightly on the right side to promote gastric emptying; the parents have positioned their infant correctly. The infant should be positioned on the right side, not the left side. When the child is in a crib, the head can be elevated, and the infant can be propped on the right side. The infant can use a pacifier if needed.

🔑 CN: Basic care and comfort; CL: Evaluate

The Client with Intussusception

28. **2.** The infant with intussusception experiences acute episodes of colic-like abdominal pain. Typically, the infant screams and draws the knees to the chest. Between these episodes of acute abdominal pain, the infant appears comfortable and normal. Feeding does not precipitate episodes of pain. Additionally, a 4-month-old infant typically would not be ingesting solid foods. Pain exhibited by crying that occurs when the infant is placed in a reclining position, as in the mother's arms, is not associated with intussusception. This type of cry may indicate that the infant wants attention, wants to be held, or needs to have a diaper change.

🔑 CN: Physiological adaptation; CL: Analyze

29. **1.** For the infant with intussusception, stools characteristically have the appearance of currant jelly because of the intestinal inflammation and hemorrhage resulting from intestinal obstruction. These stools occur later in the course of the disease process. Questions that focus on urination, vomiting, and food intake do not elicit information about the effects of intussusception.

🔑 CN: Physiological adaptation; CL: Analyze

30. 1. The first action is to check the placement of the tube to ensure that it is in the correct position. To check tube position, the nurse should aspirate the tube with a syringe. A return of gastric contents indicates that the end of the tube is in the stomach. Another method is to inject a small amount of air while auscultating with a stethoscope over the epigastric area. The tube is irrigated with normal saline to prevent electrolyte imbalances, not distilled water, and only after the position of the tube is confirmed. The suction level should not be increased because doing so could damage the mucosa. Rotating the tube could irritate or traumatize the nasal mucosa.

⚿— CN: Reduction of risk potential; CL: Synthesize

31. 2. Development of a paralytic ileus postoperatively is a functional obstruction of the bowel. Bowel sounds initially may be hyperactive, but then they diminish and cease. Measurement of urine specific gravity provides information about fluid and electrolyte status. The first stool and the amount of gastric output provide information about the return of gastric function.

⚿— CN: Physiological adaptation; CL: Analyze

32. 1. Infants who have had an interruption in their normal routine and experiences, such as hospitalization and surgery, typically manifest behavior changes when discharged. The infant's normal routine has been significantly altered, so it will take time to reestablish another routine. Calorie requirements at home will continue to be the same as those in the hospital. The infant does not need more calories at home. The surgical procedure corrected the problems, so the infant should not continue to have abdominal cramping.

⚿— CN: Physiological adaptation; CL: Create

The Client with Inguinal Hernia

33. 1. Abdominal distention and a redness of the inguinal swelling are significant findings. Their presence in conjunction with area tenderness and inability to reduce the hernia indicate an incarcerated hernia. An incarcerated hernia can lead to strangulation, necrosis, and gangrene of the bowel. Other findings associated with strangulation include irritability, anorexia, and difficulty in defecation. A strangulated hernia necessitates immediate surgical intervention. The ability to reduce the hernia and normal stooling do not indicate it is incarcerated. Irritability is nonspecific and could be caused by various factors. A palpable, thickened spermatic cord on the affected side is diagnostic of inguinal

hernia and would be an expected finding. A wet diaper indicates that urine is being excreted, a finding unrelated to inguinal hernia.

⚿— CN: Physiological adaptation; CL: Analyze

34. 3. If nonoperative reduction is successful, delaying surgery for 2 to 3 days allows the edema and inflammation in the inguinal area to subside. Thus, the area to be operated will appear more normal, helping to decrease the risk of complications. The preoperative preparation for a herniorrhaphy is minimal and is not the reason for delaying the surgery. Typically, the infant is fed until a few hours before surgery to prevent dehydration. Trusses do not prevent incarceration, and there is no reason to use a truss preoperatively.

⚿— CN: Physiological adaptation; CL: Apply

35. 2. The best way to prepare a 7-month-old infant psychologically for surgery is to have the primary caretaker stay with the child. Infants in the second 6 months of life commonly develop separation anxiety. Therefore, the priority in this case is to support the child by having the parent present. Teaching the mother what to expect may decrease her anxiety; this is important because infants sense anxiety and distress in parents, but the priority in this case is to have the parent present. Actual play and acting out life experiences are appropriate for preschool-age children. Allowing an infant to play with surgical equipment would be inappropriate and dangerous.

⚿— CN: Psychosocial integrity; CL: Synthesize

36. 1. Changing a diaper as soon as it becomes soiled helps prevent wound infection, the most common complication after inguinal hernia repair in an infant secondary to possible wound contamination with urine and stool. Because the surgical wound is unlikely to separate, an abdominal binder is unnecessary. The incision may or may not be covered with a dressing. If a dressing is not used, the **healthcare provider (HCP)** □ may apply a topical spray to protect the wound. Restraining the infant's hands is unnecessary if the diaper is applied snugly. The infant would be unable to get the hands into the diaper close to the surgical site.

⚿— CN: Safety and infection control; CL: Create

37. 3. The incision must be kept as clean and dry as possible. Therefore, daily sponge baths are given for about 1 week postoperatively. Cleaning the infant's face and diaper area should occur at least daily and continuously, not limited to a 2-week period. Because this type of surgery results in a wound that heals through primary intention, the skin will heal and cover the wound in 2 to 3 days. Therefore, it is not necessary to use sterile gauze to cleanse the incision; clean technique is acceptable. Because the incision must be kept as clean and dry, full tub baths are inappropriate.

🔑 CN: Reduction of risk potential; CL: Synthesize

The Client with Hirschsprung's Disease

38. 2. Infants with Hirschsprung's disease typically display failure to thrive, with poor weight gain due to malabsorption of nutrients. Therefore, the nurse would expect to see a child who weighs less than that which is expected for height and age. A distended, rather than a scaphoid-shaped, abdomen would be noted. Cyanosis of fingers and toes is associated with congenital heart disease. Hyperactive deep tendon reflexes are associated with upper motor neuron problems, such as cerebral palsy.

🔑 CN: Physiological adaptation; CL: Analyze

39. 3. By encouraging parents to ask questions during information-sharing sessions, the nurse can clarify misconceptions and determine the parents' understanding of information. A better understanding of what is happening allows the parents to feel some control over the situation. Assessing the adequacy of the parents' coping skills is important but secondary to encouraging them to express their concerns. The questions they ask and their interactions with the nurse may provide clues to the adequacy of their coping skills. The nurse should never give false reassurance to parents. At this point, there is no way for the nurse to know whether the child will be fine. Written materials are appropriate for augmenting the nurse's verbal communication. However, these are secondary to encouraging questions.

🔑 CN: Psychosocial integrity; CL: Synthesize

40. 3. The primary defect in Hirschsprung's disease is an absence of autonomic parasympathetic ganglion cells in the distal portion of the colon. Thus, the nerves at the end of the large colon are missing. Absence of a rectal opening refers to an imperforate anus. A tube between the trachea and esophagus refers to a tracheoesophageal fistula. Presence of a tight muscle below the stomach refers to pyloric stenosis.

🔑 CN: Physiological adaptation; CL: Evaluate

41. 3. Before intestinal surgery, dietary intake is limited to clear liquids for 24 to 48 hours. A clear liquid diet meets the child's fluid needs and avoids the formation of fecal material in the intestine. Typically, repeated saline enemas, not tap water enemas, are given to empty the bowel. Soapsuds enemas are contraindicated for infants, as are tap water enemas. A nasogastric tube may be inserted for gastric decompression. Insertion of a gastrostomy tube is outside the scope of nursing practice. Because the perineal area is not involved in the surgery, it does not need to be prepared.

🔑 CN: Physiological adaptation; CL: Create

42. In most instances, the absence of ganglionic innervation occurs in the lower portion of the sigmoid colon just above the anus.

🔑 CN: Physiological adaptation; CL: Apply

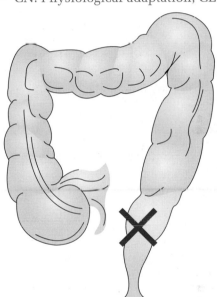

43. 2. The goal of the surgery is to remove the aganglionic portion of the intestine. The remaining intestines should have normal innervation. Colostomies are used to relieve the obstruction and allow the remaining intestines to return to normal size. A temporary loop or double-barreled colostomy has stomas for both the proximal and distal portion of the bowel. The final surgical repair is usually done when the infant is around 20 lb (9.1 kg). A new stoma is frequently swollen and bruised after surgery.

🔑 CN: Physiological adaptation; CL: Evaluate

44. 2. Typically, the stoma should remain deep red in color as long as the infant has the colostomy. A dark red to purplish color may indicate impaired circulation to the stoma.

🔑 CN: Physiological adaptation; CL: Create

45. 4. A regular diet would be recommended for the child with a colostomy; no special diet is needed. A high-fiber diet is not necessary. Fat is necessary for brain growth in the first year of life. A high-residue diet would result in bulkier stools and increased gas production, which will collect in the colostomy bag. Therefore, a high-residue diet is not indicated.

🔑 CN: Basic care and comfort;
CL: Apply

46. **2.** Toilet training is commonly more difficult for children who have undergone surgery for Hirschsprung's disease than it is for other children. This is because of the trauma to the area and the associated psychological implications. Abdominal distention is an early sign of infection, and therefore the parents need to report it to the **healthcare provider (HCP)** 📖. Typically, dietary restrictions are not required, but fiber is encouraged. Usually, the infant is placed on an age-appropriate diet. Vitamin supplementation is not necessary if the infant's dietary intake is adequate.

🔑 CN: Physiological adaptation;
CL: Evaluate

47. **3.** Popcorn is high in fiber. Foods high in fiber help the bowels move. Constipation may be managed initially with increased fiber and fluids. White bread, fruit juice, and pancakes are foods that are not high in fiber.

🔑 CN: Health promotion and maintenance;
CL: Analyze

The Client with Diarrhea, Gastroenteritis, or Dehydration

48. **3.** The infant is in need of a fluid bolus. A fluid bolus should consist of an isotonic fluid such as normal saline or lactated Ringer's. Dextrose 25% is not an appropriate bolus for dehydrated children because it could cause a fluid shift that may result in cerebral edema and death; thus, the nurse should question the prescription. D545% normal saline is an appropriate IV fluid for infants. The rate is 1.5 times maintenance for this child and is appropriate for the first 24 hours if the child is dehydrated. Once hydration is adequate, the infant's IV rate should be reduced to a maintenance rate. Vomiting is persistent, so it is appropriate for the child to be NPO. Strict I and O is an appropriate prescription for all dehydrated children.

🔑 CN: Safety and infection control;
CL: Analyze

49. **1,2,4.** Diarrhea in infants is a serious condition as it can proceed rapidly to dehydration. Clinical signs of dehydration are irritability and restlessness, weakness, stupor, loss of body weight, poor skin turgor, and sunken fontanelles. The urine output is decreased in dehydrated infants. The saliva decreases with dehydration and is not salty.

🔑 CN: Physiologic adaptation; CL: Analyze

50. **1,2,4,5.** Shigella is caused by the *Shigella* organism. Clinical manifestations of shigella include fever, nausea and vomiting, some cramping, headache, seizures, rectal prolapse, and loose, watery stools containing pus, mucus, and blood. The nurse should assess the child for these symptoms on an ongoing basis. Shigella is spread via direct contact with the organism, which is found in the stool. A stool specimen will show increased numbers of WBCs, blood, and mucus. Vomiting and loose stools can result in severe dehydration and electrolyte imbalance. Thus, the nurse should record intake, output, and daily weights. There is no need for strict isolation; masks are not needed as shigella is not transmitted by airborne methods.

🔑 CN: Physiological adaptation;
CL: Synthesize

51. **3.** The absence of tears is typically found when moderate dehydration is observed as the body attempts to conserve fluids. Other typical findings associated with moderate dehydration include a dry mouth, sunken eyes, poor skin turgor, and an increased pulse rate. Deep, rapid respirations are associated with severe dehydration. Decreased perspiration, not diaphoresis, would be seen with moderate dehydration. The specific gravity of urine increases with decreased output in the presence of dehydration.

🔑 CN: Reduction of risk potential;
CL: Analyze

52. **4.** An infant with severe diarrhea will experience some degree of dehydration. In an 8-month-old child, the anterior fontanelle has not closed. Therefore, a depressed anterior fontanelle would be an important finding. Additionally, the infant would exhibit dry mucous membranes, lethargy, hyperactive bowel sounds, dark urine, and sunken eyeballs. Skin turgor would be decreased or delayed (e.g., slow to return when pinched). Bowel sounds every 5 seconds would not be considered abnormal for an infant.

🔑 CN: Reduction of risk potential;
CL: Analyze

53. **2.** Because an infant experiencing severe diarrhea is at high risk for a fluid volume deficiency, the nurse needs to evaluate the infant's fluid balance status by weighing the infant at least every day. Body weight is the best indicator of hydration status because a higher proportion of an infant's body weight is water, compared with an adult. Initially, the infant with severe diarrhea is not allowed liquids but is given fluids intravenously. Therefore, monitoring the oral intake of formula is inappropriate. Although checking the anterior fontanelle for depression or bulging provides information about hydration status, this method is not considered the best indicator of the infant's fluid balance. Monitoring skin turgor can provide information about fluid volume status. The abdomen is commonly used to assess skin turgor in an infant because it is a large surface area and can be accessed quickly. However, weight is the best indicator of fluid balance.

⚭ CN: Physiological adaptation; CL: Synthesize

54. **8.2 mL/h**

$$4.1 \text{ kg} \times 2 \text{ mL/kg} = 8.2 \text{ mL/h}$$

⚭ CN: Pharmacological and parenteral therapies; CL: Apply

55. 2. The child is dehydrated, is not able to retain oral fluids, and continues to have diarrhea. A normal saline bolus should be given followed by maintenance of IV fluids. Antidiarrheal medications are not recommended for children and will prolong the illness. The child has gastroenteritis caused by a viral illness. IV antibiotics are not indicated for viral illnesses. Strict I&O is important in all children with gastroenteritis.

⚭ CN: Reduction of risk potential; CL: Apply

56. 1. Typically, an infant hospitalized with severe diarrhea receives fluid replacement intravenously rather than orally. Oral fluids and food are usually withheld. Although activities such as placing a mobile over the crib, speaking to the infant, or turning on the television may provide distraction for or help in calming the infant, a fussy infant receiving nothing by mouth is usually best comforted by providing a pacifier to satisfy sucking needs.

⚭ CN: Health promotion and maintenance; CL: Synthesize

57. 2. Given this infant's history of gastroenteritis, the priority problem would be fluid volume deficit. With gastroenteritis, vomiting and diarrhea occur, leading to the loss of fluids. This loss of fluids is problematic in infants because a higher proportion of their body weight is water. Pain is not a priority problem, although the nurse should continue to assess the infant for pain. There are no data to indicate impaired parenting. Impaired urinary elimination is related to the infant's fluid volume deficit resulting from vomiting and diarrhea associated with gastroenteritis. If the infant's fluid volume deficit is not corrected, then this nursing diagnosis may become the priority.

⚭ CN: Physiological adaptation; CL: Analyze

58. 1. The usual way to treat an infant hospitalized with gastroenteritis is to keep the infant nothing-by-mouth status to rest the gastrointestinal tract. The resulting fluid volume deficit is treated with intravenous fluids. When the infant's condition is controlled (e.g., when vomiting subsides), clear liquids are then started slowly. Formula and juice will be started once the infant's vomiting has subsided and the infant has demonstrated the ability to tolerate clear liquids for a period of time. In this situation, there is no need to test the infant's blood every day for anemia. Most likely, the infant's serum electrolyte levels would be monitored closely. Typically, an infant is placed in a private room because gastroenteritis is most commonly caused by a virus that is easily transmitted to others.

⚭ CN: Physiological adaptation; CL: Evaluate

59. 2. The nurse's best course of action would be to support the mother. This is best done by conveying understanding and encouraging the mother to visit or call. Telling the mother that she should not leave and that the child is very sick is critical and insensitive. Additionally, it implies guilt should the mother leave. Commenting that the child does not need anyone is not appropriate or true. Toddlers, in particular, need family members present because of the stresses associated with hospitalization. They experience separation anxiety, a normal aspect of development, and need constancy in their environment. Asking the mother to find someone else to stay with her children is inappropriate. The children at home also need the support of the mother and/or other family members to minimize the disruptions in family life resulting from the toddler's hospitalization and to maintain consistency.

⚭ CN: Psychosocial integrity; CL: Synthesize

60. **1,3,5.** Accurate intake and output recording includes noting all intake, including IV fluids; noting output, such as emesis and stool; weighing diapers; measuring weight daily; measuring urine specific gravity; monitoring serum electrolytes; and monitoring for signs of dehydration. Children who are dehydrated must receive sufficient fluid intake, but having a breast-feeding child switch to bottle-feeding will not promote intake. Restricting fluids just prior to weighing the child will not alter the accuracy of the weight, and the nurse should continue to encourage fluids for this dehydrated child.

⚭ CN: Management of care; CL: Analyze

61. 1. Potassium chloride is readily excreted in the urine. Before hanging IV fluids with potassium chloride, the nurse should ascertain whether the child can void; if not, potassium chloride may build up in the serum and cause hyperkalemia. An electrocardiogram could be done during intravenous potassium replacement therapy to evaluate for these changes. Having a stool daily is important, but because potassium is primarily excreted in the urine, the child's ability to void must be verified. Serum calcium levels do not indicate the child's ability to tolerate potassium replacement.

🔑 CN: Pharmacological and parenteral therapies; CL: Analyze

62. 3. An early sign of circulatory overload is moist rales or crackles heard when auscultating over the chest wall. Elevated blood pressure, engorged neck veins, a wide variation between fluid intake and output (with a higher intake than output), shortness of breath, increased respiratory rate, dyspnea, and cyanosis occur later.

🔑 CN: Reduction of risk potential; CL: Analyze

63. 1. After having S. *enteritidis*, some clients become chronic carriers of the causative organism and remain infectious for a long time as the organism continues to be shed from the body. During this time, the child is still considered infectious. No antitoxin is available to treat or prevent *Salmonella* infections.

🔑 CN: Physiological adaptation; CL: Evaluate

64. 1. Dietary management following rehydration for diarrhea and mild dehydration would include offering the child a regular diet. Following rehydration, there is no need for the child to be on a special diet, such as a clear liquid, full liquid, or soft diet.

🔑 CN: Basic care and comfort; CL: Evaluate

65. 3. Diarrhea related to *Salmonella* bacilli is commonly spread by raw or undercooked fowl and eggs, pet turtles, and kittens. Food poisoning caused by *Staphylococcus* species is commonly spread by inadequately cooked or refrigerated custards, cream fillings, or mayonnaise. Psittacosis, a respiratory illness, may be spread by canaries. Contaminated, unwashed fruit is associated with typhoid fever (caused by *Salmonella typhi*), a disorder rarely seen in the United States.

🔑 CN: Physiological adaptation; CL: Analyze

66. 3. The "no" behavior demonstrated by a toddler is typical of this age group as the child attempts to be self-assertive as an individual. The negativism does not demonstrate an inherited personality trait or disinterest. Rather, it reflects the developmental task of establishing autonomy. The toddler is attempting to exert control over the environment. It is too early to assess leadership qualities in a toddler.

🔑 CN: Health promotion and maintenance; CL: Analyze

67. 1. The child is demonstrating behavior associated with temper tantrums, which are relatively frequent normal occurrences during toddlerhood as the child attempts to develop a sense of autonomy. The development of autonomy requires opportunities for the child to make decisions and express individuality. Ignoring the outbursts is probably the best strategy. Doing so avoids rewarding the behavior and helps the child to learn limits, promoting the development of self-control. However, the mother should intervene in a temper tantrum if the child is likely to injure herself. Allowing the child to have what she wants occasionally would typically add to the problems associated with temper tantrums because doing so rewards the behavior and prevents the child from developing self-control. Toddlers do not possess the capacity to understand explanations about behavior. Expressing disappointment in the child's behavior or telling her that she is being a bad girl reinforces feelings of guilt and shame, thus interfering with the child's ability to develop a sense of autonomy.

🔑 CN: Health promotion and maintenance; CL: Evaluate

68. 1. Hospitalization is a traumatic time for a child, and it takes some time to readjust to the home environment. The child may regress at home for a period until she feels comfortable. Children normally do not dislike their home environment; in fact, they usually are eager to get home to familiar surroundings where they feel safe.

🔑 CN: Health promotion and maintenance; CL: Synthesize

The Client with Appendicitis

69. 2,1,4,3. The nurse should first inspect the abdomen for abnormalities. Auscultation should be done before percussion and palpation as vigorous touching may disturb the intestines. Percussion is next. Palpation is the last step as it is most likely to cause pain.

🔑 CN: Basic care and comfort; CL: Apply

70. 1,3,4. Cold is a vasoconstrictor and supplies some degree of anesthesia. The child is usually more comfortable on his side with his legs flexed to take the strain off the inflamed appendix. Limiting the child's activity puts less stress on the inflamed appendix and lessens the discomfort. Heat increases circulation to an area, causing more engorgement and pain and, possibly, rupture of the appendix. Heat is contraindicated in any situation where rupture or perforation is a possibility. A cathartic is contraindicated when appendicitis is suspected. Increasing peristalsis can cause the appendix to rupture.

⚷ CN: Physiological adaptation; CL: Synthesize

71. 2. The child is in pain and needs intervention, but before the nurse can determine how to proceed, it is essential to know the client's pain score to determine the appropriate morphine dose. In addition, the nurse cannot evaluate the effectiveness of the pain medication if there is no pain score prior to administering the medication. Changing the child's position and administering pain medication may be helpful to relieve the child's pain, but the nurse must first know the severity of the pain before determining the appropriate intervention. The nurse must perform a head-to-toe assessment, but it is not the priority in managing the child's pain.

⚷ CN: Basic care and comfort; CL: Analyze

72. 4. The nurse should use the FACES pain rating scale for children aged three or older. The visual analog and numerical scales are used preferred with adults or older children who count well. The faces, legs, activity, cry, consolability (FLACC) scale is a behavioral scale that is appropriate for very small children or nonverbal children.

⚷ CN: Basic care and comfort; CL: Analyze

73. 1. The nurse should administer the acetaminophen with codeine as the client indicates he is having pain. Although the child reports less severe pain, he is still experiencing pain. The nurse will also want the child to have less pain because he will need to be more active during the day. Assessing the child later will likely cause the pain to have increased and be more difficult to manage. While distraction is appropriate for short-term pain, such as from a needlestick or pain that the child might be able to manage himself, postoperative pain should be relieved with medication.

⚷ CN: Basic care and comfort; CL: Synthesize

74. 1. The most helpful question would be to determine the location of the pain when it started. The pain associated with appendicitis usually begins in the periumbilical area and then progresses to the right lower quadrant. After the nurse has determined the location of the pain, asking about what was done for the pain would be appropriate. Asking about the child's usual bowel movement pattern is a general question unrelated to child's condition. Children with appendicitis may have diarrhea or constipation. Additionally, knowledge about the

child's usual pattern would not be a priority because the child with appendicitis typically is not hospitalized long enough to reestablish the normal pattern. Although the characteristics of the pain are important, asking if the pain is continuous or intermittent is vague and general because the pain could be associated with numerous conditions. With appendicitis, the client's pain may begin as intermittent, but it eventually becomes continuous.

⚷ CN: Physiological adaptation; CL: Analyze

75. 3. Application of an ice bag may help to relieve pain by decreasing circulation to the area. A heating pad is contraindicated because heat may increase circulation to the appendix, possibly leading to rupture. Rectal tubes are contraindicated because they stimulate bowel motility and can exacerbate abdominal pain. Also, they would be ineffective because accumulation of gas in the lower bowel is not likely to be the cause of the child's discomfort. Because narcotics can mask the child's symptoms, such as pain and discomfort, and they also decrease bowel motility, they are not given until after a definitive diagnosis has been made.

⚷ CN: Physiological adaptation; CL: Create

76. 2. Manifestations of appendicitis include decreased or absent bowel sounds. Normally, bowel sounds are heard every 10 to 30 seconds. Therefore, bowel sounds heard twice in 2 minutes suggests appendicitis. Normally, the contour of the male adolescent abdomen is flat to slightly rounded, and tympany is typically heard when auscultating over most of the abdomen. A cremasteric reflex is normal for male adolescents.

⚷ CN: Physiological adaptation; CL: Analyze

77. 1. Sudden relief of pain in a client with appendicitis may indicate that the appendix has ruptured. Rupture relieves the pressure within the appendix but spreads the infection to the peritoneal cavity. Periumbilical pain (pain centered around the navel), vomiting, and abdominal tenderness on palpation are common findings associated with appendicitis.

⚷ CN: Physiological adaptation; CL: Analyze

78. 45 mL/h. The nurse must first calculate the daily fluid requirements for a client weighing 11.6 kg. The daily maintenance fluid volume is divided by 24 hours.

$$100 \text{ mL} \times 10 \text{ kg} = 1000 \text{ mL}$$
$$50 \text{ mL} \times 1.6 \text{ kg} = 80 \text{ mL}$$
$$1000 + 80 = 1080 \text{ mL}$$
$$1080 \text{ mL}/24 \text{ hours} = 45 \text{ mL/h}$$

⚷ CN: Pharmacological and parenteral therapies; CL: Apply

79. 1. The priority assessment after an appendectomy would be the dressing over the surgical site to determine whether there is any drainage or bleeding. If the procedure was done laparoscopically, there may be more than one incision. Any surgical dressings should be clean, dry, and intact. Once the dressing has been assessed, the nurse would assess the intravenous infusion site, assess the NG tube to be sure it is functioning, and finally, determine the degree of pain the client is experiencing.

⚠ CN: Physiological adaptation;
CL: Analyze

80. 2. After an appendectomy, the client who develops peritonitis typically has an NG tube in place. When a client has nausea, the nurse would first check to ensure that the NG tube is functioning correctly because the client's nausea may be related to a blockage of the NG tube. If the tube is clogged, it can be irrigated with normal saline. An antiemetic may be given, but only after the nurse has determined that the NG tube is functioning properly. Postoperative prescriptions usually include an antiemetic. Typically, the nurse would notify the surgeon if the client did not obtain relief from irrigation of the NG tube or administration of a prescribed antiemetic. Although taking the client's blood pressure is an important postoperative nursing activity, it is unrelated to relieving the client's nausea.

⚠ CN: Physiological adaptation;
CL: Synthesize

81. 1. After an appendectomy for a ruptured appendix, assuming the semi-Fowler's or a right side-lying position helps localize the infection. These positions promote drainage from the peritoneal cavity and decrease the incidence of subdiaphragmatic abscess.

⚠ CN: Physiological adaptation;
CL: Synthesize

82. 2. Adolescents are concerned about the immediate state and functioning of their bodies. The adolescent needs to know whether any changes (e.g., illness, trauma, surgery) will alter her lifestyle or interfere with her quest for physical perfection. Having a scar may be devastating to the adolescent. The need for plastic surgery cannot be determined at this point. The adolescent has just returned from surgery and has yet to see the scar. Healing has yet to occur. Typically, scars become smaller and fade over time. The desire for no pain is unrealistic. Although adolescents are worried about pain and how they will respond, they typically are discharged within 24 hours after an appendectomy with pain well controlled by oral analgesics. The immediate concern of adolescents is the state and functioning of their bodies. After concerns about themselves, then adolescents are concerned about their peer group and their

responses. Although the boyfriend's response will matter, this concern would be more common later in the course of the adolescent's recovery.

⚠ CN: Health promotion and maintenance;
CL: Analyze

83. 1. Adolescents struggle for independence and identity, needing to feel in control of situations and to conform to peers. Control and conformity are often manifested in appearance, including clothing, and this carries over into the hospital experience. The adolescent feels best when he is able to look and act as he normally does, for example, wearing a T-shirt and gym shorts. Adolescents normally want to interact with peers and commonly seek every opportunity to do so. Avoiding other adolescents on the nursing unit or not taking phone calls from friends might suggest ineffective coping behavior. Refusing to fill out the menu and allowing the nurse to do so demonstrate dependent behavior, not a healthy coping mechanism.

⚠ CN: Psychosocial integrity; CL: Analyze

84. 2. Part of providing client-centered care is to honor the client's preferred method of learning. The nurse should help the adolescent find accurate information about the procedure. By assisting with the information search, the nurse can verify learning. Teaching straight from a checklist does not encourage customization. If the client has requested to use the Internet, it is unlikely that written information will be read. While it is true that some information on the Internet is not accurate, the nurse can take this opportunity to help the client learn how to determine if a source is reliable.

⚠ CN: Psychosocial integrity;
CL: Synthesize

Managing Care, Quality, and Safety of Children with Health Problems of the Gastrointestinal Tract

85. 2,3,1,4. Deciding what to study and how to do it is part of the planning process. Collecting data through chart audits is part of the "do" phase. Once the chart audits are complete, the data may be "studied" or analyzed. The final step of the process, or the "act" phase, is to determine what should be done, which may include writing a new policy.

⚠ CN: Reduction of risk potential;
CL: Synthesize

86. 3. Published national standards are based on the best evidence and when available should serve as the foundation for nursing unit policies. Policies from other hospitals may or may not be evidence based. Retrospective studies and expert opinions should only be used to form policy when data from experimental studies or national standards are not available.

> ⚷ CN: Reduction of risk potential;
> CL: Synthesize

87. 3. It is the responsibility of all healthcare members to protect the client. The team member may honestly not have realized that the glove was contaminated. Therefore, the nurse needs to alert the team member to the situation. Waiting until after the procedure to address the problem puts the child at unnecessary risk for infection. Asking the parents to leave could invoke anxiety in both the child and the parents. Alerting the team member does not need to be confrontational. If done with a calm approach, the result is most likely to be gratitude instead of embarrassment.

> ⚷ CN: Reduction of risk potential;
> CL: Synthesize

88. 2. The charge nurse can anticipate needing beds for incoming victims. Any client who can go home should go home. Parents are a child's primary care givers and should not be asked to leave. If computers were not affected by the disaster, charting in the electronic health record is safer. Some routine procedures are altered during a disaster, but clients who are unstable will still need frequent assessments; reducing vital sign frequency must be considered on a case-to-case basis.

> ⚷ CN: Management of care; CL: Synthesize

89. 1. Abdominal circumference is measured to monitor for abdominal distention. An increase of 3 cm in 8 hours would require notification of the **HCP** 📖; it would indicate a substantial degree of abdominal distention, possibly from fluid or gas accumulation. Normally, after surgery, an infant experiences occasional periods of fussiness. However, as long as the infant is able to be quiet by himself or with the aid of a pacifier, the HCP does not need to be contacted. Absence of bowel sounds would be expected after surgery because of the effects of anesthesia. It takes approximately 48 hours for gastric motility to resume. New stomas are typically bright red or pink.

> ⚷ CN: Reduction of risk potential;
> CL: Synthesize

The Child with Health Problems Involving Ingestion, Nutrition, or Diet

- The Client with Toxic Substance Ingestion
- The Client with Lead Poisoning
- The Client with Celiac Disease
- The Client with Phenylketonuria
- The Client with Colic
- The Client with Obesity
- The Client with Food Sensitivity
- The Client with Failure to Thrive
- Managing Care, Quality, and Safety of Children with Health Problems Involving Ingestion, Nutrition, or Diet
- Answers, Rationales, and Test-Taking Strategies

The Client with Toxic Substance Ingestion

1. A toddler is brought to the emergency department after ingesting an undetermined amount of drain cleaner. The nurse should expect to assist with which intervention **first?**
- ☐ **1.** administering an emetic
- ☐ **2.** securing the airway
- ☐ **3.** performing gastric lavage
- ☐ **4.** inserting an indwelling urinary (Foley) catheter

2. After the acute stage following an ingestion of drain cleaner by a child, the nurse should be alert for the development of which likely complication?
- ☐ **1.** tracheal stenosis
- ☐ **2.** tracheal varices
- ☐ **3.** esophageal strictures
- ☐ **4.** esophageal diverticula

3. The parents of a 3-year-old suspect that the child has recently ingested a large amount of acetaminophen. The child does not appear in immediate distress. The nurse should anticipate doing which intervention in order of priority, from first to last? All options must be used.

1. draw acetaminophen serum levels

2. attempt to determine the exact time and amount of drug ingested

3. administer acetylcysteine IV

4. administer activated charcoal

4. When developing the plan of care for a toddler who has taken an acetaminophen overdose, which intervention should the nurse expect to include as part of the initial treatment?
- ☐ **1.** frequent blood level determinations
- ☐ **2.** gastric lavage
- ☐ **3.** tracheostomy
- ☐ **4.** electrocardiogram

5. While assessing a preschooler brought by her parents to the emergency department after ingestion of kerosene, the nurse should be alert for which complication?
- ☐ **1.** uremia
- ☐ **2.** hepatitis
- ☐ **3.** carditis
- ☐ **4.** pneumonitis

The Client with Lead Poisoning

6. Which statement by the parent of an 18-month-old child **most** indicates to the nurse that the child needs laboratory testing for lead levels?
- ☐ **1.** "My child does not always wash after playing in the dirt."
- ☐ **2.** "My child drinks two cups of milk every day."
- ☐ **3.** "My child has more temper tantrums than other kids."
- ☐ **4.** "My child is smaller than other kids of the same age."

7. In an initial screening for lead poisoning, a 2-year-old child is found to have a lead level of 10 mcg/dL (0.48 μmol/L). The nurse should:
- ☐ **1.** arrange a follow-up appointment in 6 months.
- ☐ **2.** obtain a consultation for chelation therapy.
- ☐ **3.** educate parents on ways to reduce lead in the environment.
- ☐ **4.** assure the parents this is a normal lead level.

8. When teaching the mother of a toddler diagnosed with lead poisoning, what should the nurse include as the **most** serious complication if the condition goes untreated?
- ☐ **1.** cirrhosis of the liver
- ☐ **2.** stunted growth rate
- ☐ **3.** neurologic deficits
- ☐ **4.** heart failure

9. The nurse is teaching dietary interventions to the parents of a child with an elevated blood lead level (EBLL). Which nutrient is **least** important to include in the child's diet?
- ☐ **1.** calcium
- ☐ **2.** iron
- ☐ **3.** vitamin A
- ☐ **4.** vitamin C

The Client with Celiac Disease

10. Which parent statement would suggest to the nurse that a child may have celiac disease and should be referred to a health care provider (HCP)?
- ☐ **1.** "His urine is so dark in color."
- ☐ **2.** "His stools are large and smelly."
- ☐ **3.** "His belly is so small."
- ☐ **4.** "He is so short."

11. During assessment of a child with celiac disease, the nurse would **most** likely note which physical finding?
- ☐ **1.** enlarged liver
- ☐ **2.** protuberant abdomen
- ☐ **3.** tender inguinal lymph nodes
- ☐ **4.** periorbital edema

12. After teaching the mother of a child with celiac disease about dietary management, which statement by the mother indicates successful teaching?
- ☐ **1.** "I will feed my child foods that contain wheat products."
- ☐ **2.** "I will be sure to give my child lots of milk."
- ☐ **3.** "I will plan to feed my child foods that contain rice."
- ☐ **4.** "I will be sure my child gets oatmeal every day."

13. The nurse is teaching the mother of a preschool-age child with celiac disease about a gluten-free diet. The nurse determines that the mother understands the diet if she tells the nurse she will prepare:
- ☐ **1.** eggs and orange juice.
- ☐ **2.** wheat toast and grape jelly.
- ☐ **3.** oatmeal and skim milk.
- ☐ **4.** rye toast and peanut butter.

14. Which foods would be appropriate for a 12-month-old child with celiac disease?
- ☐ **1.** oatmeal
- ☐ **2.** pancakes
- ☐ **3.** rice cereal
- ☐ **4.** waffles

15. The parent of a child with celiac disease asks, "How long must he stay on this diet?" Which response by the nurse is **best**?
- ☐ **1.** "Until the jejunal biopsy is normal."
- ☐ **2.** "Until his stools appear normal."
- ☐ **3.** "For the next 6 months."
- ☐ **4.** "For the rest of his life."

The Client with Phenylketonuria

16. When preparing to obtain a neonatal screening test for phenylketonuria (PKU), the neonate must have received which to ensure reliable results?
☐ 1. a feeding of an iron-rich formula
☐ 2. nothing by mouth for 4 hours before the test
☐ 3. initial formula or breast milk at least 24 hours before the test
☐ 4. a feeding of glucose water

17. The nurse is assessing children at risk for phenylketonuria (PKU). Which child is at greatest risk?
☐ 1. a blond, blue-eyed, fair-skinned child with eczema
☐ 2. an African American, dark-eyed child with asthma
☐ 3. a child with dark complexion who is overweight and has labile personalities
☐ 4. a red-headed child who experiences frequent contact dermatitis

18. When developing the plan of care for a child diagnosed with phenylketonuria (PKU), the nurse should establish which goal?
☐ 1. meeting the child's nutritional needs for optimal growth
☐ 2. ensuring that the special diet is started at age 3 weeks
☐ 3. maintaining serum phenylalanine level higher than 12 mg/100 mL (720 μmol/L)
☐ 4. maintaining serum phenylalanine level lower than 2 mg/100 mL (120 μmol/L)

19. When taking a diet history from the mother of a 7-year-old child with phenylketonuria, a report of an intake of which foods should cause the nurse to gather additional information?
☐ 1. diet cola
☐ 2. carrots
☐ 3. orange juice
☐ 4. bananas

20. Which foods would the nurse teach the parents of a child with phenylketonuria (PKU) to avoid? Select all that apply.
☐ 1. hamburger
☐ 2. hot dog
☐ 3. ice cream
☐ 4. juice
☐ 5. cereal

21. When teaching the mother of a child diagnosed with phenylketonuria (PKU) about its transmission, the nurse should use knowledge of which factor as the basis for the discussion?
☐ 1. chromosome translocation
☐ 2. chromosome deletion
☐ 3. autosomal recessive gene
☐ 4. X-linked recessive gene

22. A newborn diagnosed with phenylketonuria (PKU) is placed on a phenylalanine-free formula. The mother asks the nurse how long her infant will be taking this. Which response would be **most** appropriate?
☐ 1. "Until the infant is taking solid foods well."
☐ 2. "Until the child has stopped growing."
☐ 3. "Until the phenylalanine level remains below normal for 6 months."
☐ 4. "Probably for a long time, but it is not definitely known."

23. Even though several teaching sessions have been documented in the client's health record, the mother asks the nurse again what caused her child's phenylketonuria (PKU). Which statement would **best** reflect the nurse's interpretation of why the mother keeps asking for information that she has already received?
☐ 1. Because the child's condition is chronic, parents commonly want very detailed explanations about the causes of and treatments for their child's disease.
☐ 2. Parents of a chronically ill child commonly require a long time to work through the grieving process for their child's disease.
☐ 3. Parents commonly test health workers' knowledge about the causes of and treatments for their child's disease.
☐ 4. Parents commonly deal with their guilt about possibly causing their child's disease by asking challenging questions.

The Client with Colic

24. When performing the nursing history, which information would be **most** important for the nurse to obtain from the mother of an infant with suspected colic?
☐ 1. the type of formula the infant is taking
☐ 2. the infant's crying pattern
☐ 3. the infant's sleep position
☐ 4. the position of the infant during burping

25. The parents of a child with colic are asked to describe the infant's bowel movements. Which description should the nurse expect?
☐ 1. soft, yellow stools
☐ 2. frequent watery stools
☐ 3. ribbon-like stools
☐ 4. foul-smelling stools

26. The mother tells the nurse that the diagnosis of colic upsets her because she knows her infant will continue to have colicky pain. Which response by the nurse would be **most** appropriate?
- ☐ 1. "I know that your baby's crying upsets you, but she needs your undivided attention for the next few months."
- ☐ 2. "It can be difficult to listen to your baby cry so loud and so long, so try to make sure that you get some free time."
- ☐ 3. "It must be distressing to see your baby in pain, but at least she does not have an intestinal obstruction."
- ☐ 4. "The next 3 months will be a difficult time for you, but your baby will outgrow the colic by this time."

27. The nurse judges that the mother has understood the teaching about care of an infant with colic when the nurse observes the mother doing which action?
- ☐ 1. holding the infant prone while feeding
- ☐ 2. holding the infant in her lap to burp
- ☐ 3. placing the infant prone after the feeding
- ☐ 4. burping the infant during and after the feeding

The Client with Obesity

28. An 8-year-old has a body mass index (BMI) for age at the 90th percentile but has no other risk factors. The nurse should:
- ☐ 1. refer the family to a dietician.
- ☐ 2. recommend the child be reweighed in 1 year.
- ☐ 3. refer the child to a health care provider (HCP) specializing in pediatric weight loss.
- ☐ 4. recommend the child participate in a commercial diet program.

29. A parent brings a 7-month-old infant to the well-baby clinic for a check-up. The parent feeds the infant formula whenever the infant is hungry but is concerned that the infant is overweight. The nurse should instruct the parent to:
- ☐ 1. give the infant 2% milk formula and add vitamins.
- ☐ 2. use skim milk because it is high in protein and lower in calories.
- ☐ 3. decrease the amount of formula feedings to 16 oz (480 mL) daily and supplement with juice and water.
- ☐ 4. bring a 3-day record of the infant's intake back for further evaluation.

30. The nurse is providing nutrition counseling for an obese adolescent. The **most** effective method for the nurse to obtain a nutrition history from this client is to:
- ☐ 1. ask her what she knows about good nutrition.
- ☐ 2. tell her to list what she plans to eat for the next 24 hours.
- ☐ 3. ask her what she ate yesterday if it was a typical day.
- ☐ 4. telephone her mother and ask her what she ate yesterday.

31. When counseling an obese adolescent, the nurse should advise the client that which complication is the **most** common?
- ☐ 1. lifelong obesity
- ☐ 2. gastrointestinal problems
- ☐ 3. orthopedic problems
- ☐ 4. psychosocial problems

32. When developing a teaching plan for the mother of an infant about introducing solid foods into the diet, which measure should the nurse expect to include in the plan to help prevent obesity?
- ☐ 1. decreasing the amount of formula or breast milk intake as solid food intake increases
- ☐ 2. introducing the infant to the taste of vegetables by mixing them with formula or breast milk
- ☐ 3. mixing cereal and fruit in a bottle when offering solid food for the first few times
- ☐ 4. using a large-bowled spoon for feeding solid foods during the first several months

33. A pregnant mother who has brought her toddler to the clinic for a checkup asks the nurse how she can keep her next baby from becoming obese. The mother plans to bottle-feed her next child. Which information should the nurse include in the teaching plan to help the mother avoid overnourishing her infant?
- ☐ 1. recognizing clues indicating that the baby is full
- ☐ 2. establishing a regular feeding schedule
- ☐ 3. supplementing feedings with sterile water
- ☐ 4. adding more water than directed when preparing formula

The Client with Food Sensitivity

34. During a school party, a child with a known food allergy has an itchy throat, is wheezing, and is not feeling "quite right." The nurse should do what in order from first to last? All options must be used.

1. Administer the child's epinephrine.

2. Assess vital signs.

3. Position to facilitate breathing.

4. Send someone to activate the Emergency Management Systems (EMS).

5. Notify the parents.

35. After teaching the parents of a child with lactose intolerance about the disorder, the nurse determines that the teaching was effective when the mother uses which statement to describes the condition?
- ☐ 1. "The lack of an enzyme to break down lactose."
- ☐ 2. "An allergy to lactose found in milk."
- ☐ 3. "Inability to digest proteins completely."
- ☐ 4. "Inability to digest fats completely."

36. After teaching the mother of a 2-year-old child with lactose intolerance about which dairy products to include in the child's diet, which food if stated by the mother indicates effective teaching?
- ☐ 1. ice cream
- ☐ 2. creamed soups
- ☐ 3. pudding
- ☐ 4. cheese

37. The breast-feeding mother of a 1-month-old diagnosed with cow's milk sensitivity asks the nurse what she should do about feeding her infant. Which recommendation would be **most** appropriate?
- ☐ 1. "Continue to breast-feed, but eliminate all milk products from your own diet."
- ☐ 2. "Discontinue breast-feeding, and start using a predigested formula."
- ☐ 3. "Limit breast-feeding to once per day and begin feeding an iron-fortified formula."
- ☐ 4. "Change to a soy-based formula exclusively and begin solid foods."

38. The nurse teaches the parents of a preschool child diagnosed with lactose intolerance how to incorporate dairy products into their child's diet. Which statement by the parent reflects the need for more teaching?
- ☐ 1. "My child should limit milk consumption to one small glass at a time."
- ☐ 2. "It is best to drink milk alone, not with meals."
- ☐ 3. "Eating hard cheese, cottage cheese, or yogurt may cause fewer symptoms than drinking milk."
- ☐ 4. "Using lactase enzymes or milk products containing lactase may help decrease gas."

The Client with Failure to Thrive

39. The nurse is inserting a nasogastric tube in an infant to administer feedings. In the figure below, indicate the location for the correct placement of the distal end of the tube.

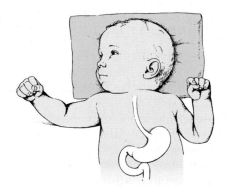

40. The nurse formulates a plan of care to address negative feeding patterns for a 5-month-old infant diagnosed with failure to thrive. To meet the short-term outcomes of the infant's plan of care, the nurse should expect to implement which intervention?
- ☐ 1. Instruct the parents in proper feeding techniques.
- ☐ 2. Give the infant high-calorie formula.
- ☐ 3. Provide consistent staff to care for the infant.
- ☐ 4. Allow the infant to sit in a highchair during feedings.

41. The health care team determines that the family of an infant with failure to thrive who is to be discharged will need follow-up care. Which approach would be the **most** effective method of follow-up?
- ☐ 1. daily phone calls from the hospital nurse
- ☐ 2. enrollment in community parenting classes
- ☐ 3. twice-weekly clinic appointments
- ☐ 4. weekly visits by a community health nurse

Managing Care, Quality, and Safety of Children with Health Problems Involving Ingestion, Nutrition, or Diet

42. When providing intermittent nasogastric feedings to an infant with failure to thrive, which method is preferred to confirm tube placement before each feeding?
☐ **1.** obtain a chest x-ray.
☐ **2.** verify that the gastric pH is less than 5.5.
☐ **3.** auscultate the stomach while instilling an air bolus.
☐ **4.** compare the tube insertion length to a standardized chart.

43. When teaching parent workshops about measures to prevent lead poisoning in children, which preventive measure should the nurse include as the **most** effective?
☐ **1.** condemning old housing developments
☐ **2.** educating the public on common sources of lead
☐ **3.** educating the public on the importance of good nutrition
☐ **4.** keeping pregnant women out of old homes that are being remodeled

44. A child with a nut allergy presents with a severe reaction for the third time in 3 months. The parent says, "I am having trouble with the food labels." The nurse should **first**:
☐ **1.** assess the parent's ability to read.
☐ **2.** refer the client to the dietician.
☐ **3.** notify the health care provider (HCP).
☐ **4.** obtain a social service consult.

Answers, Rationales, and Test-Taking Strategies

*The answers and the rationales for each question follow below, along with keys (🔑) to the client need (CN) and cognitive level (CL) for each question. In addition, you will also see a glossary icon (📖) highlighting specific terminology used on the licensing exam. As you check your answers, use the **Content Mastery and Test-Taking Skill Self-Analysis** worksheet (tear-out worksheet in back of book) to identify the reason(s) for not answering the questions correctly. For additional information about test-taking skills and strategies for answering questions, refer to pages 12–23 and pages 35–36 in Part 1 of this book.*

The Client with Toxic Substance Ingestion

1. 2. Drain cleaner almost always contains lye, which can burn the mouth, pharynx, and esophagus on ingestion. The nurse would be prepared to assist with procedures to secure the airway, which may include intubation or performing a tracheostomy. An emetic is contraindicated because, as the substance burns on ingestion, so too would it burn when vomiting. Additionally, the mucosa becomes necrotic, and vomiting could lead to perforations. Gastric lavage is contraindicated because the mucosa is burned from the ingestion of the caustic lye, causing necrosis. Gastric lavage also could lead to perforation of the necrotic mucosa. Insertion of an indwelling urinary (Foley) catheter would be indicated after the measures to remove the caustic substance have been started.

🔑 CN: Reduction of risk potential; CL: Apply

2. 3. As the burn from the lye ingestion heals, scar tissue develops and can lead to esophageal strictures, a common complication of lye ingestion. Tracheal stenosis would occur if the child had vomited and aspirated. Tracheal varices do not commonly occur after the ingestion of lye or other substances. Although very rare, esophageal diverticula may occur. Diverticula are commonly found in the colon of adults.

🔑 CN: Physiological adaptation; CL: Analyze

3. 2,4,1,3. The nurse should **first** attempt to determine exactly when and how much acetaminophen the parents think the child has taken. Determining the time of ingestion helps establish the immediate care and when lab values should be drawn. Gastric decontamination with activated charcoal is used within 4 hours of ingestion to bind the drug and help prevent toxic serum levels. Serum blood levels should be done after the gastric decontamination, but preferably not too soon after ingestion since levels drawn before 4 hours may not reflect maximum serum concentrations and will need to be repeated. The decision to administer acetylcysteine and prevent liver damage is based on serum levels.

🔑 CN: Pharmacological and parenteral therapies; CL: Synthesize

4. 2. Initial management of a child who has ingested a large amount of acetaminophen would include inducing vomiting or performing gastric lavage with or without activated charcoal to aid in the removal of the substance. Frequent blood level determinations may be obtained during the follow-up phase, but they are not done as part of the initial treatment. Tracheostomy is not typically part of the initial treatment for acetaminophen overdose. However, it may be necessary later if respiratory distress develops. Acetaminophen primarily affects the liver, not the heart. Therefore, an electrocardiogram would not be considered part of the initial treatment plan.

⚷ CN: Reduction of risk potential;
CL: Apply

5. 4. Chemical pneumonitis is the most common complication of ingestion of hydrocarbons, such as in kerosene. The pneumonitis is caused by irritation from the hydrocarbons aspirated into the lungs. Uremia is the result of renal insufficiency, which causes nitrogenous waste products to build up in the blood rather than being excreted. Hepatitis is caused by a viral infection. Carditis in a preschooler may be the result of rheumatic fever.

⚷ CN: Physiological adaptation;
CL: Analyze

The Client with Lead Poisoning

6. 1. Eating with dirty hands, especially after playing outside, can cause lead poisoning because lead is often present in soil surrounding homes. Also, children who eat lead-containing paint chips commonly develop lead poisoning. Milk is a major source of calcium, and diets high in calcium help prevent lead poisoning. Temper tantrums are characteristic of 18-month-old children as they try to assert themselves. Determining whether the child is smaller than other children the same age requires measuring height and weight and plotting them on growth charts. In addition, inadequate growth could be a result of numerous causes, such as genetics, chronic illness, or chronic drug use (e.g., prednisone).

⚷ CN: Physiological adaptation;
CL: Evaluate

7. 3. Treatment for children with minimally elevated lead levels should include family lead education, follow-up testing, and a social service consultation if needed. Waiting 6 months for a follow-up screening is too long because the effects of lead are irreversible. Oral chelation therapy is not begun until levels approach 45 mcg/dL (2.2 μmol/L). There is no such thing as a "normal" lead level because there is no beneficial action in the body.

⚷ CN: Safety and infection control;
CL: Synthesize

8. 3. The most serious and irreversible consequence of lead poisoning is neurologic changes leading to an intellectual disability. It can be expected if lead poisoning is long-standing and goes untreated. Lead poisoning also affects the hematologic and renal systems. Cirrhosis is the end stage of several chronic liver diseases, such as biliary atresia and hepatitis. Lead poisoning is not associated with stunted growth. Chronic illnesses, such as cystic fibrosis, cause slowing of the growth velocity. Heart failure is associated with congenital heart disease and rheumatic fever.

⚷ CN: Physiological adaptation; CL: Apply

9. 3. Vitamin A is not known to play a significant role in preventing EBLL. Calcium intake inhibits lead absorption. Children with EBLL levels often are anemic. While this relationship is not well understood, iron supplementation has been shown to improve developmental outcomes. Vitamin C improves iron absorption.

⚷ CN: Health promotion and maintenance;
CL: Analyze

The Client with Celiac Disease

10. 2. Celiac disease is a disorder involving intolerance to the protein gluten, which is found in wheat, rye, oats, and barley. The stools of a child with celiac disease are characteristically malodorous, pale, large (bulky), and soft (loose). Excessive flatus is common, and bouts of diarrhea may occur. Dark urine is commonly associated with concentrated urine, such as when a child has dehydration. The belly of a child with celiac disease, a malabsorption disorder, typically is protuberant. A small belly may be associated with a child who is thin. Short stature is not associated with this malabsorption disorder.

⚷ CN: Physiological adaptation;
CL: Analyze

11. 2. The intestines of a child with celiac disease fill with accumulated undigested food and flatus, causing the characteristic protuberant abdomen. Celiac disease is not usually associated with any liver dysfunction, including poor liver functioning leading to liver enlargement. Tender inguinal lymph nodes are often associated with an infection. Periorbital edema, swelling around the eyes, is associated with nephritis.

⚷ CN: Physiological adaptation;
CL: Analyze

12. 3. Damage to intestinal mucosa in celiac disease is caused by gliadin, a part of the gluten protein found in wheat, rye, barley, and oats. Foods containing these grains must be eliminated entirely from the diet of children with celiac disease. Foods containing rice and corn are a good substitute. Although an adequate intake of milk is important for any child, children with celiac disease do not need an increased milk intake.

CN: Physiological adaptation;
CL: Evaluate

13. 1. Children with celiac disease cannot digest the protein in common grains such as wheat, rye, and oats. Eggs and orange juice would be appropriate foods.

CN: Basic care and comfort; CL Evaluate

14. 3. The child with celiac disease should not eat foods containing wheat, oats, rye, or barley. Pancakes and waffles are made from flour that typically is derived from wheat and therefore should be avoided. Foods containing rice, such as rice cereal, or corn are appropriate. Pancakes and waffles are made from flour that typically is derived from wheat and therefore should be avoided.

CN: Physiological adaptation;
CL: Synthesize

15. 4. Most children with celiac disease have a lifelong sensitivity to gluten, which requires that they maintain some type of diet restriction for the rest of their lives.

CN: Physiological adaptation;
CL: Synthesize

The Client with Phenylketonuria

16. 3. PKU is an autosomal recessive disorder involving the absence of an enzyme needed to metabolize the essential amino acid phenylalanine to tyrosine. To ensure reliable results, the neonate must have ingested sufficient protein, such as breast milk or formula, for at least 24 hours. Testing the infant before that time, excessive vomiting, or poor intake can yield false-negative results. The infant does not need to fast 4 hours before the test. A loading dose of glucose water does not affect test values.

CN: Reduction of risk potential;
CL: Evaluate

17. 1. Infants with PKU are usually blond, blue-eyed, and fair and often have eczema. The other physical assessment findings are not typically found in children with PKU.

CN: Reduction of risk potential
CL: Analyze

18. 1. The goal of care is to prevent intellectual disabilities by adjusting the diet to meet the infant's nutritional needs for optimal growth. The diet needs to be started upon diagnosis, ideally within a few days of birth. Serum phenylalanine level should be maintained between 3 and 7 mg/100 mL (180 to 420 µmol/L). Significant brain damage usually occurs if the level exceeds 10 to 15 mg/100 mL (600 to 900 µmol/L). If the level drops below 2 mg/100 mL (120 µmol/L), the body begins to catabolize its protein stores, causing growth restriction.

CN: Physiological adaptation; CL: Create

19. 1. Foods with low phenylalanine levels include vegetables, fruits, and juices. Foods high in phenylalanine include meats and dairy products, which must be restricted or eliminated. Diet colas contain more phenylalanine than the fruits listed.

CN: Physiological adaptation;
CL: Analyze

20. 1,2,3. Children with PKU lack an enzyme to metabolize phenylalanine and convert it to tyrosine. Treatment is dietary management to control the amount of phenylalanine ingested. Foods with low phenylalanine levels include fruits, most vegetables, and cereals. High-protein foods have high levels of phenylalanine and include meats and dairy products.

CN: Reduction of risk potential;
CL: Create

21. 3. PKU is caused by an inborn error of metabolism. It is an autosomal recessive disorder that inhibits the conversion of phenylalanine to tyrosine. A form of Down syndrome, trisomy 21, is an example of a disorder caused by chromosomal translocation. Cri du chat is an example of a disorder caused by chromosomal deletion. Hemophilia A is an example of a disorder caused by an X-linked recessive gene.

CN: Physiological adaptation; CL: Apply

22. 4. Although it is not known how long diet therapy must continue for children with PKU, many experts suggest continuing it indefinitely because of academic difficulties and lower intelligence quotients in older children who have stopped the restrictive diet. For women, it is necessary to resume the diet before conception to lower the phenylalanine levels in the fetus and prevent complications.

CN: Physiological adaptation;
CL: Synthesize

23. 2. PKU is considered a chronic illness. Parents typically grieve about the loss of health in their child afflicted with a chronic disease. Many times, they repeat questions, as though trying to

The Client with Hydrocele

7. During a clinic visit, the mother of an infant with hydrocele states that the infant's scrotum is smaller now than when he was born. After teaching the mother about the infant's condition, which statement by the mother indicates that the teaching has been effective?
- ☐ **1.** "I guess keeping his bottom up has helped."
- ☐ **2.** "Massaging his groin area is working."
- ☐ **3.** "It seems like the fluid is being reabsorbed."
- ☐ **4.** "Keeping him quiet and in an infant seat has helped."

8. Shortly after an infant is returned to his room following hydrocele repair, the infant's parent approaches the nurse in the hall to report that the child's scrotum looks swollen and bruised. Which response by the nurse would be **most** appropriate?
- ☐ **1.** "Let me see if the surgeon has prescribed aspirin for him. If he did, I will get it right away."
- ☐ **2.** "Can you wait in his room? Then you can ask me any questions when I get there."
- ☐ **3.** "What you are describing is unusual after this type of surgery. I will let the surgeon know."
- ☐ **4.** "This is normal after this type of surgery. Let us look at it together just to be sure."

The Client with Hypospadias

9. The parents of a neonate with hypospadias and chordee wish to have him circumcised. Which explanation should the nurse incorporate into the discussion with the parents concerning the recommendation to delay circumcision?
- ☐ **1.** The associated chordee is difficult to remove during circumcision.
- ☐ **2.** The foreskin is used to repair the deformity surgically.
- ☐ **3.** The meatus can become stenosed, leading to urinary obstruction.
- ☐ **4.** The infant is too small to have a circumcision.

10. The nurse is caring for an infant with hypospadias. Identify the area where the nurse would assess for this condition.

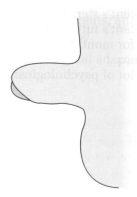

11. A 1-year-old child is scheduled for surgery to correct hypospadias and chordee. The nurse explains to the parents that this is the preferred time for surgical repair based on which factor?
- ☐ **1.** At this age, the child will experience less pain.
- ☐ **2.** The child is too young to have developed castration anxiety.
- ☐ **3.** The child will not remember the surgical experience.
- ☐ **4.** The repair is easier to perform after the child is toilet trained.

12. A 6-month-old child is discharged with a urinary stent after a procedure to repair a hypospadias. The nurse should tell the parents to:
- ☐ **1.** avoid tub baths until the stent is removed.
- ☐ **2.** measure output in the urinary bag.
- ☐ **3.** avoid giving fruit juice.
- ☐ **4.** clean the tip of the penis three times a day with soap and water.

13. After teaching the parents about the urethral catheter placed after surgical repair of their son's hypospadias, the nurse determines that the teaching was successful when the mother states that the catheter in her child's penis accomplishes which goal?
- ☐ **1.** decreases pain at the surgical site
- ☐ **2.** keeps the new urethra from closing
- ☐ **3.** measures his urine correctly
- ☐ **4.** prevents bladder spasms

14. While assessing the penis of a child who has had surgery for repair of a hypospadias, the nurse observes the appearance of the penis. The nurse should report which aspect to the surgeon?
- ☐ **1.** swollen
- ☐ **2.** dusky blue at the tip
- ☐ **3.** somewhat misshapen
- ☐ **4.** pink

15. When developing the teaching plan for the parents of a 12-month-old infant with hypospadias and chordee repair, what information is **most** important to include?
- ☐ **1.** Assist the child to become familiar with his dressings so he will leave them alone.
- ☐ **2.** Encourage the child to ambulate as soon as possible by using a favorite push toy.
- ☐ **3.** Force fluids to at least 2,500 mL/day by offering his favorite juices.
- ☐ **4.** Prevent the child from disrupting the catheters by using soft restraints.

16. The healthcare provider (HCP) prescribes a urinalysis for a child who has undergone surgical repair of a hypospadias. Which results should the nurse report to the HCP?
- ☐ **1.** urine specific gravity of 1.017
- ☐ **2.** ten red blood cells per high-powered field
- ☐ **3.** twenty-five white blood cells per high-powered field
- ☐ **4.** urine pH of 6.0

The Client with Urinary Tract Infection

17. A teenage girl has been diagnosed with a urinary tract infection. The nurse recognizes the need for teaching when the teenager states:
☐ 1. "I will not take bubble baths."
☐ 2. "I will drink plenty of water."
☐ 3. "I can drink coffee."
☐ 4. "I can drink cranberry juice."

18. A 4-year-old with a history of urinary reflux returned from surgery for bilateral urethral reimplants 2 days ago. Which assessment finding is **most** concerning?
☐ 1. intermittent bladder spasms
☐ 2. small amounts of blood-tinged urine
☐ 3. decreased oral intake
☐ 4. continuous drainage from a Foley catheter

19. The healthcare provider (HCP) has prescribed a sterile urine specimen for a 3-year-old boy with a history of recurrent urinary tract infections. The family is upset because the last time the child was catheterized, the procedure was very painful and traumatic. The nurse should tell the family:
☐ 1. "I will request a prescription for a sedative to help him relax."
☐ 2. "I cannot do anything to reduce the pain, but you can hold him during the procedure."
☐ 3. "I will get a prescription for a lidocaine lubricant with numbing medicine to make the procedure more comfortable."
☐ 4. "I can apply a topical anesthetic 20 minutes before placing the catheter."

20. The parents of a child on sulfamethoxazole and trimethoprim for a urinary tract infection report that the child has a red, blistery rash. The nurse should tell the parents to:
☐ 1. apply lotion to the affected areas.
☐ 2. discontinue the medicine and come for immediate further evaluation.
☐ 3. use sunblock while on the medication.
☐ 4. increase the child's fluid intake.

21. A recent history of which problem should alert the nurse to gather additional information about the possibility of a urinary tract infection in a 2-year-old child who is exhibiting fever and fussiness?
☐ 1. abdominal pain
☐ 2. swollen lymph glands
☐ 3. skin rash
☐ 4. back pain

22. A father of a child with a urinary tract infection calls the clinic and explains, "My wife and I are concerned because our child refuses to obey us concerning the preventions you told us about. Our child refuses to take the medication unless we buy a present. We do not want to use discipline because of the illness, but we are worried about the behavior." Which response by the nurse is **best**?
☐ 1. "I sympathize with your difficulties, but just ignore the behavior for now."
☐ 2. "I understand it is hard to discipline a child who is ill, but things need to be kept as normal as possible."
☐ 3. "I understand that things are difficult for you right now, but your child is ill and deserves special treatment."
☐ 4. "I understand your concern, but this type of behavior happens all the time; your child will get over it when feeling better."

23. A nurse is teaching the parents of a child diagnosed with a urinary tract infection secondary to vesicoureteral reflux. How should the nurse explain how the reflux contributes to the infection?
☐ 1. "It prevents complete emptying of the bladder."
☐ 2. "It causes urine backflow into the kidney."
☐ 3. "It results in painful bladder spasms."
☐ 4. "It causes painful urination."

The Client with Glomerulonephritis

24. A 15-year-old has been diagnosed with acute glomerulonephritis and has been in the hospital for 1 day. Which finding requires **immediate** action?
☐ 1. large amount of generalized edema
☐ 2. urine specific gravity of 1.030
☐ 3. large amount of albumin in the urine
☐ 4. 24-hour output of 1,500 mL

25. Which meal would be **most** appropriate for a 15-year-old with glomerulonephritis with severe hypertension?
☐ 1. egg noodles, hamburger, canned peas, milk
☐ 2. baked ham, baked potato, pear, canned carrots, milk
☐ 3. baked chicken, rice, beans, orange juice
☐ 4. hot dog on a bun, corn chips, pickle, cookie, milk

26. A 10-year-old with glomerulonephritis reports a headache and blurred vision. The nurse should **immediately**:
☐ 1. put the client to bed.
☐ 2. obtain the child's blood pressure.
☐ 3. notify the healthcare provider (HCP).
☐ 4. administer acetaminophen.

27. Which question should the nurse ask **first** when obtaining a history from the mother of a 10-year-old child with a fever, malaise, and swelling around the eyes?
☐ 1. "Has the child had a sore throat recently?"
☐ 2. "Is the child playing with friends as usual?"
☐ 3. "Does the child urinate as much as usual?"
☐ 4. "Is the urine pale in color?"

28. A school-age client admitted to the hospital because of decreased urine output and periorbital edema is diagnosed with acute poststreptococcal glomerulonephritis. Which assessment gives the nurse the **best** indication of the child's fluid balance?
☐ 1. Assess vital signs every 4 hours.
☐ 2. Monitor intake and output every 12 hours.
☐ 3. Obtain daily weight measurements.
☐ 4. Obtain serum electrolyte levels daily.

29. When developing the plan of care for a school-age child with acute poststreptococcal glomerulonephritis who has a fluid restriction of 1,000 mL/day, which fluid should the nurse consider as **most** appropriate for the client's condition and effective for preventing excessive thirst?
☐ 1. diet cola
☐ 2. ice chips
☐ 3. lemonade
☐ 4. tap water

30. The nurse is planning interventions for a school-age child hospitalized with acute poststreptococcal glomerulonephritis in need of diversional activity. Which activity should the nurse expect to include?
☐ 1. playing a card game with someone the same age
☐ 2. putting together a puzzle with mother
☐ 3. playing video games with a 4-year-old
☐ 4. watching a movie with a younger brother

31. A 10-year-old child hospitalized with acute poststreptococcal glomerulonephritis during the acute stage has elevated blood pressure and low urine output for 14 hours. The nurse should **next**:
☐ 1. assess the child's neurologic status.
☐ 2. encourage the child to drink more water.
☐ 3. advise the child to eat a low-sodium breakfast.
☐ 4. help the client to ambulate in the hallway.

32. When developing the discharge plan for a school-age child diagnosed with acute poststreptococcal glomerulonephritis, which instruction should the nurse plan to discuss?
☐ 1. Restrict dietary protein.
☐ 2. Monitor pulse rate and rhythm.
☐ 3. Prevent respiratory infections.
☐ 4. Restrict foods high in potassium.

33. An adolescent with a history of losing weight and fatigue is admitted to the hospital with a diagnosis of stage I chronic renal failure. The chart shows:

Intake and Output

Day 1: Intake 1,850 mL   Output 1,550 mL
Day 2: Intake 2,200 mL   Output 1,150 mL

Based on these findings, the nurse should:
☐ 1. continue monitoring intake and output.
☐ 2. notify the healthcare provider (HCP).
☐ 3. restrict the client's fluids.
☐ 4. increase the client's fluids.

34. A parent of a child with acute poststreptococcal glomerulonephritis (APSGN) asks how a strep infection caused the child to have a kidney problem. What is the nurse's **best** response?
☐ 1. "The streptococcal infection spread through the bloodstream to your child's kidneys."
☐ 2. "Your child made excessive antibodies to fight the infection that are now attacking the kidneys."
☐ 3. "By-products of immune complexes that fought the infection are depositing in the kidneys."
☐ 4. "The strep infection weakened your child's immune system, making him susceptible to a secondary infection."

The Client with Nephrotic Syndrome

35. A child with nephrosis is taking prednisone. The nurse should teach the caregivers to report which adverse effects? Select all that apply.
☐ 1. increased urinary output
☐ 2. hematemesis
☐ 3. respiratory infection
☐ 4. bleeding gums
☐ 5. vision problems

36. The nurse is caring for a 5-year-old boy who is taking prednisolone for nephrotic syndrome. The child is at the 75th percentile for height and has a blood pressure of 114/73 mm Hg. The nurse compares the reading to the below blood pressure levels for boys age and height percentiles.

The nurse determines that the blood pressure represents a change and notifies the healthcare provider (HCP) of the assessment of:
- ☐ **1.** hypotension.
- ☐ **2.** prehypertension.
- ☐ **3.** hypertension.
- ☐ **4.** hypertension stage II.

| | Systolic BP Reading | | | | | | | Diastolic BP Reading | | | | | | |
| | ◄—Percentile for Height—► | | | | | | | ◄—Percentile for height—► | | | | | | |
Age Percentile	5th	10th	25th	50th	75th	90th	95th	5th	10th	25th	50th	75th	90th	95th
50th	90	91	93	95	96	98	98	50	51	52	53	54	55	55
90th	104	105	106	108	110	111	112	65	66	67	68	69	69	70
95th	108	109	110	112	114	115	116	69	70	71	72	73	74	74
99th	115	116	118	120	121	123	123	77	78	79	80	81	81	82

37. The charge nurse is reviewing the laboratory results of a child admitted with nephrotic syndrome with a nurse new to the pediatric unit. The nurse is aware that teaching is required when the new nurse states that an expected finding in nephrotic syndrome is:
- ☐ **1.** hyperalbuminemia.
- ☐ **2.** elevated triglycerides.
- ☐ **3.** elevated cholesterol.
- ☐ **4.** proteinuria.

38. Which statement by the parent of a toddler diagnosed with nephrotic syndrome indicates that the parent has understood the nurse's teaching about this disease?
- ☐ **1.** "My child really likes chips and bologna. I guess we will have to find something else."
- ☐ **2.** "We will have to encourage lots of liquids. Did you say about 4 L every day?"
- ☐ **3.** "We worry about the surgery. Do you think we should do direct donation of blood?"
- ☐ **4** "We understand the need for antibiotics. I just wish the antibiotics could be given by mouth."

39. A toddler diagnosed with nephrotic syndrome has a fluid volume excess related to fluid accumulation in the tissues. Which measure should the nurse anticipate including in the child's plan of care?
- ☐ **1.** Limit visitors to 2 to 3 hours a day.
- ☐ **2.** Maintain strict bed rest.
- ☐ **3.** Test urine specific gravity every shift.
- ☐ **4.** Weigh the child before breakfast.

40. The parent of a toddler with nephrotic syndrome asks the nurse what can be done about the child's swollen eyes. Which measure should the nurse suggest?
- ☐ **1.** Apply cool compresses to the child's eyes.
- ☐ **2.** Elevate the head of the child's bed.
- ☐ **3.** Apply eyedrops every 8 hours.
- ☐ **4.** Limit the child's television watching.

41. The nurse determines that interventions for decreasing fluid retention have been effective when the nurse makes which assessment in a child with nephrotic syndrome?
- ☐ **1.** decreased abdominal girth
- ☐ **2.** increased caloric intake
- ☐ **3.** increased respiratory rate
- ☐ **4.** decreased heart rate

42. The toddler with nephrotic syndrome exhibits generalized edema. Which measure should the nurse institute for this child with impaired skin integrity related to edema?
- ☐ **1.** Ambulate every shift while awake.
- ☐ **2.** Apply lotion on opposing skin surfaces.
- ☐ **3.** Apply powder to skinfolds.
- ☐ **4.** Separate opposing skin surfaces with soft cloth.

43. A child with nephrosis is placed on prednisone. The dose is 2 mg/kg/day to be administered twice a day. The child weighs 25 lb (11.3 kg). How many milligrams will the child receive at each dose? Record your answer using one decimal place.

_____ mg.

44. The toddler with nephrotic syndrome responds to treatment and is ready to go home. When helping the family plan for home care, which instruction should the nurse include in the teaching?
- ☐ **1.** Administer pain medication as needed.
- ☐ **2.** Keep the child away from others with an infection.
- ☐ **3.** Notify the healthcare provider (HCP) if there is an increase in the child's urine output.
- ☐ **4.** Administer acetaminophen daily.

The Client with Acute or Chronic Renal Failure

45. The nurse is planning care with the parents of a child who requires continuous peritoneal dialysis. Which finding should be discussed with the healthcare provider (HCP)?
- ☐ **1.** The family lives a long distance from the medical facility.
- ☐ **2.** The child attends a large public school.
- ☐ **3.** The child reports having a previous surgery for a ruptured appendix.
- ☐ **4.** The family feels the child cannot self-regulate to wake at night and change bags.

46. While performing daily peritoneal dialysis and catheter exit site care with the mother of a child with chronic renal failure, which information would be an important step to emphasize to the mother?
- [ ] 1. Apply an occlusive dressing after cleaning the site.
- [ ] 2. Change the dressing when the peritoneal space is dry.
- [ ] 3. Examine the site for signs of infection while cleaning the area.
- [ ] 4. Pull on the catheter to hold taut while cleaning the skin.

47. When developing the discharge teaching plan for a child with chronic renal failure and the family, the nurse should emphasize restriction of which nutrient?
- [ ] 1. ascorbic acid
- [ ] 2. calcium
- [ ] 3. magnesium
- [ ] 4. phosphorus

48. After emphasizing to an adolescent with renal failure the importance of maintaining a positive self-concept, which behavior by the adolescent should the nurse identify as an indicator that the plan is working?
- [ ] 1. reports of headaches, abdominal pain, and nausea
- [ ] 2. insistence on making diet choices even if the foods chosen are restricted
- [ ] 3. verbalization of plans to quit all after-school activities when returning home
- [ ] 4. demonstration of desire to do the dressing changes and take care of the medications

49. Which diet plan would be appropriate for the nurse to discuss with the family of a child with acute renal failure?
- [ ] 1. high carbohydrate and protein
- [ ] 2. high fat and carbohydrate
- [ ] 3. low fat and protein
- [ ] 4. low carbohydrate and fat

50. An adolescent with chronic renal failure is scheduled to go home with a peritoneal dialysis catheter in place. When developing the discharge teaching plan for the client and the family focusing on psychosocial needs, which area should be a **priority** to include?
- [ ] 1. advantages of limiting social activities and contacts for the first few months
- [ ] 2. not disclosing information about the peritoneal dialysis to people outside the family
- [ ] 3. possible effect on body image of the presence of an abdominal catheter
- [ ] 4. importance of relying on parents to do the dialysis and dressing changes

51. During a home visit, the public health nurse assesses the peritoneal catheter exit site of a child with chronic renal failure. Which finding should lead the nurse to determine a client has an infection?
- [ ] 1. dialysate leakage
- [ ] 2. granulation tissue
- [ ] 3. increased time for drainage
- [ ] 4. tissue swelling

52. After teaching the parent of a young child with a peritoneal catheter about the signs and symptoms of peritonitis, the nurse determines that the parent has understood the teaching when she identifies which finding as an important sign?
- [ ] 1. cloudy dialysate drainage return
- [ ] 2. distended abdomen
- [ ] 3. shortness of breath
- [ ] 4. weight gain of 3 lb (1.36 kg) in 2 days

53. The nurse assesses the child with chronic renal failure who is receiving peritoneal dialysis for edema. Which finding is expected for this child?
- [ ] 1. absence of pulmonary crackles
- [ ] 2. increased dialysate outflow
- [ ] 3. normal blood pressure
- [ ] 4. pallor

54. The parent of a child with chronic renal failure who is receiving peritoneal dialysis at home asks the nurse what she can do if both inflow and drain times are increased. Which instructions would be **most** appropriate for the nurse to include when responding to the parent?
- [ ] 1. Assess the child for constipation.
- [ ] 2. Decrease the amount of dialysate infused for each dwell.
- [ ] 3. Incorporate the increased inflow and drain times into the dialysis schedule.
- [ ] 4. Monitor the child for shoulder pain during inflow and drain times.

55. The nurse judges that the mother understands the diet restrictions for her child with chronic renal failure who is receiving peritoneal dialysis when she reports providing a diet involving which components?
- [ ] 1. sodium and water restrictions
- [ ] 2. high protein and carbohydrates
- [ ] 3. high potassium and iron
- [ ] 4. protein and phosphorous restrictions

The Client with Wilms' Tumor

56. A 3-year-old child receiving chemotherapy after surgery for a Wilms' tumor has developed neutropenia. The parent is trying to encourage the child to eat by bringing extra foods to the room. Which food would **not** be appropriate for this child?
- [ ] 1. fudge
- [ ] 2. French fries
- [ ] 3. fresh strawberries
- [ ] 4. a milk shake

57. When assessing a 2-year-old child with Wilms' tumor, what should the nurse avoid?
- ☐ 1. measuring the child's chest circumference
- ☐ 2. palpating the child's abdomen
- ☐ 3. placing the child in an upright position
- ☐ 4. measuring the child's occipitofrontal circumference

58. Which statement by the parent of a child with Wilms' tumor tells the nurse that the parent understands what *stage II tumor* means?
- ☐ 1. "The tumor has extended beyond the kidney but was completely removed."
- ☐ 2. "Although the tumor was in the kidney, it has spread to the lung, liver, and bone."
- ☐ 3. "The tumor has extended outside the kidney to the lungs and the liver."
- ☐ 4. "The tumor was solely located in the kidney, but it was totally removed."

59. A child diagnosed with Wilms' tumor undergoes successful surgery for removal of the diseased kidney. When the child returns to the room, the nurse should place the child in which position?
- ☐ 1. modified Trendelenburg
- ☐ 2. Sims'
- ☐ 3. semi-Fowler's
- ☐ 4. supine

60. After a child undergoes nephrectomy for a Wilms' tumor, the nurse should assess the child postoperatively for which early sign of a complication?
- ☐ 1. increased abdominal distention
- ☐ 2. elevated blood pressure
- ☐ 3. increased respiratory rate
- ☐ 4. increased urine output

61. When developing the discharge plan for a child who had a nephrectomy for a Wilms' tumor, the nurse identifies outcomes to prevent damage to the child's remaining kidney and to accomplish which goal?
- ☐ 1. Minimize pain.
- ☐ 2. Prevent dependent edema.
- ☐ 3. Prevent urinary tract infection.
- ☐ 4. Minimize sodium intake.

Managing Care, Quality, and Safety of Children with Health Problems of the Urinary System

62. The nurse reads the new medication prescriptions for a 4-year-old child with nephrotic syndrome on the chart below:

Prescriptions

D/C prednisolone 40 mg PO Daily
Prednisolone 30 mg PO QOD

The nurse should:
- ☐ 1. discontinue the prednisolone 40 mg and give the 30-mg dose today.
- ☐ 2. check the medication record first to see when the last dose of prednisolone was given.
- ☐ 3. start the 30-mg dose tomorrow.
- ☐ 4. contact the prescriber for clarification.

63. The charge nurse finds the mother of a child with a chronic bladder condition requiring clean intermittent catheterization (CIC) visibly upset. The mother states, "That other nurse said parents are not allowed to perform CIC in the hospital because of increased infection risk." The charge nurse should tell the parent:
- ☐ 1. "Your child is exposed to additional bacterial in the hospital that makes CIC unsafe."
- ☐ 2. "You can catheterize your child as long as you use sterile technique."
- ☐ 3. "You can use CIC on your child. I will talk with your nurse to clarify the policy."
- ☐ 4. "I can tell you are having a conflict with this nurse. I will switch assignments."

64. The parent of an 18-year-old with chronic renal disease states, "My son has so many problems. I am really worried that he will not get the right care if he gets sick at college." The nurse should tell the parent:
- ☐ 1. "I can have his records sent to the school's health center."
- ☐ 2. "Make sure your son always carries his nephrologist's phone number."
- ☐ 3. "Your son can make an e-health history to facilitate his care if he gets sick away from home."
- ☐ 4. "Your son is going to need to learn to manage his own disease."

Answers, Rationales, and Test-Taking Strategies

The answers and the rationales for each question follow below, along with keys (🔑) to the client need (CN) and cognitive level (CL) for each question. In addition, you will also see a glossary icon (📖) highlighting specific terminology used on the licensing exam. As you check your answers, use the **Content Mastery and Test-Taking Skill Self-Analysis** *worksheet (tear-out worksheet in back of book) to identify the reason(s) for not answering the questions correctly. For additional information about test-taking skills and strategies for answering questions, refer to pages 12–23 and pages 35–36 in Part 1 of this book.*

The Client with Cryptorchidism

1. 4. Normally, the testes descend by 1 year of age; failure to do so may indicate a problem with patency or a hormonal imbalance. By age 4 weeks, descent may not have occurred. However, telling the father that lack of descent is not a cause for worry is inappropriate and uncaring. Additionally, a statement such as this may be false reassurance. By acknowledging the father's concern, the nurse indicates acceptance of his feelings. If the testes have not descended, then they will not be palpable in the scrotal sac. Surgery is not discussed until after a full assessment is completed.

🔑 CN: Health promotion and maintenance; CL: Synthesize

2. 3. A cold environment can cause the testes to retract. Cold and touch stimulate the cremasteric reflex, which causes a normal retraction of the testes toward the body. Therefore, the nurse should warm the hands and make sure that the environment also is warm. Checking the diaper for urination provides information about the infant's voiding and urinary function, not information about the testes. Giving the infant a pacifier may help to calm the infant and possibly make the examination easier, but the concern here is with the temperature of the environment. Tapping on the inguinal ring would not be helpful in assessing the infant.

🔑 CN: Health promotion and maintenance; CL: Synthesize

3. 2. The nurse needs more information about the father's perceptions and feelings before providing any information or taking action. Determining the exact nature of the father's concern rather than making an assumption about it is essential. Therefore, the nurse should identify what is observed and ask the father how he is feeling. Telling the father that everything will be fine or not to worry is inappropriate and provides false reassurance. It

also devalues the father's concern. Later on, it may be appropriate for the father to talk to a parent of a child with the same problem for support.

🔑 CN: Psychosocial integrity; CL: Synthesize

4. 3. When an anomaly is found in one system, such as the genitourinary system, that system requires a more focused assessment to reveal other conditions that also may be occurring. A bulging in the inguinal area may suggest an inguinal hernia. Also, hydrocele or an upper urinary tract anomaly may occur on the same side as the undescended testis. A neuromuscular problem, not a genitourinary problem such as undescended testes, would most likely be the cause of abnormal lower extremity reflexes. A history of frequent emesis may be caused by pyloric stenosis or viral gastroenteritis. Poor weight gain might suggest a metabolic or a feeding problem.

🔑 CN: Health promotion and maintenance; CL: Analyze

5. 2. Preoperative teaching would be directed at the parents because the child is too young to understand the teaching. Telling the child that his penis and scrotum will be "fixed," telling the child he will not see incisions after surgery, and using a doll to illustrate the surgery are appropriate interventions for a preschool-age child.

🔑 CN: Psychosocial integrity; CL: Create

6. 3. Because the incidence of testicular cancer is increased in adulthood among children who have had undescended testes, it is extremely important to teach the adolescent how to perform the testicular self-examination monthly. The undescended testicle is removed to reduce the risk of cancer in that testicle. Removal of a testis would not necessarily make the adolescent sterile because the other testicle remains. Although discussing the adolescent's future plans is important, it is not the priority at this time. Because the adolescent has been dealing with the situation for a long time, the need for a sports physical at this time should not be a cause of emotional distress requiring a lot of psychological support.

🔑 CN: Health promotion and maintenance; CL: Synthesize

The Client with Hydrocele

7. 3. A hydrocele is a collection of fluid in the tunica vaginalis of the testicle or along the spermatic cord that results from a patent processus vaginalis. As fluid is being absorbed, scrotal size decreases. Elevation of the infant's bottom, massage, or keeping the infant quiet or in an infant seat would have no effect in promoting fluid reabsorption in hydrocele.

🔑 CN: Physiological adaptation; CL: Evaluate

8. 4. Some swelling and bruising are normal postoperatively. By assessing the area with the mother, the nurse is conveying acceptance of the mother's concern. In addition, the nurse needs to inspect the area to determine if what the mother is describing is accurate. Doing so also provides an opportunity for teaching. Aspirin is not usually prescribed for children because of the link between aspirin and Reye's syndrome. Acetaminophen is commonly administered for fever or pain relief. Asking the mother to wait in the child's room ignores the mother's concerns. There is no need to notify the surgeon at this time.

CN: Psychosocial integrity;
CL: Synthesize

The Client with Hypospadias

9. 2. The condition in which the urethral opening is on the ventral side of the penis or below the glans penis is referred to as *hypospadias*. *Chordee* refers to a ventral curvature of the penis that results from a fibrous band of tissue that has replaced normal tissue. Circumcision is delayed because the foreskin, which is removed with a circumcision, often is used to reconstruct the urethra. The chordee is corrected when the hypospadias is repaired. Circumcision is performed at the same time. Urethral meatal stenosis, which can occur in circumcised infants, results from meatal ulceration, possibly leading to urinary obstruction. It is not associated with hypospadias or circumcision. The infant is not too small to have a circumcision, which is commonly performed on the first or the second day of life.

CN: Reduction of risk potential;
CL: Apply

10. In hypospadias, the urethral opening is on the ventral side of the penis.

CN: Physiological adaptation;
CL: Apply

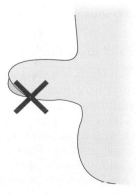

11. 2. The preferred time for surgery is between the ages of 6 and 18 months, before the child develops castration and body image anxiety. Children learn early on about society's emphasis on the importance of genitals. Pain is different for each child and is not related to the preferred time for repair of the hypospadias or chordee. Although the child will probably not remember the experience, this is not the basis for having the surgery at this age. If the condition is not repaired, the child will have difficulty with toilet training because urine is not eliminated through the tip of the penis.

CN: Physiological adaptation;
CL: Apply

12. 1. The parents should keep the penis as dry as possible until the stent is removed. Soaking in a tub bath is not recommended. Children this age typically go home voiding directly into a diaper. Infants may be started on juice at 6 months of age. Parents are advised to keep their child well hydrated after a hypospadias repair. Therefore, there is no reason to avoid juice. Cleaning the tip of the penis three times a day may cause unnecessary irritation.

CN: Safety and infection control;
CL: Synthesize

13. 2. The main purpose of the urethral catheter is to maintain patency of the reconstructed urethra. The catheter prevents the new tissue inside the urethra from healing on itself. However, the urethral catheter can cause bladder spasms. Recently, stents have been used instead of catheters. The urethral catheter will have no effect on the child's pain level. In fact, because bladder spasms are associated with its use, the child's problems of pain may actually increase. Urine output can be measured through the suprapubic catheter because it provides an alternative route for urinary elimination, thus keeping the bladder empty and pressure-free.

CN: Reduction of risk potential;
CL: Evaluate

14. 2. A dusky blue color at the tip of the penis may indicate a problem with circulation, and the nurse should notify the surgeon. Following surgery, it is normal for the penis to be swollen and pink. The penis may be misshapen and is unlikely to look normal even after reconstruction.

CN: Physiological adaptation;
CL: Analyze

15. 4. The most important consideration for a successful outcome of this surgery is maintenance of the catheters or stents. A 12-month-old infant likes to explore his environment but must be prevented from manipulating his dressings or catheters through the use of soft restraints. Allowing the infant to become familiar with the dressings will not prevent him from pulling at them. After surgery the child is allowed limited activity, possibly while sitting in the parent's lap. A 12-month-old infant may or may not be walking. If he is, most likely he will be clumsy and possibly injure himself. Although increasing fluids is important, 2,500 mL/day is an excessive amount for a 12-month-old. Fluid requirements would be 115 mL/kg.

CN: Physiological adaptation;
CL: Create

16. **3.** A normal white blood cell count in a urinalysis is 1 to 2 cells/mL. A white blood cell count of 25 per high-powered field indicates a urinary tract infection. A urine specific gravity of 1.017 is within the normal range of 1.002 to 1.030. After urologic surgery, it is not unusual for a small number of red blood cells to appear in the urine. The child's urine pH is within the normal range of 4.6 to 8.

CN: Reduction of risk potential;
CL: Analyze

The Client with Urinary Tract Infection

17. **3.** Drinking coffee and other beverages that contain caffeine can irritate the bladder and should be avoided. Bubble baths, bath oils, and hot tubs can irritate the urethra and perineal area. Drinking plenty of water will keep urine flushed through the bladder. Cranberry juice helps to acidify the urine.

CN: Health promotion and maintenance;
CL: Evaluate

18. **3.** Children with bilateral ureteral implants often have pain with urination due to bladder spasms. Some children will avoid drinking in order to avoid the pain associated with urination, thus putting the child at risk for dehydration. Intermittent bladder spasms are common after ureteral reimplant surgery and can be treated with oxybutynin to decrease discomfort. Small amounts of blood-tinged urine, bladder spasms, urinary frequency, and urinary incontinence are common following ureteral reimplant surgery.

CN: Physiological adaptation;
CL: Analyze

19. **3.** Two percent lidocaine lubricants have been found to significantly reduce the pain of urinary catheter insertion in children. If the unit does not have a standing protocol to use the lubricant, the nurse should request a prescription. A sedative would carry with it additional risks that could be avoided with the use of other methods to reduce pain. The parents should be encouraged to hold the child in addition to other pain relief methods. Frequent urination would make the use of topical anesthetics that must be left in place for a period of time impractical.

CN: Basic care and comfort;
CL: Synthesize

20. **2.** Sulfonamides have been associated with severe adverse reactions. A blistering rash may be a sign of Stevens-Johnson syndrome, a severe allergic reaction that manifests as skin lesions. This reaction is life threatening and requires immediate attention. Lotion should not be applied to skin with blisters. Sulfamethoxazole and trimethoprim may cause photosensitivity, but this usually appears as a mild red rash, not blisters. Increasing the child's fluid intake may help the urinary tract infection, but does not address the rash.

CN: Pharmacological and parenteral therapies; CL: Synthesize

21. **1.** Abdominal pain frequently accompanies urinary tract infection in children 2 years of age and older. Other associated signs and symptoms include decreased appetite, vomiting, fever, and irritability. The presence of swollen lymph glands (lymphadenopathy) is unrelated to urinary tract infections. Lymphadenopathy is associated with a systemic infection or possibly cancer. Skin rash is associated with exposure to allergens or irritants (e.g., poison ivy or harsh soaps); prolonged contact with urine (e.g., diaper dermatitis); or illnesses such as measles, rheumatic fever, or juvenile rheumatoid arthritis. Flank or back pain is associated with urinary tract infection in children older than 2 years of age and in adults.

CN: Physiological adaptation;
CL: Analyze

22. **2.** To ensure appropriate psychosocial development, a child needs to have normal patterns maintained as much as possible during illness. It is tempting to give ill children special treatment and to relax discipline. However, family routines and discipline should be kept as normal as possible. The child needs to know the limits to ensure feelings of security. When they are ill, children commonly attempt to stretch the rules and limits. If this occurs, returning to the previous well-behavior patterns will take time.

CN: Health promotion and maintenance;
CL: Synthesize

23. **1.** The reason that urinary tract infections are a problem in children with vesicoureteral reflux is that urine flows back up the ureter, past the incompetent valve, and back into the bladder after the child has finished voiding. This incomplete emptying of the bladder results in stasis of urine, providing a good medium for bacterial growth and subsequent infection. Vesicoureteral reflux does not cause bladder spasms or painful urination. However, the child may experience painful urination with a urinary tract infection.

🔑 CN: Physiological adaptation;
CL: Apply

The Client with Glomerulonephritis

24. 2. An adolescent with acute glomerulonephritis has a high urine specific gravity related to oliguria caused by inflammation of the glomeruli. The client will have periorbital edema, but not the generalized edema that occurs in nephrotic syndrome. In glomerulonephritis, there is some albumin in the urine, but there are large amounts of red blood cells, giving the urine a brown color. The urine in glomerulonephritis is scanty, averaging about 400 mL in 24 hours, which leads to fluid volume excess and hypertension.

🔑 CN: Physiological adaptation;
CL: Synthesize

25. 3. The best selection of food would include no added salt or salty food. Because sodium cannot be excreted due to the oliguria and to avoid increasing the hypertension, a low-salt diet is recommended. Most canned foods have sodium added as a preservative. Ham, hot dogs, canned peas, canned carrots, corn chips, pickles, and milk are high in sodium.

🔑 CN: Health promotion and maintenance;
CL: Synthesize

26. 2. Hypertension occurs with acute glomerulonephritis. The symptoms of headache and blurred vision may indicate an elevated blood pressure. Hypertension in acute glomerulonephritis occurs due to the inability of the kidneys to remove fluid and sodium; the fluid is reabsorbed, causing fluid volume excess. The nurse must verify that these symptoms are due to hypertension. Calling the **HCP** 📖 before confirming the cause of the symptoms would not facilitate his treatment. Putting the client to bed may help treat an elevated blood pressure, but first, the nurse must establish that high blood pressure is the cause of the symptoms. Administering acetaminophen for high blood pressure is not recommended.

🔑 CN: Physiological adaptation;
CL: Synthesize

27. 3. Most likely, the nurse suspects that the child is exhibiting signs and symptoms of glomerulonephritis, such as periorbital edema and fever. Other signs and symptoms include loss of appetite, dark-colored urine, pallor, headaches, and abdominal pain. To confirm this suspicion, the nurse would ask about the child's urinary elimination patterns.

Typically, the child with glomerulonephritis experiences a decrease in urine output. Asking about any recent sore throat would provide additional information to confirm the suspicion of glomerulonephritis, because the most common type is acute poststreptococcal glomerulonephritis, which follows a strep throat by 10 to 14 days. Frequently, the children have only mild cold symptoms and do not realize they have a streptococcal infection. Asking whether the child plays with friends as usual is important and gives the nurse information about how the child feels in general. However, this is a general question that would be appropriate to ask later on in the history. Although asking the mother about the color of the child's urine is important, the nurse needs to determine whether there is any change in the child's urinary output first.

🔑 CN: Physiological adaptation;
CL: Analyze

28. 3. The child with acute poststreptococcal glomerulonephritis experiences a problem with renal function that ultimately affects fluid balance. While intake and output, electrolytes, and vital signs all provide information about fluid status, weight is the best indicator of fluid balance.

🔑 CN: Physiological adaptation;
CL: Analyze

29. 2. The most appropriate and effective choice would be ice chips because they help moisten the mouth and lips while keeping fluid intake low. However, ice chips must still be counted as intake with the fluid restriction. Sweet beverages, such as diet cola or lemonade, commonly increase thirst. Tap water effectively relieves thirst but does not help keep fluid intake low.

🔑 CN: Physiological adaptation;
CL: Synthesize

30. 1. Generally, school-age children enjoy activities with their peers first, then family members, and lastly younger children. School-age children like to be busy but also to accomplish something. This helps to meet their task of industry versus inferiority, feeling good about what they are able to accomplish.

🔑 CN: Health promotion and maintenance;
CL: Create

31. 1. The nurse should assess the child's neurologic status because hypertensive encephalopathy is a major potential complication of the acute phase of glomerulonephritis. Seizure precautions also should be instituted. Hypertensive encephalopathy can result in transient loss of vision, hemiparesis, disorientation, and grand mal seizures. Encouraging the child to drink more water is inappropriate because the child has had a low urine output for

14 hours. Typically, in this situation, fluids would be restricted. Although a low-sodium diet is encouraged, it is not the priority action at this time. Initially, bed rest, not ambulation, is advocated during the acute phase of glomerulonephritis.

🔑 CN: Reduction of risk potential;
CL: Synthesize

32. 3. Children recovering from glomerulonephritis need to avoid exposure to all types of infections. Glomerulonephritis is caused by group A beta hemolytic streptococcus, a common cause of sore throat. As the child recovers, he or she may be susceptible to a recurrence if exposed to the organism again. During convalescence from glomerulonephritis, fluid and dietary restrictions are no longer indicated because the kidneys are now functioning normally. There is no need for the parents to assess the child's vital signs.

🔑 CN: Physiological adaptation;
CL: Synthesize

33. 2. The nurse would expect a person with a normal glomerular filtration rate (GFR) to have approximately equal inputs and outputs. Chronic renal failure has five stages. In stage I, the GFR is approximately ≥90 mL/min/1.73 m². In stage II, the GFR decreases to approximately 60 to 89 mL/min/1.73 m². The decreased urine output may indicate worsening disease and should be reported. Assessing the client's intake and output is still important, but notifying the provider is the priority. Fluids are restricted based on decreased sodium. Clients are encouraged to drink to thirst. Therefore, there is not enough information to suggest increasing or restricting fluids.

🔑 CN: Physiological adaptation;
CL: Synthesize

34. 3. APSGN is an immune complex disease. Large antigen-antibody complexes are formed that deposit in the glomerular capillary loops leading to obstruction. APSGN is considered an autoimmune disorder, not an infection. Antibodies do not attack the kidneys in this disorder.

🔑 CN: Physiologic adaptation; CL: Analyze

The Client with Nephrotic Syndrome

35. 2,3,5. Adverse effects of steroid therapy include edema of the face and trunk, increased susceptibility to infection, gastric and intestinal mucosal bleeding, sodium and water retention, and hypertension. Steroid therapy can also cause vision problems. Urinary output is decreased due to the retention of sodium. Bleeding gums do not result from steroids.

🔑 CN: Pharmacological and parenteral therapies; CL: Create

36. 3. Readings at or above the 95th percentile are considered indicative of hypertension. Here, both the systolic and diastolic readings are at the 95th percentile for a boy who is at the 75th percentile for height. This blood pressure may be a side effect of the medication or part of the disease process and needs to be reported. The charts do not define hypotension. Readings below the 90th percentile are considered normal. Blood pressures at the 90th percentile but below the 95th are considered prehypertension. Blood pressures at the 99th percentile are considered stage II hypertension and are most likely to need antihypertensive medications.

🔑 CN: Reduction of risk potential;
CL: Analyze

37. 1. The child with nephrotic syndrome would present with hypoalbuminemia due to a decrease of albumin in the bloodstream and to the increase in the glomerular permeability. Nephrotic syndrome is characterized by edema, massive proteinuria, hypoalbuminemia, hypoproteinemia, hyperlipidemia, and altered immunity.

🔑 CN: Reduction of risk potential;
CL: Evaluate

38. 1. Children with nephrotic syndrome usually require sodium restriction. Because potato chips and bologna are high in sodium, the mother's statement about finding something else reflects understanding of this need. Although fluid intake is not restricted in children with nephrotic syndrome, 4 L is an excessive amount for a toddler. The typical fluid requirement for a toddler is 115 mL/kg. Surgical intervention and antibiotic therapy are not parts of the treatment plan for nephrotic syndrome.

🔑 CN: Physiological adaptation;
CL: Evaluate

39. 4. The best indicator of fluid balance is weight. Therefore, daily weight measurements help determine fluid losses and gains. Although limiting visitors to 2 to 3 hours per day or maintaining strict bed rest would help to ensure that the child gets adequate rest, this is unrelated to the child's fluid balance. In nephrotic syndrome, urine is tested for protein, not specific gravity.

🔑 CN: Physiological adaptation;
CL: Synthesize

40. 2. The child's swollen eyes are caused by fluid accumulation. Elevating the head of the bed allows gravity to increase the downward flow of fluids in the body, away from the face. Applying cool compresses or eyedrops, or limiting television, may be comforting but will not relieve the swelling.

🔑 CN: Physiological adaptation;
CL: Synthesize

41. 1. Fluid accumulates in the abdomen and interstitial spaces owing to hydrostatic pressure changes. Increased abdominal fluid is evidenced by an increase in abdominal girth. Therefore, decreased abdominal girth is a sign of reduced fluid in the third spaces and tissues. When fluid accumulates in the abdomen and interstitial spaces, the child does not feel hungry and does not eat well. Although increased caloric intake may indicate decreased intestinal edema, it is not the best and most accurate indicator of fluid retention. Increased respiratory rate may be an indication of increasing fluid in the abdomen (ascites) causing pressure on the diaphragm. Heart rate usually stays in the normal range even with excessive fluid volume.

CN: Physiological adaptation; CL: Evaluate

42. 4. Placing soft cloth between opposing skin surfaces absorbs moisture and keeps the area dry, thus preventing any further breakdown. The child with nephrotic syndrome and severe edema is usually maintained on bed rest. Therefore, ambulation is not appropriate. Applying lotion or powder to edematous surfaces that touch increases moisture and can lead to maceration, causing further breakdown.

CN: Basic care and comfort; CL: Synthesize

43. 11.3 mg

$$11.3 \text{ kg} \times 2 \text{ mg} = 22.7 \text{ mg/day}$$
$$22.7 \text{ mg} \div 2 = 11.3 \text{ mg per dose}$$

CN: Pharmacological and parenteral therapies; CL: Apply

44. 2. A child recovering from nephrotic syndrome should be protected from infection. Therefore, the nurse would teach the parents to keep the child away from others with an infection. Because pain is not associated with this disorder, pain medication typically is not needed. The **HCP** 📖 should be notified if urine output decreases, not increases. In children recovering from nephrotic syndrome, there is no reason to administer acetaminophen daily.

CN: Reduction of risk potential; CL: Synthesize

The Client with Acute or Chronic Renal Failure

45. 3. A client who has had a ruptured appendix may have peritoneal scarring that may alter the effectiveness of treatment. Living a long distance from a medical facility is typically a reason to select peritoneal dialysis. Attending a large school is not a problem, but the school nurse needs to be included as part of the healthcare team. Typically, the treatment schedule can be planned to allow for uninterrupted sleep at night.

CN: Management of care; CL: Create

46. 3. Until it heals, the catheter exit site is particularly vulnerable to invasion by pathogenic organisms. Therefore, the site must be monitored for signs of infection. An occlusive dressing is not needed because there is no danger of air being sucked in or out of the peritoneal space. Furthermore, the catheter used is designed with a cuff so that the skin grows around the catheter, sealing off the area. Site care may be done at any time, but the child may experience abdominal discomfort if the peritoneal space is dry during site care. Holding the catheter taut or pulling on it may cause irritation of the skin at the exit site, which could lead to infection.

CN: Safety and infection control; CL: Synthesize

47. 4. With minimal or absent kidney function, the serum phosphate level rises, and the ionized calcium level falls in response. This causes increased secretion of parathyroid hormone, which releases calcium from the bones. Therefore, the intake of foods high in phosphorus is restricted. Because renal failure results in decreased erythropoietin production, an increase in ascorbic acid intake is needed. Because magnesium is minimally affected by renal failure, its intake need not be restricted.

CN: Physiological adaptation; CL: Apply

48. 4. Demonstration of desire to do the dressing changes and manage medications implies compliance with the medical regimen and acceptance of the condition, thereby indicating a positive self-image. Diffuse somatic symptoms could indicate anxiety or problems with coping, with a negative effect on self-concept. Insistence on choosing restricted foods implies that the adolescent has not accepted the diagnosis and is noncompliant, possibly indicating a negative self-concept. Social withdrawal from activities may indicate depression, possibly negatively affecting the self-concept.

CN: Physiological adaptation; CL: Evaluate

49. 2. The child with acute renal failure needs extra calories to reduce tissue catabolism, metabolic acidosis, and uremia. Using a high-fat and high-carbohydrate diet helps to supply the necessary extra calories. If the child is able to tolerate oral foods, concentrated food sources that are high in carbohydrate and fat but low in protein, potassium, and sodium may be provided.

CN: Physiological adaptation; CL: Apply

50. 3. For an adolescent, body image is a major concern. The presence of an abdominal catheter can greatly affect the client's body image. The adolescent needs opportunities to discuss feelings about altered body image due to the catheter. Adolescents need to be with their peers and to maintain social activities and contacts in order to meet the developmental tasks for this age group. The adolescent client may choose to confide in friends for both psychological health and physical safety. Because peers are most important to adolescents, they will confide in their peers before confiding in family members. Another major developmental need of the adolescent is achieving independence. Relying on the parents would interfere with the adolescent's ability to do so.

☞ CN: Psychosocial integrity; CL: Create

51. 4. Tissue swelling, pain, redness, and exudate indicate infection. Dialysate leakage is associated with improper catheter function, incomplete healing at the insertion site, or excessive instillation of dialysate. Granulation tissue indicates healing around the exit site, not infection. Increased time for drainage may indicate that the tube is kinked, suggesting an obstruction.

☞ CN: Reduction of risk potential; CL: Analyze

52. 1. Normally, dialysate drainage return should be clear. With peritonitis, large numbers of bacteria, white blood cells, and fibrin cause the dialysate to appear cloudy. Abdominal distention is unrelated to peritonitis. However, it might suggest an obstruction. Weight gain and shortness of breath are associated with fluid excess, not infection.

☞ CN: Physiological adaptation; CL: Evaluate

53. 4. With edema, pallor can occur owing to hemodilution as intestinal fluid moves to the vascular space. The child would exhibit pulmonary crackles secondary to pulmonary congestion and edema. Dialysate outflow would decrease, not increase, as the body attempts to conserve fluid. The child's blood pressure would be increased because of excessive fluid volume.

☞ CN: Physiological adaptation; CL: Analyze

54. 1. Accumulation of hard stool in the bowel can cause the distended intestine to block the holes of the catheter. Consequently, the dialysate cannot flow freely through the catheter. Decreasing the dialysate infusion may make the dialysis less effective. Altering fluid, electrolyte, and waste product removal can cause fluid and electrolyte imbalance and increased levels of blood urea nitrogen and creatinine. Incorporating the increased times into the dialysis may make the dialysis less effective because fewer cycles can be scheduled. Shoulder pain, which may occur occasionally, can be caused by air in the peritoneal space and diaphragmatic irritation. However, it is unrelated to inflow and drain times.

☞ CN: Physiological adaptation; CL: Synthesize

55. 4. Regulation of the diet is the most effective means, besides dialysis, for reducing renal excretion. Dietary phosphorus is restricted, which reduces the protein load on the kidneys. Clients are also given substances to bind phosphorus in the intestines to prevent absorption. Limited protein in the diet should include foods high in essential amino acids. Foods high in fat and carbohydrate are used to increase caloric intake. Sodium and water may not be restricted because of the continual loss of sodium and water through the dialysate. Iron-rich foods are commonly high in protein.

☞ CN: Physiological adaptation; CL: Evaluate

The Client with Wilms' Tumor

56. 3. When a client receiving chemotherapy develops neutropenia, eating uncooked fruits and vegetables may pose a health risk due to possible bacterial contamination. All other foods are either cooked or pasteurized and would not produce a health risk.

☞ CN: Safety and infection control; CL: Apply

57. 2. The abdomen of the child with Wilms' tumor should not be palpated because of the danger of disseminating tumor cells. Techniques such as measuring the occipitofrontal circumference (which is done in children younger than 18 months of age because the anterior fontanelle closes between 12 and 18 months of age), upright positioning, and measuring chest circumference are not necessarily contraindicated; however, the child with Wilms' tumor should always be handled gently and carefully.

☞ CN: Physiological adaptation; CL: Analyze

58. 1. A stage II tumor is one that extends beyond the kidney but is completely resected. The tumor staging is verified during surgery to maximize treatment protocols. The following criteria for staging are commonly used: *stage I*, tumor is limited to the kidney and completely resected; *stage II*, tumor extends beyond the kidney but is completely resected; *stage III*, residual nonhematogenous tumor is confined to the abdomen; *stage IV*, hematogenous metastasis occurs, with deposits beyond stage III (lung, bone and brain, liver); and *stage V*, bilateral renal involvement is present at diagnosis.

☞ CN: Physiological adaptation; CL: Evaluate

59. 3. The child who has undergone abdominal surgery is usually placed in a semi-Fowler's position to facilitate draining of abdominal contents and promote pulmonary expansion. The modified Trendelenburg position is used for clients in shock. The Sims' position is likely to be uncomfortable for this child because of the large transabdominal incision. The supine position, without the head elevated, puts the child at increased risk for aspiration.

⚿ CN: Reduction of risk potential;
CL: Synthesize

60. 1. Children who have undergone abdominal surgery are at risk for intestinal obstruction from a dynamic ileus. Indications of intestinal obstruction include abdominal distention, decreased or absent bowel sounds, and vomiting. Later signs of intestinal obstruction include tachycardia, fever, hypotension, increased respirations, shock, and decreased urinary output.

⚿ CN: Reduction of risk potential;
CL: Analyze

61. 3. Because the child has only one kidney, measures should be recommended to prevent urinary tract infection and injury to the remaining kidney. Severe pain and dependent edema are not associated with surgery for Wilms' tumor. Dietary sodium is not restricted because function in the remaining kidney is not impaired.

⚿ CN: Reduction of risk potential;
CL: Create

Managing Care, Quality, and Safety of Children with Health Problems of the Urinary System

62. 4. There are many problems with this medication prescription. The abbreviation QOD is ambiguous and open to various interpretations.

The abbreviation D/C may be interpreted as "discontinue" or "discharge." The prescriber should have specifically stated when to start the lower dose because the nurse could reason beginning the medication that day, the next, or even the day after that. The only safe thing to do is call for clarification.

⚿ CN: Safety and infection control;
CL: Synthesize

63. 3. The charge nurse should assure the parent that it is okay to use CIC and discuss the conversation with the nurse. It is possible that the nurse was unaware of current research findings or unit policies. The charge nurse should also determine if the parent has the supplies and uses a new catheter each time, but the insertion principles would not change. Parents are frequently taught how to do CIC while a child is in the hospital. Therefore, the rationale that it now becomes unsafe, or that sterile technique is needed, is faulty. Switching nurses will not solve the underlying problem.

⚿ CN: Management of care;
CL: Synthesize

64. 3. Access to a well-constructed e-history will facilitate care if the adolescent becomes ill while at college. Because the client is 18, legally the nurse cannot transfer the records to the school without permission. Also, the adolescent may need to seek treatment in facilities other than the health center. Instructing the adolescent to always carry the nephrologist's phone number is not bad advice, but compliance may vary and there is no guarantee the provider will be available in all instances. Telling the parent that the son must learn to manage his own disease does not address the parent's concern.

⚿ CN: Management of care;
CL: Synthesize

The Child with Neurologic Health Problems

The Client with Myelomeningocele

1. Parents bring a 10-month-old boy with myelomeningocele and hydrocephalus with a ventriculoperitoneal shunt to the emergency department. His symptoms include vomiting, poor feeding, lethargy, and irritability. What interventions by the nurse are **most** appropriate? Select all that apply.
- ☐ 1. Weigh the child.
- ☐ 2. Listen to bowel sounds.
- ☐ 3. Palpate the anterior fontanelle.
- ☐ 4. Obtain vital signs.
- ☐ 5. Assess pitch and quality of the child's cry.

2. When positioning a neonate with an unrepaired myelomeningocele, which position is **most** appropriate?
- ☐ 1. supine with the hips at 90-degree flexion
- ☐ 2. right side-lying position with the knees flexed
- ☐ 3. prone with hips in abduction
- ☐ 4. supine in semi-Fowler's position with chest and abdomen elevated

3. The nurse is teaching the parents of a child with myelomeningocele how to prevent urinary tract infections. What should the care plan include for this child? Select all that apply.
- ☐ 1. Provide meticulous skin care.
- ☐ 2. Use Crede's maneuver to empty the bladder.
- ☐ 3. Encourage frequent emptying of the bladder.
- ☐ 4. Assure adequate fluid intake.
- ☐ 5. Use tight-fitting diapers around the meatus.

4. The nurse reports to the healthcare provider (HCP) signs of increased intracranial pressure in an infant with a myelomeningocele who has which finding?
- ☐ 1. minimal lower extremity movement
- ☐ 2. a high-pitched cry
- ☐ 3. overflow voiding only
- ☐ 4. a fontanelle that bulges with crying

5. When developing the plan of care for an infant diagnosed with myelomeningocele and the parents who have just been informed of the infant's diagnosis, which action should the nurse include as the **priority** when the parents visit the infant for the first time?
- ☐ 1. Emphasize the infant's normal and positive features.
- ☐ 2. Encourage the parents to discuss their fears and concerns.
- ☐ 3. Reinforce the healthcare provider's (HCP's) explanation of the defect.
- ☐ 4. Have the parents feed their infant.

6. The mother of an infant with myelomeningocele asks if her baby is likely to have any other defects. The nurse responds based on the understanding that myelomeningocele is commonly associated with which disorder?
- ☐ 1. excessive cerebrospinal fluid within the cranial cavity
- ☐ 2. abnormally small head
- ☐ 3. congenital absence of the cranial vault
- ☐ 4. overriding of the cranial sutures

7. The parents of an infant with myelomeningocele ask the nurse about their child's future mental ability. What is the nurse's **best** response?

- ☐ 1. "About one-third have an intellectual disability, but it is too early to tell about your child."
- ☐ 2. "About two-thirds have an intellectual disability significantly retarded, and you will know soon if this will occur."
- ☐ 3. "Your child will probably be of normal intelligence since he demonstrates signs of it now."
- ☐ 4. "You will need to talk with the healthcare provider (HCP) about that, but you can ask later."

8. After placing an infant with myelomeningocele in an Isolette shortly after birth, which indicator should the nurse use as the **best** way to determine the effectiveness of this intervention?

- ☐ 1. The partial pressure of arterial oxygen remains between 94 and 100 mm Hg.
- ☐ 2. The axillary temperature remains between 97°F and 98°F (36.1°C and 36.7°C).
- ☐ 3. The bilirubin level remains stable.
- ☐ 4. Weight increases by about 1 oz (30 g) per day.

9. After surgical repair of a myelomeningocele, which position should the nurse use to prevent musculoskeletal deformity in the infant?

- ☐ 1. Place the feet in flexion.
- ☐ 2. Allow the hips to be abducted.
- ☐ 3. Maintain knees in the neutral position.
- ☐ 4. Place the legs in adduction.

10. When developing the discharge plan for the parents of an infant who has undergone a myelomeningocele repair, what information is **most** important for the nurse to include?

- ☐ 1. a list of available hospital services
- ☐ 2. schedule for daily home health care
- ☐ 3. chaplain referral for psychological support
- ☐ 4. daily care required by the infant

11. Which statement by the parent of an infant with a repaired upper lumbar myelomeningocele indicates that the parent understands the nurse's teaching at the time of discharge?

- ☐ 1. "I can apply a heating pad to his lower back."
- ☐ 2. "I will be sure to keep him away from other children."
- ☐ 3. "I will call the healthcare provider (HCP) if his urine has a funny smell."
- ☐ 4. "I will prop him on pillows to keep him from rolling over."

12. A preschooler with a history of repaired lumbar myelomeningocele is in the emergency department with wheezing and skin rash. Which questions should the nurse ask the parent **first**?

- ☐ 1. "Is your child taking any medications?"
- ☐ 2. "Who brought your child to the emergency department?"
- ☐ 3. "Is your child allergic to bananas or any other food?"
- ☐ 4. "What are you doing to treat your child's skin rash?"

The Client with Hydrocephalus

13. Before placement of a ventriculoperitoneal shunt for hydrocephalus, an infant is irritable, lethargic, and difficult to feed. To maintain the infant's nutritional status, which action would be **most** appropriate?

- ☐ 1. Feed the infant just before doing any procedures.
- ☐ 2. Give the infant small, frequent feedings.
- ☐ 3. Feed the infant in a horizontal position.
- ☐ 4. Give large, less frequent feedings.

14. Which clinical manifestation would lead the nurse to suspect an infant has hydrocephaly? Select all that apply.

- ☐ 1. depressed fontanelle
- ☐ 2. headache
- ☐ 3. vomiting
- ☐ 4. low-pitched cry
- ☐ 5. irritability
- ☐ 6. pupillary changes
- ☐ 7. bulging fontanelle

15. The nurse is providing postoperative care for an infant who had a ventriculoperitoneal shunt placed to correct hydrocephalus. Which clinical finding warrants immediate intervention?

- ☐ 1. abdominal distention
- ☐ 2. lethargy
- ☐ 3. facial edema
- ☐ 4. headache

16. Which action should the nurse take when providing postoperative nursing care to a child after insertion of a ventriculoperitoneal shunt?

- ☐ 1. Administer narcotics for pain control.
- ☐ 2. Check the urine for glucose and protein.
- ☐ 3. Monitoring for increased temperature.
- ☐ 4. Test cerebrospinal fluid leakage for protein.

17. A nurse evaluates discharge teaching as successful when the parents of a school-age child with a ventriculoperitoneal shunt insertion identify which sign as signaling a blocked shunt?
- ☐ 1. decreased urine output with stable intake
- ☐ 2. tense fontanelle and increased head circumference
- ☐ 3. elevated temperature and reddened incisional site
- ☐ 4. irritability and increasing difficulty with eating

The Client with Down Syndrome

18. The mother of a 17-year-old girl with Down syndrome tells the nurse that her daughter recently stated that she has a boyfriend. The mother is concerned that her daughter might become pregnant. Which is the **most** appropriate suggestion made by the nurse?
- ☐ 1. "I understand your concern; you may want to start your daughter on long-acting contraception."
- ☐ 2. "Women with Down syndrome are infertile, so you do not need to worry about her getting pregnant."
- ☐ 3. "I understand your concern; you may want to enroll your daughter in an abstinence program."
- ☐ 4. "I know it may be difficult, but you may want to suggest that your daughter break off the relationship."

19. A nurse is assessing a child who has a mild intellectual disability. The **best** indication of how this child is progressing can be obtained by observing him:
- ☐ 1. at school with his teacher.
- ☐ 2. at home with his family.
- ☐ 3. in the clinic with his mother.
- ☐ 4. playing soccer with his friends.

20. After talking with the parents of a child with Down syndrome, the nurse should help the parents establish which goal?
- ☐ 1. Encourage self-care skills in the child.
- ☐ 2. Teach the child something new each day.
- ☐ 3. Encourage more lenient behavior limits for the child.
- ☐ 4. Achieve age-appropriate social skills.

21. The nurse discusses with the parents how best to raise the IQ of their child with Down syndrome. Which intervention would be **most** appropriate?
- ☐ 1. Serve hearty, nutritious meals.
- ☐ 2. Give vasodilator medications as prescribed.
- ☐ 3. Let the child play with more able children.
- ☐ 4. Provide stimulating, nonthreatening life experiences.

22. When developing a teaching plan for the parents of a child with Down syndrome, the nurse focuses on activities to increase which factor for the parents?
- ☐ 1. affection for their child
- ☐ 2. responsibility for their child's welfare
- ☐ 3. understanding of their child's disability
- ☐ 4. confidence in their ability to care for their child

The Client with a Seizure Disorder

23. What should be part of the nurse's teaching plan for a child with epilepsy being discharged on a regimen of phenytoin?
- ☐ 1. Drink plenty of fluids.
- ☐ 2. Brush teeth after each meal.
- ☐ 3. Have someone be with the child during waking hours.
- ☐ 4. Report signs of infection.

24. After the nurse instructs a group of school-teachers about seizures, the teachers role-play a scenario involving a child experiencing a generalized tonic-clonic seizure. Which action, when performed **first**, indicates that the nurse's teaching has been successful?
- ☐ 1. Ask the other children what happened before the seizure.
- ☐ 2. Move the child to the nurse's office for privacy.
- ☐ 3. Remove any nearby objects that could harm the child.
- ☐ 4. Place a padded tongue blade between the child's teeth.

25. A nurse is developing a plan of care with the parents of a 6-year-old girl diagnosed with a seizure disorder. To promote growth and development, the nurse should instruct the parents that:
- ☐ 1. the child will need activity limitation and will be unable to perform as well as her peers.
- ☐ 2. there is potential for a learning disability and the child may need tutoring to reach her grade level.
- ☐ 3. the child will likely have normal intelligence and be able to attend regular school.
- ☐ 4. there will be problems associated with social stigma and parents should consider home schooling.

26. The parents of a child with occasional generalized seizures want to send the child to summer camp. The parents contact the nurse for advice on planning for the camping experience. Which type of activity should the nurse and family decide the child should avoid?
- ☐ 1. rock climbing
- ☐ 2. hiking
- ☐ 3. swimming
- ☐ 4. tennis

27. Which statement obtained from the nursing history of a toddler should alert the nurse to suspect that the child has had a febrile seizure?
- ☐ 1. The child has had a low-grade fever for several weeks.
- ☐ 2. The family history is negative for convulsions.
- ☐ 3. The seizure resulted in respiratory arrest.
- ☐ 4. The seizure occurred when the child had a respiratory infection.

28. After teaching the parents of a child with febrile seizures about methods to lower temperature other than using medication, which statement indicates successful teaching?
- ☐ 1. "We will add extra blankets when he says he is cold."
- ☐ 2. "We will wrap him in a blanket if he starts shivering."
- ☐ 3. "We will make the bath water cold enough to make him shiver."
- ☐ 4. "We will use a solution of half alcohol and half water when sponging him."

29. An adolescent girl with a seizure disorder controlled with phenytoin and carbamazepine asks the nurse about getting married and having children. Which response by the nurse would be **most** appropriate?
- ☐ 1. "You probably should not consider having children until your seizures are cured."
- ☐ 2. "Your children will not necessarily have an increased risk of seizure disorder."
- ☐ 3. "When you decide to have children, talk to the healthcare provider (HCP) about changing your medication."
- ☐ 4. "Women who have seizure disorders commonly have a difficult time conceiving."

30. When teaching an adolescent with a seizure disorder who is receiving valproic acid, which sign or symptom should the nurse instruct the client **immediately** to report to the healthcare provider (HCP)?
- ☐ 1. diarrhea
- ☐ 2. loss of appetite
- ☐ 3. jaundice
- ☐ 4. sore throat

The Client with Meningitis

31. A 3-month-old infant with meningococcal meningitis has just been admitted to the pediatric unit. Which nursing intervention has the **highest priority**?
- ☐ 1. instituting droplet precautions
- ☐ 2. administering acetaminophen
- ☐ 3. obtaining history information from the parents
- ☐ 4. orienting the parents to the pediatric unit

32. During the acute stage of meningitis, a 3-year-old child is restless and irritable. Which intervention would be **most** appropriate to institute?
- ☐ 1. limiting conversation with the child
- ☐ 2. keeping extraneous noise to a minimum
- ☐ 3. allowing the child to play in the bathtub
- ☐ 4. performing treatments quickly

33. Which sign should lead the nurse to suspect that a child with meningitis has developed disseminated intravascular coagulation?
- ☐ 1. hemorrhagic skin rash
- ☐ 2. edema
- ☐ 3. cyanosis
- ☐ 4. dyspnea on exertion

34. When interviewing the parents of a 2-year-old child, a history of which illnesses should lead the nurse to suspect pneumococcal meningitis?
- ☐ 1. bladder infection
- ☐ 2. middle ear infection
- ☐ 3. fractured clavicle
- ☐ 4. septic arthritis

35. A preschooler with pneumococcal meningitis is receiving intravenous antibiotic therapy. When discontinuing the intravenous therapy, the nurse allows the child to apply a dressing to the area where the catheter is removed. The nurse's rationale for doing so is based on the interpretation that a child in this age group has a need to accomplish which goal?
- ☐ 1. trust those caring for her
- ☐ 2. find diversional activities
- ☐ 3. protect the image of an intact body
- ☐ 4. relieve the anxiety of separation from home

36. A child with meningitis is to receive 1,000 mL of dextrose 5% in normal saline over 12 hours. At what rate in milliliters per hour should the nurse set the pump? Round your answer to the nearest whole number.

_____ mL/h.

37. Nursing care management of the child with bacterial meningitis includes which interventions? Select all that apply.
- ☐ 1. administration of IV antibiotics
- ☐ 2. intravenous fluids at 1½ times maintenance
- ☐ 3. decreasing environmental stimuli
- ☐ 4. neurologic checks every 4 hours
- ☐ 5. administration of IV anticonvulsants

38. The nurse is monitoring an infant with meningitis for signs of increased intracranial pressure (ICP). The nurse should assess the infant for which signs or symptoms? Select all that apply.
- ☐ 1. irritability
- ☐ 2. headache
- ☐ 3. mood swings
- ☐ 4. bulging fontanelle
- ☐ 5. emesis

39. A hospitalized preschooler with meningitis who is to be discharged becomes angry when the discharge is delayed. Which play activity would be **most** appropriate at this time?
☐ **1.** reading the child a story
☐ **2.** painting with watercolors
☐ **3.** pounding on a pegboard
☐ **4.** stacking a tower of blocks

The Client with Near-Drowning

40. The nurse is admitting a toddler with the diagnosis of near-drowning in a neighbor's heated swimming pool to the emergency department. The nurse should assess the child for:
☐ **1.** hypothermia.
☐ **2.** hypoxia.
☐ **3.** fluid aspiration.
☐ **4.** cutaneous capillary paralysis.

41. The nurse is caring for a lethargic 4-year-old who is a victim of a near-drowning accident. The nurse should **first**:
☐ **1.** administer oxygen.
☐ **2.** institute rewarming.
☐ **3.** prepare for intubation.
☐ **4.** start an intravenous infusion.

42. The parents of a child tell the nurse that they feel guilty because their child almost drowned. Which remark by the nurse would be **most** appropriate?
☐ **1.** "I can understand why you feel guilty, but these things happen."
☐ **2.** "Tell me a little bit more about your feelings of guilt."
☐ **3.** "You should not have taken your eyes off of your child."
☐ **4.** "You should focus on the fact that your child will be all right."

The Client with Guillain-Barré Syndrome (Infectious Polyneuritis)

43. Which assessment would be **most** important for the nurse to make initially in a school-age child being seen in the clinic who has a sore throat, muscle tenderness, arms feeling weak, and generally is not feeling well?
☐ **1.** difficulty swallowing
☐ **2.** diet intake for the last 24 hours
☐ **3.** exposure to illnesses
☐ **4.** difficulty urinating

44. Which action should be the **priority** when caring for a school-age child admitted to the pediatric unit with the diagnosis of Guillain-Barré syndrome?
☐ **1.** Assess the child's ability to follow simple commands.
☐ **2.** Evaluate the child's bilateral muscle strength.
☐ **3.** Make a game of the range-of-motion exercises.
☐ **4.** Provide the child with a diversional activity.

45. The nurse asks a school-age child with Guillain-Barré syndrome to cough and also assesses the child's speech for decreased volume and clarity. The underlying rationale for these assessments is to determine which finding?
☐ **1.** inflammation of the larynx and epiglottis
☐ **2.** increased intracranial pressure
☐ **3.** involvement of facial and cranial nerves
☐ **4.** regression to an earlier developmental phase

46. Assessment of a school-age child with Guillain-Barré syndrome reveals absent gag and cough reflexes. Which problem should receive the **highest priority** during the acute phase?
☐ **1.** risk for infection due to altered immune system
☐ **2.** ineffective breathing pattern related to neuromuscular impairment
☐ **3.** impaired swallowing related to neuromuscular impairment
☐ **4.** fluid volume deficits related to total urinary incontinence

47. A 9-year-old child with Guillain-Barré syndrome requires mechanical ventilation. Which action should the nurse take?
☐ **1.** Maintain the child in a supine position to prevent unnecessary nerve stimulation.
☐ **2.** Transfer the child to a bedside chair three times a day to prevent postural hypotension.
☐ **3.** Engage the child in vigorous passive range-of-motion exercises to prevent loss of muscle function.
☐ **4.** Turn the child slowly and gently from side to side to prevent respiratory complications.

48. The parent brings a child to the clinic after discharge from the hospital for Guillain-Barré syndrome. Which statement by the parent indicates that the discharge plan is being followed?
☐ **1.** "She and her sister argue all day."
☐ **2.** "I have to bribe her to get her to do her exercises."
☐ **3.** "I take her to the pool where she can exercise with other children."
☐ **4.** "She has missed a few of her therapy sessions because she often sleeps."

The Client with a Head Injury

49. A 12-year-old child has had a traumatic head injury from playing in a football game. He is admitted to the emergency department and transferred to the pediatric intensive care unit. He has an IV of dextrose 5% in water at 21 mL/h and nasal oxygen at 2 L/min. The nurse is assessing the child at the beginning of the shift (2300 hours) and reviews the Glasgow Coma Scale flow sheet below. The nurse notes that the child responds to pain, is making incomprehensible sounds, and has abnormal flexion of the limbs. What should the nurse do **first**?

Flow Sheet

Glasgow Coma Scale

Test	Score	Client's response
Eye Opening		
Spontaneously	4	Opens eyes spon taneously
To Speech	3	Opens eyes to verbal comma nd
To Pain	2	Opens eyes to painful stim ulus
None	1	Doesn't open eyes in response to stimulus
Motor Response		
Obeys	6	Reacts to verbal comma nd
Localizes	5	Identifi es localized pain
Withdraws	4	Flexes and withdraws from painful stimulus
Abnormal Flexion	3	Assumes a decorticate pos ition
Abnormal Extension	2	Assumes a decerebrate position
None	1	No response; lies fl accid
Verbal Response		
Oriented	5	Is oriented and c onverses
Confused	4	Is disoriented and con fused
Inappropriate Words	3	Replies randomly with i ncorrect words
Incomprehensible	2	Moans or screams
None	1	No response

Date	Time	Progress Notes
11/13	1700	GCS = 13
11/13	1800	GCS = 12
11/13	1900	GCS = 13
11/13	2000	GCS = 11
11/13	2100	GCS = 10
11/13	2200	GCS = 9

☐ 1. Notify the healthcare provider (HCP).
☐ 2. Lower the head of the bed.
☐ 3. Increase the rate of nasal oxygen.
☐ 4. Increase the rate of the IV infusion.

50. A 10-year-old with a severe head injury is unconscious and has coarse breath sounds, a temperature of 39°C (102.2°F), a heart rate of 70 bpm, a blood pressure of 130/60 mm Hg, and an intracranial pressure (ICP) of 36 mm Hg. Which action should the nurse perform **first**?
☐ 1. Administer prescribed IV mannitol.
☐ 2. Suction the child.
☐ 3. Encourage the parent to talk to the child.
☐ 4. Administer prescribed rectal acetaminophen.

51. The nurse is inserting a nasogastric (NG) tube in a child admitted with head trauma. The nurse should explain to the parents that the NG tube will be used for what purpose?
☐ 1. Administer medications.
☐ 2. Decompress the stomach.
☐ 3. Obtain gastric specimens for analysis.
☐ 4. Provide adequate nutrition.

52. A nasogastric tube is prescribed to be inserted for a child with severe head trauma. Diagnostic testing reveals that the child has a basilar skull fracture. What should the nurse do **next**?
☐ 1. Ask for the prescription to be changed to an oral gastric tube.
☐ 2. Attempt to place the tube into the duodenum.
☐ 3. Test the gastric aspirate for blood.
☐ 4. Use extra lubrication when inserting the nasogastric tube.

53. The parents of a child in a coma with a serious head injury ask the nurse if the child is going to be all right. Which response by the nurse would be **most** appropriate?
☐ 1. "Children usually do not do very well after head injuries like this."
☐ 2. "Children usually recover rapidly from head injuries."
☐ 3. "It is hard to tell this early, but we will keep you informed of the progress."
☐ 4. "That is something you will have to talk to the healthcare provider (HCP) about."

54. A parent of a child with a moderate head injury asks the nurse, "How will you know if my child is getting worse?" The nurse should tell the parents that **best** indicator of the child's brain function is:
☐ 1. the vital signs.
☐ 2. level of consciousness.
☐ 3. reactions of the pupils.
☐ 4. motor strength.

55. When developing the plan of care for a child who is unconscious after a serious head injury, in which position should the nurse expect to place the child?
☐ 1. prone with hips and knees slightly elevated
☐ 2. lying on the side, with the head of the bed elevated
☐ 3. lying on the back, in the Trendelenburg position
☐ 4. in the semi-Fowler's position, with arms at the side

56. The healthcare provider (HCP) has prescribed intravenous mannitol for a child with a head injury. The **best** indicator that the drug has been effective is:
☐ 1. increased urine output.
☐ 2. improved level of consciousness.
☐ 3. decreased intracranial pressure.
☐ 4. decreased edema.

57. The nurse assigned to telephone triage returns the call of a parent whose teenager experienced a hard tackle last night. The parent reports, "He seemed dazed after it happened, and the coach had him sit out the rest of the game, but he is fine now." What is the **most** appropriate instruction for the nurse to give?
☐ 1. "Take him immediately to the emergency department."
☐ 2. "He cannot return to play until he has been evaluated by a healthcare provider (HCP)."
☐ 3. "If he seems fine now and had no other symptom, it probably was not a concussion."
☐ 4. "Watch him closely, and call us back if you see any changes."

58. A history of which factors will complicate the recovery from a concussion? Select all that apply.
☐ 1. asthma
☐ 2. attention deficit hyperactivity disorder (ADHD)
☐ 3. depression
☐ 4. migraines
☐ 5. obesity
☐ 6. previous concussion

59. A 3-year-old is recovering from a concussion. The persistence of which finding would the nurse consider as being a normal finding for a 3-year-old?
☐ 1. lack interest in favorite toys
☐ 2. change in eating habits
☐ 3. inability to hop
☐ 4. increased temper tantrums

60. The nurse teaches an adolescent about returning to school after a concussion. Which statement by the client reflects the need for more teaching?
☐ 1. "I should limit my activities that require concentration."
☐ 2. "I must slowly return to my previous activity level as my symptoms improve."
☐ 3. "My symptoms may reemerge with exertion."
☐ 4. "Time is the most important factor in my recovery."

The Client with a Brain Tumor

61. A child with a brain tumor is less responsive to verbal commands than he was when the nurse assessed the client the previous hour. What should the nurse do **next**?
☐ 1. Raise the head of the bed.
☐ 2. Notify the healthcare provider (HCP).
☐ 3. Administer an analgesic.
☐ 4. Obtain an oximeter reading.

62. The nurse is caring for a 3-year-old client with a neuroblastoma who has been receiving chemotherapy for the last 4 weeks. His lab results indicate an Hgb of 12.5 g/dL (125 g/L), an HCT of 36.8% (0.37), a WBC of 2,000 mm³ (2 × 10⁹/L), and a platelet count of 150,000 μL (150 × 10⁹/L). Based on the child's lab values, what is the **highest priority** nursing intervention?
☐ 1. Encourage meticulous handwashing by the client and visitors.
☐ 2. Prepare to give the child a transfusion of platelets.
☐ 3. Encourage mouth care with a soft toothbrush.
☐ 4. Prepare to give the child a transfusion of packed red blood cells.

63. A 13-year-old child has seen the school nurse several times with headache, vomiting, and difficulty walking. When calling the adolescent's mother about these symptoms, what should the nurse suggest the mother do **first**?
☐ 1. Schedule an appointment with the eye healthcare provider (HCP).
☐ 2. Begin psychological counseling for her adolescent.
☐ 3. Make an appointment with the adolescent's healthcare provider (HCP).
☐ 4. Meet with the adolescent's teachers to determine academic progress.

64. A school-age child is admitted to the hospital with the diagnosis of probable infratentorial brain tumor. During the child's admission to the pediatric unit, which action should the nurse anticipate taking **first**?
☐ 1. Eliminate the child's anxiety.
☐ 2. Implement seizure precautions.
☐ 3. Introduce the child to other clients of the same age.
☐ 4. Prepare the child and parents for diagnostic procedures.

65. The nurse is giving care to an infant with a brain tumor. The nurse observes the infant arches the back (see figure). The nurse should:

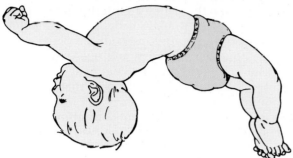

- ☐ **1.** notify the healthcare provider (HCP).
- ☐ **2.** stroke the back to release the arching.
- ☐ **3.** pad the side rails of the crib.
- ☐ **4.** place the child prone.

66. The nurse is assessing a child diagnosed with a brain tumor. Which signs and symptoms should the nurse expect the child to demonstrate? Select all that apply.
- ☐ **1.** head tilt
- ☐ **2.** vomiting
- ☐ **3.** polydipsia
- ☐ **4.** lethargy
- ☐ **5.** increased appetite
- ☐ **6.** increased pulse

67. After a child undergoes a craniotomy for an infratentorial brain tumor, the nurse should place the child in which position to prevent undue strain on the sutures?
- ☐ **1.** prone
- ☐ **2.** semi-Fowler's
- ☐ **3.** side-lying
- ☐ **4.** Trendelenburg

68. A child who was intubated after a craniotomy now shows signs of decreased level of consciousness. The healthcare provider (HCP) prescribes manual hyperventilation to keep the $PaCO_2$ between 25 and 29 mm Hg and the PaO_2 between 80 and 100 mm Hg. The nurse interprets this prescription based on the understanding that this action will accomplish which goal?
- ☐ **1.** decrease intracranial pressure
- ☐ **2.** ensure a patent airway
- ☐ **3.** lower the arousal level
- ☐ **4.** produce hypoxia

69. Which action should the nurse do **first** when noting clear drainage on the child's dressing and bed linen after a craniotomy for a brain tumor?
- ☐ **1.** Change the dressing.
- ☐ **2.** Elevate the head of the bed.
- ☐ **3.** Test the fluid for glucose.
- ☐ **4.** Notify the healthcare provider (HCP).

70. An 8-year-old child does well after infratentorial tumor removal and is transferred back to the pediatric unit. Although she had been told about having her head shaved for surgery, she is very upset. After exploring the child's feelings, which action should the nurse take?
- ☐ **1.** Ask the child if she would like to wear a hat.
- ☐ **2.** Reassure the child that her hair will grow back.
- ☐ **3.** Explain to the child's parents that her reaction is normal.
- ☐ **4.** Suggest that the parents buy the child a wig as a surprise.

71. Which statement made by the parent of a school-age child who has had a craniotomy for a brain tumor would warrant further exploration by the nurse?
- ☐ **1.** "After this, I will never let her out of my sight again."
- ☐ **2.** "I hope that she will be able to go back to school soon."
- ☐ **3.** "I wonder how long it will be before she can ride her bike."
- ☐ **4.** "Her best friend is eager to see her; I hope she will not be upset."

The Client with a Spinal Cord Injury

72. A nurse, who witnesses an accident involving an adolescent being thrown from a motorcycle, stops to help. The adolescent reports that he is now unable to move his legs. While waiting for the emergency medical service to arrive, what should the nurse do?
- ☐ **1.** Flex the adolescent's knees to relieve stress on his back.
- ☐ **2.** Leave the adolescent as he is, staying close by.
- ☐ **3.** Remove the adolescent's helmet as soon as possible.
- ☐ **4.** Assess the adolescent for abdominal trauma.

73. An adolescent sustains a T3 spinal cord injury. After insertion of an intravenous line, a nasogastric tube, and an indwelling urinary (Foley) catheter, the adolescent is admitted to the intensive care unit. What should the nurse do **next** when assessment reveals that the adolescent's feet and legs are cool to the touch?
- ☐ **1.** Cover the adolescent's legs with blankets.
- ☐ **2.** Report this finding to the healthcare provider (HCP) immediately.
- ☐ **3.** Reposition the adolescent's legs.
- ☐ **4.** Lay the adolescent flat to aid circulation.

74. During assessment of an adolescent who has sustained a recent thoracic spinal injury, the nurse auscultates the adolescent's abdomen. The nurse explains to the parents that this is necessary because clients with spinal cord injury often develop which problem?
☐ 1. abdominal cramping
☐ 2. hyperactive bowel sounds
☐ 3. paralytic ileus
☐ 4. profuse diarrhea

75. Which finding should lead the nurse to decide that spinal shock was resolving in the adolescent with a spinal cord injury?
☐ 1. atonic urinary bladder
☐ 2. flaccid paralysis
☐ 3. hyperactive reflexes
☐ 4. widened pulse pressure

76. A school-age boy with a spinal cord injury is moved to the rehabilitation unit. The nurse notes that the child tends to refuse to cooperate in care and to be hostile. The nurse interprets this behavior as indicative of which response?
☐ 1. a stage of grief reaction
☐ 2. a phase of rebellion
☐ 3. a reaction to sensory overload
☐ 4. a response to too much attention

77. Two months after an adolescent's thoracic spinal cord injury, he has a pounding headache. The nurse notes that the client's arms and face are flushed and he is diaphoretic. What should the nurse do **next**?
☐ 1. Check the patency of the urinary catheter.
☐ 2. Lower the adolescent's head below his knees.
☐ 3. Place the adolescent flat on his back.
☐ 4. Prepare to administer epinephrine subcutaneously.

Managing Care, Quality, and Safety of Children with Neurologic Health Problems

78. The nurse is admitting a child who has been diagnosed with bacterial meningitis to the pediatric unit. The nurse should implement which type of isolation?
☐ 1. standard or routine precautions
☐ 2. contact precautions
☐ 3. airborne precautions
☐ 4. droplet precautions

79. The nurse manager on a pediatric floor is updating safety recommendations for the unit. Which strategy would help reduce pediatric medication errors? Select all that apply.
☐ 1. Eliminate the pediatric satellite pharmacy.
☐ 2. Increase the number of steps in the medication administration procedure.
☐ 3. Avoid using parenteral syringes when administering liquid oral medications.
☐ 4. Limit the size of IV fluid bags that can be hung on small children.
☐ 5. Reduce the available concentrations or dose strengths of high-alert medications to the minimum.

80. The healthcare provider (HCP) prescribes carbamazepine extended release for a client with a cerebral palsy who also has a seizure disorder. The client has a gastrostomy feeding tube, and carbamazepine is on the hospital's "no crush" list. In order to administer the medication, the nurse should:
☐ 1. cut the medication into four pieces that can be placed in the feeding tube.
☐ 2. dissolve the medication in 30 mL of juice.
☐ 3. ask the pharmacist for an oral suspension.
☐ 4. contact the HCP to change the prescription.

81. When making rounds on the pediatric neurology unit, the nurse manager notes that when giving IV medications many of the staff nurses are disconnecting the flush syringe first and then clamping the intermittent infusion device. The nurse is concerned that the nurses do not understand the benefits of positive pressure technique and turbulence flow flush in preventing clots. After discussing the problem with the staff educator, which intervention would be the **most** effective way to improve the nursing practice?
☐ 1. Create a poster presentation on the topic with a required posttest.
☐ 2. Send a group e-mail discussing the importance of clamping the device first.
☐ 3. Ask each nurse if he or she is aware that his or her practice is not current.
☐ 4. Post an evidence-based article on the unit.

82. The emergency department nurse has admitted an infant with bulging fontanelles, setting sun eyes, and lethargy. Which diagnostic procedure would be **contraindicated** in this infant?
☐ 1. lumbar puncture
☐ 2. magnetic resonance imaging
☐ 3. arterial blood draw
☐ 4. computerized tomography scan

83. A 7-year-old with a history of tonic-clonic seizures has been actively seizing for 10 minutes. The child weighs 22 kg and currently has an IV of D5 NS + 20 mEq KCl/L running at 60 mL/h. The vital signs are temperature 100.4°F (38°C), heart rate 120 bpm, respiratory rate 28 breaths/min, and oxygen saturation 92%. Using the SBAR (Situation-Background-Assessment-Recommendation) technique for communication, the nurse calls the healthcare provider (HCP) with the recommendation for:
☐ **1.** rectal diazepam.
☐ **2.** IV lorazepam.
☐ **3.** rectal acetaminophen.
☐ **4.** IV fosphenytoin.

Answers, Rationales, and Test-Taking Strategies

The answers and the rationales for each question follow below, along with keys (⚷) to the client need (CN) and cognitive level (CL) for each question. In addition, you will also see a glossary icon (📖) highlighting specific terminology used on the licensing exam. As you check your answers, use the **Content Mastery and Test-Taking Skill Self-Analysis** *worksheet (tear-out worksheet in back of book) to identify the reason(s) for not answering the questions correctly. For additional information about test-taking skills and strategies for answering questions, refer to pages 12–23 and pages 35–36 in Part 1 of this book.*

The Client with Myelomeningocele

1. **1,2,4,5.** Common shunt complications are obstruction, infection, and disconnection of the tubing. The signs presented by the child indicate increased intracranial pressure from a shunt malfunction, which could be caused by an infection, such as peritonitis or meningitis. By listening to bowel sounds, the nurse will note if peritonitis might be a possibility. Intracranial pressure manifests as a bulging or taut anterior fontanel, but the posterior fontanel is typically closed. Obtaining vital signs would assess for signs of infection, such as elevated temperature or, possibly, Cushing's triad (elevated blood pressure, slow pulse, and depressed respirations). A high-pitched cry is a sign of increased intracranial pressure. Weighing the child, while it would not help identify the cause of the problem, would help determine the severity of the dehydration from vomiting.

⚷ CN: Physiological adaptation;
CL: Synthesize

2. **3.** Before surgery, the infant is kept flat in the prone position to decrease tension on the sac. This allows for optimal positioning of the hips, knees, and feet because orthopedic problems are common. The supine position is unacceptable because it causes pressure on the defect. Flexing the knees when side-lying will increase tension on the sac, as will placing the infant in semi-Fowler's position, even though the chest and abdomen are elevated.

⚷ CN: Physiological adaptation;
CL: Synthesize

3. **2,3,4.** Prevention of urinary tract infections includes adequate fluid intake, urine acidification, and frequent emptying of the bladder, with the use of Crede's maneuver if needed. While the nurse should keep the skin clean and dry, this will not prevent urinary tract infections. Keeping urine close to the meatus with a tight-fitting diaper would increase the risk for infection.

⚷ CN: Reduction of risk potential;
CL: Create

4. **2.** A Chiari malformation obstructs the flow of cerebral spinal fluid resulting in hydrocephalus. This is a common problem in infants with myelomeningocele and will require surgical intervention with a shunt. A high-pitched cry is one sign of increased intracranial pressure that may indicate the presence of a Chiari malformation and requires further evaluation. Minimal movement of the lower extremities is an expected finding associated with spinal cord damage. Overflow voiding comes from a neurogenic bladder, not increased intracranial pressure. It is normal for the fontanelle to bulge with crying.

⚷ CN: Physiological adaptation;
CL: Analyze

5. **1.** The parents should see the neonate as soon as possible, because the longer they must wait to see the neonate, the more anxiety they will feel. Because the parents are acutely aware of the deficit, the nurse should emphasize the neonate's normal and positive features during the visit. All parents, but especially those with a child who has a disability or defect, need to hear positive comments and comments that reflect how the infant is normal. Although the parents need to discuss their fears and concerns, the priority on the first visit is to emphasize the neonate's normal and positive features. Reinforcing the **HCP's** 📖 explanation of the defect may be necessary later. Reinforcing the explanation at this initial visit emphasizes the defect, not the child. The parents should spend time with or care for the neonate after birth because parent-infant contact is necessary for attachment. The parents cannot feed the neonate before the defect is repaired because the repair typically occurs within 24 hours.

The infant will be prone in an Isolette or warmed and watched closely. However, the parents can fondle and stroke the neonate.

🔑 CN: Psychosocial integrity; CL: Synthesize

6. 1. Excessive cerebrospinal fluid in the cranial cavity, called *hydrocephalus*, is the most common anomaly associated with myelomeningocele. Microcephaly, an abnormally small head, is associated with maternal exposure to rubella or cytomegalovirus. Anencephaly, a congenital absence of the cranial vault, is a different type of neural tube defect. Overriding of the sutures, possibly a normal finding after a vaginal birth, is not associated with myelomeningocele.

🔑 CN: Physiological adaptation; CL: Apply

7. 1. Approximately one-third of infants diagnosed with myelomeningocele have an intellectual disability, but the degree of disability is variable and it is difficult to predict intellectual functioning in neonates. The parents are asking for an answer now and should not be told to talk with the **HCP** 📖 later.

🔑 CN: Physiological adaptation; CL: Synthesize

8. 2. The nurse places the neonate with myelomeningocele in an Isolette shortly after birth to help to maintain the infant's temperature. Because of the defect, the neonate cannot be bundled in blankets. Therefore, it may be difficult to prevent cold stress. The Isolette can be maintained at higher than room temperature, helping to maintain the temperature of a neonate who cannot be dressed or bundled. Body temperature readings, not arterial oxygen levels, are the best indicator. Typically, an infant loses 5% to 10% of body weight before beginning to regain the weight.

🔑 CN: Reduction of risk potential; CL: Analyze

9. 2. Because of the potential for hip dislocation, the neonate's legs should be slightly abducted, hips maintained in slight to moderate abduction, and feet maintained in a neutral position. The infant's knees are flexed to help maintain the hips in abduction.

🔑 CN: Reduction of risk potential; CL: Synthesize

10. 4. The most important aspect of the discharge plan is to ensure that the parents understand what the daily care of their infant involves and to provide teaching related to carrying out this daily care. In addition to the routine care required by the infant, care also may include physical therapy to the lower extremities. Providing a list of available hospital services may be helpful to the parents, but it is not the most important aspect to include in the discharge plan. Usually, home health care is not needed because the parents are able to care for their child. A referral for counseling is initiated whenever the need arises, not just at discharge.

🔑 CN: Reduction of risk potential; CL: Synthesize

11. 3. Children with a myelomeningocele are prone to urinary tract infections (UTI), and foul-smelling urine is one symptom of a UTI. Because of the level of defect, the child may be insensitive to pressure or heat. Using a heating pad may lead to thermal injury because the child may not be able to sense if the pad is too hot. Keeping the child away from other children is unnecessary and can retard social development. Using pillows as props increases the risk of sudden infant death syndrome.

🔑 CN: Safety and infection control; CL: Evaluate

12. 3. Children with myelomeningocele are at high risk for development of latex allergy because of repeated exposure to latex products during surgery and bladder catheterizations. Cross-reactions to food items such as bananas, kiwi, chestnuts, and avocados also occur. These allergic reactions vary in severity ranging from mild (such as sneezing) to severe anaphylaxis. While the child could have allergies to medications that caused the wheezing, latex and food allergies are more common. Asking about the skin rash is not a priority when a child is wheezing. Who brought the child to the emergency department is irrelevant at this time.

🔑 CN: Reduction of risk potential; CL: Analyze

The Client with Hydrocephalus

13. 2. An infant with hydrocephalus is difficult to feed because of poor sucking, lethargy, and vomiting, which are associated with increased intracranial pressure. Small, frequent feedings given at times when the infant is relaxed and calm are tolerated best. Feeding an infant before any procedure is inappropriate because the stress of the procedure may lead to vomiting. Ideally, the infant should be held in a slightly vertical position when feeding to prevent backflow of formula into the eustachian tubes and subsequent development of ear infections. Giving large, less frequent feedings allows for rest but typically results in more vomiting.

🔑 CN: Basic care and comfort; CL: Synthesize

14. 3,5,6. Hydrocephaly is a block in the flow of cerebral spinal fluid. Hydrocephaly results in increased intracranial pressure (ICP). Vomiting, irritability, bulging fontanelle, and pupillary changes are all signs of increased intracranial pressure in an infant. A depressed fontanelle could be an indication of dehydration, not increased intracranial pressure. A headache may be present in an infant with increased ICP; however, the infant has no way of communicating this to the nurse or parent. A headache is an indication of increased ICP in a verbal child. A high-pitched cry is indicative of infants with increased intracranial pressure.

CN: Physiological adaptation;
CL: Analyze

15. 1. Abdominal distension in a pediatric client with a ventriculoperitoneal shunt can be an indication of peritonitis and requires intervention. Lethargy may be present for several days following surgery for a ventriculoperitoneal shunt. Facial and eye edema is common during the postoperative period and can be reduced by utilizing a cold compress to the eyes. Infants commonly have pain in the postoperative period that should be treated with analgesics; however, infants cannot convey that they specifically have a headache.

CN: Management of care; **CL:** Synthesize

16. 3. Monitoring the temperature allows the nurse to assess for infection, the most common and the most hazardous postoperative complication after ventriculoperitoneal shunt placement. Typically, pain after insertion of a ventriculoperitoneal shunt is mild, requiring the use of mild analgesics. Usually, narcotics are not administered because they alter the level of consciousness, making assessment of cerebral function difficult. Neither proteinuria nor glycosuria is associated with shunt placement. Cerebrospinal fluid leakage commonly occurs with head injury. It is not usually associated with shunt placement.

CN: Reduction of risk potential;
CL: Synthesize

17. 4. In a school-age child, irritability, lethargy, vomiting, difficulty with eating, and decreased level of consciousness are signs of increased intracranial pressure caused by a blocked shunt. Decreased urine output with stable fluid intake indicates fluid loss from a source other than the kidneys. A tense fontanelle and increased head circumference would be signs of a blocked shunt in an infant. Elevated temperature and redness around incisions might suggest an infection.

CN: Reduction of risk potential;
CL: Evaluate

The Client with Down Syndrome

18. 1. Children with Down syndrome range from severely intellectual disability to low-average intelligence. Thus, the adolescent's ability to make informed choices regarding sexual activity is limited. Long-acting contraception, such as an intrauterine device or a progestin implant, greatly reduces the risk of unwanted pregnancy. Most women with Down syndrome are fertile; however, children born to women with Down syndrome often have congenital defects. An abstinence program may not be effective due to the intellectual level of children with Down syndrome. Suggesting that the adolescent break off the relationship does not ensure that she will.

CN: Health promotion and maintenance;
CL: Analyze

19. 1. Watching the child relate to his teacher and schoolwork is the best indication of how he is progressing. School involves interacting with a person who is not a relative and in a situation that is not totally familiar. Observing the client in situations with family and friends shows social relationships but does not indicate how the child is learning new intellectual skills.

CN: Health promotion and maintenance;
CL: Evaluate

20. 1. The goal in working with children with intellectual disabilities is to train them to be as independent as possible, focusing on developmental skills. The child may not be capable of learning something new every day but needs to repeat what has been taught previously. Rather than encouraging more lenient behavior limits, the parents need to be strict and consistent when setting limits for the child. Most children with Down syndrome are unable to achieve age-appropriate social skills due to their disability. Rather, they are taught socially appropriate behaviors.

CN: Health promotion and maintenance;
CL: Synthesize

21. 4. Nonthreatening experiences that are stimulating and interesting to the child have been observed to help raise IQ. Practices such as serving nutritious meals or letting the child play with more able children have not been supported by research as beneficial in increasing intelligence. Vasodilator medications act to increase oxygenation to the tissues, including the brain. However, these medications do not increase the child's IQ.

CN: Health promotion and maintenance;
CL: Synthesize

22. 4. When teaching the parents of a child with Down syndrome, activities should focus on increasing the parents' confidence in their ability to care for the child. The parents must continue to work daily with their child. Most parents feel affection and a sense of responsibility for their child regardless of the child's limitations. Parents usually understand the child's disability on the cognitive level but have difficulty accepting it on the emotional level. As the parents' confidence in their caring abilities increases, their understanding of the child's disability also increases on all levels.

⚷ CN: Psychosocial integrity; CL: Create

The Client with a Seizure Disorder

23. 2. Phenytoin can cause gingival hyperplasia. Children taking phenytoin should brush their teeth after every meal and at bedtime, and visit their dentist on a regular basis. Drinking plenty of fluids is not required while taking phenytoin. A child on phenytoin does not need to be observed during waking hours because the seizures should be under control. Infections do not occur with an increased incidence in clients receiving phenytoin.

⚷ CN: Pharmacological and parenteral therapies; CL: Create

24. 3. During a generalized tonic-clonic seizure, the first priority is to keep the child safe and protect the child by removing any nearby objects that could cause injury. Although obtaining information about events surrounding the seizure is important, this information can be obtained later, once the child's safety is ensured. During a seizure, the child should not be moved. Although providing privacy is important, the child's safety is the priority. During a seizure, nothing should be forced into the client's mouth because this can cause severe damage to the teeth and mouth.

⚷ CN: Physiological adaptation; CL: Evaluate

25. 3. Most children who develop seizures after infancy are intellectually normal. A child with a seizure disorder needs the same experiences and opportunities to develop intellectual, emotional, and social abilities as any other child. Activity limitation is not needed. Learning disabilities are not associated with seizures. The child is able to attend public school, and social stigma is a rarity.

⚷ CN: Health promotion and maintenance; CL: Create

26. 1. A child who has generalized seizures should not participate in activities that are poten-

tially hazardous. Even if accompanied by a responsible adult, the child could be seriously injured if a seizure were to occur during rock climbing. Someone also should accompany the child during activities in the water. At summer camps, hiking and swimming would occur most commonly as group activities, so someone should be with the child. Tennis would be considered an appropriate, nonhazardous activity for a child with generalized seizures.

⚷ CN: Safety and infection control; CL: Synthesize

27. 4. Most febrile seizures occur in the presence of an upper respiratory infection, otitis media, or tonsillitis. Febrile seizures typically occur during a temperature rise rather than after prolonged fever. There appears to be increased susceptibility to febrile seizures within families. Infrequently, febrile seizures may lead to respiratory arrest.

⚷ CN: Physiological adaptation; CL: Analyze

28. 2. Shivering, the body's defense against rapid temperature decrease, results in an increase in body temperature. Therefore, the parents need to take measures to stop the shivering (and the resulting increase in body temperature) by increasing the room temperature or the temperature of the child's immediate environment (such as with blankets) until the shivering stops. Then, attempts are made to lower the temperature more slowly. Shivering does not necessarily correlate with being cold. Alcohol, a toxic substance, can be absorbed through the skin. Its use is to be avoided.

⚷ CN: Physiological adaptation; CL: Evaluate

29. 3. Phenytoin sodium is a known teratogenic agent, causing numerous fetal problems. Therefore, the adolescent should be advised to talk to the **HCP** 📖 to see if changing the medication is possible. Additionally, anticonvulsant requirements usually increase during pregnancy. Seizures can be controlled but cannot be cured. There is a familial tendency for seizure disorders. Seizure disorders and infertility are not related.

⚷ CN: Pharmacological and parenteral therapies; CL: Synthesize

30. 3. A toxic effect of valproic acid is liver toxicity, which may manifest with jaundice and abdominal pain. If jaundice occurs, the client needs to notify the **HCP** 📖 as soon as possible. Diarrhea and sore throat are not common side effects of this drug. Increased appetite is common with this drug.

⚷ CN: Pharmacological and parenteral therapies; CL: Analyze

The Client with Meningitis

31. 1. Instituting droplet precautions is the priority for a newly admitted infant with meningococcal meningitis. Acetaminophen may be ordered, but administering it does not take priority over instituting droplet precautions. Obtaining history information and orienting the parents to the unit do not take priority.

🔑 CN: Safety and infection control; CL: Application

32. 2. A child in the acute stage of meningitis is irritable and hypersensitive to loud noise and light. Therefore, extraneous noise should be minimized and bright lights avoided as much as possible. There is no need to limit conversations with the child. However, the nurse should speak in a calm, gentle, reassuring voice. The child needs gentle and calm bathing. Because of the acuteness of the infection, sponge baths would be more appropriate than tub baths. Although treatments need to be completed as quickly as possible to prevent overstressing the child, they should be performed carefully and at a pace that avoids sudden movements to prevent startling the child and subsequently increasing intracranial pressure.

🔑 CN: Basic care and comfort; CL: Synthesize

33. 1. Disseminated intravascular coagulation is characterized by skin petechiae and a purpuric skin rash caused by spontaneous bleeding into the tissues. An abnormal coagulation phenomenon causes the condition. Heparin therapy is often used to interrupt the clotting process. Edema would suggest a fluid volume excess. Cyanosis would indicate decreased tissue oxygenation. Dyspnea on exertion would suggest respiratory problems, such as pulmonary edema.

🔑 CN: Physiological adaptation; CL: Analyze

34. 2. Organisms that cause bacterial meningitis, such as pneumococci or meningococci, are commonly spread in the body by vascular dissemination from a middle ear infection. The meningitis may also be a direct extension from the paranasal and mastoid sinuses. The causative organism is a pneumococcus. A chronically draining ear is also frequently found. Bladder infections commonly are caused by *Escherichia coli*, unrelated to the development of pneumococcal meningitis. Pneumococcal meningitis is unrelated to a fractured clavicle or to septic arthritis, which is commonly caused by *Staphylococcus aureus*, group A streptococci, or *Haemophilus influenzae*.

🔑 CN: Physiological adaptation; CL: Analyze

35. 3. Preschool-age children worry about having an intact body and become fearful of any threat to body integrity. Allowing the child to participate in required care helps protect her image of an intact body. Development of trust is the task typically associated with infancy. Additionally, allowing the child to apply a dressing over the intravenous insertion site is unrelated to the development of trust. Finding diversional activities is not a priority need for a child in this age group. Separation anxiety is more common in toddlers than in preschoolers.

🔑 CN: Health promotion and maintenance; CL: Apply

36. 83 mL/h

$$1,000 \text{ mL} \div 12 \text{ h} = 83 \text{ mL/h}$$

🔑 CN: Pharmacological and parenteral therapies; CL: Apply

37. 1,3,4. Antibiotics are indicated for the treatment of bacterial meningitis. Clients with bacterial meningitis often have increased ICP. It is necessary to maintain adequate hydration. However, infusing fluids at 1½ maintenance can increase ICP, further risking neurologic damage due to cerebral edema. Most children with meningitis are sensitive to sound, light, and stimulation. Decreasing environmental stimuli and keeping the room dim and quiet are essential. Frequent neurologic checks are necessary to monitor any changes in the child's level of consciousness. Anticonvulsants are not indicated unless the child experiences seizures as a result of the meningitis.

🔑 CN: Physiological adaptation; CL: Apply

38. 1,4,5. Irritability, bulging fontanelle, and emesis are all signs of increased ICP in an infant. A headache may be present in an infant with increased ICP; however, the infant has no way of communicating this to the parent. A headache is an indication of increased ICP in a verbal child. An infant cannot exhibit mood swings; this is indicative of increased ICP in a child or adolescent.

🔑 CN: Reduction of risk potential; CL: Apply

39. 3. The child is angry and needs a positive outlet for expression of feelings. An emotionally tense child with pent-up hostilities needs a physical activity that will release energy and frustration. Pounding on a pegboard offers this opportunity. Listening to a story does not allow the child to express emotions. It also places the child in a passive role and does not allow the child to deal with feelings in a healthy and positive way. Activities such as painting and stacking a tower of blocks require concentration and fine movements, which could add to frustration. However, if the child then knocks the tower over, doing so may help to dispel some of the anger.

🔑 CN: Health promotion and maintenance; CL: Synthesize

The Client with Near-Drowning

40. 2. Hypoxia is the primary problem because it results in brain cell damage. Irreversible brain damage occurs after 4 to 6 minutes of submersion. Hypothermia occurs rapidly in infants and children because of their large body surface area. Hypothermia is more of a problem when the child is in cold water. Although fluid aspiration occurs in most drownings and results in atelectasis and pulmonary edema, further aggravating hypoxia, hypoxia is the primary problem. Cutaneous capillary paralysis is not a problem.

CN: Physiological adaptation;
CL: Analyze

41. 1. Near-drowning victims typically suffer hypoxia and mixed acidosis. The priority is to restore oxygenation and prevent further hypoxia. Here, the client has blunted sensorium but is not unconscious; therefore, delivery of supplemental oxygen with a mask is appropriate. Warming protocols and fluid resuscitation will most likely be needed to help correct acidosis, but these interventions are secondary to oxygen administration. Intubation is required if the child is comatose, shows signs of airway compromise, or does not respond adequately to more conservative therapies.

CN: Physiological adaptation;
CL: Synthesize

42. 2. Guilt is a common parental response. The parents need to be allowed to express their feelings openly in a nonthreatening, nonjudgmental atmosphere. Telling the parents that these things happen does not allow them to verbalize their feelings. Telling the parents that they should not have taken their eyes off the child blames them, possibly further contributing to their guilt. Telling the parents that they should not feel guilty denies the parents' feelings of guilt and is inappropriate. Telling the parents that they are lucky that the child will be okay does not remove the feelings of guilt.

CN: Psychosocial integrity;
CL: Synthesize

The Client with Guillain-Barré Syndrome (Infectious Polyneuritis)

43. 1. The child is exhibiting symptoms associated with Guillain-Barré syndrome (infectious polyneuritis). Most children with sore throat have some difficulty swallowing, so it is important for the nurse to determine the extent of difficulty to aid in determining what action is necessary. Typically, a sore throat precedes the paralysis in clients with Guillain-Barré syndrome. Muscle tenderness is an initial symptom. Distal muscle weakness follows proximal muscle weakness, ultimately progressing to paralysis. Diet history and difficulty urinating will not contribute to assessment of the cause of a sore throat or difficulty swallowing. After determining the extent of difficulty swallowing, the nurse can obtain information about exposure to illness.

CN: Health promotion and maintenance;
CL: Analyze

44. 2. With Guillain-Barré syndrome, progressive ascending paralysis occurs. Therefore, the nurse should assess the child's muscle strength bilaterally to determine the extent of involvement and progression of the illness. Assessing the child's ability to follow simple commands evaluates brain function. Range-of-motion exercises are an important part of treatment, but they are not a priority initially. Although the child may need diversional activities later, they also are not an initial priority.

CN: Physiological adaptation;
CL: Synthesize

45. 3. In a child with Guillain-Barré syndrome, decreased volume and clarity of speech and decreased ability to cough voluntarily indicate ascending progression of neural inflammation, specifically affecting the cranial nerves. Inflammation of the larynx and epiglottis is manifested by hoarseness, stridor, and dyspnea. A child with laryngeal inflammation still retains the ability to cough. Irritability, behavior changes, headache, and vomiting are common signs of increased intracranial pressure in a school-age child. Regression would be manifested by being more dependent and less able to care for self.

CN: Physiological adaptation;
CL: Apply

46. 2. An ineffective breathing pattern caused by the ascending paralysis of the disorder interferes with the child's ability to maintain an adequate oxygen supply. Therefore, this nursing diagnosis takes precedence. Additionally, as the neurologic impairment progresses, it will probably have an effect on the child's ability to maintain respirations. An increased risk for infection related to an altered immune system is not associated with Guillain-Barré syndrome. Although impaired swallowing and incontinence may occur with the ascending paralysis of this disorder, oxygenation is the priority.

CN: Physiological adaptation;
CL: Analyze

47. 4. Even in the absence of respiratory problems or distress, the child must be turned frequently to help prevent the cardiopulmonary complications associated with immobility, such as atelectasis and pneumonia. Maintaining the child in a supine position is unnecessary. Doing so does not prevent unnecessary nerve stimulation. In addition, maintaining a supine position may lead to stasis of secretions, placing the child at risk for pneumonia. Transferring the child to a chair will not prevent postural hypotension. However, doing so will increase vascular tone and help prevent respiratory and skin complications. During the acute disease phase, vigorous physiotherapy is contraindicated because the child may experience muscle pain and be hypersensitive to touch. Careful and gentle handling is essential.

∞⚯ CN: Physiological adaptation;
CL: Synthesize

48. 3. Developmentally appropriate activities and therapeutic play should be used as rehabilitation modalities. Taking the child to the pool to exercise with other children indicates that the child is participating in exercise as well as engaging with other children, thus fostering development. Arguing with the sister does not address the discharge plan. Inappropriate rewards or threats should not be used to coerce a child into compliance. Although the mother is attempting to comply with the discharge plan, bribery is an inappropriate technique to foster compliance. Missing therapy sessions delays recovery. The parents need to help set the child's schedule to ensure that she gets adequate rest to be able to follow her treatment plan.

∞⚯ CN: Physiological adaptation;
CL: Evaluate

The Client with a Head Injury

49. 1. This client is experiencing neurologic changes consistent with increasing intracranial pressure (ICP). The nurse should first notify the **HCP** 📖. The HCP may intubate the child to ensure a patent airway. The nurse should not lower the head of the bed as this will cause increased ICP. The nurse should ensure an adequate fluid balance. The HCP will likely prescribe hypertonic saline to draw fluid from the brain.

∞⚯ CN: Management of care; CL: Synthesize

50. 1. An ICP level greater than 15 mm Hg is abnormal. This child's vital signs indicate increased ICP. Mannitol is an osmotic diuretic and will decrease the child's ICP. Suctioning the child will increase the ICP. Encouraging the parent to talk to the child may be comforting but will not decrease the ICP. The priority for this child is decreasing the ICP to avoid further brain injury. The fever is

likely due to the head injury and will not decrease with acetaminophen. A cooling blanket is the most effective means of reducing a fever in a client with a head injury.

∞⚯ CN: Reduction of risk potential;
CL: Apply

51. 2. For the child with serious head trauma, a nasogastric tube is inserted initially to decompress the stomach and to prevent vomiting and aspiration. Medications would be administered intravenously in the initial period. The tube will not be used to obtain gastric specimens. Nutrition is not a priority initially. Later on, the tube may be used to administer feedings.

∞⚯ CN: Reduction of risk potential;
CL: Apply

52. 1. Because a basilar skull fracture can involve the frontal and ethmoid bones, inserting a nasogastric tube carries the risk of introducing the tube into the cranial cavity through the fracture. An oral gastric tube is preferred for a client with a basilar skull fracture. The tube would not be placed into the duodenum. Gastric aspirate is not routinely tested for blood unless there is an indication to suggest bleeding, such as a falling hemoglobin or visible blood in the drainage.

∞⚯ CN: Reduction of risk potential;
CL: Synthesize

53. 3. As a rule, children demonstrate more rapid and more complete recovery from coma than do adults. However, it is extremely difficult to predict a specific outcome. Reassuring the parents that they will be kept informed helps open lines of communication and establish trust. Telling the parents that children do not do well would be extremely negative, destroying any hope that the parents might have. Telling the parents that children recover rapidly may give the parents false hopes. Telling the parents to talk to the **HCP** 📖 ignores the parents' concerns and interferes with trust building.

∞⚯ CN: Physiological adaptation;
CL: Synthesize

54. 2. The level of consciousness (LOC) is the best indicator of brain function. If the child's condition deteriorates, the nurse would notice changes in LOC before any other changes and should notify the **healthcare provider (HCP)** 📖 that these changes are occurring. Changes in vital signs and pupils typically follow changes in LOC. Motor strength is primarily assessed as a voluntary function. With changes in levels of consciousness, there may be motor changes.

∞⚯ CN: Physiological adaptation; CL: Apply

The Client with a Spinal Cord Injury

72. 2. The adolescent's signs and symptoms suggest a spinal cord injury. A client with suspected spinal cord injury should not be moved until the spine has been immobilized. Removing the helmet could further aggravate a spinal cord injury. The nurse could assess for abdominal trauma, but only if it can be done without moving the adolescent.

☘— CN: Reduction of risk potential;
CL: Synthesize

73. 1. In spinal cord injury, temperature regulation is lost below T3. Body temperature must be maintained by adjusting room temperature or bed linens, such as covering the client's legs with blankets. Coolness of the extremities is an expected finding. Therefore, it is not necessary to notify the **HCP** ☐ immediately. Repositioning the client's legs does not alleviate the temperature regulation problem and could be harmful, considering the client's diagnosis. Moving the legs before the spine is stabilized could lead to further cord damage. Laying the client flat will not increase the warmth to the legs and feet.

☘— CN: Physiological adaptation;
CL: Synthesize

74. 3. A thoracic spinal cord injury involves the muscles of the lower extremities, bladder, and rectum. Paralytic ileus often occurs as a result of decreased gastrointestinal muscle innervation. The nurse evaluates this by auscultating the abdomen. Because the client has a thoracic spinal cord injury, the client may not feel abdominal cramping. Additionally, auscultation would provide no evidence of cramping. Hyperactive bowel sounds would be evidenced with increased peristalsis; peristalsis would probably be diminished with this injury. Profuse diarrhea, resulting from increased peristalsis, would not be an expected finding. Diarrhea would be more commonly associated with a gastrointestinal infection.

☘— CN: Physiological adaptation;
CL: Analyze

75. 3. Spinal shock causes a loss of reflex activity below the level of the injury, resulting in bladder atony and flaccid paralysis. When the reflex arc returns, it tends to be overactive, resulting in spasticity. The reflexes and bladder become hypertonic during this phase of spinal shock resolution; sensation does not return. A widened pulse pressure is not associated with resolution of spinal shock.

☘— CN: Physiological adaptation;
CL: Evaluate

76. 1. After a catastrophic injury, individuals commonly experience grief. Initially, the person experiences denial, the most common response. With gradual awareness of the situation, anger commonly occurs. The child is demonstrating anger, not rebellion, as he gradually becomes aware of his situation. Rebellion is the child's way to maintain autonomy and individuality. It is a reaction to rigid rules. Examples include refusing to follow a treatment protocol when the child had no input and running away. Sensory overload would cause the child to be irritable and tired and to have difficulty sleeping. Too much attention usually would lead to irritability, difficulty sleeping, and mood swings.

☘— CN: Psychosocial integrity; CL: Analyze

77. 1. The adolescent is exhibiting signs of autonomic dysreflexia, a generalized sympathetic response usually caused by bladder or bowel distention. Immediate treatment involves eliminating the cause. Because bladder distention is a common cause of this problem, the nurse should immediately determine the patency of the indwelling (Foley) catheter. Lowering the head below the knees would increase the blood pressure and is contraindicated because of the spinal cord injury. Lying flat will not decrease blood pressure. Epinephrine is contraindicated because it elevates blood pressure and therefore can exacerbate the problem.

☘— CN: Physiological adaptation;
CL: Synthesize

Managing Care, Quality, and Safety of Children with Neurologic Health Problems

78. 4. Bacterial meningitis is caused by one of three organisms, *H. influenzae* type b, *Neisseria meningitidis*, or *Streptococcus pneumoniae*. All three organisms may be transmitted through contact with respiratory droplets. These droplets are heavy and typically fall within 3 feet (91.4 cm) of the client. Droplet precautions require, in addition to standard (routine) precautions, that **HCPs** ☐ wear masks when coming into close contact with the client. Standard or routine precautions, previously referred to as universal precautions, are general measures used for all clients. Contact precautions are used when direct or indirect contact with the client causes disease transmission. Gowns and gloves are needed but not masks. Airborne precautions differ from droplet in that the particles are smaller and may stay suspended in the air for longer periods of time. These clients require negative pressure rooms, and all healthcare workers must wear respirators.

☘— CN: Safety and infection control;
CL: Apply

79. **3,4,5.** Using only oral syringes to administer oral medications reduces the chance that the medication will be given intravenously. The use of smart pumps alone is not enough to prevent IV fluid administration. An additional measure that pediatric floors can institute to prevent accidental fluid overload is to use smaller IV fluid bags, such as 250 mL. Whenever a medication comes in multiple concentrations and doses, there is risk of administering the wrong dose. The use of pediatric satellite pharmacies with pediatric pharmacists greatly increases the safety of medication administration. Any time steps are added to the medication administration process, there is one more place where an error might occur.

> CN: Safety and infection control;
> CL: Synthesize

80. **4.** The coating on an extended-release medication helps assure slow absorption of the medication. If the nurse crushes the medication, the medication may enter the client's system too quickly and result in toxic levels. The only appropriate action is to contact the prescriber and ask that the prescription be changed. Cutting the medication or trying to dissolve a whole tablet would have similar results as crushing it. Carbamazepine comes as an oral suspension, but it is not extended release. Therefore, a prescription would be needed to address dosing if switching to this form.

> CN: Safety and infection control;
> CL: Synthesize

81. **1.** A poster presentation is an eye-catching way to disseminate information that can be used to educate nurses on all shifts. The addition of the posttest will verify that the poster information has been received. Because of the large volume of e-mails the typical employee receives, information sent this way might be overlooked. If several nurses are observed not using the most current practice, it is quite possible many more do not understand it. Thus, a larger-scale plan is needed. Posting an article will not alone assure that the information is read.

> CN: Reduction of risk potential;
> CL: Create

82. **1.** The child is exhibiting signs and symptoms of increased intracranial pressure (ICP). A lumbar puncture is contraindicated in children with increased ICP due to the risk of herniation. Magnetic resonance imaging and a computerized tomography scan are indicated in children with suspected increased ICP. Radiology studies will allow visualization of the cause of the increased ICP, such as inflammation, a tumor, or hemorrhage. An arterial blood draw is not indicated in this client. However, there is no contraindication for performing an arterial blood draw on a child with increased ICP.

> CN: Reduction of risk potential;
> CL: Analyze

83. **2.** IV lorazepam is the benzodiazepine of choice for treating prolonged seizure activity. IV benzodiazepines act to potentiate the action of the gamma-aminobutyric acid (GABA) neurotransmitter, stopping seizure activity. If an IV is not available, rectal diazepam is the benzodiazepine of choice. The child does have a low-grade fever; however, this is likely caused by the excessive motor activity. The primary goal for the child is to stop the seizure in order to reduce neurologic damage. Benzodiazepines are used for the initial treatment of prolonged seizures. Once the seizure has ended, a loading dose of fosphenytoin or phenobarbital is given.

> CN: Pharmacological and parenteral
> therapies; CL: Apply

TEST 8

The Child with Musculoskeletal Health Problems

- The Client with Torticollis, Legg-Calvé-Perthes Disease, and Musculoskeletal Dysfunction
- The Client with Cerebral Palsy
- The Client with Duchenne's Muscular Dystrophy
- The Client with Developmental Dysplasia of the Hip
- The Client with Congenital Clubfoot
- The Client with Juvenile Idiopathic Arthritis
- The Client with a Fracture
- The Client with Osteomyelitis
- The Client with Scoliosis
- Managing Care, Quality, and Safety of Children with Musculoskeletal Health Problems
- Answers, Rationales, and Test-Taking Strategies

The Client with Torticollis, Legg-Calvé-Perthes Disease, and Musculoskeletal Dysfunction

1. In planning the discharge for a newborn diagnosed with torticollis (wry neck), the nurse should:
☐ 1. teach the parent the side effects of botulinum toxin.
☐ 2. coordinate outpatient physical therapy.
☐ 3. verify the date for corrective surgery.
☐ 4. demonstrate the use of positioning wedges for sleep.

2. A child who limps and has pain has been found to have Legg-Calvé-Perthes disease. What should the nurse expect to include in the child's plan of care?
☐ 1. initiation of pain control measures, especially at night when acute
☐ 2. promotion of ambulation despite child's discomfort in the affected hip
☐ 3. prevention of flexion in the affected hip and knee
☐ 4. avoidance of weight bearing on the head of the affected femur

3. When planning home care for the child with Legg-Calvé-Perthes disease, what should be the **primary** focus for family teaching?
☐ 1. need for intake of protein-rich foods
☐ 2. gentle stretching exercises for both legs
☐ 3. management of the corrective appliance
☐ 4. relaxation techniques for pain control

4. At the 2-week well-child visit, a parent states, "My baby seems to keep his head tilted to the right." The nurse should further assess the:
☐ 1. fontanelle.
☐ 2. cervical vertebrae.
☐ 3. trapezius muscle.
☐ 4. sternocleidomastoid muscle.

5. An adolescent tells the nurse that the area below his knee has been hurting for several weeks. The nurse should obtain history information about participation in which sport?
☐ 1. soccer
☐ 2. golf
☐ 3. diving
☐ 4. swimming

6. An adolescent is on the football team and practices in the morning and afternoon before school starts for the year. The temperature on the field has been high. The school nurse has been called to the practice field because the adolescent is now reporting that he has muscle cramps, nausea, and dizziness. Which action should the school nurse do **first**?
☐ 1. Administer cold water with ice cubes.
☐ 2. Take the adolescent's temperature.
☐ 3. Have the adolescent lie supine.
☐ 4. Move the adolescent to a cool environment.

The Client with Cerebral Palsy

7. During a developmental screening, the nurse finds that a 3-year-old child with cerebral palsy has arrested social and language development. The nurse tells the family:
- ☐ **1.** "This is a sign the cerebral palsy is progressing."
- ☐ **2.** "Your child has reached his maximum language abilities."
- ☐ **3.** "I need to refer you for more developmental testing."
- ☐ **4.** "We need to modify your therapy plan."

8. A child with spastic cerebral palsy is to begin botulinum toxin type A injections. Which treatment goals should the healthcare team set for the child related to botulinum toxin? Select all that apply.
- ☐ **1.** improved nutritional status
- ☐ **2.** decreased pain from spasticity
- ☐ **3.** improved motor function
- ☐ **4.** enhanced self-esteem
- ☐ **5.** reduced caregiver strain and improved self-care
- ☐ **6.** decreased speech impediments

9. The nurse judges that the mother understands the term *cerebral palsy* when she describes it as a term applied to impaired movement resulting from which factor?
- ☐ **1.** injury to the cerebrum caused by viral infection
- ☐ **2.** malformed blood vessels in the ventricles caused by inheritance
- ☐ **3.** nonprogressive brain damage caused by injury
- ☐ **4.** inflammatory brain disease caused by metabolic imbalances

10. When assessing the development of a 15-month-old child with cerebral palsy, which milestones should the nurse expect a typically developing toddler of this age to have achieved?
- ☐ **1.** walking up steps
- ☐ **2.** using a spoon
- ☐ **3.** copying a circle
- ☐ **4.** putting a block in a cup

11. The parent of a child with spastic cerebral palsy and a communication disorder tells the nurse, "He seems so restless. I think he is in pain." Which action is **most** indicated?
- ☐ **1.** Assess the child for pain using the faces, legs, activity, cry, consolability (FLACC) scale.
- ☐ **2.** Assess the child for pain using the pediatric FACES scale.
- ☐ **3.** Administer prescribed pain medication.
- ☐ **4.** Notify the healthcare provider (HCP) of the change in behavior.

12. The parent asks the nurse whether a child with hemiparesis due to spastic cerebral palsy will be able to walk normally because he can pull himself to a standing position. Which response by the nurse would be **most** appropriate?
- ☐ **1.** "Ask your healthcare provider what he or she thinks at your next appointment."
- ☐ **2.** "Being able to pull to a stand really only tells us his upper-body strength is good"
- ☐ **3.** "It is difficult to predict, but his ability to bear weight is a positive factor."
- ☐ **4.** "If he really wants to walk, and works hard, he probably will eventually."

13. The nurse assesses the family's ability to cope with the child's cerebral palsy. Which action should alert the nurse to the possibility of their inability to cope with the disease?
- ☐ **1.** limiting interaction with extended family and friends
- ☐ **2.** learning measures to meet the child's physical needs
- ☐ **3.** requesting teaching about cerebral palsy in general
- ☐ **4.** seeking advice on coping on social media

The Client with Duchenne's Muscular Dystrophy

14. The mother of a child with Duchenne's muscular dystrophy asks about the chance that her next child will have the disease. The nurse responds based on the understanding of what information?
- ☐ **1.** Sons have a 50% chance of being affected.
- ☐ **2.** Daughters have a 1 in 4 chance of being carriers.
- ☐ **3.** Each child has a 1 in 4 chance of developing the disease.
- ☐ **4.** Each child has a 50% chance of being a carrier.

15. A nurse is making an initial visit to a family with a 3-year-old child with early Duchenne's muscular dystrophy. Which finding is expected when assessing this child?
- ☐ **1.** contractures of the large joints
- ☐ **2.** enlarged calf muscles
- ☐ **3.** difficulty riding a tricycle
- ☐ **4.** atrophied muscles

16. The nurse observes as a child with Duchenne's muscular dystrophy attempts to rise from a sitting position on the floor. After attaining a kneeling position, the child "walks" his hands up his legs to stand. The nurse documents this as which sign?
- ☐ **1.** Galeazzi's sign
- ☐ **2.** Goodell's sign
- ☐ **3.** Goodenough's sign
- ☐ **4.** Gower's sign

17. When developing the plan of care for a child with early Duchenne's muscular dystrophy, which nursing goal is the **priority**?
☐ **1.** Encourage early wheelchair use.
☐ **2.** Foster social interactions.
☐ **3.** Maintain function of unaffected muscles.
☐ **4.** Prevent circulatory impairment.

18. When interacting with the parent of a child who has Duchenne's muscular dystrophy, the nurse observes behavior indicating that the parent may feel guilty about the child's condition. The nurse interprets this behavior as guilt stemming from which factor?
☐ **1.** the terminal nature of the disease
☐ **2.** the dependent behavior of the child
☐ **3.** the genetic mode of transmission
☐ **4.** the sudden onset of the disease

19. The nurse teaches the parent of a young child with Duchenne's muscular dystrophy about the disease and its management. Which statement by the parent indicates successful teaching?
☐ **1.** "My son will probably be unable to walk independently by the time he is 9 to 11 years old."
☐ **2.** "Muscle relaxants are effective for some children; I hope they can help my son."
☐ **3.** "When my son is a little older, he can have surgery to improve his ability to walk."
☐ **4.** "I need to help my son be as active as possible to prevent progression of the disease."

The Client with Developmental Dysplasia of the Hip

20. A 16-month-old child is seen in the clinic for a checkup for the first time. The nurse notices that the toddler limps when walking. Which would be appropriate to use when assessing this toddler for developmental dysplasia of the hip?
☐ **1.** Ortolani's maneuver
☐ **2.** Barlow's maneuver
☐ **3.** Adam's position
☐ **4.** Trendelenburg's sign

21. The nurse is assessing the infant shown in the figure. On observing the client from this angle, the nurse should document that this infant has which finding?

☐ **1.** Ortolani's "click"
☐ **2.** limited abduction
☐ **3.** Galeazzi's sign
☐ **4.** asymmetric gluteal folds

22. The nurse teaches the parents of an infant with developmental dysplasia of the hip how to handle their child in a Pavlik harness. Which care is **most** appropriate?
☐ **1.** Fit the diaper under the straps.
☐ **2.** Leave the harness off while the infant sleeps.
☐ **3.** Check for skin redness under straps every other day.
☐ **4.** Put powder on the skin under the straps every day.

23. When developing the teaching plan for parents using the Pavlik harness with their child, what should be the nurse's **initial** step?
☐ **1.** Assess the parents' current coping strategies.
☐ **2.** Determine the parents' knowledge about the device.
☐ **3.** Provide the parents with written instructions.
☐ **4.** Give the parents a list of community resources.

24. When teaching the family of an older infant who has had a spica cast applied for developmental dysplasia of the hip, which information should the nurse include when describing the abduction stabilizer bar?
☐ **1.** It can be adjusted to a position of comfort.
☐ **2.** It is used to lift the child.
☐ **3.** It adds strength to the cast.
☐ **4.** It is necessary to turn the child.

25. A parent asks the nurse about using a car seat for a toddler who is in a hip spica cast. The nurse should tell the parent:

☐ 1. "You can use a seat belt because of the spica cast."

☐ 2. "You will need a specially designed car seat for your toddler."

☐ 3. "You can still use the car seat you already have."

☐ 4. "You will need to get a special release from the police so that a car seat will not be needed."

The Client with Congenital Clubfoot

26. The nurse is discharging a baby with clubfoot who has had a cast applied. The nurse should provide additional teaching to the parents if they state:

☐ 1. "I should call if I see changes in the color of the toes under the cast."

☐ 2. "I should use a pillow to elevate my child's foot as he sleeps."

☐ 3. "My baby will need a series of casts to fix her foot."

☐ 4. "Having a cast should not prevent me from holding my baby."

27. The parents of a neonate born with congenital clubfoot express feelings of helplessness and guilt and are exhibiting anxiety about how the neonate will be treated. Which action by the nurse would be **most** appropriate initially?

☐ 1. Ask them to share these concerns with the healthcare provider (HCP).

☐ 2. Arrange a meeting with other parents whose infants have had successful clubfoot treatment.

☐ 3. Discuss the problem with the parents and the current feelings that they are experiencing.

☐ 4. Suggest that they make an appointment to talk things over with a counselor.

28. After teaching the parents of an infant with clubfoot requiring application of a plaster cast how to care for the cast, which statement would indicate that the parents have understood the teaching?

☐ 1. "If the cast becomes soiled, we will clean it with soap and water."

☐ 2. "We will elevate the leg with the cast on pillows so the leg is above heart level."

☐ 3. "We will check the color and temperature of the toes of the casted leg frequently."

☐ 4. "The petals on the edge of the cast can be removed after the first 24 hours."

The Client with Juvenile Idiopathic Arthritis

29. The parent of a preschool-age child with a tentative diagnosis of juvenile idiopathic arthritis (JIA) asks about a test to definitively diagnose JIA. The nurse's response is based on knowledge of what information?

☐ 1. The latex fixation test is diagnostic.

☐ 2. An increased erythrocyte sedimentation rate is diagnostic.

☐ 3. A positive synovial fluid culture is diagnostic.

☐ 4. No specific laboratory test is diagnostic.

30. The parents of a child just diagnosed with juvenile idiopathic arthritis (JIA) tell the nurse that the diagnosis frightens them because they know nothing about the prognosis. What information should the nurse include when teaching the parents about the disease?

☐ 1. The more joints affected, the more severe the disease will be.

☐ 2. Many affected children go into long remissions but have severe deformities.

☐ 3. The disease usually progresses to crippling rheumatoid arthritis.

☐ 4. Most affected children recover completely within a few years.

31. The mother of a 4-year-old child with juvenile idiopathic arthritis (JIA) is worried that her child will have to stop attending preschool because of the illness. Which response by the nurse would be **most** appropriate?

☐ 1. "It may be difficult for your child to attend school because of the side effects of the medications he will be prescribed."

☐ 2. "Your child should be encouraged to attend school, but he will need extra time to work out early morning stiffness."

☐ 3. "You should keep your child at home from school whenever he experiences discomfort or pain in his joints."

☐ 4. "Your child will probably need to wear splints and braces so that his joints will be supported properly."

32. A preschool-age child with juvenile idiopathic arthritis (JIA) has become withdrawn, and the mother asks the nurse what she should do. Which suggestion by the nurse would be **most** appropriate?

☐ 1. Introduce the child to other children her age who also have JIA.

☐ 2. Tell the mother to spend extra time with the child and less time with her other children.

☐ 3. Recommend that the mother send the child to see a counselor for therapy.

☐ 4. Encourage the mother to be supportive and understanding of the child.

33. Nonsteroidal anti-inflammatory drugs are the first choice in treating a child with juvenile idiopathic arthritis. Which adverse effects should the nurse include in the teaching plan for the parents? Select all that apply.
- ☐ 1. weight gain
- ☐ 2. abdominal pain
- ☐ 3. blood in the stool
- ☐ 4. folic acid deficiency
- ☐ 5. reduced blood clotting ability

34. What information should the nurse include when developing the teaching plan for the parents of a child with juvenile idiopathic arthritis who is being treated with naproxen?
- ☐ 1. Anti-inflammatory effect will occur in approximately 8 weeks.
- ☐ 2. Within 24 hours, the child will have anti-inflammatory relief.
- ☐ 3. The nurse should be called before giving the child any over-the-counter medications.
- ☐ 4. If a dose is forgotten or missed, that dose is not made up.

The Client with a Fracture

35. A 10-year-old has 5 lb (2.27 kg) of Buck's extension traction on his left leg. What finding should the nurse assess the child for? Select all that apply.
- ☐ 1. dryness of the skin, by removing the foam wraps and boot
- ☐ 2. alignment of the shoulder, hips, and knees
- ☐ 3. frayed rope near pulleys
- ☐ 4. correct amount of traction weight on fracture
- ☐ 5. pressure on the coccyx

36. A 14-year-old has just had a plaster cast placed on his lower left leg. To provide safe cast care, the nurse should:
- ☐ 1. petal the cast as soon as it is put on.
- ☐ 2. keep the child in the same position for 24 hours until the cast is dry.
- ☐ 3. use only the palms of the hand when handling the cast.
- ☐ 4. notify the healthcare provider (HCP) if the client feels heat.

37. The nurse is explaining the nature of the fracture to the parents of a 10-year-old who has a greenstick fracture. Which drawing should the nurse choose to explain the fracture to the parents?

- ☐ 1.
- ☐ 2.
- ☐ 3.
- ☐ 4.

38. A 9-year-old is given morphine for postoperative pain. As the nurse is assessing the client for pain 4 hours later, his parent leaves the room, and the child begins to cry. The nurse's initial assessment of the child's pain is that he is:
- ☐ 1. not in pain because the crying began after the parent leaves.
- ☐ 2. less tolerant of pain because he is upset.
- ☐ 3. in pain because he is crying.
- ☐ 4. not in pain because he was medicated 4 hours ago.

39. A 13-year-old is having surgery to repair a fractured left femur. As a part of the preoperative safety checklist, what should the nurse do?
- ☐ 1. Ask the teen to point to the surgery site.
- ☐ 2. Verify that the site, side, and level are marked.
- ☐ 3. Ask the parents if they have signed the operative permit.
- ☐ 4. Restate the surgery risks to the parents.

40. A child is admitted with a fracture of the femur and placed in skeletal traction. What should the nurse assess **first**?
- ☐ 1. the pull of traction on the pin
- ☐ 2. the Ace bandage
- ☐ 3. the pin sites for signs of infection
- ☐ 4. the dressings for tightness

41. The nurse is caring for a child in Bryant's traction (see figure). The nurse should:

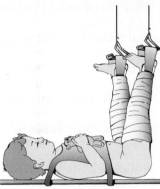

☐ **1.** adjust the weights on the legs until the buttocks rest on the bed.
☐ **2.** provide frequent skin care.
☐ **3.** place a pillow under the buttocks.
☐ **4.** remove the elastic leg wraps every 8 hours for 10 minutes.

42. A preschooler with a fractured femur of the left leg in traction tells the nurse that his leg hurts. It is too early for pain medication. The nurse should:
☐ **1.** place a pillow under the child's buttocks to provide support.
☐ **2.** remove the weight from the left leg.
☐ **3.** assess the feet for signs of neurovascular impairment.
☐ **4.** reposition the pulleys so the traction is looser.

43. The nurse in the emergency department is caring for a 3-year-old child with a fractured humerus. The child is crying and screaming, "I hate you!" Which action would be **most** appropriate?
☐ **1.** Tell the parents they will need to wait out in the lobby.
☐ **2.** Ask the charge nurse to assign this client to another nurse.
☐ **3.** Reassure the parents that this is a normal behavior under the circumstances.
☐ **4.** Ask the parents to discipline the child so that the team can treat her.

44. After a plaster cast has been applied to the arm of a child with a fractured right humerus, the nurse completes discharge teaching. The nurse should evaluate the teaching as successful when the mother agrees to seek medical advice if the child experiences which symptom?
☐ **1.** inability to extend the fingers on the right hand
☐ **2.** vomiting after the cast is applied
☐ **3.** coolness and dampness of the cast after 5 hours
☐ **4.** fussiness with statements that the cast is heavy

45. The nurse should teach the parent of a child who has a new cast for a fractured radius to do which intervention for the first few days at home?
☐ **1.** Use a hair dryer to dry the cast more quickly.
☐ **2.** Have the child refrain from strenuous activities.
☐ **3.** Check movement and sensation of the child's fingers once a day.
☐ **4.** Administer acetaminophen every 8 to 12 hours for discomfort.

46. While assessing a 3-year-old child who has had an injury to the leg, has pain, and refuses to walk, the nurse notes that the child's left thigh is swollen. What should the nurse do **next**?
☐ **1.** Assess the neurologic status of the toes.
☐ **2.** Determine the circulatory status of the upper thigh.
☐ **3.** Obtain the child's vital signs.
☐ **4.** Notify the healthcare provider (HCP) immediately.

47. Anticipating that a 3-year-old child in traction will have need for diversion, what should the nurse offer the child?
☐ **1.** a video game
☐ **2.** blocks
☐ **3.** hand puppets
☐ **4.** remote-controlled car

48. The parents of a child who requires skeletal traction are unable to visit their child for more than 1 hour a day because there are five other children at home and both parents work outside of the home. The nurse recognizes expressions of guilt in both parents. To help alleviate this guilt, the nurse should make which statement?
☐ **1.** "I am sure you feel guilty about not being able to visit often."
☐ **2.** "It is important that you visit even for 1 hour."
☐ **3.** "Not all parents can stay all the time."
☐ **4.** "Perhaps you could take turns visiting for a bit longer."

49. The child in a new hip spica cast seems to be adjusting to the cast, except that after each meal the child tells the nurse that the cast is too tight. What should the nurse plan to do?
☐ **1.** Administer a laxative prior to each meal.
☐ **2.** Offer smaller, more frequent meals.
☐ **3.** Give the child a mechanical soft diet.
☐ **4.** Offer the child more fruits and grains.

50. The nurse is helping a family plan for the discharge of their child who will be going home in a spica cast. Which information would be **most** important for the nurse to consider?
☐ **1.** The bathrooms are all on the second floor.
☐ **2.** The child's bedroom is on the second floor.
☐ **3.** A 16-year-old sister will care for the child during the day.
☐ **4.** There are three steps up to the front door.

51. The nurse is measuring a child for crutches. What factors should the nurse consider? Select all that apply.
- ☐ 1. type of gait child will be using
- ☐ 2. degree of child's elbow flexion
- ☐ 3. space above the crutch to child's axilla
- ☐ 4. weight of the child
- ☐ 5. whether child has to use the stairs

The Client with Osteomyelitis

52. During the initial assessment of a child admitted to the pediatric unit with osteomyelitis of the left tibia, when assessing the area over the tibia, which is an expected finding?
- ☐ 1. diffuse tenderness
- ☐ 2. decreased pain
- ☐ 3. increased warmth
- ☐ 4. localized edema

53. A child is to receive IV antibiotics for osteomyelitis. Before the initial dose of antibiotics can be given, the nurse confirms that a blood sample for which test has been drawn?
- ☐ 1. creatinine
- ☐ 2. culture
- ☐ 3. hemoglobin
- ☐ 4. white blood count

54. A child is being treated with vancomycin 40 mg/kg/day IV divided into three doses for osteomyelitis. The healthcare provider (HCP) has prescribed drug protocol management by pharmacy and a trough vancomycin level 30 minutes before the third dose scheduled for 09:00 hours. The laboratory report returns prior to the third dose:

Laboratory Results	
0830 Vancomycin 7 mcg/mL (4.8 µmol/L) **	Therapeutic range 10–15 mcg/mL (6.9 to 10.4 µmol/L).

The nurse should:
- ☐ 1. administer the 09:00 dose.
- ☐ 2. notify the healthcare provider (HCP).
- ☐ 3. notify the pharmacist.
- ☐ 4. draw a peak drug level.

55. The nurse is caring for a child with osteomyelitis who will be receiving high-dose intravenous antibiotic therapy for 3 to 4 weeks. What should the nurse plan to monitor?
- ☐ 1. blood glucose level
- ☐ 2. thrombin times
- ☐ 3. urine glucose level
- ☐ 4. urine specific gravity

56. To meet the developmental needs of an 8-year-old child who is confined to home with osteomyelitis, what goal should the nurse include in the care plan?
- ☐ 1. Encourage the child to communicate with schoolmates.
- ☐ 2. Encourage the parents to stay with the child.
- ☐ 3. Allow siblings to visit freely throughout the day.
- ☐ 4. Talk to the child about his interests twice daily.

57. A child with newly diagnosed osteomyelitis has nausea and vomiting. The parent wishes to give the child ginger cookies to help control the nausea. The nurse should tell the parent:
- ☐ 1. "You can try them and see how he does."
- ☐ 2. "I will need to get a prescription."
- ☐ 3. "Your child needs medication for the vomiting."
- ☐ 4. "We discourage the use of home remedies in children."

The Client with Scoliosis

58. When assessing an adolescent for scoliosis, what should the nurse ask the client to do?
- ☐ 1. Bend forward at the waist with arms hanging freely.
- ☐ 2. Lie flat on the floor and extend the legs straight from the trunk.
- ☐ 3. Sit in a chair while lifting the feet and legs to a right angle with the trunk.
- ☐ 4. Stand against a wall while pressing the length of the back against the wall.

59. The nurse determines that teaching about the correct use of a Boston brace to treat scoliosis has been effective if the child and family state they will remove the brace at which times?
- ☐ 1. when bathing, for about 1 hour per day
- ☐ 2. while eating, for a total of 3 hours a day
- ☐ 3. during school, for about 8 hours a day
- ☐ 4. when sleeping, for a total of 10 hours a day

60. When teaching the child with scoliosis being treated with a Boston brace about exercises, the nurse explains that the exercises are performed primarily for what reason?
- ☐ 1. to decrease back muscle spasms
- ☐ 2. to improve the brace's traction effect
- ☐ 3. to prevent spinal contractures
- ☐ 4. to strengthen the back and abdominal muscles

61. A 10-year-old with scoliosis has to wear a brace. The nurse should develop a teaching plan with the client to include which instruction?
- ☐ 1. Wear the brace during waking hours.
- ☐ 2. Use lotions to relieve skin irritations.
- ☐ 3. Wear a form-fitting t-shirt under the brace.
- ☐ 4. Bathe the skin under the brace once per week.

Managing Care, Quality, and Safety of Children with Musculoskeletal Health Problems

62. A child with spastic cerebral palsy receiving intrathecal baclofen therapy is admitted to the pediatric floor with vomiting and dehydration. The family tells the nurse that they were scheduled to refill the baclofen pump today but had to cancel the appointment when the child became ill. The nurse should:
- ☐ 1. explain that the medication should be discontinued during illness.
- ☐ 2. arrange for the pump to be refilled in the hospital.
- ☐ 3. reschedule the pump refill for the day of discharge.
- ☐ 4. instruct caregivers to call for a refill when the low-volume alarm sounds.

63. Which procedures can the nurse working on a pediatric floor safely delegate to the licensed practical/vocational nurse (LPN/VN)? Select all that apply.
- ☐ 1. refilling a baclofen pump
- ☐ 2. administering gastrostomy tube feedings
- ☐ 3. inserting hearing aids
- ☐ 4. giving an IV push medication
- ☐ 5. calling the morning blood sugars to the healthcare provider (HCP)

64. An 8-year-old child with juvenile idiopathic arthritis (JIA) is being admitted to the hospital for evaluation of progressively increasing symptoms. The child weighs 60 lb (27 kg) and is 50 inches (127 cm) tall. The nurse is reconciling the medications the parent brought from home with the medications prescribed. What should the nurse do? (See chart.)

Prescriptions

Home meds	Prescribed meds
Ibuprofen tablet 200 mg PO 4× day (for arthritis) Purchased over the counter	Ibuprofen tablet 200 mg PO 4× day
Cetirizine hydrochloride tablet 10 mg PO daily (for allergies) Purchased over the counter	Methotrexate tablet 10 mg PO every Monday

- ☐ 1. Have the family give the child cetirizine daily using the medication they have from home.
- ☐ 2. Explain the need to limit over-the-counter medications while in the hospital.
- ☐ 3. Request a cetirizine prescription from the healthcare provider (HCP).
- ☐ 4. Contact the HCP to question the methotrexate.

65. A 4-year-old male presents to the emergency department. His father tearfully reports that his son was on his shoulders in the driveway playing when he began to fall. When the child began to fall, the father grabbed him by the leg, swinging him toward the grass to avoid landing on the pavement. As the father swung his son, the child hit his head on the driveway and twisted his right leg. After a complete examination, it is determined that the child has a skull fracture and a spiral fracture of the femur. Which action should the nurse take?
- ☐ 1. Restrict the father's visitation.
- ☐ 2. Notify the police immediately.
- ☐ 3. Refer the father for parenting classes.
- ☐ 4. Record the father's story in the medical record.

Answers, Rationales, and Test-Taking Strategies

*The answers and rationales for each question follow below, along with keys (🔑) to the client need (CN) and cognitive level (CL) for each question. In addition, you will also see a glossary icon (📖) highlighting specific terminology used on the licensing exam. As you check your answers, use the **Content Mastery and Test-Taking Skill Self-Analysis** worksheet (tear-out worksheet in back of book) to identify the reason(s) for not answering the questions correctly. For additional information about test-taking skills and strategies for answering questions, refer to pages 10–21 and pages 31–32 in Part 1 of this book.*

The Client with Torticollis, Legg-Calvé-Perthes Disease, and Musculoskeletal Dysfunction

1. 2. Physical therapy is the most important part of the child's plan of care. Most cases of torticollis respond to gentle stretching exercises, which the parents perform daily. Regular physical therapy is needed to monitor the infant's progress. Botulinum toxin injections are not approved for children under the age of 2 and would not be an appropriate first-line treatment for an infant. Surgery is only done if physical therapy is not successful after several months. The use of wedges to position children during sleep is not recommended because they increase the risk of SIDS.

🔑 CN: Management of care; CL: Create

2. 4. Legg-Calvé-Perthes disease, also known as *coxa plana* or *osteochondrosis*, is characterized by aseptic necrosis at the head of the femur when the blood supply to the area is interrupted. Avoidance of weight bearing is especially important to prevent the head of the femur from leaving the acetabulum, thus preventing hip dislocation. Devices such as an abduction brace, a leg cast, or a harness sling are used to protect the affected joint while revascularization and bone healing occur. Surgical procedures are used in some cases. Although pain control measures may be appropriate, pain is not necessarily more acute at night. Initial therapy involves rest and non–weight bearing to help restore motion. Preventing flexion is not necessary.

🔑 CN: Physiological adaptation; CL: Create

3. 3. Because most of the child's care takes place at home, the primary focus of family teaching would be on the care and management of the corrective device. Devices such as an abduction brace, a leg cast, or a harness sling are used to protect the affected joint while revascularization and bone healing occur. As long as the child is eating a well-balanced diet, there is no need for an intake of protein-rich foods. The parents can encourage range of motion in the unaffected leg, but motion in the affected leg is limited until it heals. Once therapy has been initiated, pain is usually not a problem. The key is management of the corrective device.

🔑 CN: Reduction of risk potential; CL: Create

4. 4. The parent is describing symptoms consistent with torticollis, or wry neck syndrome. With this musculoskeletal disorder, the sternocleidomastoid muscle shortens, causing the infant to drop the head toward the affected muscle and tilt the chin upward in the opposite direction. Frequently, a lump may be felt in the affected muscle. Palpating the fontanelle is done to assess neurologic status, not musculoskeletal status. Torticollis does not involve the cervical vertebrae or trapezius muscle.

🔑 CN: Physiological adaptation; CL: Analyze

5. 1. The adolescent's problem should alert the nurse to the possibility of Osgood-Schlatter disease. This disease, found primarily in boys 10 to 15 years of age and in girls 8 to 13 years of age, occurs when the infrapatellar ligament of the quadriceps muscle is not well anchored to the tibial tubercle. Excessive activity of the quadriceps muscle results in microtrauma, which causes swelling and pain. Track, soccer, and football commonly produce this condition. Osgood-Schlatter disease is self-limited and usually responds to rest and application of ice.

🔑 CN: Physiological adaptation; CL: Analyze

6. 4. The adolescent is most likely experiencing heat exhaustion or heat collapse, which are common after vigorous exercise in a hot environment. Symptoms result from loss of fluids and include nausea, vomiting, dizziness, headache, and thirst. Treatment consists of moving the adolescent to a cool environment and giving cool liquids. Cool liquids are easier to drink than are cold liquids. Taking the adolescent's temperature would be appropriate once these actions have been completed. However, the adolescent's temperature is likely to be normal or only mildly elevated. Lying in the supine position increases the risk for aspiration if vomiting occurs in a client with nausea.

🔑 CN: Basic care and comfort; CL: Synthesize

The Client with Cerebral Palsy

7. 3. It is important to identify primary developmental delays in children with cerebral palsy and to prevent secondary and tertiary delays. The arrested development is worrisome and requires further investigation. It is possible the lack of development indicates hearing loss or may be a sign of autism. The brain damage caused by cerebral palsy is not progressive. The brain of a young child is quite plastic; assuming the child's development has peaked at age 3 would be a serious mistake. The therapy plan will need to be modified, but a better understanding of the underlying problem will lead to the greatest chance of creating a successful therapy plan.

CN: Health promotion and maintenance; CL: Synthesize

8. 2,3,4,5. Botulinum toxin injections can be used to improve many aspects of quality of life for the child with cerebral palsy. The injections can help decrease pain from spasticity. Injections improve motor status by reducing rigidity and allowing for more effective physical therapy to improve range of motion. Decreased spasms enhance self-esteem. Improved motor status facilitates the ability to provide some aspects of care, especially transfers. Botulinum does not significantly affect nutritional status or speech.

CN: Management of care; CL: Create

9. 3. The term *cerebral palsy* (CP) refers to a group of nonprogressive disorders of upper motor neuron impairment that result in motor dysfunction due to injury. In addition, a child may have speech or ocular difficulties, seizures, hyperactivity, or cognitive impairment. The condition of congenital malformed blood vessels in the ventricles is known as arteriovenous malformations. Viral infection and metabolic imbalances do not cause CP.

CN: Physiological adaptation; CL: Evaluate

10. 4. Delay in achieving developmental milestones is a characteristic of children with cerebral palsy. Ninety percent of typically developing 15-month-old children can put a block in a cup. Walking up steps typically is accomplished at 18 to 24 months. A child usually is able to use a spoon at 18 months. The ability to copy a circle is achieved at approximately 3 to 4 years of age.

CN: Health promotion and maintenance; CL: Analyze

11. 3. The parent is the child's **HCP** 📖 and may be very in tune to subtle changes in the child's behavior. If the parent thinks the child is in pain, it is very likely to be so. The nurse should administer the pain medication and evaluate if the medication affected the child's behavior. The FLACC scale may be difficult to interpret when the child has spasticity. The FACES scale requires self-report, which may not be possible in a child with a communication disorder. The HCP should be contacted regarding the change in behavior only if other available interventions are unsuccessful.

CN: Basic care and comfort; CL: Synthesize

12. 3. The nurse needs to respond honestly to the mother. Most children with hemiparesis due to spastic cerebral palsy are able to walk because the motor deficit is usually greater in the upper extremity. There is no need to refer the mother to the **HCP** 📖. Pulling to a stand requires both upper body and lower body strength. The will to walk is important, but without neurologic stability, the child may be unable to do so.

CN: Physiological adaptation; CL: Synthesize

13. 1. Limited interaction or lack of interaction with friends and family may lead the nurse to suspect a possible problem with the family's ability to cope with others' reactions and responses to a child with cerebral palsy. Learning measures to meet the child's physical needs demonstrates some understanding and acceptance of the disease. Requesting teaching about the disease suggests curiosity or a desire for understanding, thus demonstrating that the family is dealing with the situation. Participating in social media may serve as a form of support and can be a healthy coping mechanism.

CN: Psychosocial integrity; CL: Evaluate

The Client with Duchenne's Muscular Dystrophy

14. 1. Duchenne's muscular dystrophy is an X-linked recessive disorder. The gene is transmitted through female carriers to affected sons 50% of the time. Daughters have a 50% chance of being carriers.

CN: Physiological adaptation; CL: Apply

15. 3. Usually, the first clinical manifestations of Duchenne's muscular dystrophy include difficulty with typical age-appropriate physical activities such as running, riding a tricycle, and climbing stairs. Contractures of the large joints typically occur much later in the disease process. Occasionally, enlarged calves may be noted, but they are not typical findings in a child with Duchenne's muscular dystrophy. Muscular atrophy and development of small, weak muscles are later signs.

CN: Physiological adaptation; CL: Analyze

16. 4. With Gower's sign, the child walks the hands up the legs in an attempt to stand, a common approach used by children with Duchenne's muscular dystrophy when rising from a sitting to a standing position. Galeazzi's sign refers to the shortening of the affected limb in congenital hip dislocation. Goodell's sign refers to the softening of the cervix, considered a sign of probable pregnancy. Goodenough's sign refers to a test of mental age.

🔑 CN: Physiological adaptation;
CL: Analyze

17. 3. The primary nursing goal is to maintain function in unaffected muscles for as long as possible. There is no effective treatment for childhood muscular dystrophy. Children who remain active are able to forestall being confined in wheelchair. Remaining active also minimizes the risk for social isolation. Preventing rather than encouraging wheelchair use by maintaining function for as long as possible is an appropriate nursing goal. Children with muscular dystrophy become socially isolated as their condition deteriorates and they can no longer keep up with friends. Maintaining function helps prevent social isolation. Circulatory impairment is not associated with muscular dystrophy.

🔑 CN: Physiological adaptation;
CL: Create

18. 3. The guilt that mothers of children with muscular dystrophy commonly experience usually results from the fact that the disease is genetic and the mother transmitted the defective gene. Although many children die from the disease, the disease is considered chronic and progressive. As the disease progresses, the child becomes more dependent. However, guilt typically stems from the knowledge that the mother transmitted the disease to her son rather than the dependency of the child. The disease onset is usually gradual, not sudden.

🔑 CN: Psychosocial integrity;
CL: Analyze

19. 1. Muscular dystrophy is a progressive disease. Children who are affected by this disease usually are unable to walk independently by age 9 to 11 years. There is no effective treatment for childhood muscular dystrophy. Although children who remain active are able to avoid wheelchair confinement for a longer period, activity does not prevent disease progression.

🔑 CN: Physiological adaptation;
CL: Evaluate

The Client with Developmental Dysplasia of the Hip

20. 4. A Trendelenburg's sign is seen in children with developmental dysplasia of the hip who are walking. Weight bearing causes the pelvis to tilt downward on the unaffected side instead of upward as it would normally. Ortolani's maneuver is used during the neonatal period to assess developmental dysplasia of the hip in infants. With the infant quiet, relaxed, and lying on the back, the hips and knees are flexed at right angles. The knees are moved to abduction, and pressure is exerted. If the femoral head moves forward, then it is dislocated. Barlow's maneuver is used to assess developmental dysplasia of the hip in infants. As the femur is moved into or out of the acetabulum, a "clunk" is heard, indicating dislocation. Adam's position is used to evaluate for structural scoliosis. The child bends forward with feet together and arms hanging freely or with palms together.

🔑 CN: Reduction of risk potential;
CL: Analyze

21. 4. This infant with congenital hip dysplasia has asymmetric gluteal folds. The Ortolani's "click" occurs when the nurse feels the femur sliding into the acetabulum with a "click." Limited abduction may be observed during an attempt to abduct the infant's thighs. Galeazzi's sign reveals femoral foreshortening and is observed by flexing the thighs.

🔑 CN: Health promotion and maintenance;
CL: Analyze

22. 1. The Pavlik harness is worn over a diaper. Knee socks are also worn to prevent the straps and foot and leg pieces from rubbing directly on the skin. For maximum results, the infant needs to wear the harness continuously. The skin should be inspected several times a day, not every other day, for signs of redness or irritation. Lotions and powders are to be avoided because they can cake and irritate the skin.

🔑 CN: Reduction of risk potential;
CL: Synthesize

23. 2. Assessing the learner's knowledge level is the initial step in any teaching plan to promote the maximum amount of learning. This assessment also provides the nurse with a starting point for teaching. Assessing coping strategies can provide important information to the development of the teaching plan but is not the initial step. Giving parents written instructions or a list of community resources is appropriate once the parents' knowledge level has been determined and teaching has begun.

🔑 CN: Reduction of risk potential;
CL: Create

24. 3. The abduction bar is incorporated into the cast to increase the cast's strength and maintain the legs in alignment. The bar cannot be removed or adjusted, unless the cast is removed and a new cast is applied. The bar should never be used to lift or turn the client because doing so may weaken the cast.

⚷ CN: Reduction of risk potential; CL: Synthesize

25. 2. The toddler in a hip spica cast needs a specially designed car seat. The one that the mother already has will not be appropriate because of the need for the car seat to accommodate the cast and abductor bar.

⚷ CN: Safety and infection control; CL: Synthesize

The Client with Congenital Clubfoot

26. 2. Elevating the extremity at different points during the day is helpful to prevent edema, but pillows should not be used in the crib because they increase the risk of sudden infant death syndrome (SIDS). A change in the color of the toes is a sign of impaired circulation and requires medical evaluation. Children typically need a series of 5 to 10 casts to correct the deformity. Infants with clubfeet still need frequent holding like any other newborn.

⚷ CN: Safety and infection control; CL: Evaluate

27. 3. When an infant is born with an unexpected anomaly, parents are faced with questions, uncertainties, and possible disappointments. They may feel inadequate, helpless, and anxious. The nurse can help the parents initially by assessing their concerns and providing appropriate information to help them clarify or resolve the immediate problems. Referring the parents to the **healthcare provider (HCP)** 📖 is not necessary at this time. The nurse can assist the parents by listening to their concerns. Having them talk with other parents would be helpful a little bit later, once the nurse assesses their concerns and discusses the problem and the parents' current feelings. If the parents continue to have difficulties expressing and working through their feelings, referral to a counselor would be appropriate.

⚷ CN: Psychosocial integrity; CL: Synthesize

28. 3. A cast that is too tight can cause a tourniquet effect, compromising the neurovascular integrity of the extremity. Manifestations of neurovascular impairment include pain, edema, pulselessness, coolness, altered sensation, and inability to move the distal exposed extremity. The toes of the casted extremity should be assessed frequently to evaluate for changes in neurovascular integrity. Wetting a plaster cast with water and soap softens the plaster, which may alter the cast's effectiveness. There is no reason to elevate the casted extremities when a child with clubfoot is being treated with nonsurgical measures. The legs would be elevated if swelling were present. Petals, which are applied to cover the rough edges of the cast, are to be left in place to minimize the risk for skin irritation from the cast edges.

⚷ CN: Reduction of risk potential; CL: Evaluate

The Client with Juvenile Idiopathic Arthritis

29. 4. The nurse's response to the father is based on the knowledge that there is no definitive test for JIA. The latex fixation test, which is commonly used to diagnose arthritis in adults, is negative in 90% of children. The erythrocyte sedimentation rate may or may not be increased during active disease. This test identifies the presence of inflammation only. Synovial fluid cultures are done to rule out septic arthritis, not to diagnose JIA.

⚷ CN: Reduction of risk potential; CL: Analyze

30. 1. With JIA, the more joints affected, the more severe the disease is likely to be and the less likely the symptoms will totally resolve. Approximately one-third of the children will continue to have the disease into adulthood, and approximately one-sixth will experience severe, crippling deformities.

⚷ CN: Physiological adaptation; CL: Apply

31. 2. Socialization is important for this preschool-age child, and activity is important to maintain function. Because children with JIA commonly experience most problems in the early morning after arising, they need more time to "warm up." Adverse effects may or may not occur. The child's normal routine needs to be maintained as much as possible. Although splints and braces may be needed, they are worn during periods of rest, not activity, to maintain function.

⚷ CN: Physiological adaptation; CL: Synthesize

32. 4. Because the child is dealing with grief and loss associated with a chronic illness, parents need to be supportive and understanding. The child needs to feel valued and worthwhile. Introducing the child to others of the same age who also have

JIA most probably would be ineffective because preschoolers are developmentally egocentric. Although the child needs to feel valued, the mother's spending more time with the child and less time with her other children is inappropriate because the child with JIA may experience secondary gain from the illness if the family interaction patterns are altered. Also, this action reinforces the child's withdrawal behavior. Psychological counseling is not needed at this time because the child's reaction is normal.

⚷ CN: Psychosocial integrity;
CL: Synthesize

33. 2,3,5. Adverse effects from nonsteroidal anti-inflammatory drugs include abdominal pain, blood in stool, and reduced clotting ability. Weight gain is common with corticosteroids. Folic acid deficiency is associated with methotrexate therapy.

⚷ CN: Pharmacological and parenteral therapies; CL: Apply

34. 3. The first group of drugs typically prescribed is the nonsteroidal anti-inflammatory drugs, which include naproxen. Once therapy is started, it takes hours or days for relief from pain to occur. However, it takes 3 to 4 weeks for the anti-inflammatory effects to occur, including reduction in swelling and less pain with movement. Naproxen is included in only a few over-the-counter medications, but aspirin is in several. The family should check with the nurse before giving any over-the-counter medications. Toxicity or GI bleeding may occur when nonsteroidal anti-inflammatory drugs are combined. The missed dose will need to be made up to maintain the serum level and to maintain therapeutic effectiveness of the drug.

⚷ CN: Pharmacological and parenteral therapies; CL: Apply

The Client with a Fracture

35. 2,3,4,5. Buck's traction provides a skin traction that keeps the extremity in straight alignment and can be observed by noting a straight line formed between the shoulder, hips, and knees. The rope must be intact to maintain the prescribed traction from the weights. The correct amount of traction must be maintained to keep the fractured femur in correct alignment. Because the client is in a recumbent position, the nurse should also inspect the skin on the back and buttocks for integrity. The nurse should not remove the client's wraps and boot unless he or she has a **healthcare provider's (HCP's)** 📖 prescription to do so.

⚷ CN: Physiological adaptation;
CL: Analyze

36. 3. The wet plaster cast should be handled using only the palms of the hands to prevent indentations of the cast surface. Petaling a cast should be done only when the edges of the cast are rough and are causing irritation to the client's skin. The nurse should not keep the child in the same position until the cast is dry. Doing so would prohibit proper toileting and elimination and would produce undue pressure on the coccyx. The cast typically emits heat as it dries, so notifying a **healthcare provider (HCP)** 📖 is not necessary in this instance. If needed, a fan can be used to circulate the room air.

⚷ CN: Health promotion and maintenance;
CL: Evaluate

37. 3. The nurse should show the parents the figure of the greenstick fracture as noted in answer 3 in which the fracture does not completely cross through the bone. Answer A is a plastic deformation, or a bend in the bone. Answer B is a buckle. Answer D is a complete fracture.

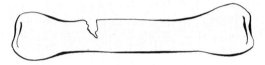

⚷ CN: Physiological adaptation;
CL: Synthesize

38. 2. Emotional or physical stress lowers a person's tolerance of pain. The parent's presence may have distracted him, and when the parent left, it caused him to focus on the pain he was having. Crying does not automatically indicate pain. The nurse must further assess the client for pain. Although an analgesic was given 4 hours before, pain may be present.

⚷ CN: Physiological adaptation;
CL: Analyze

39. 2. As part of a surgery safety checklist, the nurse must verify that the site, side, and level are marked. Pointing to the area is not sufficient identification of the surgery site. The nurse must verify the form has been signed by reviewing the form. The surgeon holds primary responsibility for explaining the risks of surgery.

⚷ CN: Safety and infection control;
CL: Synthesize

40. 1. Skeletal traction applies the pull directly to the skeletal structure by tongs, pin, or wire. The nurse should assess the pull of the traction on the pin first. This is critical to the success of the traction. Once this is assessed, then the pin sites are assessed for signs of infection. The dressings would be examined after the pull of the traction, neurovascular status, and pin sites were assessed. The Ace wrap is used to anchor skin traction nonadherent straps, not skeletal traction.

> CN: Reduction of risk potential;
> CL: Synthesize

41. 2. The traction is positioned correctly; the nurse should provide frequent skin care to the back and shoulder areas. The hips and buttocks should be lifted off the bed to provide countertraction; the nurse should not adjust the weights. The nurse should not place a pillow under the buttocks as this would prevent countertraction. The elastic wraps should remain on the legs unless removal is prescribed by the **healthcare provider (HCP)** 📖.

> CN: Physiological adaptation;
> CL: Synthesize

42. 3. The nurse should assess the client frequently for signs of neurovascular impairment of the feet, such as pallor, coldness, numbness, or tingling. Pillows are not placed under the buttocks because the pillows would alter the alignment of the traction. Weights provide traction and should not be removed. Pulleys help to maintain optimal alignment of the traction and therefore should be left alone.

> CN: Basic care and comfort;
> CL: Synthesize

43. 3. Explaining to the parents that this is a normal reaction under the circumstances is most appropriate. The child's outburst is related to the child's fears of the unknown. The child is scared and anxious and needs the parents for support. Asking the parents to wait outside would only add to the child's fear and anxiety. The reaction is normal for a child her age and does not usually call for a change in staff assignments. Asking the parents to discipline their child for her behavior is inappropriate. The nurse needs to handle the situation.

> CN: Health promotion and maintenance;
> CL: Synthesize

44. 1. Inability to extend the fingers of the involved arm may indicate neurologic impairment caused by pressure on soft tissue. It is not unusual for a child to vomit after experiencing a traumatic injury. It may take up to 72 hours for a plaster cast to dry. Until the cast dries, the dampness causes the sensation of coolness. The cast will seem heavy until the child adjusts to the extra weight. The child may exhibit fussiness (such as whining, crying, or clinging) as a result of numerous causes, such as placement of the cast, the hospital experience, or pain. These reactions are normal and do not warrant medical advice.

> CN: Reduction of risk potential;
> CL: Evaluate

45. 2. For the first few days after application of a plaster or fiberglass cast, the child should not engage in strenuous activities, to minimize swelling that would cause the cast to become too tight. Use of a hair dryer to complete the drying of the cast is not encouraged because the hair dryer only dries the outside of the cast. Movement and sensation of the fingers need to be checked several times a day for the first few days. Typically, the parent would be instructed to administer acetaminophen every 4 to 6 hours, not every 8 to 12 hours, for discomfort.

> CN: Reduction of risk potential;
> CL: Synthesize

46. 1. Because the nurse suspects a possible fracture based on the child's presentation, assessing the neurologic and circulatory status of the toes, the tissues distal to the fracture, is important. Soft tissue contusions, which accompany femur fractures, can result in severe hemorrhage into the tissue and subsequent circulatory and neurologic impairment. Once this information has been obtained, vital signs can be assessed, and the nurse can notify the **healthcare provider (HCP)** 📖 and report the findings. In fractures, circulation impairment will occur distal to the injury.

> CN: Physiological adaptation;
> CL: Synthesize

47. 3. Hand puppets would enable a 3-year-old child in traction to act out feelings within the constraints imposed by the traction. A 3-year-old needs creative play. The video game would make the child too active in bed and does not meet the child's developmental need for creative play. Blocks would be more appropriate for a younger child. Remote-controlled cars are appropriate for older children but can present a fall risk to others if used in a hospital.

> CN: Health promotion and maintenance;
> CL: Synthesize

48. 2. Stressing the importance of the parents' visiting when they can helps to alleviate the guilt they feel. It allows the parents to feel that they are doing what they can. Acknowledging the guilt gives the parents an opportunity to talk about it but does not help alleviate it. Comparing the parents with other parents does not alleviate guilt feelings. The parents need reinforcement that what they are doing is appropriate. Suggesting that the parents take turns visiting implies that they should feel guilty because they may not be doing all they could.

> CN: Psychosocial integrity;
> CL: Synthesize

49. 2. A hip spica cast encircles the abdomen. When the child eats a large meal, abdominal pressure increases, causing the cast to feel tight. Therefore, the nurse should plan to offer smaller, more frequent meals to minimize abdominal distention. If the child's appetite were decreased in conjunction with a feeling of fullness, the nurse might suspect that the child was becoming constipated and plan to use laxatives or a higher-fiber diet. A mechanical soft diet is indicated when the child has difficulty chewing food adequately. Giving the child more fruits and grains would contribute to abdominal distention and problems with the cast tightness after eating.

🔑 CN: Reduction of risk potential;
CL: Synthesize

50. **2.** The child with a hip spica cast who is going home and has a bedroom on the second floor of the home needs to have the bed moved to an area that is more central to family life. Negotiating a flight of steps at least twice a day (on awakening in the morning and before going to bed at night) with a child in a hip spica cast would be difficult and most likely dangerous. Because the child in a hip spica cast will need to use a bedpan or urinal, the bathrooms can be on any floor. Because the family is involved in the discharge, the 16-year-old sister should be taught appropriate care along with the rest of the family. The child can be carried up and down the three steps to the house the few times necessary after discharge.

🔑 CN: Safety and infection control;
CL: Create

51. **2,3.** To ensure proper fit of crutches, the child's elbow flexion should be 20 degrees, and the area above the top of the crutch to the child's axilla should be 1 to 1½ inches (2.5 to 3.8 cm). The type of gait, weight of the child, and use of stairs are not factors in the measurement.

🔑 CN: Reduction of risk potential;
CL: Apply

The Client with Osteomyelitis

52. **3.** Findings associated with osteomyelitis commonly include pain over the area, increased warmth, localized tenderness, and diffuse swelling over the involved bone. The area over the affected bone is red.

🔑 CN: Physiological adaptation;
CL: Analyze

53. **2.** Cultures are used to determine exactly what organism is causing the inflammation. From the culture, sensitivities to various antibiotics may be determined. If the antibiotics are given before obtaining the culture, the antibiotics may inhibit the growth of the organism in the culture medium. This may lead to a delay in the most appropriate treatment. Unless a child has a known renal problem, baseline creatinine levels are not typically needed. However,

levels may be needed during treatment depending on the medication. A complete blood count (CBC) with hemoglobin and white blood cell count is typically prescribed for any suspected infection, but these tests do not identify the causative organism.

🔑 CN: Reduction of risk potential;
CL: Apply

54. **3.** The vancomycin level is not therapeutic and will need to be adjusted. Drug management by the pharmacy is prescribed. Thus, the nurse should notify the pharmacist to adjust the dose. This is very frequently done in institutions with pediatric clinical pharmacists. Giving subtherapeutic doses may prolong care. If needed, the pharmacist would notify the care provider. Peak levels are not prescribed on this client.

🔑 CN: Pharmacological and parenteral therapies; CL: Synthesize

55. **4.** Long-term, high-dose antibiotic therapy can adversely affect renal, hepatic, and hematopoietic function. Urine specific gravity would provide valuable information about the kidneys' ability to concentrate or dilute urine, thereby suggesting renal impairment. Blood glucose levels reveal how well the client's body is using glucose. Thrombin times reveal information about the clotting mechanism. Urine glucose levels reveal information about the body's use and excretion of glucose.

🔑 CN: Pharmacological and parenteral therapies; CL: Analyze

56. **1.** Encouraging contact with schoolmates allows the school-age child to maintain and develop socialization with peers, an important developmental task of this age group. Although having family visits and interacting with the child are important, they do not meet the child's developmental needs. Talking to the child about his interests is important, but encouraging contact with schoolmates is crucial to maintain and develop socialization with peers.

🔑 CN: Health promotion and maintenance;
CL: Create

57. **1.** Some clients find ginger cookies or "snaps" help relieve nausea. Ginger, in small doses such as would be found in the cookies, has few side effects. There is no reason that the parent should not try this dietary intervention; however, the nurse must monitor the client's response. If the child has a diet as tolerated prescription, there is no need for an additional prescription. Ultimately, the child may need an antiemetic medication, but dietary strategies are often successful in treating vomiting related to osteomyelitis. Making a universal statement disregarding home remedies is not a client-centered approach.

🔑 CN: Physiological adaptation;
CL: Synthesize

The Client with Scoliosis

58. 1. Scoliosis, a lateral deviation of the spine, is assessed by having the client bend forward at the waist with arms hanging freely and then looking for lateral curvature of the spine and a rib hump. The other positions will not reveal the deviation of the spine.

CN: Health promotion and maintenance; CL: Analyze

59. 1. One of the most effective spinal braces for correcting scoliosis, the Boston brace should be worn for at least 16 to 23 hours a day, except when carrying out personal hygiene measures.

CN: Reduction of risk potential; CL: Evaluate

60. 4. Exercises are prescribed for the child with scoliosis wearing a Boston brace to help strengthen spinal and abdominal muscles and provide support. Typically, children wearing a Boston brace do not have muscle spasms. Performing exercises provides no effect on the brace's traction ability. Spinal contractures do not occur when a Boston brace is worn.

CN: Physiological adaptation; CL: Apply

61. 3. A form-fitting t-shirt can be worn under the brace to prevent skin irritation and collect perspiration. Braces are worn 23 hours each day. Lotions may cause irritation and should not be used. The skin under the brace should be bathed daily to help prevent irritation from the brace. The brace can be removed for bathing so all the skin can be bathed.

CN: Physiological adaptation; CL: Create

Managing Care, Quality, and Safety of Children with Musculoskeletal Health Problems

62. 2. To prevent a baclofen withdraw, pump refills are scheduled several days before anticipated low-volume alarms. The nurse should make it a high priority to have the pump refilled as soon as possible. Discontinuing baclofen suddenly can result in a high fever, muscle rigidity, change in level of consciousness, and even death. Waiting until the child leaves the hospital for a refill may lead to a low dose or withdrawal. Waiting for the low-volume alarm puts the client at risk because medication and team members who can refill the pump may not be readily available under all circumstances.

CN: Management of care; CL: Synthesize

63. 2,3. In general, **LPN/VNs** 📖 may perform skills related to feeding, oral medication administration, and activities of daily living, such as insertion of a hearing aid. Refilling a baclofen pump constitutes administering an intrathecal medication and is beyond the scope of practice for LPN/VNs in most areas. Some institutions allow LPN/VNs to give IV push medicines; however, special training is required. Communicating with the **healthcare provider (HCP)** 📖 would require discussion of the client's assessments and evaluations, which fall under the RN scope of practice.

CN: Management of care; CL: Synthesize

64. 3. If the child was taking cetirizine for allergies, the nurse should contact the **HCP** 📖 for a prescription to continue the medication in the hospital. The provider should either prescribe the medication or provide a valid reason to discontinue its use. Advising the family to take a home supply of medications increases the risk of adverse reactions because the provider would be unaware of potential medication interactions. Many allergy medications that formerly required a prescription are now available over the counter, and because parents use them, the nurse should be aware of the interactions and risks. The nurse does not need to question the methotrexate prescription as this medication is being added to treat the JIA.

CN: Safety and infection control; CL: Synthesize

65. 4. The father's story is consistent with the injuries incurred by the child; therefore, the nurse should document the cause of injury. There is no need to restrict the father's visitation because the injuries sustained by the child are consistent with the explanation given. The police only need to be notified if there is suspicion of child abuse. The injuries incurred by this child appear to be accidental. There is no need to refer the father for parenting classes. The father appears to be upset about the accident and will not likely repeat such reckless behavior. However, the nurse should educate the father regarding child safety.

CN: Management of care; CL: Analyze

The Child with Dermatologic and Endocrine Health Problems

- The Client with Skin Disorders
- The Client with Burns
- The Client with a Thyroid Problem
- The Client with Insulin-Dependent Diabetes Mellitus
- The Client with Polycystic Ovarian Syndrome
- Managing Care, Quality, and Safety of Children with Dermatologic and Endocrine Health Problems
- Answers, Rationales, and Test-Taking Strategies

The Client with Skin Disorders

1. A 17-year-old female with severe nodular acne is considering treatment with isotretinoin. Prior to beginning the medication, the nurse explains that the client will be required to:
- ☐ 1. enroll in a risk management plan.
- ☐ 2. have proof of a mental health evaluation.
- ☐ 3. begin an effective form of birth control when starting the medication.
- ☐ 4. temporarily give up sports.

2. When teaching an adolescent with facial acne about skin care, the nurse should instruct the adolescent to:
- ☐ 1. wash the face twice a day with mild soap and water.
- ☐ 2. remove whiteheads and comedones after washing the face with antibacterial soap.
- ☐ 3. apply vitamin E ointment twice daily to the affected skin.
- ☐ 4. apply tretinoin daily in the morning and expose the face to the sun.

3. A 9-month-old infant with eczema has lesions that are secondarily infected. Which recommendation is the **most** appropriate to help the parents best meet the needs of the child?
- ☐ 1. Prevent siblings from being in close contact.
- ☐ 2. Send the child to day care as usual.
- ☐ 3. Play video games for several hours each evening.
- ☐ 4. Play with the child every day.

4. After the nurse teaches the mother of a child with atopic dermatitis how to bathe her child, which statement by the mother indicates effective teaching?
- ☐ 1. "I let my child play in the tub for 30 minutes every night."
- ☐ 2. "My child loves the bubble bath I put in the tub."
- ☐ 3. "When my child gets out of the tub I just pat the skin dry."
- ☐ 4. "I make sure my child has a bath every night."

5. A 5-year-old child brought to the clinic with several superficial sores on the front of the left leg is diagnosed with impetigo. Which instructions should the nurse give the parent?
- ☐ 1. Wash the child's legs once a day with a mild soap.
- ☐ 2. Cover the sores with loose gauze.
- ☐ 3. Allow the child to go back to school after 24 hours of treatment.
- ☐ 4. Have the child return to the clinic the next week for a follow-up examination.

6. When developing the teaching plan for the mother of a 2-year-old child diagnosed with scabies, what information should the nurse expect to include?
- ☐ 1. The floors of the house should be cleaned with a damp mop.
- ☐ 2. The child should be held frequently.
- ☐ 3. Itching should cease in a few days.
- ☐ 4. The entire family should be treated.

The Client with Burns

7. A 10-year-old has just spilled hot liquid on his arm, and a 4-inch (10-cm) area on his forearm is severely burned. His mother calls the emergency department. What should the nurse advise the mother to do?
- ☐ 1. Keep the child warm.
- ☐ 2. Cover the burned area with an antibiotic cream.
- ☐ 3. Apply cool water to the burned area.
- ☐ 4. Call 911 to transport the child to the hospital.

8. A school-age child who has received burns over 60% of his body is to receive 2,000 mL of IV fluid over the next 8 hours. At what rate (in milliliters per hour) should the nurse set the infusion pump? Round your answer to a whole number.

_____ mL/h.

9. Which interventions would be **most** appropriate to institute when a school-age child with burns becomes angry and combative when it is time to change the dressings and apply mafenide acetate?
- ☐ 1. Ensure parental support during the dressing changes.
- ☐ 2. Allow the child to assist in removing the dressings and applying the cream.
- ☐ 3. Give the child permission to cry during the procedure.
- ☐ 4. Allow the child to schedule the time for dressing changes.

10. A 5-year-old child with burns on the trunk and arms has no appetite. The nurse and the parent develop a plan of care to stimulate the child's appetite. Which suggestion made by the parent would indicate the need for additional teaching?
- ☐ 1. deciding that she will feed the child herself
- ☐ 2. withholding dessert and treats unless meals are eaten
- ☐ 3. offering the child finger foods that the child likes
- ☐ 4. serving smaller and more frequent meals

11. After teaching the parent of a child with severe burns about the importance of specific nutritional support in burn management, which selection of foods, if chosen by the parent from the child's diet menu, indicate the need for further instruction?
- ☐ 1. bacon, lettuce, and tomato sandwich; milk; and celery and carrot sticks
- ☐ 2. cheeseburger, cottage cheese and pineapple salad, chocolate milk, and a brownie
- ☐ 3. chicken nuggets, orange and grapefruit sections, and a vanilla milkshake
- ☐ 4. beef, bean, and cheese burrito; a banana; fruit-flavored yogurt; and skim milk

12. When caring for a child with moderate burns from the waist down, what should the nurse do when positioning the child?
- ☐ 1. Place the child in a position of comfort.
- ☐ 2. Allow the child to lie on the abdomen.
- ☐ 3. Ensure the application of leg splints.
- ☐ 4. Have the child flex the hips and knees.

The Client with a Thyroid Problem

13. An adolescent is to receive radioactive iodine for Graves' disease. Which statement by the client reflects the need for more teaching?
- ☐ 1. "I plan to talk on Facebook since I have to keep several feet (meters) from my friends for 3 days."
- ☐ 2. "Taking radioactive iodine will not affect my ability to have children in the future."
- ☐ 3. "The advantage of radioactive iodine is that I will not need future medication for my disease."
- ☐ 4. "I should try to use a separate bathroom from the rest of my family for several days."

14. Which clinical manifestations would lead the nurse to suspect that an infant has hypothyroidism? Select all that apply.
- ☐ 1. cool extremities
- ☐ 2. umbilical hernia
- ☐ 3. increased appetite
- ☐ 4. muscle weakness
- ☐ 5. lethargy
- ☐ 6. tachycardia

15. The nurse should instruct the family of a child with newly diagnosed hyperthyroidism to:
- ☐ 1. keep their home warmer than usual.
- ☐ 2. encourage plenty of outdoor activities.
- ☐ 3. promote interactions with one friend instead of groups.
- ☐ 4. limit bathing to prevent skin irritation.

16. An 11-year-old child has been diagnosed with Graves' disease and is to start drug therapy. Which instruction should the nurse include in the teaching plan for the child's parent and teacher?
- ☐ 1. Continue with the same amount of schoolwork and homework.
- ☐ 2. Understand that mood swings are rare with this disorder.
- ☐ 3. Limit the amount of food that is offered to the child.
- ☐ 4. Provide the child with a calm, nonstimulating environment.

The Client with Insulin-Dependent Diabetes Mellitus

17. A student with type 1 diabetes tells the nurse she is feeling light-headed. The student's blood sugar is 60 mg/dL (3.3 mmol/L). Using the 15-15 rule, the nurse should give:
- ☐ 1. 15 mL of juice and give another 15 mL in 15 minutes.
- ☐ 2. 15 g of carbohydrate and retest the blood sugar in 15 minutes.
- ☐ 3. 15 g of carbohydrate and 15 g of protein.
- ☐ 4. 15 oz of juice and retest in 15 minutes.

18. An overweight adolescent has been diagnosed with type 2 diabetes. To increase the client's self-efficacy to manage the disease, the nurse should:
- ☐ 1. provide the client with a written daily food and exercise plan.
- ☐ 2. discuss eliminating junk food in the home with the parents.
- ☐ 3. arrange for the school nurse to weigh the child weekly.
- ☐ 4. utilize a peer with type 2 diabetes to role model lifestyle changes.

19. After 6 months of treatment with diet and exercise, a 12-year-old with type 2 diabetes still has a fasting blood glucose level of 140 mg/dL (7.8 mmol/L). The healthcare provider (HCP) has decided to begin metformin. The adolescent asks how the medication works. The nurse should tell the client that the medicine decreases the glucose production and:
☐ 1. replaces natural insulin.
☐ 2. helps the body make more insulin.
☐ 3. increases insulin sensitivity.
☐ 4. decreases carbohydrate adsorption.

20. The nurse is evaluating a child's skills in self-administering insulin (see figure). The nurse should:

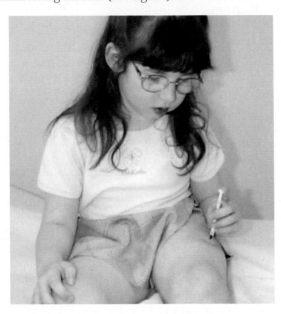

☐ 1. have the child use both hands on the syringe.
☐ 2. ask the child to place the needle at a 45-degree angle.
☐ 3. tell the child to use a site lower on her thigh.
☐ 4. remind the child to rotate sites.

21. A 14-year-old is using glargine and lispro to manage type 1 diabetes. The prescription for sliding scale lispro reads:

Lispro subcutaneous give units according to sliding scale:

Blood glucose: 70–150 mg/dL (3.9–8.3 mmol/L) = 0 units
151–200 mg/dL (8.4 –11.1 mmol/L) = 1 unit
201–250 mg/dL (11.2 – 13.9 mmol/L) = 2 units
251–300 mg/dL (13.93 – 16.65 mmol/L) = 3 units
301–350 mg/dL (17 – 19.4 mmol/L) = 4 units
Call for Blood glucose > 350 (19.4 mmol/L)
In addition give 1 unit for every
15 g of carbohydrate.

The morning blood glucose is 202 mg/dL (11.2 mmol/L), and the client is going to eat two carbohydrate exchanges. The nurse has the client administer how many units of lispro?

_____ units. Round your answer to a whole number.

22. An 8-year-old with diabetes is placed on an intermediate-acting insulin and regular insulin before breakfast and before dinner. She will receive a snack of milk and cereal at bedtime. The snack will:
☐ 1. help her regain lost weight.
☐ 2. provide carbohydrates for immediate use.
☐ 3. prevent late night hypoglycemia.
☐ 4. help her stay on her diet.

23. A nurse is teaching an 8-year-old with diabetes and her parents about managing diabetes during illness. The nurse determines the parents understand the instruction when they indicate that when the child is ill they will provide:
☐ 1. more calories.
☐ 2. more insulin.
☐ 3. less insulin.
☐ 4. less protein and fat.

24. A nurse is assessing an 8-year-old with diabetes who is experiencing hyperglycemia. Which symptoms indicate that the hyperglycemia requires immediate intervention? Select all that apply.
☐ 1. weakness
☐ 2. thirst
☐ 3. shakiness
☐ 4. hunger
☐ 5. headache
☐ 6. dizziness

25. The nurse talks to an adolescent about how she can tell her friends about her new diagnosis of diabetes. Which behavior by the adolescent indicates that the adolescent has responded positively to the discussion?
☐ 1. She asks the nurse for material on diabetes for a school paper.
☐ 2. She introduces the nurse to her friends as "the one who taught me all about my diabetes."
☐ 3. She says, "I will try to tell my friends, but they will probably quit hanging out with me."
☐ 4. She asks her friends what they think about someone who has a lifelong illness.

26. An adolescent with insulin-dependent diabetes is being taught the importance of rotating the sites of insulin injections. The nurse should judge that the teaching was successful when the adolescent identifies which complication that can result from using the same site?
☐ 1. destruction of the fat tissue and poor absorption
☐ 2. destruction of nerves and painful neuritis
☐ 3. destruction of the tissue and too-rapid insulin uptake
☐ 4. development of resistance to insulin and need for increased amounts

The Client with Polycystic Ovarian Syndrome

27. A 16-year-old has been diagnosed with polycystic ovarian syndrome (PCOS). Which statement indicates the need for more teaching?
- ☐ 1. "High levels of male hormones contribute to my PCOS."
- ☐ 2. "I am at risk for type 2 diabetes."
- ☐ 3. "Maintaining a healthy weight is an important part of my treatment plan."
- ☐ 4. "Untreated PCOS will make getting pregnant impossible."

28. A 15-year-old female client suspects that she might have polycystic ovarian syndrome (PCOS). Which symptoms would be consistent with PCOS? Select all that apply.
- ☐ 1. primary amenorrhea
- ☐ 2. obesity
- ☐ 3. increased body hair
- ☐ 4. acne
- ☐ 5. darkened skin in body fold
- ☐ 6. enlarged breast

29. A 17-year-old with polycystic ovarian syndrome (PCOS) has been placed on metformin. The nurse determines the client needs more teaching about metformin if she states the medication helps achieve which outcome?
- ☐ 1. reduced androgen levels
- ☐ 2. normalization of the menstrual cycle
- ☐ 3. increased insulin levels
- ☐ 4. reduced blood glucose levels

30. A 16-year-old female with polycystic ovarian syndrome (PCOS) is extremely upset, saying, "I am so embarrassed by hair on my face. I just do not fit in." Which intervention is **most** needed?
- ☐ 1. Refer the client to a hair removal specialist.
- ☐ 2. Screen the client for depression.
- ☐ 3. Provide more information on causes and treatment options.
- ☐ 4. Suggest the client join a support group.

Managing Care, Quality, and Safety of Children with Dermatologic and Endocrine Health Problems

31. The parent of a 17-year-old boy, who is hospitalized for complications related to type I diabetes, requests to review the adolescent's medical record. The client reported receiving mental health counseling during the admission history but did not want his parent to know. The nurse is uncertain of how to protect the adolescent's privacy and accommodate the parent's request. Who is the **most** appropriate person to consult?
- ☐ 1. the unit nurse manager
- ☐ 2. the health care provider (HCP)
- ☐ 3. the organization's privacy officer
- ☐ 4. the customer service representative

32. The charge nurse on the pediatric floor has assigned a 6-year-old girl with newly diagnosed type 1 diabetes and an 8-year-old girl recovering from ketoacidosis to the same semiprivate room. The 6-year-old's mother is upset because the parent staying with the other child is male and believes the arrangement violates her social norms. The nurse should:
- ☐ 1. explain to the parents that this room arrangement facilitates teaching.
- ☐ 2. reassign the children to different rooms.
- ☐ 3. offer the parent another place to sleep.
- ☐ 4. refer the parent to the customer service representative.

33. A 7-year-old client with type 1 diabetes is sick with the flu. What is the **most** important information for the nurse to convey regarding diabetes management during illness?
- ☐ 1. Blood glucose needs to be checked more frequently during illness.
- ☐ 2. Children require less insulin when they are sick with the flu.
- ☐ 3. Urine ketones should be checked every other day during illness.
- ☐ 4. Increase intake of fluids high in carbohydrate to prevent diarrhea.

34. Which nursing intervention should be done **first** when managing a pediatric client admitted to the emergency department with severe diabetic ketoacidosis (DKA)?
- ☐ 1. Begin an insulin drip to lower the client's blood glucose level.
- ☐ 2. Correct any fluid deficit using an isotonic saline solution.
- ☐ 3. Draw a blood glucose level and serum electrolyte panel.
- ☐ 4. Secure the client's airway to ensure adequate ventilation.

35. The mother of an 8-year-old with diabetes tells the nurse that she does not want the school to know about her daughter's condition. The nurse should reply:
- ☐ 1. "Your daughter will most likely tell her teacher even if you do not."
- ☐ 2. "What is it that concerns you about having the school know about your daughter's condition?"
- ☐ 3. "It would be fine not to tell your daughter's friends, but the teacher must know."
- ☐ 4. "In order to keep your daughter safe, it is necessary for all adults in the school to know her condition."

Answers, Rationales, and Test-Taking Strategies

The answers and rationales for each question follow below, along with keys (⚷➤) to the client need (CN) and cognitive level (CL) for each question. In addition, you will also see a glossary icon (📖) highlighting specific terminology used on the licensing exam. As you check your answers, use the **Content Mastery and Test-Taking Skill Self-Analysis** *worksheet (tear-out worksheet in back of book) to identify the reason(s) for not answering the questions correctly. For additional information about test-taking skills and strategies for answering questions, refer to pages 12–23 and pages 35–36 in Part 1 of this book.*

The Client with Skin Disorders

1. 1. Because of the risk of birth defects with isotretinoin, risk management plans require all clients to meet certain requirements to obtain the medication. Providers are advised to closely monitor clients for signs of depression, but a mental health evaluation is not universally required. It is not sufficient to begin a single form of birth control after starting the medication. Women of childbearing age must use two forms of effective birth control for 2 months before, during, and 1 month after taking the drug. Isotretinoin may cause muscle aches, and extreme exercise should be avoided, but general participation in sports should be considered on an individual basis.

⚷➤ CN: Safety and infection control; CL: Synthesize

2. 1. Washing the face once or twice a day with a mild soap removes fatty acids from the skin. Acne is an inflammation of the sebaceous glands that produce sebum. Washing the face with mild soap and water keeps the sebaceous glands from becoming plugged. Excessive washing or squeezing the eruptions can cause rupture of these glands, spreading the sebum and causing further inflammation. Applying vitamin E to the lesions does not reduce the inflammation and, due to the greasiness of the preparation, may plug the ducts. Isotretinoin should be applied at night. Exposure to the sun can result in sunburn and an increased risk of skin cancer and should be avoided. Sunscreen with a sun protection factor of at least 15 must be applied before the client can be exposed to the sun.

⚷➤ CN: Physiological adaptation; CL: Synthesize

3. 4. The parents can best meet the needs of their 9-month-old infant by playing with the child every day. All infants need time with their parents to develop trust and thus attain optimal development. The parents of a child with a chronic problem may need more guidance to meet the child's needs because of the focus on medical problems. The child's lesions are secondarily infected and therefore should not be contagious. Siblings do not need to stay away. Even with lesions that are infected, the child can still attend day care, but the child needs attention from the parents as well. Playing video games for several hours is not appropriate for a 9-month-old infant.

⚷➤ CN: Health promotion and maintenance; CL: Synthesize

4. 3. Atopic dermatitis is a chronic pruritic dermatitis that usually begins in infancy. Many of the children diagnosed with it have a family history of eczema, allergies, or asthma. Atopic dermatitis is best treated with hydrating the skin, controlling the pruritus, and preventing secondary infection. Patting the skin dry removes less natural skin moisturizer and thus maintains skin hydration. Playing in the tub for 30 minutes each night would deplete the skin of its natural moisturizers, thereby leading to increased pruritus and dry skin. Bubble baths are to be avoided in children with atopic dermatitis because they may act as an irritant, possibly exacerbating the condition. Also, bubble baths deplete the skin of its natural moisturizers. The issue is not whether the child bathes every night. Rather, the goal is to decrease dryness and itching.

⚷➤ CN: Physiological adaptation; CL: Evaluate

5. 3. Impetigo involving several superficial lesions is usually treated topically, including washing the affected areas, removing crusts, and applying antibiotic ointment several times a day. The child can return to day care or school after being treated for 24 hours. The lesions do not need to be covered, and they can remain open to the air. There is no need for follow-up unless the lesions have not resolved or have become more severe.

⚷➤ CN: Physiological adaptation; CL: Create

6. 4. Scabies is caused by the scabies mite, *Sarcoptes scabiei*. The mite burrows into the stratum corneum of the epidermis, where the female deposits eggs and fecal material. These burrows are linear. Scabies is highly contagious. The length of time from infestation to physical symptoms is 30 to 60 days, so everyone in close contact with the child will need to be treated. The bed linens and the child's clothing should be washed in hot water and dried on the hot setting. It is not necessary to damp mop the floors to prevent the spread of scabies. The child should be held minimally until treatment is completed. Family members should wash their hands after contact with the child. Itching lasts for 2 to 3 weeks until the stratum corneum is replaced.

    CN: Safety and infection control; CL: Create

The Client with Burns

7. 3. To prevent further injury to the skin, the mother should apply cool water to the burn site. Doing so causes vasoconstriction, retards further damage to tissues, and decreases fluid loss. Keeping the child warm promotes vasodilation, increases fluid loss, and decreases blood pressure and, thus, circulation to the area. Applying ointment to the burn is contraindicated because it does not allow healing to occur and may need to be removed in the hospital. Only a clean cloth should be used to cover the wound to prevent contamination or decrease pain or chilling. If only the arm is burned, a call to 911 for emergency care is not necessary, but the mother should seek health care services immediately.

    CN: Health promotion and maintenance; CL: Synthesize

8. 250 mL/h

$$2,000 \text{ mL} \div 8 \text{ h} = 250 \text{ mL/h}$$

    CN: Pharmacological and parenteral therapies; CL: Apply

9. 2. Expressions of anger and combativeness are often the result of loss of control and a feeling of powerlessness. Some control over the situation is regained by allowing the child to participate in care. Although having parental support during the dressing changes may be helpful, this action does nothing to allow the child control. Giving the child permission to cry may help with verbalizing feelings, but doing so does nothing to provide the child with control over the situation. Although allowing the child to determine the time for dressing changes may provide a sense of control over the situation, doing so is inappropriate because the dressing changes need to be performed as prescribed to ensure effectiveness and healing.

    CN: Physiological adaptation; CL: Synthesize

10. 2. Withholding certain foods until the child complies is punitive and rarely successful. Allowing the mother to feed the child, serving smaller and more frequent meals, and offering finger foods are all acceptable interventions for a 5-year-old child. This is true whether the child is well or ill.

    CN: Basic care and comfort; CL: Evaluate

11. 1. Hypoproteinemia is common after severe burns. The child's diet should be high in protein to compensate for protein loss and to promote tissue healing. The child will also require a diet that is high in calories and rich in iron. The menu of bacon, lettuce, and tomato sandwich; milk; and celery sticks is lacking in sufficient protein and calories.

    CN: Physiological adaptation; CL: Evaluate

12. 3. A child with moderate burns is at high risk for contractures. A position of comfort would encourage contracture formation. Therefore, splints need to be applied to maintain proper positioning and joint function, thereby preventing contractures and loss of function. Allowing the child to lie on the abdomen or with the hips and knees flexed often encourages contracture formation.

    CN: Reduction of risk potential; CL: Synthesize

The Client with a Thyroid Problem

13. 3. Most clients will need lifelong thyroid replacement after treatments with radioactive iodine. Most clients are treated as outpatients. To reduce the risk of exposure to radioactivity to others, clients are advised to avoid public places for at least 1 day and maintain a prudent distance from others for 2 to 3 days. Additionally, clients are advised to avoid close contact with pregnant women and children for 5 to 11 days. The use of radioiodine to treat Graves' disease has not been found to affect long-term fertility. Clients are taught not to share food, utensils, and towels. Use of a private bathroom is desirable. Clients are also instructed to flush the toilet more than one time after each use.

    CN: Safety and infection control; CL: Evaluate

14. 1,2,4,5. Hypothyroidism is a disorder in which the levels of active thyroid hormone are decreased. Clinical manifestations include cool extremities, mottling, umbilical hernia, lethargy, constipation, muscle weakness, and a hoarse cry. Hyperthyroidism occurs when thyroid hormone levels are increased. Clinical manifestations include increased appetite, goiter, irritability, prominent eyes, and tachycardia.

    CN: Physiological adaptation; CL: Analysis

15. 3. Children with hyperthyroidism experience emotional lability that may strain interpersonal relationships. Focusing on one friend is easier than adapting to group dynamics until the child's condition improves. Because of their high metabolic rate, children with hyperthyroidism feel too warm.

Bright sunshine may be irritating because of disease-related ophthalmopathy. Sweating is common, and bathing should be encouraged.

🔑 CN: Physiological adaptation;
CL: Synthesize

16. 4. Because it takes approximately 2 weeks before the response to drug treatment occurs, much of the child's care focuses on managing the child's physical symptoms. Signs and symptoms of the disorder include inability to sit still or concentrate, increased appetite with weight loss, emotional lability, and fatigue. Nursing care is directed toward ensuring that the mother and teacher know how to handle the child, suggesting a shortened school day, a nonstimulating environment, and decreased stress and workload. The child should be encouraged to eat a well-balanced diet.

🔑 CN: Physiological adaptation;
CL: Create

The Client with Insulin-Dependent Diabetes Mellitus

17. 2. The 15-15 rule is a general guideline for treating hypoglycemia where the client consumes 15 g of carbohydrate and repeats testing the blood sugar in 15 minutes. Fifteen grams of carbohydrate equals 60 calories and is roughly equal to ½ cup (120 mL) of juice or soda, six to eight Life Savers, or a tablespoon of honey or sugar. The general recommendation is if the blood sugar is still low, the client may repeat the sequence. Fifteen milliliters of juice would only provide 8 calories. This would not be sufficient carbohydrates to treat the hypoglycemia. Protein does not treat insulin-related hypoglycemia; however, a protein-starch snack may be offered after the blood glucose improves. Fifteen ounces of juice would be approximately 440 mL—almost four times the recommended 4 oz (120 mL) of juice.

🔑 CN: Physiological adaptation;
CL: Synthesize

18. 4. Self-efficacy, or the belief that one can act in a way to produce a desired outcome, can be promoted through the observation of role models. Peers are particularly effective role models because clients can more readily identify with them and believe they are capable of similar behaviors. Providing a written plan alone does not promote self-efficacy. Having parents eliminate junk food and having the school nurse weigh the adolescent can be part of the plan, but these actions do not empower the client.

🔑 CN: Management of care;
CL: Synthesize

19. 3. Metformin is currently approved by the FDA and Health Canada to treat type 2 diabetes in children. The medication decreases glucogenesis in the liver and increases insulin sensitivity in the peripheral tissues. Only insulin can actually replace insulin. This treatment is reserved for clients with type 1 diabetes or those with type 2 who do not respond to diet, exercise, and an oral diabetic agent. Other oral medications used to treat diabetes augments insulin production or decreases carbohydrate absorption, but those medications are primarily used in adults.

🔑 CN: Pharmacological and parenteral therapies; CL: Apply

20. 4. The child is using the correct injection technique, and the nurse can remind the child to rotate sites. The nurse should also reinforce that the child has used the correct technique and praise the child for doing so. If the child can manipulate the plunger of the syringe with one hand, this is appropriate. Insulin is administered at a 90-degree angle as shown. The child should identify appropriate sites on the thighs as one handbreadth below the hip and above the knee; the child is using appropriate sites.

🔑 CN: Health promotion and maintenance;
CL: Apply

21. Four units. Each carbohydrate food exchange has 15 g of carbohydrate. Two units are needed to cover the current blood glucose, and 2 units are needed to cover the anticipated carbohydrate intake.

🔑 CN: Pharmacological and parenteral therapies; CL: Apply

22. 3. Intermediate-acting insulin peaks in 6 to 8 hours, which would occur during sleep. A bedtime snack is needed to prevent late night hypoglycemia. The snack is not given to help regain weight. Milk contains fat and protein, which cause delayed absorption into the bloodstream, and maintains the blood glucose level at night when the intermediate-acting insulin will peak. The snack is not used to provide carbohydrates for immediate use because an intermediate-acting insulin, unlike regular insulin, does not peak immediately. The snack has nothing to do with a diet.

🔑 CN: Psychosocial integrity; CL: Apply

23. 2. The child needs more insulin during an illness, because the cells become more insulin resistant during illness and need more insulin to achieve a normal blood glucose level. Glucose levels rise with illness; therefore, more food calories are not needed. During an acute illness, simple carbohydrates and fluids are usually tolerated best.

🔑 CN: Physiological adaptation; CL: Evaluate

24. 1,2,6. Weakness, thirst, and dizziness are symptoms related to dehydration caused by excretion of large amounts of glucose and water in the urine. The nurse should notify the **healthcare provider (HCP)** 📖. Shakiness, hunger, headache, and irritability are related to hypoglycemia and result from the brain and other cells being starved for nutrients.

↝ CN: Physiological adaptation; CL: Analyze

25. 2. The ability to talk about her diabetes indicates that the adolescent feels good enough about herself to share her problem with her peers. Asking for reference material does not specifically indicate that the client's self-esteem has improved or that she has accepted her diagnosis. Saying that her friends will probably desert her if she tells them about the illness indicates that the adolescent still needs to work on her self-esteem and her feelings about the disease. Asking her friends what they think of someone with a lifelong illness would not indicate that the nurse's interventions targeted toward improving self-esteem have been successful. Rather, this statement demonstrates the adolescent's uncertainty about herself.

↝ CN: Psychosocial integrity; CL: Evaluate

26. 1. Repeated use of the same injection site can result in atrophy of the fat in the subcutaneous tissue and lead to poor insulin absorption. The neuritis that develops from diabetes is related to microvascular changes that occur. Subcutaneous tissue is not destroyed, and insulin is not rapidly absorbed. Resistance to insulin is caused by an immune response to the insulin protein.

↝ CN: Pharmacological and parenteral therapies; CL: Evaluate

The Client with Polycystic Ovarian Syndrome

27. 4. While pregnancy may be difficult for some clients, the nurse must work to prevent the false conception that a sexually active teen with PCOS does not need to use a reliable form of birth control. PCOS is associated with high levels of androgens and excessive insulin. It is the excess insulin that is thought to increase androgen production. Clients with PCOS are at risk for type 2 diabetes. Initial treatment focuses on weight management and exercise. These measures often reduce insulin production and restore normal menstrual cycles.

↝ CN: Physiologic adaptation; CL: Evaluate

28. 2,3,4,5. PCOS is associated with obesity, increased body or facial hair (hirsutism), acne, and darkening of the skin usually in body folds (acanthosis nigricans). When a female has never had a menstrual cycle, it is referred to as primary amenorrhea. PCOS is associated with irregular menstrual cycles and/or secondary amenorrhea, not primary amenorrhea. High androgen levels frequently lead to decreased versus enlarged breast size.

↝ CN: Physiologic adaptation; CL: Analyze

29. 3. Metformin works by decreasing the production of glucose in the liver and improving insulin sensitivity. These two mechanisms reduce insulin and blood glucose level. Reducing insulin levels reduces androgens and helps to restore menstruation.

↝ CN: Pharmacology and parental therapies; CL: Evaluate

30. 2. Many clients with PCOS suffer from depression. As depression is associated with a significant risk of suicide, the priority would be to determine if the client has symptoms of depression requiring further evaluation and treatment. Referrals to a hair removal specialist and possibly a support group would be appropriate, but only after determining if the client needs a referral for a major mood disorder. Providing more information on causes and treatment options is better saved for when the client is less distraught.

↝ CN: Psychosocial integrity; CL: Analyze

Managing Care, Quality, and Safety of Children with Dermatologic and Endocrine Health Problems

31. 3. Confidentiality legislation specifies that institutions designate a "privacy officer" who is responsible for developing and implementing privacy policies. This would be the very best resource for the nurse to contact. Depending on the nurse manager's experience, he or she may or may not know the answer and may have to consult the privacy officer. While **HCPs** 📖 would have an understanding of confidentiality laws, it is unlikely they understand the specifics of nursing policies. The customer service representatives typically address client concerns or complaints. At this time, the family has not voiced a complaint.

↝ CN: Management of care; CL: Apply

32. 2. Sleeping in the same room with a person of the opposite sex may be viewed as a violation of norms by persons of conservative faiths. If at all possible, the charge nurse should reassign the family to a different room. While it makes sense to have two clients with similar educational needs in the same room, it is likely that the arrangement would be distressing enough to create a learning barrier. Offering the mother another place to sleep deprives the child of her parent at night. The customer service representative would only need to be involved if it became impossible to accommodate the mother's needs.

🔑 CN: Management of care; CL: Synthesize

33. 1. Blood sugar levels can go up during the flu; therefore, blood glucose levels should be monitored every 3 to 4 hours during flu. Because glucose levels are higher when a client has the flu, clients should continue to take diabetes medications as ordered. If blood sugar level is over 240 mg/dL, ketones should be checked. If ketones are present, the client should be encouraged to drink calorie-free fluids and eat small meals.

🔑 CN: Management of care; CL: Synthesize

34. 4. Treating pediatric clients with severe DKA is a medical emergency; therefore, attending to the airway, breathing, and circulation is the first priority. Once the airway is secured, the healthcare team should estimate the level of dehydration and begin replacement fluids of normal saline. An insulin drip

should be started after the initial 1 to 2 hours of treatment at a rate of 0.1 units/kg/h. Blood glucose should be tested every 1 to 2 hours until the client is stable, then it should be every 6 hours. Additionally, serum electrolytes should be drawn every 1 to 2 hours until the client is stable, then every 4 to 6 hours.

🔑 CN: Management of care; CL: Synthesis

35. 2. The nurse's first response should be to obtain more information about the mother's concerns. It is true that the child may have a diabetic reaction anywhere at school, and it is advisable that her teacher, classmates, and other adults know about her diabetes in order to help her; however, it is ultimately the client and her parents who will make the decision about informing the school. The nurse can facilitate a dialogue that will help the mother reach this decision. Dictating to the mother does not explain any rationale for the necessity of the information. Telling the mother that her daughter will tell the school does not address the mother's concerns.

🔑 CN: Safety and infection control; CL: Synthesize

The Nursing Care of Adults with Medical and Surgical Health Problems

TEST 1

The Client with Cardiac Health Problems

- **The Client with Acute Coronary Syndromes**
- **The Client with Heart Failure**
- **The Client with Valvular Heart Disease**
- **The Client with Hypertension**
- **The Client with Atrial Fibrillation and Other Dysrhythmias**
- **The Client Requiring Rapid Response or Cardiopulmonary Resuscitation**
- **Managing Care, Quality, and Safety for Clients with Cardiac Health Problems**
- **Answers, Rationales, and Test-Taking Strategies**

The Client with Acute Coronary Syndromes

1. A client returns from a left heart catheterization. The right groin was used for catheter access. In which location should the nurse palpate the distal pulse on this client?
- ☐ 1. anterior to the right tibia
- ☐ 2. dorsal surface of the right foot
- ☐ 3. posterior to the right knee
- ☐ 4. right midinguinal area

2. A client is admitted with chest pain and kept overnight for stress testing the next morning. Prior to sending the client to the stress test, the nurse reviews the results of the laboratory reports (see lab report). The nurse should report which elevated laboratory value to the healthcare provider (HCP) prior to the stress test?
- ☐ 1. cholesterol level
- ☐ 2. erythrocyte sedimentation rate
- ☐ 3. prothrombin time
- ☐ 4. troponin

3. A client has chest pain rated at 8 on a 10-point visual analog scale. The 12-lead electrocardiogram reveals ST elevation in the inferior leads, and troponin levels are elevated. What should the nurse do **first**?
- ☐ 1. Monitor daily weights and urine output.
- ☐ 2. Limit visitation by family and friends.
- ☐ 3. Provide client education on medications and diet.
- ☐ 4. Reduce pain and myocardial oxygen demand.

4. A client with chest pain is prescribed intravenous nitroglycerin. Which assessment is of **greatest** concern for the nurse initiating the nitroglycerin drip?
- ☐ 1. Serum potassium is 3.5 mEq/L (3.5 mmol/L).
- ☐ 2. Blood pressure is 88/46 mm Hg.
- ☐ 3. ST elevation is present on the electrocardiogram.
- ☐ 4. Heart rate is 61 bpm.

5. The nurse is caring for a client diagnosed with an anterior myocardial infarction 2 days ago. Upon assessment, the nurse identifies a systolic murmur at the apex. The nurse should **first**:
☐ 1. assess for changes in vital signs.
☐ 2. draw an arterial blood gas.
☐ 3. evaluate heart sounds with the client leaning forward.
☐ 4. obtain a 12-lead electrocardiogram.

6. A client with acute chest pain is receiving IV morphine sulfate. Which is an expected effect of morphine? Select all that apply.
☐ 1. reduces myocardial oxygen consumption
☐ 2. promotes reduction in respiratory rate
☐ 3. prevents ventricular remodeling
☐ 4. reduces blood pressure and heart rate
☐ 5. reduces anxiety and fear

7. A client is receiving an IV infusion of heparin sodium at 1,200 units/h. The dilution is 25,000 units/500 mL. How many milliliters per hour will this client receive? Round your answer to a whole number.

_____ mL/h.

8. An older adult has chest pain and shortness of breath. The healthcare provider (HCP) prescribes nitroglycerin tablets. What should the nurse instruct the client to do?
☐ 1. Put the tablet under the tongue until it is absorbed.
☐ 2. Swallow the tablet with 120 mL of water.
☐ 3. Chew the tablet until it is dissolved.
☐ 4. Place the tablet between the cheek and gums until it disappears.

9. The nurse has completed an assessment on a client with a decreased cardiac output. Which findings should receive the **highest priority**?
☐ 1. BP 110/62 mm Hg, atrial fibrillation with HR 82, bilateral basilar crackles
☐ 2. confusion, urine output 15 mL over the last 2 hours, orthopnea
☐ 3. SpO_2 92 on 2 L nasal cannula, respirations 20, 1+ edema of lower extremities
☐ 4. weight gain of 1 kg in 3 days, BP 130/80, mild dyspnea with exercise

10. The nurse notices that a client's heart rate decreases from 63 to 50 bpm on the monitor. The nurse should **first**:
☐ 1. administer atropine 0.5 mg IV push.
☐ 2. auscultate for abnormal heart sounds.
☐ 3. prepare for transcutaneous pacing.
☐ 4. take the client's blood pressure.

11. When preparing a client for a cardiac angiogram, what actions should the nurse take? Select all that apply.
☐ 1. Determine if the client has an allergy to liquid contrast material.
☐ 2. Inform the client that an intravenous infusion will be started before the procedure.
☐ 3. Remind the client to have nothing to eat or drink 8 hours before the procedure.
☐ 4. Instruct the client to remain still during the procedure.
☐ 5. Explain that the client will receive a fast-acting acting anesthetic.

12. A client is admitted with a myocardial infarction and atrial fibrillation. While auscultating the heart, the nurse notes an irregular heart rate and hears an extra heart sound at the apex after the S_2 that remains constant throughout the respiratory cycle. The nurse should document these findings as:
☐ 1. heart rate irregular with S_3.
☐ 2. heart rate irregular with S_4.
☐ 3. heart rate irregular with aortic regurgitation.
☐ 4. heart rate irregular with mitral stenosis.

13. A 60-year-old comes into the emergency department with crushing substernal chest pain that radiates to the shoulder and left arm. The admitting diagnosis is acute myocardial infarction (MI). Admission prescriptions include oxygen by nasal cannula at 4 L/min, complete blood count (CBC), a chest radiograph, a 12-lead electrocardiogram (ECG), and 2 mg of morphine sulfate given IV. The nurse should **first**:
☐ 1. administer the morphine.
☐ 2. obtain a 12-lead ECG.
☐ 3. obtain the blood work.
☐ 4. prescribe the chest radiograph.

14. An older adult had a myocardial infarction (MI) 4 days ago. At 0930, the client's blood pressure is 102/64 mm Hg. After reviewing the client's progress notes (see chart), the nurse should **first**:

Nurses Progress Notes

Date	1/10
Time	0030
Urinary output for the last 4 hours	90 mL
Capillary refill	>3 seconds
Blood pressure	128/82
Extremities	Cool
	D. Smith, RN

☐ 1. give a fluid challenge/bolus.
☐ 2. notify the healthcare provider (HCP).
☐ 3. assist the client to walk.
☐ 4. administer furosemide as prescribed.

15. When administering a thrombolytic drug to the client who is experiencing a myocardial infarction (MI) and who has premature ventricular contractions, the expected outcome of the drug is to:
- ☐ 1. promote hydration.
- ☐ 2. dissolve clots.
- ☐ 3. prevent kidney failure.
- ☐ 4. treat dysrhythmias.

16. The nurse is assessing a client who has had a myocardial infarction (MI). The nurse notes the cardiac rhythm on the monitor (see the electrocardiogram strip). The nurse should:
- ☐ 1. notify the healthcare provider (HCP).
- ☐ 2. call the rapid response team.
- ☐ 3. assess the client for changes in the rhythm.
- ☐ 4. administer lidocaine as prescribed.

17. The nurse is assessing a client who has had a stent inserted in a coronary artery via the right femoral artery. The client is receiving intravenous heparin sodium at 1,000 units per hour. During the second postprocedure check, the nurse notes that the puncture site at the groin has begun to steadily ooze blood. The nurse should **first**:
- ☐ 1. don gloves and apply direct pressure over the site.
- ☐ 2. observe and document the bleeding.
- ☐ 3. notify the healthcare provider (HCP).
- ☐ 4. prepare protamine sulfate for intravenous administration.

18. A client admitted for a myocardial infarction (MI) develops cardiogenic shock. An arterial line is inserted. Which prescription from the healthcare provider should the nurse verify before implementing?
- ☐ 1. Call for urine output < 30 mL/h for 2 consecutive hours.
- ☐ 2. Administer metoprolol 5 mg IV push.
- ☐ 3. Prepare for a pulmonary artery catheter insertion.
- ☐ 4. Titrate dobutamine to keep systolic BP > 100 mm Hg.

19. The nurse is monitoring a client admitted with a myocardial infarction (MI) who is at risk for cardiogenic shock. The nurse should report which changes noted from the client's chart to the healthcare provider (HCP)?

Nurses Progress Notes

	1300	1500	
BP	110/70	100/65	
T	98.7 (37.1)	99 (37.2)	
HR	70	75	
R	20	26	
Urine output	90 mL/h	20 mL/h	

- ☐ 1. urine output
- ☐ 2. heart rate
- ☐ 3. blood pressure
- ☐ 4. respiratory rate

20. The healthcare provider (HCP) prescribes continuous IV nitroglycerin infusion for the client with myocardial infarction. The nurse should:
- ☐ 1. obtain an infusion pump for the medication.
- ☐ 2. take the blood pressure every 4 hours.
- ☐ 3. monitor urine output hourly.
- ☐ 4. obtain serum potassium levels daily.

21. The client is admitted to the telemetry unit due to chest pain. The client has polysubstance abuse, and the nurse assesses that the client is anxious and irritable and has moist skin. What should the nurse do in order of priority from first to last? All options must be used.

1. Obtain a history of which drugs the client has used recently.

2. Administer the prescribed dose of morphine.

3. Position electrodes on the chest.

4. Take vital signs.

22. A client is scheduled for insertion of a coronary stent with right groin access. Which teaching points should the nurse include in this client's preoperative teaching plan? Select all that apply.

☐ 1. "If you have a hearing aid, you will need to remove it prior to leaving for the procedure."

☐ 2. "If you have chest pain during this procedure, please tell the staff when or if this should occur."

☐ 3. "The stitches at your right groin will be able to be removed in 7 to 10 days following the procedure."

☐ 4. "You will be given general anesthesia and will be asleep for throughout this procedure."

☐ 5. "You will need to remain flat during the procedure and for 3 to 6 hours after the procedure."

☐ 6. "You will need to keep your right leg in a flexed position for 1 to 2 hours following the procedure."

23. The nurse is assessing a client who has had a myocardial infarction. The nurse notes the cardiac rhythm shown on the electrocardiogram strip. The nurse interprets this rhythm as:

☐ 1. atrial fibrillation.

☐ 2. ventricular tachycardia.

☐ 3. premature ventricular contractions.

☐ 4. sinus tachycardia.

24. While caring for a client who has sustained a myocardial infarction (MI), the nurse notes eight premature ventricular contractions (PVCs) in 1 minute on the cardiac monitor. The client is receiving an IV infusion of 5% dextrose in water (D_5W) at 125 mL/h and oxygen at 2 L/min. The nurse should **first**:

☐ 1. increase the IV infusion rate to 150 mL/h.

☐ 2. notify the healthcare provider (HCP).

☐ 3. increase the oxygen concentration to 4 L/min.

☐ 4. administer a prescribed analgesic.

25. Which is an expected outcome for a client on the 2nd day of hospitalization after a myocardial infarction (MI)? The client:

☐ 1. continues to have severe chest pain.

☐ 2. can identify risk factors for MI.

☐ 3. participates in a cardiac rehabilitation walking program.

☐ 4. can perform personal self-care activities without pain.

26. Which is an expected outcome when a client is receiving an IV administration of furosemide?

☐ 1. increased blood pressure

☐ 2. increased urine output

☐ 3. decreased pain

☐ 4. decreased premature ventricular contractions

27. The nurse is preparing to measure central venous pressure (CVP). Mark the spot on the torso indicating the location for leveling the transducer.

28. A client has had a pulmonary artery catheter inserted. In performing hemodynamic monitoring with the catheter, the nurse should wedge the catheter to gain information about:

☐ 1. cardiac output.

☐ 2. right atrial blood flow.

☐ 3. left end-diastolic pressure.

☐ 4. cardiac index.

29. After a myocardial infarction, the hospitalized client is taught to move the legs while resting in bed. What is the expected outcome of this exercise?

☐ 1. Prepare the client for ambulation.

☐ 2. Promote urinary and intestinal elimination.

☐ 3. Prevent thrombophlebitis and blood clot formation.

☐ 4. Decrease the likelihood of pressure ulcer formation.

30. Which is the **most** appropriate diet for a client during the acute phase of myocardial infarction?

☐ 1. liquids as desired

☐ 2. small, easily digested meals

☐ 3. three regular meals per day

☐ 4. nothing by mouth

31. The nurse is caring for a client who recently experienced a myocardial infarction and has been started on clopidogrel. The nurse should develop a teaching plan that includes which points? Select all that apply.

☐ 1. The client should report unexpected bleeding or bleeding that lasts a long time.

☐ 2. The client should take clopidogrel with food.

☐ 3. The client may bruise more easily and may experience bleeding gums.

☐ 4. Clopidogrel works by preventing platelets from sticking together and forming a clot.

☐ 5. The client should drink a glass of water after taking clopidogrel.

32. Which client is at **greatest** risk for coronary artery disease?
- ☐ 1. a 32-year-old female with mitral valve prolapse who quit smoking 10 years ago
- ☐ 2. a 43-year-old male with a family history of CAD and cholesterol level of 158 (8.8 mmol/L)
- ☐ 3. a 56-year-old male with an HDL of 60 (3.3 mmol/L) who takes atorvastatin
- ☐ 4. a 65-year-old female who is obese with an LDL of 188 (10.4 mmol/L)

33. The client has been managing angina episodes with nitroglycerin. Which finding indicates that the therapeutic effect of the drug has been achieved?
- ☐ 1. decreased chest pain
- ☐ 2. increased blood pressure
- ☐ 3. decreased blood pressure
- ☐ 4. decreased heart rate

34. A client has risk factors for coronary artery disease, including smoking cigarettes, eating a diet high in saturated fat, and leading a sedentary lifestyle. The nurse can coach this client to improve health by:
- ☐ 1. explaining how the risk factors lead to poor health.
- ☐ 2. withholding praise until the client changes the risky behavior.
- ☐ 3. helping the client establish a wellness vision to reduce the health risks.
- ☐ 4. instilling mild fear into the client about the potential outcomes of the risky health behaviors.

35. Alteplase recombinant, or tissue plasminogen activator (t-PA), a thrombolytic enzyme, is administered during the first 6 hours after onset of myocardial infarction (MI) to:
- ☐ 1. control chest pain.
- ☐ 2. reduce coronary artery vasospasm.
- ☐ 3. control the arrhythmias associated with MI.
- ☐ 4. revascularize the blocked coronary artery.

36. When monitoring a client who is receiving tissue plasminogen activator (t-PA), the nurse should have resuscitation equipment available because reperfusion of the cardiac tissue can result in:
- ☐ 1. cardiac arrhythmias.
- ☐ 2. hypertension.
- ☐ 3. seizure.
- ☐ 4. hypothermia.

37. Prior to administering tissue plasminogen activator (t-PA), the nurse should assess the client for which contradiction to administering the drug?
- ☐ 1. age > 60 years
- ☐ 2. history of cerebral hemorrhage
- ☐ 3. history of heart failure
- ☐ 4. cigarette smoking

38. A middle-aged client being admitted to the hospital has a history of hypertension and informs the nurse that his father died from a heart attack at age 60. The client reports having "indigestion." The nurse connects the client to a cardiac monitor, which reveals eight premature ventricular contractions (PVCs) per minute. The nurse should **next**:
- ☐ 1. call the healthcare provider (HCP).
- ☐ 2. start an IV line.
- ☐ 3. obtain a portable chest radiograph.
- ☐ 4. draw blood for laboratory studies.

39. A 68-year-old client on day 2 after hip surgery has no cardiac history but reports having chest heaviness. The nurse should **first**:
- ☐ 1. inquire about the onset, duration, severity, and precipitating factors of the heaviness.
- ☐ 2. administer oxygen via nasal cannula.
- ☐ 3. offer pain medication for the chest heaviness.
- ☐ 4. inform the healthcare provider (HCP) of the chest heaviness.

40. Following diagnosis of angina pectoris, a client reports being unable to walk up two flights of stairs without pain. Which instruction would **most** likely help the client prevent this problem?
- ☐ 1. Climb the steps early in the day.
- ☐ 2. Rest for at least an hour before climbing the stairs.
- ☐ 3. Take a nitroglycerin tablet before climbing the stairs.
- ☐ 4. Lie down after climbing the stairs.

41. The client who experiences angina has been told to follow a low-cholesterol diet. Which meal would be **best**?
- ☐ 1. hamburger, salad, and milk shake
- ☐ 2. baked liver, green beans, and coffee
- ☐ 3. spaghetti with tomato sauce, salad, and coffee
- ☐ 4. fried chicken, green beans, and skim milk

42. Which symptom should the nurse teach the client with unstable angina to report **immediately** to the healthcare provider (HCP)?
- ☐ 1. a change in the pattern of the chest pain
- ☐ 2. pain during sexual activity
- ☐ 3. pain during an argument
- ☐ 4. pain during or after a physical activity

43. A client with unstable angina is scheduled to have a cardiac catheterization. The nurse explains to the client that this procedure is being used to:
- ☐ 1. open and dilate blocked coronary arteries.
- ☐ 2. assess the extent of arterial blockage.
- ☐ 3. bypass obstructed vessels.
- ☐ 4. assess the functional adequacy of the valves and heart muscle.

44. The nurse is caring for a client who has just returned from having a percutaneous transluminal balloon angioplasty with femoral artery access. In which order, from first to last, should the nurse obtain information about the client? All options must be used.

1. vital signs and oxygen saturation

2. pedal pulses

3. color and sensation of extremity

4. catheterization site

45. Which is **not** a risk factor for the development of atherosclerosis?
- ☐ 1. family history of early heart attack
- ☐ 2. late onset of puberty
- ☐ 3. total blood cholesterol level > 220 mg/dL (12.2 mmol/L)
- ☐ 4. elevated fasting blood glucose concentration

46. As an initial step in treating a client with angina, the healthcare provider (HCP) prescribes nitroglycerin tablets, 0.3 mg, given sublingually. This drug's principal effects are produced by:
- ☐ 1. antispasmodic effects on the pericardium.
- ☐ 2. causing an increased myocardial oxygen demand.
- ☐ 3. vasodilation of peripheral vasculature.
- ☐ 4. improved conductivity in the myocardium.

47. A client has a throbbing headache when nitroglycerin is taken for angina. The nurse should instruct the client that:
- ☐ 1. acetaminophen or ibuprofen can be taken for this common side effect.
- ☐ 2. nitroglycerin should be avoided if the client is experiencing this serious side effect.
- ☐ 3. taking the nitroglycerin with a few glasses of water will reduce the problem.
- ☐ 4. the client should lie in a supine position to alleviate the headache.

48. How should the nurse instruct the client with unstable angina to use sublingual nitroglycerin tablets when chest pain occurs? "Sit down and then:
- ☐ 1. take one tablet every 2 to 5 minutes until the pain stops."
- ☐ 2. take one tablet and rest for 15 minutes. Call the healthcare provider if pain persists after 15 minutes."
- ☐ 3. take one tablet; then if the pain persists, take additional two tablets in 5 minutes. Call the healthcare provider if pain persists after 15 minutes."
- ☐ 4. take one tablet. If pain persists after 5 minutes, call 911."

49. A client with angina is taking nifedipine. What instruction should the nurse give the client?
- ☐ 1. Monitor blood pressure monthly.
- ☐ 2. Perform daily weights.
- ☐ 3. Inspect gums daily.
- ☐ 4. Limit intake of green leafy vegetables.

50. The nurse is developing a teaching plan for a client who will be starting a prescription for simvastatin 40 mg/day. What instructions should the nurse give the client? Select all that apply.
- ☐ 1. "Take once a day in the morning."
- ☐ 2. "If you miss a dose, take it when you remember it."
- ☐ 3. "Limit greens such as lettuce in the diet to prevent bleeding."
- ☐ 4. "Be sure to take the pill with food."
- ☐ 5. "Report muscle pain or tenderness to your healthcare provider."
- ☐ 6. "Continue to follow a diet that is low in saturated fats."

The Client with Heart Failure

51. Captopril, furosemide, and metoprolol are prescribed for a client with systolic heart failure. The client's blood pressure is 136/82 mm Hg, and the heart rate is 65 bpm. Prior to medication administration at 0900, the nurse reviews the following lab tests (see chart). What should the nurse do **first**?

Laboratory Results	
Sodium	140 mEq/L (140 mmol/L)
Potassium	6.8 mEq/L (6.8 mmol/L)
BUN	18 mg/dL (6.4 mmol/L)
Creatinine	1.0 mg/dL (76.3 µmol/L)
Hemoglobin	12 g/dL (120 g/L)
Hematocrit	37% (0.37)

- ☐ 1. Administer the medications.
- ☐ 2. Call the healthcare provider (HCP).
- ☐ 3. Withhold the captopril.
- ☐ 4. Question the metoprolol dose.

52. A client with chronic heart failure has atrial fibrillation and a left ventricular ejection fraction of 15%. The client is taking warfarin. The expected outcome of this drug is to:
☐ 1. decrease circulatory overload.
☐ 2. improve the myocardial workload.
☐ 3. prevent thrombus formation.
☐ 4. regulate cardiac rhythm.

53. A client has a history of heart failure and has been prescribed furosemide, digoxin, and potassium chloride. The client has nausea, blurred vision, headache, and weakness. The nurse notes that the client is confused. The telemetry strip shows first-degree atrioventricular block. The nurse should assess the client for signs of:
☐ 1. hyperkalemia.
☐ 2. digoxin toxicity.
☐ 3. fluid deficit.
☐ 4. pulmonary edema.

54. The nurse should assess the client with left-sided heart failure for which findings? Select all that apply.
☐ 1. dyspnea
☐ 2. jugular vein distention (JVD)
☐ 3. crackles
☐ 4. right upper quadrant pain
☐ 5. oliguria
☐ 6. decreased oxygen saturation levels

55. Which are indications that a client with a history of left-sided heart failure is developing pulmonary edema? Select all that apply.
☐ 1. distended jugular veins
☐ 2. dependent edema
☐ 3. anorexia
☐ 4. coarse crackles
☐ 5. tachycardia

56. An older adult with a history of heart failure is admitted to the emergency department with pulmonary edema. On admission, what should the nurse assess **first**?
☐ 1. blood pressure
☐ 2. skin breakdown
☐ 3. serum potassium level
☐ 4. urine output

57. The nurse is caring for an older adult with mild dementia admitted with heart failure. What nursing care will be helpful for this client in reducing potential confusion related to hospitalization and change in routine? Select all that apply.
☐ 1. Reorient frequently to time, place, and situation.
☐ 2. Put the client in a quiet room furthest from the nursing station.
☐ 3. Perform necessary procedures quickly.
☐ 4. Arrange for familiar pictures or special items at bedside.
☐ 5. Limit the client's visitors.
☐ 6. Spend time with the client, establishing a trusting relationship.

58. The nurse is assessing a client with chronic heart failure who is demonstrating neurohormonal compensatory mechanisms. Which are expected findings on assessment? Select all that apply.
☐ 1. decreased cardiac output
☐ 2. increased heart rate
☐ 3. vasoconstriction in skin, GI tract, and kidneys
☐ 4. decreased pulmonary perfusion
☐ 5. fluid overload

59. Furosemide 40 mg intravenous push (IVP) is prescribed. Furosemide 10 mg/mL is available. How much should the nurse administer? Round your answer to a whole number.
_____ mL.

60. Which position is **best** for a client with heart failure who has orthopnea?
☐ 1. semisitting (low Fowler's position) with legs elevated on pillows
☐ 2. lying on the right side (Sims' position) with a pillow between the legs
☐ 3. sitting upright (high Fowler's position) with legs resting on the mattress
☐ 4. lying on the back with the head lowered (Trendelenburg's position) and legs elevated

61. What is the major goal of nursing care for a client with heart failure and pulmonary edema?
☐ 1. Increase cardiac output.
☐ 2. Improve respiratory status.
☐ 3. Decrease peripheral edema.
☐ 4. Enhance comfort.

62. A client with heart failure is receiving digoxin intravenously. The nurse should determine the effectiveness of the drug by assessing:
☐ 1. dilated coronary arteries.
☐ 2. increased myocardial contractility.
☐ 3. decreased cardiac arrhythmias.
☐ 4. decreased electrical conductivity in the heart.

63. Furosemide is administered intravenously to a client with heart failure. How soon after administration should the nurse begin to see evidence of the drug's desired effect?
☐ 1. 5 to 10 minutes
☐ 2. 30 to 60 minutes
☐ 3. 2 to 4 hours
☐ 4. 6 to 8 hours

64. The nurse teaches a client with heart failure to take oral furosemide in the morning. The **primary** reason for this is to prevent:
☐ 1. electrolyte imbalances.
☐ 2. nausea or vomiting.
☐ 3. excretion of excessive fluids accumulated during the night.
☐ 4. sleep disturbances during the night.

65. The nurse should teach the client that signs of digoxin toxicity include:
☐ 1. rash over the chest and back.
☐ 2. increased appetite.
☐ 3. visual disturbances such as seeing yellow spots.
☐ 4. elevated blood pressure.

66. The nurse should assess the client for digoxin toxicity if serum levels indicate that the client has a:
☐ 1. low sodium level.
☐ 2. high glucose level.
☐ 3. high calcium level.
☐ 4. low potassium level.

67. Which food should the nurse teach a client with heart failure to limit when following a 2-g sodium diet?
☐ 1. apples
☐ 2. canned tomato juice
☐ 3. whole wheat bread
☐ 4. beef tenderloin

68. A client receiving a loop diuretic should be encouraged to eat which foods? Select all that apply.
☐ 1. angel food cake
☐ 2. banana
☐ 3. dried fruit
☐ 4. orange juice
☐ 5. peppers

69. When assessing an older adult, the nurse finds the apical impulse below the fifth intercostal space. The nurse should further assess the client for:
☐ 1. left atrial enlargement.
☐ 2. left ventricular enlargement.
☐ 3. right atrial enlargement.
☐ 4. right ventricular enlargement.

70. The nurse is admitting an older adult to the hospital. The echocardiogram report revealed left ventricular enlargement. The nurse notes 2+ pitting edema in the ankles when getting the client into bed. Based on this finding, what should the nurse do **first**?
☐ 1. Assess respiratory status.
☐ 2. Draw blood for laboratory studies.
☐ 3. Insert a Foley catheter.
☐ 4. Weigh the client.

71. The nurse's discharge teaching plan for the client with heart failure should emphasize the importance of:
☐ 1. maintaining a high-fiber diet.
☐ 2. walking 2 miles (3.2 km) every day.
☐ 3. obtaining daily weights at the same time each day.
☐ 4. remaining sedentary for most of the day.

72. The nurse is teaching a client with heart failure how to avoid complications and future hospitalizations. The nurse is confident that the client has understood the teaching when the client identifies which potential complications? Select all that apply.
☐ 1. becoming increasingly short of breath at rest
☐ 2. weight gain of 2 lb (0.9 kg) or more in 1 day
☐ 3. high intake of sodium for breakfast
☐ 4. having to sleep sitting up in a reclining chair
☐ 5. weight loss of 2 lb (0.9 kg) in 1 day

The Client with Valvular Heart Disease

73. A client has returned from the cardiac catheterization laboratory after a balloon valvuloplasty for mitral stenosis. Which finding requires **immediate** nursing action?
☐ 1. There is a low, grade 1 intensity mitral regurgitation murmur.
☐ 2. SpO$_2$ is 94% on 2 L of oxygen via nasal cannula.
☐ 3. Client has become more somnolent.
☐ 4. Urine output decreased from 60 mL/h to 40 mL over the last hour.

74. An older client with diabetes who has been maintained on metformin has been scheduled for a cardiac catheterization. The nurse should verify that the healthcare provider (HCP) has written a prescription to:
☐ 1. limit the amount of protein in the diet prior to the cardiac catheterization.
☐ 2. withhold the metformin prior to the cardiac catheterization.
☐ 3. administer the metformin with only a sip of water prior to the cardiac catheterization.
☐ 4. give the metformin before breakfast.

75. A client with aortic stenosis has increasing dyspnea and dizziness. Identify the area where the nurse would place the stethoscope to assess a murmur from aortic stenosis.

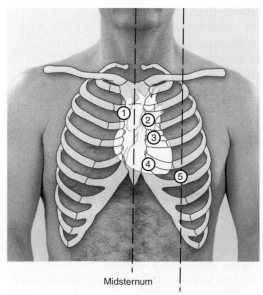

Midsternum

Midclavicular line

76. A client is scheduled for a cardiac catheterization. The nurse should do which preprocedure tasks? Select all that apply.
- ☐ 1. Administer all prescribed oral medications.
- ☐ 2. Check for iodine sensitivity.
- ☐ 3. Verify that written consent has been obtained.
- ☐ 4. Withhold food and oral fluids before the procedure.
- ☐ 5. Insert a urinary drainage catheter.

77. Which is the **most** important initial post-procedure nursing assessment for a client who has had a cardiac catheterization?
- ☐ 1. Monitor the laboratory values.
- ☐ 2. Observe neurologic function every 15 minutes.
- ☐ 3. Observe the puncture site for swelling and bleeding.
- ☐ 4. Monitor skin warmth and turgor.

78. A client experiences initial indications of dizziness after having an IV infusion of lidocaine hydrochloride started. The nurse should further assess the client when the client reports having:
- ☐ 1. palpitations.
- ☐ 2. tinnitus.
- ☐ 3. urinary frequency.
- ☐ 4. lethargy.

79. A pulmonary artery catheter is inserted in a client with severe mitral stenosis and regurgitation. The nurse administers furosemide to treat pulmonary congestion and begins a nitroprusside drip as prescribed. The nurse notices a sudden drop in the pulmonary artery diastolic pressure and pulmonary artery wedge pressure. The nurse should **first** assess:
- ☐ 1. 12-lead EKG.
- ☐ 2. blood pressure.
- ☐ 3. lung sounds.
- ☐ 4. urine output.

80. A client has mitral stenosis and will have a valve replacement. The nurse is instructing the client about health maintenance prior to surgery. Inability to follow which prescription would pose the **greatest** health hazard to this client at this time?
- ☐ 1. medication therapy
- ☐ 2. diet modification
- ☐ 3. activity restrictions
- ☐ 4. dental care

81. In preparing the client and the family for a postoperative stay in the intensive care unit (ICU) after open-heart surgery, the nurse should explain that:
- ☐ 1. the client will remain in the ICU for 5 days.
- ☐ 2. the client will sleep most of the time while in the ICU.
- ☐ 3. noise and activity within the ICU are minimal.
- ☐ 4. the client will receive medication to relieve pain.

82. A client who has undergone a mitral valve replacement has had a mediastinal chest tube inserted. The client has persistent bleeding from the sternal incision during the early postoperative period. What actions should the nurse take? Select all that apply.
- ☐ 1. Administer warfarin.
- ☐ 2. Check the postoperative CBC, INR, PTT, and platelet levels.
- ☐ 3. Confirm availability of blood products.
- ☐ 4. Monitor the mediastinal chest tube drainage.
- ☐ 5. Start a dopamine drip for a systolic BP < 100 mm Hg.

83. The **most** effective measure the nurse can use to prevent wound infection when changing a client's dressing after coronary artery bypass surgery is to:
- ☐ 1. observe careful handwashing procedures.
- ☐ 2. clean the incisional area with an antiseptic.
- ☐ 3. use prepackaged sterile dressings to cover the incision.
- ☐ 4. place soiled dressings in a waterproof bag before disposing of them.

84. Which measure should the nurse institute to help prevent complications associated with excessive calcium excretion following cardiac surgery to replace an aortic valve?
- ☐ 1. Ensure a liberal fluid intake.
- ☐ 2. Provide an alkaline-ash diet.
- ☐ 3. Prevent constipation.
- ☐ 4. Enrich the client's diet with dairy products.

85. The nurse should teach the client who is receiving warfarin sodium that:
- ☐ 1. partial thromboplastin time values determine the dosage of warfarin sodium.
- ☐ 2. protamine sulfate is used to reverse the effects of warfarin sodium.
- ☐ 3. international normalized ratio (INR) is used to assess effectiveness.
- ☐ 4. warfarin sodium will facilitate clotting of the blood.

86. Good dental care is an important measure in reducing the risk of endocarditis. What should a teaching plan to promote good dental care in a client with mitral stenosis instruct the client to do? Select all that apply.
- ☐ 1. Brush the teeth at least twice a day.
- ☐ 2. Avoid use of an electric toothbrush.
- ☐ 3. Take an antibiotic prior to oral surgery.
- ☐ 4. Floss the teeth at least once a day.
- ☐ 5. Have regular dental checkups.
- ☐ 6. Rinse the mouth with an antibiotic mouthwash once a day.

87. Before a client's discharge after mitral valve replacement surgery, the nurse should evaluate the client's understanding of postsurgery activity restrictions. The client should avoid which activity until after the 1-month postdischarge appointment with the surgeon?
☐ **1.** showering
☐ **2.** lifting anything heavier than 10 lb (4.5 kg)
☐ **3.** a program of gradually progressive walking
☐ **4.** light housework

88. Three days after mitral valve replacement surgery, the client tells the nurse there is a "clicking" noise coming from the chest incision. The nurse's response should reflect the understanding that the client may be experiencing:
☐ **1.** anxiety related to altered body image.
☐ **2.** depression related to altered health status.
☐ **3.** altered tissue perfusion.
☐ **4.** lack of knowledge regarding the postoperative course.

The Client with Hypertension

89. Metoprolol is added to the pharmacologic therapy of a diabetic female diagnosed with stage 2 hypertension who has been initially treated with furosemide and ramipril. An expected therapeutic effect is:
☐ **1.** decrease in heart rate.
☐ **2.** lessening of fatigue.
☐ **3.** improvement in blood sugar levels.
☐ **4.** increase in urine output.

90. Which set of postural vital signs (BP in mm Hg and heart rate in beats per minute) indicate inadequate blood volume?
☐ **1.** Supine 124/76, 88
Sitting 124/74, 92
Standing 122/74, 92
☐ **2.** Supine 120/70, 70
Sitting 102/64, 86
Standing 100/60, 92
☐ **3.** Supine 138/86, 74
Sitting 136/84, 80
Standing 134/82, 82
☐ **4.** Supine 100/70, 72
Sitting 100/68, 74
Standing 98/68, 80

91. A client is taking clonidine for treatment of hypertension. The nurse should teach the client about which common adverse effects of this drug? Select all that apply.
☐ **1.** dry mouth
☐ **2.** hyperkalemia
☐ **3.** impotence
☐ **4.** pancreatitis
☐ **5.** sleep disturbance

92. A client with hypertensive emergency is being treated with sodium nitroprusside. In a dilution of 50 mg/250 mL, how many micrograms of sodium nitroprusside are in each milliliter? Round your answer to a whole number.
_____ mcg.

93. The nurse is discussing medications with a client with hypertension who has a prescription for furosemide daily. The client needs further education when the client states:
☐ **1.** "I know I should not drive after taking my furosemide."
☐ **2.** "I should be careful not to stand up too quickly when taking furosemide."
☐ **3.** "I should take the furosemide in the morning instead of before bed."
☐ **4.** "I need to be sure to also take the potassium supplement that the doctor prescribed along with my furosemide."

94. In teaching the client with hypertension to avoid orthostatic hypotension, the nurse should teach the client to follow which instructions? Select all that apply.
☐ **1.** Plan regular times for taking medications.
☐ **2.** Arise slowly from bed.
☐ **3.** Avoid standing still for long periods.
☐ **4.** Avoid excessive alcohol intake.
☐ **5.** Avoid hot baths.

95. The nurse is teaching a client with hypertension about taking atenolol. The nurse should instruct the client to:
☐ **1.** avoid sudden discontinuation of the drug.
☐ **2.** monitor the blood pressure annually.
☐ **3.** follow a 2-g sodium diet.
☐ **4.** discontinue the medication if severe headaches develop.

96. The nurse teaches a client who has recently been diagnosed with hypertension about following a low-calorie, low-fat, low-sodium diet. Which of the following menu selections would **best** meet the client's needs?
☐ **1.** mixed green salad with blue cheese dressing, crackers, and cold cuts
☐ **2.** ham sandwich on rye bread and an orange
☐ **3.** baked chicken, an apple, and a slice of white bread
☐ **4.** hot dogs, baked beans, and celery and carrot sticks

97. A client who has diabetes is taking metoprolol for hypertension. What should the nurse instruct the client to do? Select all that apply.
☐ 1. Take the tablets with food at same time each day.
☐ 2. Do not crush or chew the tablets.
☐ 3. Notify the healthcare provider (HCP) if pulse is 82 beats/min.
☐ 4. Have a blood glucose level drawn every 6 to 12 months during therapy.
☐ 5. Use an appropriate decongestant if needed.
☐ 6. Report any fainting spells to the HCP.

98. A client diagnosed with primary (essential) hypertension is taking chlorothiazide. The nurse determines teaching about this medication is effective when the client makes which statement? "I will: (Select all that apply.)
☐ 1. take my weight daily at the same time each day."
☐ 2. not drink alcoholic beverages while on this medication."
☐ 3. reduce salt intake in my diet."
☐ 4. reduce my dosage if I have severe dizziness."
☐ 5. use sunscreen if I have prolonged exposure to sunlight."
☐ 6. take the drug late in the evening."

99. Which would **most** likely assist the client with hypertension in maintaining an exercise program?
☐ 1. Give the client a written exercise program.
☐ 2. Explain the exercise program to the client's spouse.
☐ 3. Reassure the client that he or she can do the exercise program.
☐ 4. Tailor a program to the client's needs and abilities.

100. Which would be **most** helpful when coaching a client to stop smoking?
☐ 1. Review the negative effects of smoking on the body.
☐ 2. Discuss the effects of passive smoking on environmental pollution.
☐ 3. Establish the client's daily smoking pattern.
☐ 4. Explain how smoking worsens high blood pressure.

101. When teaching a client about propranolol hydrochloride, the nurse should base the information on the knowledge that propranolol:
☐ 1. blocks beta-adrenergic stimulation and thus causes decreased heart rate, myocardial contractility, and conduction.
☐ 2. increases norepinephrine secretion and thus decreases blood pressure and heart rate.
☐ 3. is a potent arterial and venous vasodilator that reduces peripheral vascular resistance and lowers blood pressure.
☐ 4. is an angiotensin-converting enzyme inhibitor that reduces blood pressure by blocking the conversion of angiotensin I to angiotensin II.

102. What is the **most** important long-term goal for an obese client with hypertension who smokes?
☐ 1. Take medications as prescribed.
☐ 2. Stop smoking.
☐ 3. Make a commitment to long-term lifestyle changes.
☐ 4. Lose weight.

The Client Atrial Fibrillation and Other Dysrhythmias

103. Cardiac telemetry shows that a client who is up to the bathroom has converted from normal sinus rhythm with a rate of 72 beats/min to atrial fibrillation with a ventricular response rate of 100 beats/min. In what order from first to last should the nurse perform these interventions? All options must be used.

1. Assess vital signs.
2. Assist the client to the bed.
3. Initiate intravenous access.
4. Obtain a stat 12-lead electrocardiogram.

104. A client admitted with normal sinus rhythm converts to the following rhythm on the cardiac monitor.

For which symptoms should the nurse assess the client? Select all that apply.
☐ 1. carotid bruit
☐ 2. light-headedness
☐ 3. nausea
☐ 4. palpitations
☐ 5. shortness of breath
☐ 6. systolic murmur

105. A client is admitted to the hospital for evaluation of recurrent episodes of ventricular tachycardia as observed on Holter monitoring. The client is scheduled for electrophysiology studies (EPS) the following morning. Which statement should the nurse include in a teaching plan for this client?

☐ 1. "You will continue to take your medications until the morning of the test."

☐ 2. "You might be sedated during the procedure and will not remember what has happened."

☐ 3. "This test is a noninvasive method of determining the effectiveness of your medication regimen."

☐ 4. "During the procedure, the healthcare provider will insert a special wire to increase the heart rate and produce the irregular beats that caused your signs and symptoms."

106. During physical assessment, the nurse should further assess the client for signs of atrial fibrillation when palpation of the radial pulse reveals:

☐ 1. two regular beats followed by one irregular beat.

☐ 2. an irregular rhythm with pulse rate > 100.

☐ 3. pulse rate below 60 bpm.

☐ 4. a weak, thready pulse.

107. When teaching a client about self-care following placement of a new permanent pacemaker to the left upper chest, the nurse should include which information? Select all that apply.

☐ 1. Take and record daily pulse rate.

☐ 2. Avoid air travel because of airport security alarms.

☐ 3. Immobilize the affected arm for 4 to 6 weeks.

☐ 4. Avoid using a microwave oven.

☐ 5. Avoid lifting anything heavier than 3 lb (1.36 kg).

108. A client has been admitted to the coronary care unit. The nurse observes third-degree heart block at a rate of 35 bpm on the client's cardiac monitor. The client has a blood pressure of 90/60 mm Hg. The nurse should **first**:

☐ 1. prepare for transcutaneous pacing.

☐ 2. prepare to defibrillate the client at 200 J.

☐ 3. administer an IV lidocaine infusion.

☐ 4. schedule the operating room for insertion of a permanent pacemaker.

109. A client has atrial fibrillation and a heart rate of 165 bpm. In which order from first to last should the nurse implement these prescriptions? All options must be used.

1. Administer oxygen via nasal cannula.

2. Gather supplies for an IV insertion.

3. Place client on a cardiac monitor (ECG).

4. Obtain vital signs including BP, P, R, T, and O$_2$ saturation.

110. A client is scheduled for the insertion of an implantable cardioverter-defibrillator (ICD). The spouse expresses anxiety about what would happen if the device discharges during physical contact. What should the nurse tell the spouse?

☐ 1. Physical contact should be avoided whenever possible.

☐ 2. They will not feel the countershock.

☐ 3. The shock would feel like a "tingle," but it would not cause any harm.

☐ 4. A warning device sounds before countershock, so there is time to move away.

111. An older adult is admitted to the telemetry unit for placement of a permanent pacemaker because of sinus bradycardia. What is a **priority** goal for the client within 24 hours after insertion of a permanent pacemaker?

☐ 1. Maintain skin integrity.

☐ 2. Maintain cardiac conduction stability.

☐ 3. Decrease cardiac output.

☐ 4. Increase activity level.

112. The client who had a permanent pacemaker implanted 2 days earlier is being discharged from the hospital. The nurse knows that the client understands the discharge plan when the client:

☐ 1. selects a low-cholesterol diet to control coronary artery disease.

☐ 2. states a need for bed rest for 1 week after discharge.

☐ 3. verbalizes safety precautions needed to prevent pacemaker malfunction.

☐ 4. explains signs and symptoms of myocardial infarction (MI).

113. An 85-year-old client is admitted to the emergency department (ED) at 2000 hours with syncope, shortness of breath, and reported palpitations (see nurse's notes below). At 2015, the nurse places the client on the ECG monitor and identifies the following rhythm (see below). What should the nurse do? Select all that apply.

Nurse's Progress Notes

Admitted to emergency department	2000
Pulse	150
BP	90/62
Oxygen saturation	92% on room air
RR	22
Progress notes	Client has shortness of breath and states, "My heart is jumping out of my chest and hurts some. I am having trouble catching my breath. I don't want to faint again."
	R. Black, RN

☐ 1. Apply oxygen.
☐ 2. Prepare to defibrillate the client.
☐ 3. Monitor vital signs.
☐ 4. Have the client sign consent for cardioversion as prescribed.
☐ 5. Teach the client about warfarin treatment and the need for frequent blood testing.
☐ 6. Draw blood for a CBC count and thyroid function study.

The Client Requiring Rapid Response or Cardiopulmonary Resuscitation

114. Upon assessment of third-degree heart block on the monitor, what should the nurse do **first**?
☐ 1. Call a code.
☐ 2. Begin cardiopulmonary resuscitation.
☐ 3. Place transcutaneous pacing pads on the client.
☐ 4. Prepare for defibrillation.

115. The nurse observes the cardiac rhythm (see below) for a client who is being admitted with a myocardial infarction. What should the nurse do **first**?

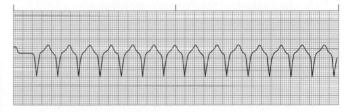

☐ 1. Prepare for immediate cardioversion.
☐ 2. Begin cardiopulmonary resuscitation (CPR).
☐ 3. Check for a pulse.
☐ 4. Prepare for immediate defibrillation.

116. A client who has been given cardiopulmonary resuscitation (CPR) is transported by ambulance to the hospital's emergency department, where the admitting nurse quickly assesses the client's condition. The **most** effective way to evaluate adequate oxygenation is to determine if:
☐ 1. there is a pulse.
☐ 2. pupils are reacting to light.
☐ 3. mucous membranes are pink.
☐ 4. systolic blood pressure is at least 80 mm Hg.

117. A client is given amiodarone in the emergency department for a dysrhythmia. Which finding indicates the drug is having the desired effect?
☐ 1. The ventricular rate is increasing.
☐ 2. The absent pulse is now palpable.
☐ 3. The number of premature ventricular contractions is decreasing.
☐ 4. The fine ventricular fibrillation changes to coarse ventricular fibrillation.

118. During cardiopulmonary resuscitation (CPR) for an adult, the rescuer's hands should be placed two fingers' width above the lower end of the sternum. Which organ would be **most** likely at risk for laceration by forceful compressions over the xiphoid process?
☐ 1. lung
☐ 2. liver
☐ 3. stomach
☐ 4. diaphragm

119. When performing external chest compressions on an adult during cardiopulmonary resuscitation (CPR), the rescuer should depress the sternum:
☐ 1. 0.5 inch (1 cm).
☐ 2. 1 inch (2.5 cm).
☐ 3. 1.5 inches (4 cm).
☐ 4. 2 inches (5 cm).

120. If a client is receiving rescue breaths, and the chest wall fails to rise during cardiopulmonary resuscitation, the rescuer should **first**:
☐ 1. try using a bag mask device.
☐ 2. decrease the rate of compressions.
☐ 3. intubate the client.
☐ 4. reposition the airway.

121. During rescue breathing in cardiopulmonary resuscitation (CPR), the victim will exhale by:
☐ 1. normal relaxation of the chest.
☐ 2. gentle pressure of the rescuer's hand on the upper chest.
☐ 3. the pressure of cardiac compressions.
☐ 4. turning the head to the side.

122. The rapid response team has been called to manage an unwitnessed cardiac arrest in a client's hospital room. The estimated maximum time a person can be without cardiopulmonary function and still not experience permanent brain damage is:
☐ 1. 1 to 2 minutes.
☐ 2. 4 to 6 minutes.
☐ 3. 8 to 10 minutes.
☐ 4. 12 to 15 minutes.

123. A nurse is helping a suspected choking victim. The nurse should perform the Heimlich maneuver when the victim:
☐ 1. starts to become cyanotic.
☐ 2. cannot speak due to airway obstruction.
☐ 3. can make only minimal vocal noises.
☐ 4. is coughing vigorously.

124. When performing the Heimlich maneuver on a conscious adult victim, the rescuer delivers inward and upward thrusts specifically:
☐ 1. above the umbilicus.
☐ 2. at the level of the xiphoid process.
☐ 3. over the victim's midabdominal area.
☐ 4. below the xiphoid process and above the umbilicus.

125. The monitor technician informs the nurse that the client has started having premature ventricular contractions every other beat. What should the nurse do **first**?
☐ 1. Activate the rapid response team.
☐ 2. Assess the client's orientation and vital signs.
☐ 3. Call the healthcare provider (HCP).
☐ 4. Administer a bolus of lidocaine.

126. A client returns to the nursing unit following successful synchronized cardioversion using transthoracic chest wall patches. The nurse should assess which when the client returns to the room? Select all that apply.
☐ 1. vital signs
☐ 2. skin of chest wall
☐ 3. arterial puncture site
☐ 4. level of consciousness
☐ 5. cardiac rhythm

127. The nurse is preparing to defibrillate a client on a cardiac monitor who is in ventricular fibrillation (see photo). What should the nurse do?

☐ 1. Move the paddle in the nurse's left hand to the midline.
☐ 2. Move the paddle in the nurse's right hand to above the client's nipple.
☐ 3. Grasp the handles of the paddles to allow visibility of the black markings on the paddle.
☐ 4. After pressing the charge button and "calling all clear," push the shock button.

128. The nurse is caring for a client who has become unresponsive, the blood pressure is 80/40 mm Hg, and SpO$_2$ is 90% on 50% face mask. The nurse should:
☐ 1. begin chest compressions.
☐ 2. call the rapid response team.
☐ 3. remove the family from the room.
☐ 4. ventilate the client with a bag mask device.

Managing Care, Quality, and Safety for Clients with Cardiac Health Problems

129. A nurse working the day shift on a cardiac unit receives the following shift report:

1. Client 1: Admitted yesterday morning with hypokalemia. Awaiting repeat electrolyte lab results drawn at 06:00.

2. Client 2: Experienced chest pain at 06:30. Pain resolved after 2 sublingual nitroglycerin tablets.

3. Client 3: Scheduled for oral antihypertensive medications at 0900. Incontinent of urine during the night.

4. Client 4: Scheduled for coronary artery bypass surgery at 0800. The client's family is in the client's room.

At the conclusion of shift report, it is 0730. Put the clients in the order from first to last in which the nurse should plan to assess them. All options must be used.

130. Which activity would be appropriate to delegate to unlicensed assistive personnel (UAP) for a client diagnosed with a myocardial infarction who is stable?
☐ **1.** Evaluate the lung sounds.
☐ **2.** Help the client identify risk factors for CAD.
☐ **3.** Provide teaching on a 2-g sodium diet.
☐ **4.** Record the intake and output.

131. The unlicensed assistive personnel (UAP) reports to the nurse that a client is "feeling short of breath." The client's blood pressure was 124/78 mm Hg 2 hours ago with a heart rate of 82 bpm; the unlicensed assistive personnel reports that blood pressure is now 84/44 mm Hg with a heart rate of 54 bpm, and the client stated, "I just do not feel good." What actions should the nurse take? Select all that apply.
☐ **1.** Confirm the client's vital signs, and complete a quick assessment.
☐ **2.** Inform the charge nurse of the change in condition, and initiate the hospital's rapid/emergency response team.
☐ **3.** Make a quick check on other assigned clients before spending the amount of time required to take care of this client.
☐ **4.** Position the client in semi-Fowler's position.
☐ **5.** Stay with the client, and reassure the client.
☐ **6.** Call the healthcare provider (HCP), and report the situation using SBAR format.

132. The nurse is assessing a client with heart failure whose blood pressure and weight are being monitored remotely. The nurse reviews data obtained within the last 3 days.

	April 3	April 4	April 5
Weight	160 (72 kg)	162 (73 kg)	165 (74 kg)
Blood Pressure	120/80	130/88	140/90

The nurse calls the client to follow up. The nurse should **first** ask the client:
☐ **1.** "How are you feeling today?"
☐ **2.** "Are you having shortness of breath?"
☐ **3.** "Did you calibrate the scales before using them?"
☐ **4.** "How much fluid did you drink during the last 24 hours?"

133. The nurse is tracking data on a group of clients with heart failure who have been discharged from the hospital and are being followed at a clinic. Which data are the **best** indicators that nursing interventions of monitoring and teaching have been effective?
☐ **1.** Ninety percent of clients have not gained weight.
☐ **2.** Seventy-five percent of the clients viewed the educational DVD.
☐ **3.** Eighty percent of the clients reported that they are taking their medications.
☐ **4.** Five percent of the clients required hospitalization in the last 90 days.

134. The nurse in the intensive care unit is giving a report to the nurse in a cardiac step-down unit about a client who had coronary artery bypass surgery. Which is the **most** effective way to assure essential information about the client is reported?

☐ 1. Give the report face-to-face with both nurses in a quiet room.

☐ 2. Audiotape the report for future reference and documentation.

☐ 3. Use a printed checklist with information individualized for the client.

☐ 4. Document essential transfer information in the client's medical record.

135. The nurse is planning care for a group of elderly clients who are affected by orthostatic hypotension. What should the nurse do? Select all that apply.

☐ 1. Assist the clients to stand to help prevent falls.

☐ 2. Teach clients how to gradually change their position.

☐ 3. Request a prescription for antihypertensive medications for clients at high risk.

☐ 4. Conduct "fall risk" assessments.

☐ 5. Consider the use of sequential compression devices (SCDs) for high-risk clients.

☐ 6. Place clients on bed rest.

136. The nurse is caring for a group of clients on a medical-surgical nursing unit. Which task(s) could the nurse delegate to unlicensed assistive personnel (UAP)? Select all that apply.

☐ 1. Assess pedal pulses on a client who just returned from a cardiac angiogram.

☐ 2. Administer oxygen via nasal cannula to a client with a saturation of 89%.

☐ 3. Administer acetaminophen to a client with a pain level of "5" out of "10."

☐ 4. Perform vital signs and oxygen saturation on a client returning from the catheterization lab.

☐ 5. Obtain intake and outputs on a client experiencing heart failure.

Answers, Rationales, and Test-Taking Strategies

*The answers and the rationales for each question follow below, along with keys (🗝) to the client need (CN) and cognitive level (CL) for each question. In addition, you will also see a glossary icon (📖) highlighting specific terminology used on the licensing exam. As you check your answers, use the **Content Mastery and Test-Taking Skill Self-Analysis** worksheet (tear-out worksheet in back of book) to identify the reason(s) for not answering the questions correctly. For additional information about test-taking skills and strategies for answering questions, refer to pages 12–23 and pages 35–36 in Part 1 of this book.*

The Client with Acute Coronary Syndromes

1. 2. To best monitor that the client's circulation remains intact, the dorsal surface of the right foot should be palpated. When the left side of the heart is catheterized, the cannula enters via an artery. In this instance, the right femoral artery was accessed. While all options assess arterial points of the right leg, the dorsal surface of the right foot (the pedal pulse) is the most distal. If this pulse point is present and unchanged from before the procedure, the other pulse points should also be intact.

🗝 CN: Physiological adaptation; CL: Apply

2. 4. The elevated troponin level should be reported to the **HCP** 📖 prior to the stress test as this change indicates myocardial damage. Sending the client to walk on a treadmill for stress testing would be contraindicated with evidence of recent myocardial injury and could further extend the damage. The other blood levels are helpful but not critical to this client's welfare at this point in time.

🗝 CN: Reduction of risk potential; CL: Analyze

3. 4. Nursing management for a client with a myocardial infarction should focus on pain management and decreasing myocardial oxygen demand. Fluid status should be closely monitored. Client education should begin once the client is stable and amenable to teaching. Visitation should be based on client comfort and maintaining a calm environment.

🗝 CN: Physiological adaptation; CL: Synthesize

4. 2. Nitroglycerin is a vasodilator that will lower blood pressure. The client is having chest pain, and the ST elevation indicates injury to the myocardium, which may benefit from nitroglycerin. The potassium and heart rate are within normal range.

🗝 CN: Pharmacological and parenteral therapies; CL: Analyze

5. 1. The nurse should first obtain vital signs as changes in the vital signs will reflect the severity of the sudden drop in cardiac output: decrease in blood pressure, increase in heart rate, and increase in respirations. Infarction of the papillary muscles is a potential complication of an MI causing ineffective closure of the mitral valve during systole. Mitral regurgitation results when the left ventricle contracts and blood flows backward into the left atrium, which is heard at the fifth intercostal space, left midclavicular line. The murmur worsens during expiration and in the supine or left-side position and can best be heard when the client is in these positions, not with the client leaning forward. A 12-lead ECG views the electrical activity of the heart; an echocardiogram views valve function.

CN: Physiological adaptation; **CL:** Synthesize

6. 1,4,5. Morphine sulfate acts as an analgesic and sedative. It also reduces myocardial oxygen consumption, blood pressure, and heart rate. Morphine also reduces anxiety and fear due to its sedative effects and by slowing the heart rate. It can depress respirations; however, such an effect may lead to hypoxia, which should be avoided in the treatment of chest pain. Angiotensin-converting enzyme inhibitor drugs, not morphine, may help to prevent ventricular remodeling.

CN: Pharmacological and parenteral therapies; **CL:** Evaluate

7. 24 mL/h

First, calculate how many units are in each milliliter of the medication:

$$\frac{25,000 \text{ units}}{500 \text{ mL}} = \frac{50 \text{ units}}{1 \text{ mL}}$$

Next, calculate how many milliliters the client receives per hour:

$$\frac{1,200 \text{ units}}{1 \text{ hour}} \div \frac{50 \text{ units}}{1 \text{ mL}}$$

$$= \frac{\overset{24}{\cancel{1,200}} \text{ units}}{1 \text{ hour}} \times \frac{1 \text{ mL}}{\underset{1}{\cancel{50}} \text{ units}} = 24 \text{ mL/h}$$

CN: Pharmacological and parenteral therapies; **CL:** Apply

8. 1. The client is having symptoms of a myocardial infarction. The first action is to prevent platelet formation and block prostaglandin synthesis. The client should place the tablet under the tongue and wait until it is absorbed. Nitroglycerin tablets are not effective if chewed, swallowed, or placed between the cheek and gums.

CN: Physiological adaptation; **CL:** Apply

9. 2. A low urine output and confusion are signs of decreased tissue perfusion. Orthopnea is a sign of left-sided heart failure. Crackles, edema, and weight gain should be monitored closely, but the levels are not as high a priority. With atrial fibrillation, there is a loss of atrial kick, but the blood pressure and heart rate are stable.

CN: Physiological adaptation; **CL:** Analyze

10. 4. The nurse should first assess the client's tolerance to the drop in heart rate by checking the blood pressure and level of consciousness and determine if atropine is needed. If the client is symptomatic, atropine and transcutaneous pacing are interventions for symptomatic bradycardia. Once the client is stable, further physical assessments can be done.

CN: Physiological adaptation; **CL:** Synthesize

11. 1,2,3,4. When preparing the client for a cardiac angiogram, the nurse should determine if the client has an allergy to the liquid contrast medium used in the procedure. Contrast dyes contain iodine, and the administration of a dye could lead to an anaphylactic response in clients who are allergic to the dye. An intravenous infusion will be started before the procedure to administer the contrast dye. The client should not eat or drink for 8 hours prior to the procedure. The client may experience a flushing sensation, but this is a normal response and does not indicate a life-threatening reaction. The client may receive light sedation, but not an anesthetic as the client must be awake to follow instructions. The client should be instructed to remain still during the procedure.

CN: Reduction of risk potential; **CL:** Apply

12. 1. An S_3 heart sound occurs early in diastole as the mitral and tricuspid valves open and blood rushes into the ventricles. To distinguish an S_3 from a physiologic S_2 split, a split S_2 occurs during inspiration and S_3 remains constant during the respiratory cycle. Its pitch is softer and best heard with the bell at the apex, and it is one of the first clinical findings in left ventricular failure. An S_4 is heard in late diastole when atrial contraction pumps volume into a stiff, noncompliant ventricle. An S_4 is not heard in a client with atrial fibrillation because there is no atrial contraction. Murmurs are sounds created by turbulent blood flow through an incompetent or stenotic valve.

CN: Physiological adaptation; **CL:** Analyze

13. 1. Although obtaining the ECG, chest radiograph, and blood work are all important, the nurse's priority action should be to relieve the crushing chest pain. Therefore, administering morphine sulfate is the priority action.

CN: Physiological adaptation; **CL:** Synthesize

14. 2. All of the 1200 hour assessments are signs of decreased cardiac output and can be an ominous sign in a client who has recently experienced an MI; the nurse should notify the **HCP** 📖 of these changes. Cardiac output and blood pressure may continue to fall to dangerous levels, which can induce further coronary ischemia and extension of the infarct. While the client is currently hypotensive, giving a fluid challenge/bolus can precipitate increased workload on a damaged heart and extend the myocardial infarction. Exercise or walking for this client will increase both the heart rate and stroke volume, both of which will increase cardiac output, but the increased cardiac output will increase oxygen needs especially in the heart muscle and can induce further coronary ischemia and extension of the infarct. The client is hypotensive. Although the client has decreased urinary output, this is the body's response to a decreasing cardiac output, and it is not appropriate to administer furosemide.

🔑 CN: Physiological adaptation;
CL: Synthesize

15. 2. Thrombolytic drugs are administered within the first 6 hours after onset of an MI to lyse clots and reduce the extent of myocardial damage.

🔑 CN: Pharmacological and parenteral therapies; CL: Evaluate

16. 3. The client is experiencing a single PVC. PVCs are characterized by a QRS of longer than 0.12 second and by a wide, notched, or slurred QRS complex. There is no P wave related to the QRS complex, and the T wave is usually inverted. PVCs are potentially serious and can lead to ventricular fibrillation or cardiac arrest when they occur more than 6 to 10 in an hour in clients with myocardial infarction. The nurse should continue to monitor the client and note if the PVCs are increasing. It is not necessary to notify the **HCP** 📖 or call the **rapid response team** 📖 at this point. Lidocaine is not indicated from the data on this ECG.

🔑 CN: Reduction of risk potential;
CL: Synthesize

17. 1. The nurse should first don gloves and apply direct pressure over the site to stop blood loss from the femoral artery. While the nurse will later observe the site for further bleeding and record the extent of bleeding, this is not the first action that is needed. If the bleeding cannot be controlled, the healthcare provider who performed the procedure should be contacted, but first, an attempt to manually stop the bleeding with direct pressure is warranted. Protamine sulfate is the antidote for heparin sodium, but this is not an initial action to control the bleeding.

🔑 CN: Reduction of risk potential.
CL: Synthesize

18. 2. Metoprolol is indicated in the treatment of hemodynamically stable clients with an acute MI to reduce cardiovascular mortality. Cardiogenic shock causes severe hemodynamic instability, and a beta-blocker will further depress myocardial contractility. The metoprolol should be discontinued. The decrease in cardiac output will impair perfusion to the kidneys. Cardiac output, hemodynamic measurements, and appropriate interventions can be determined with a PA catheter. Dobutamine will improve contractility and increase the cardiac output that is depressed in cardiogenic shock.

🔑 CN: Physiological adaptation;
CL: Synthesize

19. 1. Oliguria occurs during cardiogenic shock because there is reduced blood flow to the kidneys. Typical signs of cardiogenic shock include low blood pressure, rapid and weak pulse, decreased urine output, and signs of diminished blood flow to the brain, such as confusion and restlessness. Cardiogenic shock is a serious complication of MI, with a mortality rate approaching 90%. Fever is not a typical sign of cardiogenic shock. The other changes in vital signs on the client's chart are not as significant as the decreased urinary output.

🔑 CN: Reduction of risk potential;
CL: Analyze

20. 1. IV nitroglycerin infusion requires an infusion pump for precise control of the medication. Blood pressure monitoring would be done with a continuous system and more frequently than every 4 hours. Hourly urine outputs are not always required. Obtaining serum potassium levels is not associated with nitroglycerin infusion.

🔑 CN: Pharmacological and parenteral therapies; CL: Synthesize

21. 3,4,2,1. The nurse should first connect the client to the monitor by attaching the electrodes. Electrocardiography can be used to identify myocardial ischemia and infarction, rhythm and conduction disturbances, chamber enlargement, electrolyte imbalances, and the effects of drugs on the client's heart. The nurse next obtains vital signs to establish a baseline. Next, the nurse should administer the morphine; morphine is the drug of choice in relieving myocardial infarction (MI) pain; it may cause a transient decrease in blood pressure. When the client is stable, the nurse can obtain a history of the client's drug use.

🔑 CN: Reduction of risk potential;
CL: Synthesize

22. 2,5. It is important for clients to wear hearing aids to this procedure so that they can hear the questions posed to them by the healthcare team. Chest pain often occurs when the balloon within the stent is inflated and deployed into the coronary artery. It is expected and brief but should still be reported by the client. During the procedure and for a prescribed amount of time after the procedure, the client will need to remain flat in bed with the right leg straight, not flexed, to prevent bleeding from the access site. The site is not routinely stitched. It is a puncture rather than an incision requiring sutures. The client may be given intravenous medication to help with comfort, but the client is kept awake to answer questions and to hear instructions and explanations. General anesthesia is not given.

> 🔑 CN: Reduction of risk potential; CL: Create

23. 4. Sinus tachycardia is characterized by normal conduction and a regular rhythm, but with a rate exceeding 100 bpm. A P wave precedes each QRS, and the QRS is usually normal.

> 🔑 CN: Reduction of risk potential; CL: Analyze

24. 2. PVCs are often a precursor of life-threatening arrhythmias, including ventricular tachycardia and ventricular fibrillation. An occasional PVC is not considered dangerous, but if PVCs occur at a rate greater than five or six per minute in the post-MI client, the **HCP** 📖 should be notified immediately. More than six PVCs per minute is considered serious and usually calls for decreasing ventricular irritability by administering medications such as lidocaine hydrochloride. Increasing the IV infusion rate would not decrease the number of PVCs. Increasing the oxygen concentration should not be the nurse's first course of action; rather, the nurse should notify the HCP promptly. Administering a prescribed analgesic would not decrease ventricular irritability.

> 🔑 CN: Physiological adaptation; CL: Synthesize

25. 4. By day 2 of hospitalization after an MI, clients are expected to be able to perform personal care without chest pain. Severe chest pain should not be present on day 2 after an MI. Day 2 of hospitalization may be too soon for clients to be able to identify risk factors for MI or to begin a walking program; however, the client may be sitting up in a chair as part of the cardiac rehabilitation program.

> 🔑 CN: Physiological adaptation; CL: Evaluate

26. 2. Furosemide is a loop diuretic that acts to increase urine output. Furosemide does not increase blood pressure, decrease pain, or decrease arrhythmias.

> 🔑 CN: Pharmacological and parenteral therapies; CL: Evaluate

27.

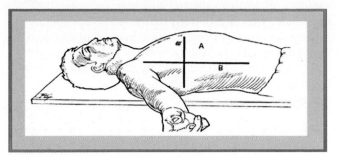

Correct location: The zero point on the CVP transducer needs to be at the level of the right atrium. The right atrium is located at the midaxillary line at the fourth intercostal space. The phlebostatic axis is determined by drawing an imaginary vertical line from the fourth intercostal space at the sternal border to the right side of the chest (A). A secondary imaginary line is drawn horizontally at the level of the midpoint between the anterior and posterior surfaces of the chest (B). The phlebostatic axis is located at the intersection of points A and B.

> 🔑 CN: Physiologic adaptation; CL: Apply

28. 3. When wedged, the catheter is "pointing" indirectly at the left end-diastolic pressure. The pulmonary artery wedge pressure is measured when the tip of the catheter is slowly inflated and allowed to wedge into a branch of the pulmonary artery. Once the balloon is wedged, the catheter reads the pressure in front of the balloon. During diastole, the mitral valve is open, reflecting left ventricular end-diastolic pressure. Cardiac output is the amount of blood ejected by the heart in 1 minute and is determined through thermodilution and not wedge pressure. Cardiac index is calculated by dividing the client's cardiac output by the client's body surface area and is considered a more accurate reflection of the individual client's cardiac output. Right atrial blood pressure is not measured with the pulmonary artery catheter.

> 🔑 CN: Physiologic adaptation; CL: Apply

29. 3. Encouraging the client to move the legs while in bed is a preventive strategy taught to all clients who are hospitalized and on bed rest to promote venous return. The muscular action aids in venous return and prevents venous stasis in the lower extremities. These exercises are not intended to prepare the client for ambulation. These exercises are not associated with promoting urinary and intestinal elimination. These exercises are not performed to decrease the risk of pressure ulcer formation.

> 🔑 CN: Physiological adaptation; CL: Apply

30. 2. Recommended dietary principles in the acute phase of MI include avoiding large meals because small, easily digested foods are better tolerated. Fluids are given according to the client's needs, and sodium restrictions may be prescribed, especially for clients with manifestations of heart failure. Cholesterol restrictions may be prescribed as well. Clients are not prescribed diets of liquids only or restricted to nothing by mouth unless their condition is very unstable.

   CN: Physiological adaptation; CL: Apply

31. 1,3,4. Clopidogrel is generally well absorbed and may be taken with or without food; it should be taken at the same time every day, and, while food may help prevent potential GI upset, food has no effect on absorption of the drug. Bleeding is the most common adverse effect of clopidogrel; the client must understand the importance of reporting any unexpected, prolonged, or excessive bleeding including blood in urine or stool. Increased bruising and bleeding gums are possible side effects of clopidogrel; the client should be aware of this possibility. Plavix is an antiplatelet agent used to prevent clot formation in clients that have experienced or are at risk for myocardial infarction, ischemic stroke, peripheral artery disease, or acute coronary syndrome. It is not necessary to drink a glass of water after taking clopidogrel.

   CN: Pharmacological and parenteral therapies; CL: Create

32. 4. The woman who is 65 years old, is overweight, and has an elevated LDL is at greatest risk. Total cholesterol >200 (11.1 mmol/L), LDL >100 (5.5 mmol/L), HDL <40 (2.2 mmol/L) in men, HDL <50 (2.8 mmol/L) in women, men 45 years and older, women 55 years and older, smoking, and obesity increase the risk of CAD. Atorvastatin reduces LDL and decreases risk of CAD. The combination of postmenopausal, obesity, and high LDL places this client at greatest risk.

   CN: Health promotion and maintenance; CL: Analyze

33. 1. Nitroglycerin acts to decrease myocardial oxygen consumption. Vasodilation makes it easier for the heart to eject blood, resulting in decreased oxygen needs. Decreased oxygen demand reduces pain caused by heart muscle not receiving sufficient oxygen. While blood pressure may decrease ever so slightly due to the vasodilation effects of nitroglycerin, it is only secondary and not related to the angina the client is experiencing. Increased blood pressure would mean the heart would work harder, increasing oxygen demand and thus angina. Decreased heart rate is not an effect of nitroglycerin.

   CN: Pharmacological and parenteral therapy; CL: Evaluate

34. 3. In health coaching, unlike traditional client education techniques in which the nurse provides information, the goal of coaching is to encourage the client to explore the reasons for the behavior and establish a vision for health behavior and the way he or she can make changes to improve their health behavior and reduce or eliminate health risks. When coaching a client, the nurse does not provide information, withhold praise, or instill fear.

   CN: Psychosocial integrity; CL: Synthesize

35. 4. The thrombolytic agent t-PA, administered intravenously, lyses the clot blocking the coronary artery. The drug is most effective when administered within the first 6 hours after onset of MI. The drug does not reduce coronary artery vasospasm; nitrates are used to promote vasodilation. Arrhythmias are managed by antiarrhythmic drugs. Surgical approaches are used to open the coronary artery and re-establish a blood supply to the area.

   CN: Pharmacological and parenteral therapies; CL: Apply

36. 1. Cardiac arrhythmias are commonly observed with administration of t-PA. Cardiac arrhythmias are associated with reperfusion of the cardiac tissue. Hypotension is commonly observed with administration of t-PA. Seizures and hypothermia are not generally associated with reperfusion of the cardiac tissue.

   CN: Reduction of risk potential; CL: Synthesize

37. 2. A history of cerebral hemorrhage is a contraindication to administration of t-PA because the risk of hemorrhage may be further increased. Age > 60 years, history of heart failure, and cigarette smoking are not contraindications.

   CN: Pharmacological and parenteral therapies; CL: Apply

38. 2. Advanced cardiac life support recommends that at least one or two IV lines be inserted in one or both of the antecubital spaces. Calling the **HCP** 📖, obtaining a portable chest radiograph, and drawing blood for the laboratory are important but secondary to starting the IV line.

   CN: Physiological adaptation; CL: Synthesize

39. 1. Further assessment is needed in this situation. It is premature to initiate other actions until further data have been gathered. Inquiring about the onset, duration, location, severity, and precipitating factors of the chest heaviness will provide pertinent information to convey to the **HCP** 📖.

   CN: Reduction of risk potential; CL: Synthesize

40. 3. Nitroglycerin may be used prophylactically before stressful physical activities such as stair climbing to help the client remain pain free. Climbing the stairs early in the day would have no impact on decreasing pain episodes. Resting before or after an activity is not as likely to help prevent an activity-related pain episode.

CN: Reduction of risk potential; CL: Synthesize

41. 3. Pasta, tomato sauce, salad, and coffee would be the best selection for the client following a low-cholesterol diet. Hamburgers, milk shakes, liver, and fried foods tend to be high in cholesterol.

CN: Basic care and comfort; CL: Apply

42. 1. The client should report a change in the pattern of chest pain. It may indicate increasing severity of coronary artery disease. Pain occurring during stress or sexual activity would not be unexpected, and the client may be instructed to take nitroglycerin to prevent this pain. Pain during or after an activity such as lawn mowing also would not be unexpected; the client may be instructed to take nitroglycerin to prevent this pain or may be restricted from doing such activities.

CN: Reduction of risk potential; CL: Apply

43. 2. Cardiac catheterization is done in clients with angina primarily to assess the extent and the severity of the coronary artery blockage. A decision about medical management, angioplasty, or coronary artery bypass surgery will be based on the catheterization results. Coronary bypass surgery would be used to bypass obstructed vessels. Although cardiac catheterization can be used to assess the functional adequacy of the valves and heart muscle, in this case the client has unstable angina and therefore would need the procedure to assess the extent of arterial blockage.

CN: Reduction of risk potential; CL: Apply

44. 1,2,4,3. When a client returns from having a transluminal balloon angioplasty with femoral access, the nurse should first obtain baseline vital signs and oxygen saturation to determine evidence of bleeding or decreased tissue perfusion. The nurse should next assess the pedal pulses to determine if the client has adequate peripheral tissue perfusion. Next the nurse should inspect the catheterization site and then determine color and sensation in the affected leg.

CN: Physiologic integrity; CL: Analyze

45. 2. Late onset of puberty is not generally considered to be a risk factor for the development of atherosclerosis. Risk factors for atherosclerosis include family history of atherosclerosis, cigarette smoking, hypertension, high blood cholesterol level, male gender, diabetes mellitus, obesity, and physical inactivity.

CN: Physiological adaptation; CL: Apply

46. 3. Nitroglycerin produces peripheral vasodilation, which reduces myocardial oxygen consumption and demand. Vasodilation in coronary arteries and collateral vessels may also increase blood flow to the ischemic areas of the heart. Nitroglycerin decreases myocardial oxygen demand. Nitroglycerin does not have an effect on pericardial spasticity or conductivity in the myocardium.

CN: Pharmacological and parenteral therapies; CL: Apply

47. 1. Headache is a common side effect of nitroglycerin that can be alleviated with aspirin, acetaminophen, or ibuprofen. The sublingual nitroglycerin needs to be absorbed in the mouth, which will be disrupted with drinking. Lying flat will increase blood flow to the head and may increase pain and exacerbate other symptoms, such as shortness of breath.

CN: Physiological adaptation; CL: Synthesize

48. 4. The nurse should instruct the client that correct protocol for using sublingual nitroglycerin involves immediate administration when chest pain occurs. Sublingual nitroglycerin appears in the bloodstream within 2 to 3 minutes and is metabolized within about 10 minutes. The client should sit down and place the tablet under the tongue. If the chest pain is not relieved within 5 minutes, the client should call 911. Although some **healthcare providers (HCPs)** may recommend taking a second or third tablet spaced 5 minutes apart and then calling for emergency assistance, it is not appropriate to take two tablets at once. Nitroglycerin acts within 2 to 3 minutes, and the client should not wait 15 minutes to take further action. The client should call 911 to obtain emergency help rather than calling the HCP.

CN: Pharmacological and parenteral therapies; CL: Synthesize

49. 3. The client taking nifedipine should inspect the gums daily to monitor for gingival hyperplasia. This is an uncommon adverse effect but one that requires monitoring and intervention if it occurs. The client taking nifedipine might be taught to monitor blood pressure, but more often than monthly. These clients would not generally need to perform daily weights or limit intake of green leafy vegetables.

CN: Pharmacological and parenteral therapies; CL: Synthesize

50. 2,5,6. Simvastatin is used in combination with diet and exercise to decrease elevated total cholesterol. The client should take simvastatin in the evening, and the nurse should instruct the client that if a dose is missed, to take it as soon as remembered, but not to take at the same time as the next scheduled dose. It is not necessary to take the pill with food. The client does not need to limit greens (limiting greens is appropriate for clients taking warfarin), but the nurse should instruct the client to avoid grapefruit and grapefruit juice, which can increase the amount of the drug in the bloodstream. A serious side effect is myopathy, and the client should report muscle pain or tenderness to the **healthcare provider (HCP)** 📖.

🗝 CN: Pharmacology; CL: Create

The Client with Heart Failure

51. 3. The nurse should withhold the dose of captopril; captopril is an ACE inhibitor, and a side effect of the medication is hyperkalemia. The BUN and creatinine, which are normal, should be viewed prior to administration since renal insufficiency is another potential side effect of an ACE-I. The heart rate is within normal limits. The nurse should question the dose of metoprolol if the client's heart rate is bradycardic. The hemoglobin and hematocrit are normal for a female. The nurse should report the high potassium level and that the captopril was withheld.

🗝 CN: Pharmacological and parenteral therapies; CL: Synthesize

52. 3. Warfarin is an anticoagulant, which is used in the treatment of atrial fibrillation and decreased left ventricular ejection fraction (<20%) to prevent thrombus formation and release of emboli into the circulation. The client may also take other medication as needed to manage the heart failure. Warfarin does not reduce circulatory load or improve myocardial workload. Warfarin does not affect cardiac rhythm.

🗝 CN: Reduction of risk potential; CL: Evaluate

53. 2. Early symptoms of digoxin toxicity include anorexia, nausea, and vomiting. Visual disturbances can also occur, including double or blurred vision and visual halos. Hypokalemia is a common cause of digoxin toxicity associated with arrhythmias because low serum potassium can enhance ectopic pacemaker activity. Although vomiting can lead to fluid deficit, given the client's history, the vomiting is likely due to the adverse effects of digoxin toxicity. Pulmonary edema is manifested by dyspnea and coughing.

🗝 CN: Pharmacological and parenteral therapies; CL: Analyze

54. 1,3,5,6. Dyspnea, crackles, oliguria, and decreased oxygen saturation are signs and symptoms related to pulmonary congestion and inadequate tissue perfusion associated with left-sided heart failure. JVD and right upper quadrant pain along with ascites and edema are usually associated with congestion of the peripheral tissues and viscera in right-sided heart failure.

🗝 CN: Physiological adaptation; CL: Apply

55. 4,5. Signs of pulmonary edema are identical to those of acute heart failure. Signs and symptoms are generally apparent in the respiratory system and include coarse crackles, severe dyspnea, and tachypnea. Severe tachycardia occurs due to sympathetic stimulation in the presence of hypoxemia. Blood pressure may be decreased or elevated, depending on the severity of the edema. Jugular vein distention, dependent edema, and anorexia are symptoms of right-sided heart failure.

🗝 CN: Physiological adaptation; CL: Analyze

56. 1. It is a priority to assess blood pressure first because people with pulmonary edema typically experience severe hypertension that requires early intervention. The client probably does not have skin breakdown, but when the client is stable and when the nurse obtains a complete health history, the nurse should inspect the client's skin for any signs of breakdown; however, when the client is stable, the nurse should inspect the skin. Potassium levels are not the first priority. The nurse should monitor urine output after the client is stable.

🗝 CN: Reduction of risk potential; CL: Analyze

57. 1,4,6. It is not unusual for the elderly client to become somewhat confused when "relocated" to the hospital, and this may be more difficult for those with known dementia. Frequent reorientation delivered patiently and calmly along with placing familiar items nearby so the client can see them may help decrease confusion related to hospitalization. Establishing a trusting relationship is important with every client but may be more so with this client. Putting the client in a room further from the nursing station may decrease extra noise for the client but will also make it more difficult to observe the client and maintain a safe environment. Procedures should be explained to the client prior to proceeding and should not be rushed. Visits by family and friends may help to keep the client oriented.

🗝 CN: Basic care and comfort; CL: Synthesize

58. 1,2,3,5. Heart failure can be a result of several cardiovascular conditions, which will affect the heart's ability to pump effectively. The body attempts to compensate through several neurohormonal mechanisms. Decreased cardiac output stimulates the aortic and carotid baroreceptors, which activates the sympathetic nervous system to release norepinephrine and epinephrine. This early response increases the heart rate and contractility. It also has some negative effects, including vasoconstriction of the skin, GI tract, and kidneys. Decreased renal perfusion (due to low CO and vasoconstriction) activates the renin-angiotensin-aldosterone process resulting in the release of antidiuretic hormone. This causes fluid retention in an attempt to increase blood pressure and, therefore, cardiac output. In the damaged heart, this causes fluid overload. There is no parasympathetic response. Decreased pulmonary perfusion can be a result of fluid overload or concomitant pulmonary disease.

CN: Physiologic adaptation; CL: Analyze

59. 4 mL. Desired amount (D) divided by what is available (H) times quantity (Q) = amount to administer. D = 40 mg divided by H = 10 mg/mL equals 40 divided by 10 = 4 mL.

CN: Pharmacological and parenteral therapies; CL: Apply

60. 3. Sitting almost upright in bed with the feet and legs resting on the mattress decreases venous return to the heart, thus reducing myocardial workload. Also, the sitting position allows maximum space for lung expansion. Low Fowler's position would be used if the client could not tolerate high Fowler's position for some reason. Lying on the right side would not be a good position for the client in heart failure. The client in heart failure would not tolerate Trendelenburg's position.

CN: Reduction of risk potential; CL: Synthesize

61. 1. Increasing cardiac output is the main goal of therapy for the client with heart failure or pulmonary edema. Pulmonary edema is an acute medical emergency requiring immediate intervention. Respiratory status and comfort will be improved when cardiac output increases to an acceptable level. Peripheral edema is not typically associated with pulmonary edema.

CN: Reduction of risk potential; CL: Apply

62. 2. Digoxin is a cardiac glycoside with positive inotropic activity. This inotropic activity causes increased strength of myocardial contractions and thereby increases output of blood from the left ventricle. Digoxin does not dilate coronary arteries. Although digoxin can be used to treat arrhythmias and does decrease the electrical conductivity of the myocardium, these are not primary reasons for its use in clients with heart failure and pulmonary edema.

CN: Pharmacological and parenteral therapies; CL: Evaluate

63. 1. After intravenous injection of furosemide, diuresis normally begins in about 5 minutes and reaches its peak within about 30 minutes. Medication effects last 2 to 4 hours. When furosemide is given intramuscularly or orally, drug action begins more slowly and lasts longer than when it is given intravenously.

CN: Pharmacological and parenteral therapies; CL: Evaluate

64. 4. When diuretics are given early in the day, the client will void frequently during the daytime hours and will not need to void frequently during the night. Therefore, the client's sleep will not be disturbed. Taking furosemide in the morning has no effect on preventing electrolyte imbalances or retarding rapid drug absorption. The client should not accumulate excessive fluids throughout the night.

CN: Pharmacological and parenteral therapies; CL: Apply

65. 3. Colored vision and seeing yellow spots are symptoms of digoxin toxicity. Abdominal pain, anorexia, nausea, and vomiting are other common symptoms of digoxin toxicity. Additional signs of toxicity include arrhythmias, such as atrial fibrillation or bradycardia. Rash, increased appetite, and elevated blood pressure are not associated with digoxin toxicity.

CN: Pharmacological and parenteral therapies; CL: Apply

66. 4. A low serum potassium level (hypokalemia) predisposes the client to digoxin toxicity. Because potassium inhibits cardiac excitability, a low serum potassium level would mean that the client would be prone to increased cardiac excitability. Sodium, glucose, and calcium levels do not affect digoxin or contribute to digoxin toxicity.

CN: Pharmacological and parenteral therapies; CL: Analyze

67. 2. Canned foods and juices such as tomato juice are typically high in sodium and should be avoided in a sodium-restricted diet. Canned foods and juices in which sodium has been removed or limited are available. The client should be taught to read labels carefully. Apples and whole wheat breads are not high in sodium. Beef tenderloin would have less sodium than canned foods or tomato juice.

CN: Reduction of risk potential; CL: Apply

68. 2,3,4. Hypokalemia is a side effect of loop diuretics. Bananas, dried fruit, and oranges are examples of food high in potassium. Angel food cake and peppers are low in potassium.

CN: Pharmacological and parenteral therapies; CL: Apply

69. 2. A normal apical impulse is found over the apex of the heart and is typically located and auscultated in the left fifth intercostal space in the midclavicular line. An apical impulse located or auscultated below the fifth intercostal space or

include ensuring a liberal fluid intake (unless contraindicated). A diet rich in acid should be provided to keep the urine acidic, which increases the solubility of calcium. Preventing constipation is not associated with excessive calcium excretion. Limiting foods rich in calcium, such as dairy products, will help in preventing renal calculi.

CN: Physiological adaptation;
CL: Synthesize

85. 3. INR is the value used to assess effectiveness of the warfarin sodium therapy. INR is the prothrombin time ratio that would be obtained if the thromboplastin reagent from the World Health Organization was used for the plasma test. It is now the recommended method to monitor effectiveness of warfarin sodium. Generally, the INR for clients administered warfarin sodium should range from 2 to 3. In the past, prothrombin time was used to assess effectiveness of warfarin sodium and was maintained at 1.5 to 2.5 times the control value. Partial thromboplastin time is used to assess the effectiveness of heparin therapy. Fresh frozen plasma or vitamin K is used to reverse warfarin sodium's anticoagulant effect, whereas protamine sulfate reverses the effects of heparin. Warfarin sodium will help to prevent blood clots.

CN: Pharmacological and parenteral therapies; CL: Apply

86. 1,4,5. Daily dental care including brushing the teeth twice a day and flossing once a day and frequent checkups by a dentist who is informed about the client's condition are required to maintain good oral health. The client can use a regular toothbrush; it is not necessary to avoid use of an electric toothbrush. Taking antibiotics prior to certain dental procedures is recommended only if the client has a prosthetic valve or a heart transplant. It is not necessary to use an antibiotic mouthwash.

CN: Reduction of risk potential;
CL: Create

87. 2. Most cardiac surgical clients have median sternotomy incisions, which take about 3 months to heal. Measures that promote healing include avoiding heavy lifting, performing muscle reconditioning exercises, and using caution when driving. Showering or bathing is allowed as long as the incision is well approximated with no open areas or drainage. Activities should be gradually resumed on discharge.

CN: Safety and infection control;
CL: Evaluate

88. 1. Verbalized concerns from this client may stem from anxiety over the changes in the body after open-heart surgery. Although the client may experience depression related to altered health status or may have a lack of knowledge regarding

the postoperative course, the client is pointing out the changes in the body image. The client is not concerned about altered tissue perfusion.

CN: Psychosocial integrity; CL: Analyze

The Client with Hypertension

89. 1. The effect of a beta-blocker is a decrease in heart rate, contractility, and afterload, which leads to a decrease in blood pressure. The client at first may have an increase in fatigue when starting the beta-blocker. The mechanism of action does not improve blood sugar or urine output.

CN: Pharmacological and parenteral therapies; CL: Evaluate

90. 2. There was a significant change in both blood pressure and heart rate with position change. This indicates inadequate blood volume to sustain normal values. Normal postural changes allow for an increase in heart rate of 5 to 20 bpm, a possible slight decrease of <5 mm Hg in the systolic blood pressure, and a possible slight increase of <5 mm Hg in the diastolic blood pressure.

CN: Management of care; CL: Analyze

91. 1,3,5. Clonidine is a central-acting adrenergic antagonist. It reduces sympathetic outflow from the central nervous system. Dry mouth, impotence, and sleep disturbances are possible adverse effects. Hyperkalemia and pancreatitis are not anticipated with use of this drug.

CN: Pharmacological and parenteral therapies; CL: Apply

92. 200 mcg

First, calculate the number of milligrams per milliliter:

$$\frac{50 \text{ mg}}{250 \text{ mL}} = \frac{1 \text{ mg}}{5 \text{ mL}} = \frac{0.2 \text{ mg}}{1 \text{ mL}}$$

Next, calculate the number of micrograms in each milligram:

$$0.2 \text{ mg} \times \frac{1{,}000 \text{ mcg}}{1 \text{ mg}} = 200 \text{ mcg}$$

CN: Pharmacological and parenteral therapies; CL: Apply

93. 1. Furosemide is a diuretic often prescribed for clients with hypertension or heart failure; the drug should not affect a client's ability to drive safely. Furosemide may cause orthostatic hypotension, and clients should be instructed to be careful when changing from supine to sitting to standing position. Diuretics should be taken in the morning if possible to prevent sleep disturbance due to the need to get up to void. Furosemide is a loop diuretic that is not potassium sparing; clients should take potassium supplements as prescribed and have their serum potassium levels checked at prescribed intervals.

⌚ CN: Pharmacological and parenteral therapies; CL: Evaluate

94. 2,3. Changing positions slowly and avoiding long periods of standing may limit the occurrence of orthostatic hypotension. Scheduling regular medication times is important for blood pressure management, but this aspect is not related to the development of orthostatic hypotension. Excessive alcohol intake and hot baths are associated with vasodilation.

⌚ CN: Reduction of risk potential; CL: Create

95. 1. Atenolol is a beta-adrenergic antagonist indicated for management of hypertension. Sudden discontinuation of this drug is dangerous because it may exacerbate symptoms. The medication should not be discontinued without a prescription. Blood pressure needs to be monitored more frequently than annually in a client who is newly diagnosed and treated for hypertension. Clients are not usually placed on a 2-g sodium diet for hypertension.

⌚ CN: Pharmacological and parenteral therapies; CL: Synthesize

96. 3. Processed and cured meat products, such as cold cuts, ham, and hot dogs, are all high in both fat and sodium and should be avoided on a low-calorie, low-fat, low-salt diet. Dietary restrictions of all types are complex and difficult to implement with clients who are basically asymptomatic.

⌚ CN: Basic care and comfort; CL: Apply

97. 1,2,4,6. Metoprolol is a beta-adrenergic blocker indicated for hypertension, angina, and myocardial infarction. The tablets should be taken with food at same time each day; they should not be chewed or crushed. The **HCP** 📖 should be notified if pulse falls below 50 for several days. Blood glucose should be checked regularly during therapy since increased episodes of hypoglycemia may occur. It may mask evidence of hypoglycemia such as palpitations, tachycardia, and tremor. Use of any OTC decongestants, asthma and cold remedies, and herbal preparations must be avoided. Fainting spells may occur due to exercise or stress, and the dosage of the drug may need to be reduced or discontinued.

⌚ CN: Pharmacological and parenteral therapies; CL: Create

98. 1,2,3,5. Chlorothiazide causes increased urination and decreased swelling (if there is edema) and weight loss. It is important to check and record weight two to three times per week at same time of day with similar amount of clothing. Clients should not drink alcoholic beverages or take other medications without the approval of the **healthcare provider (HCP)** 📖. Reducing sodium intake in the diet helps diuretic drugs to be more effective and allows smaller doses to be taken. Smaller doses are less likely to cause adverse effects, and therefore, excessive table salt as well as salty foods should be avoided. Chlorothiazide is a diuretic that is prescribed for lower blood pressure and may cause dizziness and faintness when the client stands up suddenly. This can be prevented or decreased by changing positions slowly. If dizziness is severe, the HCP must be notified. Diuretics may cause sensitivity to sunlight; hence the need to avoid prolonged exposure to sunlight, use sunscreens, and wear protective clothing. Chlorothiazide causes increased urination and must be taken early in the day to decrease nighttime trips to the bathroom. Fewer bathroom trips mean less interference with sleep and less risk of falls. The client should not change the dosage without consulting the HCP.

⌚ CN: Pharmacological and parenteral therapies; CL: Evaluate

99. 4. Tailoring or individualizing a program to the client's lifestyle has been shown to be an effective strategy for changing health behaviors. Providing a written program, explaining the program to the client's spouse, and reassuring the client that he or she can do the program may be helpful but are not as likely to promote adherence as individualizing the program.

⌚ CN: Psychosocial integrity; CL: Synthesize

100. 3. A plan to reduce or stop smoking begins with establishing the client's personal daily smoking pattern and activities associated with smoking. It is important that the client understands the associated health and environmental risks, but this knowledge has not been shown to help clients change their smoking behavior.

⌚ CN: Psychosocial integrity; CL: Synthesize

101. 1. Propranolol is a beta-adrenergic blocking agent. Actions of propranolol include reducing heart rate, decreasing myocardial contractility, and slowing conduction. Propranolol does not increase norepinephrine secretion, cause vasodilation, or block conversion of angiotensin I to angiotensin II.

⌚ CN: Pharmacological and parenteral therapies; CL: Apply

102. 3. In most instances, clients with hypertension require lifelong treatment and their hypertension cannot be managed successfully without changes in health behavior. The client must first commit to making these long-term changes. The changes will involve taking medications, stopping smoking, and losing weight, but the client must first accept the need for a lifelong management and establish a vision and plan to control the hypertension.

🔑 CN: Psychosocial integrity;
CL: Synthesize

The Client with Atrial Fibrillation and Other Dysrhythmias

103. 2,1,3,4. To decrease myocardial workload and promote timely intervention, the client should be assisted to the bed. Assessing vital signs provides the data needed to determine client tolerance. Early initiation of an intravenous access will enable timely medication administration if it is emergently needed. While a 12-lead electrocardiogram is needed, it can be obtained after the IV is initiated.

🔑 CN: Physiological adaptation;
CL: Synthesize

104. 2,4,5. This ECG strip indicates the client has atrial fibrillation. There is no P wave and PR interval; these are replaced with a fine wavy lines. In atrial fibrillation, the ventricular rate may be normal, slow, or fast. Clients with atrial fibrillation may have palpitations secondary to a fast and irregular atrial rhythm. Because atrial fibrillation also may result in a sudden decrease in cardiac output, the client may also experience light-headedness and shortness of breath. A carotid bruit, nausea, and a systolic murmur are not manifestations of new-onset atrial fibrillation.

🔑 CN: Physiological adaptation;
CL: Analyze

105. 4. The purpose of EPS is to study the heart's electrical system. During this invasive procedure, a special wire is introduced into the heart to produce dysrhythmia. To prepare for this procedure, the client should be NPO for 6 to 8 hours before the test, and all antidysrhythmics are held for at least 24 hours before the test in order to study the dysrhythmia without the influence of medications. Because the client's verbal responses to the rhythm changes are extremely important, sedation is avoided if possible.

🔑 CN: Physiological integrity; CL: Create

106. 2. Characteristics of atrial fibrillation include pulse rate >100 bpm, totally irregular rhythm, and no definite P waves on the ECG. During assessment,

the nurse is likely to note the irregular rate and should report it to the **healthcare provider (HCP)** 📖. A weak, thready pulse is characteristic of a client in shock. Two regular beats followed by an irregular beat may indicate a premature ventricular contraction.

🔑 CN: Reduction of risk potential;
CL: Analyze

107. 1,5. The nurse must teach the client how to take and record the pulse daily. The client should be instructed to avoid lifting the operative-side arm above shoulder level for 1 week postinsertion. It takes up to 2 months for the incision site to heal and full range of motion to return. The client should avoid heavy lifting until approved by the **healthcare provider (HCP)** 📖. The pacemaker metal casing does not set off airport security alarms, so there are no travel restrictions. Prolonged immobilization is not required. Microwave ovens are safe to use and do not alter pacemaker function.

🔑 CN: Reduction of risk potential;
CL: Create

108. 1. Transcutaneous pacemaker therapy provides an adequate heart rate to a client in an emergency situation. Defibrillation and a lidocaine infusion are not indicated for the treatment of third-degree heart block. Transcutaneous pacing is used temporarily until a transvenous or permanent pacemaker can be inserted.

🔑 CN: Physiological adaptation;
CL: Synthesize

109. 1,3,4,2. Because atrial fibrillation causes a decrease in cardiac output, the heart rate increases in response to this drop. As a result of an increased heart rate, the oxygen demands of the heart increase. It is important for oxygen to be administered first to help compensate for the increased oxygen demand and cardiac workload. Placing the client on a cardiac monitor will help confirm a diagnosis of atrial fibrillation. Performing vital signs will determine the client's response to the abnormal rhythm and responses to treatment. If the rhythm is determined to be atrial fibrillation, it will be necessary for an IV to be inserted so medication can be administered.

🔑 CN: Physiological integrity;
CL: Synthesize

110. 3. The spouse can have physical contact with the client, but if the ICD were to discharge while the spouse had contact with the client, the spouse would feel a "tingle" but would not be harmed. There is not a warning device on the ICD.

🔑 CN: Management of care;
CL: Synthesize

111. 2. Maintaining cardiac conduction stability to prevent arrhythmias is a priority immediately after artificial pacemaker implantation. The client should have continuous electrocardiographic monitoring until proper pacemaker functioning is verified. Skin integrity, while important, is not an immediate concern. The pacemaker is used to increase heart rate and cardiac output, not decrease it. The client should limit activity for the first 24 to 48 hours after pacemaker insertion. The client should also restrict movement of the affected extremity for 24 hours.

CN: Reduction of risk potential; CL: Synthesize

112. 3. Education is a major component of the discharge plan for a client with an artificial pacemaker. The client with a permanent pacemaker needs to be able to state specific information about safety precautions, such as to refrain from lifting more than 3 lb (1.35 kg) or stretching and bending. The client should know how to count the pulse and do so daily or as instructed by the **healthcare provider (HCP)** . The client will not necessarily be placed on a low-cholesterol diet. The client should resume activities and does not need to remain on bed rest. The client should know signs and symptoms of an MI but is not at risk because of the pacemaker.

CN: Basic care and comfort; CL: Evaluate

113. 1,3,4. The client has atrial fibrillation and will have an irregularly irregular pulse and will commonly be tachycardic, with rapid ventricular responses (heart rates) typically in the 110 to 140 range, but rarely over 150 to 170. The goal of treatment is the restoration of sinus rhythm. With a heart rate >150 and symptoms such as shortness of breath, dizziness and syncope, and chest pain, synchronized cardioversion will most likely be the treatment of choice. With more controlled heart rates and more minor signs and symptoms, chemical conversion with drugs such as diltiazem and digoxin prior to other interventions such as synchronized cardioversion with appropriate anticoagulation may be attempted. Because of the decreased cardiac output, monitoring is essential. Obtaining consent for cardioversion requires a prescription from a **healthcare provider (HCP)** , but with the current heart rate, having cardioversion is a very strong possibility for this client. Defibrillation is used for ventricular fibrillation, not atrial fibrillation. Teaching the client about warfarin will be a possibility, but not an immediate intervention. Clients in continued atrial fibrillation usually require some form of anticoagulation. Drawing labs for CBCs to detect anemia or infection, and thyroid function studies (to determine thyrotoxicosis, a rare, but not-to-be-missed cause, especially in older adults), serum electrolytes, and BUN/creatinine (looking for electrolyte disturbances or renal failure) are commonly drawn for determining the cause of the atrial fibrillation; they are not an immediate action.

CN: Physiological adaptation; CL: Synthesize

The Client Requiring Rapid Response or Cardiopulmonary Resuscitation

114. 3. Transcutaneous pads should be placed on the client with third-degree heart block. For a client who is symptomatic, transcutaneous pacing is the treatment of choice. The hemodynamic stability and pulse should be assessed prior to calling a code or initiating CPR. Defibrillation is performed for ventricular fibrillation or ventricular tachycardia with no pulse.

CN: Management of care; CL: Synthesize

115. 3. This ECG strip indicates the client has ventricular tachycardia. The nurse should first check the client for the presence of a pulse. The presence of a pulse determines the treatment for ventricular tachycardia. It is also important to assess the client's heart rate and level of consciousness. Cardioversion may be used to treat hemodynamically unstable tachycardias. Assessment of instability is required before cardioversion. It is not appropriate to begin CPR unless the pulse is absent. Defibrillation is used to treat ventricular fibrillation or pulseless ventricular tachycardia.

CN: Physiological adaptation; CL: Synthesize

116. 2. Pupillary reaction is the best indication of whether oxygenated blood has been reaching the client's brain. Pupils that remain widely dilated and do not react to light may indicate lack of oxygenation and that serious brain damage may have occurred. The pulse rate may be normal, mucous membranes may still be pink, and systolic blood pressure may be 80 mm Hg or higher, yet there can be inadequate oxygenation to the brain.

CN: Reduction of risk potential; CL: Evaluate

117. 3. Amiodarone is used for the treatment of premature ventricular contractions, ventricular tachycardia with a pulse, atrial fibrillation, and atrial flutter. Amiodarone is not used as initial therapy for a pulseless dysrhythmia.

CN: Pharmacological and parenteral therapies; CL: Evaluate

118. 2. Because of its location near the xiphoid process, the liver is the organ most easily damaged from pressure exerted over the xiphoid process during CPR. The pressure on the victim's chest wall should be sufficient to compress the heart but not so great as to damage internal organs. Injury may result, however, even when CPR is performed properly.

    CN: Reduction of risk potential; CL: Apply

119. 4. An adult's sternum must be depressed 2 inches (5 cm) with each compression to ensure adequate heart compression.

    CN: Reduction of risk potential; CL: Apply

120. 4. If the chest wall is not rising with rescue breaths, the head should be repositioned first to ensure that the airway is adequately opened. A bag mask device allows for delivery of 100% oxygen but is difficult to manage if there is just one rescuer; ideally, two persons are used to operate the bag mask device, one to maintain the seal and the other to provide the ventilations. Compressions should be maintained at 100 per minute.

    CN: Physiological adaptation; CL: Synthesize

121. 1. The exhalation phase of ventilation is a passive activity that occurs during CPR as part of the normal relaxation of the victim's chest. No action by the rescuer is necessary.

    CN: Reduction of risk potential; CL: Apply

122. 2. After a person is without cardiopulmonary function for 4 to 6 minutes, permanent brain damage is almost certain. To prevent permanent brain damage, it is important to begin CPR promptly after a cardiopulmonary arrest.

    CN: Reduction of risk potential; CL: Apply

123. 2. The Heimlich maneuver should be administered only to a victim who cannot make *any* sounds due to airway obstruction. If the victim can whisper words or cough, some air exchange is occurring and the emergency medical system should be called instead of attempting the Heimlich maneuver. Cyanosis may accompany or follow choking; however, the Heimlich maneuver should only be initiated when the victim cannot speak.

    CN: Reduction of risk potential; CL: Apply

124. 4. The thrusts should be delivered below the xiphoid process, but above the umbilicus, to minimize the risk of internal injuries.

    CN: Reduction of risk potential; CL: Apply

125. 2. The priority action is to assess the client and determine whether the rhythm is life threatening. More information, including vital signs, should be obtained, and the nurse should notify the **HCP** . A bolus of lidocaine may be prescribed to treat this arrhythmia. This is not a code-type situation unless the client has been determined to be in a life-threatening situation.

    CN: Physiological adaptation; CL: Synthesize

126. 1,2,4,5. Vital signs give an important initial assessment of this client's status. The client may experience burns from the patches and current used for the cardioversion. Therefore, it is important to assess the skin of the chest wall for redness or burns. Because conscious sedation is used for this procedure, assessing the client's level of consciousness also is an important initial step. Attaching the client to cardiac monitoring is also important to assess rhythm abnormalities. There is no arterial puncture associated with the procedure.

    CN: Reduction of risk potential; CL: Synthesize

127. 4. The paddles are in the correct position. The nurse can push the shock button to defibrillate the client.

    CN: Physiological adaptation; CL: Apply

128. 2. The **rapid response team** should be called immediately to evaluate and treat the client. There is no indication at this time for manual ventilations or chest compressions. If the family is not interfering in client care, it can be reassuring to the family to see that all possible care is being provided.

    CN: Management of care; CL: Synthesize

Managing Care, Quality, and Safety for Clients with Cardiac Health Problems

129. 2,4,3,1. Even though the chest pain experienced by Client 2 is resolved, it was recent and requires reassessment. Client 4 is scheduled to leave for major surgery very soon. The nurse should check this client and the client's chart and make certain that everything is ready so as to not delay the surgery. Client 3 has scheduled medications for blood pressure control. While not experiencing any acute problems, this medication should be administered as scheduled. Client 1 is stable at this time and can be seen last.

    CN: Management of care; CL: Create

130. **4.** UAP 📖 are able to measure and record intake and output. The nurse is responsible for client teaching, physical assessments, and evaluating the information collected on the client.

🔑 CN: Management of care; CL: Synthesize

131. **1,2,4,5,6.** The nurse must have assessment data and verify vital signs if necessary in order to determine the action that is required. If there is a significant change in the client's condition, the charge nurse should be notified in order to help the nurse with both this client and the nurse's other assigned clients if necessary; most acute care facilities have a **rapid response team** 📖 that can also help assess and intervene with basic standing orders if necessary. Positioning the client in semi-Fowler's is a nursing action that may assist in breathing and relieve shortness of breath. It is important for the nurse to reassure the client by staying calm and remaining with the client. The nurse must notify the **HCP** 📖 about the change in client's condition; the nurse must have all information available and present it in a concise and accurate manner using SBAR format including a recommendation for treatment if indicated. The nurse should stay with this client and delegate checking on other assigned clients to the charge nurse or **UAP** 📖.

🔑 CN: Management of care; CL: Synthesize

132. **2.** The client has gained 5 lb (2.3 kg) in 3 days with a steady increase in blood pressure. The client is exhibiting signs of heart failure, and if the client is short of breath, this will be another sign. Asking how the client is feeling is too general, and a more focused question will quickly determine the client's current health status. The scales should be calibrated periodically, but a 5-lb (2.3-kg) weight gain, along with increased blood pressure, is not likely due to problems with the scale. The weight gain is likely due to fluid retention, not drinking too much fluid.

🔑 CN: Management of care; CL: Analyze

133. **4.** The goals of managing clients outside of the hospital are for the clients to maintain health and prevent readmission; thus, interventions, such as monitoring and teaching, appear to have contributed to the low readmission rate in this group of clients. Although it is important that clients do not gain weight, view educational material, and continue to take their medication, the primary indicator of effectiveness of the program is the lack of rehospitalization.

🔑 CN: Management of care; CL: Evaluate

134. **3.** Using an individualized, printed checklist ensures that all key information is reported; the checklist can then serve as a record to which nurses can refer later. Giving a verbal report leaves room for error in memory; using an audiotape or a **medical record** 📖 requires nurses to spend unnecessary time retrieving information.

🔑 CN: Safety and infection control; CL: Evaluate

135. **1,2,4,5.** Orthostatic hypotension is a drop in blood pressure that occurs when changing position, usually to a more upright position. Orthostatic hypotension often occurs in elderly clients, and it is a common cause of falls. Nurses must assess clients for orthostatic hypotension and assist all clients with orthostatic hypotension in standing to help prevent falls. Lower limb compression devices aid in prevention of decreased orthostatic systolic blood pressure and reduce symptoms in elderly clients with progressive orthostatic hypotension. Nurses must teach clients how to gradually change their position, and they must conduct "fall risk" assessments. Sequential compression devices may be helpful to high-risk clients and should be considered when developing the care plan. Antihypertensive medications are not necessary for clients with orthostatic hypertension and may precipitate dangerous drops in blood pressure. The clients should be encouraged to be ambulatory.

🔑 CN: Reduction of risk potential; CL: Synthesize

136. **4,5.** Performing vital signs and obtaining intake and outputs are tasks that can be delegated to UAP 📖. Assessing pedal pulses and administering medications and oxygen are skills that require nursing judgments.

🔑 CN: Management of care; CL: Analyze

The Client with Vascular Disease

The Client with Peripheral Artery Disease

1. What instructions should the nurse give a client experiencing signs and symptoms related to decreased arterial insufficiency? Select all that apply.

☐ **1.** Avoid smoking and exposure to the cold.

☐ **2.** Take acetaminophen if experiencing pain at night.

☐ **3.** Take aspirin or clopidogrel as prescribed.

☐ **4.** Use additional bed clothes at night.

☐ **5.** Wear tight socks to keep feet warm.

2. The nurse is caring for a client who has just had an ankle-brachial index (ABI) test. The left arm blood pressure was 160/80 mm Hg, and a palpable systolic blood pressure of the left lower extremity was 130/60 mm Hg. These findings suggest that the client has:

☐ **1.** mild peripheral artery disease.

☐ **2.** moderate peripheral artery disease.

☐ **3.** no apparent occlusion in the left lower extremity.

☐ **4.** severe peripheral artery disease.

3. A client is admitted for a revascularization procedure for arteriosclerosis in the left iliac artery. To promote circulation in the extremities, the nurse should:

☐ **1.** position the client on a firm mattress.

☐ **2.** keep the involved extremity warm with blankets.

☐ **3.** position the left leg at or below the body's horizontal plane.

☐ **4.** encourage the client to raise and lower the leg four times every hour.

4. A sedentary, obese, middle-aged client is recovering from surgery to remove an embolus in the right iliac artery. The nurse should develop a discharge plan with the client that will focus on participating in which activities? Select all that apply.

☐ **1.** aerobic activity

☐ **2.** strength training

☐ **3.** weight control

☐ **4.** stress management

☐ **5.** wearing supportive athletic shoes

5. The nurse is assessing the pulse in a client with aortoiliac disease. On the illustration below, indicate the pulse site that will give the nurse the **most** useful data.

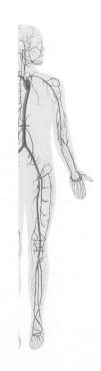

6. The nurse is assessing a 48-year-old client with a history of smoking during a routine clinic visit. The client, who exercises regularly, reports having pain in the calf during exercise that disappears at rest. Which finding requires further evaluation?
- ☐ **1.** heart rate 57 bpm
- ☐ **2.** SpO$_2$ of 94% on room air
- ☐ **3.** blood pressure 134/82 mm Hg
- ☐ **4.** ankle-brachial index of 0.65

7. A client with peripheral artery disease has undergone a right femoral-popliteal bypass graft. The blood pressure has decreased from 124/80 mm Hg to 88/62 mm Hg. What should the nurse assess **first**?
- ☐ **1.** IV fluid infusion rate
- ☐ **2.** pedal pulses
- ☐ **3.** nasal cannula flow rate
- ☐ **4.** capillary refill

8. An obese client taking warfarin has dry skin due to decreased arterial blood flow. What should the nurse instruct the client to do? Select all that apply.
- ☐ **1.** Apply lanolin or petroleum jelly to intact skin.
- ☐ **2.** Follow a reduced-calorie, reduced-fat diet.
- ☐ **3.** Inspect the involved areas daily for new ulcerations.
- ☐ **4.** Limit activities of daily living (ADLs).
- ☐ **5.** Use an electric razor to shave.

9. The nurse is caring for a client with peripheral artery disease who has recently been prescribed clopidogrel. The nurse understands that more teaching is necessary when the client states:
- ☐ **1.** "I should not be surprised if I bruise easier or if my gums bleed a little when brushing my teeth."
- ☐ **2.** "It does not really matter if I take this medicine with or without food, whatever works best for my stomach."
- ☐ **3.** "I should stop taking my medicine if it makes me feel weak and dizzy."
- ☐ **4.** "The doctor prescribed this medicine to make my platelets less likely to stick together and help prevent clots from forming."

10. A client is receiving cilostazol for peripheral artery disease causing intermittent claudication. The nurse determines this medication is effective when the client reports:
- ☐ **1.** "I am having fewer aches and pains."
- ☐ **2.** "I do not have headaches anymore."
- ☐ **3.** "I am able to walk further without leg pain."
- ☐ **4.** "My toes are turning grayish black in color."

11. The client with peripheral artery disease reports both legs hurt when walking. What should the nurse instruct the client to do?
- ☐ **1.** Avoid walking when the pain occurs.
- ☐ **2.** Rest frequently with the legs elevated.
- ☐ **3.** Wear support stockings.
- ☐ **4.** Enroll in a supervised exercise training program.

12. The nurse is assessing a client with peripheral artery insufficiency. Where should the nurse palpate the client's pulse to identify tibioperoneal artery involvement on the right side of the body?

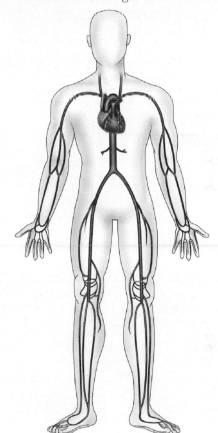

13. The nurse is obtaining the pulse of a client who has had a femoral-popliteal bypass surgery 6 hours ago (see below). Which assessment provides the **most** accurate information about the client's postoperative status?

☐ **1.**

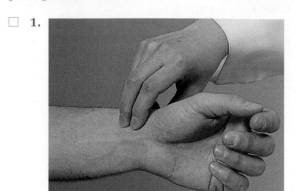

☐ **2.**

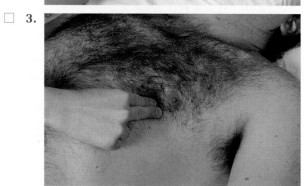

☐ **3.**

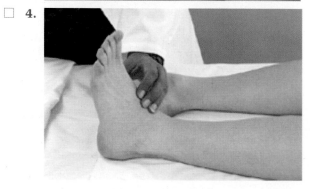

☐ **4.**

14. The nurse is assessing the lower extremities of the client with peripheral artery disease. Which findings are expected? Select all that apply.
☐ **1.** hairy legs
☐ **2.** mottled skin
☐ **3.** pink skin
☐ **4.** coolness
☐ **5.** moist skin

15. The nurse is unable to palpate the client's left pedal pulses. What should the nurse do **first**?
☐ **1.** Auscultate the pulses with a stethoscope.
☐ **2.** Call the healthcare provider (HCP).
☐ **3.** Use a Doppler ultrasound device.
☐ **4.** Inspect the lower left extremity.

16. When assessing an individual with peripheral artery disease, which clinical manifestation would indicate complete arterial obstruction in the lower left leg?
☐ **1.** aching pain in the left calf
☐ **2.** burning pain in the left calf
☐ **3.** numbness and tingling in the left leg
☐ **4.** coldness of the left foot and ankle

17. A client has returned to the surgical care unit after having femoral-popliteal bypass grafting. Indicate in which order from first to last the nurse should conduct assessment of this client. All options must be used.

1. postoperative pain

2. peripheral pulses

3. urine output

4. incision site

18. A client with heart failure has bilateral +4 edema of the right ankle that extends up to midcalf. The client is sitting in a chair in no evident distress with the legs in a dependent position. The nurse should **first**:
☐ **1.** assist the client to the bed.
☐ **2.** request a prescription for support stockings.
☐ **3.** elevate the client's legs on a foot stool.
☐ **4.** take the client's blood pressure.

19. The nurse is assessing a client who has a history of peripheral artery disease. The nurse observes that the left great toe is black. The discoloration is likely a result of:
- ☐ **1.** atrophy.
- ☐ **2.** contraction.
- ☐ **3.** gangrene.
- ☐ **4.** rubor.

20. A client has peripheral artery disease of both lower extremities. The client tells the nurse, "I have really tried to manage my condition well." Which example indicates the client is using appropriate care management strategies?
- ☐ **1.** The client rests with the legs elevated above the level of the heart.
- ☐ **2.** The client walks slowly but steadily for 30 minutes twice a day.
- ☐ **3.** The client limits activity to walking around the house.
- ☐ **4.** The client wears antiembolism stockings at all times when out of bed.

21. A client is scheduled to have an arteriogram. During the arteriogram, the client reports having nausea, tingling, and dyspnea. The nurse's **immediate** action should be to:
- ☐ **1.** administer epinephrine.
- ☐ **2.** inform the healthcare provider (HCP).
- ☐ **3.** administer oxygen.
- ☐ **4.** inform the client that the procedure is almost over.

22. A client with peripheral artery disease has chronic, severe bilateral pretibial and ankle edema; the client is on complete bed rest. To maintain skin integrity, what should the nurse do?
- ☐ **1.** Administer pain medication.
- ☐ **2.** Ensure fluid intake of 3,000 mL per 24 hours.
- ☐ **3.** Turn the client every 1 to 2 hours.
- ☐ **4.** Maintain hygiene.

23. A client who has been diagnosed with peripheral artery disease is being discharged. The client needs further instruction if the client states he or she will:
- ☐ **1.** avoid heating pads.
- ☐ **2.** not cross the legs.
- ☐ **3.** wear leather shoes.
- ☐ **4.** use iodine on an injured site.

24. A client with peripheral artery disease has femoral-popliteal bypass surgery. The **primary** goal of the plan of care after surgery is to:
- ☐ **1.** maintain circulation.
- ☐ **2.** prevent infection.
- ☐ **3.** relieve pain.
- ☐ **4.** provide education.

25. The nurse is instructing a client who is at risk for peripheral artery disease how to use knee-length elastic stockings (support hose). What instructions should the teaching plan include? Select all that apply.
- ☐ **1.** Apply the elastic stockings before getting out of bed.
- ☐ **2.** Remove the stockings if swelling occurs.
- ☐ **3.** Remove the stockings every 8 hours, elevate the feet, and reapply in 15 minutes.
- ☐ **4.** Once the stockings have been pulled over the calf, roll the remaining stocking down to make a cuff.
- ☐ **5.** Keep the stockings in place for 48 hours, and reapply using a clean pair of stockings.

26. A client is scheduled to undergo right axillary-to-axillary artery bypass surgery. Immediately following surgery, to prevent infection, the nurse should:
- ☐ **1.** assess the temperature in the right arm.
- ☐ **2.** monitor the radial pulse in the right arm.
- ☐ **3.** protect the extremity from cold.
- ☐ **4.** avoid using the arm for a venipuncture.

27. One goal in caring for a client with arterial occlusive disease is to promote vasodilation in the affected extremity. To achieve this goal, the nurse should encourage the client to:
- ☐ **1.** avoid eating low-fat foods.
- ☐ **2.** elevate the legs above the heart.
- ☐ **3.** stop smoking.
- ☐ **4.** begin a jogging program.

28. The nurse is caring for a client with peripheral artery disease who has just returned from having a percutaneous transluminal balloon angioplasty. Which of these findings require **immediate** attention from the nurse?
- ☐ **1.** a change in the intensity of the pulse from the baseline
- ☐ **2.** pain "2 out of 10" at the catheterization site
- ☐ **3.** shiny skin and a hairless appearance on the affected leg
- ☐ **4.** the presence of an ulcer on the limb of the catheterization site

29. Which instructions should be included in the plan of care for a client who had a left femoral-popliteal bypass yesterday? Select all that apply.
- ☐ **1.** Turn frequently, and use pillows to support the incision.
- ☐ **2.** Encourage the client to change positions frequently to prevent atelectasis.
- ☐ **3.** Place the left leg in a knee-flexed position to promote oxygenation.
- ☐ **4.** Place the client in supine position, and elevate the leg above the heart to prevent edema.
- ☐ **5.** Encourage the client to walk short distances to promote circulation.
- ☐ **6.** Encourage the client to maintain bed rest to prevent stress on suture line.

30. The client with peripheral artery disease has been prescribed diltiazem. The nurse should determine the effectiveness of this medication by assessing the client for:
☐ 1. relief of anxiety.
☐ 2. sedation.
☐ 3. vasoconstriction.
☐ 4. vasodilation.

31. A client is receiving pentoxifylline for intermittent claudication. The nurse should determine the effectiveness of the drug by asking if the client:
☐ 1. has less pain in the legs.
☐ 2. can wiggle the toes.
☐ 3. is urinating more frequently.
☐ 4. is less dizzy.

32. A client with peripheral artery disease, coronary artery disease, and chronic obstructive pulmonary disease takes theophylline 200 mg twice daily every day and digoxin 0.5 mg once a day. The healthcare provider (HCP) now prescribes pentoxifylline. To prevent adverse effects, the nurse should monitor the client's:
☐ 1. digoxin level.
☐ 2. partial thromboplastin time (PTT).
☐ 3. serum cholesterol level.
☐ 4. theophylline level.

33. A client with a history of coronary artery disease (CAD) has been diagnosed with peripheral artery disease. The healthcare provider (HCP) started the client on pentoxifylline once daily. Approximately 1 hour after receiving the initial dose of pentoxifylline, the client reports having chest pain. The nurse should **first**:
☐ 1. initiate the rapid response team.
☐ 2. contact the healthcare provider.
☐ 3. have the client rest in bed.
☐ 4. start an intravenous infusion of normal saline.

34. A client with peripheral artery disease is recovering from surgery to insert an aortofemoral-popliteal bypass graft. When developing a postoperative education plan, which question by the nurse will provide the **most** helpful information?
☐ 1. "How did you manage your health before admission?"
☐ 2. "How far could you walk without pain before surgery?"
☐ 3. "What is your home environment like?"
☐ 4. "Do you have problems with urine retention?"

35. The client with peripheral artery disease and a history of hypertension is to be discharged on a low-fat, low-cholesterol, low-sodium diet. Which should be the nurse's **first** step in planning the dietary instructions?
☐ 1. Determine the client's knowledge level about cholesterol.
☐ 2. Ask the client to name foods high in fat, cholesterol, and salt.
☐ 3. Explain the importance of complying with the diet.
☐ 4. Assess the family's food preferences.

The Client with Peripheral Vascular Disease Having an Amputation

36. While the nurse is providing preoperative teaching for a client with peripheral vascular disease who is to have a below-the-knee amputation, the client says, "I hate the idea of being an invalid after they cut off my leg." The nurse's **most** therapeutic response should be:
☐ 1. "Focusing on using your one good leg will make your recovery easier."
☐ 2. "Tell me more about how you are feeling."
☐ 3. "We will talk more about this after your surgery."
☐ 4. "You are fortunate to have a wife who can take care of you."

37. The client asks the nurse, "Why can't the doctor tell me exactly how much of my leg they're going to take off? Don't you think I should know that?" The nurse responds, knowing that the final decision on the level of the amputation will depend primarily on:
☐ 1. the need to remove as much of the leg as possible.
☐ 2. the adequacy of the blood supply to the tissues.
☐ 3. the ease with which a prosthesis can be fitted.
☐ 4. considering how to fit a prosthesis.

38. A client has undergone an amputation of three toes and a femoral-popliteal bypass. The nurse should teach the client that after surgery, which leg position is contraindicated while sitting in a chair?
☐ 1. crossing the legs
☐ 2. elevating the legs
☐ 3. flexing the ankles
☐ 4. extending the knees

39. The nurse is monitoring a client after an above-the-knee amputation and notes that blood has saturated through the distal part of the dressing. What should the nurse do **immediately**?
☐ 1. Apply a tourniquet.
☐ 2. Assess vital signs.
☐ 3. Call the healthcare provider (HCP).
☐ 4. Elevate the involved extremity with a large pillow.

40. The client has had a below-the-knee amputation secondary to arterial occlusive disease. The nurse is instructing the client in residual limb care. Which statement by the client indicates that the client understands how to implement the plan of care?
- ☐ 1. "I should inspect the incision carefully when I change the dressing every other day."
- ☐ 2. "I should wash the incision, dry it, and apply moisturizing lotion daily."
- ☐ 3. "I should rewrap the stump as often as needed."
- ☐ 4. "I should elevate the stump on pillows to decrease swelling."

The Client with an Aneurysm

41. The nurse is developing a discharge teaching plan for a client who had a graft insertion for an abdominal aortic aneurysm 4 days ago. The nurse reviews the client's chart for information about the client's history. Key findings are noted in the chart below.

History and Physical

1) Smokes four cigars a month.
2) Vital signs: blood pressure, ranges from 150/76–170/98 mm Hg; heart rate, 90–100 bpm; respirations, 12–18 bpm; temperature, 99.9°F (37.8°C).
3) +1 bilateral ankle edema.

Based on the data and expected outcomes, which should the nurse emphasize in the teaching plan?
- ☐ 1. food intake
- ☐ 2. fluid volume
- ☐ 3. skin integrity
- ☐ 4. tissue perfusion

42. A client is admitted with a 6.5-cm thoracic aneurysm. The nurse records findings from the initial assessment in the client's chart, as shown below.

Vital Signs

Date	05/07	
Time	1000	
Blood pressure	160/90 mm Hg	
Heart rate	74 bpm	
Respirations	20/min	
		G. Fuentes, RN

At 1030, the client has sharp midchest pain after having a bowel movement. What should the nurse do **first**?
- ☐ 1. Assess the client's vital signs.
- ☐ 2. Administer pain medication as prescribed.
- ☐ 3. Assess the client's neurologic status.
- ☐ 4. Contact the healthcare provider (HCP).

43. A client with an enlarged abdominal aorta admitted to the emergency department has severe back pain, nausea, blood pressure of 90/40 mm Hg, heart rate 128 bpm, and respirations 28/minute. In which order from first to last should the nurse implement these prescriptions? All options must be used.

1. Monitor intake and output.

2. Establish an intravenous infusion.

3. Administer pain medication.

4. Insert a nasogastric tube.

44. A client had a repair of a thoracoabdominal aneurysm 2 days ago. Which findings should the nurse consider unexpected and report to the healthcare provider (HCP) **immediately**?
- ☐ 1. abdominal pain at 5 on a scale of 0 to 10 for the last 2 days
- ☐ 2. heart rate of 100 bpm after ambulating 200 feet (0.06 km)
- ☐ 3. urine output of 2,000 mL in 24 hours
- ☐ 4. weakness and numbness in the lower extremities

45. A client is admitted to the emergency department with severe abdominal pain. A radiograph reveals a large abdominal aortic aneurysm. The **primary** goal at this time is to:
- ☐ 1. maintain circulation.
- ☐ 2. manage pain.
- ☐ 3. prepare the client for emergency surgery.
- ☐ 4. teach postoperative breathing exercises.

46. A client has sudden, severe pain in the back and chest, accompanied by shortness of breath. The client describes the pain as a "tearing" sensation. The healthcare provider (HCP) suspects the client is experiencing a dissecting aortic aneurysm. The emergency supply cart is brought into the room because one complication of a dissecting aneurysm is:
- ☐ 1. cardiac tamponade.
- ☐ 2. stroke.
- ☐ 3. pulmonary edema.
- ☐ 4. myocardial infarction.

47. The nurse is planning care for a client who has just returned to the medical-surgical unit following repair of an aortic aneurysm. The nurse **first** should assess the client for:
☐ 1. decreased urinary output.
☐ 2. electrolyte imbalance.
☐ 3. anxiety.
☐ 4. wound infection.

48. A client underwent surgery to repair an abdominal aortic aneurysm. The surgeon made an incision that extends from the xiphoid process to the pubis. At 1200 hours 2 days after surgery, the client has abdominal distention. The nurse checks the progress notes in the client's medical record, as shown below.

Nurses Progress Notes

Date	Time	Progress Notes
07/07	2200	The client is receiving D₅W, 1,000 mL every 8 h. The NG tube is attached to low suction and draining well. The client has been NPO except ice chips. The client has had 10 mg morphine for pain at 6 AM E. Levine, RN

What is **most** likely contributing to the client's abdominal distention?
☐ 1. nasogastric (NG) tube
☐ 2. ice chips
☐ 3. IV fluid intake
☐ 4. morphine

49. A client is discharged after an aortic aneurysm repair with a synthetic graft to replace part of the aorta. The nurse should instruct the client to notify the healthcare provider (HCP) before having:
☐ 1. blood drawn.
☐ 2. an IV line inserted.
☐ 3. major dental work.
☐ 4. an x-ray examination.

50. The nurse is assessing a client who had an abdominal aortic aneurysm repair 2 hours ago. Which finding warrants further evaluation?
☐ 1. absent bowel sounds and mild abdominal distention
☐ 2. a BUN of 26 mg/dL (26 mmol/L) and creatinine of 1.2 mg/dL (1.2 μmol/L)
☐ 3. an arterial blood pressure of 80/50 mm Hg
☐ 4. +1 pedal pulses in bilateral lower extremities

51. The nurse is planning care for a client who had an abdominal aortic aneurysm repair 3 days ago. The nurse is reviewing the progress notes below.

Nurses Progress Notes

Date	Time	Progress Notes
2/20	0900	Temperature is 36.8°C; Pulse is 138; BP is 86/44 mm Hg; CVP is 2 mm Hg Robin Brown, RN
2/20	1100	Urine output is 20 ml/hr for the last 2 hours; Hgb is 7.8 gm/dL, IV of D5½ normal saline is infusing at 74 cc/hr Robin Brown, RN

Two units of PRBCs have been prescribed for transfusion. What should the nurse do **first**?
☐ 1. Administer furosemide.
☐ 2. Increase the drip rate of IV fluids.
☐ 3. Initiate a dopamine drip.
☐ 4. Transfuse PRBCs.

The Client with Raynaud's Phenomenon

52. When instructing a client who has been newly diagnosed with Raynaud's phenomenon about management of care, the nurse should discuss which topic?
☐ 1. scheduling a sympathectomy procedure for the next visit
☐ 2. using a beta-blocker medication
☐ 3. follow-up monitoring for development of connective tissue disease
☐ 4. benefit of an angioplasty to the affected extremities

53. A client has been diagnosed with Raynaud's phenomenon on the tip of the nose and fingertips. The healthcare provider (HCP) has prescribed reserpine to determine if the client will obtain relief. The client often works outside in cold weather and also smokes two packs of cigarettes per day. Which directions should be included in the discharge plan for this client? Select all that apply.
☐ 1. Stop smoking.
☐ 2. Wear a face covering and gloves in the winter.
☐ 3. Place fingertips in cool water to rewarm them.
☐ 4. Find employment that can be done in a warm environment.
☐ 5. Report signs of orthostatic hypotension.

54. A nurse assesses a 40-year-old female client with Raynaud's phenomenon involving her right hand. The nurse records the information in the progress notes, as shown below. From these findings, the nurse should develop a plan with the client to **first** manage:

Progress Notes

Date	Time	Progress Notes
06/10	1500	The client has a palpable but faint right radial pulse. Capillary refill on all five digits < 8 s. No observable swelling. The client is reporting numbness in the tips of all five digits. The skin is warm, dry, and red.
		G. Fuentes, RN

☐ 1. acute pain.
☐ 2. numbness.
☐ 3. lack of circulation.
☐ 4. potential for skin breakdown.

55. Which group is at **greatest** risk for Raynaud's phenomenon?
☐ 1. young women
☐ 2. old women
☐ 3. old men
☐ 4. young men

56. The client with Raynaud's phenomenon has coldness and numbness in the fingers. Which is an **early** sign of vasoconstriction?
☐ 1. cyanosis
☐ 2. gangrene
☐ 3. pallor
☐ 4. rubor

57. During an initial assessment of a client diagnosed with Raynaud's phenomenon, the nurse notes a sudden color change from pink to white in the fingers. The nurse should **first** assess:
☐ 1. appearance of cyanosis.
☐ 2. radial pulse.
☐ 3. SpO_2 of the affected fingers.
☐ 4. blood pressure.

58. The nurse should instruct a client who has been diagnosed with Raynaud's phenomenon to:
☐ 1. immerse the hands in cold water during an episode.
☐ 2. wear light garments when the temperature gets below 50°F (10°C).
☐ 3. wear gloves when handling ice or frozen foods.
☐ 4. live in a cold climate.

59. In order to prevent recurrent vasospastic episodes with Raynaud's phenomenon, what should the nurse instruct the client to do?
☐ 1. Keep the hands and feet elevated as much as possible.
☐ 2. Use a vibrating massage device on the hands.
☐ 3. Wear gloves when obtaining food from the refrigerator.
☐ 4. Increase coffee intake to two cups per day.

60. A client with Raynaud's phenomenon is prescribed diltiazem. The intended outcome is:
☐ 1. decreased heart rate.
☐ 2. conversion to normal sinus rhythm.
☐ 3. reduced episodes of finger numbness.
☐ 4. increased SpO_2.

61. When giving discharge instructions to the client with Raynaud's phenomenon, the nurse should explain that the expected outcome of taking a beta-adrenergic blocking medication is to control the symptoms by:
☐ 1. decreasing the influence of the sympathetic nervous system on the tissues in the hands and feet.
☐ 2. decreasing the pain by producing analgesia.
☐ 3. increasing the blood supply to the affected area.
☐ 4. increasing monoamine oxidase.

62. A client with Raynaud's phenomenon is considering having a sympathectomy. This nurse should tell the client that the surgery is performed:
☐ 1. in the early stages of the disease to prevent further circulatory disturbances.
☐ 2. when the disease is controlled by medication.
☐ 3. when the client is unable to control stress-related vasospasm.
☐ 4. when all other treatment alternatives have failed.

The Client with Peripheral Venous Disease: Thrombophlebitis, Deep Vein Thrombosis, and Embolus Formation

63. A client is being treated for deep vein thrombosis (DVT) in the left femoral artery. The healthcare provider (HCP) has prescribed 60 mg of enoxaparin subcutaneously. Before administering the drug, the nurse checks the client's laboratory results, noted below.

Laboratory Results	
Test	**Result**
Prothrombin time	12.5s
INR	2.0s
Platelet count	50,000/µL (50 × 10^9/L)

Based on these results, what should the nurse do?
- [ ] 1. Contact the pharmacist for a lower dose of the medication.
- [ ] 2. Administer the medication as prescribed.
- [ ] 3. Assess the client for signs of bruising on the extremities.
- [ ] 4. Withhold the dose of the medication and contact the healthcare provider (HCP).

64. A client with deep vein thrombosis suddenly develops dyspnea, tachypnea, and chest discomfort. What should the nurse do **first**?
- [ ] 1. Elevate the head of the bed 30 to 45 degrees.
- [ ] 2. Encourage the client to cough and deep breathe.
- [ ] 3. Auscultate the lungs to detect abnormal breath sounds.
- [ ] 4. Contact the healthcare provider (HCP).

65. A client with a recent diagnosis of deep vein thrombosis (DVT) has sudden onset of shortness of breath and chest pain that increases with a deep breath. The nurse should **first**:
- [ ] 1. assess the oxygen saturation.
- [ ] 2. call the healthcare provider (HCP).
- [ ] 3. administer morphine sulfate, 2 mg IV.
- [ ] 4. perform range-of-motion exercises in the involved leg.

66. The nurse is caring for a client with venous thrombosis of the left lower extremity. To prevent further tissue damage, it is important for the nurse to observe for which finding?
- [ ] 1. blood pressure and heart rate changes
- [ ] 2. gradual or acute loss of sensory and motor function
- [ ] 3. metabolic acidosis
- [ ] 4. swelling in the left lower extremity

67. A client with venous thrombus reports having pain in the legs. What should the nurse do **first**?
- [ ] 1. Elevate the foot of the bed.
- [ ] 2. Elevate the legs by using a pillow under the knees.
- [ ] 3. Encourage adequate fluid intake.
- [ ] 4. Massage the lower legs.

68. A 45-year-old client had a complete abdominal hysterectomy with bilateral salpingo-oophorectomy 2 days ago. The client's abdominal dressing is dry and intact. While sitting up in the chair, the client has severe pain and numbness in her left leg. The nurse should **first**:
- [ ] 1. administer pain medication.
- [ ] 2. assess edema in the left leg.
- [ ] 3. assess color and temperature of the left leg.
- [ ] 4. encourage the client to change her position.

69. A client who is being discharged after a hospitalization for thrombophlebitis will be riding home in a car. During the 2-hour ride, what should the nurse advise the client to do?
- [ ] 1. Perform arm circles while riding in the car.
- [ ] 2. Perform ankle pumps and foot range-of-motion exercises.
- [ ] 3. Elevate the legs while riding in the car.
- [ ] 4. Take an ambulance home.

70. A client with a cerebral embolus is receiving streptokinase. The nurse should evaluate the client for which expected therapeutic outcomes of this drug therapy?
- [ ] 1. improved cerebral perfusion
- [ ] 2. decreased vascular permeability
- [ ] 3. dissolved emboli
- [ ] 4. prevention of cerebral hemorrhage

71. A client who weighs 187 lb (85 kg) has a prescription to receive enoxaparin 1 mg/kg. This drug is available in a concentration of 30 mg/0.3 mL. What dose would the nurse administer in milliliters? Record your answer to two decimal points.
_____ mL.

72. A client is on complete bed rest. The nurse should initiate measures to prevent which complication of bed rest?
- [ ] 1. air embolus
- [ ] 2. fat embolus
- [ ] 3. stress fractures
- [ ] 4. thrombophlebitis

73. Knee-high sequential compression devices have been prescribed for a newly admitted client. The client reports new pain localized in the right calf area that is noted to be slightly reddened and warm to touch upon initial assessment. What should the nurse do **first**?
- ☐ 1. Offer analgesics as prescribed, and apply the compression devices.
- ☐ 2. Leave the compression devices off, and contact the healthcare provider (HCP) to report the assessment findings.
- ☐ 3. Massage the area of discomfort before applying the compression devices.
- ☐ 4. Leave the compression devices off, and report assessment findings to the oncoming shift.

74. A client is receiving an IV infusion of 5% dextrose in water (D_5W). The skin around the IV insertion site is red, warm to touch, and painful. The nurse should **first**:
- ☐ 1. administer acetaminophen.
- ☐ 2. change the D_5W to normal saline.
- ☐ 3. discontinue the IV.
- ☐ 4. place a warm compress on the area.

75. The nurse is planning care for a client on complete bed rest. The plan of care should include all **except**:
- ☐ 1. turning every 2 hours.
- ☐ 2. passive and active range-of-motion exercises.
- ☐ 3. use of thromboembolic disease (TED) support hose.
- ☐ 4. maintaining the client in the supine position.

76. The client is admitted with left lower leg pain, a positive Homans' sign, and a temperature of 100.4°F (38°C). The nurse should assess the client further for signs of:
- ☐ 1. aortic aneurysm.
- ☐ 2. deep vein thrombosis (DVT) in the left leg.
- ☐ 3. IV drug abuse.
- ☐ 4. intermittent claudication.

77. A client is admitted with a diagnosis of thrombophlebitis and deep vein thrombosis of the right leg. A loading dose of heparin has been given in the emergency department, and IV heparin will be continued for the next several days. The nurse should develop a plan of care for this client that will involve:
- ☐ 1. administering aspirin as prescribed.
- ☐ 2. encouraging green leafy vegetables in the diet.
- ☐ 3. monitoring the client's prothrombin time (PT).
- ☐ 4. monitoring the client's activated partial thromboplastin time (aPTT) and international normalized ratio (INR).

78. In order to prevent deep vein thrombosis (DVT) following abdominal surgery, the nurse should:
- ☐ 1. limit fluids to 1,000 mL in 24 hours.
- ☐ 2. encourage deep breathing.
- ☐ 3. assist the client to remain sedentary.
- ☐ 4. use pneumatic compression stockings.

79. A client diagnosed with a deep vein thrombosis has heparin sodium infusing at 1,500 units/h. The concentration of heparin is 25,000 units/500 mL. If the infusion remains at the same rate for a full 12-hour shift, how many milliliters of fluid will infuse? Round your answer to a whole number.

_____ mL.

80. The nurse interviews a 22-year-old female client who is scheduled for abdominal surgery the following week. The client is obese and uses estrogen-based oral contraceptives. This client is at high risk for development of:
- ☐ 1. atherosclerosis.
- ☐ 2. diabetes.
- ☐ 3. Raynaud's disease.
- ☐ 4. thrombophlebitis.

81. A client weighs 300 lb (136 kg) and has a history of deep vein thrombosis and thrombophlebitis. When coaching a client about behaviors to maintain health, the nurse determines that the client has understood the nurse's instructions when the client states a willingness to:
- ☐ 1. limit exercise that involves walking.
- ☐ 2. lose weight by following a reduced-calorie, balanced diet.
- ☐ 3. perform leg lifts every 4 hours to strengthen hamstring muscles.
- ☐ 4. wear knee-high stockings, rolled at the top to hold the stockings up.

82. Which instructions should the nurse include when developing a teaching plan for a client being discharged from the hospital on anticoagulant therapy after having deep vein thrombosis (DVT)? Select all that apply.
- ☐ 1. Check urine for bright blood and a dark smoky color.
- ☐ 2. Walk daily as a good exercise.
- ☐ 3. Use garlic and ginger, which may decrease bleeding time.
- ☐ 4. Perform foot/leg exercises and walking around the airplane cabin when on long flights.
- ☐ 5. Prevent DVT because of risk of pulmonary emboli.
- ☐ 6. Avoid surface bumps because the skin is prone to injury.

83. A client has an emergency embolectomy for an embolus in the femoral artery. After the client returns from the recovery room, in what order, from first to last, should the nurse provide care? All options must be used.

1. Administer pain medication.

2. Draw blood for laboratory studies.

3. Regulate the IV infusion.

4. Monitor the pulses.

5. Inspect the dressing.

84. A client with deep vein thrombosis has been receiving warfarin for 2 months. The client is to go to an anticoagulant monitoring laboratory every 3 weeks. The last visit to the laboratory was 2 weeks ago. The client reports bleeding gums, increased bruising, and dark stools. What should the nurse instruct the client to do?
- ☐ 1. Decrease the dose of the warfarin.
- ☐ 2. Return to laboratory for analysis of prothrombin times.
- ☐ 3. Decrease the amount of vitamin K in the diet.
- ☐ 4. Notify the healthcare provider (HCP) about the bleeding.

The Client with Varicose Veins

85. A client is talking with the nurse about unsightly varicose veins and their discomfort. What information should the nurse provide to the client?
- ☐ 1. Avoid walking to reduce the discomfort.
- ☐ 2. Keep the legs elevated when sitting or lying down.
- ☐ 3. Sclerotherapy can be used for cosmetic improvement.
- ☐ 4. Contact a surgeon to perform a femoral-popliteal bypass graft.

86. The nurse is teaching a group of women about risk for varicose veins. Which client is at risk for varicose veins?
- ☐ 1. a client who has had a cerebrovascular accident
- ☐ 2. a client who has had anemia
- ☐ 3. a client who has had thrombophlebitis
- ☐ 4. a client who has had transient ischemic attacks

87. A client is to have sclerotherapy to treat varicose veins. The nurse should instruct the client that this procedure:
- ☐ 1. causes the veins to fade and disappear.
- ☐ 2. ensures that varicosities will not occur again.
- ☐ 3. requires a short hospitalization for complete recovery.
- ☐ 4. results in bruising lasting for 2 weeks.

88. A clinically obese client with moderately painful varicose veins chooses self-care options for managing the varicosities. The nurse should coach the client to follow which healthcare practices? Select all that apply.
- ☐ 1. Lose weight.
- ☐ 2. Wear compression stockings.
- ☐ 3. Apply lotion to the veins.
- ☐ 4. Elevate the legs.
- ☐ 5. Sleep with pillows under the knees.

The Client with Stasis Ulcers

89. A well-nourished client is admitted with a stasis ulcer. The nurse assesses the ulcer and finds excavation of the skin surface as a result of sloughing of inflammatory necrotic tissue. The healthcare provider (HCP) has prescribed the ulcer to be flushed with a fibrinolytic agent. Which goals are appropriate for this client? Select all that apply.
- ☐ 1. Increase oxygen to the tissues.
- ☐ 2. Prevent direct trauma to the ulcer.
- ☐ 3. Improve nutrition.
- ☐ 4. Prevent infection.
- ☐ 5. Reduce pain.

90. A client has had a stasis ulcer of the left ankle with 2+ pitting edema for 2 years. The client is taking chlorothiazide. The desired outcome of this drug for this client is:
- ☐ 1. improved capillary circulation.
- ☐ 2. decreased blood pressure.
- ☐ 3. wound healing.
- ☐ 4. absence of infection.

91. The nurse assesses a client with a 5 × 2 stasis ulcer just above the left malleolus. The wound is open with irregular, reddened, swollen edges, and there is a moderate amount of yellowish tan drainage coming from the wound. The client verbalizes pressure-type pain and rates the discomfort at 7 on a scale of 0 to 10. To maintain tissue integrity, the **primary** nursing goal should focus on:
☐ 1. administering prescribed analgesics.
☐ 2. applying lanolin lotions to the left ankle stasis ulcer.
☐ 3. encouraging the client to sit up in a chair four times per day.
☐ 4. keeping pressure of bed linens off the area.

92. In preparation for being discharged to home, the nurse is teaching a client with a chronic right ankle stasis ulcer about wound care. The client needs further teaching when the client states: "I will:
☐ 1. make an appointment with a physical therapist."
☐ 2. apply a home herb mixture to the wound to promote healing."
☐ 3. be patient with the healing process."
☐ 4. eat a balanced diet."

Managing Care, Quality, and Safety for Clients with Vascular Disease

93. The nurse has received a change of shift report about clients. Which client should the nurse assess **first**?
☐ 1. a client with chronic heart failure with right upper quadrant fullness
☐ 2. a client in atrial fibrillation with a heart rate of 90 with a "fluttering" feeling
☐ 3. a client with peripheral artery disease (PAD) just returning from an angiogram
☐ 4. a client who had coronary artery bypass surgery 2 days ago who reports having incisional pain of "3" out of "10"

94. A client with a history of hypertension and peripheral vascular disease underwent an aorto-bifemoral bypass graft. Preoperative medications included pentoxifylline, metoprolol, and furosemide. On postoperative day 1, the 1200 vital signs are as follows: temperature 98.9°F (37.2°C), heart rate 132 bpm, respiratory rate 20 breaths/min, and blood pressure 126/78 mm Hg. Urine output is 50 to 70 mL/h. The hemoglobin and the hematocrit are stable. The medications have not been prescribed for administration after surgery. Using the SBAR (Situation-Background-Assessment-Recommendation) technique for communication, the nurse contacts the healthcare provider (HCP) and recommends to:
☐ 1. continue the pentoxifylline.
☐ 2. increase the IV fluids.
☐ 3. restart the metoprolol.
☐ 4. resume the furosemide.

95. The nurse is planning care for a client who had surgery for abdominal aortic aneurysm repair 2 days ago. The pain medication and the use of relaxation and imagery techniques are not relieving the client's pain, and the client refuses to get out of bed to ambulate as prescribed. The nurse contacts the healthcare provider (HCP), explains the situation, and provides information about drug dose, frequency of administration, the client's vital signs, and the client's score on the pain scale. The nurse requests a prescription for a different, or stronger, pain medication. The HCP tells the nurse that the current prescription for pain medication is sufficient for this client and that the client will feel better in several days. The nurse should **next**:
☐ 1. explain to the HCP that the current pain medication and other strategies are not helping the client and it is making it difficult for the client to ambulate as prescribed.
☐ 2. ask the surgical resident to write a prescription for a stronger pain medication.
☐ 3. wait until the next shift and ask the nurse on that shift to contact the HCP.
☐ 4. report the incident to the team leader.

96. The nurse is making the client assignment for a group of clients. The personnel include the registered nurse (RN), a licensed practical/vocational nurse (LPN/VN), and an unlicensed assistive personnel (UAP). Which client would the nurse assign to the LPN/VN?
☐ 1. a client who is undergoing femoropopliteal bypass graft surgery this morning and needs the preoperative check list completed
☐ 2. a stable client with thrombophlebitis of the lower left extremity with limited mobility and requiring a complete bed bath
☐ 3. a client with a palpable abdominal mass, painful lower extremities, and a decreasing BP
☐ 4. a client with intermittent claudication who needs frequent assistance with getting out of bed and ambulating

97. The nurse is obtaining a blood sample for a partial thromboplastin time test prescribed for a client who is taking heparin. It is 0500 when drawing the blood. What should the nurse do? Select all that apply.
☐ 1. Awake the client.
☐ 2. Check the armband for client identification number and compare with the prescription.
☐ 3. Label the sample vial in front of the client.
☐ 4. Verify the room number with the room assignment.
☐ 5. Ask the client to state his/her name.

98. A client has acute arterial occlusion. The healthcare provider (HCP) has prescribed IV heparin. **Before** starting the medication, the nurse should:

☐ 1. review the blood coagulation laboratory values.
☐ 2. test the client's stools for occult blood.
☐ 3. count the client's apical pulse for 1 minute.
☐ 4. check the 24-hour urine output record.

99. The nurse is caring for a client who has a below-the-knee amputation. The client has been somewhat confused since returning from surgery last evening but has no history of falls. The client is receiving intravenous antibiotics intermittently through a peripheral IV and has prescriptions to be up with physical therapy only. Using the Morse Fall Risk Scale (see scale), what is this client's total score and risk level?

Morse Fall Risk/Scale

Item	Scale		Scoring
1. History of falling; immediate or within 3 months	No	0	
	Yes	25	
2. Secondary diagnosis	No	0	
	Yes	15	
3 Ambulatory aid			
Bed rest/nurse assist		0	
Crutches/cane/walker		15	
Furniture		30	
4. IV/Heparin Lock	No	0	
	Yes	20	
5. Gait/Transferring			
Normal/bedrest/ immobile Weak		0	
		10	
Impaired		20	
6. Mental status			
Oriented to own ability		0	
Forgets limitations		15	

☐ 1. 20, low risk
☐ 2. 30, medium risk
☐ 3. 40, medium risk
☐ 4. 50, high risk

Answers, Rationales, and Test-Taking Strategies

*The answers and rationales for each question follow below, along with keys (⚷) to the client need (CN) and cognitive level (CL) for each question. In addition, you will also see a glossary icon (📖) highlighting specific terminology used on the licensing exam. As you check your answers, use the **Content Mastery and Test-Taking Skill Self-Analysis** worksheet (tear-out worksheet in back of book) to identify the reason(s) for not answering the questions correctly. For additional information about test-taking skills and strategies for answering questions, refer to pages 12–23 and pages 35–36 in Part 1 of this book.*

The Client with Peripheral Artery Disease

1. 1,3,4. Smoking and exposure to the cold cause vasoconstriction and should be avoided. Aspirin and clopidogrel should be taken as prescribed for the antiplatelet properties. Using extra bed clothes at night provides warmth, which increases vasodilation. The presence of pain should be investigated as it could indicate increasing arterial insufficiency. Tight socks should be avoided as they could impair circulation.

⚷ CN: Health promotion and maintenance; CL: Synthesis

2. 1. The ABI test is a noninvasive test that compares the systolic blood pressure in the arm with that of the ankle. It may be done before or after exercise. The client's highest brachial systolic pressure is divided by the left ankle systolic blood pressure to get 0.81. This score is between 0.71 and 0.90, which suggests mild peripheral artery disease. Moderate peripheral artery disease would yield a score of 0.41 to 0.70. Severe peripheral artery disease would result in a score of 0.00 to 0.40.

⚷ CN: Physiological adaptation; CL: Analyze

3. 3. Keeping the involved extremity at or below the body's horizontal plane will facilitate tissue perfusion and prevent tissue damage. The nurse should avoid placing the affected extremity on a hard surface, such as a firm mattress, to avoid pressure ulcers. In addition, the involved extremity should be free from heavy overlying bed linens. The nurse should handle the involved extremity in a gentle fashion to prevent friction or pressure. Raising the leg would cause occlusion to the iliac artery, which is contrary to the goal to promote arterial circulation.

⚷ CN: Physiological adaptation; CL: Synthesize

4. 1,3. Discharge teaching begins when the client enters the hospital. One of the risk factors for clot formation is a sedentary lifestyle, and the client should engage in daily aerobic activity, such as biking or swimming (non–weight bearing). The client is also overweight and should plan to control the weight through dietary counseling or attending weight management programs in the community. Strength training is beneficial by increasing strength and lean body mass, but not helpful in preventing vascular disease. Stress management is not a focus based on the client's needs at this time. It is not necessary to wear special supportive shoes; comfortable shoes for walking are adequate.

⚷ CN: Health promotion and maintenance; CL: Create

5. The nurse should assess the femoral artery. Weak or absent femoral pulses are symptomatic of aortoiliac disease.

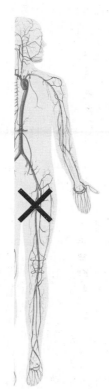

⚷ CN: Physiological adaptation; CL: Analyze

6. 4. An ankle-brachial index of 0.65 suggests moderate arterial vascular disease in a client who is experiencing intermittent claudication. A Doppler ultrasound is indicated for further evaluation. The bradycardic heart rate is acceptable in an athletic client with a normal blood pressure. The SpO_2 is acceptable; the client has a smoking history.

⚷ CN: Physiological adaptation; CL: Analyze

7. 2. With each set of vital signs, the nurse should assess the dorsalis pedis and posterior tibial pulses. The nurse needs to ensure adequate perfusion to the lower extremity with the drop in blood pressure. IV fluids, nasal cannula setting, and capillary refill are important to assess; however, priority is to determine the cause of drop in blood pressure and that adequate perfusion through the new graft is maintained.

⚷ CN: Reduction of risk potential; CL: Analyze

8. 1,2,3,5. Maintaining skin integrity is important in preventing chronic ulcers and infections. The client should be taught to inspect the skin on a daily basis. The client should reduce weight to promote circulation; a diet lower in calories and fat is appropriate. Because the client is receiving warfarin, the client is at risk for bleeding from cuts. To decrease the risk of cuts, the nurse should suggest that the client use an electric razor. The client with decreased arterial blood flow should be encouraged to participate in ADLs. In fact, the client should be encouraged to consult an exercise physiologist for an exercise program that enhances the aerobic capacity of the body.

⚷ CN: Health promotion and maintenance; CL: Synthesize

9. 3. Weakness, dizziness, and headache are common adverse effects of clopidogrel, and the client should report these to the **healthcare provider (HCP)** 📖 if they are problematic; in order to decrease risk of clot formation, the drug must be taken regularly and should not be stopped or taken intermittently. The main adverse effect of clopidogrel is bleeding, which often occurs as increased bruising or bleeding when brushing teeth. Clopidogrel is well absorbed, and while food may help decrease potential gastrointestinal upset, the drug may be taken with or without food. Clopidogrel is an antiplatelet agent used to prevent clot formation in clients who have experienced or are at risk for myocardial infarction, ischemic stroke, peripheral artery disease, or acute coronary syndrome.

⚷ CN: Pharmacological and parenteral therapies; CL: Evaluate

10. 3. Cilostazol is indicated for management of intermittent claudication. Symptoms usually improve within 2 to 4 weeks of therapy. Intermittent claudication prevents clients from walking for long periods of time. Cilostazol inhibits platelet aggregation induced by various stimuli and improving blood flow to the muscles and allowing the client to walk long distances without pain. Peripheral artery disease causes pain mainly of the leg muscles. "Aches and pains" does not specify exactly where the pain is occurring. Headaches may occur as a side effect of this drug, and the client should report this information to the **healthcare provider (HCP)** 📖. Peripheral artery disease causes decreased blood supply to the peripheral tissues and may cause gangrene of the toes; the drug is effective when the toes are warm to the touch and the color of the toes is similar to the color of the body.

   🔑 CN: Pharmacological and parenteral therapies; CL: Evaluate

11. 4. Decreased blood flow is a common characteristic of all peripheral artery disease. When the demand for oxygen to the working muscles becomes greater than the supply, pain is the outcome. The nurse should suggest that the client enroll in a supervised exercise training program that will assist the client to gradually increase walking distances without pain. Not walking and resting will not increase blood flow to the legs. Support stockings may be prescribed, but the client should improve the capacity to walk and obtain exercise.

   🔑 CN: Reduction of risk potential; CL: Apply

12. The nurse palpates the dorsalis pedis; if the pulse is obtained in that artery, the tibioperoneal artery is patent.

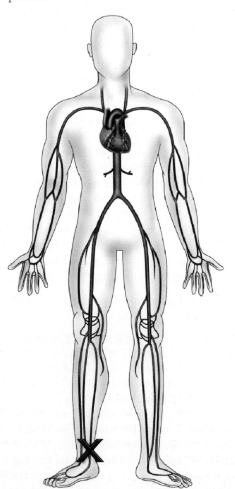

13. 4.

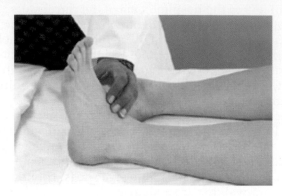

The presence of a strong dorsalis pedis pulse indicates that there is circulation to the extremity distal to the surgery indicating that the graft between the femoral and popliteal artery is allowing blood to circulate effectively. Answer 1 shows the nurse obtaining the radial pulse; answer 2 shows the femoral pulse, which is proximal to the surgery site and will not indicate circulation distal to the surgery site. Answer 3 shows the nurse obtaining an apical pulse.

   🔑 CN: Reduction of risk potential; CL: Analyze

14. 2,4. Reduction of blood flow to a specific area results in decreased oxygen and nutrients. As a result, the skin may appear mottled. The skin will also be cool to the touch. Loss of hair and dry skin are other signs that the nurse may observe in a client with peripheral artery disease of the lower extremities.

   🔑 CN: Health promotion and maintenance; CL: Analyze

15. 3. When pedal pulses are not palpable, the nurse should obtain a Doppler ultrasound device. Auscultation is not likely to be helpful if the pulse is not palpable. Inspection of the lower extremity can be done simultaneously when palpating, but the nurse should first try to locate a pulse by Doppler. Calling the **HCP** 📖 may be necessary if there is a change in the client's condition.

   🔑 CN: Physiological adaptation; CL: Synthesize

16. 4. Coldness in the left foot and ankle is consistent with complete arterial obstruction. Other expected findings would include paralysis and pallor. Aching pain, a burning sensation, or numbness and tingling are earlier signs of tissue hypoxia and ischemia and are commonly associated with incomplete obstruction.

   🔑 CN: Physiological adaptation; CL: Analyze

17. **2,4,3,1.** Because assessment of the presence and quality of the pedal pulses in the affected extremity is essential after surgery to make sure that the bypass graft is functioning, this step should be done **first**. The nurse should next ensure that the dressing is intact and then that the client has adequate urine output. Lastly, the nurse should determine the client's level of pain.

CN: Physiological adaptation; CL: Synthesize

18. **3.** Decreasing venous congestion in the extremities is a desired outcome for clients with heart failure. The nurse should elevate the client's legs. It is not necessary for the client to return to bed. Support stockings are not indicated at this time. The client is not having difficulty breathing or other signs of distress; it is not necessary to take the vital signs.

CN: Health promotion and maintenance; CL: Synthesize

19. **3.** The term *gangrene* refers to blackened, decomposing tissue that is devoid of circulation. Chronic ischemia and death of the tissue can lead to gangrene in the affected extremity. Injury, edema, and decreased circulation lead to infection, gangrene, and tissue death. Atrophy is the shrinking of tissue, and contraction is joint stiffening secondary to disuse. The term *rubor* denotes a reddish color of the skin.

CN: Physiological adaptation; CL: Analyze

20. **2.** Slow, steady walking is a recommended activity for clients with peripheral vascular disease because it stimulates the development of collateral circulation. The client with PVD should not remain inactive. Elevating the legs above the heart or wearing antiembolism stockings is a strategy for alleviating venous congestion and may worsen peripheral artery disease.

CN: Basic care and comfort; CL: Evaluate

21. **2.** Clients may have an immediate or a delayed reaction to the radiopaque dye. The HCP 📖 should be notified immediately because the symptoms suggest an allergic reaction. Treatment may involve administering oxygen and epinephrine. Explaining that the procedure is over does not address the current symptoms.

CN: Physiological adaptation; CL: Synthesize

22. **3.** The client is at greater risk for skin breakdown in the lower extremities related to the edema and to remaining in one position, which increases capillary pressure. Turning the client every 1 to 2 hours promotes vasodilation and prevents vascular compression. Administering pain medication will not have an effect on skin integrity. Encouraging

fluids is not a direct intervention for maintaining skin integrity, although being well hydrated is a goal for most clients. Maintaining hygiene does influence skin integrity but is secondary in this situation.

CN: Physiological adaptation; CL: Synthesize

23. **4.** The client should avoid using iodine or over-the-counter medications. Iodine is a highly toxic solution. An individual who has known PVD should be seen by a **healthcare provider (HCP)** 📖 for treatment to avoid infection. The client with PVD should avoid heating pads and crossing the legs, and should wear leather shoes. A heating pad can cause injury, which, because of the decreased blood supply, can be difficult to heal. Crossing the legs can further impede blood flow. Leather shoes provide better protection.

CN: Health promotion and maintenance; CL: Evaluate

24. **1.** Maintaining circulation in the affected extremity after surgery is the focus of care. The graft can become occluded, and the client must be assessed frequently to determine whether the graft is patent. Preventing infection and relieving pain are important but are secondary to maintaining graft patency. Education should have taken place in the preoperative phase and then continued during the recovery phase.

CN: Physiological adaptation; CL: Synthesize

25. **1,3.** Elastic stockings (support hose) are used to promote circulation by preventing pooling of blood in the feet and legs. The stockings should be applied in the morning before the client gets out of bed. The stockings should be applied smoothly to avoid wrinkles, but the top should not be rolled down to avoid constriction of circulation. The stockings should be removed every 8 hours, and the client should elevate the legs for 15 minutes and reapply the stockings. Clean stockings should be applied daily or as needed.

CN: Health promotion and maintenance; CL: Create

26. **4.** If surgery is scheduled, the nurse should avoid venipunctures in the affected extremity. The goal should be to prevent unnecessary trauma and possible infection in the affected arm. Disruptions in skin integrity and even minor skin irritations can cause the surgery to be canceled. The nurse can continue to monitor the temperature and radial pulse in the affected arm; however, doing so is not the **priority**. Keeping the client warm is important but is not the **priority** at this time.

CN: Reduction of risk potential; CL: Analyze

27. 3. Nicotine causes vasospasm and impedes blood flow. Stopping smoking is the most significant lifestyle change the client can make. The client should eat low-fat foods as part of a balanced diet. The legs should not be elevated above the heart because this will impede arterial flow. The legs should be in a slightly dependent position. Jogging is not necessary and probably is not possible for many clients with arterial occlusive disease. A rehabilitation program that includes daily walking is suggested.

🔑 CN: Health promotion and maintenance; CL: Synthesize

28. 1. A change in the intensity of a pulse may be indicative of arterial closure and warrants immediate attention; the nurse should notify the **healthcare provider (HCP)** 📖 immediately. A pain level of 2 out of 10 is not uncommon from the catheter insertion site especially after the placement of a stent. Shiny and hairless skin is expected in clients with PAD. A client undergoing a catheterization may experience pain at the catheterization site as large-bore sheaths are placed in the femoral artery. Because people with PAD have poor circulation in their lower extremities, it is possible for them to develop leg ulcers. However, it is unlikely that the percutaneous transluminal balloon angioplasty caused this.

🔑 CN: Physiological adaptation; CL: Analyze

29. 1,2,5. Turning frequently promotes circulation, while using pillows for support will prevent stress to the suture line. Short periods of different leg/body positions will not impair postoperative oxygen levels. The client should only be in a knee-flexed position when walking and not at rest. Prolonged sitting is discouraged, and it may cause pain and edema. It is not recommended that the leg be placed in a dependent position as this promotes edema. Placing a client in a supine position with the leg elevated above the heart is recommended only if the client develops edema.

🔑 CN: Physiological adaptation; CL: Synthesize

30. 4. Diltiazem is a calcium channel blocker that blocks the influx of calcium into the cell. In this situation, the primary use of diltiazem is to promote vasodilation and prevent spasms of the arteries. As a result of the vasodilation, blood, oxygen, and nutrients can reach the muscle and tissues. Diltiazem is not an antianxiety agent and does not promote sedation. It also does not cause vasoconstriction, which would be contraindicated for the client with peripheral vascular disease.

🔑 CN: Pharmacological and parenteral therapies; CL: Evaluate

31. 1. Although pentoxifylline's precise mechanism of action is unknown, its therapeutic effect is to increase blood flow, and the client should have improved circulation in the legs as evident by less pain. The client does not have nerve impairment and should be able to wiggle the toes. Urination is not improved by taking pentoxifylline. Dizziness is a side effect of the drug, not an intended outcome.

🔑 CN: Pharmacological and parenteral therapies; CL: Evaluate

32. 4. Pentoxifylline can potentiate the effects of theophylline and increase the risk of theophylline toxicity. Therefore, the nurse should monitor the client's theophylline level. Pentoxifylline does not interact with digoxin. Pentoxifylline can interact with heparin, and the client's PTT would need to be monitored closely if the client were taking heparin. It does not affect cholesterol levels.

🔑 CN: Pharmacological and parenteral therapies; CL: Analyze

33. 2. Angina is an adverse reaction to pentoxifylline, which should be used cautiously in clients with CAD. The nurse should report the client's symptoms to the **HCP** 📖, who may prescribe nitroglycerin and possibly discontinue the pentoxifylline. The client should rest until the chest pain subsides. It is not necessary at this point to initiate the **rapid response team** 📖 or start an intravenous infusion. The client's reports of symptoms should never be dismissed.

🔑 CN: Physiological adaptation; CL: Synthesize

34. 1. Assessing the individual's health behavior before surgery will help the nurse and client develop strategies to manage the postoperative course. Asking open-ended questions will elicit the most helpful information. The client's ability to walk will be improved after surgery. The client should report any changes in urination, but urinary retention is not expected before or after surgery.

🔑 CN: Health promotion and maintenance; CL: Create

35. 4. Before beginning dietary interventions, the nurse must assess the client's pattern of food intake, lifestyle, food preferences, and ethnic, cultural, and financial influences. With this information, the nurse can then discuss the client's knowledge about cholesterol, foods high in fat, cholesterol and sodium, and coach the client about the importance of following the diet plan.

🔑 CN: Basic care and comfort; CL: Synthesize

The Client with Peripheral Vascular Disease Having an Amputation

36. 2. Encouraging the client who is undergoing amputation to verbalize feelings is the **most** therapeutic nursing intervention. By eliciting concerns, the nurse may be able to provide information to help the client cope. The nurse should avoid value-laden responses, such as "You will still have one good leg," that may make the client feel guilty or hostile and block further communication. The nurse should not ignore the client's expressed concerns, nor should the nurse reinforce the client's concern about invalidism and dependency or assume that his wife is willing to care for him.

CN: Psychosocial integrity;
CL: Synthesize

37. 2. The level of amputation commonly cannot be accurately determined until surgery, when the surgeon can directly assess the adequacy of the circulation of the residual limb. A longer residual limb facilitates prosthesis fitting and will make it easier for the client to walk. However, although these aspects will be considered in the final decision, they are not the primary factors influencing the decision.

CN: Physiological adaptation;
CL: Synthesize

38. 1. Leg crossing is contraindicated because it causes adduction of the hips and decreases the flow of blood into the lower extremities. This may result in increased pressure in the graft in the affected leg. Elevating the legs, flexing the ankles, and extending the knees are not necessarily contraindicated.

CN: Reduction of risk potential;
CL: Synthesize

39. 2. The client should be evaluated for hemodynamic stability and extent of bleeding prior to calling the **HCP** 📖. Direct pressure can be used prior to applying a tourniquet if there is significant bleeding. To avoid flexion contractures, which can delay rehabilitation, elevation of the surgical limb is contraindicated.

CN: Reduction of risk potential;
CL: Synthesize

40. 3. The purpose of wrapping the residual limb is to shape the residual limb to accept a prosthesis and bear weight. The compression bandaging should be worn at all times for many weeks after surgery and should be reapplied as needed to keep it free of wrinkles and snug. The dressing should be changed daily to allow for inspection of the stump incision. No lotions should be applied to the stump unless specifically prescribed by the **healthcare provider (HCP)** 📖. The stump should not be elevated on pillows because this will contribute to the formation of flexion contractures. Contractures will prevent the client from wearing a prosthesis and ambulating.

CN: Physiological adaptation;
CL: Evaluate

The Client with an Aneurysm

41. 4. The underlying pathophysiology in this client is atherosclerosis. The findings from the assessment indicate the risk factors of smoking and high blood pressure. Therefore, tissue perfusion is a **priority** for health-promoting education. The data do not support education that focuses on food or fluid intake. Although edema is a potential problem and could contribute to poor skin integrity, the edema will likely be resolved by the aneurysm repair.

CN: Physiological adaptation;
CL: Synthesize

42. 1. The size of the thoracic aneurysm is rather large, so the nurse should anticipate rupture. A sudden incidence of pain may indicate leakage or rupture. The blood pressure and heart rate will provide useful information in assessing for hypovolemic shock. The nurse needs more data before initiating other interventions. After assessment of vital signs, neurologic status, and pain, the nurse can then contact the **HCP** 📖.

CN: Physiological adaptation;
CL: Synthesize

43. 2,4,3,1. The data suggest an abdominal aortic aneurysm that is leaking or rupturing. When implementing the prescriptions, the nurse should **first** establish an intravenous infusion with a large-bore needle for immediate volume replacement. Next, the nurse should insert the nasogastric tube to relieve the nausea and vomiting and decompress the stomach. The nurse next should administer pain medication. Last, the nurse should monitor intake and output; with hypovolemia, the urine output will be diminished.

CN: Physiological adaptation;
CL: Synthesize

44. 4. One of the complications of a thoracoabdominal aneurysm repair is spinal cord injury. Therefore, it is important for the nurse to assess for signs and symptoms of neurologic changes at and below the site where the aneurysm was repaired. The client is expected to have moderate pain following surgery. An elevated heart rate is expected after physical exertion. It is important to monitor urine output following aneurysm surgery, but a urine output of 2,000 mL in 24 hours is adequate following surgery.

CN: Safety and infection control;
CL: Synthesize

45. 3. The primary goal is to prepare the client for emergency surgery. The goal would be to prevent rupture of the aneurysm and potential death. Circulation is maintained, unless the aneurysm ruptures. When the client is prepared for surgery, the nurse should place the client in a recumbent position to promote circulation, teach the client about postoperative breathing exercises, and administer pain medication if prescribed.

CN: Physiological adaptation;
CL: Synthesize

46. 1. Cardiac tamponade is a life-threatening complication of a dissecting thoracic aneurysm. The sudden, painful "tearing" sensation is typically associated with the sudden release of blood, and the client may experience cardiac arrest. Stroke, pulmonary edema, and myocardial infarction are not common complications of a dissecting aneurysm.

CN: Physiological adaptation; CL: Apply

47. 1. Following surgical repair of an aortic aneurysm, there is a potential for an alteration in renal perfusion, manifested by decreased urine output. The altered renal perfusion may be related to renal artery embolism, prolonged hypotension, or prolonged aortic cross-clamping during surgery. Electrolyte imbalance and anxiety do not present imminent risk for this client; signs of wound infection are generally not evident immediately following surgery, but the nurse should monitor the incision on an ongoing basis.

CN: Physiological adaptation;
CL: Analyze

48. 4. The client is experiencing paralytic ileus. One of the adverse effects of morphine used to manage pain is decreased GI motility. Bowel manipulation and immobility also contribute to a postoperative ileus. Insertion of an NG tube generally prevents a postoperative ileus. The ice chips and IV fluids will not affect the ileus.

CN: Basic care and comfort; CL: Analyze

49. 3. The client with a synthetic graft may need to be treated with prophylactic antibiotics before undergoing major dental work. This reduces the danger of systemic infection caused by bacteria from the oral cavity. Venous access for drawing blood, IV line insertion, and x-rays do not contribute to the risk of infection.

CN: Pharmacological and parenteral therapies; CL: Synthesize

50. 3. A blood pressure of 80/50 mm Hg in a client who has just had surgical repair of an abdominal aortic aneurysm warrants further evaluation as this indicates decreased perfusion to the brain, heart, and kidneys. A BUN of 26 and a creatinine of 1.2 are normal findings. While +1 pedal pulses may be an abnormal finding, it is not uncommon, and it is important to compare this finding to previous assessments and note if this is a change of the strength of the pedal pulses. Absent bowel sound and mild abdominal distension are expected for a client immediately following surgery. However, this finding should be monitored as it could indicate a paralytic ileus.

CN: Physiological adaptation;
CL: Analyze

51. 4. A blood transfusion is required postoperatively with significant blood loss from surgery or bleeding. Data from the progress notes indicate the client is hypovolemic and has a low hemoglobin level, which warrants transfusion at this time rather than IV fluids. The nurse must continue to assess the client for signs of bleeding. Correction of hypovolemia precedes a dopamine infusion. The transfusion should improve the hemodynamics, and the hemoglobin and hematocrit are reassessed post transfusion. The client has fluid volume deficit, so furosemide is not needed at this time.

The Client with Raynaud's Phenomenon

52. 3. Clients with Raynaud's phenomenon should receive routine follow-up to monitor symptoms and to assess for the development of connective tissue or autoimmune diseases associated with Raynaud's. Beta-blockers are not considered first-line drug therapy. A sympathectomy is considered only in advanced cases. There is no benefit to an angioplasty, which is used for atherosclerotic vascular disease.

CN: Health promotion and maintenance;
CL: Create

53. 1,2,5. Vasospastic disorder (Raynaud's disease) is a form of intermittent arteriolar vasoconstriction that results in coldness, pain, and pallor of the fingertips, toes, or tip of the nose, and a rebound circulation with redness and pain. The nurse should instruct the client to stop smoking because nicotine is a vasoconstrictor. An adverse effect of reserpine is orthostatic hypotension. The client should report dizziness and low blood pressure as it may be necessary to consider stopping the drug. The client should prevent vasoconstriction by covering affected parts when in cold environments. The nurse can teach the client to rewarm exposed extremities by using warm water or placing them next to the body, such as under the axilla. It is not realistic to ask this client to change jobs at this time.

CN: Health promotion and maintenance;
CL: Create

54. 2. The client has numbness in the fingertips, and the nurse should **first** help the client regain sensory perception and discuss strategies for prevention of injury. The client does not have acute pain. The client does have adequate circulation and is not at risk for skin breakdown at this time.

🔑 CN: Physiological adaptation; CL: Analyze

55. 1. Vasospastic disorder (Raynaud's disease) is more common in young women and is associated with collagen diseases such as rheumatoid arthritis and lupus.

🔑 CN: Physiological adaptation; CL: Analyze

56. 3. Initially, the vasoconstriction effect produces pallor or a whitish coloring, followed by cyanosis (bluish) and finally rubor (red). Gangrene is the end result of complete arterial occlusion; the skin is blackened and without a blood supply.

🔑 CN: Reduction of risk potential; CL: Analyze

57. 2. Decreased perfusion from vasospasm induces color changes in the extremity. The degree of decreased perfusion should be assessed by taking the radial pulse. Color changes progressively to blue with cyanosis and then red when reperfusion occurs. The SpO$_2$ requires adequate perfusion for accuracy. A blood pressure will cause further constriction and reduction of perfusion in the extremity.

🔑 CN: Physiological adaptation; CL: Analyze

58. 3. Extreme changes in temperature can precipitate a vasospastic episode and should be avoided by clients with vasospastic disorder (Raynaud's disease). The client should be encouraged to wear gloves when handling frozen foods or ice. The client should immerse the involved extremity in warm water during an episode to promote vasodilation and relaxation of the small arteries that are in spasm. The client can help prevent vasospasm brought on by temperature changes by wearing warm clothes. Living in a cold climate will exacerbate the symptoms.

🔑 CN: Health promotion and maintenance; CL: Synthesize

59. 3. Loose warm clothing should be worn to protect from the cold. Wearing gloves when handling cold objects will help prevent vasospasms. Vibrating equipment and typing contribute to vasospasm. Tobacco and caffeine should be avoided. Elevation will decrease arterial perfusion during vasospasms.

🔑 CN: Health promotion and maintenance; CL: Synthesize

60. 3. Calcium channel blockers are first-line drug therapy for the treatment of vasospasms with Raynaud's phenomenon when other therapies are ineffective. Diltiazem relaxes smooth muscles and improves peripheral perfusion, thereby reducing finger numbness. Diltiazem decreases heart rate and is used to treat atrial fibrillation, but these are not associated with Raynaud's. When vasospasms are prevented, an accurate SpO$_2$ can be measured in the affected extremity; however, SpO$_2$ is a measurement of systemic oxygenation not influenced by diltiazem.

🔑 CN: Pharmacological and parenteral therapies; CL: Evaluate

61. 1. Beta-adrenergic medications block the beta-adrenergic receptors. Therefore, the expected outcome of the medication is to decrease the influence of the sympathetic nervous system on the blood vessels in the hands. Beta-adrenergic blockers have no analgesic effects. Increasing blood supply to the affected area is an indirect effect of beta-adrenergic blockers. They do not increase monoamine oxidase, which does not play a role in Raynaud's disease.

🔑 CN: Pharmacological and parenteral therapies; CL: Apply

62. 4. Sympathectomy is scheduled only after other treatment alternatives have been explored and have failed. Medication and stress management are beneficial strategies to prevent advancement of the disease process. If the disease is controlled by medication, there is no reason for surgery.

🔑 CN: Physiological adaptation; CL: Apply

The Client with Peripheral Venous Disease: Thrombophlebitis, Deep Vein Thrombosis, and Embolus Formation

63. 4. Based on the laboratory findings, prothrombin time and INR are at acceptable anticoagulation levels for the treatment of DVT. However, the platelets are below the acceptable level. Clients taking enoxaparin are at risk for thrombocytopenia. Because of the low platelet level, the nurse should withhold the enoxaparin and contact the **HCP** 📖. The nurse should not administer the drug until the HCP has been contacted. The HCP, not the pharmacist, will make the decision about the dose of the enoxaparin. The decision about administering the drug will be based on laboratory results, not evidence of bruising or bleeding.

🔑 CN: Pharmacological and parenteral therapies; CL: Synthesize

64. 1. Elevating the head of the bed facilitates breathing because the lungs are able to expand as the diaphragm descends. Coughing and deep breathing do not alleviate the symptoms of a pulmonary embolus, nor does lung auscultation. The **HCP** 📖 must be kept informed of changes in a client's status, but the priority in this case is alleviating the symptoms.

🗝 CN: Reduction of risk potential; CL: Synthesize

65. 1. A client with deep vein thrombosis (DVT) is at high risk for a pulmonary embolism from an embolus traveling to the lung. Sudden onset of symptoms and worsening of chest pain with a deep breath suggest a pulmonary embolism. The nurse assesses the client and obtains oxygen saturation levels prior to calling the **HCP** 📖 and administering morphine. Range of motion is a preventive measure for DVT and is not appropriate that this time.

🗝 CN: Reduction of risk potential; CL: Synthesize

66. 2. Acute arterial occlusion is a sudden interruption of blood flow. The interruption can be the result of complete or partial obstruction. Acute pain, loss of sensory and motor function, and a pale, mottled, numb extremity are the most dramatic and observable changes that indicate a life-threatening interruption of tissue perfusion. Blood pressure and heart rate changes may be associated with the acute pain episode. Metabolic acidosis is a complication of irreversible ischemia. Swelling may result but may also indicate venous stasis or arterial insufficiency.

🗝 CN: Physiological adaptation; CL: Analyze

67. 1. Venous stasis can increase pain. Therefore, proper positioning in bed with the foot of the bed elevated or when sitting up in a chair can help promote venous drainage, reduce swelling, and reduce the amount of pain the client might experience. Placing a pillow under the knees causes flexion of the joint, resulting in a dependent position of the lower leg and causing a decrease in blood flow. Fluids are encouraged to maintain normal fluid and electrolyte balance but do little to relieve pain. Therapeutic massage to the legs is discouraged because of the danger of breaking up the clot.

🗝 CN: Basic care and comfort; CL: Synthesize

68. 3. The client is likely suffering from an embolus as a result of abdominal surgery. The nurse should inspect the left leg for color and temperature changes associated with tissue perfusion. Administering pain medication without gathering more information about the pain can mask important signs and symptoms. Although assessing for edema is important, it is not critical to this situation. Encouraging the client to change her position does not adequately address the need for gathering more data.

🗝 CN: Reduction of risk potential; CL: Synthesize

69. 2. Performing active ankle and foot range-of-motion exercises periodically during the ride home will promote muscular contraction and provide support to the venous system. It is the muscular action that facilitates return of the blood from the lower extremities, especially when in the dependent position. Arm circle exercises will not promote circulation in the leg. It is not necessary for the client to elevate the legs as long as the client does not occlude blood flow to the legs and does the leg exercises. It is not necessary to take an ambulance because the client is able to sit in the car safely.

🗝 CN: Reduction of risk potential; CL: Synthesize

70. 3. Thrombolytic agents such as streptokinase are used for clients with a history of thrombus formation, cerebrovascular accidents, and chronic atrial fibrillation. The thrombolytic agents act by dissolving emboli. Thrombolytic agents do not directly improve perfusion or increase vascular permeability, nor do they prevent cerebral hemorrhage.

🗝 CN: Pharmacological and parenteral therapies; CL: Evaluate

71. 0.85 mL. The prescription is for the client to receive enoxaparin 1 mg/kg. Therefore, the client is to receive 85 mg. The desired dose in milliliters then can be calculated by using the formula of desired dose (D) divided by dose or strength of dose on hand (H) times volume (V).

$$85 (mg) \times 0.3\, mL = 25.5\, mg/mL$$

$$25.5\, mg \div 30 = 0.85\, mL$$

🗝 CN: Pharmacological and parenteral therapies; CL: Apply

72. 4. Thrombophlebitis is an inflammation of a vein. The underlying etiology involves stasis of blood, increased blood coagulability, and vessel wall injury. The symptoms of thrombophlebitis are pain, swelling, and deep muscle tenderness. Air embolus is a result of air entering the vascular system. Fat embolus is associated with the presence of intracellular fat globules in the lung parenchyma and peripheral circulation after long-bone fractures. Stress fractures are associated with the musculoskeletal system.

🗝 CN: Health promotion and maintenance; CL: Analyze

73. **2.** Localized pain, tenderness, redness, and warmth may be symptoms of deep vein thrombosis (DVT), information the nurse should report to the **HCP** []; the compression devices should not be applied until further evaluation is completed as intermittent compression may dislodge a thrombus. Massaging the area may dislodge a thrombus and is not recommended. The nurse may offer PRN analgesics if the client requires pain management, but the compression devices should not be applied until further evaluation is completed. Diagnosis and treatment of DVT should be discussed with the HCP as soon as possible; the nurse should not wait until the next shift to report findings as a DVT can become life threatening if a thrombus travels to the lung and becomes a pulmonary embolus.

    CN: Reduction of risk potential; CL: Synthesize

74. **3.** The first action should be to discontinue the IV. The nurse should restart the IV elsewhere and then apply a warm compress to the affected area. The nurse should administer acetaminophen or an anti-inflammatory agent only if prescribed by the **healthcare provider (HCP)** []. The type of infusion cannot be changed without an HCP's prescription, and such a change would not help in this case.

    CN: Reduction of risk potential; CL: Synthesize

75. **4.** Three factors contribute to the formation of venous thrombus and thrombophlebitis: damage to the inner lining of the vein (prolonged pressure), hypercoagulability of the blood, and venous stasis. Bed rest and immobilization are associated with decreased blood flow and venous pooling in the lower extremities. Keeping the client in the supine position would not be appropriate. Turning the client every 1 to 2 hours, passive and active range-of-motion exercises, and use of TED hose help prevent venous stasis in the lower extremities.

    CN: Reduction of risk potential; CL: Create

76. **2.** The client demonstrates classic symptoms of DVT, and the nurse should continue to assess the client. Signs and symptoms of an aortic aneurysm include abdominal pain and a pulsating abdominal mass. Clients with drug abuse demonstrate confusion and decreased levels of consciousness. Claudication is an intermittent pain in the leg.

    CN: Psychosocial integrity; CL: Analyze

77. **4.** Heparin dosage is usually determined by the **healthcare provider (HCP)** [] based on the client's aPTT and INR laboratory values. Therefore, the nurse monitors these values to prevent complications. Administering aspirin when the client is on heparin is contraindicated. Green leafy vegetables are high in vitamin K and therefore are not recommended for clients receiving heparin. Monitoring of the client's PT is done when the client is receiving warfarin sodium.

    CN: Pharmacological and parenteral therapies; CL: Create

78. **4.** The use of pneumatic compression stockings is an intervention used to prevent DVT. Other strategies include early ambulation, leg exercises if the client is confined to bed, adequate fluid intake, and administering anticoagulant medication as prescribed. Deep breathing would be encouraged postoperatively, but it does not prevent DVT.

    CN: Health promotion and maintenance; CL: Synthesize

79. 360 mL

$$25{,}000 \text{ U} / 500 \text{ mL} = 50 \text{ U} / \text{mL}$$
$$1 \text{ mL} / 50 \text{ U} \times 1500 \text{ U} / \text{h} = 30 \text{ mL} / \text{h} \times 12 \text{ h}$$
$$= 360 \text{ mL}$$

    CN: Pharmacological and parenteral therapies; CL: Apply

80. **4.** The data suggest an increased risk of thrombophlebitis. The risk factors in this situation include abdominal surgery, obesity, and use of estrogen-based oral contraceptives. Risk factors for atherosclerosis include genetics, older age, and a high-cholesterol diet. Risk factors for diabetes include genetics and obesity. Risk factors for vasospastic disorders include cold climate, age (16 to 40), and immunologic disorders.

    CN: Reduction of risk potential; CL: Analyze

81. **2.** The client is at risk for development of varicose veins. Therefore, prevention is key in the treatment plan. Maintaining ideal body weight is the goal. In order to achieve this, the client should consume a balanced diet and participate in a regular exercise program. Performing leg lifts improves muscle strength, but it is more important for the client to increase exercise by walking. Wearing support stockings is helpful to promote circulation, but the client should not roll the stockings at the top to hold the stockings up as this will decrease circulation at the knees.

    CN: Reduction of risk potential; CL: Evaluate

82. 1,2,4,5,6. Clients with resolving DVT being sent home on anticoagulant therapy need instructions about assessing and preventing bleeding episodes and preventing a recurrence of DVT. Blood in the urine (hematuria) is often one of the first symptoms of anticoagulant overdose. Fresh blood in the urine is red; however, blood in the urine may also be a dark smoky color. Daily ambulation is an excellent activity to keep the venous blood circulating and thus to prevent blood clots from forming in the lower extremities. Garlic and ginger increase the bleeding time and should not be used when a client is on anticoagulant therapy. Clients who have had previous DVTs should avoid activities that cause stagnation and pooling of venous blood. Prolonged sitting coupled with change of air pressure without foot or leg exercises or ambulation in the cabin are activities that prevent venous return. Instructing the client about prevention measures is important because clients with DVT are at high risk for pulmonary emboli (PE), which can be fatal. The client can be taught risk factors for DVT and PE. In addition, recommendations for prevention of these events also are standard protocol in practice and should be shared with the client for home care purposes. Older adults should be monitored closely for bleeding because the skin becomes thinner and the capillaries become more fragile with the aging process.

⚷ CN: Health promotion and maintenance; CL: Create

83. 4,5,3,1,2. The nurse should first monitor the popliteal and the pedal pulses in the affected extremity after arterial embolectomy. Monitoring peripheral pulses below the site of occlusion checks the arterial circulation in the involved extremity. The nurse should next inspect the dressing to be sure that the client is not bleeding at the surgical site. The nurse should next regulate the IV infusion to prevent fluid overload. Then the nurse should assess pain and administer pain medications as prescribed. Last, the nurse can obtain blood for laboratory studies.

⚷ CN: Physiological adaptation; CL: Synthesize

84. 2. These symptoms suggest that the client is receiving too much warfarin; the client should return to the laboratory and have a blood sample drawn to determine the prothrombin levels and have the dosage of warfarin adjusted. The diet can influence clotting, but the client needs to first have the prothrombin levels checked. It is not necessary to contact the HCP 🖵; the client should return to the laboratory first, and the results of the prothrombin time will be reported to the HCP.

⚷ CN: Pharmacological and parenteral therapies; CL: Evaluate

The Client with Varicose Veins

85. 2. The nurse instructs the client to elevate the legs to improve venous return and alleviate discomfort. Walking is encouraged to increase venous return. Sclerotherapy or laser treatment is done for cosmetic reasons, but it does not improve circulation. Surgery may be performed for severe venous insufficiency or recurrent thrombophlebitis in the varicosities. Femoral-popliteal bypass graft is a surgical intervention for arterial disease.

⚷ CN: Health promotion and maintenance; CL: Synthesize

86. 3. Secondary varicosities can result from previous thrombophlebitis of the deep femoral veins, with subsequent valvular incompetence. Cerebrovascular accident, anemia, and transient ischemic attacks are not associated with an increased risk of varicose veins.

⚷ CN: Health promotion and maintenance; CL: Analyze

87. 1. Sclerotherapy involves injecting small- and medium-sized varicose veins with a solution that scars and closes those veins. In a few weeks, the veins should fade and disappear. This procedure does not require anesthesia and can be done in a **healthcare provider's (HCP's)** 🖵 office. Varicose veins can reoccur regardless of the procedure. Bruising is more likely following vein stripping or catheter-assisted procedures.

⚷ CN: Physiological adaptation; CL: Application

88. 1,2,4. To manage varicose veins, the nurse should coach the client to lose weight to relieve pressure on the veins, wear compression stockings to promote circulation, and elevate the legs when sitting or lying down. Applying lotion to the veins will keep the skin moist, but does not promote venous circulation. Pillows under the knees will obstruct circulation.

⚷ CN: Health promotion and maintenance; CL: Create

The Client with Stasis Ulcers

89. 1,2,4,5. The underlying pathophysiology in stasis ulcers of the skin surface is a result of inadequate oxygen and other nutrients to the tissues because of edema and decreased circulation. The nurse should first initiate care that will increase oxygen and improve tissue integrity. It is also important to prevent trauma to the tissues and prevent infections, which result from decreased microcirculation that limits the body's response to infection. Stasis ulcers are painful. The nurse can administer prescribed analgesics 30 minutes before changing the dressing. There is no indication that the client's overall nutrition needs to be improved.

🔑 CN: Physiological adaptation; CL: Create

90. 1. The result of chronic venous stasis is swelling and edema and superficial varicose veins. Diuretics will help reduce the swelling, thus improving capillary circulation. Although diuretics may decrease blood pressure, that is not the intended outcome of this drug. The nurse should teach the client to prevent infection and monitor wound healing, but these are not the primary outcomes of chlorothiazide.

🔑 CN: Pharmacological and parenteral therapies; CL: Evaluate

91. 4. The nurse should keep bed linens off of the stasis ulcer to decrease the amount of pressure that the linens exert upon the lower extremity and prevent further tissue breakdown. Administering prescribed analgesics would be an intervention for reducing the pain. Applying lanolin lotions to the left ankle ulcer will not promote healing. Encouraging the client to sit up in a chair four times per day is an intervention to promote activity. The nurse would elevate the involved extremity while the client is sitting up to reduce venous stasis and capillary pressure.

🔑 CN: Health promotion and maintenance; CL: Synthesize

92. 2. The nurse should first determine how the client will apply an herb mixture to the ulcer. The nurse should then encourage the client to consult the **healthcare provider (HCP)** 📖 because home remedies may be beneficial or may interfere with the medical treatment plan. In many cultures, home remedies are commonly used and may be helpful. The nurse must be sensitive to these traditions and cultural beliefs. The other statements demonstrate that the client understands the plan of care for the ulcer.

🔑 CN: Pharmacological and parenteral therapies; CL: Evaluate

Managing Care, Quality, and Safety for Clients with Vascular Disease

93. 3. It is important for the nurse to assess the client with peripheral artery disease (PAD) returning from an angiogram. It will be important to make baseline assessments on this client. A client with atrial fibrillation with a heart rate of 90 bpm is not an abnormal finding. A "fluttering feeling" is expected in a client with atrial fibrillation. A client with heart failure experiencing right upper quadrant fullness does not require urgent attention; the client might be experiencing signs and symptoms of hepatomegaly.

🔑 CN: Management of care; CL: Analyze

94. 3. The client is experiencing a rebound tachycardia from abrupt withdrawal of the beta-blocker. The beta-blocker should be restarted due to the tachycardia, history of hypertension, and the desire to reduce the risk of postoperative myocardial morbidity. The bypass surgery should correct the claudication and need for pentoxifylline. The furosemide and increase in fluids are not indicated since the client's urine output and blood pressure are satisfactory and there is no indication of bleeding. The nurse should also determine the potassium level before starting the furosemide.

🔑 CN: Management of care; CL: Synthesize

95. 1. The nurse is the client's advocate in planning for pain relief. When presented with a communications conflict, the nurse should first restate the concern, providing as much information as needed. If the **HCP** 📖 still does not offer an acceptable solution for pain management, the nurse can then discuss the situation with the hospitalist on the team and report the incident to the team leader. Waiting until the next shift to handle the problem does not contribute to the goal of managing the client's pain.

🔑 CN: Safety and infection control; CL: Synthesize

96. 1. The **LPN/VN** 📖 can complete the assessment sheet and care for the client before surgery. Clients who are stable and requiring complete care or frequent assistance with basic care needs along with vital signs and intake and output recordings can be assigned to a **UAP** 📖. An unstable client requiring critical assessments receives care from the **RN** 📖.

🔑 CN: Management of Care; CL: Synthesize

97. 1,2,3,5. When obtaining blood samples, the nurse must use two acceptable sources of identification (the client states his/her name; the nurse verifies the client's name and identification number of the armband); verifying a room number is not acceptable as clients can be easily reassigned to other rooms. The client must be awake to state his/her name. Blood samples must be labeled in front of the client.

🔑 CN: Safety and infection control; CL: Synthesize

98. 1. Before starting a heparin infusion, it is essential for the nurse to know the client's baseline blood coagulation values (hematocrit, hemoglobin, and red blood cell and platelet counts). In addition, the partial thromboplastin time should be monitored closely during the process. The client's stools would be tested only if internal bleeding is suspected. Although monitoring vital signs such as apical pulse is important in assessing potential signs and symptoms of hemorrhage or potential adverse reactions to the medication, vital signs are not the most important data to collect before administering the heparin. Intake and output are not important assessments for heparin administration unless the client has fluid and volume problems or kidney disease.

⚏⚊ CN: Safety and infection control;
CL: Synthesize

99. 4. Several variables make this client a high fall risk including secondary diagnosis of diabetes (15); intermittent IV antibiotics (20); and mental status changes (15) possibly due to anesthesia, pain, or recent limb loss. This client's assessment may clearly change as the effects of anesthesia wear off, pain is controlled, and the client becomes accustomed to ambulating with a prosthesis; because assessments may be continually changing, in most acute care facilities, a fall risk is completed every 24 hours and, sometimes, every shift.

⚏⚊ CN: Safety and infection control;
CL: Apply

The Client with Hematologic Health Problems

- The Client with Red Blood Cell Disorders
- The Client with Platelet Disorders
- The Client with White Blood Cell Disorders
- The Client with Lymphoma
- The Client Who Is in Shock
- Managing Care, Quality, and Safety for Clients with Hematologic Health Problems
- Answers, Rationales, and Test-Taking Strategies

The Client with Red Blood Cell Disorders

1. The nurse is assisting with a bone marrow aspiration and biopsy. In which order, from first to last, should the nurse complete these tasks? All options must be used.

| 1. Position the client in a side-lying position. |

| 2. Clean the skin with an antiseptic solution. |

| 3. Verify the client has signed an informed consent. |

| 4. Apply ice to the biopsy site. |

| |

| |

| |

| |

2. A client with iron deficiency anemia is refusing to take the prescribed oral iron medication because the medication is causing nausea; the client is also constipated. What actions should the nurse take? Select all that apply.
- ☐ 1. Suggest that the client use ginger when taking the medication.
- ☐ 2. Ask the client what is causing the nausea.
- ☐ 3. Tell the client to use stool softeners to minimize constipation.
- ☐ 4. Offer to administer the medication by an intramuscular injection.
- ☐ 5. Suggest that the client take the iron with orange juice.

3. A client had a mastectomy followed by chemotherapy 6 months ago. She reports that she is now "unable to concentrate at her card game" and "it seems harder and harder to finish her errands because of exhaustion." Based on this information, the nurse should suggest that the client:
- ☐ 1. take frequent naps.
- ☐ 2. limit activities.
- ☐ 3. increase fluid intake.
- ☐ 4. avoid contact with others.

4. A client is to have a transfusion of packed red blood cells from a designated donor. The client asks if any diseases can be transmitted by this donor. The nurse should inform the client that which diseases can be transmitted by a designated donor? Select all that apply.
- ☐ 1. Epstein-Barr virus
- ☐ 2. human immunodeficiency virus (HIV)
- ☐ 3. cytomegalovirus (CMV)
- ☐ 4. hepatitis A
- ☐ 5. malaria

5. The nurse is preparing to teach a client with iron deficiency anemia about the diet to follow after discharge. Which food should be included in the diet?
- ☐ 1. eggs
- ☐ 2. lettuce
- ☐ 3. citrus fruits
- ☐ 4. cheese

6. The nurse should instruct the client with vitamin B_{12} deficiency to eat which foods to obtain the **best** supply of vitamin B_{12}?
- ☐ 1. whole grains
- ☐ 2. green leafy vegetables
- ☐ 3. meats and dairy products
- ☐ 4. broccoli and Brussels sprouts

7. The nurse has just admitted a 35-year-old female client who has a serum vitamin B_{12} concentration of 800 pg/mL (590 pmol/L). Which laboratory findings should alert the nurse to focus the health history to obtain specific information about drug or alcohol use?
- ☐ 1. total bilirubin, 0.3 mg/dL (5.1 µmol/L)
- ☐ 2. serum creatinine, 0.5 mg/dL (44.2 µmol/L)
- ☐ 3. hemoglobin, 16 g/dL (160 g/L)
- ☐ 4. folate, 1.5 ng/mL (3.4 nmol/L)

8. Which lab values should the nurse report to the healthcare provider (HCP) when the client has anemia?
- ☐ 1. Schilling test result, elevated
- ☐ 2. intrinsic factor, absent
- ☐ 3. sedimentation rate, 16 mm/h
- ☐ 4. red blood cells (RBCs) within normal range

9. The nurse is developing a teaching plan for the client with aplastic anemia. Which is **most** important to include the plan?
- ☐ 1. Eat animal protein and dark green, leafy vegetables every day.
- ☐ 2. Avoid exposure to others with acute infections.
- ☐ 3. Practice yoga and meditation to decrease stress and anxiety.
- ☐ 4. Get 8 hours of sleep at night, and take naps during the day.

10. A client had a resection of the terminal ileum 3 years ago. While obtaining a health history and physical assessment, the nurse finds that the client has weakness, shortness of breath, and a sore tongue. Which additional information from the client indicates a need for client teaching?
- ☐ 1. "I have been drinking plenty of fluids."
- ☐ 2. "I have been gargling with warm salt water for my sore tongue."
- ☐ 3. "I have regular bowel movements on most days."
- ☐ 4. "I take a vitamin B_{12} tablet every day."

11. A client who follows a vegetarian diet was referred to a dietitian for nutritional counseling for anemia. Which client outcome indicates that the client does **not** understand nutritional counseling? The client:
- ☐ 1. adds dried fruit to cereal and baked goods.
- ☐ 2. cooks tomato-based foods in iron pots.
- ☐ 3. drinks coffee or tea with meals.
- ☐ 4. adds vitamin C to all meals.

12. A client was admitted to the hospital with iron deficiency anemia and blood-streaked emesis. Which question is **most** appropriate for the nurse to ask in determining the extent of the client's activity intolerance?
- ☐ 1. "What daily activities were you able to do 6 months ago compared with the present?"
- ☐ 2. "How long have you had this problem?"
- ☐ 3. "Have you been able to keep up with all your usual activities?"
- ☐ 4. "Are you more tired now than you used to be?"

13. A healthcare provider (HCP) prescribes vitamin B_{12} for a client with pernicious anemia. Which sites are appropriate for the nurse to administer vitamin B_{12} to an adult? Select all that apply.
- ☐ 1. median cutaneous
- ☐ 2. greater femur trochanter
- ☐ 3. acromion muscle
- ☐ 4. ventrogluteal
- ☐ 5. upper back
- ☐ 6. dorsogluteal

14. Which position would **most** help to decrease a client's discomfort when the client's spouse injects vitamin B_{12} using the ventrogluteal site?
- ☐ 1. lying on the side with legs extended
- ☐ 2. lying on the abdomen with toes pointed inward
- ☐ 3. leaning over the edge of a low table with hips flexed
- ☐ 4. standing upright with the feet one shoulder-width apart

15. A client is admitted from the emergency department after falling down a flight of stairs at home. The client's vital signs are stable, and the history states that the client had a gastric stapling 2 years ago. The client jokes about being clumsy lately and tripping over things. The nurse should gather additional information by asking the client which questions? Select all that apply.
- ☐ 1. "Are you experiencing numbness in your extremities?"
- ☐ 2. "How much vitamin B_{12} are you getting?"
- ☐ 3. "Are you feeling depressed?"
- ☐ 4. "Do you feel safe at home?"
- ☐ 5. "Are you getting sufficient iron in your diet?"

16. A client has fatigue, temperature of 99.5°F (37.5°C), dark bronze skin, and dark urine. Hemoglobin is 9 g/dL (90 g/L); hematocrit is 49 (0.49), and red blood cells are 2.75 million/µL (2.75×10^{12}/L). What should the nurse do **first**?
- ☐ 1. Initiate an intake and output record.
- ☐ 2. Place the client on bed rest.
- ☐ 3. Place the client on contact isolation.
- ☐ 4. Keep the client out of sunlight.

17. When a client is receiving a cephalosporin, the nurse must monitor the client for which finding?
- ☐ 1. drug-induced hemolytic anemia
- ☐ 2. purpura
- ☐ 3. infectious emboli
- ☐ 4. ecchymosis

18. A client is to have a Schilling's test. The nurse should:
- ☐ 1. administer methylcellulose.
- ☐ 2. start a 24- to 48-hour urine specimen collection.
- ☐ 3. maintain nothing-by-mouth (NPO) status.
- ☐ 4. start a 72-hour stool specimen collection.

19. A client with pernicious anemia is receiving vitamin B$_{12}$. The nurse should evaluate the client for which expected outcomes of vitamin B$_{12}$?
- ☐ **1.** increased energy
- ☐ **2.** healed tongue and lips
- ☐ **3.** absence of paresthesias
- ☐ **4.** improved clotting time

20. A client with pernicious anemia asks why it is necessary to take vitamin B$_{12}$ injections forever. Which is the nurse's **best** response?
- ☐ **1.** "The reason for your vitamin deficiency is an inability to absorb the vitamin because the stomach is not producing sufficient acid."
- ☐ **2.** "The reason for your vitamin deficiency is an inability to absorb the vitamin because the stomach is not producing sufficient amounts of a factor that allows the vitamin to be absorbed."
- ☐ **3.** "The reason for your vitamin deficiency is an excessive excretion of the vitamin because of kidney dysfunction."
- ☐ **4.** "The reason for your vitamin deficiency is an increased requirement for the vitamin because of rapid red blood cell production."

21. The nurse is assessing a client's activity tolerance. Which report from a treadmill test indicates an abnormal response?
- ☐ **1.** pulse rate increased by 20 bpm immediately after the activity
- ☐ **2.** respiratory rate decreased by 5 breaths/min
- ☐ **3.** diastolic blood pressure increased by 7 mm Hg
- ☐ **4.** pulse rate within 6 bpm of resting pulse after 3 minutes of rest

22. In a postoperative client, the hematocrit decreased from 36% (0.36) to 34% (0.34) on the 3rd day even though the red blood cell (RBC) count and hemoglobin value remained stable at 4.5 million/μL (4.5 × 10^{12}/L) and 11.9 g/dL (119 g/L), respectively. The nurse should **next**:
- ☐ **1.** check the dressing and drains for frank bleeding.
- ☐ **2.** call the healthcare provider (HCP).
- ☐ **3.** continue to monitor vital signs.
- ☐ **4.** start oxygen at 2 L/min per nasal cannula.

23. The nurse is administering packed red blood cells (PRBCs) to a client. The nurse should **first:**
- ☐ **1.** discontinue the IV catheter if a blood transfusion reaction occurs.
- ☐ **2.** administer the PRBCs through a percutaneously inserted central catheter line with a 20-gauge needle.
- ☐ **3.** flush PRBCs with 5% dextrose and 0.45% normal saline solution.
- ☐ **4.** stay with the client during the first 15 minutes of infusion.

24. What directions should the nurse provide to a young female adult with sickle cell anemia? Select all that apply.
- ☐ **1.** Drink plenty of fluids when outside in hot weather.
- ☐ **2.** Avoid being in high altitudes where less oxygen is available.
- ☐ **3.** Be aware that since she is homozygous for HbS, she carries the sickle cell trait.
- ☐ **4.** Know that pregnancy with sickle cell disease increases the risk of a crisis.
- ☐ **5.** Avoid flying on commercial airlines.

25. The nurse is teaching a client and his family about the client's new diagnosis of hemochromatosis. Which information should the nurse include in the teaching plan?
- ☐ **1.** Hemochromatosis is an autoimmune disorder that affects the *HFE* gene.
- ☐ **2.** Individuals who are heterozygous for hemochromatosis rarely develop the disease.
- ☐ **3.** Individuals who are homozygous for hemochromatosis are carriers of hemochromatosis.
- ☐ **4.** Men are at greater risk for hemochromatosis.

26. A client is having a blood transfusion reaction. What must the nurse do in order of priority from first to last? All options must be used.

1. Notify the healthcare provider (HCP) and blood bank.

2. Complete the appropriate Transfusion Reaction Form(s).

3. Stop the transfusion.

4. Keep the IV open with normal saline infusion.

27. Which safety measures would be **most** important to implement when caring for a client who is receiving 2 units of packed red blood cells (PRBCs)? Select all that apply.

☐ 1. Verify that the ABO and Rh of the two units are the same.

☐ 2. Infuse a unit of PRBCs in <4 hours.

☐ 3. Stop the transfusion if a reaction occurs, but keep the line open.

☐ 4. Take vital signs every 15 minutes while the unit is transfusing.

☐ 5. Inspect the blood bag for leaks, abnormal color, and clots.

☐ 6. Use a 22-gauge catheter for optimal flow of a blood transfusion.

28. A client who had received 25 mL of packed red blood cells (PRBCs) has low back pain and pruritus. After stopping the infusion, the nurse should take what action **next**?

☐ 1. Administer prescribed antihistamine and an antipyretic.

☐ 2. Collect blood and urine samples and send to the lab.

☐ 3. Administer prescribed diuretics.

☐ 4. Administer prescribed vasopressors.

29. A client is to receive epoetin injections. What laboratory value should the nurse assess before giving the injection?

☐ 1. hematocrit

☐ 2. partial thromboplastin time

☐ 3. hemoglobin concentration

☐ 4. prothrombin time

30. When beginning IV erythropoietin therapy, what actions should the nurse take? Select all that apply.

☐ 1. Check the hemoglobin levels before administering subsequent doses.

☐ 2. Shake the vial thoroughly to mix the concentrated white, milky solution.

☐ 3. Keep the multidose vial refrigerated between scheduled twice-a-day doses.

☐ 4. Administer the medication through the IV line without other medications.

☐ 5. Adjust the initial doses according to the client's changes in blood pressure.

☐ 6. Instruct the client to avoid driving and performing hazardous activity during the initial treatment.

31. A client is afraid of receiving vitamin B_{12} injections because of potential toxic reactions. Which is the nurse's **best** response to relieve these fears?

☐ 1. "Vitamin B_{12} will cause ringing in the ears before a toxic level is reached."

☐ 2. "Vitamin B_{12} may cause a very mild rash initially."

☐ 3. "Vitamin B_{12} cause mild nausea but nothing toxic."

☐ 4. "Vitamin B_{12} is generally free of toxicity because it is water soluble."

32. A client with iron deficiency anemia is having trouble selecting food from the hospital menu. Which foods should the nurse suggest to meet the client's need for iron? Select all that apply.

☐ 1. eggs

☐ 2. brown rice

☐ 3. dark green vegetables

☐ 4. tea

☐ 5. oatmeal

33. A client with macrocytic anemia has a burn on the foot and reports watching television while lying on a heating pad. Which action should be the nurse's **first** response?

☐ 1. Assess for potential abuse.

☐ 2. Check for diminished sensations.

☐ 3. Document the findings.

☐ 4. Clean and dress the area.

34. Which is a late symptom of polycythemia vera?

☐ 1. headache

☐ 2. dizziness

☐ 3. pruritus

☐ 4. shortness of breath

35. When a client is diagnosed with aplastic anemia, the nurse should assess the client for changes in which physiologic functions?

☐ 1. bleeding tendencies

☐ 2. intake and output

☐ 3. peripheral sensation

☐ 4. bowel function

The Client with Platelet Disorders

36. A healthcare provider (HCP) prescribes 0.5 mg of protamine sulfate for a client who is showing signs of bleeding after receiving a 100-unit dose of heparin. The nurse should expect the effects of the protamine sulfate to be noted in how many minutes?

☐ 1. 5 minutes

☐ 2. 10 minutes

☐ 3. 20 minutes

☐ 4. 30 minutes

37. The nurse is to administer subcutaneous heparin to an underweight older adult. What facts should the nurse keep in mind when administering this medication? Select all that apply.

☐ 1. Administer in the anterior area of the iliac crest.

☐ 2. The onset is immediate.

☐ 3. Use a 27-G, 5/8-inch (1.6-mm) needle.

☐ 4. Cephalosporin potentiates the effects of heparin.

☐ 5. Verify the dose with another nurse according to agency policy.

38. The nurse should instruct the client with a platelet count of 31,000/μL (31 × 10⁹/L) to:
- ☐ **1.** pad sharp surfaces to avoid minor trauma when walking.
- ☐ **2.** assess for spontaneous petechiae in the extremities.
- ☐ **3.** wear a mask when in crowds of people.
- ☐ **4.** check for blood in the urine.

39. A 25-year-old woman with a history of systemic lupus erythematosus was admitted with a severe viral respiratory tract infection and diffuse petechiae. Based on these data, it is **most** important that the nurse further evaluate the client's recent:
- ☐ **1.** quality and quantity of food intake.
- ☐ **2.** type and amount of fluid intake.
- ☐ **3.** extent of weakness and fatigue.
- ☐ **4.** length and amount of menstrual flow.

40. When a client with thrombocytopenia has a severe headache, what does the nurse interpret that this may indicate?
- ☐ **1.** stress of the disease
- ☐ **2.** cerebral bleeding
- ☐ **3.** migraine headache
- ☐ **4.** sinus congestion

41. The nurse evaluates that the client correctly understands how to report signs and symptoms of bleeding when the client says:
- ☐ **1.** "Petechiae are large, red skin bruises."
- ☐ **2.** "Ecchymoses are large, purple skin bruises."
- ☐ **3.** "Purpura is an open cut on the skin."
- ☐ **4.** "Abrasions are small pinpoint red dots on the skin."

42. The nurse should instruct the client with a platelet count of <150,000/μL (150 × 10⁹/L) to avoid which activity?
- ☐ **1.** walking for more than 10 minutes
- ☐ **2.** straining to have a bowel movement
- ☐ **3.** visiting with young children
- ☐ **4.** sitting in semi-Fowler's position

43. A client who is taking acetylsalicylic acid (ASA) caplets develops prolonged bleeding from a superficial skin injury on the forearm. The nurse should tell the client to do which action **first**?
- ☐ **1.** Place the forearm under a running stream of lukewarm water.
- ☐ **2.** Pat the injury with a dry washcloth.
- ☐ **3.** Wrap the entire forearm from the wrist to the elbow.
- ☐ **4.** Apply an ice pack for 20 minutes.

44. A client's bone marrow report reveals normal stem cells and precursors of platelets (megakaryocytes) in the presence of decreased circulating platelets. The nurse recognizes a knowledge deficit when the client says:
- ☐ **1.** "I need to stop flossing and throw away my hard toothbrush."
- ☐ **2.** "I am glad that my report turned out normal."
- ☐ **3.** "Now I know why I have all these bruises."
- ☐ **4.** "I should not jump off that last step anymore."

45. A client with thrombocytopenia has developed a hemorrhage. The nurse should assess the client for which finding?
- ☐ **1.** tachycardia
- ☐ **2.** bradycardia
- ☐ **3.** decreased P_{aCO_2}
- ☐ **4.** narrowed pulse pressure

46. The client with idiopathic thrombocytopenic purpura (ITP) asks the nurse why it is necessary to take steroids. The nurse should base the response on which information?
- ☐ **1.** Steroids destroy the antibodies and prolong the life of platelets.
- ☐ **2.** Steroids neutralize the antigens and prolong the life of platelets.
- ☐ **3.** Steroids increase phagocytosis and increase the life of platelets.
- ☐ **4.** Steroids alter the spleen's recognition of platelets and increase the life of platelets.

47. A client is to be discharged on prednisone. Which statement indicates that the client understands important concepts about the medication therapy?
- ☐ **1.** "I need to take the medicine in divided doses at morning and bedtime."
- ☐ **2.** "I am to take 40 mg of prednisone for 2 months and then stop."
- ☐ **3.** "I need to wear or carry identification that I am taking prednisone."
- ☐ **4.** "Prednisone will give me extra protection from colds and flu."

48. When teaching the client older than age 50 who is receiving long-term prednisone therapy, what should the nurse suggest to the client?
- ☐ **1.** Take the prednisone with food.
- ☐ **2.** Take over-the-counter antiemetics.
- ☐ **3.** Exercise three to four times a week.
- ☐ **4.** Eat foods that are low in potassium.

49. The nurse is preparing a teaching plan about increased exercise for a female client who is receiving long-term corticosteroid therapy. What type of exercise is **most** appropriate for this client?
- ☐ **1.** floor exercises
- ☐ **2.** stretching
- ☐ **3.** running
- ☐ **4.** walking

50. The nurse is teaching a female client with a history of acquired thrombocytopenia about how to prevent and control hemorrhage. Which statement indicates that the client needs further instruction?
☐ 1. "I can apply direct pressure over small cuts for at least 5 to 10 minutes to stop a venous bleed."
☐ 2. "I can count the number of tissues saturated to detect blood loss during a nosebleed."
☐ 3. "I can take hormones to decrease blood loss during menses."
☐ 4. "I can count the number of sanitary napkins to detect excess blood loss during menses."

51. A client has been on long-term prednisone therapy. What should the nurse instruct the client to include in her diet? Select all that apply.
☐ 1. carbohydrates
☐ 2. protein
☐ 3. trans fat
☐ 4. potassium
☐ 5. calcium
☐ 6. vitamin D

52. Platelets should **not** be administered when:
☐ 1. the platelet bag is cold.
☐ 2. the platelets are 2 days old.
☐ 3. the platelet bag is at room temperature.
☐ 4. the platelets are 12 hours old.

53. The nurse is preparing to administer platelets. The nurse should:
☐ 1. check the ABO compatibility.
☐ 2. administer the platelets slowly.
☐ 3. gently rotate the bag.
☐ 4. use a whole-blood tubing set.

54. Which indicates that a client has achieved the goal of correctly demonstrating deep breathing for an upcoming splenectomy? The client:
☐ 1. breathes in through the nose and out through the mouth.
☐ 2. breathes in through the mouth and out through the nose.
☐ 3. uses diaphragmatic breathing in the lying, sitting, and standing positions.
☐ 4. takes a deep breath in through the nose, holds it for 5 seconds, and blows out through pursed lips.

55. A client is scheduled for an elective splenectomy. The **last** thing the nurse should do before the client goes to surgery is to determine that the client has:
☐ 1. voided completely.
☐ 2. signed the consent.
☐ 3. vital signs recorded.
☐ 4. name band on wrist.

56. When receiving a client from the postanesthesia care unit after a splenectomy, which should the nurse assess **next** after obtaining vital signs?
☐ 1. nasogastric drainage
☐ 2. urinary catheter
☐ 3. dressing
☐ 4. need for pain medication

57. A client who had a splenectomy yesterday has a nasogastric (NG) tube. The expected outcome of using the NG tube is to:
☐ 1. move the stomach away from where the spleen was removed.
☐ 2. irrigate the operative site.
☐ 3. decrease abdominal distention.
☐ 4. assess for the gastric pH as peristalsis returns.

58. A client who had a splenectomy is being discharged. The nurse should instruct the client to:
☐ 1. not drive a car for 6 weeks.
☐ 2. alternate rest and activity.
☐ 3. make an appointment for the staples to be removed.
☐ 4. report early signs of infection.

59. The nurse should assess a client at risk for acute disseminated intravascular coagulation (DIC) for which early sign?
☐ 1. severe shortness of breath
☐ 2. bleeding without history or cause
☐ 3. orthopnea
☐ 4. hematuria

60. Which is contraindicated for a client diagnosed with disseminated intravascular coagulation (DIC)?
☐ 1. treating the underlying cause
☐ 2. administering heparin
☐ 3. administering warfarin sodium
☐ 4. replacing depleted blood products

61. A client with disseminated intravascular coagulation develops clinical manifestations of microvascular thrombosis. The nurse should assess the client for:
☐ 1. hemoptysis.
☐ 2. focal ischemia.
☐ 3. petechiae.
☐ 4. hematuria.

62. Which is a finding associated with internal bleeding with disseminated intravascular coagulation?
☐ 1. bradycardia
☐ 2. hypertension
☐ 3. increasing abdominal girth
☐ 4. petechiae

The Client with White Blood Cell Disorders

63. A young adult is diagnosed with infectious mononucleosis. The white blood cell (WBC) count is 19,000/μL (19 × 10⁹/L). The client has a strepto-coccal throat infection, enlarged spleen, and aching muscles. Which instructions should the nurse include in discharge planning with the client? Select all that apply.
☐ **1.** Stay on bed rest until the temperature is normal.
☐ **2.** Gargle with warm saline while the throat is irritated.
☐ **3.** Increase intake of fluids until the infection subsides.
☐ **4.** Wear a mask if others are present.
☐ **5.** Avoid contact sports while the spleen is enlarged.

64. The daily white blood cell (WBC) count in a client with aplastic anemia drops overnight from 3,900 to 2,900/μL (3.9 to 2.9 × 10⁹/L). Which is the appropriate nursing intervention?
☐ **1.** Continue monitoring the client.
☐ **2.** Call the laboratory to verify the report.
☐ **3.** Document the finding.
☐ **4.** Call the healthcare provider (HCP), and request that the client be placed in reverse isolation.

65. A client who had an exploratory laparotomy 3 days ago has a white blood cell (WBC) differential with a shift to the left. The nurse instructs unlicensed assistive personnel (UAP) to report which clinical manifestation of this laboratory report?
☐ **1.** swelling around the incision
☐ **2.** redness around the incision
☐ **3.** elevated temperature
☐ **4.** purulent wound drainage

66. The nurse is developing a care plan with a client who has leukemia. What instructions should the nurse include in the plan? Select all that apply.
☐ **1.** Monitor temperature and report elevation.
☐ **2.** Recognize signs and symptoms of infection.
☐ **3.** Avoid crowds.
☐ **4.** Maintain integrity of skin and mucous membranes.
☐ **5.** Take a baby aspirin each day.

67. A client with neutropenia has an absolute neutrophil count (ANC) of 900 (0.9 × 10⁹/L). What is the client's risk of infection?
☐ **1.** normal risk
☐ **2.** moderate risk
☐ **3.** high risk
☐ **4.** extremely high risk

68. Which nursing action is **most** important in preventing cross-contamination?
☐ **1.** changing gloves immediately after use
☐ **2.** standing 2 feet (61 cm) from the client
☐ **3.** speaking minimally when in the room
☐ **4.** wearing protective coverings

69. What should the nurse teach the client with neutropenia and the family to avoid?
☐ **1.** using suppositories or enemas
☐ **2.** using a high-efficiency particulate air (HEPA) filter mask
☐ **3.** performing perianal care after every bowel movement
☐ **4.** performing oral care after every meal

70. A client with granulocytopenia has many visitors. The **most** important measure to prevent infection is for the visitors to:
☐ **1.** visit only if they do not have a cold.
☐ **2.** wash their hands.
☐ **3.** leave the children at home.
☐ **4.** not to kiss the client.

71. A nurse is obtaining consent for a bone marrow aspiration. Which actions should the nurse take? Select all that apply.
☐ **1.** Witness the client signing the consent form.
☐ **2.** Evaluate that the client understands the procedure.
☐ **3.** Explain the risks of the procedure to the client.
☐ **4.** Verify that the client is signing the consent form of his or her own free will.
☐ **5.** Determine that the client understands postprocedure care.

72. A client is about to undergo bone marrow aspiration of the sternum. What should the nurse tell the client?
☐ **1.** "You may feel a solution being wiped over your entire front from your neck down to your navel and out to your shoulders."
☐ **2.** "You will not feel the local anesthetic being applied because it will be sprayed on."
☐ **3.** "You will feel a pulling type of discomfort for a few seconds."
☐ **4.** "After the needle is removed, you will feel a bandage being applied around your chest."

73. Twenty-four hours after a bone marrow aspiration, the nurse evaluates which client outcome as an appropriate one?
☐ **1.** The client maintains bed rest.
☐ **2.** There is redness and swelling at the aspiration site.
☐ **3.** The client requests a strong analgesic for pain.
☐ **4.** There is no bleeding at the aspiration site.

74. A client states, "I do not want any more tests. Who cares what kind of leukemia I have? I just want to be treated now." Which is the nurse's **best** response?
☐ 1. "I am sure you are frustrated and want to be well now."
☐ 2. "Your treatment can be more effective if it is based on more specific information about your disease."
☐ 3. "Now, you know the tests are necessary and that you are just upset right now."
☐ 4. "I understand how you feel."

75. During the induction stage for treatment of leukemia, the nurse should remove which items that the family has brought into the room?
☐ 1. a prayer book
☐ 2. a picture
☐ 3. a bouquet of flowers
☐ 4. a hairbrush

76. The nurse understands that the client who is undergoing induction therapy for leukemia needs additional instruction when the client makes which statement?
☐ 1. "I will pace my activities with rest periods."
☐ 2. "I cannot wait to get home to my cat!"
☐ 3. "I will use warm saline gargle instead of brushing my teeth."
☐ 4. "I must report a temperature of 100°F (37.7°C)."

77. A client with chronic myelogenous leukemia is taking imatinib. The nurse should instruct the client to report which adverse effect of this drug?
☐ 1. edema
☐ 2. numbness and tingling in extremities
☐ 3. bloody stools
☐ 4. persistent cough

78. A client with acute lymphocytic leukemia is receiving vincristine. Prior to infusing the drug, the nurse administers diphenhydramine. The nurse should inform the client that the expected outcome of using diphenhydramine in this situation is to:
☐ 1. promote sleep, while the vincristine is infusing.
☐ 2. decrease incidence of a reaction to the vincristine.
☐ 3. potentiate the action of the vincristine.
☐ 4. reduce anxiety associated with the vincristine infusion.

79. A female client is receiving chemotherapy and is experiencing pancytopenia. Which laboratory result **most** warrants that the nurse immediately contact the healthcare provider (HCP)?
☐ 1. platelet count of 12,000/mm³
☐ 2. WBC count of 4,000/mm³
☐ 3. absolute neutrophil count of 1,500/mm³
☐ 4. hemoglobin of 12 g/100 mL

80. A nurse is administering an IV antineoplastic agent when the client says, "My arm is burning by the IV site." What should the nurse do **first**?
☐ 1. Slow the infusion rate and check the IV site.
☐ 2. Call the healthcare provider (HCP) to report the incident.
☐ 3. Stop infusing the medication.
☐ 4. Place a warm, moist pack on the IV site area.

81. A client who is receiving a blood transfusion suddenly experiences chills and a temperature of 101°F (38°C). The client also has a headache and appears flushed. In what order, from first to last, should the nurse perform the actions? All options must be used.

1. Obtain a blood culture from the client.

2. Send the blood bag and administration set to the blood bank.

3. Stop the blood infusion.

4. Infuse normal saline to keep the vein open.

82. A client undergoing antineoplastic therapy is prescribed subcutaneous epoetin. The nurse evaluates that the drug is effective when:
☐ 1. biopsies no longer show malignancy.
☐ 2. hemoglobin levels rise.
☐ 3. nausea and vomiting stop.
☐ 4. a scan shows tumor shrinkage.

83. The goal of nursing care for a client with acute myeloid leukemia (AML) is to prevent:
☐ 1. cardiac arrhythmias.
☐ 2. liver failure.
☐ 3. renal failure.
☐ 4. hemorrhage.

84. At what age is an individual **most** at risk for acquiring acute lymphocytic leukemia (ALL)?
☐ 1. 4 to 12 years
☐ 2. 20 to 30 years
☐ 3. 40 to 50 years
☐ 4. 60 to 70 years

85. The client with acute lymphocytic leukemia (ALL) is at risk for infection. What action should the nurse take?
☐ **1.** Place the client in a private room.
☐ **2.** Have the client wear a mask.
☐ **3.** Have staff wear gowns and gloves.
☐ **4.** Restrict visitors.

86. The nurse is planning care with a client with acute leukemia who has mucositis. The nurse should advise the client that after every meal and every 4 hours while awake, the client should use:
☐ **1.** lemon-glycerin swabs.
☐ **2.** a commercial mouthwash.
☐ **3.** saline.
☐ **4.** a commercial toothpaste and brush.

87. The client with acute leukemia and the healthcare team establish mutual client outcomes of improved tidal volume and activity tolerance. Which measure would be **least** likely to promote these outcomes?
☐ **1.** ambulating in the hallway
☐ **2.** sitting up in a chair
☐ **3.** lying in bed and taking deep breaths
☐ **4.** using a stationary bicycle in the room

88. The nurse is evaluating the client's understanding about combination chemotherapy. Which statement by the client about reasons for using combination chemotherapy indicates the need for **further** explanation?
☐ **1.** "Combination chemotherapy is used to interrupt cell growth cycle at different points."
☐ **2.** "Combination chemotherapy is used to destroy cancer cells and treat side effects simultaneously."
☐ **3.** "Combination chemotherapy is used to decrease resistance."
☐ **4.** "Combination chemotherapy is used to minimize the toxicity from using high doses of a single agent."

89. In providing care to the client with leukemia who has developed thrombocytopenia, the nurse assesses the most common sites for bleeding. Which is **not** a common site?
☐ **1.** biliary system
☐ **2.** gastrointestinal tract
☐ **3.** brain and meninges
☐ **4.** pulmonary system

90. The nurse's **best** explanation for why the severely neutropenic client is placed in reverse isolation is that reverse isolation helps prevent the spread of organisms:
☐ **1.** to the client from sources outside the client's environment.
☐ **2.** from the client to healthcare personnel, visitors, and other clients.
☐ **3.** by using special techniques to dispose of contaminated materials.
☐ **4.** by using special techniques to handle the client's linens and personal items.

The Client with Lymphoma

91. Which clinical manifestation does the nurse **most** likely observe in a client with Hodgkin's disease?
☐ **1.** difficulty swallowing
☐ **2.** painless, enlarged cervical lymph nodes
☐ **3.** difficulty breathing
☐ **4.** a feeling of fullness over the liver

92. The nurse is developing a care plan for a client who has had radiation therapy for Hodgkin's lymphoma. What is the primary goal of care for this client?
☐ **1.** Maintain fluid balance.
☐ **2.** Obtain sufficient exercise.
☐ **3.** Prevent infection.
☐ **4.** Avoid depression.

93. A client with a suspected diagnosis of Hodgkin's disease is to have a lymph node biopsy. What should the nurse make sure that personnel involved with the procedure do?
☐ **1.** Maintain sterile technique.
☐ **2.** Use a mask, gloves, and a gown when assisting with the procedure.
☐ **3.** Send the specimen to the laboratory when someone is available to take it.
☐ **4.** Ensure that all instruments used are placed in a sealed and labeled container.

94. The client with Hodgkin's disease undergoes an excisional cervical lymph node biopsy under local anesthesia. After the procedure, what does the nurse assess **first**?
☐ **1.** vital signs
☐ **2.** the incision
☐ **3.** the airway
☐ **4.** neurologic signs

95. When assessing the client with Hodgkin's disease, the nurse should observe the client for which finding?
☐ **1.** herpes zoster infections
☐ **2.** discolored teeth
☐ **3.** hemorrhage
☐ **4.** hypercellular immunity

96. The client with Hodgkin's disease develops B symptoms. What do these manifestations indicate?
☐ **1.** The client has a low-grade fever (temperature lower than 100°F [37.8°C]).
☐ **2.** The client has a weight loss of 5% or less of body weight.
☐ **3.** The client has night sweats.
☐ **4.** The client probably has not progressed to an advanced stage.

97. The nurse is developing a discharge plan with a client who has lymphoma. What should the nurse emphasize to the client?
☐ 1. Use analgesics as needed.
☐ 2. Take a shower with perfumed shower gel.
☐ 3. Wear a mask when outside of the home.
☐ 4. Take an antipyretic every morning.

98. The client asks the nurse to explain what it means that Hodgkin's disease is diagnosed at stage 1A. What describes the involvement of the disease?
☐ 1. involvement of a single lymph node
☐ 2. involvement of two or more lymph nodes on the same side of the diaphragm
☐ 3. involvement of lymph node regions on both sides of the diaphragm
☐ 4. diffuse disease of one or more extralymphatic organs

99. A client is undergoing a bone marrow aspiration and biopsy. What is the **best** way for the nurse to help the client and two upset family members handle anxiety during the procedure?
☐ 1. Allow the client's family to stay as long as possible.
☐ 2. Stay with the client without speaking.
☐ 3. Encourage the client to take slow, deep breaths to relax.
☐ 4. Allow the client time to express feelings.

100. The nurse explains to the client with Hodgkin's disease that a bone marrow biopsy will be taken after the aspiration. What should the nurse explain about the biopsy?
☐ 1. "Your biopsy will be performed before the aspiration because enough tissue may be obtained so that you will not have to go through the aspiration."
☐ 2. "You will feel a pressure sensation when the biopsy is taken but should not feel actual pain; if you do, tell the healthcare provider so that you can be given extra numbing medicine."
☐ 3. "You may hear a crunch as the needle passes through the bone, but when the biopsy is taken, you will feel a suction-type pain that will last for just a moment."
☐ 4. "You will be shaved and cleaned with an antiseptic agent, after which the healthcare provider will inject a needle without making an incision to aspirate out the bone marrow."

101. A client with advanced Hodgkin's disease is admitted to hospice because death is imminent. The goal of nursing care at this time is to:
☐ 1. reduce the client's fear of pain.
☐ 2. support the client's wish to discontinue further therapy.
☐ 3. prevent feelings of isolation.
☐ 4. help the client overcome feelings of social inadequacy.

102. The client is a survivor of non-Hodgkin's lymphoma. Which statement indicates the client needs additional information?
☐ 1. "Regular screening is very important for me."
☐ 2. "The survivor rate is directly proportional to the incidence of second malignancy."
☐ 3. "The survivor rate is indirectly proportional to the incidence of second malignancy."
☐ 4. "It is important for survivors to know the stage of the disease and their current treatment plan."

The Client Who Is in Shock

103. What is the **most** important goal of nursing care for a client who is in shock?
☐ 1. Manage fluid overload.
☐ 2. Manage increased cardiac output.
☐ 3. Manage inadequate tissue perfusion.
☐ 4. Manage vasoconstriction of vascular beds.

104. Which finding indicates hypovolemic shock in an adult who has had a 15% blood loss?
☐ 1. pulse rate <60 bpm
☐ 2. respiratory rate of 4 breaths/min
☐ 3. pupils unequally dilated
☐ 4. systolic blood pressure <90 mm Hg

105. Which finding is the **best** indication that fluid replacement for the client in hypovolemic shock is adequate?
☐ 1. urine output >30 mL/h
☐ 2. systolic blood pressure >110 mm Hg
☐ 3. diastolic blood pressure >90 mm Hg
☐ 4. respiratory rate of 20 breaths/min

106. Which finding is a risk factor for hypovolemic shock?
☐ 1. hemorrhage
☐ 2. antigen-antibody reaction
☐ 3. gram-negative bacteria
☐ 4. vasodilation

107. Which is a **priority** assessment for the client in shock who is receiving an IV infusion of packed red blood cells and normal saline solution?
☐ 1. fluid balance
☐ 2. anaphylactic reaction
☐ 3. pain
☐ 4. altered level of consciousness

108. The client who does not respond adequately to fluid replacement has a prescription for an IV infusion of dopamine hydrochloride at 5 mcg/kg/min. To determine that the drug is having the desired effect, the nurse should assess the client for:
☐ 1. increased renal and mesenteric blood flow.
☐ 2. increased cardiac output.
☐ 3. vasoconstriction.
☐ 4. reduced preload and afterload.

109. A client is receiving dopamine hydrochloride for treatment of shock. What action should the nurse take?
- ☐ 1. Administer pain medication concurrently.
- ☐ 2. Monitor blood pressure continuously.
- ☐ 3. Evaluate arterial blood gases at least every 2 hours.
- ☐ 4. Monitor for signs of infection.

110. A client who has been taking warfarin has been admitted with severe acute rectal bleeding and the following laboratory results: international normalized ratio (INR), 8; hemoglobin, 11 g/dL (110 g/L); and hematocrit, 33% (0.33). In which order, from first to last, should the nurse implement the healthcare provider's prescriptions? All options must be used.

1. Give 1 unit fresh frozen plasma (FFP).

2. Administer vitamin K 2.5 mg by mouth.

3. Schedule the client for sigmoidoscopy.

4. Administer IV dextrose 5% in 0.45% normal saline.

111. When assessing a client for early septic shock, the nurse should assess the client for which finding?
- ☐ 1. cool, clammy skin
- ☐ 2. warm, flushed skin
- ☐ 3. increased blood pressure
- ☐ 4. hemorrhage

112. A client with toxic shock has been receiving ceftriaxone sodium, 1 g every 12 hours. In addition to culture and sensitivity studies, what other laboratory finding should the nurse monitor?
- ☐ 1. serum creatinine
- ☐ 2. spinal fluid analysis
- ☐ 3. arterial blood gases
- ☐ 4. serum osmolality

113. Which nursing intervention is **most** important in preventing septic shock?
- ☐ 1. administering IV fluid replacement therapy as prescribed
- ☐ 2. obtaining vital signs every 4 hours for all clients
- ☐ 3. monitoring red blood cell counts for elevation
- ☐ 4. maintaining asepsis of indwelling urinary catheters

114. Which finding is an indication of a complication of septic shock?
- ☐ 1. anaphylaxis
- ☐ 2. acute respiratory distress syndrome (ARDS)
- ☐ 3. chronic obstructive pulmonary disease (COPD)
- ☐ 4. mitral valve prolapse

Managing Care, Quality, and Safety for Clients with Hematologic Health Problems

115. A nurse is taking care of two clients who have a prescription to receive a blood transfusion of packed red blood cells at the same time. The first client's blood pressure dropped from the preoperative value of 120/80 mm Hg to a postoperative value of 100/50 mm Hg. The second client is hospitalized because he developed dehydration and anemia following pneumonia. After checking the patency of their IV lines and vital signs, what should the nurse do **next**?
- ☐ 1. Call for both clients' blood transfusions at the same time.
- ☐ 2. Ask another nurse to verify the compatibility of both units at the same time.
- ☐ 3. Call for and hang the first client's blood transfusion.
- ☐ 4. Ask another nurse to call for and hang the blood for the second client.

116. When a blood transfusion is terminated following a reaction, what actions must the nurse take? Select all that apply.
- ☐ 1. Send freshly collected urine samples to the laboratory.
- ☐ 2. Return the remainder of the blood component unit to the blood bank.
- ☐ 3. Return the intravenous administration set to the blood bank.
- ☐ 4. Alert Risk Management about the incident.
- ☐ 5. Report the incident to the Infection Control Manager.

117. The nurse is administering a medication to a client with myeloid leukemia and does not know the use, dose, or side effects. To obtain the **most** up-to-date information about this drug, what should the nurse do?
- ☐ 1. Check a commercially published drug guide.
- ☐ 2. Read a pharmacology textbook.
- ☐ 3. Consult the drug guide provided by the clinical agency.
- ☐ 4. Review information at the drug manufacturer's website.

118. The charge nurse on a hematology/oncology unit is reviewing the policy for using abbreviations with the staff. The charge nurse should emphasize which information about why dangerous abbreviations need to be eliminated? Select all that apply.
- ☐ 1. to ensure efficient and accurate communication
- ☐ 2. to prevent medication errors
- ☐ 3. to ensure client safety
- ☐ 4. to make it easier for clients to understand the medication prescriptions
- ☐ 5. to make data entry into a computerized health record easier

119. The nurse should remind the unlicensed assistive personnel (UAP) that the **most** important goal in the care of the neutropenic client in isolation is:
- ☐ 1. listening to the client's feelings of concern.
- ☐ 2. completing the client's care in a calm manner.
- ☐ 3. completing all of the client's care at one time.
- ☐ 4. instructing the client to dispose of the tissue used after blowing the nose.

Answers, Rationales, and Test-Taking Strategies

*The answers and rationales for each question follow below, along with keys (🔑) to the client need (CN) and cognitive level (CL) for each question. In addition, you will also see a glossary icon (📖) highlighting specific terminology used on the licensing exam. As you check your answers, use the **Content Mastery and Test-Taking Skill Self-Analysis** worksheet (tear-out worksheet in back of book) to identify the reason(s) for not answering the questions correctly. For additional information about test-taking skills and strategies for answering questions, refer to pages 12–23 and pages 35–36 in Part 1 of this book.*

The Client with Red Blood Cell Disorders

1. 3,1,2,4. First, the nurse must verify that the client has voluntarily signed a **consent** 📖 form before the procedure begins and check that the client understands the procedure. The nurse then positions the client in a side-lying, or *lateral decubitus*, position with the affected side up. Then, the nurse should clean the skin site and surrounding area with an antiseptic solution before the **healthcare provider (HCP)** 📖 numbs the site and collects the specimen. When the procedure is finished, the nurse must apply ice to the biopsy site to reduce pain.

🔑 CN: Management of care; CL: Synthesize

2. 1,2,5. Nausea and vomiting are common adverse effects of oral iron preparations. The nurse should first ask the client why the client does not want to take the oral medication and then suggest ways to decrease the nausea and vomiting. Ginger may help minimize the nausea, and the client can try this remedy and evaluate its effectiveness. Iron should be taken on an empty stomach but can be taken with orange juice. The client can evaluate if this helps the nausea. Stool softeners should not be used in clients with iron deficiency anemia. Instead, constipation can be prevented by following a high-fiber diet. Administering iron intramuscularly is done only if other approaches are not effective.

🔑 CN: Health promotion and maintenance; CL: Synthesize

3. 1. This client is likely experiencing fatigue and should increase her periods of rest. The fatigue may be caused by anemia from depletion of red blood cells due to the chemotherapy. Asking the client to limit her activities may cause the client to become withdrawn. The information given does not support limiting activity. Increasing fluid intake will not reduce the fatigue. The information does not indicate that the client is immunosuppressed and should avoid contact with others.

🔑 CN: Physiological adaptation; CL: Synthesize

4. 1,2,3. Using designated donors does not decrease the risk of contracting infectious diseases, such as the Epstein-Barr virus, HIV, or CMV. Hepatitis A is transmitted by the oral-fecal route, not the blood route; however, hepatitis B and C can be contracted from a designated donor. Malaria is transmitted by mosquitoes.

🔑 CN: Safety and infection control; CL: Apply

5. 1. For the client with iron deficiency anemia, a rich source of iron is needed in the diet, and eggs are high in iron. Other foods high in iron include organ and muscle (dark) meats; shellfish, shrimp, and tuna; enriched, whole-grain, and fortified cereals and breads; legumes, nuts, dried fruits, and beans; oatmeal; and sweet potatoes. Dark green, leafy vegetables and citrus fruits are good sources of vitamin C. Cheese is a good source of calcium.

🔑 CN: Reduction of risk potential; CL: Apply

6. 3. Good sources of vitamin B_{12} include meats and dairy products. Whole grains are a good source of thiamine. Green, leafy vegetables are good sources of niacin, folate, and carotenoids (precursors of vitamin A). Broccoli and Brussels sprouts are good sources of ascorbic acid (vitamin C).

🔑 CN: Reduction of risk potential; CL: Apply

7. 4. Normal range of folic acid is 1.8 to 9 ng/mL (4.1 to 20.4 nmol/L), and normal range of vitamin B_{12} is 200 to 900 pg/mL (147.6 to 664 pmol/L). A low folic acid level in the presence of a normal vitamin B_{12} level is indicative of a primary folic acid deficiency anemia. Factors that affect the absorption of folic acid are drugs such as methotrexate, oral contraceptives, antiseizure drugs, and alcohol. The total bilirubin, serum creatinine, and hemoglobin values are within normal limits.

CN: Physiological adaptation;
CL: Analyze

8. 2. The defining characteristic of pernicious anemia, a megaloblastic anemia, is lack of the intrinsic factor, which results from atrophy of the stomach wall. Without the intrinsic factor, vitamin B_{12} cannot be absorbed in the small intestine, and folic acid needs vitamin B_{12} for deoxyribonucleic acid synthesis of RBCs. The gastric analysis is done to determine the primary cause of the anemia. An elevated excretion of the injected radioactive vitamin B_{12}, which is protocol for the first and second stages of the Schilling test, indicates that the client has the intrinsic factor and can absorb vitamin B_{12} in the intestinal tract. A sedimentation rate of 16 mm/h is normal for both men and women and is a nonspecific test to detect the presence of inflammation; it is not specific to anemias. An RBC value within the normal range does not indicate an anemia.

CN: Physiological adaptation;
CL: Synthesize

9. 2. Clients with aplastic anemia are severely immunocompromised and at risk for infection and possible death related to bone marrow suppression and pancytopenia. Strict aseptic technique and reverse isolation are important measures to prevent infection. Although diet, reduced stress, and rest are valued in supporting health, the potentially fatal consequence of an acute infection places it as a priority for teaching the client about health maintenance. Animal meat and dark green leafy vegetables, good sources of vitamin B_{12} and folic acid, should be included in the daily diet. Yoga and meditation are good complementary therapies to reduce stress. Eight hours of rest and naps are good for spacing and pacing activity and rest.

CN: Reduction of risk potential;
CL: Synthesize

10. 4. Vitamin B_{12} combines with intrinsic factor in the stomach and is then carried to the ileum, where it is absorbed into the bloodstream. In this situation, vitamin B_{12} cannot be absorbed regardless of the amount of oral intake of sources of vitamin B_{12}, such as animal protein or vitamin B_{12} tablets. Vitamin B_{12} needs to be injected every month because the ileum has been surgically removed. Warm salt water is used to soothe sore mucous membranes. Crohn's disease and a small-bowel resection may cause several loose stools a day, but the client does not report having this problem.

CN: Physiological adaptation;
CL: Analyze

11. 3. Coffee and tea increase gastrointestinal motility and inhibit the absorption of nonheme iron. Clients are instructed to add dried fruits to dishes at every meal because dried fruits are a nonheme or nonanimal iron source. Cooking in iron cookware, especially acid-based foods such as tomatoes, adds iron to the diet. Clients are instructed to add a rich supply of vitamin C to every meal because the absorption of iron is increased when food with vitamin C or ascorbic acid is consumed.

CN: Reduction of risk potential;
CL: Evaluate

12. 1. It is difficult to determine activity intolerance without objectively comparing activities from one time frame to another. Because iron deficiency anemia can occur gradually and individual endurance varies, the nurse can best assess the client's activity tolerance by asking the client to compare activities 6 months ago and at present. Asking a client how long a problem has existed is a very open-ended question that allows for too much subjectivity for any definition of the client's activity tolerance. Also, the client may not even identify that a "problem" exists. Asking the client whether he is staying abreast of usual activities addresses whether the tasks were completed, not the tolerance of the client while the tasks were being completed or the resulting condition of the client after the tasks were completed. Asking the client if he is more tired now than usual does not address his activity tolerance. Tiredness is a subjective evaluation and again can be distorted by factors such as the gradual onset of the anemia or the endurance of the individual.

CN: Reduction of risk potential;
CL: Analyze

13. 4,6. A client with pernicious anemia has lost the ability to absorb vitamin B_{12} either because of the lack of an acidic gastric environment or the lack of the intrinsic factor. Vitamin B_{12} must be administered by a deep intramuscular route. The ventrogluteal and dorsogluteal locations are the most acceptable sites for a deep intramuscular injection. The other sites are not acceptable.

CN: Pharmacological and parenteral therapies; CL: Apply

14. 2. To promote comfort when injecting at the ventrogluteal site, the position of choice is with the client lying on the abdomen with toes pointed inward. This positioning promotes muscle relaxation, which decreases the discomfort of making an injection into a tense muscle. Lying on the side with legs extended will not provide the greatest muscle relaxation. Leaning over the edge of a table with the hips flexed and standing upright with the feet apart will increase muscular tension.

⚷━ CN: Physiological adaptation; CL: Apply

15. 1,2,3,4. The nurse should ask the client about symptoms related to pernicious anemia because the client had the stomach stapled 2 years ago and shows no history of supplemental vitamin B_{12}. Numbness and tingling relate to a loss of intrinsic factor from the gastric stapling. Intrinsic factor is necessary for absorption of vitamin B_{12}. The nurse should suspect pernicious anemia if the client is not taking supplemental vitamin B_{12}. Other signs and symptoms of pernicious anemia include cognitive problems and depression. The nurse also should ask about the client's support at home in case the fall was not an accident. Pernicious anemia is not related to dietary intake of iron.

⚷━ CN: Reduction of risk potential;
CL: Analyze

16. 1. The nurse should prepare to start an intake and output record because the client is exhibiting clinical manifestations of anemia with jaundice and is demonstrating a fluid imbalance. The client does not need to be on bed rest at this point. The client is not contagious and does not need to be placed in contact isolation. The changes in the color of the skin and urine are related to the jaundice and will not be affected by sunlight.

⚷━ CN: Physiological adaptation;
CL: Synthesize

17. 1. Drug-induced hemolytic anemia is acquired, antibody-mediated, RBC destruction precipitated by medications, such as cephalosporins, sulfa drugs, rifampin, methyldopa, procainamide, quinidine, and thiazides. Purpura is a condition with various manifestations characterized by hemorrhages into the skin, mucous membranes, internal organs, and other tissues. Infectious emboli are clumps of bacteria present in blood or lymph. Ecchymoses are skin discolorations due to extravasations of blood into the skin or mucous membranes.

⚷━ CN: Reduction of risk potential;
CL: Analyze

18. 2. Urinary vitamin B_{12} levels are measured after the ingestion of radioactive vitamin B_{12}. A 24- to 48-hour urine specimen is collected after administration of an oral dose of radioactively tagged vitamin B_{12} and an injection of nonradioactive vitamin B_{12}. In a healthy state of absorption, excess vitamin B_{12} is excreted in the urine; in a malabsorptive state or when the intrinsic factor is missing, vitamin B_{12} is excreted in the feces. Methylcellulose is a bulk-forming agent. Laxatives interfere with the absorption of vitamin B_{12}. The client is NPO 8 to 12 hours before the test but is not NPO during the test. A stool collection is not a part of the Schilling test. If stool contaminates the urine collection, the results will be altered.

⚷━ CN: Pharmacological and parenteral therapies; CL: Analyze

19. 3. Pernicious anemia is caused by a lack of vitamin B_{12}. Primary symptoms include neuropathy with paresthesias of hands and feet. The nurse assesses the client to determine the effectiveness of the monthly dose of vitamin B_{12}, which is to reverse the deficiency and the related symptoms. Improved energy is associated with treatment for iron deficiency anemia. Healing of cracked lips and tongue is an outcome of taking folic acid for folic acid deficiency. Delayed clotting time is associated with hemophilia; the clotting time is not affected by vitamin B_{12}.

⚷━ CN: Pharmacological and parenteral therapies; CL: Evaluate

20. 2. Most clients with pernicious anemia have deficient production of intrinsic factor in the stomach. Intrinsic factor attaches to the vitamin in the stomach and forms a complex that allows the vitamin to be absorbed in the small intestine. The stomach is producing enough acid, there is not an excessive excretion of the vitamin, and there is not a rapid production of red blood cells in this condition.

⚷━ CN: Physiological adaptation;
CL: Synthesize

21. 2. The normal physiologic response to activity is an increased metabolic rate over the resting basal rate. The decrease in respiratory rate indicates that the client is not strong enough to complete the mechanical cycle of respiration needed for gas exchange. The postactivity pulse is expected to increase immediately after activity but by no more than 50 bpm if it is strenuous activity. The diastolic blood pressure is expected to rise but by no more than 15 mm Hg. The pulse returns to within 6 bpm of the resting pulse after 3 minutes of rest.

⚷━ CN: Physiological adaptation;
CL: Evaluate

22. 3. The nurse should continue to monitor the client because this value reflects a normal physiologic response. The **HCP** 📖 does not need to be called, and oxygen does not need to be started based on these laboratory findings. Immediately after surgery, the client's hematocrit reflects a falsely high value related to the body's compensatory response to the stress of sudden loss of fluids and blood. Activation of the intrinsic pathway and the renin-angiotensin cycle via antidiuretic hormone produces vasoconstriction and retention of fluid for the first 1 to 2 days postoperatively. By the 2nd to 3rd day, this response decreases, and the client's hematocrit level is more reflective of the amount of RBCs in the plasma. Fresh bleeding is a less likely occurrence on the third postoperative day but is not impossible; however, the nurse should have expected to see a decrease in the RBC count and hemoglobin value accompanying the hematocrit.

CN: Physiological adaptation; CL: Synthesize

23. 4. The most likely time for a blood transfusion reaction to occur is during the first 15 minutes or first 50 mL of the infusion. If a blood transfusion reaction does occur, it is imperative to keep an established IV line so that medication can be administered to prevent or treat cardiovascular collapse in case of anaphylaxis. PRBCs should be administered through a 19-gauge or larger needle; a peripherally inserted central catheter line is not recommended, in order to avoid a slow flow. RBCs will hemolyze in dextrose or lactated Ringer's solution and should be infused with only normal saline solution.

CN: Pharmacological and parenteral therapies; CL: Synthesize

24. 1,2,4. The nurse should teach the client to drink plenty of fluids to avoid becoming dehydrated. The client should avoid being in high altitudes, such as mountains above 5,000 feet (1,524 m), where less oxygen is available and may precipitate a sickle cell crisis. The nurse should alert young women with sickle cell anemia that pregnancy increases the risk of a crisis. People who are homozygous for HbS have sickle cell anemia; the heterozygous form is the sickle cell carrier trait. A client with sickle cell anemia may fly on commercial airlines; the airplane is pressurized and has an adequate oxygen level.

CN: Health promotion and maintenance; CL: Synthesize

25. 2. The nurse should teach the client and family that individuals who are heterozygous for hemochromatosis rarely develop the disease. Men and women are equally at risk for hemochromatosis, but men are diagnosed earlier because women do not usually have manifestations until menopause. Hemochromatosis is the most common genetic disorder in Canada and the United States. Individuals who are homozygous for hemochromatosis received a defective gene from each parent. Those with homozygous genes may develop the disease.

CN: Health promotion and maintenance; CL: Synthesize

26. 3,4,1,2. When the client is having a blood transfusion reaction, the nurse should first stop the transfusion and then keep the IV open with normal saline infusion. Next, the nurse should notify the HCP and blood bank and then complete the required form(s) regarding the transfusion reaction.

CN: Physiological adaptation; CL: Synthesize

27. 2,3,5. The American Association of Blood Banks and Canadian Blood Services recommend that two qualified people, such as two **registered nurses (RN)**, compare the name and number on the identification bracelet with the tag on the blood bag. Verifying that the two units are the same is not a recommendation. Rather, the verification is always with the client, not with bags of blood. A unit of blood should infuse in 4 hours or less to avoid the risk of septicemia since no preservatives are used. When a blood transfusion reaction occurs, the blood transfusion should be stopped immediately, but the IV line should be kept open so that emergency medications and fluids can be administered.

The unit of PRBCs should be inspected for contamination by looking for leaks, abnormal color, clots, and excessive air bubbles. When a unit of PRBCs is being transfused, vital signs are assessed before the transfusion begins, after the first 15 minutes and then every hour until 1 hour after the transfusion has been completed. When PRBCs are being administered, a 20-gauge or larger needle is needed to avoid destroying the red blood cells (RBCs) passing through the lumen and to allow for maximal flow rate.

CN: Pharmacological and parenteral therapies; CL: Synthesize

28. 2. ABO- and Rh-incompatible blood causes an antigen-antibody reaction that produces hemolysis or agglutination of red blood cells (RBCs). At the first indication of any sign/symptom of reaction, the blood transfusion is stopped. Blood and urine samples are obtained from the client and sent to the lab along with the remaining untransfused blood. Hemoglobin in the urine and blood samples taken at the time of the reaction provides evidence of a hemolytic blood transfusion reaction. Antihistamine, aspirin, diuretics, and vasopressors may be administered with different types of transfusion reactions.

CN: Reduction of risk potential; CL: Synthesize

29. 1. Epoetin is a recombinant DNA form of erythropoietin, which stimulates the production of red blood cells (RBCs) and therefore causes the hematocrit to rise. The elevation in hematocrit causes an elevation in the blood pressure; therefore, the blood pressure is a vital sign that should be

of hemorrhage that occurred and the period of time over which it occurred. Bradycardia is a late symptom of hemorrhage; it occurs after the client is no longer able to compromise and is debilitating further into shock. If bradycardia is left untreated, the client will die from cardiovascular collapse. Decreased $Paco_2$ is a late symptom of hemorrhage, after transport of oxygen to the tissue has been affected. A narrowed pulse pressure is not an early sign of hemorrhage.

🔑 CN: Physiological adaptation;
CL: Analyze

46. 4. ITP is treated with steroids to suppress the splenic macrophages from phagocytizing the antibody-coated platelets, which are recognized as foreign bodies, so that the platelets live longer. The steroids also suppress the binding of the autoimmune antibody to the platelet surface. Steroids do not destroy the antibodies on the platelets, neutralize antigens, or increase phagocytosis.

🔑 CN: Pharmacological and parenteral therapies; CL: Apply

47. 3. The client needs to wear or carry information containing the name of the drug, dosage, **healthcare provider (HCP)** 📖 and contact information, and emergency instructions because additional corticosteroid drug therapy would be needed during emergency situations. Prednisone should be taken in the morning because it can cause insomnia and because exogenous corticosteroid suppression of the adrenal cortex is less when it is administered in the morning. Prednisone must never be stopped suddenly. It must be tapered off to allow for the adrenal cortex to recover from drug-induced atrophy so that it can resume its function. Prednisone suppresses the immune response and masks infections. It does not provide extra protection against infection.

🔑 CN: Pharmacological and parenteral therapies; CL: Evaluate

48. 1. Nausea, vomiting, and peptic ulcers are gastrointestinal adverse effects of prednisone, so it is recommended that clients take the prednisone with food. In some instances, the client may be advised to take a prescribed antacid prophylactically. The client should never take over-the-counter drugs without notifying the **healthcare provider (HCP)** 📖 who prescribed the prednisone. The client should ask the HCP about the amount and kind of exercise because of the need to establish baseline physical values before starting an exercise program and because of the increased potential for comorbidity with increasing age. The client should eat foods that are high in potassium to prevent hypokalemia.

🔑 CN: Pharmacological and parenteral therapies; CL: Synthesize

49. 4. The best exercise for females who are on long-term corticosteroid therapy is a low-impact, weight-bearing exercise such as walking or weight lifting. Floor exercises do not provide for the weight bearing. Stretching is appropriate but does not offer sufficient weight bearing. Running provides for weight bearing but is hard on the joints and may cause bleeding.

🔑 CN: Pharmacological and parenteral therapies; CL: Synthesize

50. 2. The client needs further teaching if she thinks that the number of tissues saturated represents all of the blood lost during a nosebleed. During a nosebleed, a significant amount of blood can be swallowed and go undetected. It is important that clients with severe thrombocytopenia do not take a nosebleed lightly. Clients with thrombocytopenia can apply pressure for 5 to 10 minutes over a small, superficial cut. Clients with thrombocytopenia can take hormones to suppress menses and control menstrual blood loss. Clients can also count the number of saturated sanitary napkins to approximate blood loss during menses. Some authorities estimate that a completely soaked sanitary napkin holds 50 mL.

🔑 CN: Reduction of risk potential; CL: Evaluate

51. 2,4,5,6. Adverse effects of prednisone are weight gain, retention of sodium and fluids with hypertension and cushingoid features, a low serum albumin level, suppressed inflammatory processes with masked symptoms, and osteoporosis. A diet high in protein, potassium, calcium, and vitamin D is recommended. Carbohydrates would elevate glucose and further compromise a client's immune status. Trans fat does not counteract the adverse effects of steroids such as prednisone.

🔑 CN: Pharmacological and parenteral therapies; CL: Synthesize

52. 1. Platelets cannot survive cold temperatures. The platelets should be stored at room temperature and last for no more than 5 days.

🔑 CN: Pharmacological and parenteral therapies; CL: Synthesize

53. 3. The bag containing platelets needs to be gently rotated to prevent clumping. ABO compatibility is not a necessary requirement, but human leukocyte antigen (HLA) matching of lymphocytes may be completed to avoid development of anti-HLA antibodies when multiple platelet transfusions are necessary. Platelets should be administered as fast as can be tolerated by the client to avoid aggregation. Most institutions use tubing especially for platelets instead of tubing for blood and blood products.

🔑 CN: Pharmacological and parenteral therapies; CL: Synthesize

54. 4. The correct technique for deep breathing postoperatively to avoid atelectasis and pneumonia is to take in a deep breath through the nose, hold it for 5 seconds, and then blow it out through pursed lips. The goal is to fully expand and empty the lungs for pulmonary hygiene.

CN: Reduction of risk potential; CL: Evaluate

55. 3. An elective surgical procedure is scheduled in advance so that all preparations can be completed ahead of time. The vital signs are the final check that must be completed before the client leaves the room so that continuity of care and assessment is provided for. The first assessment that will be completed in the preoperative holding area or operating room will be the client's vital signs. The client should have emptied the bladder before receiving preoperative medications so that the bladder is empty when it is time for transport into the operating room. The client should have signed the **consent** before the transport time so that if there were any questions or concerns, there was time to meet with the surgeon. Also, the consent form must be signed before any sedative medications are given. The client's name band should be placed as soon as the client arrives in the perioperative setting, and it remains in place through discharge.

CN: Physiological adaptation; CL: Analyze

56. 3. After a splenectomy, the client is at high risk for hypovolemia and hemorrhage. The dressing should be checked often; if drainage is present, a circle should be drawn around the drainage and the time noted to help determine how fast bleeding is occurring. The nasogastric tube should be connected, but this can wait until the dressing has been checked. A urinary catheter is not needed. The last pain medication administration and the client's current pain level should be communicated in the exchange report. Checking for hemorrhage is a greater priority than assessing pain level.

CN: Physiological adaptation; CL: Analyze

57. 3. A splenectomy may involve manipulation of the upper abdominal organs, such as diaphragm, stomach, liver, spleen, and small intestines. Manipulation of these organs and resulting inflammation lead to a slowed peristalsis. An NG tube is placed to decrease abdominal distention in the immediate postoperative phase. The stomach does not need to be manipulated away from the spleen postoperatively, nor would an NG tube accomplish this. The NG tube drains gastric contents and air in the stomach; it is not in the operative site and therefore cannot be used to irrigate it. The gastric juices are not checked as an indicator that peristalsis has returned; instead, bowel sounds are auscultated in all four quadrants to indicate the return of peristalsis.

CN: Physiological adaptation; CL: Apply

58. 4. Clients who have had a splenectomy are especially prone to infection. The reduction of immunoglobulin M leaves the client especially at risk for immunologic deficiency infections. All clients who have had major abdominal surgery usually receive discharge instructions not to drive because the stomach muscles are not strong enough to brake hard or quickly after the abdominal muscles have been separated. All clients need to pace activity and rest when going home after major surgery. Rest and sleep allow the growth hormone to repair the tissue, and activity allows the energy and strength to build endurance and muscle strength. An appointment is usually made to see the surgeon in the office 1 week after discharge for follow-up and to remove sutures or staples if this has not already been done.

CN: Reduction of risk potential; CL: Synthesize

59. 2. There is no well-defined sequence for acute DIC other than that the client starts bleeding without a history or cause and does not stop bleeding. Later signs may include severe shortness of breath, hypotension, pallor, petechiae, hematoma, orthopnea, hematuria, vision changes, and joint pain.

CN: Physiological adaptation; CL: Analyze

60. 3. DIC has not been found to respond to oral anticoagulants such as warfarin sodium. Treatments for DIC are controversial but include treating the underlying cause, administering heparin, and replacing depleted blood products.

CN: Pharmacological and parenteral therapies; CL: Synthesize

61. 2. Clinical manifestations of microvascular thrombosis are those that represent a blockage of blood flow and oxygenation to the tissue that results in eventual death of the organ. Examples of microvascular thrombosis include acute respiratory distress syndrome, focal ischemia, superficial gangrene, oliguria, azotemia, cortical necrosis, acute ulceration, delirium, and coma. Hemoptysis, petechiae, and hematuria are signs of hemorrhage.

CN: Physiological adaptation; CL: Analyze

62. 3. As blood collects in the peritoneal cavity, it causes dilation and distention, which is reflected in increased abdominal girth. The client would be tachycardic and hypotensive. Petechiae reflect bleeding in the skin.

CN: Physiological adaptation; CL: Analyze

The Client with White Blood Cell Disorders

63. **1,2,3,5.** The nurse should teach this client to stay on bed rest as long as there is a fever, gargle with warm saline, and increase oral fluids to prevent dehydration from the elevated temperature. The client with an enlarged spleen should avoid contact sports due to the increased risk of injury due to the enlargement. The client does not need to wear a mask, but should observe handwashing procedures.

CN: Basic care and comfort; CL: Create

64. **4.** The client will need a prescription from the **healthcare provider (HCP)** 📖 to be placed in reverse (protective) isolation because the normal defenses are ineffective and place the client at risk for infection (leukopenia, <5,000 cells/μL [5 × 10⁹/L]). The faster the decrease in WBCs, the greater the bone marrow suppression and the more susceptible the client is to infection from not only pathogenic but also nonpathogenic organisms. The client will continue to be monitored, the laboratory may be called, and the report will be placed on the chart, but protection of the client must be instituted immediately.

CN: Physiological adaptation;
CL: Synthesize

65. **3.** A shift to the left means that more immature than mature WBCs are at the site of inflammation or infection. Immature WBCs are less effective at phagocytosis and do not produce classic signs of inflammation, such as pus, redness, swelling, or heat. Fever is the only sign; therefore, it is a significant sign of infection in a client with immature or depressed WBCs.

CN: Physiological adaptation;
CL: Analyze

66. **1,2,3,4.** Nursing care of a client with leukemia includes managing and preventing infection, maintaining integrity of skin and mucous membranes, instituting measures to prevent bleeding, and monitoring for bleeding. Aspirin is an anticoagulant; bleeding tendencies, such as petechiae, ecchymosis, epistaxis, gingival bleeding, and retinal hemorrhages, are likely due to thrombocytopenia.

CN: Reduction of risk potential;
CL: Create

67. **2.** A client is at moderate risk when the ANC is <1,000 (1 × 10⁹/L). The ANC decreases proportionately to the increased risk for infection. Normal risk for infection is when the ANC is 1,500 (1.5 × 10⁹/L) or greater. High risk for infection is when the ANC is <500 (0.5 × 10⁹/L). An ANC of 100 (0.1 × 10⁹/L) or less is life threatening.

CN: Physiological adaptation;
CL: Analyze

68. **1.** Bedside rails, call bells, drug administration controls operated by the client, and other surface areas are frequently touched by caregivers with used gloves. Changing gloves immediately after use protects the client from contamination by organisms. Cross-contamination is a break in technique of serious consequence to the severely compromised client. Standing 2 feet (61 cm) from the client, speaking minimally, and wearing protective covering shirts are not required in standard interventions for risk of infection.

CN: Safety and infection control;
CL: Synthesize

69. **1.** The neutropenic client is at risk for infection, especially bacterial infection of the respiratory and gastrointestinal tracts. Breaks in the mucous membranes, such as those that could be caused by the insertion of a suppository or enema tube, would be a break in the first line of the body's defense and a direct port of entry for infection. The client with neutropenia is encouraged to wear an HEPA filter mask and to use an incentive spirometer for pulmonary hygiene. The client needs to know the importance of completing meticulous total body hygiene daily, including perianal care after every bowel movement, to decrease the flora at normal body orifices. The client also needs to know the importance of performing oral care after every meal and every 4 hours while the client is awake to decrease the bacterial buildup in the oropharynx.

CN: Health promotion and maintenance;
CL: Synthesize

70. **2.** Washing hands before, during, and after care has a significant effect in reducing infections. It is advisable to avoid introducing a cold or children's germs and to avoid kissing the client, but the primary prevention technique is handwashing.

CN: Health promotion and maintenance;
CL: Synthesize

71. **1,2,4,5.** The nurse can serve as a witness for **consent** 📖 for procedures. The nurse also ascertains whether the client has an understanding that is consistent with the procedure listed on the form, determines that the client is signing the consent of his or her own free will, and determines that the client understands postprocedure care. The nurse's role does not include explaining the risks of the procedure; that responsibility belongs to the person who is to perform the procedure, such as the **healthcare provider (HCP)** 📖 .

CN: Management of care; CL: Synthesize

72. **3.** As the bone marrow is being aspirated, the client will feel a suction or pulling type of sensation or discomfort that lasts a few seconds. A systemic premedication may be given to decrease this discomfort. A small area over the sternum is cleaned with an antiseptic. It is unnecessary to paint the entire anterior chest. The local anesthetic is injected through the subcutaneous tissue to numb the tissue for the larger-bore needle that is used for aspiration and biopsy. After the needle is removed, pressure is held over the aspiration site for 5 to 10 minutes to achieve hemostasis. A small dressing is applied; a large pressure dressing, such as an Ace bandage, would restrict the expansion of the lungs and is not used.

⚭ CN: Psychosocial adaptation; CL: Apply

73. 4. After a bone marrow aspiration, the puncture site should be checked every 10 to 15 minutes for bleeding. For a short period after the procedure, bed rest may be prescribed. Signs of infection, such as redness and swelling, are not anticipated at the aspiration site. A mild analgesic may be prescribed for pain, but if the client has pain longer than 24 hours, the nurse should assess the client for internal bleeding or increased pressure at the puncture site, which may be the cause of the pain, and should consult the **healthcare provider (HCP)** 📖.

⚭ CN: Physiological adaptation; CL: Evaluate

74. 2. The nurse is an advocate for the client with leukemia who can be empowered with knowledge of the treatment. Immunologic, cytogenic, morphologic, histochemical, and other means are used to identify cell subtypes and stages of leukemia cell development for very specific and optimal treatment. The nurse should not label the client's feeling, such as frustration or emotional; only the client can identify her own feelings. Chastising the client is not helpful. It disavows the client's emotional state and responses to her diagnosis and involved treatment. Unless nurses have had leukemia, they cannot possibly know how the client feels even though they may be trying to offer her empathy.

⚭ CN: Psychosocial adaptation; CL: Synthesize

75. 3. The induction phase of chemotherapy is an aggressive treatment to kill leukemia cells. The client is severely immunocompromised and severely at risk for infection. Flowers, herbs, and plants should be avoided during this time. The client's Bible, pictures, and other personal belongings can be cleaned before being brought into the room to prevent client contact with pathogenic and nonpathogenic organisms.

⚭ CN: Safety and infection control; CL: Synthesize

76. 2. The nurse identifies that the client does not understand that contact with animals must be avoided because they carry infection and the induction therapy will destroy the client's white blood cells (WBCs). The induction therapy will cause anemia, and the client will experience fatigue and will have to pace activities with rest periods. Platelet production will be decreased, and the client will be at risk for bleeding tendencies; oral hygiene will have to be provided by using a warm saline gargle instead of brushing the teeth and gums. The client will be at risk for infection owing to the decrease in WBC production and should report a temperature of 100°F (37.8°C) or higher.

⚭ CN: Safety and infection control; CL: Evaluate

77. 1. Imatinib works by inhibiting the proliferation of abnormal cells. Adverse effects include edema and GI irritation. Typical effects of this drug do not include numbness and tingling, bloody stools, or persistent cough. If the client has these symptoms, they may relate to disease occurrence or recurrence.

⚭ CN: Pharmacological and parenteral therapies; CL: Apply

78. 2. Diphenhydramine is an antihistamine. This drug helps reduce the incidence of an allergic response by blocking the release of histamine. Diphenhydramine also possesses anticholinergic effects and can reduce the incidence of nausea and vomiting for clients receiving chemotherapy. Although diphenhydramine may promote sleep, it is not the primary reason for its administration in this instance. Diphenhydramine will not reduce anxiety or potentiate the action of the vincristine.

⚭ CN: Pharmacological and parenteral therapies; CL: Apply

79. 1. Pancytopenia means a decrease in all blood components. Because a platelet count of <15,000/mm³ can result in spontaneous bleeding, the nurse notifies the **HCP** 📖 of this laboratory result. Neutrophils are a type of WBC. An absolute neutrophil count between 1,000 and 1,800/mm³ suggests mild neutropenia and represents a low risk of infection. Although references vary, normal range for WBC counts is 5,000 to 11,000/mm³, and a female's normal hemoglobin (Hgb) value is roughly 12 to 16 g/100 mL. Therefore, the WBC count and Hgb levels are a bit low, but not critical.

⚭ CN: Pharmacological and parenteral therapies; CL: Analyze

80. 3. Antineoplastic agents can cause severe tissue damage if they extravasate; therefore, the nurse immediately stops the infusion and then notifies the **HCP** 📖. If extravasation has occurred, it may be appropriate to apply ice packs to the site. Ice packs cause desired vasoconstriction; warm, moist packs cause vasodilation. Ice packs should not remain in place for more than 15 to 20 minutes because rebound vasodilation can occur; the ice packs are removed for a short time and then reapplied as needed.

🔑 CN: Pharmacological and parenteral Therapies; CL: Synthesize

81. 3,4,1,2. The client is experiencing a septic reaction to the blood transfusion. The nurse first stops the infusion and notifies the **HCP** 📖 and blood bank; then, the nurse uses an infusion of normal saline to keep the vein open and follows by obtaining a sample of the client's blood for a blood culture. Lastly, the nurse sends the blood bag and the administration set to the blood bank for culture.

🔑 CN: Pharmacological and parenteral Therapies; CL: Synthesize

82. 2. Epoetin stimulates erythropoiesis and the production of RBCs. This is important for clients taking antineoplastics because they often suffer bone marrow depression as a side effect of antineoplastic therapy. Epoetin does not affect tissue malignancy or tumor size. Nausea and vomiting are commonly associated with antineoplastics, but these are treated with antiemetics.

🔑 CN: Pharmacological parenteral therapies; CL: Evaluate

83. 4. Bleeding and infection are the major complications and causes of death for clients with AML. Bleeding is related to the degree of thrombocytopenia, and infection is related to the degree of neutropenia. Cardiac arrhythmias rarely occur as a result of AML. Liver or renal failure may occur, but neither is a major cause of death in AML.

🔑 CN: Reduction of risk potential; CL: Synthesize

84. 1. The peak incidence of ALL is at 4 years of age. ALL is uncommon after 15 years of age. The median age at incidence of CML is 40 to 50 years. The peak incidence of AML occurs at 60 years of age. Two-thirds of cases of chronic lymphocytic leukemia occur in clients older than 60 years of age.

🔑 CN: Physiological adaptation; CL: Analyze

85. 1. Clients with ALL are at risk for infection due to granulocytopenia. The nurse should place the client in a private room. Strict handwashing procedures should be enforced and will be the most effective way to prevent infection. It is not necessary to have the client wear a mask. The client is not contagious, and the staff does not need to wear gloves. The client can have visitors; however, they should be screened for infection and use handwashing procedures.

🔑 CN: Physiological adaptation; CL: Synthesize

86. 3. Simple rinses with saline or a baking soda and water solution are effective and moisten the oral mucosa. Commercial mouthwashes and lemon glycerin swabs contain glycerin and alcohol, which are drying to the mucosa and should be avoided. Brushing after each meal is recommended, but every 4 hours may be too traumatic. During acute leukemia, the neutrophil and platelet counts are often low, and a soft-bristle toothbrush, instead of the client's usual brush, should be used to prevent bleeding gums.

🔑 CN: Reduction of risk potential; CL: Synthesize

87. 3. The client with acute leukemia experiences fatigue and deconditioning. Lying in bed and taking deep breaths will not help achieve the goals. The client must get out of bed to increase activity tolerance and improve tidal volume. Ambulating in the hall (using an HEPA filter mask if neutropenic) is a sensible activity and helps improve conditioning. Sitting up in a chair facilitates lung expansion. Using a stationary bicycle in the room allows the client to increase activity as tolerated.

🔑 CN: Reduction of risk potential; CL: Synthesize

88. 2. Combination chemotherapy does not mean two groups of drugs, one to kill the cancer cells and one to treat the adverse effects of the chemotherapy. Combination chemotherapy means that multiple drugs are given to interrupt the cell growth cycle at different points, decrease resistance to a chemotherapy agent, and minimize the toxicity associated with use of a high dose of a single agent (i.e., by using multiple agents with different toxicities).

🔑 CN: Pharmacological and parenteral therapies; CL: Evaluate

89. 1. The biliary system is not especially prone to hemorrhage. Thrombocytopenia (a low platelet count) leaves the client at risk for a potentially life-threatening spontaneous hemorrhage in the gastrointestinal, respiratory, and intracranial cavities.

🔑 CN: Physiological adaptation; CL: Analyze

90. 1. The primary purpose of reverse isolation is to reduce transmission of organisms to the client from sources outside the client's environment.

🔑 CN: Safety and infection control; CL: Apply

The Client with Lymphoma

91. 2. Painless and enlarged cervical lymph nodes, tachycardia, weight loss, weakness and fatigue, and night sweats are signs of Hodgkin's disease. Difficulty swallowing and breathing may occur, but only with mediastinal node involvement. Hepatomegaly is a late-stage manifestation.

CN: Physiological adaptation;
CL: Analyze

92. 3. The client with Hodgkin's lymphoma who has had radiation therapy is prone to infection; therefore, the primary goal is to prevent infection. The nurse instructs the client to perform frequent hand hygiene, avoid crowded areas, and report a temperature over 100°F (37.7°C). Maintaining fluid balance, exercising, and maintaining mental health are also important, but not the primary goal at this time.

CN: Safety and infection control;
CL: Synthesize

93. 1. The nurse must ensure that sterile technique is used when a biopsy is obtained because the client is at high risk for infection. In most cases, a lymph node biopsy is sent immediately to the laboratory once it is placed in a specific solution in a closed container. It is not necessary to wear a gown and mask when obtaining the specimen. It is not necessary to use special handling procedures for the instruments used.

CN: Management of care; **CL:** Apply

94. 3. Assessing for an open airway is always first. The procedure involves the neck; the anesthesia may have affected the swallowing reflex, or the inflammation may have closed in on the airway, leading to ineffective air exchange. Once a patent airway is confirmed and an effective breathing pattern established, the circulation is checked. Vital signs and the incision are assessed as soon as possible, but only after it is established that the airway is patent and the client is breathing normally. A neurologic assessment is completed as soon as possible after other important assessments.

CN: Physiological adaptation;
CL: Synthesize

95. 1. Herpes zoster infections are common in clients with Hodgkin's disease. Discoloring of the teeth is not related to Hodgkin's disease but rather to the ingestion of iron supplements or some antibiotics such as tetracycline. Mild anemia is common in Hodgkin's disease, but the platelet count is not affected until the tumor has invaded the bone marrow. A cellular immunity defect occurs in Hodgkin's disease in which there is little or no reaction to skin sensitivity tests. This is called anergy.

CN: Physiological adaptation;
CL: Analyze

96. 3. A temperature higher than 100.4°F (38°C), profuse night sweats, and an unintentional weight loss of 10% of body weight represent the cluster of clinical manifestations known as the B symptoms. Forty percent of clients with Hodgkin's disease have B symptoms, and B symptoms are more common in advanced stages of the disease.

CN: Physiological adaptation;
CL: Analyze

97. 1. Analgesics are used as needed to relieve painful encroachment of enlarged lymph nodes. Perfumed shower gel will increase pruritus. Wearing a mask does not protect the client from infection if pathogens are not spread by airborne droplets. Antipyretics should be used to treat fever symptomatically after infection is ruled out.

CN: Health promotion and maintenance;
CL: Create

98. 1. In the staging process, the designations A and B signify that symptoms were or were not present when Hodgkin's disease was found, respectively. The Roman numerals I through IV indicate the extent and location of involvement of the disease. Stage I indicates involvement of a single lymph node; stage II, two or more lymph nodes on the same side of the diaphragm; stage III, lymph node regions on both sides of the diaphragm; and stage IV, diffuse disease of one or more extralymphatic organs.

CN: Physiological adaptation; **CL:** Apply

99. 3. Encouraging the client to take slow, deep breaths during uncomfortable parts of procedures is the best method of decreasing the stress response of tightening and tensing the muscles. Slow, deep breathing affects the level of carbon dioxide in the brain to increase the client's sense of well-being. Allowing the client's family to stay may be appropriate if the family has a calming effect on the client, but this family is upset and may contribute to the client's stress. Silence can be therapeutic, but when the client is faced with a potentially life-threatening diagnosis and a new, invasive procedure, taking deep breaths will be more effective in reducing the stress response. Expressing feelings is important, but deep breathing will promote relaxation; the nurse can encourage the client to express feelings when the procedure is completed.

CN: Psychosocial adaptation;
CL: Synthesize

100. 2. A biopsy needle is inserted through a separate incision in the anesthetized area. The client will feel a pressure sensation when the biopsy is taken but should not feel actual pain. The client should be instructed to inform the **healthcare provider (HCP)** 📖 if pain is felt so that more anesthetic agent can be administered to keep the client comfortable. The biopsy is performed after the aspiration and from a slightly different site so that the tissue is not disturbed by either test. The client will feel a suction-type pain for a moment when the aspiration is being performed, not the biopsy. A small incision is made for the biopsy to accommodate the larger-bore needle. This may require a stitch.

🔑 CN: Psychosocial adaptation;
CL: Synthesize

101. 3. Terminally ill clients most often describe feelings of isolation because they tend to be ignored, they are often left out of conversations (especially those dealing with the future), and they sense the attitudes of discomfort that many people feel in their presence. Helpful nursing measures include taking the time to be with the client, offering opportunities to talk about feelings, and answering questions honestly.

🔑 CN: Psychosocial adaptation;
CL: Synthesize

102. 2. It is incorrect that the survivor rate is directly proportional to the incidence of second malignancy. The survivor rate is indirectly proportional to the incidence of second malignancy, and regular screening is very important to detect a second malignancy, especially acute myeloid leukemia or myelodysplastic syndrome. Survivors should know the stage of the disease and their current treatment plan so that they can remain active participants in their health care.

🔑 CN: Physiological adaptation;
CL: Evaluate

The Client Who Is in Shock

103. 3. Nursing interventions and collaborative management are focused on correcting and maintaining adequate tissue perfusion. Inadequate tissue perfusion may be caused by hemorrhage, as in hypovolemic shock; by decreased cardiac output, as in cardiogenic shock; or by massive vasodilation of the vascular bed, as in neurogenic, anaphylactic, and septic shock. Fluid deficit, not fluid overload, occurs in shock.

🔑 CN: Physiological adaptation;
CL: Synthesize

104. 4. Typical signs and symptoms of hypovolemic shock include systolic blood pressure <90 mm Hg, narrowing pulse pressure, tachycardia, tachypnea, cool and clammy skin, decreased urine output, and mental status changes, such as irritability or anxiety. Unequal dilation of the pupils is related to central nervous system injury or possibly to a previous history of eye injury.

🔑 CN: Physiological adaptation;
CL: Analyze

105. 1. Urine output provides the most sensitive indication of the client's response to therapy for hypovolemic shock. Urine output should be consistently >35 mL/h. Blood pressure is a more accurate reflection of the adequacy of vasoconstriction than of tissue perfusion. Respiratory rate is not a sensitive indicator of fluid balance in the client recovering from hypovolemic shock.

🔑 CN: Pharmacological and parenteral therapies; CL: Evaluate

106. 1. Causes of hypovolemic shock include external fluid loss, such as hemorrhage; internal fluid shifting, such as ascites and severe edema; and dehydration. Massive vasodilation is the initial phase of vasogenic or distributive shock, which can be further subdivided into three types of shock: septic, neurogenic, and anaphylactic. A severe antigen-antibody reaction occurs in anaphylactic shock. Gram-negative bacterial infection is the most common cause of septic shock. Loss of sympathetic tone (vasodilation) occurs in neurogenic shock.

🔑 CN: Physiological adaptation;
CL: Analyze

107. 2. The client who is receiving a blood product requires astute assessment for signs and symptoms of allergic reaction and anaphylaxis, including pruritus (itching), urticaria (hives), facial or glottal edema, and shortness of breath. If such a reaction occurs, the nurse should stop the transfusion immediately, but leave the IV line intact, and notify the **healthcare provider (HCP)** 📖. Usually, an antihistamine (such as diphenhydramine hydrochloride) is administered. Epinephrine and corticosteroids may be administered in severe reactions. Fluid balance is not an immediate concern during the blood administration. The administration should not cause pain unless it is extravasating out of the vein, in which case the IV administration should be stopped. Administration of a unit of blood should not affect the level of consciousness.

🔑 CN: Pharmacological and parenteral therapies; CL: Analyze

108. 2. At medium doses (4 to 8 mcg/kg/min), dopamine hydrochloride slightly increases the heart rate and improves contractility to increase cardiac output and improve tissue perfusion. When given at low doses (0.5 to 3.0 mcg/kg/min), dopamine increases renal and mesenteric blood flow. At high doses (8 to 10 mcg/kg/min), dopamine produces vasoconstriction, which is an undesirable effect. Dopamine is not given to affect preload and afterload.

🔑 CN: Pharmacological and parenteral therapies; CL: Evaluate

109. 2. The client who is receiving dopamine hydrochloride requires continuous blood pressure monitoring with an invasive or noninvasive device. The nurse may titrate the IV infusion to maintain a systolic blood pressure of 90 mm Hg. Administration of a pain medication concurrently with dopamine hydrochloride, which is a potent sympathomimetic with dose-related alpha-adrenergic agonist, beta 1-selective adrenergic agonist, and dopaminergic blocking effects, is not an essential nursing action for a client who is in shock with already low hemodynamic values. Arterial blood gas concentrations should be monitored according to the client's respiratory status and acid-base balance status and are not directly related to the dopamine hydrochloride dosage. Monitoring for signs of infection is not related to the nursing action for the client receiving dopamine hydrochloride.

CN: Pharmacological and parenteral therapies; CL: Synthesize

110. 4,1,2,3. Analysis of the client's laboratory results indicates that an INR of 8 is increased beyond therapeutic ranges. The client is also experiencing severe acute rectal bleeding and has a hemoglobin level in the low range of normal and a hematocrit reflecting fluid volume loss. The nurse should first establish an IV line and administer the dextrose in saline. Next, the nurse should administer the FFP. FFP contains concentrated clotting factors and provides an immediate reversal of the prolonged INR. Vitamin K 2.5 mg PO should be given next because it reverses the warfarin by returning the PT to normal values. However, the reversal process occurs over 1 to 2 hours. Lastly, the nurse can schedule the client for the sigmoidoscopy.

CN: Pharmacological and parenteral therapies; CL: Synthesize

111. 2. Warm, flushed skin from a high cardiac output with vasodilation occurs in warm shock or the hyperdynamic phase (first phase) of septic shock. Other signs and symptoms of early septic shock include fever with restlessness and confusion; normal or decreased blood pressure with tachypnea and tachycardia; increased or normal urine output; and nausea and vomiting or diarrhea. Cool, clammy skin occurs in the hypodynamic or cold phase (later phase). Hemorrhage is not a factor in septic shock.

CN: Physiological adaptation; CL: Analyze

112. 1. The nurse monitors the blood levels of antibiotics, white blood cells, serum creatinine, and blood urea nitrogen because of the decreased perfusion to the kidneys, which are responsible for filtering out the ceftriaxone sodium. It is possible that the clearance of the antibiotic has been decreased enough to cause toxicity. Increased levels of these laboratory values should be reported to the healthcare provider (HCP) ▭ immediately. A spinal fluid analysis is done to examine cerebral spinal fluid, but there is no indication of central nervous system involvement in this case. Arterial blood gases are used to determine actual blood gas levels and assess acid-base balance. Serum osmolality is used to monitor fluid and electrolyte balance.

CN: Pharmacological and parenteral therapies; CL: Analyze

113. 4. Maintaining asepsis of indwelling urinary catheters is essential to prevent infection. Preventing septic shock is a major focus of nursing care because the mortality rate for septic shock is as high as 90% in some populations. Very young and elderly clients (those younger than age 2 or older than age 65) are at increased risk for septic shock. Administering IV fluid replacement therapy, obtaining vital signs every 4 hours on all clients, and monitoring red blood cell counts for elevation do not pertain to septic shock prevention.

CN: Safety and infection control; CL: Synthesize

114. 2. ARDS is a complication associated with septic shock. ARDS causes respiratory failure and may lead to death, even after the client has recovered from shock. Anaphylaxis is a type of distributive or vasogenic shock. COPD is a functional category of pulmonary disease that consists of persistent obstruction of bronchial airflow and involves chronic bronchitis and chronic emphysema. Mitral valve prolapse is a condition in which the mitral valve is pushed back too far during ventricular contraction.

CN: Physiological adaptation; CL: Analyze

Managing Care, Quality, and Safety for Clients with Hematologic Health Problems

115. 3. When two clients are to receive blood at the same time, the nurse should call for and hang the clients' transfusions separately to avoid error. The nurse should call for and hang the first client's blood first because this client has experienced a change in blood pressure over a short period of time. The nurse should next call and hang the second client's blood transfusion as there is no indication that this client is unstable at this time. The nurse should not call for both units of transfusions at the same time due to the increased risk of misidentification. The nurse should not verify compatibility of both units at the same time due to the increased risk of misidentification. It is not necessary to involve two nurses because the second client can wait until the nurse has time to hang the blood.

CN: Management of care; CL: Synthesize

116. **1,2,3,4.** If a blood transfusion is terminated, the nurse must send a freshly collected blood sample to the blood bank and a urine sample to the laboratory; the nurse must send the blood component unit with the attached administration set and completed Transfusion Reaction Form to the blood bank. It is not necessary to inform Infection Control, but the Risk Management department should be notified, since a transfusion reaction may be a significant liability issue.

    CN: Reduction of risk potential;
CL: Synthesize

117. **3.** The most current pharmacology information is found in the clinical agency's drug guide, which may be available on electronic sources that are frequently updated and can be transmitted to a handheld device or by logging into the Internet or hospital's intranet, if available. A commercially published drug guide and pharmacology textbooks are outdated once published and, therefore, may not have current information. The manufacturer's website has the potential for bias.

    CN: Safety and infection control;
CL: Apply

118. **1,2,3.** Abbreviations can be misinterpreted and all healthcare professionals should avoid the use of easily misunderstood abbreviations. The purpose of avoiding abbreviations is not to make it easier for clients to understand the medication prescriptions or to make data entry easier.

    CN: Safety and infection control;
CL: Synthesize

119. **4.** The most common source of infection and microbial colonization in neutropenic clients is their own nonpathogenic normal flora. Attention to personal hygiene, such as oral, pulmonary, urinary, and rectal care, is essential. It is important to acknowledge the client's concerns and fears and to provide organized, calm, compassionate care, but it is more important to teach the client how to prevent an infection that could be life threatening.

    CN: Health promotion and maintenance;
CL: Synthesize

The Client with Respiratory Health Problems

- ■ The Client with an Upper Respiratory Tract Infection
- ■ The Client Undergoing Nasal Surgery
- ■ The Client with Cancer of the Larynx
- ■ The Client with Pneumonia
- ■ The Client with Tuberculosis
- ■ The Client with Chronic Obstructive Pulmonary Disease
- ■ The Client with Asthma
- ■ The Client with Lung Cancer
- ■ The Client with Chest Trauma
- ■ The Client with Acute Respiratory Distress Syndrome
- ■ Managing Care, Quality, and Safety of Clients with Respiratory Health Problems
- ■ Answers, Rationales, and Test-Taking Strategies

The Client with an Upper Respiratory Tract Infection

1. A nurse is completing the health history for a client who has been taking Echinacea for a head cold. The client asks, "Why is this not helping me feel better?" Which response by the nurse would be the **most** accurate?
- ☐ 1. "There is limited information as to the effectiveness of herbal products."
- ☐ 2. "Antibiotics are the agents needed to treat a head cold."
- ☐ 3. "The head cold should be gone within the month."
- ☐ 4. "Combining herbal products with prescription antiviral medications is sure to help you."

2. A nurse is teaching a client about taking antihistamines. Which information should the nurse include in the teaching plan? Select all that apply.
- ☐ 1. Operating machinery and driving may be dangerous while taking antihistamines.
- ☐ 2. Continue taking antihistamines even if nasal infection develops.
- ☐ 3. The effect of antihistamines is not felt until a day later.
- ☐ 4. Do not use alcohol with antihistamines.
- ☐ 5. Increase fluid intake to 2,000 mL/day.

3. A nurse instructs a client with allergic rhinitis about the correct technique for using an intranasal inhaler. Which statement indicates that the client understands the instructions?
- ☐ 1. "I should limit the use of the inhaler to early morning and bedtime use."
- ☐ 2. "It is important to not shake the canister because that can damage the spray device."
- ☐ 3. "I should hold one nostril closed while I insert the spray into the other nostril."
- ☐ 4. "The inhaler tip is inserted into the nostril and pointed toward the inside nostril wall."

4. Which is an expected outcome for a client recovering from an upper respiratory tract infection? The client will:
- ☐ 1. maintain a fluid intake of 800 mL every 24 hours.
- ☐ 2. experience chills only once a day.
- ☐ 3. cough productively without chest discomfort.
- ☐ 4. experience less nasal obstruction and discharge.

5. The nurse teaches the client how to instill nose drops. Which technique is correct?
- ☐ 1. The client uses sterile technique when handling the dropper.
- ☐ 2. The client blows the nose gently before instilling drops.
- ☐ 3. The client uses a new dropper for each instillation.
- ☐ 4. The client sits in a semi-Fowler's position for 2 minutes.

6. The nurse should include which instructions in the teaching plan for a client with chronic sinusitis? Select all that apply.
☐ 1. Avoid the use of caffeinated beverages.
☐ 2. Perform postural drainage every day.
☐ 3. Take a hot shower in the morning and evening.
☐ 4. Report a temperature of 102°F (38.9°C) or higher.
☐ 5. Limit fluid intake to 1,000 mL per 24 hours.

7. A client with allergic rhinitis asks the nurse what to do to decrease rhinorrhea. Which instruction would be appropriate for the nurse to give the client?
☐ 1. "Use your nasal decongestant spray regularly to help clear your nasal passages."
☐ 2. "Ask the healthcare provider for antibiotics. Antibiotics will help decrease the secretion."
☐ 3. "It is important to increase your activity. A daily brisk walk will help promote drainage."
☐ 4. "Keep a diary of when your symptoms occur. This can help you identify what precipitates your attacks."

8. Guaifenesin 300 mg four times a day has been prescribed as an expectorant. The dosage strength of the liquid is 200 mg/5 mL. How many milliliters should the nurse administer for each dose? Record your answer using one decimal place.

_____ mL.

9. Pseudoephedrine has been prescribed as a nasal decongestant. What is a possible adverse effect of this drug?
☐ 1. constipation
☐ 2. bradycardia
☐ 3. diplopia
☐ 4. restlessness

The Client Undergoing Nasal Surgery

10. A healthcare provider (HCP) has just inserted nasal packing for a client with epistaxis. The client is taking ramipril for hypertension. What should the nurse instruct the client to do?
☐ 1. Use 81 mg of aspirin daily for relief of discomfort.
☐ 2. Omit the next dose of ramipril.
☐ 3. Remove the packing if there is difficulty swallowing.
☐ 4. Avoid rigorous aerobic exercise.

11. A client had surgery for a deviated nasal septum. Which finding indicates that bleeding is occurring even if the nasal drip pad remains dry and intact?
☐ 1. nausea
☐ 2. repeated swallowing
☐ 3. increased respiratory rate
☐ 4. increased pain

12. A client who has undergone outpatient nasal surgery is ready for discharge and has nasal packing in place. The nurse should instruct the client to:
☐ 1. avoid activities that elicit Valsalva's maneuver.
☐ 2. take aspirin to control nasal discomfort.
☐ 3. avoid brushing the teeth until the nasal packing is removed.
☐ 4. apply heat to the nasal area to control swelling.

13. Which statement indicates to the nurse that a client has understood the discharge instructions provided after nasal surgery?
☐ 1. "I should not shower until my packing is removed."
☐ 2. "I will take stool softeners and modify my diet to prevent constipation."
☐ 3. "Coughing every 2 hours is important to prevent respiratory complications."
☐ 4. "It is important to blow my nose each day to remove the dried secretions."

14. The nurse is giving preoperative instructions to a client who will be undergoing rhinoplasty. The nurse should instruct the client that:
☐ 1. after surgery, nasal packing will be in place for 7 to 10 days.
☐ 2. normal saline nose drops will need to be administered preoperatively.
☐ 3. the results of the surgery will be immediately obvious postoperatively.
☐ 4. aspirin-containing medications should not be taken for 2 weeks before surgery.

15. Following nasal surgery, what should the nurse do **first**?
☐ 1. Assess the client's pain.
☐ 2. Inspect the area for periorbital ecchymosis.
☐ 3. Assess respiratory status.
☐ 4. Measure intake and output.

16. After nasal surgery, the client expresses concern about how to decrease facial pain and swelling while recovering at home. Which instruction would be **most** effective for decreasing pain and edema?
☐ 1. Take analgesics every 4 hours around the clock.
☐ 2. Use corticosteroid nasal spray as needed to control symptoms.
☐ 3. Use a bedside humidifier while sleeping.
☐ 4. Apply cold compresses to the area.

17. A client is being discharged with nasal packing in place. The nurse should instruct the client to:
☐ 1. perform frequent mouth care.
☐ 2. use normal saline nose drops daily.
☐ 3. sneeze and cough with mouth closed.
☐ 4. gargle every 4 hours with salt water.

18. The nurse is teaching a client how to manage a nosebleed. What instruction should the nurse give the client?
- ☐ 1. "Tilt your head backward, and pinch your nose."
- ☐ 2. "Lie down flat, and place an ice compress over the bridge of the nose."
- ☐ 3. "Blow your nose gently with your neck flexed."
- ☐ 4. "Sit down, lean forward, and pinch the soft portion of your nose."

19. An elderly client had posterior packing inserted to control a severe nosebleed. After insertion of the packing, the nurse should observe the client for which finding?
- ☐ 1. vertigo
- ☐ 2. Bell's palsy
- ☐ 3. hypoventilation
- ☐ 4. loss of gag reflex

The Client with Cancer of the Larynx

20. Following surgery for a radical neck dissection for laryngeal cancer, the **priority** for nursing care is:
- ☐ 1. maintaining complete bed rest until postsurgical swelling decreases.
- ☐ 2. taking vital signs once a shift until the client is stable.
- ☐ 3. starting a clear liquid diet at 48 hours.
- ☐ 4. suctioning the laryngectomy tube as often as needed.

21. A client who has had a total laryngectomy appears withdrawn and depressed. The client keeps the curtain drawn, refuses visitors, and indicates a desire to be left alone. Which nursing intervention would be **most** therapeutic for the client?
- ☐ 1. discussing the behavior with the spouse to determine the cause
- ☐ 2. exploring future plans
- ☐ 3. respecting the need for privacy
- ☐ 4. encouraging expression of feelings nonverbally and in writing

22. The nurse is suctioning a client who had a laryngectomy. What is the **maximum** amount of time the nurse should suction the client?
- ☐ 1. 10 seconds
- ☐ 2. 20 seconds
- ☐ 3. 25 seconds
- ☐ 4. 30 seconds

23. When suctioning a tracheostomy tube 3 days following insertion, what should the nurse do?
- ☐ 1. Use a sterile catheter each time the client is suctioned.
- ☐ 2. Clean the catheter in sterile water after each use, and reuse for no longer than 8 hours.
- ☐ 3. Protect the catheter in sterile packaging between suctioning episodes.
- ☐ 4. Use a clean catheter with each suctioning, and disinfect it in hydrogen peroxide between uses.

24. The client with a laryngectomy does not want to be observed by the family because the opening in the throat is "disgusting." The nurse should:
- ☐ 1. initiate teaching about the care of a stoma.
- ☐ 2. explain that the stoma will not always look as it does now.
- ☐ 3. inform the client of the benefits of family support at this time.
- ☐ 4. explore why the client believes the stoma is "disgusting."

25. The nurse team leader is making rounds and observes the client who had a tracheostomy tube inserted 2 days ago (see figure). The nursing policy manual recommends use of the gauze pad. The nurse should:

- ☐ 1. make sure the gauze pad is dry and the client is in a comfortable position.
- ☐ 2. ask the unlicensed assistive personnel (UAP) to tie the tracheostomy tube ties in the back of the client's neck.
- ☐ 3. reposition the gauze pad around the stoma with the open end downward.
- ☐ 4. ask a registered nurse (RN) to change the ties and position another gauze pad around the stoma.

26. To reduce the risk of laryngeal cancer in employees in a factory that uses respiratory irritants, what instructions should the nurse give the employees? Select all that apply.
- ☐ 1. Stop smoking.
- ☐ 2. Use a portable HEPA air purifier in the home.
- ☐ 3. Limit alcohol intake.
- ☐ 4. Brush teeth after every meal.
- ☐ 5. Avoid raising the voice to be heard over the noise in the factory.

27. A client has had hoarseness for more than 2 weeks. The nurse should:
- ☐ 1. refer the client to a healthcare provider (HCP) for a prescription for an antibiotic.
- ☐ 2. instruct the client to gargle with salt water at home.
- ☐ 3. assess the client for dysphagia.
- ☐ 4. instruct the client to take a throat analgesic.

28. A client has just returned from the postanesthesia care unit after undergoing a laryngectomy. Which instruction should the nurse include in the plan of care?
- ☐ 1. Maintain the head of the bed at 30 to 40 degrees.
- ☐ 2. Teach the client how to use esophageal speech.
- ☐ 3. Initiate small feedings of soft foods.
- ☐ 4. Irrigate drainage tubes as needed.

29. Which goal is an expected outcome for a client recovering from a total laryngectomy? The client will:
- ☐ 1. regain the ability to taste and smell food.
- ☐ 2. demonstrate appropriate care of the gastrostomy tube.
- ☐ 3. communicate feelings about body image changes.
- ☐ 4. demonstrate sterile suctioning technique for stoma care.

30. What instruction should the nurse give the client who underwent a laryngectomy and is now going home?
- ☐ 1. Perform mouth care every morning and evening.
- ☐ 2. Provide adequate humidity in the home.
- ☐ 3. Maintain a soft, bland diet.
- ☐ 4. Limit physical activity to shoulder and neck exercises.

The Client with Pneumonia

31. The nurse is caring for a client with bacterial pneumonia. The effectiveness of the client's oxygen therapy can be **best** determined by the:
- ☐ 1. absence of cyanosis.
- ☐ 2. client's respiratory rate.
- ☐ 3. arterial blood gas values.
- ☐ 4. client's level of consciousness.

32. An elderly client admitted with pneumonia and dementia has attempted several times to pull out the IV and Foley catheter. After trying other options, the nurse obtains a prescription for bilateral soft wrist restraints. Which nursing action is **most** appropriate?
- ☐ 1. Perform circulation checks to bilateral upper extremities each shift.
- ☐ 2. Attach the ties of the restraints to the bed frame.
- ☐ 3. Reevaluate the need for restraints and document weekly.
- ☐ 4. Ensure the restraint prescription has been signed by the healthcare provider (HCP) within 72 hours.

33. A 79-year-old client is admitted to the hospital with a diagnosis of bacterial pneumonia. While obtaining the client's health history, the nurse learns that the client has osteoarthritis, follows a vegetarian diet, and is very concerned with cleanliness. Which client information would **most** likely be a predisposing factor for the diagnosis of pneumonia?
- ☐ 1. age
- ☐ 2. osteoarthritis
- ☐ 3. vegetarian diet
- ☐ 4. daily bathing

34. Which findings are significant data to gather from a client who has been diagnosed with pneumonia? Select all that apply.
- ☐ 1. quality of breath sounds
- ☐ 2. presence of bowel sounds
- ☐ 3. occurrence of chest pain
- ☐ 4. amount of peripheral edema
- ☐ 5. color of nail beds

35. A client with bacterial pneumonia is to be started on IV antibiotics. Which diagnostic test must be completed before antibiotic therapy begins?
- ☐ 1. urinalysis
- ☐ 2. sputum culture
- ☐ 3. chest radiograph
- ☐ 4. red blood cell count

36. When caring for the client who is receiving an aminoglycoside antibiotic, the nurse should monitor which laboratory value?
- ☐ 1. serum sodium
- ☐ 2. serum potassium
- ☐ 3. serum creatinine
- ☐ 4. serum calcium

37. The healthcare provider has prescribed penicillin for a client admitted to the hospital for treatment of pneumonia. Prior to administering the first dose of penicillin, the nurse should ask the client:
- ☐ 1. "Do you have a history of seizures?"
- ☐ 2. "Do you have any cardiac history?"
- ☐ 3. "Have you had any recent infections?"
- ☐ 4. "Have you had a previous allergy to penicillin?"

38. A client with pneumonia has a temperature of 102.6°F (39.2°C), is diaphoretic, and has a productive cough. The client is able to ambulate. What should the nurse do?
- ☐ 1. Change the client's position every 4 hours.
- ☐ 2. Use nasotracheal suctioning to clear secretions.
- ☐ 3. Change the bedsheets frequently.
- ☐ 4. Offer the use of a bedpan every 2 hours.

39. Bed rest is prescribed for a client with pneumonia during the acute phase of the illness. The nurse should determine the effectiveness of bed rest by assessing the client's:
- ☐ 1. decreased cellular demand for oxygen.
- ☐ 2. reduced episodes of coughing.
- ☐ 3. diminished pain when breathing deeply.
- ☐ 4. ability to expectorate secretions more easily.

40. A client with pneumonia is experiencing pleuritic chest pain. The nurse should assess the client for:

☐ **1.** a mild but constant aching in the chest.
☐ **2.** severe midsternal pain.
☐ **3.** moderate pain that worsens on inspiration.
☐ **4.** muscle spasm pain that accompanies coughing.

41. Which nursing action would **most** likely be successful in reducing pleuritic chest pain in a client with pneumonia?

☐ **1.** Encourage the client to breathe shallowly.
☐ **2.** Have the client practice abdominal breathing.
☐ **3.** Offer the client incentive spirometry.
☐ **4.** Teach the client to splint the rib cage when coughing.

42. The nurse administers two 325-mg aspirin every 4 hours to a client with pneumonia. The nurse should evaluate the outcome of administering the drug by assessing the client for which findings? Select all that apply.

☐ **1.** decreased pain when breathing
☐ **2.** prolonged clotting time
☐ **3.** decreased temperature
☐ **4.** decreased respiratory rate
☐ **5.** increased ability to expectorate secretions

43. Which mental status change may occur when a client with pneumonia is first experiencing hypoxia?

☐ **1.** coma
☐ **2.** apathy
☐ **3.** irritability
☐ **4.** depression

44. The client with pneumonia develops mild constipation, and the nurse administers docusate sodium as prescribed. This drug works by:

☐ **1.** softening the stool.
☐ **2.** lubricating the stool.
☐ **3.** increasing stool bulk.
☐ **4.** stimulating peristalsis.

45. Which finding is an expected outcome for an elderly client following treatment for bacterial pneumonia?

☐ **1.** a respiratory rate of 25 to 30 breaths/min
☐ **2.** the ability to perform activities of daily living without dyspnea
☐ **3.** a maximum loss of 5 to 10 lb (2 to 5 kg) of body weight
☐ **4.** chest pain that is minimized by splinting the rib cage

The Client with Tuberculosis

46. A client newly diagnosed with tuberculosis (TB) is being admitted with the prescription for "isolation precautions for tuberculosis." The nurse should assign the client to which type of room?

☐ **1.** a room at the end of the hall for privacy
☐ **2.** a private room to implement airborne precautions
☐ **3.** a room near the nurses' station to ensure confidentiality
☐ **4.** a room with windows to allow sunlight

47. The nurse is reviewing the history and physical and healthcare provider (HCP) prescriptions on the medical record of a newly admitted client.

History and Physical Tab	
Subjective:	19-year-old reports a constant cough for the past "few weeks" with "dark" sputum for the past few days. Has night sweats, 10-lb (4.5-kg) weight loss in the past month, and "always" being tired. He took one Tylenol about an hour prior to arrival.
Objective:	
BP	120/64
HR	84/reg
Resp	26/unlabored/slight wheezing in right lower lobe posteriorly
O² Sat	92%
Temp	99.9°F (37.7°C) oral
Skin	Warm, slightly diaphoretic
Nonproductive cough at this time	
Assessment:	Possible respiratory infection
Physician prescriptions tab	
	Chest x-ray
	Sputum specimen
	Oxygen at 2 L per nasal cannula

The nurse should **first:**

☐ **1.** initiate airborne precautions.
☐ **2.** apply oxygen at 2 L per nasal cannula.
☐ **3.** collect a sputum sample.
☐ **4.** reassess vital signs.

48. A client is receiving streptomycin in the treatment regimen of tuberculosis. The nurse should assess for:

☐ **1.** decreased serum creatinine.
☐ **2.** difficulty swallowing.
☐ **3.** hearing loss.
☐ **4.** IV infiltration.

49. The nurse is reconciling the prescriptions for a client diagnosed recently with pulmonary tuberculosis who is being admitted to the hospital for a total hip replacement. (See medication prescription sheet.) The client asks if it is necessary to take all of these medications while in the hospital. The nurse should:

Medication Prescription

isoniazid (INH), 300 mg PO daily

Rifampin (Rifadin), 600 mg PO daily

Pyridoxine (vitamin B₆), 10 mg PO daily

ethambutol, 400 mg PO daily

pyrazinamide, 1.5 g PO daily.

Dr. Smith 6-29-15

☐ 1. request that the healthcare provider (HCP) review the prescriptions for a duplication between isoniazid and ethambutol.
☐ 2. inform the client that all drugs will be discontinued until the client can eat solid foods.
☐ 3. ask the pharmacist to check for drug interactions between the rifampin and isoniazid.
☐ 4. tell the client that it is important to continue to take the medications because the combination of drugs prevents bacterial resistance.

50. The client with tuberculosis is to be discharged home with nursing follow-up. Which aspect of nursing care will have the **highest priority**?
☐ 1. offering the client emotional support
☐ 2. teaching the client about the disease and its treatment
☐ 3. coordinating various agency services
☐ 4. assessing the client's environment for sanitation

51. The nurse is reading the results of a tuberculin skin test (see figure). The nurse should interpret the results as:

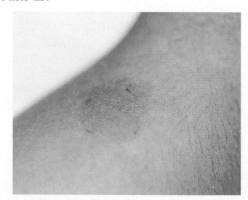

☐ 1. negative.
☐ 2. needing to be repeated.
☐ 3. positive.
☐ 4. false.

52. Which technique for administering the Mantoux test is correct?
☐ 1. Hold the needle and syringe almost parallel to the client's skin.
☐ 2. Pinch the skin when inserting the needle.
☐ 3. Aspirate before injecting the medication.
☐ 4. Massage the site after injecting the medication.

53. A client had a Mantoux test result of an 8-mm induration. The test is considered positive when the client:
☐ 1. lives in a long-term care facility.
☐ 2. has no known risk factors.
☐ 3. is immunocompromised.
☐ 4. works as a healthcare provider (HCP) in a hospital.

54. Which family member exposed to tuberculosis would be at **highest** risk for contracting the disease?
☐ 1. 45-year-old mother
☐ 2. 17-year-old daughter
☐ 3. 8-year-old son
☐ 4. 76-year-old grandmother

55. The nurse is teaching a client who has been diagnosed with tuberculosis how to avoid spreading the disease to family members. Which statements indicate that the client has understood the nurse's instructions? Select all that apply.
☐ 1. "I will need to dispose of my old clothing when I return home."
☐ 2. "I should always cover my mouth and nose when sneezing."
☐ 3. "It is important that I isolate myself from family when possible."
☐ 4. "I should use paper tissues to cough in and dispose of them promptly."
☐ 5. "I will avoid crowds."

56. A client has a positive reaction to the Mantoux test. The nurse interprets this reaction to mean that the client has:
☐ 1. active tuberculosis.
☐ 2. been exposed to *Mycobacterium tuberculosis*.
☐ 3. developed a resistance to tubercle bacilli.
☐ 4. developed passive immunity to tuberculosis.

57. A client with tuberculosis is taking isoniazid (INH). To help prevent development of peripheral neuropathies, the nurse should instruct the client to:
☐ 1. adhere to a low-cholesterol diet.
☐ 2. supplement the diet with pyridoxine (vitamin B₆).
☐ 3. get extra rest.
☐ 4. avoid excessive sun exposure.

58. The nurse should caution sexually active female clients taking isoniazid (INH) that the drug:
☐ 1. increases the risk of vaginal infection.
☐ 2. has mutagenic effects on ova.
☐ 3. decreases the effectiveness of hormonal contraceptives.
☐ 4. inhibits ovulation.

59. Clients who have had active tuberculosis are at risk for recurrence. Which condition increases that risk?
- ☐ **1.** cool and damp weather
- ☐ **2.** active exercise and exertion
- ☐ **3.** physical and emotional stress
- ☐ **4.** rest and inactivity

60. In which areas of the United States and Canada is the incidence of tuberculosis **highest**?
- ☐ **1.** rural farming areas
- ☐ **2.** inner-city areas
- ☐ **3.** areas where clean water standards are low
- ☐ **4.** suburban areas with significant industrial pollution

61. The nurse should include which instruction when developing a teaching plan for a client who is receiving isoniazid and rifampin for treatment of tuberculosis?
- ☐ **1.** Take the medication with antacids.
- ☐ **2.** Double the dosage if a drug dose is missed.
- ☐ **3.** Increase intake of dairy products.
- ☐ **4.** Avoid alcohol.

62. A client who has been diagnosed with tuberculosis has been placed on drug therapy. The medication regimen includes rifampin. Which instruction should the nurse give the client about potential adverse effects of rifampin? Select all that apply.
- ☐ **1.** Have eye examinations every 6 months.
- ☐ **2.** Maintain follow-up monitoring of liver enzymes.
- ☐ **3.** Decrease protein intake in the diet.
- ☐ **4.** Avoid alcohol intake.
- ☐ **5.** The urine may have an orange color.

63. The nurse is providing follow-up care to a client with tuberculosis who does not regularly take the prescribed medication. Which nursing action would be **most** appropriate for this client?
- ☐ **1.** Ask the client's spouse to supervise the daily administration of the medications.
- ☐ **2.** Visit the client weekly to verify compliance with taking the medication.
- ☐ **3.** Notify the healthcare provider (HCP) of the client's noncompliance, and request a different prescription.
- ☐ **4.** Remind the client that tuberculosis can be fatal if it is not treated promptly.

The Client with Chronic Obstructive Pulmonary Disease

64. A client with newly diagnosed chronic obstructive disease is to be discharged home with oxygen per nasal prongs. Which teaching points should the nurse include in this client's discharge plan? Select all that apply.
- ☐ **1.** Apply Vaseline or petroleum jelly on lips and nose to prevent dryness and irritation.
- ☐ **2.** Avoid areas where people are smoking cigarettes or cigars.
- ☐ **3.** Increase oxygen flow at night during hours of sleep.
- ☐ **4.** Place gauze between the ears and oxygen tubing to prevent skin irritation.
- ☐ **5.** Request a large, pressurized oxygen tank for use during car travel.
- ☐ **6.** Avoid use of a microwave oven when using oxygen.

65. A nurse is reviewing the medications used by a client who has chronic bronchitis and a history of high blood pressure and prostate enlargement. The nurse should verify that the client understands how to use which medications? Select all that apply.
- ☐ **1.** albuterol and ipratropium by metered-dose inhaler
- ☐ **2.** guaifenesin with dextromethorphan liquid
- ☐ **3.** generic pseudoephedrine tablets
- ☐ **4.** lisinopril tablets
- ☐ **5.** tamsulosin

66. Which information should the nurse include in a teaching plan for the client newly diagnosed with chronic obstructive pulmonary disease? Select all that apply.
- ☐ **1.** Pulmonary rehabilitation programs offer very little benefit.
- ☐ **2.** Pneumococcal vaccination is contraindicated for clients with lung disease.
- ☐ **3.** High humidity may increase your work of breathing.
- ☐ **4.** A bronchodilator with metered-dose inhaler should be readily available.
- ☐ **5.** Smoking cessation is important to slow or stop disease progression.

67. A nurse is assessing a client with chronic emphysema. Which finding requires immediate intervention?
- ☐ **1.** using pursed-lip breathing and prolonged expiration
- ☐ **2.** circumoral cyanosis
- ☐ **3.** crackles auscultated posteriorly halfway up the left lung
- ☐ **4.** appearance of a "barrel chest"

68. The nurse is assessing a client with COPD. Which requires immediate intervention?
☐ 1. distant heart sounds
☐ 2. diminished lung sounds
☐ 3. inability to speak
☐ 4. pursed-lip breathing

69. The nurse is instructing a client with chronic obstructive pulmonary disease (COPD) how to do pursed-lip breathing. In which order from first to last should the nurse explain the steps to the client? All options must be used.

| 1. "Breathe in normally through your nose for two counts (while counting to yourself, one, two)." |
| 2. "Relax your neck and shoulder muscles." |
| 3. "Pucker your lips as if you were going to whistle." |
| 4. "Breathe out slowly through pursed lips for four counts (while counting to yourself, one, two, three, four)." |

| |
| |
| |
| |

70. The nurse reviews an arterial blood gas report for a client with chronic obstructive pulmonary disease (COPD). The results are as follows: pH 7.35; Pco_2 62 (8.25 kPa); Po_2 70 (9.31 kPa); HCO_3 34 mEq/L (34 mmol/L). The nurse should **first**:
☐ 1. apply a 100% nonrebreather mask.
☐ 2. assess the vital signs.
☐ 3. reposition the client.
☐ 4. prepare for intubation.

71. When developing a discharge plan to manage the care of a client with chronic obstructive pulmonary disease (COPD), the nurse should advise the client to expect to:
☐ 1. develop respiratory infections easily.
☐ 2. maintain current status.
☐ 3. require less supplemental oxygen.
☐ 4. show permanent improvement.

72. The client with chronic obstructive pulmonary disease (COPD) is taking theophylline. The nurse should instruct the client to report which signs of theophylline toxicity? Select all that apply.
☐ 1. nausea
☐ 2. vomiting
☐ 3. seizures
☐ 4. insomnia
☐ 5. vision changes

73. Which statement indicates that the client with chronic obstructive pulmonary disease (COPD) who has been discharged to home understands the care plan?
☐ 1. The client will avoid direct contact with family and friends.
☐ 2. The client states actions to reduce pain.
☐ 3. The client will use oxygen via a nasal cannula at 5 L/min.
☐ 4. The client agrees to call the healthcare provider (HCP) if dyspnea on exertion increases.

74. When instructing clients on how to decrease the risk of developing chronic obstructive pulmonary disease (COPD), the nurse should emphasize which instruction?
☐ 1. Participate regularly in aerobic exercises.
☐ 2. Maintain a high-protein diet.
☐ 3. Avoid exposure to people with known respiratory infections.
☐ 4. Abstain from cigarette smoking.

75. Which is an expected outcome of pursed-lip breathing for clients with emphysema?
☐ 1. to promote oxygen intake
☐ 2. to strengthen the diaphragm
☐ 3. to strengthen the intercostal muscles
☐ 4. to promote carbon dioxide elimination

76. Which is a **priority** goal for the client with chronic obstructive pulmonary disease (COPD)?
☐ 1. maintaining functional ability
☐ 2. minimizing chest pain
☐ 3. increasing carbon dioxide levels in the blood
☐ 4. treating infectious agents

77. When teaching a client with chronic obstructive pulmonary disease to conserve energy, the nurse should teach the client to lift objects:
☐ 1. while inhaling through an open mouth.
☐ 2. while exhaling through pursed lips.
☐ 3. after exhaling but before inhaling.
☐ 4. while taking a deep breath and holding it.

78. The nurse is teaching a client with chronic obstructive pulmonary disease (COPD) to assess for signs and symptoms of right-sided heart failure. Which signs and symptoms should be included in the teaching plan?
- ☐ 1. clubbing of nail beds
- ☐ 2. hypertension
- ☐ 3. peripheral edema
- ☐ 4. increased appetite

79. The nurse assesses the respiratory status of a client who is experiencing an exacerbation of chronic obstructive pulmonary disease (COPD) secondary to an upper respiratory tract infection. Which findings are expected?
- ☐ 1. normal breath sounds
- ☐ 2. prolonged inspiration
- ☐ 3. normal chest movement
- ☐ 4. coarse crackles and rhonchi

80. A client with chronic obstructive pulmonary disease (COPD) is experiencing dyspnea and has a low PaO_2 level. The nurse plans to administer oxygen as prescribed. Which statement is true concerning oxygen administration to a client with COPD?
- ☐ 1. High oxygen concentrations will cause coughing and dyspnea.
- ☐ 2. High oxygen concentrations may inhibit the hypoxic stimulus to breathe.
- ☐ 3. Increased oxygen use will cause the client to become dependent on the oxygen.
- ☐ 4. Administration of oxygen is contraindicated in clients who are using bronchodilators.

81. Which diet would be **most** appropriate for a client with chronic obstructive pulmonary disease (COPD)?
- ☐ 1. low-fat, low-cholesterol diet
- ☐ 2. bland, soft diet
- ☐ 3. low-sodium diet
- ☐ 4. high-calorie, high-protein diet

82. The nurse administers theophylline to a client. When evaluating the effectiveness of this medication, the nurse should assess the client for:
- ☐ 1. suppression of the client's respiratory infection
- ☐ 2. decrease in bronchial secretions
- ☐ 3. less difficulty breathing
- ☐ 4. thinning of tenacious, purulent sputum

83. The nurse is planning to teach a client with chronic obstructive pulmonary disease how to cough effectively. Which instruction should be included?
- ☐ 1. Take a deep abdominal breath, bend forward, and cough three or four times on exhalation.
- ☐ 2. Lie flat on the back, splint the thorax, take two deep breaths, and cough.
- ☐ 3. Take several rapid, shallow breaths, and then cough forcefully.
- ☐ 4. Assume a side-lying position, extend the arm over the head, and alternate deep breathing with coughing.

The Client with Asthma

84. The nurse observes a client using a metered-dose inhaler (MDI) to aid in management of asthma. Which actions indicate that the client needs further instruction? Select all that apply.
- ☐ 1. shakes the MDI before using
- ☐ 2. exhales before starting to use the MDI
- ☐ 3. inspires rapidly when dispensing the medication from the MDI
- ☐ 4. holds the breath for 3 seconds after inhaling with the MDI
- ☐ 5. cleans the inhaler and canister in soapy water before using again in rapid succession

85. A client with a history of asthma is admitted to the emergency department. The nurse notes that the client is dyspneic, with a respiratory rate of 35 breaths/min, nasal flaring, and use of accessory muscles. Auscultation of the lung fields reveals greatly diminished breath sounds. What should the nurse do **first**?
- ☐ 1. Initiate oxygen therapy as prescribed, and reassess the client in 10 minutes.
- ☐ 2. Draw blood for an arterial blood gas.
- ☐ 3. Encourage the client to relax and breathe slowly through the mouth.
- ☐ 4. Administer bronchodilators as prescribed.

86. A client is experiencing an acute asthmatic attack. Prior to treatment with levalbuterol, respirations were 40 breaths/min, pulse 132 beats/min, oxygen saturation 86% on room air, and with audible wheezing. Which findings indicate achievement of the desired outcome of asthma treatment?
- ☐ 1. decreased peak expiratory flow (PEF) rate
- ☐ 2. wheezing inaudible with diminished breath sounds
- ☐ 3. pulse 96 bpm and SpO_2 92% on room air
- ☐ 4. inspiratory cycle twice as long as the expiratory cycle

87. For a client with asthma, the healthcare provider (HCP) prescribes albuterol, two puffs twice a day via MDI, and beclomethasone, two puffs twice a day via MDI. The nurse should instruct the client to administer:
- ☐ 1. medications 1 hour apart, two times a day.
- ☐ 2. albuterol first and follow with beclomethasone two times a day.
- ☐ 3. albuterol on awakening and alternate the medications every 4 hours.
- ☐ 4. beclomethasone inhaler first and follow with albuterol.

88. A client experiencing a severe asthma attack has the following arterial blood gas results: pH 7.33; P_{CO_2} 48 mm Hg (6.4 kPa); P_{O_2} 58 mm Hg (7.7 kPa); HCO_3 26 mEq/L (26 mmol/L). Which prescriptions should the nurse implement **first**?

☐ **1.** albuterol nebulizer
☐ **2.** chest x-ray
☐ **3.** ipratropium inhaler
☐ **4.** sputum culture

89. A client with acute asthma is prescribed short-term corticosteroid therapy. Which is the expected outcome for the use of steroids in clients with asthma?

☐ **1.** promote bronchodilation
☐ **2.** act as an expectorant
☐ **3.** have an anti-inflammatory effect
☐ **4.** prevent development of respiratory infections

90. The nurse is teaching the client how to use a metered-dose inhaler (MDI) to administer a corticosteroid. Which observation indicates that the client is using the MDI correctly? Select all that apply.

☐ **1.** The inhaler is held upright.
☐ **2.** The head is tilted down while inhaling the medicine.
☐ **3.** The client waits 5 minutes between puffs.
☐ **4.** The client rinses the mouth with water following administration.
☐ **5.** The client lies supine for 15 minutes following administration.

91. A client is prescribed metaproterenol via a metered-dose inhaler, two puffs every 4 hours. The nurse instructs the client to report which adverse effect?

☐ **1.** irregular heartbeat
☐ **2.** constipation
☐ **3.** pedal edema
☐ **4.** decreased pulse rate

92. A client who has been taking flunisolide nasal spray, two inhalations a day, for treatment of asthma has painful, white patches in the mouth. What should the nurse tell the client?

☐ **1.** "This is an anticipated adverse effect of your medication. It should go away in a couple of weeks."
☐ **2.** "You are using your inhaler too much, and it has irritated your mouth."
☐ **3.** "You have developed a fungal infection from your medication. It will need to be treated with an antifungal agent."
☐ **4.** "Be sure to brush your teeth and floss daily. Good oral hygiene will treat this problem."

93. A nurse is teaching a client to use a metered-dose inhaler (MDI) to administer bronchodilator medication. Indicate the correct order of the steps from first to last the client should take to use the MDI appropriately. All options must be used.

1. Shake the inhaler immediately before use.

2. Hold the breath for 10 seconds, and then exhale.

3. Activate the MDI on inhalation.

4. Breathe out through the mouth.

94. What is an expected outcome for an adult client with well-controlled asthma?

☐ **1.** Chest x-ray demonstrates minimal hyperinflation.
☐ **2.** Temperature remains lower than 100°F (37.8°C).
☐ **3.** Arterial blood gas analysis demonstrates a decrease in PaO_2.
☐ **4.** Breath sounds are clear.

95. Which instruction should the nurse include in the discharge teaching plan for a client with asthma?

☐ **1.** Incorporate physical exercise as tolerated into the daily routine.
☐ **2.** Monitor peak flow numbers after meals and at bedtime.
☐ **3.** Eliminate stressors in the work and home environment.
☐ **4.** Use sedatives to ensure uninterrupted sleep at night.

96. The nurse should teach the client with asthma to avoid which of the **most** common precipitating factors of an acute asthma attack?

☐ **1.** occupational exposure to toxins
☐ **2.** Valsalva maneuver
☐ **3.** exposure to cigarette smoke
☐ **4.** exercising in cold temperatures

97. When assessing a client with asthma, which findings would **most** likely indicate the presence of a respiratory infection?

☐ **1.** cough productive of yellow sputum
☐ **2.** bilateral expiratory wheezing
☐ **3.** chest tightness
☐ **4.** respiratory rate of 30 breaths/min

98. The nurse is caring for a client who has asthma. The nurse should conduct a focused assessment to detect:

- ☐ **1.** increased forced expiratory volume.
- ☐ **2.** normal breath sounds.
- ☐ **3.** inspiratory and expiratory wheezing.
- ☐ **4.** morning headaches.

The Client with Lung Cancer

99. The nurse has assisted the healthcare provider (HCP) at the bedside with insertion of a left subclavian, triple lumen catheter in a client admitted with lung cancer. Suddenly, the client becomes restless and tachypneic. The nurse should:

- ☐ **1.** assess breath sounds.
- ☐ **2.** remove the catheter.
- ☐ **3.** insert a peripheral IV.
- ☐ **4.** reposition the client.

100. A recently extubated client has shortness of breath. The nurse reports the client's discomfort and the results of the recently prescribed arterial blood gas analysis to the healthcare provider (HCP). After reviewing the report of the complete blood count (see report), the nurse should also report which results to the HCP?

- ☐ **1.** PT
- ☐ **2.** hemoglobin and hematocrit
- ☐ **3.** monocytes
- ☐ **4.** platelets

Laboratory Values

Complete Blood Count (CBC) with Differential				
Test Results	**Current Results**	**Previous Results**	**Units**	**Reference Interval**
White Blood Count (WBC)	3.6	3.4	×10³/mm³	5.0–10.0
Red Blood Count (RBC)	3.20	3.6	×10⁶/mm³	4.1–5.3
Hemoglobin (Hgb)	9.6	10.5	g/dL	12.0–18.0
Hematocrit (Hct)	30.5	32.6	%	37.0–52.0
Platelets	302	300	×10³/mm³	150–400
Polys (neutrophils)	36	34	%	45–76
Lymphocytes	68	70	%	17–44
Monocytes	7	8	%	3–10
Eosinophils	2	3	%	0–4
Basophils	0.6	0.6	%	0.2
Polys (absolute)	0.34	0.36	×10³/mm³	1.8–7.8
Lymphocytes (absolute)	1.0	1.0	×10³/mm³	0.7–4.5
Monocytes (absolute)	0.1	0.1	×10³/mm³	0.1–1.0
Eosinophils (absolute)	0.1	0.1	×10³/mm³	0.0–0.4
Basophils (absolute)	0.0	0.0	×10³/mm³	0.0–0.2
Hemoglobin A1c				
Test Results	**Current Results**	**Previous Results**	**Units**	**Reference Interval**
HA1c	7.4		%	<7
Prothrombin				
Test Results	**Current Results**	**Previous Results**	**Units**	**Reference Interval**
PT	13	12	s	10–12 s

101. A female client diagnosed with lung cancer is to have a left lower lobectomy. What **increases** the client's risk of developing postoperative pulmonary complications?
☐ 1. Height is 5 feet, 7 inches (170.2 cm) and weight is 110 lb (49.9 kg).
☐ 2. The client tends to keep her real feelings to herself.
☐ 3. She ambulates and can climb one flight of stairs without dyspnea.
☐ 4. The client is 58 years of age.

102. The nurse in the perioperative area is preparing a client for surgery and notices that the client looks sad. The client says, "I am scared of having cancer. It is so horrible, and I brought it on myself. I should have quit smoking years ago." What would be the nurse's **best** response to the client?
☐ 1. "It is okay to be scared. What is it about cancer that you are afraid of?"
☐ 2. "It is normal to be scared. I would be, too. We will help you through it."
☐ 3. "Do not be so hard on yourself. You do not know if your smoking caused the cancer."
☐ 4. "Do you feel guilty because you smoked?"

103. A client who underwent a left lower lobectomy has been out of surgery for 48 hours. The client is receiving morphine sulfate via a patient-controlled analgesia (PCA) system and reports having pain in the left thorax that worsens when coughing. After checking the PCA system, the nurse should **next**:
☐ 1. let the client rest, so that the client is not stimulated to cough.
☐ 2. encourage the client to take deep breaths to help control the pain.
☐ 3. reassure the client that the machine is working and will administer medication to relieve the pain.
☐ 4. obtain a more detailed assessment of the client's pain using a pain scale.

104. Which factor is a **priority** to evaluate when completing discharge planning for a client who has had a lobectomy for treatment of lung cancer?
☐ 1. the support available to assist the client at home
☐ 2. the distance the client lives from the hospital
☐ 3. the client's ability to do home blood pressure monitoring
☐ 4. the client's knowledge of the causes of lung cancer

105. What is an instruction the nurse can give to help people prevent lung cancer?
☐ 1. Encourage cigarette smokers to have yearly chest radiographs.
☐ 2. Instruct people about techniques for smoking cessation.
☐ 3. Recommend that people have their houses and apartments checked for asbestos leakage.
☐ 4. Encourage people to install central air filters in their homes.

106. After a thoracotomy, the nurse instructs the client to perform deep-breathing exercises. What is an expected outcome of these exercises?
☐ 1. The elevated diaphragm enlarges the thorax and increases the lung surface available for gas exchange.
☐ 2. There is increased blood flow to the lungs to allow them to recover from the trauma of surgery.
☐ 3. The rate of airflow to the remaining lobe is controlled so that it will not become hyperinflated.
☐ 4. The alveoli expand and increase the lung surface available for ventilation.

107. Following a thoracotomy, the client has pain of 9 on a 10-point scale. Thirty minutes after administering the highest dose of the prescribed pain medication, the nurse should:
☐ 1. reposition the client.
☐ 2. reassess the client.
☐ 3. reassure the client.
☐ 4. readjust the pain medication dosage as needed.

108. While assessing a thoracotomy incisional area from which a chest tube exits, the nurse feels a crackling sensation under the fingertips along the entire incision. What should the nurse do **next**?
☐ 1. Lower the head of the bed, and call the healthcare provider (HCP).
☐ 2. Prepare an aspiration tray.
☐ 3. Mark the area with a skin pencil at the outer periphery of the crackling.
☐ 4. Turn off the suction of the chest drainage system.

109. When teaching a client to deep breathe effectively after a lobectomy, what should the nurse instruct the client to do?
☐ 1. Contract the abdominal muscles; take a slow, deep breath through the nose; hold it for 3 to 5 seconds; and then exhale.
☐ 2. Contract the abdominal muscles, take a deep breath through the mouth, and exhale slowly as if trying to blow out a candle.
☐ 3. Relax the abdominal muscles; take a slow, deep breath through the nose; and hold it for 3 to 5 seconds.
☐ 4. Relax the abdominal muscles, take a deep breath through the mouth, and exhale slowly over 10 seconds.

110. Which instruction should the nurse give the client who has undergone chest surgery to prevent shoulder ankylosis?
- [ ] **1.** Turn from side to side.
- [ ] **2.** Raise and lower the head.
- [ ] **3.** Raise the arm on the affected side over the head.
- [ ] **4.** Flex and extend the elbow on the affected side.

111. When caring for a client with a chest tube and water seal drainage system, the nurse should:
- [ ] **1.** verify that the air vent on the water seal drainage system is capped when the suction is off.
- [ ] **2.** strip the chest drainage tubes at least every 4 hours if excessive bleeding occurs.
- [ ] **3.** ensure that the chest tube is clamped when moving the client out of the bed.
- [ ] **4.** make sure that the drainage apparatus is always below the client's chest level.

112. A client has a chest tube attached to a water seal drainage system, and the nurse notes that the fluid in the chest tube and in the water seal column has stopped fluctuating. The nurse should determine that:
- [ ] **1.** the lung has fully expanded.
- [ ] **2.** the lung has collapsed.
- [ ] **3.** the chest tube is in the pleural space.
- [ ] **4.** the mediastinal space has decreased.

113. The nurse observes a constant gentle bubbling in the water seal column of a water seal chest drainage system. The nurse should:
- [ ] **1.** continue monitoring as usual; this is expected.
- [ ] **2.** check the connectors between the chest and drainage tubes and where the drainage tube enters chest drainage system.
- [ ] **3.** decrease the suction and continue observing the system for changes in bubbling during the next several hours.
- [ ] **4.** notify the healthcare provider (HCP).

114. A client who underwent a lobectomy and has a water seal chest drainage system is breathing with a little more effort and at a faster rate than 1 hour ago. The client's pulse rate is also increased. The nurse should:
- [ ] **1.** check the tubing to ensure that the client is not lying on it or kinking it.
- [ ] **2.** increase the suction.
- [ ] **3.** lower the drainage bottles 2 to 3 feet (61 to 91.4 cm) below the level of the client's chest.
- [ ] **4.** ensure that the chest tube has two clamps on it to prevent air leaks.

115. The nurse is assessing a client who has a chest tube connected to a water seal chest tube drainage system. According to the illustration shown, what should the nurse do?
- [ ] **1.** Clamp the chest tube near the insertion site to prevent air from entering the pleural cavity.
- [ ] **2.** Notify the healthcare provider (HCP) of the amount of chest tube drainage.
- [ ] **3.** Add water to maintain the water seal.
- [ ] **4.** Lower the drainage system to maintain gravity flow.

116. What should be readily available at the bedside of a client with a chest tube in place?
- [ ] **1.** a tracheostomy tray
- [ ] **2.** another sterile chest tube
- [ ] **3.** a bottle of sterile water
- [ ] **4.** a spirometer

117. The nurse is preparing to assist with the removal of a chest tube. Which dressing is appropriate at the site from which the chest tube is removed?
- [ ] **1.** adhesive strips
- [ ] **2.** petrolatum gauze
- [ ] **3.** dry 4 × 4 gauze
- [ ] **4.** no dressing is necessary

The Client with Chest Trauma

118. A nurse should interpret which finding as an early sign of a tension pneumothorax in a client with chest trauma?
- [ ] **1.** diminished bilateral breath sounds
- [ ] **2.** muffled heart sounds
- [ ] **3.** respiratory distress
- [ ] **4.** tracheal deviation

119. A nurse is to administer 10 mg of morphine sulfate to a client with three fractured ribs. The available concentration for this drug is 15 mg/mL. How many milliliters should the nurse administer? Round to one decimal point.

_____ mL.

120. A young adult is admitted to the emergency department after an automobile accident. The client has severe pain in the right chest from contact with the steering wheel. What should the nurse do **first**?
- ☐ 1. Reduce the client's anxiety.
- ☐ 2. Maintain adequate oxygenation.
- ☐ 3. Decrease chest pain.
- ☐ 4. Maintain adequate circulating volume.

121. A client with rib fractures and a pneumothorax has a chest tube inserted that is connected to a water seal chest tube drainage system. The nurse notes that the fluid in the water seal column is fluctuating with each breath that the client takes. What is the significance of this fluctuation?
- ☐ 1. An obstruction is present in the chest tube.
- ☐ 2. The client is developing subcutaneous emphysema.
- ☐ 3. The chest tube system is functioning properly.
- ☐ 4. There is a leak in the chest tube system.

122. Which finding would suggest pneumothorax in a trauma victim?
- ☐ 1. pronounced crackles
- ☐ 2. inspiratory wheezing
- ☐ 3. dullness on percussion
- ☐ 4. absent breath sounds

123. For a client with rib fractures and a pneumothorax, the healthcare provider (HCP) prescribes morphine sulfate, 1 to 2 mg/h, given IV as needed for pain. The nursing care goal is to provide adequate pain control so that the client can breathe effectively. Which finding indicates the goal has been met?
- ☐ 1. pain rating of 0 to 2 on a scale of 0 to 10 by the client
- ☐ 2. decreased client anxiety
- ☐ 3. respiratory rate of 26 breaths/min
- ☐ 4. PaO$_2$ of 70 mm Hg (9.31 kPa)

124. A client undergoes surgery to repair lung injuries. Postoperative prescriptions include the transfusion of one unit of packed red blood cells at a rate of 60 mL/h. How long will this transfusion take to infuse?
- ☐ 1. 2 hours
- ☐ 2. 4 hours
- ☐ 3. 6 hours
- ☐ 4. 8 hours

125. The primary reason for infusing blood at a rate of 60 mL/h is to help prevent:
- ☐ 1. emboli formation.
- ☐ 2. fluid volume overload.
- ☐ 3. red blood cell hemolysis.
- ☐ 4. allergic reaction.

126. A client has been in an automobile accident, and the nurse is assessing the client for possible pneumothorax. The nurse should assess the client for:
- ☐ 1. sudden, sharp chest pain.
- ☐ 2. wheezing breath sounds over affected side.
- ☐ 3. hemoptysis.
- ☐ 4. cyanosis.

127. The healthcare provider (HCP) has inserted a chest tube in a client with a pneumothorax. The nurse should evaluate the effectiveness of the chest tube:
- ☐ 1. for administration of oxygen.
- ☐ 2. to promote formation of lung scar tissue.
- ☐ 3. to insert antibiotics into the pleural space.
- ☐ 4. to remove air and fluid.

128. The nurse is preparing the client diagnosed with pleural effusion for a left-sided thoracentesis. The x-ray shows fluid in the pleural cavity. During the preparation for the procedure, the client asks where the healthcare provider (HCP) will "put the needle." Select the appropriate site from the diagram.

129. A client is undergoing a thoracentesis. What should the nurse monitor the client for during and immediately after the procedure? Select all that apply.
- ☐ 1. pneumothorax
- ☐ 2. subcutaneous emphysema
- ☐ 3. tension pneumothorax
- ☐ 4. pulmonary edema
- ☐ 5. infection

130. When assessing a client with chest trauma, the nurse notes that the client is taking small breaths at first, then bigger breaths, and then a couple of small breaths, then 10 to 20 seconds of no breaths. The nurse should record the breathing pattern as:
- [ ] 1. Cheyne-Stokes respiration.
- [ ] 2. hyperventilation.
- [ ] 3. obstructive sleep apnea.
- [ ] 4. Biot's respiration.

The Client with Acute Respiratory Distress Syndrome

131. The nurse has placed the intubated client with acute respiratory distress syndrome (ARDS) in prone position for 30 minutes. Which factors would require the nurse to discontinue prone positioning and return the client to the supine position? Select all that apply.
- [ ] 1. The family is coming in to visit.
- [ ] 2. The client has increased secretions requiring frequent suctioning.
- [ ] 3. The SpO_2 and Po_2 have decreased.
- [ ] 4. The client is tachycardic with drop in blood pressure.
- [ ] 5. The face has increased skin breakdown and edema.

132. To improve the oxygenation of a client with acute respiratory distress syndrome (ARDS) who is receiving mechanical ventilation, the nurse should place the client in which position?
- [ ] 1. supine
- [ ] 2. semi-Fowler's
- [ ] 3. lateral side
- [ ] 4. prone

133. A client with acute respiratory distress syndrome (ARDS) has fine crackles at lung bases, and the respirations are shallow at a rate of 28 breaths/min. The client is restless and anxious. In addition to monitoring the arterial blood gas results, what should the nurse do? Select all that apply.
- [ ] 1. Monitor serum creatinine and blood urea nitrogen levels.
- [ ] 2. Administer a sedative.
- [ ] 3. Keep the head of the bed flat.
- [ ] 4. Administer humidified oxygen.
- [ ] 5. Auscultate the lungs.

134. Which nursing interventions would be **most** likely to prevent the development of acute respiratory distress syndrome (ARDS)?
- [ ] 1. teaching cigarette smoking cessation
- [ ] 2. maintaining adequate serum potassium levels
- [ ] 3. monitoring clients for signs of hypercapnia
- [ ] 4. replacing fluids adequately during hypovolemic states

135. The nurse interprets which finding as an early sign of acute respiratory distress syndrome (ARDS) in a client at risk?
- [ ] 1. elevated carbon dioxide level
- [ ] 2. hypoxia not responsive to oxygen therapy
- [ ] 3. metabolic acidosis
- [ ] 4. severe, unexplained electrolyte imbalance

136. A client with acute respiratory distress syndrome (ARDS) is showing signs of increased dyspnea. The nurse reviews a report of blood gas values that recently arrived (see report).

Laboratory Results

Blood Chemistry	Result
pH	7.35
$PaCO_2$	25 mm Hg (3.3 kPa)
Hco_3^-	22 mEq/L (22 mmol/L)
PaO_2	95 mm Hg (12.6 kPa)

Which finding is abnormal?
- [ ] 1. pH
- [ ] 2. $PaCO_2$
- [ ] 3. HCO_3
- [ ] 4. PaO_2

137. A client with acute respiratory distress syndrome (ARDS) is on a ventilator. The client's peak inspiratory pressures and spontaneous respiratory rate are increasing, and the Po_2 is not improving. Using the SBAR (Situation-Background-Assessment-Recommendation) technique for communication, the nurse calls the healthcare provider (HCP) with the recommendation for:
- [ ] 1. initiating IV sedation.
- [ ] 2. starting a high-protein diet.
- [ ] 3. providing pain medication.
- [ ] 4. increasing the ventilator rate.

138. A client, diagnosed with acute pancreatitis 5 days ago, is experiencing respiratory distress. Which finding should the nurse report to the healthcare provider (HCP)?
- [ ] 1. arterial oxygen level of 46 mm Hg (6.1 kPa)
- [ ] 2. respirations of 12 breaths/min
- [ ] 3. lack of adventitious lung sounds
- [ ] 4. oxygen saturation of 96% on room air

139. A client has the following arterial blood gas values: pH, 7.52; PaO_2, 50 mm Hg (6.7 kPa); $PaCO_2$, 28 mm Hg (3.72 kPa); HCO_3^- 24 mEq/L (24 mmol/L). Based upon the client's PaO_2, which conclusion would be accurate?

☐ 1. The client is severely hypoxic.

☐ 2. The oxygen level is low but poses no risk for the client.

☐ 3. The client's PaO_2 level is within normal range.

☐ 4. The client requires oxygen therapy with very low oxygen concentrations.

140. Which action should the nurse anticipate in a client who has been diagnosed with acute respiratory distress syndrome (ARDS)?

☐ 1. tracheostomy

☐ 2. use of a nasal cannula

☐ 3. mechanical ventilation

☐ 4. insertion of a chest tube

141. Which condition can place a client at risk for acute respiratory distress syndrome (ARDS)?

☐ 1. septic shock

☐ 2. chronic obstructive pulmonary disease

☐ 3. asthma

☐ 4. heart failure

142. Which assessment is **most** appropriate for determining the correct placement of an endotracheal tube in a mechanically ventilated client?

☐ 1. assessing the client's skin color

☐ 2. monitoring the respiratory rate

☐ 3. verifying the amount of cuff inflation

☐ 4. auscultating breath sounds bilaterally

143. To promote effective airway clearance in a client with acute respiratory distress, what should the nurse do?

☐ 1. Administer oxygen every 2 hours.

☐ 2. Turn the client every 4 hours.

☐ 3. Administer sedatives to promote rest.

☐ 4. Suction if cough is ineffective.

144. Which complication is associated with mechanical ventilation?

☐ 1. gastrointestinal hemorrhage

☐ 2. immunosuppression

☐ 3. increased cardiac output

☐ 4. pulmonary emboli

Managing Care, Quality, and Safety of Clients with Respiratory Health Problems

145. The nurse has received a change of shift report on clients. Which client should the nurse assess **first**?

☐ 1. a client with COPD with a PaO_2 of 56 mm Hg who is being discharged home on oxygen

☐ 2. a client with asthma with respirations of 36 breaths/min whose wheezing has diminished

☐ 3. a client with asthma who has a heart rate of 90 bpm and whose beta-blocker is scheduled to be administered now

☐ 4. a client who is scheduled for an angiogram now and is ready to be transported

146. The nurse is caring for a group of clients on a pulmonary unit. The nurse can delegate which task to unlicensed assistive personnel (UAP)?

☐ 1. Assisting a client with adjusting his or her nasal cannula

☐ 2. Making adjustments to flow rates based on client responses

☐ 3. Monitoring a client for adverse effects of oxygen therapy

☐ 4. Assessing a client for the best method of oxygen delivery

147. A confused client with carbon monoxide poisoning experiences dizziness when ambulating to the bathroom. The nurse should:

☐ 1. put all four side rails up on the bed.

☐ 2. ask the unlicensed assistive personnel (UAP) to place restraints on the client's upper extremities.

☐ 3. request that the client's roommate put the call light on when the client is attempting to get out of bed.

☐ 4. check on the client at regular intervals to ascertain the need to use the bathroom.

148. The nurse should use which type of precautions for a client being admitted to the hospital with suspected tuberculosis?

☐ 1. hand hygiene

☐ 2. contact precautions

☐ 3. droplet precautions

☐ 4. airborne precautions

149. A client has developed a hospital-acquired pneumonia. When preparing to administer cephalexin 500 mg, the nurse notices that the pharmacy sent cefazolin. What should the nurse do? Select all that apply.
- ☐ 1. Administer the cefazolin.
- ☐ 2. Verify the medication prescription as written by the healthcare provider (HCP).
- ☐ 3. Contact the pharmacy and speak to a pharmacist.
- ☐ 4. Request that cephalexin be sent promptly.
- ☐ 5. Return the cefazolin to the pharmacy.

150. A nurse receives the taped change-of-shift report for assigned clients and prioritizes client rounds. In what order from first to last should the nurse assess these clients? All options must be used.

1. a client who has an endotracheal tube and who will be transferred to a long-term respiratory care unit that day

2. a client with type 2 diabetes who had a cerebrovascular accident 4 days ago

3. a client with cellulitis of the left lower extremity with a fever of 100.8°F (38.2°C)

4. a client receiving D5W IV at 125 mL/h with 75 mL remaining

151. The nurse is a member of a team that is planning a client-centered, community-based approach to care of clients with chronic obstructive pulmonary disease (COPD). In which areas should the team focus on improving quality of care and delivery? Select all that apply.
- ☐ 1. the community
- ☐ 2. clinical information systems
- ☐ 3. delivery system design
- ☐ 4. administrative leadership
- ☐ 5. acute care setting

152. The nurse is caring for a client admitted for pneumonia with a history of hypertension and heart failure. The client has reported at least one fall in the last 3 months. The client may ambulate with assistance, has a saline lock in place, and has demonstrated appropriate use of the call light to request assistance. Using the Morse Fall Scale (see chart), what is this client's total score and risk level?

Morse Fall Scale

Item	Scale		Scoring
1. History of falling; immediate or within 3 months	No	0	
	Yes	25	
2. Secondary diagnosis	No	0	
	Yes	15	
3. Ambulatory aid			
Bed rest/nurse assist		0	
Crutches/cane/walker		15	
Furniture		30	
4. IV/Heparin Lock	No	0	
	Yes	20	
5. Gait/Transferring			
Normal/bedrest/ immobile Weak		0	
		10	
Impaired		20	
6. Mental status			
Oriented to own ability		0	
Forgets limitations		15	

- ☐ 1. 20, low risk
- ☐ 2. 30, medium risk
- ☐ 3. 40, medium risk
- ☐ 4. 60, high risk

153. The nurse is caring for a client who has been placed on droplet precautions. Which protective gear is required to take care of this client? Select all that apply.
- ☐ 1. gloves
- ☐ 2. gown
- ☐ 3. surgical mask
- ☐ 4. glasses
- ☐ 5. respirator

154. While making rounds, the nurse finds a client with COPD sitting in a wheelchair, slumped over a lunch tray. After determining the client is unresponsive and calling for help, the nurse's **first** action should be to:
- ☐ 1. push the "code blue" (emergency response) button.
- ☐ 2. call the rapid response team.
- ☐ 3. open the client's airway.
- ☐ 4. call for a defibrillator.

155. The nurse is caring for a client with pneumonia who is confused about time and place and has intravenous fluids infusing. Despite the nurse's attempt to reorient the client and then provide distraction, the client has begun to pull at the IV tubing. After increasing the frequency of observation, in which order should the nurse implement interventions to ensure the client's safety? All options must be used.

1. Review the client's medications for interactions that may cause or increase confusion.
2. Assess the client's respiratory status including oxygen saturation.
3. Ensure the client does not need toileting or pain medications.
4. Contact the healthcare provider (HCP), and request a prescription for soft wrist restraints.

156. The nurse's assignment consists of four clients. After receiving shift report, in which order from first to last should the nurse assess these clients? All options must be used.

1. an 85-year-old client with bacterial pneumonia, temperature of 102.2°F (42°C), and shortness of breath
2. a 60-year-old client with chest tubes who is 2 days postoperative following a thoracotomy for lung cancer and is requesting something for pain
3. a 35-year-old client with suspected tuberculosis who has a cough
4. a 56-year-old client with emphysema who has a scheduled dose of a bronchodilator due to be administered, with no report of acute respiratory distress

157. The unlicensed assistive personnel (UAP) reports to the registered nurse (RN) that a client admitted with pneumonia is very diaphoretic. The nurse reviews the vital signs in the medical record obtained by the UAP. What should the nurse do? Select all that apply.

Vital Signs			
Time	0800	1000	1200
Temperature	38.3°C		38.8°C
Pulse	90	104	118
Respirations	16	18	24
Blood Pressure	112/74	110/68	116/78
SpO$_2$	93%	92%	92%

☐ 1. Assure the client is maintaining complete bed rest.
☐ 2. Check the urine output.
☐ 3. Ask the client to drink more fluids.
☐ 4. Notify the healthcare provider (HCP).
☐ 5. Administer acetaminophen as prescribed.

Answers, Rationales, and Test-Taking Strategies

*The answers and rationales for each question follow below, along with keys (🔑) to the client need (CN) and cognitive level (CL) for each question. In addition, you will also see a glossary icon (📖) highlighting specific terminology used on the licensing exam. As you check your answers, use the **Content Mastery and Test-Taking Skill Self-Analysis** worksheet (tearout worksheet in back of book) to identify the reason(s) for not answering the questions correctly. For additional information about test-taking skills and strategies for answering questions, refer to pages 12–23 and pages 35–36 in Part 1 of this book.*

The Client with an Upper Respiratory Tract Infection

1. 1. At this time, there is no strong research evidence to warrant recommendations of herbal products for management of colds; further study is needed to show evidence of therapeutic effects and indications. Antibiotics are effective against bacteria; the head cold may have a viral cause. An uncomplicated upper respiratory tract infection subsides within 2 to 3 weeks. There may be a drug-drug interaction with herbal products and prescriptions.

🔑 CN: Basic care and comfort; CL: Synthesize

2. 1,4,5. Antihistamines have an anticholinergic action and a drying effect and reduce nasal, salivary, and lacrimal gland hypersecretion (runny nose, tearing, and itching eyes). An adverse effect is drowsiness, so operating machinery and driving are not recommended. There is also an additive depressant effect when alcohol is combined with antihistamines, so alcohol should be avoided during antihistamine use. The client should ensure adequate fluid intake of at least 2,000 mL (about eight glasses) per day due to the drying effect of the drug. Antihistamines have no antibacterial action, and are not used to treat nasal infections. The effect of antihistamines is prompt, not delayed.

> CN: Pharmacological and parenteral therapies; CL: Create

3. 3. When using an intranasal inhaler, it is important to close off one nostril while inhaling the spray into the other nostril to ensure the best inhalation of the spray. Use of the inhaler is not limited to mornings and bedtime. The canister should be shaken immediately before use. The inhaler tip should be inserted into the nostril and pointed toward the outside nostril wall to maximize inhalation of the medication.

> CN: Pharmacological and parenteral therapies; CL: Evaluate

4. 4. A client recovering from an upper respiratory tract infection should report decreasing or no nasal discharge and obstruction. Daily fluid intake should be increased to more than 1 L every 24 hours to liquefy secretions. The temperature should be below 100°F (37.8°C) with no chills or diaphoresis. A productive cough with chest pain indicates a pulmonary infection, not an upper respiratory tract infection.

> CN: Physiological adaptation; CL: Evaluate

5. 2. The client should blow the nose before instilling nose drops. Instilling nose drops is a clean technique. The dropper should be cleaned after each administration, but it does not need to be changed. The client should assume a position that will allow the medication to reach the desired area; this is usually a supine position.

> CN: Pharmacological and parenteral therapies; CL: Evaluate

6. 3,4. The client with chronic sinusitis should be instructed to take hot showers in the morning and evening to promote drainage of secretions. There is no need to limit caffeine intake. Performing postural drainage will inhibit removal of secretions, not promote it. Clients should elevate the head of the bed to promote drainage. Clients should report all temperatures higher than 100.4°F (38°C) because a temperature that high can indicate infection. The client

should increase, not limit, fluid intake; a 24-hour fluid intake of 2,000 to 3,000 mL would be appropriate.

> CN: Reduction of risk potential; CL: Synthesize

7. 4. It is important for clients with allergic rhinitis to determine the precipitating factors so that they can be avoided. Keeping a diary can help identify these triggers. Nasal decongestant sprays should not be used regularly because they can cause a rebound effect. Antibiotics are not appropriate for allergic rhinitis because an infection is not present. Increasing activity will not control the client's symptoms; in fact, walking outdoors may increase them if the client is allergic to pollen.

> CN: Health promotion and maintenance; CL: Synthesize

8. 7.5 mL.

$$300\,mg\,/\,X = 200\,mg\,/\,5\,mL$$
$$X = 7.5\,mL.$$

> CN: Pharmacological and parenteral therapies; CL: Apply

9. 4. Adverse effects of pseudoephedrine are experienced primarily in the cardiovascular system and through sympathetic effects on the central nervous system (CNS). The most common CNS adverse effects include restlessness, dizziness, tension, anxiety, insomnia, and weakness. Common cardiovascular adverse effects include tachycardia, hypertension, palpitations, and arrhythmias. Constipation and diplopia are not adverse effects of pseudoephedrine. Tachycardia, not bradycardia, is an adverse effect of pseudoephedrine.

> CN: Pharmacological and parenteral therapies; CL: Analyze

The Client Undergoing Nasal Surgery

10. 4. Epistaxis, or nosebleed, is a common, sudden emergency. Commonly, no apparent explanation for the bleeding is known. With significant blood loss, systemic symptoms, such as vertigo, increased pulse, shortness of breath, decreased blood pressure, and pallor, will occur. Because aerobic exercise may increase blood pressure and increased blood pressure can cause epistaxis, the client with hypertension should avoid it. Aspirin inhibits platelet aggregation, reducing the ability of the blood to clot. The client should continue to take his antihypertension medication, ramipril. Posterior nasal packing should be left in place for 1 to 3 days.

> CN: Health promotion and maintenance; CL: Synthesize

11. 2. Because of the dense nasal packing, bleeding may not be apparent through the nasal drip pad. Instead, the blood may run down the throat, causing the client to swallow frequently. The back of the throat, where the blood will be apparent, can be assessed with a flashlight. An accumulation of blood in the stomach can cause nausea and vomiting, but nausea would not be the initial indicator of bleeding. An increased respiratory rate occurs in shock but is not an early sign of bleeding in a client who has undergone nasal surgery. Increased pain warrants further assessment but is not an indicator of bleeding.

CN: Reduction of risk potential; CL: Analyze

12. 1. The client should be instructed to avoid any activities that cause Valsalva's maneuver (e.g., constipation, vigorous coughing, exercise) in order to reduce bleeding and stress on suture lines. The client should not take aspirin because of its antiplatelet properties, which may cause bleeding. Oral hygiene is important to rid the mouth of old dried blood and to enhance the client's appetite. Cool compresses, not heat, should be applied to decrease swelling and control discoloration of the area.

CN: Physiological adaptation; CL: Create

13. 2. Constipation can cause straining during defecation, which can induce bleeding. Showering is not contraindicated. The client should take measures to prevent coughing, which can cause bleeding. The client should avoid blowing the nose for 48 hours after the packing is removed. Thereafter, the client should blow the nose gently, using the open-mouth technique to minimize bleeding in the surgical area.

CN: Physiological adaptation; CL: Evaluate

14. 4. Aspirin-containing medications should be discontinued for 2 weeks before surgery to decrease the risk of bleeding. Nasal packing is usually removed the day after surgery. Normal saline nose drops are not routinely administered preoperatively. The results of the surgery will not be obvious immediately after surgery because of edema and ecchymosis.

CN: Reduction of risk potential; CL: Create

15. 3. Immediately after nasal surgery, ineffective breathing patterns may develop as a result of the nasal packing and nasal edema. Nasal packing may dislodge, leading to obstruction. Assessing for airway obstruction is a priority. Assessing for pain is important, but it is not as high a priority as assessment of the airways. It is too early to detect ecchymosis. Measuring intake and output is not typically a **priority** nursing assessment after nasal surgery.

CN: Physiological adaptation; CL: Analyze

16. 4. Applying cold compresses helps to decrease facial swelling and pain from edema. Analgesics may decrease pain, but they do not decrease edema. A corticosteroid nasal spray would not be administered postoperatively because it can impair healing. Use of a bedside humidifier promotes comfort by providing moisture for nasal mucosa, but it does not decrease edema.

CN: Basic care and comfort; CL: Synthesize

17. 1. Frequent mouth care is important to provide comfort and encourage eating. Mouth care promotes moist mucous membranes. Nose drops cannot be used with nasal packing in place. When sneezing and coughing, the client should do so with the mouth open to decrease the chance of dislodging the packing. Gargling should not be attempted with packing in place.

CN: Basic care and comfort; CL: Create

18. 4. The client should assume a sitting position and lean forward. Firm pressure should be applied to the soft portion of the nose for approximately 10 minutes. Tilting the head backward can cause the client to swallow blood, which can obscure the amount of bleeding and also can lead to nausea. Ice compresses may be applied, but the client should not lie flat. Blowing the nose is to be avoided because it can increase bleeding.

CN: Reduction of risk potential; CL: Synthesize

19. 3. Posterior packing may alter the respiratory status of the client, especially in elderly clients, causing hypoventilation. Clients should be observed carefully for changes in level of consciousness, respiratory rate, and heart rate and rhythm after the insertion of the packing. Vertigo does not occur as a result of the insertion of posterior packing. Bell's palsy, a disorder of the seventh cranial nerve, is not associated with epistaxis or nasal packing. Loss of gag reflex does not occur as a result of the insertion of posterior packing.

CN: Reduction of risk potential; CL: Analyze

The Client with Cancer of the Larynx

20. 4. The nurse must maintain patency of the airway with frequent suctioning of the laryngectomy tube that can become occluded from secretions, blood, and mucus plugs. Once the client is hemodynamically stable, getting out of bed should be encouraged to prevent postoperative complications. Vital signs should be monitored more frequently in a postoperative client. A swallow study is done at approximately 5 to 7 days after surgery, prior to starting oral intake.

CN: Physiological adaptation; CL: Synthesize

21. 4. The client has undergone body changes and permanent loss of verbal communication. He may feel isolated and insecure. The nurse can encourage him to express his feelings and use this information to develop an appropriate plan of care. Discussing the client's behavior with his wife may not reveal his feelings. Exploring future plans is not appropriate at this time because more information about the client's behavior is needed before proceeding to this level. The nurse can respect the client's need for privacy while also encouraging him to express his feelings.

CN: Psychosocial adaptation; CL: Synthesize

22. 1. A client should be suctioned for no longer than 10 seconds at a time. Suctioning for longer than 10 seconds may reduce the client's oxygen level so much that the client becomes hypoxic.

CN: Reduction of risk potential; CL: Apply

23. 1. The recommended technique is to use a sterile catheter each time the client is suctioned. There is a danger of introducing organisms into the respiratory tract when strict aseptic technique is not used. Reusing a suction catheter is not consistent with aseptic technique. The nurse does not use a clean catheter when suctioning a tracheostomy or a laryngectomy; it is a sterile procedure.

CN: Reduction of risk potential; CL: Apply

24. 4. Changes in body image are expected after a laryngectomy, and the nurse should first explore what is upsetting the client the most at this time. Many clients are concerned about how their family members will respond to the physical changes that have occurred as a result of a laryngectomy, but discussing the importance of family support is not helpful; instead, the nurse should allow the client to communicate any negative feelings or concerns that exist because of the surgery. The client's feelings are not related to a knowledge deficit, and therefore, it is too early to begin teaching about stoma care. It is also not helpful to offer reassurances about the change in appearance; the client will require time to adjust to the changed body image.

CN: Psychosocial adaptation; CL: Synthesize

25. 1. The tracheostomy tube, ties, and gauze pad are positioned correctly; the nurse team leader should be sure the client is comfortable. The tracheostomy tube ties should be tied in a square knot on the side of the neck and alternate sides of the neck when the ties are changed. The full part of the gauze square should be placed under the tracheostomy tube to absorb drainage. There is no indication the ties need to be changed; an additional gauze pad is not necessary; if necessary, the current gauze square should be changed rather than adding an additional pad.

CN: Basic care and comfort; CL: Evaluate

26. 1,3. The primary risk factors for laryngeal cancer are smoking and alcohol abuse. Smoking cessation is most successful with a support group or counseling. Heavy drinking should be avoided since the risk increases with amount of alcohol consumption. HEPA filters help trap small particles and allergens to reduce allergy symptoms and asthma. Poor oral hygiene is not a risk factor, nor is overusing the voice.

CN: Health promotion and maintenance; CL: Create

27. 3. Hoarseness occurring longer than 2 weeks is a warning sign of laryngeal cancer. The nurse should first assess other signs, such as a lump in the neck or throat, persistent sore throat or cough, earache, pain, and difficulty swallowing (dysphagia). Gargling with salt water may lead to increased irritation. There is no indication of infection warranting an antibiotic. An oral analgesic would provide only temporary relief of discomfort if hoarseness is accompanied by a sore throat.

CN: Physiological adaptation; CL: Synthesize

28. 1. Immediately after surgery, the client should be maintained in a position with the head of the bed elevated 30 to 40 degrees (semi-Fowler's position) to decrease tissue edema, facilitate breathing, and decrease pain related to edema formation. Immediately postoperatively, the client should be provided alternative means of communicating, such as a communication board. As healing progresses and edema subsides, a speech therapist should work with the client to explore various voice restoration options, such as the use of a voice prosthesis, electrolarynx, artificial larynx, or esophageal speech. Food is not initiated in the immediate postoperative phase; enteral feedings are usually used to meet nutritional needs until edema subsides. Irrigation of the drainage tubes is an inappropriate action.

CN: Basic care and comfort; CL: Synthesize

29. 3. It is important that the client be able to communicate his or her feelings about the body image changes that have occurred as a result of surgery. Open communication helps promote adjustment. The client may not regain the ability to taste and smell food because of no longer breathing through the nose or because of radiation therapy treatments, or both. A gastrostomy tube would not typically be placed after a total laryngectomy, nor would it be necessary for the client to demonstrate sterile suctioning technique for stoma care. The client would use clean technique.

🔑 CN: Physiological adaptation;
CL: Evaluate

30. 2. Adequate humidity should be provided in the home to help keep secretions moist. A bedside humidifier is recommended. A high fluid intake is also important to liquefy secretions. Mouth care is important to prevent drying of mucous membranes and should be performed frequently throughout the day, especially before and after meals, to help stimulate appetite. The client may eat any food that can be chewed and swallowed comfortably. The client may resume physical activity as tolerated.

🔑 CN: Reduction of risk potential;
CL: Synthesize

The Client with Pneumonia

31. 3. The client's ABG levels are the most sensitive indicator of the effectiveness of the client's oxygen therapy. Cyanosis is a late sign of decreased oxygenation and is not a reliable indicator. The client's respiratory rate and level of consciousness may be altered because of other problems not related to the client's oxygenation.

🔑 CN: Physiological adaptation;
CL: Evaluate

32. 2. Restraints should be secured to the bed frame, not the side rails, to ensure that the side rails can be raised and lowered safely. Circulation checks, reevaluating need for restraints, and documentation should be done every 1 to 2 hours. Medical restraint prescriptions must be renewed and signed by an **HCP** 📖 every 24 hours.

🔑 CN: Safety and infection control;
CL: Synthesize

33. 1. The client's age is a predisposing factor for pneumonia; pneumonia is more common in elderly or debilitated clients. Other predisposing factors include smoking, upper respiratory tract infections, malnutrition, immunosuppression, and the presence of a chronic illness. Osteoarthritis, a nutritionally sound vegetarian diet, and frequent bathing are not predisposing factors for pneumonia.

🔑 CN: Reduction of risk potential;
CL: Analyze

34. 1,3,5. A respiratory assessment, which includes auscultating breath sounds and assessing the color of the nail beds, is a priority for clients with pneumonia. Assessing for the presence of chest pain is also an important respiratory assessment as chest pain can interfere with the client's ability

to breathe deeply. Auscultating bowel sounds and assessing for peripheral edema may be appropriate assessments, but these are not priority assessments for the client with pneumonia.

🔑 CN: Physiological adaptation;
CL: Analyze

35. 2. A sputum specimen is obtained for culture to determine the causative organism. After the organism is identified, an appropriate antibiotic can be prescribed. Beginning antibiotic therapy before obtaining the sputum specimen may alter the results of the test. Urinalysis, a chest radiograph, and a red blood cell count do not need to be obtained before initiation of antibiotic therapy for pneumonia.

🔑 CN: Reduction of risk potential;
CL: Apply

36. 3. It is essential to monitor serum creatinine in the client receiving an aminoglycoside antibiotic because of the potential of this type of drug to cause acute tubular necrosis. Aminoglycoside antibiotics do not affect serum sodium, potassium, or calcium levels.

🔑 CN: Pharmacological and parenteral therapies; CL: Analyze

37. 4. The nurse should determine if the client is allergic to penicillin prior to administering the drug. History of seizures, recent infections, and a cardiac history are not contraindications for this client to receive penicillin. While important to know, recent infections will not preclude this client receiving penicillin at this time.

🔑 CN: Pharmacological and parenteral therapies; CL: Apply

38. 3. Frequent changes of the bedsheets are appropriate for this client because of the diaphoresis. Diaphoresis produces general discomfort, and the client should be kept dry to promote comfort and prevent skin irritation. The client should change position every 2 hours. Nasotracheal suctioning is not indicated with the client's productive cough. The client can ambulate to the bathroom, but the nurse should offer assistance as needed.

🔑 CN: Basic care and comfort;
CL: Synthesize

39. 1. Exudate in the alveoli interferes with ventilation and the diffusion of gases in clients with pneumonia. During the acute phase of the illness, it is essential to reduce the body's need for oxygen at the cellular level; bed rest is the most effective method for doing so. Bed rest does not decrease coughing or promote clearance of secretions, and it does not reduce pain when taking deep breaths.

🔑 CN: Physiological adaptation;
CL: Evaluate

40. 3. Chest pain in pneumonia is generally caused by friction between the pleural layers. It is more severe on inspiration than on expiration, secondary to chest wall movement. Pleuritic chest pain is usually described as sharp, not mild or aching. Pleuritic chest pain is not localized to the sternum, and it is not the result of a muscle spasm.

➤ CN: Physiological adaptation; CL: Analyze

41. 4. The pleuritic pain is triggered by chest movement and is particularly severe during coughing. Splinting the chest wall will help reduce the discomfort of coughing. Deep breathing is essential to prevent further atelectasis. Abdominal breathing is not as effective in decreasing pleuritic chest pain as is splinting of the rib cage. Incentive spirometry facilitates effective deep breathing but does not decrease pleuritic chest pain.

➤ CN: Physiological adaptation; CL: Synthesize

42. 1,3. Aspirin is administered to clients with pneumonia because it is an analgesic that helps control chest discomfort and an antipyretic that helps reduce fever. Aspirin has an anticoagulant effect, but that is not the reason for prescribing it for a client with pneumonia, and the use of the drug will be short term. Aspirin does not affect the respiratory rate and does not facilitate expectoration of secretions.

➤ CN: Pharmacological and parenteral therapies; CL: Evaluate

43. 3. Clients who are experiencing hypoxia characteristically exhibit irritability, restlessness, or anxiety as initial mental status changes. As the hypoxia becomes more pronounced, the client may become confused and combative. Coma is a late clinical manifestation of hypoxia. Apathy and depression are not symptoms of hypoxia.

➤ CN: Physiological adaptation; CL: Analyze

44. 1. Docusate sodium is a stool softener that allows fluid and fatty substances to enter the stool and soften it. Docusate sodium does not lubricate the stool, increase stool bulk, or stimulate peristalsis.

➤ CN: Pharmacological and parenteral therapies; CL: Apply

45. 2. An expected outcome for a client recovering from pneumonia would be the ability to perform activities of daily living without experiencing dyspnea. A respiratory rate of 25 to 30 breaths/min indicates the client is experiencing tachypnea, which would not be expected on recovery. A weight loss of 5 to 10 lb (2.27 to 4.53 kg) is undesirable;

the expected outcome would be to maintain normal weight. A client who is recovering from pneumonia should experience decreased or no chest pain.

➤ CN: Management of care; CL: Evaluate

The Client with Tuberculosis

46. 1. Implementing airborne precautions for possible TB requires a private room assignment. In addition to isolating the client by using a private room, engineering controls can help prevent the spread of TB; a room at the end of the hall will aid in controlling airflow direction and can prevent contamination of air in adjacent areas. Confidentiality is provided for every client, regardless of the client's room location. Sunlight is not a component of isolation precautions.

➤ CN: Physiological adaptation; CL: Apply

47. 1. There is a high risk and potential for tuberculosis, and airborne precautions should be implemented immediately to prevent the spread of infection. After initiating precautions, the nurse can start the oxygen, check the vital signs, and collect the sputum specimen.

➤ CN: Safety and infection control; CL: Synthesize

48. 3. Streptomycin can cause toxicity to the eighth cranial nerve, which is responsible for hearing, balance, and body position sense. Nephrotoxicity is a side effect that would be indicated with an increase in creatinine. Streptomycin does not cause difficulty in swallowing. Streptomycin is given via intramuscular injection.

➤ CN: Pharmacological and parenteral therapies; CL: Analyze

49. 4. The nurse should tell the client that it is necessary to take all of these medications because combination drug therapy prevents bacterial resistance; they will be administered throughout the hospitalization to maintain blood levels. The HCP 📖 will review the prescriptions per hospital policy because the client is being admitted to the hospital; there is no duplication between any of the drugs being prescribed for this client. It is not necessary to ask the pharmacist to check for drug interactions as these drugs are commonly used together.

➤ CN: Pharmacologic and parenteral therapy; CL: Synthesize

50. 2. Ensuring that the client is well educated about tuberculosis is the highest **priority**. Education of the client and family is essential to help the client understand the need for completing the prescribed drug therapy to cure the disease. Offering the client emotional support, coordinating various agency services, and assessing the environment may be part of the care for the client with tuberculosis; however, these interventions are of less importance than education about the disease process and its treatment.

⚷ CN: Basic care and comfort; CL: Synthesize

51. 3. The tuberculin test is positive. The test should be interpreted 2 to 3 days after administering the purified protein derivative (PPD) by measuring the size of the firm, raised area (induration). Positive responses indicate that the client may have been exposed to the tuberculosis bacteria. A negative response is indicated by the absence of a firm, raised area, or an area that is <5 mm in diameter. Since the test is positive, it is not necessary to redo the test. The test is positive, not false.

⚷ CN: Physiological adaptation; CL: Analyze

52. 1. The Mantoux test is administered via intradermal injection. The appropriate technique for an intradermal injection includes holding the needle and syringe almost parallel to the client's skin, keeping the skin slightly taut when the needle is inserted, and inserting the needle with the bevel side up. There is no need to aspirate, a technique that assesses for incorrect placement in a blood vessel, when giving an intradermal injection. The injection site is not massaged.

⚷ CN: Pharmacological and parenteral therapies; CL: Apply

53. 3. An induration (palpable raised hardened area of skin) of more than 5 to 15 mm (depending upon the person's risk factors) to 10 Mantoux units is considered a positive result, indicating TB infection. An induration of >5 mm is found in HIV-positive individuals, those with recent contacts with persons with TB, persons with nodular or fibrotic changes on chest x-ray consistent with old healed TB, or clients with organ transplants or immunosuppressed. An induration of >10 mm is positive, and the client may be a recent arrival (<5 years) from high-prevalent countries, injection drug user, resident or an employee of high-risk congregate settings (e.g., prisons, long-term care facilities, hospitals, homeless shelters), or mycobacteriology lab personnel. An induration of >10 mm is also considered positive in persons with clinical conditions that place them at high risk (e.g., diabetes, prolonged corticosteroid therapy, leukemia, end-stage renal disease, chronic malabsorption syndromes, low body weight), a child <4 years of age, or a child or adolescents exposed to adults in high-risk categories.

⚷ CN: Physiological adaptation; CL: Analyze

54. 4. Elderly persons are believed to be at higher risk for contracting tuberculosis because of decreased immunocompetence. Other high-risk populations in the United States and Canada include the urban poor, clients with acquired immunodeficiency syndrome, and minority groups.

⚷ CN: Safety and infection control; CL: Analyze

55. 2,4. When teaching the client how to avoid the transmission of tubercle bacilli, it is important for the client to understand that the organism is transmitted by droplet infection. Therefore, covering the mouth and nose when sneezing, using paper tissues to cough in with prompt disposal, indicates that the client has understood the nurse's instructions about preventing the spread of airborne droplets. It is not essential to discard clothing, nor does the client need to be isolated from family members. The client does not need to avoid crowds.

⚷ CN: Health promotion and maintenance; CL: Evaluate

56. 2. A positive Mantoux skin test indicates that the client has been exposed to tubercle bacilli. Exposure does not necessarily mean that active disease exists. A positive Mantoux test does not mean that the client has developed resistance. Unless involved in treatment, the client may still develop active disease at any time. Immunity to tuberculosis is not possible.

⚷ CN: Reduction of risk potential; CL: Analyze

57. 2. INH competes for the available vitamin B_6 in the body and leaves the client at risk for development of neuropathies related to vitamin deficiency. Supplemental vitamin B_6 is routinely prescribed. Following a low-cholesterol diet, getting extra rest, and avoiding excessive sun exposure will not prevent the development of peripheral neuropathies.

⚷ CN: Pharmacological and parenteral therapies; CL: Synthesize

58. 3. INH interferes with the effectiveness of hormonal contraceptives, and female clients of childbearing age should be counseled to use an alternative form of birth control while taking the drug. INH does not increase the risk of vaginal infection, nor does it affect the ova or ovulation.

⚷ CN: Pharmacological and parenteral therapies; CL: Apply

59. 3. Tuberculosis can be controlled but never completely eradicated from the body. Periods of intense physical or emotional stress increase the likelihood of recurrence. Clients should be taught to recognize the signs and symptoms of a potential recurrence. Weather and activity levels are not related to recurrences of tuberculosis.

🔑 CN: Physiological adaptation;
CL: Analyze

60. 2. Statistics show that of the four geographic areas described, most cases of tuberculosis are found in inner-core residential areas of large cities, where health and sanitation standards tend to be low. Substandard housing, poverty, and crowded living conditions also generally characterize these city areas and contribute to the spread of the disease. Farming areas have a low incidence of tuberculosis. Variations in water standards and industrial pollution are not correlated to tuberculosis incidence.

🔑 CN: Safety and infection control;
CL: Analyze

61. 4. Isoniazid and rifampin are hepatotoxic. The client should be warned to limit intake of alcohol during drug therapy. The drug should be taken on an empty stomach. If antacids are needed for gastrointestinal distress, they should be taken 1 hour before or 2 hours after the drug is administered. The client should not double the dose of the drug because of potential toxicity. The client taking the drug should avoid foods that are rich in tyramine, such as cheese and dairy products, or the client may develop hypertension.

🔑 CN: Pharmacological and parenteral therapies; CL: Create

62. 2,4,5. A potential adverse effect of rifampin is hepatotoxicity. Clients should be instructed to avoid alcohol intake while taking rifampin and keep follow-up appointments for periodic monitoring of liver enzyme levels to detect liver toxicity. Rifampin causes the urine to turn an orange color, and the client should understand that this is normal. It is not necessary to restrict protein intake in the diet or have the eyes examined due to rifampin therapy.

🔑 CN: Pharmacological and parenteral therapies; CL: Create

63. 1. Directly observed therapy (DOT) can be implemented with clients who are not compliant with drug therapy. In DOT, a responsible person, who may be a family member or an **HCP** 📖, observes the client taking the medication. Visiting the client, changing the prescription, or threatening the client will not ensure compliance if the client will not or cannot follow the prescribed treatment.

🔑 CN: Safety and infection control;
CL: Synthesize

The Client with Chronic Obstructive Pulmonary Disease

64. 2,4. Close proximity to smoking, fire, and small electrical appliances can be a fire hazard and should be avoided. The use of gauze is helpful in preventing skin irritation from the constant pressure and friction of the oxygen tubing. Typically, oxygen needs are lower at rest and during sleep. Increasing oxygen flow should be done at the discretion of the prescribing healthcare provider and not the client. Water-soluble lubricants are considered safer than petroleum-based lubricants. Small liquid oxygen tanks are easier to transport during travel than pressurized tanks. Use of microwave ovens for cooking is considered safe for those using supplemental oxygen.

🔑 CN: Reduction of risk potential
CL: Create

65. 2,3. The cough reflex for these clients promotes airway clearance. While the guaifenesin may thin secretions and facilitate expectoration, dextromethorphan suppresses the cough and should not be used with chronic bronchitis. Pseudoephedrine can increase blood pressure and increase urinary retention with an enlarged prostate and should be avoided. The albuterol and ipratropium is expected, since it promotes bronchial dilation. Lisinopril is an ACE inhibitor and useful in reducing blood pressure. The tamsulosin is commonly prescribed to treat benign prostate hypertrophy.

🔑 CN: Reduction of risk potential; CL: Synthesize

66. 3,4,5. High humidity has been shown to increase the work of breathing. Carrying a metered-dose inhaler can facilitate early intervention if bronchospasm and shortness of breath should occur. Smoking cessation is difficult to achieve but very important in preventing COPD progression. Pulmonary rehabilitation programs are a great source of support for health promotion and maintenance for clients with COPD. Both the pneumococcal and influenza vaccines can help protect against respiratory infections.

🔑 CN: Reduction of risk potential;
CL: Create

67. 3. Crackles auscultated in the lung field indicate excessive fluid, a problem that requires immediate intervention. Pursed-lip breathing and a prolonged expiratory phase, circumoral cyanosis, and increased anterior-posterior diameter of the chest (resulting in "barrel chest") are not unusual findings for clients with emphysema.

🔑 CN: Physiological adaptation;
CL: Analyze

68. **4.** Inability to speak could indicate respiratory distress. Pursed-lip breathing, while it is an abnormal finding, is not indicative of respiratory distress. Distant heart sounds could indicate heart failure but are not indicative of any distress. Diminished lung sounds may be normal for this client, and do not require immediate intervention.

🔑 CN: Physiological adaptation;
CL: Analyze

69. **2,1,3,4.** The nurse should first instruct the client to relax the neck and the shoulders and then take several normal breaths. After taking a breath in, the client should pucker the lips and finally breathe out through pursed lips.

🔑 CN: Health promotion and maintenance;
CL: Apply

70. **2.** Clients with chronic COPD have CO_2 retention, and the respiratory drive is stimulated when the Po_2 decreases. The heart rate, respiratory rate, and blood pressure should be evaluated to determine if the client is hemodynamically stable. Symptoms, such as dyspnea, should also be assessed. After assessing the vital signs, the nurse should assist the client as needed to assume the most comfortable position for breathing. Oxygen supplementation, if indicated, should be titrated upward in small increments. There is no indication that the client is experiencing respiratory distress requiring intubation.

🔑 CN: Physiological adaptation;
CL: Synthesize

71. **1.** A client with COPD is at high risk for development of respiratory infections. COPD is slowly progressive; therefore, maintaining current status and establishing a goal that the client will require less supplemental oxygen are unrealistic expectations. Treatment may slow progression of the disease, but permanent improvement is highly unlikely.

🔑 CN: Management of care; CL: Synthesize

72. **1,2,3,4.** The therapeutic range for serum theophylline is 10 to 20 mcg/mL (55.5 to 111 µmol/L). At higher levels, the client will experience signs of toxicity such as nausea, vomiting, seizures, and insomnia. The nurse should instruct the client to report these signs and to keep appointments to have theophylline blood levels monitored. If the theophylline level is below the therapeutic range, the client may be at risk for more frequent exacerbations of the disease.

🔑 CN: Physiological Integrity; CL: Apply

73. **4.** Increasing dyspnea on exertion indicates that the client may be experiencing complications of COPD. Therefore, the client should notify the **HCP** 📖. It is not necessary to avoid being around others. Pain is not a common symptom of COPD. Clients with COPD use low-flow oxygen supplementation (1 to 2 L/min)

to avoid suppressing the respiratory drive, which, for these clients, is stimulated by hypoxia.

🔑 CN: Basic care and comfort; CL: Evaluate

74. **4.** Cigarette smoking is the primary cause of COPD. Other risk factors include exposure to environmental pollutants and chronic asthma. Participating in an aerobic exercise program, although beneficial, will not decrease the risk of COPD. Insufficient protein intake and exposure to people with respiratory infections do not increase the risk of COPD.

🔑 CN: Health promotion and maintenance;
CL: Synthesize

75. **4.** Pursed-lip breathing prolongs exhalation and prevents air trapping in the alveoli, thereby promoting carbon dioxide elimination. By prolonging exhalation and helping the client relax, pursed-lip breathing helps the client learn to control the rate and depth of respiration. Pursed-lip breathing does not promote the intake of oxygen, strengthen the diaphragm, or strengthen intercostal muscles.

🔑 CN: Physiological adaptation;
CL: Evaluate

76. **1.** A priority goal for the client with COPD is to manage the signs and symptoms of the disease process so as to maintain the client's functional ability. Chest pain is not a typical symptom of COPD. The carbon dioxide concentration in the blood is increased to an abnormal level in clients with COPD; it would not be a goal to increase the level further. Preventing infection would be a goal of care for the client with COPD.

🔑 CN: Basic care and comfort;
CL: Synthesize

77. **2.** Exhaling requires less energy than does inhaling. Therefore, lifting while exhaling saves energy and reduces perceived dyspnea. Pursing the lips prolongs exhalation and provides the client with more control over breathing. Lifting after exhaling but before inhaling is similar to lifting with the breath held. This should not be recommended because it is similar to Valsalva's maneuver, which can stimulate cardiac arrhythmias.

🔑 CN: Basic care and comfort;
CL: Synthesize

78. **3.** Right-sided heart failure is a complication of COPD that occurs because of pulmonary hypertension. Signs and symptoms of right-sided heart failure include peripheral edema, jugular venous distention, hepatomegaly, and weight gain due to increased fluid volume. Clubbing of nail beds is associated with conditions of chronic hypoxemia. Hypertension is associated with left-sided heart failure. Clients with heart failure have decreased appetites.

🔑 CN: Physiological adaptation;
CL: Synthesize

79. 4. Exacerbations of COPD are commonly caused by respiratory infections. Coarse crackles and rhonchi would be auscultated as air moves through airways obstructed with secretions. In COPD, breath sounds are diminished because of an enlarged anteroposterior diameter of the chest. Expiration, not inspiration, becomes prolonged. Chest movement is decreased as lungs become overdistended.

CN: Physiological adaptation; CL: Analyze

80. 2. Clients who have a long history of COPD may retain carbon dioxide (CO_2). Gradually, the body adjusts to the higher CO_2 concentration, and the high levels of CO_2 no longer stimulate the respiratory center. The major respiratory stimulant then becomes hypoxemia. Administration of high concentrations of oxygen eliminates this respiratory stimulus and leads to hypoventilation. Oxygen can be drying if it is not humidified, but it does not cause coughing and dyspnea. Increased oxygen use will not create an oxygen dependency; clients should receive oxygen as needed. Oxygen is not contraindicated with the use of bronchodilators.

CN: Physiological adaptation; CL: Apply

81. 4. The client should eat high-calorie, high-protein meals to maintain nutritional status and prevent weight loss that results from the increased work of breathing. The client should be encouraged to eat small, frequent meals. A low-fat, low-cholesterol diet is indicated for clients with coronary artery disease. The client with COPD does not necessarily need to follow a sodium-restricted diet, unless otherwise medically indicated. There is no need for the client to eat bland, soft foods.

CN: Basic care and comfort; CL: Synthesize

82. 3. Theophylline is a bronchodilator that is administered to relax airways and decrease dyspnea. Theophylline is not used to treat infections and does not decrease or thin secretions.

CN: Pharmacological and parenteral therapies; CL: Evaluate

83. 1. The goal of effective coughing is to conserve energy, facilitate removal of secretions, and minimize airway collapse. The client should assume a sitting position with feet on the floor if possible. The client should bend forward slightly and, using pursed-lip breathing, exhale. After resuming an upright position, the client should use abdominal breathing to slowly and deeply inhale. After repeating this process three or four times, the client should take a deep abdominal breath, bend forward, and cough three or four times upon exhalation ("huff" cough). Lying flat does not enhance lung expansion; sitting upright promotes full expansion of the thorax. Shallow breathing does not facilitate removal of secretions, and forceful coughing promotes collapse of airways. A side-lying position does not allow for adequate chest expansion to promote deep breathing.

CN: Basic care and comfort; CL: Create

The Client with Asthma

84. 3,4,5. Utilization of an MDI requires the following actions: shaking the MDI before use; exhaling prior to dispensing the medication; taking a deep breath to ensure the medication is distributed in the lungs and holding it for 10 seconds or as long as possible to disperse the medication into the lungs; and allowing 30 seconds between puffs to provide an adequate amount of inhalation medication. The client should rinse the plastic parts of the MDI and wipe them dry; the canister should not become wet.

CN: Pharmacological and parenteral therapies; CL: Evaluate

85. 4. In an acute asthma attack, diminished or absent breath sounds can be an ominous sign indicating lack of air movement in the lungs and impending respiratory failure. The client requires immediate intervention with inhaled bronchodilators, IV corticosteroids, and, possibly, IV theophylline. Administering oxygen and reassessing the client 10 minutes later would delay needed medical intervention, as would drawing blood for an arterial blood gas analysis. It would be futile to encourage the client to relax and breathe slowly without providing the necessary pharmacologic intervention.

CN: Management of care; CL: Synthesize

86. 3. Quick-acting bronchodilators are used in acute asthma to improve airflow and relieve symptoms; following treatment, tachycardia resolves as gas exchange and work of breathing are improved. SpO2 and PEF rates improve, and wheezing from a constricted airway resolves. The normal inspiratory to expiratory ratio is 1:2.

CN: Physiological adaptation; CL: Evaluate

87. 2. The nurse instructs the client to administer the bronchodilator first (the beta-2 agonist always leads) in order to open the airway and allow for improved delivery of the corticosteroid to the lung tissue, which follows after 1 minute between puffs. Using a spacer device with an MDI provides the best delivery of medication to the lungs.

CN: Pharmacological and parenteral therapies; CL: Synthesize

88. 1. The arterial blood gas reveals a respiratory acidosis with hypoxia. A quick-acting bronchodilator, albuterol, should be administered via nebulizer to improve gas exchange. Ipratropium is a maintenance treatment for bronchospasm that can be used with albuterol. A chest x-ray and sputum sample can be obtained once the client is stable.

CN: Physiological adaptation;
CL: Synthesize

89. 3. Corticosteroids have an anti-inflammatory effect and act to decrease edema in the bronchial airways and decrease mucus secretion. Corticosteroids do not have a bronchodilator effect, act as expectorants, or prevent respiratory infections.

CN: Pharmacological and parenteral therapies; CL: Evaluate

90. 1,4. The client should shake the inhaler and hold it upright when administering the drug. The head should be tilted back slightly. The client should wait about 30 seconds between puffs. The mouth should be rinsed following the use of a corticosteroid MDI to decrease the likelihood of developing an oral infection. The client does not need to lie supine; instead, the client will likely to be able to breathe more freely if sitting upright.

CN: Pharmacological and parenteral therapies; CL: Evaluate

91. 1. Irregular heartbeats should be reported promptly to the care provider. Metaproterenol may cause irregular heartbeat, tachycardia, or anginal pain because of its adrenergic effect on beta-adrenergic receptors in the heart. It is not recommended for use in clients with known cardiac disorders. Metaproterenol does not cause constipation, pedal edema, or bradycardia.

CN: Pharmacological and parenteral therapies; CL: Analyze

92. 3. Use of oral inhalant corticosteroids such as flunisolide can lead to the development of oral thrush, a fungal infection. Once developed, thrush must be treated by antifungal therapy; it will not resolve on its own. Fungal infections can develop even without overuse of the corticosteroid inhaler. Although good oral hygiene can help prevent development of a fungal infection, it cannot be used alone to treat the problem.

CN: Pharmacological and parenteral therapies; CL: Synthesize

93. 1,4,3,2. When using inhalers, clients should first shake the inhaler to activate the MDI and then breathe out through the mouth. Next, the client should activate the MDI while inhaling, hold the breath for 5 to 10 seconds, and then exhale normally.

CN: Pharmacological and parenteral therapies; CL: Apply

94. 4. Between attacks, breath sounds should be clear on auscultation with good airflow present throughout lung fields. Chest x-rays should be normal. The client should remain afebrile. Arterial blood gases should be normal.

CN: Physiological adaptation;
CL: Evaluate

95. 1. Physical exercise is beneficial and should be incorporated as tolerated into the client's schedule. Peak flow numbers should be monitored daily, usually in the morning (before taking medication). Peak flow does not need to be monitored after each meal. Stressors in the client's life should be modified but cannot be totally eliminated. Although adequate sleep is important, it is not recommended that sedatives be routinely taken to induce sleep.

CN: Reduction of risk potential;
CL: Create

96. 3. A common precipitator of asthma attacks is exposure to cigarette and cigar smoke. The client should avoid being in environments where there is exposure to smoke. Environmental exposure to toxins or heavy particulate matter can trigger asthma attacks; however, far fewer asthmatics are exposed to such toxins than are exposed to smoke. Valsalva's maneuver (holding the breath while defecating or bearing down) is associated with causing cardiac arrhythmias. Rarely, asthmatic attacks are triggered by exercising in cold weather.

CN: Reduction of risk potential;
CL: Synthesize

97. 1. A cough productive of yellow sputum is the most likely indicator of a respiratory infection. The other signs and symptoms—wheezing, chest tightness, and increased respiratory rate—are all findings associated with an asthma attack and do not necessarily mean an infection is present.

CN: Physiological adaptation;
CL: Analyze

98. 3. The hallmark signs of asthma are chest tightness, audible wheezing, and coughing. Inspiratory and expiratory wheezing is the result of bronchoconstriction. Even between exacerbations there may be some soft wheezing, so a finding of normal breath sounds would be expected in the absence of asthma. The expected finding is decreased forced expiratory volume (forced expiratory flow [FEF] is the flow [or speed] of air coming out of the lung during the middle portion of a forced expiration) due to bronchial constriction. Morning headaches are found in more advanced cases of COPD and signal nocturnal hypercapnia or hypoxemia.

CN: Physiological adaptation;
CL: Analyze

The Client with Lung Cancer

99. 1. The nurse should first assess for bilateral breath sounds since a complication of central line insertion is a pneumothorax, which would cause an increase in respiratory rate and drop in oxygen, causing irritability. The nurse should also assess blood pressure and heart rate for the complication of bleeding. A chest x-ray will be performed to determine correct placement and complications. A central line was most likely placed because peripheral IV access was not available or adequate for the client. Repositioning may be considered after assessments are done.

CN: Physiological adaptation;
CL: Synthesize

100. 2. The nurse should review the CBC with differential to evaluate the client's hemoglobin and hematocrit, which are abnormal and should be reported to the **HCP** 📖. Anemia leads to decreased oxygen-carrying capacity of the blood. A client unable to compensate for the anemia may experience a profound sense of dyspnea. There has been a significant drop in the hemoglobin and hematocrit since the previous report, and these should be reported to the HCP. The monocytes are within normal range. A_1C is a laboratory test evaluating glycosylated hemoglobin and is in the normal range. This test is used to diagnose diabetes and/or monitor diabetic glucose control over time. PT is a coagulation study reflecting liver function and clotting time and is in the normal range.

CN: Physiological adaptation;
CL: Synthesize

101. 1. Risk factors for postoperative pulmonary complications include malnourishment, which is indicated by this client's height and weight. It is thought that emotional responses can affect overall health; however, not verbalizing one's feelings is not a contributing factor in postoperative pulmonary complications. The client's current activity level and age do not place her at increased risk for complications.

CN: Physiological adaptation;
CL: Analyze

102. 1. Acknowledging the basic feeling the client expresses—fear—and asking an open-ended question allow the client to explain any fears. The other options dismiss the client's feelings and may give false reassurance or label the client's feelings. The client should be encouraged to explore feelings about a cancer diagnosis.

CN: Psychosocial adaptation;
CL: Synthesize

103. 4. Systematic pain assessment is necessary for adequate pain management in the postoperative client. Guidelines from a variety of healthcare agencies and nursing groups recommend that institutions adopt a pain assessment scale to assist in facilitating pain management. Even though the client is receiving morphine sulfate by PCA, and the pump is working, the nurse should continue to assess the client. The concern is not to eliminate coughing but to control pain adequately. Coughing is necessary to prevent postoperative atelectasis and pneumonia. Breathing exercises may help control pain in some circumstances; however, most clients with thoracic surgery require parenteral opioid analgesics in the early postoperative period. Although it is necessary that the PCA device be checked periodically, reassuring the client is not sufficient, so further assessment is needed.

CN: Basic care and comfort;
CL: Synthesize

104. 1. Because clients are discharged as soon as possible from the hospital, it is essential to evaluate the support they have to assist them with self-care at home. The distance the client lives from the hospital is not a critical factor in discharge planning. There are no data indicating that home blood pressure monitoring is needed. Knowledge of the causes of lung cancer, although important, is not the most essential area to evaluate given the client's postoperative status.

CN: Psychosocial adaptation;
CL: Synthesize

105. 2. Epidermoid cancer involving the larger bronchi is almost entirely associated with heavy cigarette smoking. The American and Canadian Cancer Societies report that smoking is responsible for more than 80% of lung cancers in men and women. The prevalence of lung cancer is related to the duration and intensity of the smoking, so nurses can best prevent lung cancer by persuading clients to stop smoking. Chest radiographs aid in detection of lung cancer; they do not prevent it. Exposure to asbestos has been implicated as a risk factor for lung cancer, but cigarette smoking is the major risk factor. There are no data to support the use of home air filters in the prevention of lung cancer.

CN: Health promotion and maintenance;
CL: Synthesize

106. 4. Deep breathing helps prevent microatelectasis and pneumonitis and also helps force air and fluid out of the pleural space into the chest tubes. More than half of the ventilatory process is accomplished by the rise and fall of the diaphragm. The diaphragm is the major muscle of respiration; deep breathing causes it to descend, not elevate, thereby increasing the ventilating surface. Deep breathing increases blood flow to the lungs; however, the primary reason for deep breathing is to expand alveoli and prevent atelectasis. The remaining lobe naturally hyperinflates to fill the space created by the resected lobe. This is an expected phenomenon.

🔑 CN: Physiological adaptation; CL: Evaluate

107. 2. It is essential that the nurse evaluate the effects of pain medication after the medication has had time to act; reassessment is necessary to determine the effectiveness of the pain management plan. Although it is prudent to check for discomfort related to positioning when assessing the client's pain, repositioning the client immediately after administering pain medication is not necessary. Verbally reassuring the client after administering pain medication may be useful to help instill confidence in the treatment plan; however, it is not as important as evaluating the effectiveness of the medication. Readjusting the pain medication dosage as needed according to the client's condition is essential, but the effectiveness of the medication must be evaluated first.

🔑 CN: Physiological adaptation; CL: Synthesize

108. 3. This crackling sensation is subcutaneous emphysema. Subcutaneous emphysema is not an unusual finding and is not dangerous if confined, and the nurse should mark the area to detect if the area is expanding. Progression can be serious, especially if the neck is involved; a tracheotomy may be needed at that point. If emphysema progresses noticeably in 1 hour, the **HCP** 📖 should be notified. Lowering the head of the bed will not arrest the progress or provide any further information. A tracheotomy tray would be useful if subcutaneous emphysema progresses to the neck. Subcutaneous emphysema may progress if the chest drainage system does not adequately remove air and fluid; therefore, the system should not be turned off.

🔑 CN: Physiological adaptation; CL: Synthesize

109. 1. The recommended procedure for teaching clients postoperatively to deep breathe includes contracting (pulling in) the abdominal muscles and taking a slow, deep breath through the nose. This breath is held 3 to 5 seconds, which facilitates alveolar ventilation by improving the inspiratory phase of ventilation. Exhaling slowly as if trying to blow out a candle is a technique used in pursed-lip breathing to facilitate exhalation in clients with chronic obstructive pulmonary disease. It is

recommended that the abdominal muscles be contracted, not relaxed, to promote deep breathing. The client should breathe through the nose.

🔑 CN: Physiological adaptation; CL: Synthesize

110. 3. A client who has undergone chest surgery should be taught to raise the arm on the affected side over the head to help prevent shoulder ankylosis. This exercise helps restore normal shoulder movement, prevents stiffening of the shoulder joint, and improves muscle tone and power. Turning from side to side, raising and lowering the head, and flexing and extending the elbow on the affected side do not exercise the shoulder joint.

🔑 CN: Basic care and comfort; CL: Synthesize

111. 4. The drainage apparatus is always kept below the client's chest level to prevent backflow of fluid into the pleural space. The air vent must always be open in the closed chest drainage system to allow air from the client to escape. Stripping a chest tube causes excessive negative intrapleural pressure and is not recommended. Clamping a chest tube when moving a client is not recommended.

🔑 CN: Physiological adaptation; CL: Synthesize

112. 1. Cessation of fluid fluctuation in the tubing can mean one of several things: the lung has fully expanded and negative intrapleural pressure has been reestablished, the chest tube is occluded, or the chest tube is not in the pleural space. Fluid fluctuation occurs because during inspiration, intrapleural pressure exceeds the negative pressure generated in the water seal system. Therefore, drainage moves toward the client. During expiration, the pleural pressure exceeds that generated in the water seal system, and fluid moves away from the client. When the lung is collapsed or the chest tube is in the pleural space, fluid fluctuation is likely to be noted. The chest tube is not inserted in the mediastinal space.

🔑 CN: Physiological adaptation; CL: Analyze

113. 2. There should never be constant bubbling in the water seal system; normally, the bubbling is intermittent. Constant bubbling in the water seal bottle indicates an air leak, which means that less negative pressure is being exerted on the pleural space. Decreasing the suction will not reduce the leak. It is not necessary to notify the **HCP** 📖 until the system has been checked and the problem identified.

🔑 CN: Physiological adaptation; CL: Synthesize

114. 1. In this case, there may be some obstruction to the flow of air and fluid out of the pleural space, causing air and fluid to collect and build up pressure. This prevents the remaining lung from reexpanding and can cause a mediastinal shift to the opposite side. The nurse's first response is to assess the tubing for kinks or obstruction. Increasing the suction is not done without a **healthcare provider's** 📖 prescription. The normal position of the drainage bottles is 2 to 3 feet (61 to 91.4 cm) below chest level. Clamping the tubes obstructs the flow of air and fluid out of the pleural space and should not be done.

🔑 CN: Physiological adaptation; CL: Synthesize

115. 4. To promote chest tube drainage, the drainage system must be lower than the client's lungs. The amount of drainage is not abnormal; it is not necessary to notify the **HCP** 📖. The nurse should chart the amount and color of drainage every 4 to 8 hours. The chest tube does not need to be clamped; the tubing connection is intact. There is sufficient water to maintain a water seal.

🔑 CN: Physiological adaptation; CL: Synthesize

116. 3. A bottle of sterile water should be readily available and in view when a client has a chest tube so that the tube can be immediately submersed in the water if the chest tube system becomes disconnected. The chest tube should be reconnected to the water seal system as soon as a sterile functioning system can be reestablished. There is no need for a tracheostomy tray, another chest tube, or a spirometer to be placed at the bedside for emergency use.

🔑 CN: Physiological adaptation; CL: Apply

117. 2. Gauze saturated with petrolatum is placed over the site to make an airtight seal to prevent air leakage during the healing process. Dry dressings or adhesive strips are not used. An airtight dressing is needed until the insertion site is healed.

🔑 CN: Management of care; CL: Apply

The Client with Chest Trauma

118. 3. Respiratory distress or arrest is a universal finding of a tension pneumothorax. Unilateral, diminished, or absent breath sounds is a common finding. Tracheal deviation is an inconsistent and late finding. Muffled heart sounds are suggestive of pericardial tamponade.

🔑 CN: Physiological adaptation; CL: Analyze

119. 0.7 mL

$$10\,mg : X\,mL = 15\,mg : 1\,mL$$
$$15\,mg \times X\,mL = 10\,mg \times 1\,mL$$
$$15X = 10$$
$$X = 0.6667$$
$$X = 0.67\,mL$$

🔑 CN: Pharmacological and parenteral therapies; CL: Apply

120. 2. Blunt chest trauma may lead to respiratory failure, and maintenance of adequate oxygenation is the priority for the client. Decreasing the client's anxiety is related to maintaining effective respirations and oxygenation. Although pain is distressing to the client and can increase anxiety and decrease respiratory effectiveness, pain control is secondary to maintaining oxygenation. Maintaining adequate circulatory volume is also secondary to maintaining adequate oxygenation.

🔑 CN: Physiological adaptation; CL: Synthesize

121. 3. Fluctuation of fluid in the water seal column with respirations indicates that the system is functioning properly. If an obstruction were present in the chest tube, fluid fluctuation would be absent. Subcutaneous emphysema occurs when air pockets can be palpated beneath the client's skin around the chest tube insertion site. A leak in the system is indicated when continuous bubbling occurs in the water seal column.

🔑 CN: Physiological adaptation; CL: Analyze

122. 4. Pneumothorax means that there is air in the pleural space causing pressure on the lung and the lung will collapse. The nurse will hear no sounds of air movement on auscultation. Movement of air through mucus produces crackles. Wheezing occurs when airways become obstructed. Dullness on percussion indicates increased density of lung tissue, usually caused by accumulation of fluid.

🔑 CN: Physiological adaptation; CL: Evaluate

123. 1. If the client reports no pain, then the objective of adequate pain relief has been met. Decreased anxiety is not related only to pain control; it could also be related to other factors. A respiratory rate of 26 breaths/min is not within normal limits, nor is the PaO_2 of 70 mm Hg (9.31 kPa), but these values are not measures of pain relief.

🔑 CN: Physiological adaptation; CL: Evaluate

124. 2. One unit of packed red blood cells is about 250 mL. If the blood is delivered at a rate of 60 mL/h, it will take about 4 hours to infuse the entire unit. The transfusion of a single unit of packed red blood cells should not exceed 4 hours to prevent the growth of bacteria and minimize the risk of septicemia.

CN: Pharmacological and parenteral therapies; CL: Apply

125. 2. Too rapid infusion of blood, or any intravenous fluid, can cause fluid volume overload and related problems such as pulmonary edema. Emboli formation, red blood cell hemolysis, and allergic reaction are not related to rapid infusion.

CN: Pharmacological and parenteral therapies; CL: Apply

126. 1. Pneumothorax signs and symptoms include sudden, sharp chest pain, tachypnea, and tachycardia. Other signs and symptoms include diminished or absent breath sounds over the affected lung, anxiety, and restlessness. Hemoptysis and cyanosis are not typically present with a moderate pneumothorax.

CN: Physiological adaptation; CL: Analyze

127. 4. A chest tube is inserted to reexpand the lung and remove air and fluid. Oxygen is not administered through a chest tube. Chest tubes are not inserted to promote scar tissue formation. Antibiotics are not used to treat a pneumothorax.

CN: Basic care and comfort; CL: Evaluate

128. The fluid typically localizes at the base of the thorax.

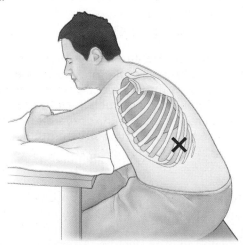

CN: Management of care; CL: Synthesize

129. 1,2,3,4. Following a thoracentesis, the nurse should assess the client for possible complications of the procedure such as pneumothorax, tension pneumothorax, and subcutaneous emphysema, which can occur because of the needle entering the chest cavity. Pulmonary edema could occur if a large volume was aspirated causing a significant

mediastinal shift. Although infection is a possible complication, signs of infection will not be evident immediately after the procedure.

CN: Management of care; CL: Synthesize

130. 1. Cheyne-Stokes respiration is defined as a regular cycle that starts with normal breaths, which increase and then decrease followed by a period of apnea. It can be related to heart failure or a dysfunction of the respiratory center of the brain. Hyperventilation is associated with an increased rate and depth of respirations. Obstructive sleep apnea is recurring episodes of upper airway obstruction and reduced ventilation. Biot's respiration, also known as "cluster breathing," is periods of normal respirations followed by varying periods of apnea.

CN: Health promotion and maintenance; CL: Analyze

The Client with Acute Respiratory Distress Syndrome

131. 3,4,5. The prone position is used to improve oxygenation, ventilation, and perfusion. The importance of placing clients with ARDS in prone positioning should be explained to the family. The positioning allows for mobilization of secretions, and the nurse can provide suctioning. Clinical judgment must be used to determine the length of time in the prone position. If the client's hemodynamic status, oxygenation, or skin is compromised, the client should be returned to the supine position for evaluation. Facial edema is expected with the prone position, but the skin breakdown is of concern.

CN: Physiological adaptation; CL: Synthesize

132. 4. Prone positioning is used to improve oxygenation in clients with ARDS who are receiving mechanical ventilation. The positioning allows for recruitment of collapsed alveolar units, improvement in ventilation, reduction in shunting, mobilization of secretions, and improvement in functional reserve capacity (FRC). When the client is supine, side-to-side repositioning should be done every 2 hours with the head of the bed elevated at least 30 degrees.

CN: Physiological adaptation; CL: Synthesize

133. 1,4,5. Acute respiratory distress syndrome (ARDS) may cause renal failure and superinfection, so the nurse should monitor urine output and urine chemistries. Treatment of hypoxemia can be complicated because changes in lung tissue leave less pulmonary tissue available for gas exchange, thereby causing inadequate perfusion. Humidified oxygen may be one means of promoting oxygenation. The client has crackles in the lung bases, so the nurse should continue to assess breath sounds. Sedatives should be used with caution in clients with ARDS. The nurse should try other measures to relieve the client's restlessness and anxiety. The head of the bed should be elevated to 30 degrees to promote chest expansion and prevent atelectasis.

🔑 CN: Management of care; CL: Create

134. 4. One of the major risk factors for development of ARDS is hypovolemic shock. Adequate fluid replacement is essential to minimize the risk of ARDS in these clients. Teaching smoking cessation does not prevent ARDS. An abnormal serum potassium level and hypercapnia are not risk factors for ARDS.

🔑 CN: Physiological adaptation; CL: Synthesize

135. 2. A hallmark of early ARDS is refractory hypoxemia. The client's PaO_2 level continues to fall, despite higher concentrations of administered oxygen. Elevated carbon dioxide and metabolic acidosis occur late in the disorder. Severe electrolyte imbalances are not indicators of ARDS.

🔑 CN: Physiological adaptation; CL: Analyze

136. 2. The normal range for $PaCO_2$ is 35 to 45 mm Hg (4.7 to 6 kPa). Thus, this client's $PaCO_2$ level is low. The client is experiencing respiratory alkalosis (carbonic acid deficit) due to hyperventilation. The nurse should report this finding to the **healthcare provider (HCP)** 📖 because it requires intervention. The increase in ventilation decreases the $PaCO_2$ level, which leads to decreased carbonic acid and alkalosis. The bicarbonate level is normal in uncompensated respiratory alkalosis along with the normal PaO_2 level. Normal serum pH is 7.35 to 7.45; in uncompensated respiratory alkalosis, the serum pH is >7.45.

🔑 CN: Reduction of risk potential; CL: Analyze

137. 1. The client may be fighting the ventilator breaths. Sedation is indicated to improve compliance with the ventilator in an attempt to lower peak inspiratory pressures. The workload of breathing does indicate the need for increased protein calories; however, this will not correct the respiratory problems with high pressures and respiratory rate. There is no indication that the client is experiencing pain. Increasing the rate on the ventilator is not indicated with the client's increased spontaneous rate.

🔑 CN: Physiological adaptation; CL: Synthesize

138. 1. Manifestations of adult respiratory distress syndrome (ARDS) secondary to acute pancreatitis include respiratory distress, tachypnea, dyspnea, fever, dry cough, fine crackles heard throughout lung fields, possible confusion and agitation, and hypoxemia with arterial oxygen level below 50 mm Hg. The nurse should report the arterial oxygen level of 46 mm Hg (6.1 kPa) to the **HCP** 📖. A respiratory rate of 12 is normal and not considered a sign of respiratory distress. Adventitious lung sounds, such as crackles, are typically found in clients with ARDS. Oxygen saturation of 96% is satisfactory and does not represent hypoxemia or low arterial oxygen saturation.

🔑 CN: Physiologic adaptation; CL: Synthesize

139. 1. Normal PaO_2 level ranges from 80 to 100 mm Hg (10.7 to 13.3 kPa). When PaO_2 falls to 50 mm Hg (6.7 kPa), the nurse should be alert for signs of hypoxia and impending respiratory failure. An oxygen level this low poses a severe risk for respiratory failure. The client will require oxygenation at a concentration that maintains the PaO_2 at 55 to 60 mm Hg (7.3 to 8 kPa) or more.

🔑 CN: Physiological adaptation; CL: Analyze

140. 3. Endotracheal intubation and mechanical ventilation are required in ARDS to maintain adequate respiratory support. Endotracheal intubation, not a tracheostomy, is usually the initial method of maintaining an airway. The client requires mechanical ventilation; nasal oxygen will not provide adequate oxygenation. Chest tubes are used to remove air or fluid from intrapleural spaces.

🔑 CN: Physiological adaptation; CL: Apply

141. 1. The two risk factors most commonly associated with the development of ARDS are gram-negative septic shock and gastric content aspiration. Nurses should be particularly vigilant in assessing a client for onset of ARDS if the client has experienced direct lung trauma or a systemic inflammatory response syndrome (which can be caused by any physiologic insult that leads to widespread inflammation). Chronic obstructive pulmonary disease, asthma, and heart failure are not direct causes of ARDS.

🔑 CN: Reduction of risk potential; CL: Apply

142. 4. Auscultation for bilateral breath sounds is the most appropriate method for determining cuff placement. The nurse should also look for the symmetrical rise and fall of the chest and should note the location of the exit mark on the tube. Assessments of skin color, respiratory rate, and the amount of cuff inflation cannot validate the placement of the endotracheal tube.

🔑 CN: Basic care and comfort; CL: Evaluate

143. 4. The nurse should suction the client if the client is not able to cough up secretions and clear the airway. Administering oxygen will not promote airway clearance. The client should be turned every 2 hours to help move secretions; every 4 hours is not often enough. Administering sedatives to promote rest is contraindicated in acute respiratory distress because sedatives can depress respirations.

🔑 CN: Physiological adaptation;
CL: Synthesize

144. 1. Gastrointestinal hemorrhage occurs in about 25% of clients receiving prolonged mechanical ventilation because of the development of stress ulcers. Clients who are receiving steroid therapy and those with a previous history of ulcers are most likely to be at risk. Other possible complications include incorrect ventilation, oxygen toxicity, fluid imbalance, decreased cardiac output, pneumothorax, infection, and atelectasis.

🔑 CN: Physiological adaptation;
CL: Analyze

Managing Care, Quality, and Safety of Clients with Respiratory Health Problems

145. 2. Respirations of 36 breaths/min and diminished wheezing are indicative of respiratory distress. This finding takes precedence over a client scheduled for an angiogram, a client with a heart rate if 90 bpm needing a scheduled beta-blocker, or a client with a PaO_2 of 56 mm Hg, which is indicated for a client being discharged home on oxygen.

🔑 CN: Management of care; CL: Synthesize

146. 1. UAP 📖 can assist a client with the adjustment of his or her oxygen delivery device. Making adjustments based on client responses, monitoring for adverse effects, and assessing for the best methods of oxygen delivery are skills that require nursing judgments and can only be performed by a nurse.

🔑 CN: Management of care; CL: Analyze

147. 4. Confusion and vertigo are risk factors for falls. Measures must be taken to minimize the risk of injury. The nurse or **UAP** 📖 should check on the client regularly to determine needs regarding elimination. Restraints, including bed rails and extremity restraints, should be used only to ensure the person's safety or the safety of others, and there must be a written prescription from a **healthcare provider (HCP)** 📖 before using them. The nurse should never ask the roommate of a client to be responsible for the client's safety.

🔑 CN: Safety and infection control;
CL: Synthesize

148. 4. Airborne precautions prevent transmission of infectious agents that remain infectious over long distances when suspended in the air (e.g., *Mycobacterium tuberculosis*, measles, varicella virus [chickenpox], and possibly SARS-CoV). The preferred placement is in an isolation single-client room that is equipped with special air handling and ventilation. A negative pressure room, or an area that exhausts room air directly outside or through HEPA filters, should be used if recirculation is unavoidable. While hand hygiene is important, it is not sufficient to prevent transmission of tuberculosis. Contact precautions are for clients with known or suspected infections or evidence of syndromes that represent an increased risk for contact transmission. Droplet precautions are intended to prevent transmission of pathogens spread through close respiratory or mucous membrane contact with respiratory secretions. Because these pathogens do not remain infectious over long distances in a healthcare facility, special air handling and ventilation are not required to prevent droplet transmission.

🔑 CN: Safety and infection control;
CL: Synthesize

149. 2,3,4,5. One of the "five rights" of drug administration is "right medication." Cefazolin was not the medication prescribed. The pharmacist is the professional resource and serves as a check to ensure that clients receive the right medication. Returning unwanted medications to the pharmacy will decrease the opportunity for a medication error by the nurse who follows the current nurse.

🔑 CN: Safety and infection control;
CL: Synthesize

150. 1,3,4,2. Because two major complications of endotracheal tube intubation, inadvertent extubation and aspiration, can be catastrophic events, assessment of this client is the first priority. Cellulitis is a serious infection as there is inflammation of subcutaneous tissues; third spacing of fluid may promote the formation of a fluid volume deficit, which can be exacerbated by the fever due to insensible fluid loss. The nurse should assess this client next to determine current vital signs and fluid status. The nurse should assess the client with the IV fluids next because the new bag of fluids will need to be hung in 30 to 40 minutes. IV therapy necessitates that the client be assessed for signs and symptoms of adequate hydration (moist mucous membranes, elastic skin turgor, vital signs within normal limits, adequate urine output, and level of consciousness within normal limits), and the IV access site needs to be assessed. From the information provided, there is no indication that the client who had the cerebrovascular accident is unstable. Thus, this client is the last **priority** for assessment.

🔑 CN: Management of care; CL: Synthesize

151. 1,2,3. The process of changing a healthcare system from an acute care model to a community-based care model uses continuous quality improvement (CQI) methods. The goal is to improve the health of chronically ill clients. Areas for improvement include health systems, delivery system design, decision support, clinical information systems, self-management support, and the community. This system requires healthcare services that are client centered and coordinated among members of the healthcare team and the client and the family. These changes do not focus on the administrative leadership or the care in the acute care setting alone.

🔑 CN: Management of care; CL: Synthesize

152. 4. Several factors designate this client as a high fall risk based on the Morse Fall Scale: history of falling (25), secondary diagnosis (15), plus IV access (20). The client's total score is 60. There is also concern that the client's gait is at least weak if not impaired due to hospitalization for pneumonia, which may add to the client's fall risk. After evaluating the client's risk, the nurse must develop a plan and take action to maximize the client's safety.

🔑 CN: Safety and infection control;
CL: Analyze

153. 1,2,3,4. Gloves, gown, surgical mask, and eye protection/glasses are worn to protect healthcare workers and to help prevent the spread of infection when clients are placed in droplet isolation. Because droplets are too heavy to be airborne, a respirator is not required when caring for a client in droplet precautions.

🔑 CN: Safety and infection control; CL: Apply

154. 3. The nurse has already called for help and established unresponsiveness, so the first action is to open the client's airway; opening the airway may result in spontaneous breathing and will help the nurse determine whether or not further intervention is required. Pushing the "code blue" button may not be the appropriate action if the client is breathing and becomes responsive once the airway is open. A quick assessment upon opening the client's airway will help the nurse to determine if the **rapid response team** 📖 is needed. Calling for a defibrillator may not be the necessary or appropriate action once the client's airway has been opened.

🔑 CN: Safety and infection control;
CL: Synthesize

155. 2,3,1,4. The nurse should first assess the client's respiratory status to determine if there is a physiological reason for the client's confusion. Other physiological factors to assess include pain and elimination. Safety needs including medication interactions should then be evaluated. Requesting restraints in order to maintain client safety should be used as a last resort.

🔑 CN: Safety and infection control;
CL: Synthesize

156. 1,2,4,3. The elderly client with pneumonia, an elevated temperature, and shortness of breath is the most acutely ill client described and should be the client with the highest priority. The elevated temperature and the shortness of breath can lead to a decrease in the client's oxygen levels and can predispose the client to dehydration and confusion. Then the nurse should assess the client with the thoracotomy who is requesting pain medication and administer any needed medication. The client with emphysema should be the next priority so that the bronchodilator can be administered on schedule as close as possible. The nurse would then assess the client with suspected tuberculosis and a cough.

🔑 CN: Management of care; CL: Synthesize

157. 2,3,5. A client with pneumonia experiencing diaphoresis is at risk for dehydration and increased temperature and heart rate. The fluid status, intake, and urine output should be monitored closely. The client is febrile, causing an increase in heart rate. Fluid volume deficit may also increase the heart rate. The underlying cause of the tachycardia can be treated with acetaminophen and increased intake of fluids. Bed rest limits lung expansion, and sitting up and deep breathing should be encouraged in a client with pneumonia. The blood pressure is stable enough to allow the client to get out of bed to the chair, with assistance to ensure safety. It is not necessary to notify the **HCP** 📖.

🔑 CN: Physiological adaptation;
CL: Synthesize

TEST 5

The Client with Upper Gastrointestinal Tract Health Problems

- The Client with Disorders of the Oral Cavity
- The Client with Peptic Ulcer Disease
- The Client with Cancer of the Stomach
- The Client with Gastroesophageal Reflux Disease
- Managing Care, Quality, and Safety of Clients with Upper Gastrointestinal Tract Health Problems
- Answers, Rationales, and Test-Taking Strategies

The Client with Disorders of the Oral Cavity

1. A nurse is caring for a client who has just returned from surgery to treat a fractured mandible. The jaws are wired. Which items should always be available at this client's bedside? Select all that apply.
- [ ] 1. nasogastric tube
- [ ] 2. wire cutters
- [ ] 3. oxygen cannula
- [ ] 4. suction equipment
- [ ] 5. code cart

2. The nurse is teaching a client with stomatitis about mouth care. Which instruction is **most** appropriate?
- [ ] 1. Drink hot tea at frequent intervals.
- [ ] 2. Gargle with antiseptic mouthwash.
- [ ] 3. Use an electric toothbrush.
- [ ] 4. Eat a soft, bland diet.

3. A client who has a history of bacterial endo-carditis is scheduled to have oral surgery to remove a tooth. What should the nurse instruct the client to do?
- [ ] 1. Gargle with a saline solution prior to the appointment.
- [ ] 2. Rinse the mouth with mouthwash the night before and day of the surgery.
- [ ] 3. Contact the health provider to request a sedative.
- [ ] 4. Be sure the dentist prescribes a prophylactic antibiotic prior to the oral surgery.

4. Amoxicillin trihydrate 300 mg PO has been prescribed for a client with an oral infection. The medication is available in a liquid suspension that is available as 250 mg/5 mL. How many milliliters should the nurse administer? Record your answer using a whole number.

_____ mL.

5. During the assessment of a client's mouth, the nurse notes the absence of saliva. The client reports having pain behind the ear. The client has been nothing-by-mouth (NPO) for several days but now can have liquids. The nurse should:
- [ ] 1. request a prescription for an antifungal mouthwash.
- [ ] 2. instruct the client to brush the gums as well as the teeth.
- [ ] 3. encourage the client to suck on hard candy.
- [ ] 4. give the client a hydrogen peroxide–based mouthwash.

6. The nurse is preparing a community presentation on oral cancer. Which is a **primary** risk factor for oral cancer that the nurse should include in the presentation?
- [ ] 1. use of alcohol
- [ ] 2. frequent use of mouthwash
- [ ] 3. lack of vitamin B_{12}
- [ ] 4. lack of regular teeth cleaning by a dentist

7. A client has early signs of oral cancer. To conduct a focused assessment, what should the nurse do? Select all that apply.
- [ ] 1. inspect the mouth for infection and inflammation
- [ ] 2. inquire about loss of sense of taste
- [ ] 3. determine presence of dysphagia
- [ ] 4. monitor the client's height and weight
- [ ] 5. ask if the client is urinating regularly
- [ ] 6. monitor for frequent usage of narcotics

8. Following surgery to set a fractured mandible, the client has swelling at the surgery site. The **priority** for nursing care is to:
- [ ] 1. prevent nausea and vomiting.
- [ ] 2. maintain a patent airway.
- [ ] 3. provide frequent oral hygiene.
- [ ] 4. establish a way for the client to communicate.

9. A client who has had the jaws wired begins to vomit. The nurse should **first**:
- [ ] 1. insert a nasogastric (NG) tube and connect it to suction.
- [ ] 2. use wire cutters to cut the wire.
- [ ] 3. suction the client's airway as needed.
- [ ] 4. administer an antiemetic intravenously.

The Client with Peptic Ulcer Disease

10. A client is admitted to the hospital after vomiting bright red blood and is diagnosed with a bleeding duodenal ulcer. The client develops a sudden, sharp pain in the midepigastric region along with a rigid, board-like abdomen. After obtaining the client's vital signs, what should the nurse do **next**?
- [ ] 1. Administer pain medication as prescribed.
- [ ] 2. Raise the head of the bed.
- [ ] 3. Prepare to insert a nasogastric tube.
- [ ] 4. Notify the healthcare provider (HCP).

11. When obtaining a nursing history from a client with a suspected gastric ulcer, which signs and symptoms should the nurse assess? Select all that apply.
- [ ] 1. epigastric pain at night
- [ ] 2. relief of epigastric pain after eating
- [ ] 3. vomiting
- [ ] 4. weight loss
- [ ] 5. melena

12. The nurse is caring for a client who has had a gastroscopy. Which findings indicate that the client is developing a complication related to the procedure? Select all that apply.
- [ ] 1. The client has a sore throat.
- [ ] 2. The client has a temperature of 100°F (37.8°C).
- [ ] 3. The client appears drowsy following the procedure.
- [ ] 4. The client has epigastric pain.
- [ ] 5. The client experiences hematemesis.

13. A client admitted to the hospital with peptic ulcer disease tells the nurse about having black, tarry stools. The nurse should:
- [ ] 1. encourage the client to increase fluid intake.
- [ ] 2. advise the client to avoid iron-rich foods.
- [ ] 3. place the client on contact precautions.
- [ ] 4. report the finding to the healthcare provider (HCP).

14. A client with peptic ulcer disease is taking ranitidine. What is the expected outcome of this drug?
- [ ] 1. heal the ulcer
- [ ] 2. protect the ulcer surface from acids
- [ ] 3. reduce acid concentration
- [ ] 4. limit gastric acid secretion

15. A client with a peptic ulcer reports epigastric pain that frequently causes the client to wake up during the night. The nurse should instruct the client to do which activities? Select all that apply.
- [ ] 1. Obtain adequate rest to reduce stimulation.
- [ ] 2. Eat small, frequent meals throughout the day.
- [ ] 3. Take all medications on time as prescribed.
- [ ] 4. Sit up for 1 hour when awakened at night.
- [ ] 5. Stay away from crowded areas.

16. A client with peptic ulcer disease reports being nauseated most of the day and now feeling light-headed and dizzy. Based upon these findings, which nursing actions would be **most** appropriate for the nurse to take? Select all that apply.
- [ ] 1. administering an antacid hourly until nausea subsides
- [ ] 2. monitoring the client's vital signs
- [ ] 3. notifying the healthcare provider (HCP) of the client's symptoms
- [ ] 4. initiating oxygen therapy
- [ ] 5. reassessing the client in an hour

17. The nurse is teaching a client with a peptic ulcer about the diet that should be followed after discharge. The nurse should explain that the diet should include:
- [ ] 1. bland foods.
- [ ] 2. high-protein foods.
- [ ] 3. any foods that are tolerated.
- [ ] 4. a glass of milk with each meal.

18. A client diagnosed with peptic ulcer disease (PUD) has an *H. pylori* infection. The client is following a 2-week drug regimen that includes clarithromycin along with omeprazole and amoxicillin. The nurse should instruct the client to:
- [ ] 1. alternate the use of the drugs.
- [ ] 2. take the drugs at different times during the day.
- [ ] 3. discontinue all drugs if nausea occurs.
- [ ] 4. take the drugs for the entire 2-week period.

19. A client with peptic ulcer disease (PUD) is admitted to the hospital for a gastric resection. The client reports a sudden sharp pain in the midepigastric area that radiates to the shoulder. The nurse should **first**:
- [ ] 1. establish an IV line.
- [ ] 2. administer pain medication.
- [ ] 3. notify the surgeon.
- [ ] 4. call for a stat ECG.

20. A client is to take one daily dose of ranitidine at home to treat a peptic ulcer. The client understands proper drug administration of ranitidine when the client will take the drug:
- [ ] 1. before meals.
- [ ] 2. with meals.
- [ ] 3. at bedtime.
- [ ] 4. when pain occurs.

21. A client has been taking aluminum hydroxide 30 mL six times per day at home to treat a peptic ulcer. The client has been unable to have a bowel movement for 3 days. Based on this information, the nurse would determine that the **most** likely cause of the client's constipation is because the client:
- ☐ **1.** has not been including enough fiber in the diet.
- ☐ **2.** needs to increase the daily exercise.
- ☐ **3.** is experiencing an adverse effect of the aluminum hydroxide.
- ☐ **4.** has developed a gastrointestinal obstruction.

22. A client is taking an antacid for treatment of a peptic ulcer. Which statement **best** indicates that the client understands how to correctly take the antacid?
- ☐ **1.** "I should take my antacid before I take my other medications."
- ☐ **2.** "I need to decrease my intake of fluids so that I do not dilute the effects of my antacid."
- ☐ **3.** "My antacid will be most effective if I take it whenever I experience stomach pains."
- ☐ **4.** "It is best for me to take my antacid 1 to 3 hours after meals."

23. Which is an expected outcome for a client with peptic ulcer disease? The client will:
- ☐ **1.** demonstrate appropriate use of analgesics to control pain.
- ☐ **2.** explain the rationale for eliminating alcohol from the diet.
- ☐ **3.** verbalize the importance of monitoring hemoglobin and hematocrit every 3 months.
- ☐ **4.** eliminate engaging in contact sports.

The Client with Cancer of the Stomach

24. The nurse should assess the client who is being admitted to the hospital with upper GI bleeding for which finding? Select all that apply.
- ☐ **1.** dry, flushed skin
- ☐ **2.** decreased urine output
- ☐ **3.** tachycardia
- ☐ **4.** widening pulse pressure
- ☐ **5.** rapid respirations
- ☐ **6.** thirst

25. A client with cancer of the stomach had a total gastrectomy 2 days earlier. Which indicates the client is ready to try a liquid diet? The client:
- ☐ **1.** is hungry.
- ☐ **2.** has not requested pain medication for 8 hours.
- ☐ **3.** has frequent bowel sounds.
- ☐ **4.** has had a bowel movement.

26. Within 6 hours following a subtotal gastrectomy, the drainage from the client's NG tube is bright red. The nurse should **first**:
- ☐ **1.** clamp the NG tube.
- ☐ **2.** remove the existing NG tube.
- ☐ **3.** irrigate the NG tube with iced saline.
- ☐ **4.** chart the finding in the client's medical record.

27. A client has been diagnosed with adenocarcinoma of the stomach and is scheduled to undergo a subtotal gastrectomy (Billroth II procedure). During preoperative teaching, the nurse is reinforcing information about the surgical procedure. The nurse should instruct the client that the procedure will result in:
- ☐ **1.** enlargement of the pyloric sphincter.
- ☐ **2.** anastomosis of the gastric stump to the jejunum.
- ☐ **3.** removal of the duodenum.
- ☐ **4.** repositioning of the vagus nerve.

28. Since the diagnosis of stomach cancer, the client has been having trouble sleeping and is frequently preoccupied with thoughts about how life will change. The client says, "I wish my life could stay the same." Based on this information, the nurse should understand that the client:
- ☐ **1.** is having difficulty coping.
- ☐ **2.** has a sleep disorder.
- ☐ **3.** is grieving.
- ☐ **4.** is anxious.

29. After a subtotal gastrectomy, the drainage in the nasogastric tube is expected to be what color for about 12 to 24 hours after surgery?
- ☐ **1.** dark brown
- ☐ **2.** bile green
- ☐ **3.** bright red
- ☐ **4.** cloudy white

30. Following a subtotal gastrectomy, a client has a nasogastric (NG) tube connected to low suction. The nurse should:
- ☐ **1.** irrigate the tube with 30 mL of sterile water every hour, if needed.
- ☐ **2.** reposition the tube if it is not draining well.
- ☐ **3.** monitor the client for nausea, vomiting, and abdominal distention.
- ☐ **4.** change to high suction if the drainage is sluggish on low suction.

31. A client who is recovering from gastric surgery is receiving IV fluids to be infused at 100 mL/h. The IV tubing delivers 15 gtt/mL. The nurse should infuse the solution at a flow rate of how many drops per minute to ensure that the client receives 100 mL/h? Record your answer using a whole number.

_____ gtt/min.

32. Following a gastrectomy, the nurse should place the client in which position?
- [ ] **1.** prone
- [ ] **2.** supine
- [ ] **3.** low Fowler's
- [ ] **4.** right or left Sims

33. To reduce the risk of dumping syndrome, the nurse should teach the client to:
- [ ] **1.** sit upright for 30 minutes after meals.
- [ ] **2.** drink liquids with meals, avoiding caffeine.
- [ ] **3.** avoid milk and other dairy products.
- [ ] **4.** decrease the carbohydrate content of meals.

34. A client who is recovering from a subtotal gastrectomy experiences dumping syndrome. The client asks the nurse, "When will I be able to eat three meals a day again like I used to?" Which response by the nurse is **most** appropriate?
- [ ] **1.** "Eating six meals a day is time-consuming, isn't it?"
- [ ] **2.** "You will have to eat six small meals a day for the rest of your life."
- [ ] **3.** "You will be able to tolerate three meals a day before you are discharged."
- [ ] **4.** "Most clients can resume their normal meal patterns in about 6 to 12 months."

35. After surgery for gastric cancer, a client is scheduled to undergo radiation therapy. The nurse should include which information in the teaching plan?
- [ ] **1.** nutritional intake
- [ ] **2.** management of alopecia
- [ ] **3.** exercise and activity levels
- [ ] **4.** access to community resources

36. One month following a subtotal gastrectomy for cancer, the nurse is evaluating the nursing care goal related to improved nutrition. What indicates that the client has attained the goal? The client has:
- [ ] **1.** regained weight loss.
- [ ] **2.** resumed normal dietary intake of three meals a day.
- [ ] **3.** controlled nausea and vomiting through regular use of antiemetics.
- [ ] **4.** achieved adequate nutritional status through oral or parenteral feedings.

The Client with Gastroesophageal Reflux Disease

37. Which instruction should the nurse include in the teaching plan for a client who is experiencing gastroesophageal reflux disease (GERD)?
- [ ] **1.** Limit caffeine intake to two cups of coffee per day.
- [ ] **2.** Do not lie down for 2 hours after eating.
- [ ] **3.** Follow a low-protein diet.
- [ ] **4.** Take medications with milk to decrease irritation.

38. The client is scheduled to have an upper gastrointestinal tract series of x-rays. Following the x-rays, the nurse should instruct the client to:
- [ ] **1.** take a laxative.
- [ ] **2.** follow a clear liquid diet.
- [ ] **3.** administer an enema.
- [ ] **4.** take an antiemetic.

39. A client who has been diagnosed with gastroesophageal reflux disease (GERD) has heartburn. To decrease the heartburn, the nurse should instruct the client to **eliminate** which item from the diet?
- [ ] **1.** lean beef
- [ ] **2.** air-popped popcorn
- [ ] **3.** hot chocolate
- [ ] **4.** raw vegetables

40. The client with gastroesophageal reflux disease (GERD) has a chronic cough. This symptom may indicate:
- [ ] **1.** development of laryngeal cancer.
- [ ] **2.** irritation of the esophagus.
- [ ] **3.** esophageal scar tissue formation.
- [ ] **4.** aspiration of gastric contents.

41. Bethanechol has been prescribed for a client with gastroesophageal reflux disease (GERD). The nurse should assess the client for which adverse effect?
- [ ] **1.** constipation
- [ ] **2.** urinary urgency
- [ ] **3.** hypertension
- [ ] **4.** dry oral mucosa

42. The nurse is developing a care management plan with a client who has been diagnosed with gastroesophageal reflux disease (GERD). What should the nurse instruct the client to do? Select all that apply.
- [ ] **1.** Avoid a diet high in fatty foods.
- [ ] **2.** Avoid beverages that contain caffeine.
- [ ] **3.** Eat three meals a day, with the largest meal being at dinner in the evening.
- [ ] **4.** Avoid all alcoholic beverages.
- [ ] **5.** Lie down after consuming each meal for 30 minutes.
- [ ] **6.** Use over-the-counter (OTC) antisecretory agents rather than prescriptions.

43. Which dietary measures would be useful in preventing esophageal reflux?
- [ ] **1.** eating small, frequent meals
- [ ] **2.** increasing fluid intake
- [ ] **3.** avoiding air swallowing with meals
- [ ] **4.** adding a bedtime snack to the dietary plan

44. The nurse is obtaining a health history from a client who has a sliding hiatal hernia associated with reflux. The nurse should ask the client about the presence of which symptom?
- [ ] **1.** heartburn
- [ ] **2.** jaundice
- [ ] **3.** anorexia
- [ ] **4.** stomatitis

45. Which risk factor would **most** likely contribute to the development of a hiatal hernia?
☐ 1. having a sedentary desk job
☐ 2. being 5 feet, 3 inches tall (160 cm) and weighing 190 lb (86.2 kg)
☐ 3. using laxatives frequently
☐ 4. being 40 years old

46. Which nursing interventions would **most** likely promote self-care behaviors in the client with a hiatal hernia?
☐ 1. Introduce the client to other people who are successfully managing their care.
☐ 2. Include the client's daughter in the teaching so that she can help implement the plan.
☐ 3. Ask the client to identify other situations in which the client changed healthcare habits.
☐ 4. Provide reassurance that the client will be able to implement all aspects of the plan successfully.

47. The client has been taking magnesium hydroxide (milk of magnesia) to control hiatal hernia symptoms. The nurse should assess the client for which condition most commonly associated with the ongoing use of magnesium-based antacids?
☐ 1. anorexia
☐ 2. weight gain
☐ 3. diarrhea
☐ 4. constipation

48. Which lifestyle modification should the nurse encourage the client with a hiatal hernia to include in activities of daily living?
☐ 1. daily aerobic exercise
☐ 2. eliminating smoking and alcohol use
☐ 3. balancing activity and rest
☐ 4. avoiding high-stress situations

49. In developing a teaching plan for the client with a hiatal hernia, the nurse's assessment of which work-related factors would be **most** useful?
☐ 1. number and length of breaks
☐ 2. body mechanics used in lifting
☐ 3. temperature in the work area
☐ 4. cleaning solvents used

50. The nurse instructs the client on health maintenance activities to help control symptoms from a hiatal hernia. Which statement would indicate that the client has understood the instructions?
☐ 1. "I will avoid lying down after a meal."
☐ 2. "I can still enjoy my potato chips and cola at bedtime."
☐ 3. "I wish I did not have to give up swimming."
☐ 4. "If I wear a girdle, I will have more support for my stomach."

51. The nurse should instruct the client to avoid which drug while taking metoclopramide hydrochloride?
☐ 1. antacids
☐ 2. antihypertensives
☐ 3. anticoagulants
☐ 4. alcohol

52. A client is taking cimetidine to treat a hiatal hernia. The nurse should evaluate the client to determine that the drug has been effective in preventing which health problem?
☐ 1. esophageal reflux
☐ 2. dysphagia
☐ 3. esophagitis
☐ 4. ulcer formation

53. The client asks the nurse if surgery is needed to correct a hiatal hernia. Which reply by the nurse would be **most** accurate?
☐ 1. "Surgery is usually required, although medical treatment is attempted first."
☐ 2. "Hiatal hernia symptoms can usually be successfully managed with diet modifications, medications, and lifestyle changes."
☐ 3. "Surgery is not performed for this type of hernia."
☐ 4. "A minor surgical procedure to reduce the size of the diaphragmatic opening will probably be planned."

Managing Care, Quality, and Safety of Clients with Upper Gastrointestinal Tract Health Problems

54. A client has returned from surgery during which the jaws were wired as treatment for a fractured mandible. The client is in stable condition. The nurse is instructing the unlicensed assistive personnel (UAP) on how to properly position the client. Which instructions about positioning would be appropriate for the nurse to give the UAP?
☐ 1. Keep the client in a side-lying position with the head slightly elevated.
☐ 2. Do not reposition the client without the assistance of a registered nurse (RN).
☐ 3. The client can assume any position that is comfortable.
☐ 4. Keep the client's head elevated on two pillows at all times.

55. The nurse has been assigned to provide care for four clients. In what order, from first to last, should the nurse assess these clients? All options must be used.

| 1. a client awaiting surgery for a hiatal hernia repair at 1100 |

| 2. a client with suspected gastric cancer who is on nothing-by-mouth (NPO) status for tests |

| 3. a client with peptic ulcer disease experiencing a sudden onset of acute stomach pain |

| 4. a client who is requesting pain medication 2 days after surgery to repair a fractured jaw |

| |

| |

| |

| |

56. The nurse is caring for a client who has just had an upper GI endoscopy. The client's vital signs must be taken every 30 minutes for 2 hours after the procedure. The nurse assigns an unlicensed assistive personnel (UAP) to take the vital signs. One hour later, the UAP reports the client, who was previously afebrile, has developed a temperature of 101.8°F (38.8°C). The nurse should:
- ☐ 1. promptly assess the client for potential perforation.
- ☐ 2. tell the assistant to change thermometers and retake the temperature.
- ☐ 3. plan to give the client acetaminophen to lower the temperature.
- ☐ 4. ask the UAP to bathe the client with tepid water.

57. Which hospitalized client is at risk to develop parotitis?
- ☐ 1. a 50-year-old client with nausea and vomiting who is on nothing-by-mouth status
- ☐ 2. a 75-year-old client with diabetes who has ill-fitting dentures
- ☐ 3. an 80-year-old client who has poor oral hygiene and is dehydrated
- ☐ 4. a 65-year-old client with lung cancer who has a feeding tube in place

58. The nurse instructs the unlicensed assistive personnel (UAP) on how to provide oral hygiene for clients who cannot perform this task for themselves. Which technique should the nurse ask the UAP to incorporate into the client's daily care?
- ☐ 1. Assess the oral cavity each time mouth care is given and record observations.
- ☐ 2. Use a soft toothbrush to brush the client's teeth after each meal.
- ☐ 3. Swab the client's tongue, gums, and lips with a soft foam applicator every 2 hours.
- ☐ 4. Rinse the client's mouth with mouthwash several times a day.

59. The nurse is developing standards of care for a client with gastroesophageal reflux disease and wants to review current evidence for practice. Which resource will provide the **most** helpful information?
- ☐ 1. a review in the Cochrane Library
- ☐ 2. a literature search in a database, such as the Cumulative Index to Nursing and Allied Health Literature (CINAHL)
- ☐ 3. an online nursing textbook
- ☐ 4. the policy and procedure manual at the healthcare agency

60. The nurse in the intensive care unit is giving a report to the nurse in the postsurgical unit about a client who had a gastrectomy. The **most** effective way to assure essential information about the client is reported is to:
- ☐ 1. give the report face to face with both nurses in a quiet room.
- ☐ 2. audiotape the report for future reference and documentation.
- ☐ 3. use a checklist with information individualized for the client.
- ☐ 4. document essential transfer information in the client's electronic health record.

61. A nurse is delegating activities to unlicensed assistive personnel (UAP). Which activities can be appropriately delegated? Select all that apply.
- ☐ 1. Assist client with oral care prior to breakfast.
- ☐ 2. Ask about location, quality, and radiation of pain.
- ☐ 3. Observe and document effect of medication after given by the nurse.
- ☐ 4. Measure and record intake and output throughout the shift.
- ☐ 5. Determine if client is oriented to person, place, and time and report to nurse.
- ☐ 6. Change a simple dry dressing on a client's coccyx while bathing.

Answers, Rationales, and Test-Taking Strategies

*The answers and rationales for each question follow below, along with keys (🔑) to the client need (CN) and cognitive level (CL) for each question. In addition, you will also see a glossary icon (📖) highlighting specific terminology used on the licensing exam. As you check your answers, use the **Content Mastery and Test-Taking Skill Self-Analysis** worksheet (tear-out worksheet in back of book) to identify the reason(s) for not answering the questions correctly. For additional information about test-taking skills and strategies for answering questions, refer to pages 12–23 and pages 35–36 in Part 1 of this book.*

The Client with Disorders of the Oral Cavity

1. 2,4. Following surgery for a fractured mandible, the client's jaws will be wired. The nurse should be prepared to intervene quickly in case the client develops respiratory distress or begins to choke or vomit. Wire cutters or scissors should always be available in case the wires need to be cut in a medical emergency. Suction equipment should be available to help clear the client's airway if necessary. It is not necessary to keep a nasogastric tube or oxygen cannula at the client's bedside. Cardiopulmonary arrest is unlikely, so a code cart is not needed at the bedside.

🔑 CN: Safety and infection control; CL: Apply

2. 4. Clients with stomatitis (inflammation of the mouth) have significant discomfort, which impacts their ability to eat and drink. They will be most comfortable eating soft, bland foods and avoiding temperature extremes in their food and liquids. Gargling with an antiseptic mouthwash will be irritating to the mucosa. Mouth care should include gentle brushing with a soft toothbrush and flossing.

🔑 CN: Basic care and comfort; CL: Synthesize

3. 4. Clients who are at risk for developing infective endocarditis due to cardiac conditions such as a history of bacterial endocarditis must take prophylactic antibiotics before any dental procedure that may cause bleeding. Gargling with saline or using mouthwash is not sufficient to prevent infection. The client will not need a sedative prior to the surgery.

🔑 CN: Reduction of risk potential; CL: Synthesize

4. 6 mL. To administer 300 mg PO, the nurse will need to administer 6 mL. The following formula is used to calculate the correct dosage:

$$300 \text{ mg}/X \text{ mL} = 250 \text{ mg}/5 \text{ mL}.$$

🔑 CN: Pharmacological and parenteral therapies; CL: Apply

5. 3. The lack of saliva, pain near the area of the ear, and the prolonged NPO status of the client are indications that the client may be developing parotitis, or inflammation of the parotid gland. Parotitis usually develops with dehydration combined with poor oral hygiene or when clients have been NPO for an extended period. Preventive measures include the use of sugarless hard candy or gum to stimulate saliva production, adequate hydration, and frequent mouth care. The client does not have indications of stomatitis (inflammation of the mouth), which produces excessive salivation and a sore mouth. The client does not have indications of oral candidiasis (thrush), which causes bluish white mouth lesions, and the nurse does not need to request a prescription for an antifungal mouthwash. There are no indications that the client has gingivitis, which can be recognized by the inflamed gingiva and bleeding that occur during toothbrushing, and while the client should brush the teeth and gums, increasing salivation to prevent parotitis is the priority at this time.

🔑 CN: Basic care and comfort; CL: Synthesize

6. 1. Chronic and excessive use of alcohol can lead to oral cancer. Smoking and use of smokeless tobacco are other significant risk factors. Additional risk factors include chronic irritation such as a broken tooth or ill-fitting dentures, poor dental hygiene, overexposure to sun (lip cancer), and syphilis. Use of mouthwash, lack of vitamin B_{12}, and lack of regular teeth cleaning appointments have not been implicated as primary risk factors for oral cancer.

🔑 CN: Health promotion and maintenance; CL: Analyze

7. 1,3,4. The nurse is conducting a focused assessment of the client's mouth and ability to obtain nutrition. Therefore, the nurse focuses on inspecting the mouth for infection or inflammation, determining if the client has difficulty swallowing, and assuring nutrition by weighing the client and noting weight loss or gain. A sign of oral cancer is numbness of the tongue; losing a sense of taste is not an early sign of oral cancer. Urinary output, while important, is not a part of a focused assessment for this health problem. The client may have pain, and for a more general assessment, the nurse can inquire about use of pain medications.

🔑 CN: Reduction of risk potential; CL: Synthesize

8. 2. The priority of care in the immediate post-operative phase is to maintain a patent airway. The nurse should observe the client carefully for signs of respiratory distress. If the client becomes nauseated, antiemetics should be administered to decrease the chance of vomiting with obstruction of the airway and aspiration of vomitus. Providing frequent oral hygiene and an alternative means of communication are important aspects of nursing care, but maintaining a patent airway is most important.

🔑 CN: Physiological adaptation;
CL: Synthesize

9. 3. The nurse's first action is to clear the client's airway as necessary. Inserting an NG tube or administering an antiemetic may prevent future vomiting episodes, but these procedures are not helpful when the client is actually vomiting. Cutting the wires is done only as a last resort or in case of respiratory or cardiac arrest.

🔑 CN: Physiological adaptation;
CL: Synthesize

The Client with Peptic Ulcer Disease

10. 4. The client is experiencing a perforation of the ulcer, and the nurse should notify the HCP immediately. The body reacts to perforation of an ulcer by immobilizing the area as much as possible. This results in board-like abdominal rigidity, usually with extreme pain. Perforation is a medical emergency requiring immediate surgical intervention because peritonitis develops quickly after perforation. Administering pain medication is not the first action, although the nurse later should institute measures to relieve pain. Elevating the head of the bed will not minimize the perforation. A nasogastric tube may be used following surgery.

🔑 CN: Physiological adaptation;
CL: Synthesize

11. 3,4,5. Vomiting and weight loss are common with gastric ulcers. The client may also have blood in the stools (melena) from gastric bleeding. Clients with a gastric ulcer are most likely to have a burning epigastric pain that occurs about 1 hour after eating. Eating frequently aggravates the pain. Clients with duodenal ulcers are more likely to have pain that occurs during the night and is frequently relieved by eating.

🔑 CN: Physiological adaptation;
CL: Analyze

12. 2,4,5. Following a gastroscopy, the nurse should monitor the client for complications, which include perforation and the potential for aspiration. An elevated temperature, epigastric pain, or the vomiting of blood (hematemesis) are all indications of a possible perforation and should be reported promptly. A sore throat is a common occurrence following a gastroscopy. Clients are usually sedated to decrease anxiety, and the nurse would anticipate that the client will be drowsy following the procedure.

🔑 CN: Reduction of risk potential;
CL: Analyze

13. 4. Black, tarry stools are an important warning sign of bleeding in peptic ulcer disease. Digested blood in the stool causes it to be black; the odor of the stool is very offensive. The nurse should instruct the client to report the incidence of black stools promptly to the HCP. Increasing fluids or avoiding iron-rich foods will not change the stool color or consistency if the stools contain digested blood. Until other information is available, it is not necessary to initiate contact precautions.

🔑 CN: Reduction of risk potential;
CL: Synthesize

14. 4. Histamine-2 (H2) receptor antagonists, such as ranitidine, reduce gastric acid secretion. Antisecretories, or proton pump inhibitors, such as omeprazole, help ulcers heal quickly in 4 to 8 weeks. Cytoprotective drugs, such as sucralfate, protect the ulcer surface against acid, bile, and pepsin. Antacids reduce acid concentration and help reduce symptoms.

🔑 CN: Pharmacological and parenteral therapies; CL: Evaluate

15. 1,2,3,4. The nurse should encourage the client to reduce stimulation that may enhance gastric secretion. The nurse can also advise the client to utilize health practices that will prevent recurrences of ulcer pain, such as avoiding fatigue and elimination of smoking. Eating small, frequent meals helps to prevent gastric distention if not actively bleeding and decreases distention and release of gastrin. Medications should be administered promptly to maintain optimum levels. After awakening during the night, the client should eat a small snack and return to bed, keeping the head of the bed elevated for an hour after eating. It is not necessary to stay away from crowded areas.

🔑 CN: Physiological adaptation;
CL: Synthesize

16. 2,3. The symptoms of nausea and dizziness in a client with peptic ulcer disease may be indicative of hemorrhage and should not be ignored. The appropriate nursing actions at this time are for the nurse to monitor the client's vital signs and notify the HCP of the client's symptoms. To administer an antacid hourly or to wait 1 hour to reassess the client would be inappropriate; prompt intervention is essential in a client who is potentially experiencing a gastrointestinal hemorrhage. The nurse would notify the HCP of assessment findings and then initiate oxygen therapy if prescribed by the HCP.

CN: Physiological adaptation; CL: Synthesize

17. 3. Diet therapy for ulcer disease is a controversial issue. There is no scientific evidence that diet therapy promotes healing. Most clients are instructed to follow a diet that they can tolerate. There is no need for the client to ingest only a bland or high-protein diet. Milk may be included in the diet, but it is not recommended in excessive amounts.

CN: Basic care and comfort; CL: Apply

18. 4. The use of the triple-therapy approach to the *H. pylori* infection has proved effective; therefore, the nurse advises the client to take the drugs as prescribed for the duration of the prescription. The nurse instructs the client to avoid alternating the use of the drugs and to take all medication at the same time, three times a day unless otherwise noted by the **healthcare provider (HCP)** 📖. Drugs have very few side effects; however, the nurse instructs the client to continue taking medications and contact the HCP if adverse effects occur.

CN: Pharmacological and parenteral therapies; CL: Synthesize

19. 3. The sharp, sudden midepigastric pain indicates the client may have a perforated ulcer. The nurse notifies the surgeon and may then obtain prescriptions for pain medication and IV fluids. It is not necessary to first obtain an ECG because the pain from ulcer perforation is different from that of chest pain that may indicate coronary artery syndrome (crushing pain radiating to the jaw).

CN: Physiological adaptation; CL: Synthesize

20. 3. Ranitidine blocks secretion of hydrochloric acid. Clients who take only one daily dose of ranitidine are usually advised to take it at bedtime to inhibit nocturnal secretion of acid. Clients who take the drug twice a day are advised to take it in the morning and at bedtime. It is not necessary to take the drug before meals. The client should take the drug regularly, not just when pain occurs.

CN: Pharmacological and parenteral therapies; CL: Evaluate

21. 3. It is most likely that the client is experiencing an adverse effect of the antacid. Antacids with aluminum salt products, such as aluminum hydroxide, form insoluble salts in the body. These precipitate and accumulate in the intestines, causing constipation. Increasing dietary fiber intake or daily exercise may be a beneficial lifestyle change for the client but is not likely to relieve the constipation caused by the aluminum hydroxide. Constipation, in isolation from other symptoms, is not a sign of a bowel obstruction.

CN: Pharmacological and parenteral therapies; CL: Analyze

22. 4. Antacids are most effective if taken 1 to 3 hours after meals and at bedtime. When an antacid is taken on an empty stomach, the duration of the drug's action is greatly decreased. Taking antacids 1 to 3 hours after a meal lengthens the duration of action, thus increasing the therapeutic action of the drug. Antacids should be administered about 2 hours after other medications to decrease the chance of drug interactions. It is not necessary to decrease fluid intake when taking antacids. If antacids are taken more frequently than recommended, the likelihood of developing adverse effects increases. Therefore, the client should not take antacids as often as desired to control pain.

CN: Pharmacological and parenteral therapies; CL: Evaluate

23. 2. Alcohol is a gastric irritant that should be eliminated from the intake of the client with peptic ulcer disease. Analgesics are not used to control ulcer pain; many analgesics are gastric irritants. The client's hemoglobin and hematocrit typically do not need to be monitored every 3 months, unless gastrointestinal bleeding is suspected. The client can maintain an active lifestyle and does not need to eliminate contact sports as long as they are not stress inducing.

CN: Reduction of risk potential; CL: Evaluate

The Client with Cancer of the Stomach

24. 2,3,5,6. The client who is experiencing upper GI bleeding is at risk for developing hypovolemic shock from blood loss. Therefore, the signs and symptoms the nurse should expect to find are those related to hypovolemia, including decreased urine output, tachycardia, rapid respirations, and thirst. The client's skin would be cool and clammy, not dry, and flushed. The client would also be likely to develop hypotension, which would lead to a narrowing pulse pressure, not a widening pulse pressure.

CN: Physiological adaptation; CL: Analyze

25. 3. The client can begin eating with a liquid diet when bowel sounds return, usually in 2 to 3 days. The client may be hungry but cannot have oral fluids or foods until intestinal motility has been established. The client may continue to have postoperative pain for several days; because receiving a liquid diet does not depend on the client being pain free, the nurse can continue to offer pain medication. The client does not have to experience a bowel movement to receive fluids and food.

☞ CN: Physiological adaptation; CL: Synthesize

26. 4. NG drainage is expected to be bright red during the first 12 hours after surgery and then darken within 24 hours. The nurse notes the color of the drainage on the **medical record** and then monitors the change of color of the drainage throughout the immediate postoperative period. To prevent stress on the suture line, NG suction is applied and patency of the tube maintained. Removal of the NG tube may traumatize the surgical site. The NG tube is irrigated only if the **healthcare provider (HCP)** prescribes irrigation because there is danger of injury to the suture line; saline at room temperature is usually prescribed.

☞ CN: Physiological adaptation; CL: Synthesize

27. 2. A Billroth II procedure bypasses the duodenum and connects the gastric stump directly to the jejunum. The pyloric sphincter is removed, along with some of the stomach fundus.

☞ CN: Physiological adaptation; CL: Apply

28. 3. The information presented indicates the client is grieving about the changes that will occur as a result of the diagnosis of gastric cancer. The information does not indicate the client is having difficulty coping or experiencing insomnia. The client is not demonstrating signs of anxiety.

☞ CN: Psychosocial adaptation; CL: Analyze

29. 1. About 12 to 24 hours after a subtotal gastrectomy, gastric drainage is normally brown, which indicates digested blood. Bile green or cloudy white drainage is not expected during the first 12 to 24 hours after a subtotal gastrectomy. Drainage during the first 6 to 12 hours contains some bright red blood, but large amounts of blood or excessive bloody drainage should be reported to the **healthcare provider (HCP)** promptly.

☞ CN: Reduction of risk potential; CL: Apply

30. 3. Nausea, vomiting, or abdominal distention indicates that gas and secretions are accumulating within the gastric pouch due to impaired peristalsis or edema at the operative site and may indicate that the drainage system is not working properly. Saline is used to irrigate NG tubes. Hypotonic solutions such as water increase electrolyte loss. In addition, a **healthcare provider's (HCP)** prescription is needed to irrigate the NG tube because this procedure could disrupt the suture line. After gastric surgery, only the surgeon repositions the NG tube because of the danger of rupturing or dislodging the suture line. The amount of suction varies with the type of tube used and is prescribed by the HCP. High suction may create too much tension on the gastric suture line.

☞ CN: Reduction of risk potential; CL: Synthesize

31. 25 gtt/min. To administer IV fluids at 100 mL/h using tubing that has a drip factor of 15 gtt/mL, the nurse should use the following formula: 100 mL/60 minutes × 15 gtts/1 mL = 25 gtt/min.

☞ CN: Pharmacological and parenteral therapies; CL: Apply

32. 3. A client who has had abdominal surgery is best placed in a low Fowler's position postoperatively. This positioning relaxes abdominal muscles and provides for maximum respiratory and cardiovascular function. The prone, supine, or Sims position would not be tolerated by a client who has had abdominal surgery, nor do those positions support respiratory or cardiovascular functioning.

☞ CN: Physiological adaptation; CL: Synthesize

33. 4. Carbohydrates are restricted, but protein, including meat and dairy products, is recommended because it is digested more slowly. Lying down for 30 minutes after a meal is encouraged to slow movement of the food bolus. Fluids are restricted to reduce the bulk of food. There is no need to avoid caffeine.

☞ CN: Basic care and comfort; CL: Synthesize

34. 4. The symptoms related to dumping syndrome that occur after a gastrectomy usually disappear by 6 to 12 months after surgery. Most clients can begin to resume normal meal patterns after signs of the dumping syndrome have stopped. Acknowledging that eating six meals a day is time-consuming does not address the client's question and makes an assumption about the client's concerns. It is not necessarily true that a six-meal-a-day dietary pattern will be required for the rest of the client's life. Clients will not be able to eat three meals a day before hospital discharge.

☞ CN: Physiological adaptation; CL: Synthesize

35. 1. Clients who have had gastric surgery are prone to postoperative complications, such as dumping syndrome and postprandial hypoglycemia, which can affect nutritional intake. Vitamin absorption can also be an issue, depending on the extent of the gastric surgery. Radiation therapy to the upper gastrointestinal area also can affect nutritional intake by causing anorexia, nausea, and esophagitis. The client would not be expected to develop alopecia. Exercise and activity levels as well as access to community resources are important teaching areas, but nutritional intake is a priority need.

CN: Reduction of risk potential;
CL: Synthesize

36. 4. An appropriate expected outcome is for the client to achieve optimal nutritional status through the use of oral feedings or total parenteral nutrition (TPN). TPN may be used to supplement oral intake, or it may be used alone if the client cannot tolerate oral feedings. The client would not be expected to regain lost weight within 1 month after surgery or to tolerate a normal dietary intake of three meals a day. Nausea and vomiting would not be considered an expected outcome of gastric surgery, and regular use of antiemetics would not be anticipated.

CN: Physiological adaptation;
CL: Evaluate

The Client with Gastroesophageal Reflux Disease

37. 2. The nurse should instruct the client to not lie down for about 2 hours after eating to prevent reflux. Caffeinated beverages decrease pressure in the lower esophageal sphincter, and milk increases gastric acid secretion, so these beverages should be avoided. The client is encouraged to follow a high-protein, low-fat diet and avoid foods that are irritating.

CN: Reduction of risk potential;
CL: Synthesize

38. 1. The client should take a laxative after an upper gastrointestinal series to stimulate a bowel movement. This examination involves the administration of barium, which must be promptly eliminated from the body because it may harden and cause an obstruction. A clear liquid diet would have no effect on stimulating removal of the barium. The client should not have nausea, and an antiemetic would not be necessary; additionally, the antiemetic will decrease peristalsis and increase the likelihood of eliminating the barium. An enema would be ineffective because the barium is too high in the gastrointestinal tract.

CN: Reduction of risk potential;
CL: Synthesize

39. 3. With GERD, eating substances that decrease lower esophageal sphincter pressure causes heartburn. A decrease in the lower esophageal sphincter pressure allows gastric contents to reflux into the lower end of the esophagus. Foods that can cause a decrease in esophageal sphincter pressure include fatty foods, chocolate, caffeinated beverages, peppermint, and alcohol. A diet high in protein and low in fat is recommended for clients with GERD. Lean beef, popcorn, and raw vegetables would be acceptable.

CN: Physiological adaptation;
CL: Synthesize

40. 4. Clients with GERD can develop pulmonary symptoms, such as coughing, wheezing, and dyspnea, that are caused by the aspiration of gastric contents. GERD does not predispose the client to the development of laryngeal cancer. Irritation of the esophagus and esophageal scar tissue formation can develop as a result of GERD. However, GERD is more likely to cause painful and difficult swallowing.

CN: Physiological adaptation; **CL:** Analyze

41. 2. Bethanechol, a cholinergic drug, may be used in GERD to increase lower esophageal sphincter pressure and facilitate gastric emptying. Cholinergic adverse effects may include urinary urgency, diarrhea, abdominal cramping, hypotension, and increased salivation. To avoid these adverse effects, the client should be closely monitored to establish the minimum effective dose.

CN: Pharmacological and parenteral therapies; **CL:** Analyze

42. 1,2,4. No specific diet is necessary, but foods that cause reflux are avoided, including fatty foods (which decrease the rate of gastric emptying) and foods that decrease lower esophageal sphincter (LES) pressure such as chocolate, peppermint, coffee, and tea. The client should also avoid alcohol. The client should not lie down for 3 to 4 hours after eating. Antisecretory agents decrease the secretion of hydrochloric acid (HCl) by the stomach; some are available in both OTC and prescription formulations, but the OTC preparations have lower drug dosages compared with prescription drugs. Cimetidine, ranitidine, famotidine, and nizatidine are available in both formulations.

CN: Physiological adaptation;
CL: Synthesize

43. **1.** Esophageal reflux worsens when the stomach is overdistended with food. Therefore, an important measure is to eat small, frequent meals. Fluid intake should be decreased during meals to reduce abdominal distention. Avoiding air swallowing does not prevent esophageal reflux. Food intake in the evening should be strictly limited to reduce the incidence of nighttime reflux, so bedtime snacks are not recommended.

CN: Basic care and comfort; CL: Synthesize

44. **1.** Heartburn, the most common symptom of a sliding hiatal hernia, results from reflux of gastric secretions into the esophagus. Regurgitation of gastric contents and dysphagia are other common symptoms. Jaundice, which results from a high concentration of bilirubin in the blood, is not associated with hiatal hernia. Anorexia is not a typical symptom of hiatal hernia. Stomatitis is inflammation of the mouth.

CN: Physiological adaptation; CL: Analyze

45. **2.** Any factor that increases intra-abdominal pressure, such as obesity, can contribute to the development of hiatal hernia. Other factors include abdominal straining, frequent heavy lifting, and pregnancy. Hiatal hernia is also associated with older age and occurs in women more frequently than in men. Having a sedentary desk job, using laxatives frequently, or being 40 years old is not likely to be a contributing factor in development of a hiatal hernia.

CN: Reduction of risk potential; CL: Analyze

46. **3.** Self-responsibility is the key to individual health maintenance. Using examples of situations in which the client has demonstrated self-responsibility can be reinforcing and supporting. The client has ultimate responsibility for personal health habits. Meeting other people who are managing their care and involving family members can be helpful, but individual motivation is more important. Reassurance can be helpful but is less important than individualization of care.

CN: Basic care and comfort; CL: Synthesize

47. **3.** The magnesium salts in magnesium hydroxide are related to those found in laxatives and may cause diarrhea. Aluminum salt products can cause constipation. Many clients find that a combination product is required to maintain normal bowel elimination. The use of magnesium hydroxide does not cause anorexia or weight gain.

CN: Pharmacological and parenteral therapies; CL: Analyze

48. **2.** Smoking and alcohol use both reduce esophageal sphincter tone and can result in reflux. They therefore should be avoided by clients with hiatal hernia. Daily aerobic exercise, balancing activity and rest, and avoiding high-stress situations may increase the client's general health and well-being, but they are not directly associated with hiatal hernia.

CN: Health promotion and maintenance; CL: Synthesize

49. **2.** Bending, especially after eating, can cause gastroesophageal reflux. Lifting heavy objects increases intra-abdominal pressure. Assessing the client's lifting techniques enables the nurse to evaluate the client's knowledge of factors contributing to hiatal hernia and how to prevent complications. Number and length of breaks, temperature in the work area, and cleaning solvents used are not directly related to treatment of hiatal hernia.

CN: Basic care and comfort; CL: Create

50. **1.** A client with a hiatal hernia should avoid the recumbent position immediately after meals to minimize gastric reflux. Bedtime snacks, as well as high-fat foods and carbonated beverages, should be avoided. Excessive vigorous exercise also should be avoided, especially after meals, but there is no reason why the client must give up swimming. Wearing tight, constrictive clothing such as a girdle can increase intra-abdominal pressure and thus lead to reflux of gastric juices.

CN: Basic care and comfort; CL: Evaluate

51. **4.** Metoclopramide hydrochloride can cause sedation. Alcohol and other central nervous system depressants add to this sedation. A client who is taking this drug should be cautioned to avoid driving or performing other hazardous activities for a few hours after taking the drug. Clients may take antacids, antihypertensives, and anticoagulants while on metoclopramide.

CN: Pharmacological and parenteral therapies; CL: Synthesize

52. **3.** Cimetidine is a histamine receptor antagonist that decreases the quantity of gastric secretions. It may be used in hiatal hernia therapy to prevent or treat the esophagitis and heartburn associated with reflux. Cimetidine is not used to prevent reflux, dysphagia, or ulcer development.

CN: Pharmacological and parenteral therapies; CL: Apply

53. **2.** Most clients can be treated successfully with a combination of diet restrictions, medications, weight control, and lifestyle modifications. Surgery to correct a hiatal hernia, which commonly produces complications, is performed only when medical therapy fails to control the symptoms.

🔑 CN: Reduction of risk potential;
CL: Synthesize

Managing Care, Quality, and Safety of Clients with Upper Gastrointestinal Tract Health Problems

54. 1. Immediately after surgery, the client should be placed on the side with the head slightly elevated. This position helps facilitate removal of secretions and decreases the likelihood of aspiration should vomiting occur. An **RN** 📖 does not need to be present to reposition the client, unless the client's condition warrants the presence of the nurse. Although it is important to elevate the head, there is no need to keep the client's head elevated on two pillows unless that position is comfortable for the client.

🔑 CN: Reduction of risk potential;
CL: Synthesize

55. 3,4,2,1. The client with peptic ulcer disease who is experiencing a sudden onset of acute stomach pain should be assessed first by the nurse. The sudden onset of stomach pain could be indicative of a perforated ulcer, which would require immediate medical attention. It is also important for the nurse to thoroughly assess the nature of the client's pain. The client with the fractured jaw is experiencing pain and should be assessed next. The nurse should then assess the client who is NPO for tests to ensure NPO status and comfort. Last, the nurse can assess the client before surgery.

🔑 CN: Management of care; CL: Synthesize

56. 1. A sudden spike in temperature following an endoscopic procedure may indicate perforation of the GI tract. The nurse should promptly conduct a further assessment of the client, looking for further indicators of perforation, such as a sudden onset of acute upper abdominal pain; a rigid, board-like abdomen; and developing signs of shock. Telling the assistant to change thermometers is not an appropriate action and only further delays the appropriate action of assessing the client. The nurse would not administer acetaminophen without further assessment of the client or without a **healthcare provider's (HCP's)** 📖 prescription; a suspected perforation would require that the client be placed on nothing-by-mouth status. Asking the assistant to bathe the client before any assessment by the nurse is inappropriate.

🔑 CN: Management of care; CL: Synthesize

57. 3. Parotitis is inflammation of the parotid gland. Although any of the clients listed could develop parotitis, given the data provided, the one most likely to develop parotitis is the elderly client who is dehydrated with poor oral hygiene. Any client who experiences poor oral hygiene is at risk for developing parotitis. To help prevent parotitis, it is essential for the nurse to ensure the client receives oral hygiene at regular intervals and has an adequate fluid intake.

🔑 CN: Reduction of risk potential;
CL: Analyze

58. 2. A soft toothbrush should be used to brush the client's teeth after every meal and more often as needed. Mechanical cleaning is necessary to maintain oral health, stimulate gingiva, and remove plaque. Assessing the oral cavity and recording observations are the responsibilities of the nurse, not of the **UAP** 📖. Swabbing with a safe foam applicator does not provide enough friction to clean the mouth. Mouthwash can be a drying irritant and is not recommended for frequent use.

🔑 CN: Basic care and comfort;
CL: Synthesize

59. 1. The Cochrane Library provides systematic reviews of healthcare interventions and will provide the best resource for evidence for nursing care. The CINAHL offers key word searches to published articles in nursing and allied health literature, but not reviews. A nursing textbook has information about nursing care, which may include evidence-based practices, but textbooks may not have the most up-to-date information. While the policy and procedure manual may be based on evidence-based practices, the most current practices will be found in evidence-based reviews of literature.

🔑 CN: Management of care; CL: Apply

60. 3. Using a checklist assures that all key information is reported; the checklist can then serve as a record to which nurses can refer later. Giving a verbal report leaves room for error in memory; using an audiotape or an electronic health record requires nurses to spend unnecessary time retrieving information.

🔑 CN: Safety and infection control;
CL: Apply

61. 1,4. Though still responsible for follow-up to make sure oral care is completed and accurate intake and output is ongoing, these are appropriate tasks to delegate to **UAP** 📖. Evaluating level of consciousness (orientation), pain, and the effect of medications given by the nurse requires nursing judgment and should not be delegated to UAP. While UAP often assist clients with bathing, dressing changes are not delegated to UAP as the wound should be assessed by a nurse while changing the dressing.

🔑 CN: Management of care; CL: Synthesize

The Client with Lower Gastrointestinal Tract Health Problems

- The Client with Cancer of the Colon
- The Client with Hemorrhoids
- The Client with Inflammatory Bowel Disease
- The Client with an Intestinal Obstruction
- The Client with an Ileostomy
- The Client Receiving Total Parenteral Nutrition
- The Client with Diverticular Disease
- The Client with Appendicitis
- The Client with an Inguinal Hernia
- Managing Care, Quality, and Safety of Clients with Lower Gastrointestinal Tract Health Problems
- Answers, Rationales, and Test-Taking Strategies

The Client with Cancer of the Colon

1. Which guideline reflects the current American and Canadian Cancer Societies' recommendations for screening for colon cancer in individuals who are **not** at high risk?
- ☐ **1.** Annual digital rectal examination should begin at age 40.
- ☐ **2.** Annual fecal testing for occult blood should begin at age 50.
- ☐ **3.** Individuals should obtain a baseline barium enema at age 40.
- ☐ **4.** Individuals should obtain a baseline colonoscopy at age 45.

2. A client refuses to look at or care for her colostomy. Which statement by the nurse would be **most** appropriate?
- ☐ **1.** "It has been 4 days since your surgery, and you will soon be discharged. You have to learn to care for your colostomy before you leave the hospital."
- ☐ **2.** "I think we will need to teach your husband to care for your colostomy if you are not going to be able to do it."
- ☐ **3.** "I understand how you are feeling. It is important for you to feel attractive, and you think having a colostomy changes your attractiveness."
- ☐ **4.** "I can see that you are upset. Would you like to share your concerns with me?"

3. The nurse should teach clients about which potential risk factor for the development of colon cancer?
- ☐ **1.** chronic constipation
- ☐ **2.** long-term use of laxatives
- ☐ **3.** history of smoking
- ☐ **4.** history of inflammatory bowel disease

4. A client had a colon resection yesterday. The client's hemoglobin was 14.1 g/dL yesterday and today it is 7.2 g/dL. The client's oxygen saturation is 87%. After reviewing the chart (see chart) and notifying the healthcare provider (HCP), the nurse should **first**:

Prescriptions
1000 mL normal saline every 8 hours at 125 gtts/h
Vital signs every 4 hours
Morphine sulfate 10 mg IV every 4 hours as needed for pain
Nothing by mouth
Oxygen 2–4 L/min per mask

- ☐ **1.** Take the vital signs every hour.
- ☐ **2.** Increase the saline infusion to 150 gtts/h.
- ☐ **3.** Administer oxygen at 2 L/min.
- ☐ **4.** Determine when last pain medication was administered.

5. A client with colon cancer is having a barium enema. The nurse should instruct the client to take which type of medication after the procedure is completed?
- ☐ 1. laxative
- ☐ 2. anticholinergic
- ☐ 3. antacid
- ☐ 4. demulcent

6. A client has a nasogastric tube inserted at the time of abdominal-perineal resection with permanent colostomy for colon cancer. This tube will most likely be removed when the client demonstrates:
- ☐ 1. absence of nausea and vomiting.
- ☐ 2. passage of mucus from the rectum.
- ☐ 3. passage of flatus and feces from the colostomy.
- ☐ 4. absence of stomach drainage for 24 hours.

7. The client with colon cancer has an abdominal-perineal resection with a colostomy. To promote hygiene following surgery, what should the nurse do?
- ☐ 1. Maintain the client in a semi-Fowler's position.
- ☐ 2. Assist the client with warm sitz baths.
- ☐ 3. Administer 30 mL of milk of magnesia to stimulate peristalsis.
- ☐ 4. Remove the ostomy pouch as needed so the stoma can be assessed.

8. The nurse assesses the client's stoma during the initial postoperative period. What observation should the nurse report to the healthcare provider (HCP) **immediately**?
- ☐ 1. The stoma is slightly edematous.
- ☐ 2. The stoma is dark red to purple.
- ☐ 3. The stoma oozes a small amount of blood.
- ☐ 4. The stoma does not expel stool.

9. While changing the client's colostomy bag and dressing, the nurse determines that the client is ready to participate in self-care when the client:
- ☐ 1. asks if the healthcare provider (HCP) will change the dressing soon.
- ☐ 2. asks about the supplies used during the dressing change.
- ☐ 3. talks about the news on the television.
- ☐ 4. is upset about the way the night nurse changed the dressing.

10. Which skin preparation would be **best** to apply around the client's colostomy?
- ☐ 1. adhesive skin barrier
- ☐ 2. petroleum jelly
- ☐ 3. cornstarch
- ☐ 4. antiseptic cream

11. When planning diet teaching for the client with a colostomy, the nurse should develop a plan that emphasizes which dietary instruction?
- ☐ 1. Foods containing roughage should not be eaten.
- ☐ 2. Liquids are best limited to prevent diarrhea.
- ☐ 3. Clients should experiment to find the diet that is best for them.
- ☐ 4. A high-fiber diet will produce a regular passage of stool.

12. What is an expected outcome for a client during the first 2 weeks who is recovering from an abdominal-perineal resection with a colostomy? The client will:
- ☐ 1. maintain a fluid intake of 3,000 mL/day.
- ☐ 2. eliminate fiber from the diet.
- ☐ 3. limit physical activity to light exercise.
- ☐ 4. accept that sexual activity will be diminished.

13. A client with colon cancer has developed ascites. The nurse should conduct a focused assessment for which signs and symptoms? Select all that apply.
- ☐ 1. respiratory distress
- ☐ 2. bleeding
- ☐ 3. fluid and electrolyte imbalance
- ☐ 4. weight gain
- ☐ 5. infection

14. A client has 4,000 mL removed via paracentesis. When the nurse weighs the client after the procedure, how many kilograms is an expected weight loss? Record your answer in whole numbers.
_____ kg.

15. Two days following a colon resection, an elderly client shows new onset of confusion. When contacting the healthcare provider (HCP), the nurse should make which recommendation?
- ☐ 1. "Do you want a CT scan to rule out stroke?"
- ☐ 2. "May we have a prescription for restraining this client?"
- ☐ 3. "Shall I collect and send a urine sample for culture and sensitivity?"
- ☐ 4. "Would you like a stat potassium level done?"

16. The nurse is caring for a 70-year-old male client after a colectomy. The client has received chemotherapy prior to surgery and has hypertension and diabetes mellitus. Which factors put this client at risk for sepsis? Select all that apply.
- ☐ 1. age
- ☐ 2. abdominal surgery
- ☐ 3. gender
- ☐ 4. diabetes mellitus
- ☐ 5. weight

The Client with Hemorrhoids

17. A 36-year-old female client has been diagnosed with hemorrhoids. Which factor in the client's history would **most** likely be a primary cause of her hemorrhoids?
- ☐ **1.** her age
- ☐ **2.** three vaginal delivery pregnancies
- ☐ **3.** her job as a schoolteacher
- ☐ **4.** varicosities in her legs

18. The nurse instructs the client who has had a hemorrhoidectomy not to use sitz baths until at least 12 hours postoperatively to avoid inducing which complication?
- ☐ **1.** hemorrhage
- ☐ **2.** rectal spasm
- ☐ **3.** urine retention
- ☐ **4.** constipation

19. The nurse teaches the client who has had rectal surgery the proper timing for a cleansing sitz baths. The client has understood the teaching when the client states that it is **most** important to take a sitz bath:
- ☐ **1.** first thing each morning.
- ☐ **2.** as needed for discomfort.
- ☐ **3.** after a bowel movement.
- ☐ **4.** at bedtime.

The Client with Inflammatory Bowel Disease

20. A client has been placed on long-term sulfasalazine therapy for treatment of ulcerative colitis. The nurse should encourage the client to eat which foods to help avoid the nutrient deficiencies that may develop as a result of this medication?
- ☐ **1.** citrus fruits
- ☐ **2.** green, leafy vegetables
- ☐ **3.** eggs
- ☐ **4.** milk products

21. A client who has had ulcerative colitis for the past 5 years is admitted to the hospital with an exacerbation of the disease. Which factor is of **greatest** significance in causing an exacerbation of ulcerative colitis?
- ☐ **1.** a demanding and stressful job
- ☐ **2.** changing to a modified vegetarian diet
- ☐ **3.** beginning a weight-training program
- ☐ **4.** walking 2 miles (3.2 km) every day

22. A client who is experiencing an exacerbation of ulcerative colitis is receiving IV fluids that are to be infused at 125 mL/h. The IV tubing delivers 15 gtt/mL. How quickly should the nurse infuse the fluids in drops per minute to infuse the fluids at the prescribed rate? Record your answer using a whole number.

_____ gtt/min.

23. Which goal for the client's care should take **priority** during the first days of hospitalization for an exacerbation of ulcerative colitis?
- ☐ **1.** promoting self-care and independence
- ☐ **2.** managing diarrhea
- ☐ **3.** maintaining adequate nutrition
- ☐ **4.** promoting rest and comfort

24. The client with ulcerative colitis is to be on bed rest with bathroom privileges. When evaluating the effectiveness of this level of activity, the nurse should determine if the client has:
- ☐ **1.** conserved energy.
- ☐ **2.** reduced intestinal peristalsis.
- ☐ **3.** obtained needed rest.
- ☐ **4.** minimized stress.

25. A client has had an exacerbation of ulcerative colitis with cramping and diarrhea persisting longer than 1 week. The nurse should assess the client for which complication?
- ☐ **1.** heart failure
- ☐ **2.** deep vein thrombosis
- ☐ **3.** hypokalemia
- ☐ **4.** hypocalcemia

26. A client who has ulcerative colitis says to the nurse, "I cannot take this anymore; I am constantly in pain, and I cannot leave my room because I need to stay by the toilet. I do not know how to deal with this." Based on these comments, the nurse should determine the client is experiencing:
- ☐ **1.** extreme fatigue.
- ☐ **2.** disturbed thought.
- ☐ **3.** a sense of isolation.
- ☐ **4.** difficulty coping.

27. A client newly diagnosed with ulcerative colitis who has been placed on steroids asks the nurse why steroids are prescribed. The nurse should tell the client:
- ☐ **1.** "Ulcerative colitis can be cured by the use of steroids."
- ☐ **2.** "Steroids are used in severe flare-ups because they can decrease the incidence of bleeding."
- ☐ **3.** "Long-term use of steroids will prolong periods of remission."
- ☐ **4.** "The side effects of steroids outweigh their benefits to clients with ulcerative colitis."

28. A client who has ulcerative colitis has persistent diarrhea and has lost 12 lb (5.5 kg) since the exacerbation of the disease. Which approach will be **most** effective in helping the client meet nutritional needs?
- ☐ **1.** continuous enteral feedings
- ☐ **2.** following a high-calorie, high-protein diet
- ☐ **3.** total parenteral nutrition (TPN)
- ☐ **4.** eating six small meals a day

29. A client with ulcerative colitis is to take sulfasalazine. Which instructions should the nurse give the client about taking this medication at home? Select all that apply.
☐ 1. Drink enough fluids to maintain a urine output of at least 1,200 to 1,500 mL/day.
☐ 2. Discontinue therapy if symptoms of acute intolerance develop, and notify the healthcare provider (HCP).
☐ 3. Stop taking the medication if the urine turns orange-yellow.
☐ 4. Avoid activities that require alertness.
☐ 5. If dose is missed, skip and continue with the next dose.

30. The nurse has a prescription to administer sulfasalazine 2 g. The medication is available in 500-mg tablets. How many tablets should the nurse administer?

_____ tablets.

31. Which diet would be **most** appropriate for the client with ulcerative colitis?
☐ 1. high-calorie, low-protein
☐ 2. high-protein, low-residue
☐ 3. low-fat, high-fiber.
☐ 4. low-sodium, high-carbohydrate

32. A client who has a history of Crohn's disease is admitted to the hospital with fever, diarrhea, cramping, abdominal pain, and weight loss. The nurse should monitor the client for:
☐ 1. hyperalbuminemia.
☐ 2. thrombocytopenia.
☐ 3. hypokalemia.
☐ 4. hypercalcemia.

33. A client with Crohn's disease has concentrated urine; decreased urinary output; dry skin with decreased turgor; hypotension; and weak, thready pulses. What should the nurse do **first**?
☐ 1. Encourage the client to drink at least 1,000 mL/day.
☐ 2. Provide parenteral rehydration therapy as prescribed.
☐ 3. Turn and reposition every 2 hours.
☐ 4. Monitor vital signs every shift.

34. Which is a **priority** focus of care for a client experiencing an exacerbation of Crohn's disease?
☐ 1. encouraging regular ambulation
☐ 2. promoting bowel rest
☐ 3. maintaining current weight
☐ 4. decreasing episodes of rectal bleeding

The Client with an Intestinal Obstruction

35. A nurse is assessing a client who has been admitted with a diagnosis of an obstruction in the small intestine. The nurse should assess the client for which signs and symptoms? Select all that apply.
☐ 1. projectile vomiting
☐ 2. significant abdominal distention
☐ 3. copious diarrhea
☐ 4. rapid onset of dehydration
☐ 5. increased bowel sounds

36. A client is admitted with a bowel obstruction. The client has nausea, vomiting, and crampy abdominal pain. The healthcare provider (HCP) has written the following prescriptions: for the client to be up ad lib, have narcotics for pain, have a nasogastric tube inserted if needed, and for IV, Ringer's lactate and hyperalimentation fluids. What should the nurse do in order of priority from first to last? All options must be used.

1. Assist with ambulation to promote peristalsis.

2. Insert a nasogastric tube.

3. Administer IV Ringer's lactate.

4. Start an infusion of hyperalimentation fluids.

37. The healthcare provider (HCP) prescribes intestinal decompression with a Cantor tube for a client with an intestinal obstruction. In order to determine effectiveness of intestinal decompression, the nurse should evaluate the client to determine if:
☐ 1. intestinal fluid and gas have been removed.
☐ 2. the client has had a bowel movement.
☐ 3. the client's urinary output is adequate.
☐ 4. the client can sit up without pain.

38. After insertion of a nasoenteric tube, the nurse should place the client in which position?
☐ 1. supine
☐ 2. right side-lying
☐ 3. semi-Fowler's
☐ 4. upright in a bedside chair

39. What should the nurse tell the client who is preparing for insertion of a nasoduodenal tube? Select all that apply.
☐ 1. The nose and throat will be numbed with a viscous anesthetic.
☐ 2. The tube will be placed at the bedside.
☐ 3. X-rays with the use of a contrast dye will be used to verify placement.
☐ 4. The client will be closely monitored for 30 minutes following the procedure.
☐ 5. The tube will be taped to the nose.

40. The client with an intestinal obstruction continues to have acute pain even though the nasoenteric tube is patent and draining. The nurse should **first**:
☐ 1. reassure the client that the nasoenteric tube is functioning.
☐ 2. assess the client for signs of peritonitis.
☐ 3. administer an opioid as prescribed.
☐ 4. reposition the client on the left side.

41. Before abdominal surgery for an intestinal obstruction, the nurse monitors the client's urine output and finds that the total output for the past 2 hours was 35 mL. The nurse then assesses the client's total intake and output over the last 24 hours and notes 2,000 mL of IV fluid for intake, 500 mL of drainage from the nasogastric tube, and 700 mL of urine for a total output of 1,200 mL. These findings indicate:
☐ 1. decreased renal function.
☐ 2. the nasogastric tube is not draining well.
☐ 3. extension of the obstruction.
☐ 4. inadequate fluid replacement.

The Client with an Ileostomy

42. The nurse is teaching the client how to care for an ileostomy. The client asks the nurse how long to wear the pouch before changing it. The nurse should tell the client:
☐ 1. "The pouch is changed only when it leaks."
☐ 2. "You can wear the pouch for about 4 to 7 days."
☐ 3. "You should change the pouch every evening before bedtime."
☐ 4. "It depends on your activity level and your diet."

43. A client is scheduled for an ileostomy. Which would be **most** helpful in preparing the client psychologically for the surgery?
☐ 1. Include family members in preoperative teaching sessions.
☐ 2. Encourage the client to ask questions about managing an ileostomy.
☐ 3. Provide a brief, thorough explanation of all preoperative and postoperative procedures.
☐ 4. Invite a member of the ostomy association to visit the client.

44. Two weeks before a client was scheduled for an ileostomy, and the nurse should instruct the client to:
☐ 1. stop taking drugs that will interfere with clotting (aspirin, ibuprofen).
☐ 2. follow a low-residue diet.
☐ 3. abstain from having sex.
☐ 4. report having a temperature above 99°F (37.2°C).

45. Immediately after having surgery to create an ileostomy, which goal has the **highest priority**?
☐ 1. providing relief from constipation
☐ 2. assisting the client with self-care activities
☐ 3. maintaining fluid and electrolyte balance
☐ 4. minimizing odor formation

46. The client asks the nurse, "Is it really possible to lead a normal life with an ileostomy?" Which action by the nurse would be the **most** effective to address this question?
☐ 1. Have the client talk with a member of the clergy about these concerns.
☐ 2. Tell the client to worry about those concerns after surgery.
☐ 3. Arrange for a person with an ostomy to visit the client preoperatively.
☐ 4. Notify the surgeon of the client's question.

47. Three weeks after the client has had an ileostomy, the nurse is following up with instruction about using a skin barrier around the stoma at all times. The client has been applying the skin barrier correctly when:
☐ 1. there is no odor from the stoma.
☐ 2. the client is adequately hydrated.
☐ 3. there is no skin irritation around the stoma.
☐ 4. the client only changes the ostomy pouch once a day.

48. What observation should the nurse instruct the client with an ileostomy to report **immediately**?
☐ 1. passage of liquid stool from the stoma
☐ 2. occasional presence of undigested food in the effluent
☐ 3. absence of drainage from the ileostomy for 6 or more hours
☐ 4. temperature of 99.8°F (37.7°C)

49. The nurse finds the client who has had an ileostomy crying. The client explains to the nurse, "I am upset because I know I will not be able to have children now that I have an ileostomy." Which response by the nurse is **best**?
☐ 1. "Many women with ileostomies decide to adopt. Perhaps you could consider that option?"
☐ 2. "Having an ileostomy does not necessarily mean that you cannot bear children. Let us talk about your concerns."
☐ 3. "I can understand your reasons for being upset. Having children must be important to you."
☐ 4. "I am sure you will adjust to this situation with time. Try not to be too upset."

50. Which statement about ileostomy care indicates that the client understands the discharge instruction?
- ☐ 1. "I should be able to resume weight lifting in 2 weeks."
- ☐ 2. "I can return to work in 2 weeks."
- ☐ 3. "I need to drink at least 3,000 mL a day of fluid."
- ☐ 4. "I will need to avoid getting my stoma wet while bathing."

51. A client with a well-managed ileostomy has sudden onset of abdominal cramps, vomiting, and watery discharge from the ileostomy. The nurse should:
- ☐ 1. tell the client to take an antiemetic.
- ☐ 2. encourage the client to increase fluid intake to 3 L/day to replace fluid lost through vomiting.
- ☐ 3. instruct the client to take 30 mL of milk of magnesia to stimulate a bowel movement.
- ☐ 4. notify the healthcare provider (HCP).

The Client Receiving Total Parenteral Nutrition

52. The nurse is changing the subclavian dressing of a client who is receiving total parenteral nutrition. When assessing the catheter insertion site, the nurse notes the presence of yellow drainage from around the sutures that are anchoring the catheter. What should the nurse do **first**?
- ☐ 1. Clean the insertion site and redress the area.
- ☐ 2. Document assessment findings in the client's chart.
- ☐ 3. Request a prescription to obtain a culture of the drainage.
- ☐ 4. Check the client's temperature.

53. Total parenteral nutrition (TPN) is prescribed for a client who has recently had a small and large bowel resection and who is currently not taking anything by mouth. The nurse should:
- ☐ 1. administer TPN through a nasogastric or gastrostomy tube.
- ☐ 2. handle TPN using strict aseptic technique.
- ☐ 3. auscultate for the presence of bowel sounds prior to administering TPN.
- ☐ 4. designate a peripheral intravenous (IV) site for TPN administration.

54. Using a sliding scale schedule, the nurse is preparing to administer an evening dose of regular insulin to a client who is receiving total parenteral nutrition (TPN). The nurse should base the dosage on the:
- ☐ 1. glucometer reading of the client's glucose level obtained immediately before administering the insulin.
- ☐ 2. fasting blood glucose level obtained earlier in the day.
- ☐ 3. amount of TPN fluid the client has received since the last dose of insulin.
- ☐ 4. client's dietary intake for the evening meal and snack.

55. A client with inflammatory bowel disease is receiving total parenteral nutrition (TPN). The basic component of the client's TPN solution is **most** likely to be:
- ☐ 1. an isotonic dextrose solution.
- ☐ 2. a hypertonic dextrose solution.
- ☐ 3. a hypotonic dextrose solution.
- ☐ 4. a colloidal dextrose solution.

56. A nurse is assisting with the removal a of central venous access device (CVAD). The nurse should:
- ☐ 1. turn the client to the left side.
- ☐ 2. have the client exhale slowly and evenly.
- ☐ 3. elevate the head of the bed.
- ☐ 4. instruct the client to take a deep breath and hold it.

57. TPN is prescribed for a client with Crohn's disease. The TPN solution is having an intended outcome when:
- ☐ 1. the client's nutritional needs are met.
- ☐ 2. the client does not have metabolic acidosis.
- ☐ 3. the client is hydrated.
- ☐ 4. the client is in a negative nitrogen balance.

58. A client is receiving total parenteral nutrition (TPN) solution. The nurse should assess a client's ability to metabolize the TPN solution adequately by monitoring the client for which sign? Select all that apply.
- ☐ 1. tachycardia
- ☐ 2. hypertension
- ☐ 3. elevated blood urea nitrogen concentration
- ☐ 4. hyperglycemia

59. To prevent complications associated with TPN administered through a central line, the nurse should:
- ☐ 1. use strict aseptic technique for all dressing changes.
- ☐ 2. secure all connections of the system.
- ☐ 3. encourage bed rest.
- ☐ 4. cover the insertion site with a moisture-proof dressing.

60. The nurse administers fat emulsion solution during TPN as prescribed based on the understanding that this type of solution:
☐ 1. provides essential fatty acids.
☐ 2. provides extra carbohydrates.
☐ 3. promotes effective metabolism of glucose.
☐ 4. maintains a normal body weight.

61. Which finding indicates a complication after the first few days of TPN therapy?
☐ 1. glycosuria
☐ 2. a 1- to 2-lb (0.45- to 0.9-kg) weight gain
☐ 3. decreased appetite
☐ 4. elevated temperature

62. Which adverse effects occur when there is too rapid an infusion of TPN solution?
☐ 1. negative nitrogen balance
☐ 2. circulatory overload
☐ 3. hypoglycemia
☐ 4. hypokalemia

The Client with Diverticular Disease

63. Following the acute stage of diverticulosis, which foods should the nurse encourage a client to incorporate into the diet? Select all that apply.
☐ 1. bran cereal
☐ 2. broccoli
☐ 3. tomato juice
☐ 4. navy beans
☐ 5. cheese

64. When a client has an acute attack of diverticulitis, the nurse should **first**:
☐ 1. prepare the client for a colonoscopy.
☐ 2. encourage the client to eat a high-fiber diet.
☐ 3. assess the client for signs of peritonitis.
☐ 4. encourage the client to drink a glass of water every 2 hours.

65. A barium enema is not prescribed as a diagnostic test for a client with diverticulitis because a barium enema:
☐ 1. can perforate an intestinal abscess.
☐ 2. would greatly increase the client's pain.
☐ 3. is of minimal diagnostic value in diverticulitis.
☐ 4. is too lengthy a procedure for the client to tolerate.

66. The nurse should teach the client with diverticulitis to integrate which measure into a daily routine at home?
☐ 1. using enemas to relieve constipation
☐ 2. decreasing fluid intake to increase the formed consistency of the stool
☐ 3. eating a high-fiber diet when symptomatic with diverticulitis
☐ 4. refraining from straining and lifting activities

67. After instructing a client with diverticulosis about appropriate self-care activities, which comment by the client indicates effective teaching? Select all that apply.
☐ 1. "With careful attention to my diet, my diverticulosis can be cured."
☐ 2. "Using a cathartic laxative weekly is okay to control bowel movements."
☐ 3. "I should follow a diet that is high in fiber."
☐ 4. "It is important for me to drink at least 2,000 mL of fluid every day."
☐ 5. "I should exercise regularly."

68. A client with diverticular disease is receiving psyllium hydrophilic mucilloid. The drug has been effective when the client:
☐ 1. passes stool without cramping.
☐ 2. does not have diarrhea.
☐ 3. has firm, well-formed stool.
☐ 4. does not expel gas.

69. A client with diverticulitis has developed peritonitis following diverticular rupture. When assessing the client, what should the nurse do? Select all that apply.
☐ 1. Percuss the abdomen to note tympany.
☐ 2. Percuss the liver to note lack of dullness.
☐ 3. Monitor the vital signs for fever.
☐ 4. Assess presence of excessive thirst.
☐ 5. Auscultate bowel sounds to note frequency.

The Client with Appendicitis

70. A nurse is providing wound care to a client 1 day following an appendectomy. A drain was inserted into the incisional site during surgery. When providing wound care, the nurse should:
☐ 1. remove the dressing and leave the incision open to air.
☐ 2. remove the drain if wound drainage is minimal.
☐ 3. gently irrigate the drain to remove exudate.
☐ 4. clean the area around the drain moving away from the drain.

71. An adult with appendicitis has severe abdominal pain. Which action will be the **most** effective to assist the client to manage pain prior to surgery?
☐ 1. Place the client in semi-Fowler's position with the knees to the chest.
☐ 2. Apply moist heat to the abdomen.
☐ 3. Teach client to massage the painful area.
☐ 4. Provide distraction with music.

72. Postoperative nursing care for a client after an appendectomy should include:
☐ 1. administering sitz baths four times a day.
☐ 2. noting the first bowel movement after surgery.
☐ 3. limiting the client's activity to bathroom privileges.
☐ 4. measuring abdominal girth every 2 hours.

73. A client who had an appendectomy for a perforated appendix returns from surgery with a drain inserted in the incisional site. The purpose of the drain is to:
☐ 1. provide access for wound irrigation.
☐ 2. promote drainage of wound exudates.
☐ 3. minimize development of scar tissue.
☐ 4. decrease postoperative discomfort.

The Client with an Inguinal Hernia

74. A client who has a history of an inguinal hernia is admitted to the hospital with sudden, severe abdominal pain, vomiting, and abdominal distention. The nurse should assess the client further for which complication?
☐ 1. peritonitis
☐ 2. incarcerated hernia
☐ 3. strangulated hernia
☐ 4. intestinal perforation

75. The nurse is providing discharge instructions for a client who had an inguinal herniorrhaphy. The nurse should teach the client to:
☐ 1. cough and deep breathe every 2 hours.
☐ 2. apply warm, moist heat to the groin.
☐ 3. sneeze with mouth closed.
☐ 4. avoid lifting items weighing more than 5 lb.

76. After an inguinal herniorrhaphy, the nurse should assess the male client carefully for which complication?
☐ 1. hypostatic pneumonia
☐ 2. deep vein thrombosis
☐ 3. paralytic ileus
☐ 4. urine retention

Managing Care, Quality, and Safety for Clients with Lower Gastrointestinal Tract Health Problems

77. A client has anemia resulting from bleeding from ulcerative colitis and is to receive two units of packed red blood cells (PRBCs). The client is receiving an infusion of total parenteral nutrition (TPN). In preparing to administer the PRBCs, what should the nurse do to ensure client comfort and safety?
☐ 1. Discontinue the TPN infusion.
☐ 2. Start an IV infusion of normal saline.
☐ 3. Administer PRBCs in the same IV as the TPN.
☐ 4. Wait until the TPN infusion is completed, and use the same IV line to infuse the PRBCs.

78. The nurse is assigning clients for the evening shift. Which clients are appropriate for the nurse to assign to a licensed practical/vocational nurse (LPN/VN) to provide client care? Select all that apply.
☐ 1. a client with Crohn's disease who is receiving total parenteral nutrition (TPN)
☐ 2. a client who had inguinal hernia repair surgery 3 hours ago; vital signs are stable
☐ 3. a client with an intestinal obstruction who needs a Cantor tube inserted
☐ 4. a client with diverticulitis who needs teaching about take home medications
☐ 5. a client who is experiencing an exacerbation of ulcerative colitis

79. When planning care for a client with ulcerative colitis who is experiencing an exacerbation of symptoms, which client care activities can the nurse appropriately delegate to an unlicensed assistive personnel (UAP)? Select all that apply.
☐ 1. assessing the client's bowel sounds
☐ 2. providing skin care following bowel movements
☐ 3. evaluating the client's response to antidiarrheal medications
☐ 4. maintaining intake and output records
☐ 5. obtaining the client's weight

80. The nurse is caring for a client 1 day after having a colectomy. The client is lethargic and difficult to arouse; the temperature is 101.5°F (38.6°C), blood pressure is 92/36 mm Hg (MAP 55), and heart rate is 114 bpm with SpO2 of 88% on oxygen at 2 L/min/nasal cannula (previously 94%). A saline lock has been established and is patent. Which prescription should the nurse implement **first**?
☐ 1. Obtain stat portable chest x-ray.
☐ 2. Administer vancomycin intravenously.
☐ 3. Draw blood cultures.
☐ 4. Insert an indwelling urinary catheter.

81. The nurse is taking care of a client with *Clostridium difficile* (*C. difficile*). To prevent the spread of infection, what should the nurse do? Select all that apply.
☐ 1. Wear a particulate respirator.
☐ 2. Wear sterile gloves when providing care.
☐ 3. Cleanse hands with alcohol-based hand sanitizer.
☐ 4. Wash hands with soap and water.
☐ 5. Wear a protective gown when in the client's room.

82. The nurse discovers that a client's TPN solution was running at an incorrect rate and is now 2 hours behind schedule. Which action is **most** appropriate for the nurse to take to correct the problem?
☐ 1. Readjust the solution to infuse the desired amount.
☐ 2. Continue the infusion at the current rate, but run the next bottle at an increased rate.
☐ 3. Double the infusion rate for 2 hours.
☐ 4. Notify the healthcare provider (HCP).

83. The nurse is to administer ampicillin 500 mg orally to a client with a ruptured appendix. The nurse checks the capsule in the client's medication box, which is located inside of the client's room. The dosage of the medication is not labeled, but the nurse recognizes the color and shape of the capsule. The nurse should **next**:
☐ 1. administer the medication to maintain blood levels of the drug.
☐ 2. ask another registered nurse (RN) to verify that the capsule is ampicillin.
☐ 3. contact the pharmacy to bring a properly labeled medication.
☐ 4. notify the unit manager to report the problem.

84. On the 2nd day following an abdominal-perineal resection, the nurse notes that the wound edges are not approximated and one-half of the incision has torn apart. What should the nurse do **first**?
☐ 1. Flush the wound with sterile water.
☐ 2. Apply an abdominal binder.
☐ 3. Cover the wound with a sterile dressing moistened with normal saline.
☐ 4. Apply strips of tape.

85. A client has received numerous different antibiotics and now is experiencing diarrhea. The healthcare provider (HCP) has prescribed a transmission-based precaution. The nurse should institute:
☐ 1. airborne precautions.
☐ 2. contact precautions.
☐ 3. droplet precautions.
☐ 4. needlestick precautions.

86. The healthcare provider (HCP) has prescribed ciprofloxacin for a client who takes warfarin. What should the nurse instruct the client to do? Select all that apply.
☐ 1. Split the tablets and stir them in food.
☐ 2. Avoid exposure to sunlight.
☐ 3. Eliminate caffeine from the diet.
☐ 4. Report unusual bleeding.
☐ 5. Increase fluid intake to 3,000 mL/day.

Answers, Rationales, and Test-Taking Strategies

The answers and rationales for each question follow below, along with keys (☒⚊) to the client need (CN) and cognitive level (CL) for each question. In addition, you will also see a glossary icon (▢) highlighting specific terminology used on the licensing exam. As you check your answers, use the **Content Mastery and Test-Taking Skill Self-Analysis** *worksheet (tear-out worksheet in back of book) to identify the reason(s) for not answering the questions correctly. For additional information about test-taking skills and strategies for answering questions, refer to pages 12–23 and pages 35–36 in Part 1 of this book.*

The Client with Cancer of the Colon

1. 2. Annual fecal testing for occult blood should begin at age 50. Annual digital rectal examinations are recommended in men beginning at age 50 to screen for prostate cancer. Baseline barium enemas or colonoscopies are recommended at age 50. Baseline barium enemas and colonoscopies are not performed on individuals in their 40s unless they experience signs or symptoms that indicate the need for such diagnostic testing or are considered to be at high risk.

☒⚊ CN: Health promotion and maintenance; CL: Apply

2. 4. It is important for the nurse to recognize that individuals go through a grieving process when adjusting to a colostomy. The nurse should be accepting and provide the client with opportunities to share her concerns and feelings when she is ready. Lecturing the client about the need to learn how to care for the colostomy is not productive nor is attempting to shame her into caring for the colostomy by implying her husband will have to provide the care if she does not. It is not possible for the nurse to understand what the client is feeling.

☒⚊ CN: Psychosocial adaptation; CL: Synthesize

3. 4. A history of inflammatory bowel disease is a risk factor for colon cancer. Other risk factors include age (older than 40 years), history of familial polyposis, colorectal polyps, and high-fat or low-fiber diet.

☒⚊ CN: Reduction of risk potential; CL: Analyze

4. 3. This client has decreased oxygen saturation and also decreased hemoglobin, which puts the client at great risk for cardiac ischemia. The nurse should start the oxygen as prescribed. The nurse can take the vital signs more frequently once the oxygen flow has been started. It is not appropriate to increase the rate of the intravenous infusion, and it would be necessary to request a prescription to do so. After starting the oxygen, the nurse can ask the client about the current pain level.

CN: Physiological Adaptation;
CL: Synthesize

5. 1. After a barium enema, a laxative is ordinarily prescribed. This is done to promote elimination of the barium. Retained barium predisposes the client to constipation and fecal impaction. Anticholinergic drugs decrease gastrointestinal motility. Antacids decrease gastric acid secretion. Demulcents soothe mucous membranes of the gastrointestinal tract and are used to treat diarrhea.

CN: Reduction of risk potential;
CL: Synthesize

6. 3. A sign indicating that a client's colostomy is open and ready to function is passage of feces and flatus. When this occurs, gastric suction is ordinarily discontinued, and the client is allowed to start taking fluids and food orally. Absence of bowel sounds would indicate that the tube should remain in place because peristalsis has not yet returned.

CN: Physiological adaptation;
CL: Analyze

7. 2. Appropriate nursing interventions after an abdominal-perineal resection with a colostomy include assisting the client with warm sitz baths three to four times a day to clean the perineal incision. The client will be more comfortable assuming a side-lying position because of the perineal incision. It would be inappropriate to administer milk of magnesia to stimulate colostomy activity. Stool passage will begin as peristalsis returns. It is not necessary or desirable to change the ostomy pouch daily to assess the stoma. The ostomy pouch should be transparent to allow easy observation of the stoma and drainage.

CN: Physiological adaptation;
CL: Synthesize

8. 2. A dark red to purple stoma indicates inadequate blood supply. Mild edema and slight oozing of blood are normal in the early postoperative period. The colostomy would typically not begin functioning until 2 to 4 days after surgery.

CN: Physiological adaptation;
CL: Analyze

9. 2. A client who displays interest in the procedure and asks about supplies used for dressings may be ready to participate in self-care. Inquiring about when the HCP 🔲 will change the dressing does not indicate the client's readiness to change the dressing. Discussing news events and discussing a dressing change are behaviors that avoid the subject of the colostomy.

CN: Basic care and comfort; CL: Analyze

10. 1. An adhesive skin barrier is effective for protecting the skin around a colostomy to keep the skin healthy and prevent skin irritation from stoma drainage. Petroleum jelly, cornstarch, and antiseptic creams do not protect the skin adequately and may prevent an adequate seal between the skin and the colostomy bag.

CN: Basic care and comfort; CL: Apply

11. 3. It is best to adjust the diet of a client with a colostomy in a manner that suits the client rather than trying special diets. Severe restriction of roughage is not recommended. The client is encouraged to drink 2 to 3 L of fluid per day. A high-fiber diet may produce loose stools.

CN: Basic care and comfort; CL: Create

12. 1. An expected outcome is that the client will maintain a fluid intake of 3,000 mL/day unless contraindicated. There is no need to eliminate fiber from the diet; the client can eat whatever foods are desired, avoiding those that are bothersome. Physical activity does not need to be limited to light exercise. The client can resume normal activities as tolerated, usually within 6 to 8 weeks. The client's sexual activity may be affected, but it does not need to be diminished.

CN: Physiological adaptation;
CL: Evaluate

13. 1,3. Ascites limits the movement of the diaphragm leading to respiratory distress. Fluid shift from the intravascular space precipitates fluid and electrolyte imbalances. Weight gain is not a direct consequence of ascites, but weight loss may result in decreased albumin levels. Decreased albumin in the intravascular space results in decreased oncotic pressure, precipitating movement of fluid out of space. A client with ascites is not at increased risk for infection unless a peritoneal tap is done to remove fluid. The risk of bleeding is a result of alterations in liver enzymes affecting coagulation.

CN: Physiological adaptation;
CL: Analyze

14. 4 kg. A liter of water weighs 1 kg. Therefore, the client should have a weight of 4 kilograms less than preprocedure weight.

☞ CN: Physiological adaptation; CL: Apply

15. 3. Sending a urine sample for culture and sensitivity is most warranted. An older adult often has confusion when experiencing a bladder infection. While stroke is always a concern, particularly in the older adult, the presenting information most supports a bladder infection and perhaps early-onset urosepsis. Restraining the client may be needed at some point in time, but finding the cause of the client's new onset of confusion has greatest priority. Potassium is usually related to cardiac rhythm irritability rather than confusion.

☞ CN: Physiological adaptation; CL: Analysis

16. 1,2,4. Known risk factors for sepsis include age (<1 year and >65 years old), chronic illness, and invasive procedures. Immunosuppression and malnourishment are also risk factors. There is no correlation between gender or age and risk for sepsis. Nurses must be aware of risk factors and monitor clients at risk closely for any signs of sepsis.

☞ CN: Reduction of risk potential; CL: Apply

The Client with Hemorrhoids

17. 2. Hemorrhoids are associated with prolonged sitting or standing, portal hypertension, chronic constipation, and prolonged increased intra-abdominal pressure, as associated with pregnancy and the strain of vaginal childbirth. Her job as a schoolteacher does not require prolonged sitting or standing. Age and leg varicosities are not related to the development of hemorrhoids.

☞ CN: Reduction of risk potential; CL: Analyze

18. 1. Applying heat during the immediate postoperative period may cause hemorrhage at the surgical site. Moist heat may relieve rectal spasms after bowel movements. Urine retention caused by reflex spasm may also be relieved by moist heat. Increasing fiber and fluid in the diet can help prevent constipation.

☞ CN: Physiological adaptation; CL: Apply

19. 3. Adequate cleaning of the anal area is difficult but essential. After rectal surgery, sitz baths assist in this process, so the client should take a sitz bath after a bowel movement. Other times are dictated by client comfort.

☞ CN: Reduction of risk potential; CL: Evaluate

The Client with Inflammatory Bowel Disease

20. 2. In long-term sulfasalazine therapy, the client may develop folic acid deficiency. The client can take folic acid supplements, but the nurse should also encourage the client to increase the intake of folic acid in the client's diet. Green, leafy vegetables are a good source of folic acid. Citrus fruits, eggs, and milk products are not good sources of folic acid.

☞ CN: Pharmacological and parenteral therapies; CL: Apply

21. 1. Stressful and emotional events have been clearly linked to exacerbations of ulcerative colitis, although their role in the etiology of the disease has been disproved. A modified vegetarian diet or an exercise program is an unlikely cause of the exacerbation.

☞ CN: Physiological adaptation; CL: Apply

22. 31 gtt/min. To administer IV fluids at 125 mL/h using tubing that has a drip factor of 15 gtt/mL, the nurse should use the formula:

$$125 \text{ mL}/60 \text{ min} \times 15 \text{ gtt}/1 \text{ mL} = 31 \text{ gtt/min}$$

☞ CN: Pharmacological and parenteral therapies; CL: Apply

23. 2. Diarrhea is the primary symptom in an exacerbation of ulcerative colitis, and decreasing the frequency of stools is the first goal of treatment. The other goals are ongoing and will be best achieved by halting the exacerbation. The client may receive antidiarrheal agents, antispasmodic agents, bulk hydrophilic agents, or anti-inflammatory drugs.

☞ CN: Physiological adaptation; CL: Synthesize

24. 2. Although modified bed rest does help conserve energy and promotes comfort, its primary purpose in this case is to help reduce the hypermotility of the colon. Remaining on bed rest does not by itself reduce stress, and if the client is having stress, the nurse can plan with the client to use strategies that will help the client manage the stress.

☞ CN: Physiological adaptation; CL: Evaluate

25. 3. Excessive diarrhea causes significant depletion of the body's stores of sodium and potassium as well as fluid. The client should be closely monitored for hypokalemia and hyponatremia. Ulcerative colitis does not place the client at risk for heart failure, deep vein thrombosis, or hypocalcemia.

☞ CN: Reduction of risk potential; CL: Analyze

26. **4.** It is not uncommon for clients with ulcerative colitis to become apprehensive and have difficulty coping with the frequency of stools and the presence of abdominal cramping. During these acute exacerbations, clients need emotional support and encouragement to verbalize their feelings about their chronic health concerns and assistance in developing effective coping methods. The client has not expressed feelings of fatigue or isolation or demonstrated disturbed thought processes.

🔑 CN: Psychosocial adaptation;
CL: Analyze

27. **2.** Steroids are effective in management of the acute symptoms of ulcerative colitis. Steroids do not cure ulcerative colitis, which is a chronic disease. Long-term use is not effective in prolonging the remission and is not advocated. Clients should be assessed carefully for side effects related to steroid therapy, but the benefits of short-term steroid therapy usually outweigh the potential adverse effects.

🔑 CN: Pharmacological and parenteral therapies; CL: Apply

28. **3.** Food will be withheld from the client with severe symptoms of ulcerative colitis to rest the bowel. To maintain the client's nutritional status, the client will be started on TPN. Enteral feedings or dividing the diet into six small meals does not allow the bowel to rest. A high-calorie, high-protein diet will worsen the client's symptoms.

🔑 CN: Physiological adaptation; CL: Apply

29. **1,2,4.** Sulfasalazine may cause dizziness, and the nurse should caution the client to avoid driving or other activities that require alertness until response to medication is known. If symptoms of acute intolerance (cramping, acute abdominal pain, bloody diarrhea, fever, headache, rash) occur, the client should discontinue therapy and notify the **HCP** 🖥 immediately. Fluid intake should be sufficient to maintain a urine output of at least 1,200 to 1,500 mL daily to prevent crystalluria and stone formation. The nurse can also inform the client that this medication may cause orange-yellow discoloration of urine and skin, which is not significant and does not require the client to stop taking the medication. The nurse should instruct the client to take missed doses as soon as remembered unless it is almost time for the next dose.

🔑 CN: Pharmacological and parenteral therapies; CL: Synthesize

30. **4 tablets.** To administer 2 g sulfasalazine, the nurse will need to administer four tablets. The following formula is used to calculate the correct dosage:

The first step is to convert grams into milligrams:

$$1 \text{ g}/1,000 \text{ mg} = 2 \text{ g}/X \text{ mg}$$
$$X = 2,000 \text{ mg}$$

Then, $2,000 \text{ mg}/X \text{ tablets} = 500 \text{ mg}/1 \text{ tablet}$
$$X = 4 \text{ tablets}$$

🔑 CN: Pharmacological and parenteral therapies; CL: Apply

31. **2.** Clients with ulcerative colitis should follow a well-balanced high-protein, high-calorie, low-residue diet, avoiding such high-residue foods as whole-wheat grains, nuts, and raw fruits and vegetables. Clients with ulcerative colitis need more protein for tissue healing and should avoid excess roughage. There is no need for clients with ulcerative colitis to follow low-sodium diets.

🔑 CN: Basic care and comfort; CL: Apply

32. **3.** Hypokalemia is the most expected laboratory finding owing to the diarrhea. Hypoalbuminemia can also occur in Crohn's disease; however, the client's potassium level is of greater importance at this time because a low potassium level can cause cardiac arrest. Anemia is an expected development, but thrombocytopenia is not. Calcium levels are not affected.

🔑 CN: Physiological adaptation;
CL: Analyze

33. **2.** Initially, the extracellular fluid (ECF) volume with isotonic IV fluids should be administered until adequate circulating blood volume and renal perfusion are achieved. Vital signs should be monitored as parenteral and oral rehydration are achieved. Oral fluid intake should be >1,000 mL/day. Turning and repositioning the client at regular intervals aid in the prevention of skin breakdown, but it is first necessary to rehydrate this client.

🔑 CN: Physiological adaptation;
CL: Synthesize

34. **2.** A priority goal of care during an acute exacerbation of Crohn's disease is to promote bowel rest. This is accomplished through decreasing activity, encouraging rest, and initially placing client on nothing-by-mouth status while maintaining nutritional needs parenterally. Regular ambulation is important, but the priority is bowel rest. The client will probably lose some weight during the acute phase of the illness. Diarrhea is nonbloody in Crohn's disease, and episodes of rectal bleeding are not expected.

🔑 CN: Physiological adaptation;
CL: Synthesize

The Client with an Intestinal Obstruction

35. **1,4,5.** Signs and symptoms of intestinal obstructions in the small intestine may include projectile vomiting and rapidly developing dehydration and electrolyte imbalances. The client will also have increased bowel sounds, usually high pitched and tinkling. The client would not normally have diarrhea and would have minimal abdominal distention. Pain is intermittent, being relieved by vomiting. Intestinal obstructions in the large intestine usually evolve slowly and produce persistent pain, and vomiting is less common. Clients with a large intestine obstruction may develop obstipation and significant abdominal distention.

🔑 CN: Physiological adaptation;
CL: Analyze

36. **1,3,2,4.** The nurse should first help the client ambulate to try to induce peristalsis; this may be effective and require the least amount of invasive procedures. Next, the nurse should initiate IV fluid therapy to correct fluid and electrolyte imbalances (sodium and potassium) with Ringer's lactate to correct interstitial fluid deficit. Nasogastric (NG) decompression of the GI tract to reduce gastric secretions and nasointestinal tubes may also be used as necessary. Lastly, hyperalimentation can be used to correct protein deficiency from chronic obstruction, paralytic ileus, or infection.

🔑 CN: Physiological adaptation;
CL: Synthesize

37. **1.** Intestinal decompression is accomplished with a Cantor, Harris, or Miller-Abbott tube. These 6- to 10-foot (180- to 300-cm) tubes are passed into the small intestine to the obstruction. They remove accumulated fluid and gas, relieving the pressure. The client will not have an adequate bowel movement until the obstruction is removed. The pressure from the distended intestine should not obstruct urinary output. While the client may be able to more easily sit up, and the pain caused by the intestinal pressure will be less, these are not the primary indicators for successful intestinal decompression.

🔑 CN: Physiological adaptation;
CL: Evaluate

38. **2.** The client is placed in a right side-lying position to facilitate movement of the mercury-weighted tube through the pyloric sphincter. After the tube is in the intestine, the client is turned from side to side or encouraged to ambulate to facilitate tube movement through the intestinal loops. Placing the client in the supine or semi-Fowler's position or having the client sitting out of bed in a chair will not facilitate tube progression.

🔑 CN: Reduction of risk potential; CL: Apply

39. **1,3,4,5.** A nasoduodenal tube is used primarily for feeding. The tube is inserted in endoscopy or radiology. Prior to insertion of the tube, the client's nose and throat will be numbed with a viscous anesthetic such as lidocaine. The tube placement is verified by contrast x-rays, and the client is observed for 30 minutes after the insertion to be sure the client does not have an allergic reaction, puncture to the lung, or bleeding. The tube is taped to the nose.

🔑 CN: Reduction of risk potential;
CL: Apply

40. **2.** The client's pain may be indicative of peritonitis, and the nurse should assess for signs and symptoms, such as a rigid abdomen, elevated temperature, and increasing pain. Reassuring the client is important, but accurate assessment of the client is essential. The full assessment should occur before pain relief measures are employed. Repositioning the client to the left side will not resolve the pain.

🔑 CN: Reduction of risk potential;
CL: Synthesize

41. **4.** Considering that there is usually 1 L of insensible fluid loss, this client's output exceeds his intake (intake, 2,000 mL; output, 2,200 mL), indicating deficient fluid volume. The kidneys are concentrating urine in response to low circulating volume, as evidenced by a urine output of <30 mL/h. This indicates that increased fluid replacement is needed. Decreasing urine output can be a sign of decreased renal function, but the data provided suggest that the client is dehydrated. Pain does not affect urine output. There are no data to suggest that the obstruction has worsened.

🔑 CN: Reduction of risk potential;
CL: Analyze

The Client with an Ileostomy

42. **2.** Unless the pouch leaks, the client can wear the ileostomy pouch for about 4 to 7 days. If leakage occurs, it is important to promptly change the pouch to avoid skin irritation. It is not necessary to change the pouch daily or in the evening. Diet and activity typically do not affect the schedule for changing the pouch.

🔑 CN: Basic care and comfort;
CL: Synthesize

43. **3.** Providing explanations of preoperative and postoperative procedures helps the client prepare and understand what to expect. It also provides an opportunity for the client to share concerns. Including family members in the teaching sessions is beneficial but does not focus on the client's psychological preparation. Encouraging the client to ask questions about managing the ileostomy may be rushing the client psychologically into accepting the change in body image and function. The client may need time to first handle the stress of surgery and then observe the care of the ileostomy by others before it is appropriate to begin discussing self-management. The nurse should gently explore whether the client is ready to ask questions about management throughout the hospitalization. The client should have the opportunity to express concerns and to agree to an ostomy association visitor before an invitation is extended.

CN: Psychosocial adaptation; CL: Synthesize

44. 1. The nurse should instruct the client to stop taking drugs that would interfere with clotting, such as aspirin or ibuprofen. The client should follow a high-fiber diet with increased fluids during the 2-week preoperative period. It is not necessary to abstain from sex. The client does not need to report having a temperature above 99°F (37.2°C) to the **healthcare provider (HCP)** as this is within normal limits; however, if the temperature is higher, this could indicate an infection, and the client should notify the HCP.

CN: Pharmacological and parenteral therapies; CL: Apply

45. 3. A high-priority outcome after ileostomy surgery is the maintenance of fluid and electrolyte balance. The client will experience continuous liquid to semiliquid stools. The client should be engaged in self-care activities, and minimizing odor formation is important; however, these goals do not take priority over maintaining fluid and electrolyte balance.

CN: Physiological adaptation; CL: Synthesize

46. 3. If the client agrees, having a visit by a person who has successfully adjusted to living with an ileostomy would be the most helpful measure. This would let the client actually see that typical activities of daily living can be pursued postoperatively. Someone who has felt some of the same concerns can answer the client's questions. A visit from the clergy may be helpful to some clients but would not provide this client with the information sought. Disregarding the client's concerns is not helpful. Although the **healthcare provider (HCP)** should know about the client's concerns, this in itself will not reassure the client about life after an ileostomy.

CN: Psychosocial adaptation; CL: Synthesize

47. 3. Because of high concentrations of digestive enzymes, ileostomy effluent is irritating to skin and can cause excoriation and ulceration. Some form of protection must be used to keep the effluent from contacting the skin. A skin barrier does not decrease odor formation; odor is controlled by diet. The barrier does not affect the client's hydration status, and the nurse can encourage the client to have an adequate daily intake of fluids. Pouches are usually worn for 4 to 7 days before being changed.

CN: Basic care and comfort; CL: Evaluate

48. 3. Any sudden decrease in drainage or onset of severe abdominal pain should be reported to the **healthcare provider (HCP)** immediately because it could mean that an obstruction has developed. The ileostomy drains liquid stool at frequent intervals throughout the day. Undigested food may be present at times. A temperature of 99.8°F (37.7°C) is not necessarily abnormal or a cause for concern.

CN: Reduction of risk potential; CL: Synthesize

49. 2. The fact that the client has an ileostomy does not necessarily mean that she cannot get pregnant and bear children. It may be recommended, however, that the number of pregnancies be limited. Women of childbearing age should be encouraged to discuss their concerns with their **healthcare provider (HCP)**. Discussing their concerns about sexual functioning and pregnancy will help decrease fears and anxiety. Empathizing or telling the woman that she can adopt does not address her concerns. Her current fears may be based on erroneous understanding. Telling the client that she will adjust to the situation ignores her concerns.

CN: Psychosocial adaptation; CL: Synthesize

50. 3. To maintain an adequate fluid balance, the client needs to drink at least 3,000 mL/day. Heavy lifting should be avoided; the **healthcare provider (HCP)** will indicate when the client can participate in sports again. The client will not resume working as soon as 2 weeks after surgery. Water does not harm the stoma, so the client does not have to worry about getting it wet.

CN: Physiological adaptation; CL: Evaluate

51. 4. Sudden onset of abdominal cramps, vomiting, and watery discharge with no stool from an ileostomy are likely indications of an obstruction. It is imperative that the **healthcare provider (HCP)** examine the client immediately. Although the client is vomiting, the client should not take an antiemetic until the HCP has examined the client. If an obstruction is present, ingesting fluids or taking milk of magnesia will increase the severity of symptoms. Oral intake is avoided when a bowel obstruction is suspected.

CN: Reduction of risk potential; CL: Synthesize

The Client Receiving Total Parenteral Nutrition

52. **3.** The nurse should first obtain a prescription to obtain a culture specimen. The presence of drainage is a potential indication of an infection and the catheter may need to be removed. A culture specimen should be obtained and sent for analysis so that treatment can be promptly initiated. Since removing the catheter will be required in the presence of an infection, the nurse would not clean and redress the area. While the body temperature may increase indicating an infection, a culture needs to be obtained to identify the causative organism. After the culture report is obtained, the nurse should notify the **healthcare provider (HCP)** 📖 and document all assessments and client care activities in the client's record.

🔑 CN: Safety and infection control; CL: Synthesize

53. **2** Total parenteral nutrition (TPN) is a hypertonic, high-calorie, high-protein intravenous (IV) fluid that should be provided for clients who do not have functional gastrointestinal track motility, in order to better meet metabolic needs of the client and to support optimal nutrition and healing. TPN is prescribed once daily, based on the client's current electrolyte and fluid balance, and must be handled with strict aseptic technique (due to the high glucose content, it is a perfect medium for bacterial growth). Also, because of the high tonicity, TPN must be administered through a central venous access, not a peripheral IV line. There is no specific need to auscultate for bowel sounds to determine whether TPN can safely be administered.

🔑 CN: Pharmacological and parenteral therapies; CL: Synthesize

54. **1.** When using a sliding scale insulin schedule, the nurse obtains a glucometer reading of the client's blood glucose level immediately before giving the insulin and bases the dosage on those findings. The fasting blood glucose level obtained earlier in the day is not relevant to an evening sliding scale insulin dosage. The nurse cannot calculate insulin dosage by assessing the amount of TPN intake or dietary intake.

🔑 CN: Pharmacological and parenteral therapies; CL: Synthesize

55. **2.** The TPN solution is usually a hypertonic dextrose solution. The greater the concentration of dextrose in the solution, the greater the tonicity. Hypertonic dextrose solutions are used to meet the body's calorie demands in a volume of fluid that will not overload the cardiovascular system. An isotonic dextrose solution (e.g., 5% dextrose in water) or a hypotonic dextrose solution will not provide enough calories to meet metabolic needs. Colloids are plasma expanders and blood products and are not used in TPN.

🔑 CN: Pharmacological and parenteral therapies; CL: Apply

56. **4.** The client should be asked to perform the Valsalva maneuver (take a deep breath and hold it) during insertion and removal of a CVAD. This increases central venous pressure during the procedure and prevents air embolism. Trendelenburg is the preferred position for CVAD insertion and removal. If not possible, supine position is sufficient for CVAD removal. The client should hold the breath, not exhale.

🔑 CN: Physiological integrity; CL: Apply

57. **1.** The goal of TPN is to meet the client's nutritional needs. TPN is not used to treat metabolic acidosis; ketoacidosis can actually develop as a result of administering TPN. TPN is a hypertonic solution containing carbohydrates, amino acids, electrolytes, trace elements, and vitamins. It is not used to meet the hydration needs of clients. TPN is administered to provide a positive nitrogen balance.

🔑 CN: Pharmacological and parenteral therapies; CL: Evaluate

58. **4.** During TPN administration, the client should be monitored regularly for hyperglycemia. The client may require small amounts of insulin to improve glucose metabolism. The client should also be observed for signs and symptoms of hypoglycemia, which may occur if the body overproduces insulin in response to a high glucose intake or if too much insulin is administered to help improve glucose metabolism. Tachycardia or hypertension is not indicative of the client's ability to metabolize the solution. An elevated blood urea nitrogen concentration is indicative of renal status and fluid balance.

🔑 CN: Pharmacological and parenteral therapies; CL: Analyze

59. **1,2,4.** Complications associated with administration of TPN through a central line include infection and air embolism. To prevent these complications, strict aseptic technique is used for all dressing changes, the insertion site is covered with an air-occlusive dressing, and all connections of the system must be secure. Ambulation and activities of daily living are encouraged and not limited during the administration of TPN.

🔑 CN: Pharmacological and parenteral therapies; CL: Synthesize

60. **1.** The administration of fat emulsion solution provides additional calories and essential fatty acids to meet the body's energy needs. Fatty acids are lipids, not carbohydrates. Fatty acids do not aid in the metabolism of glucose. Although they are necessary for meeting the complete nutritional needs of the client, fatty acids do not necessarily help a client maintain normal body weight.

🔑 CN: Pharmacological and parenteral therapies; CL: Apply

61. 4. An elevated temperature can be an indication of an infection at the insertion site or in the catheter. Vital signs should be taken every 2 to 4 hours after initiation of TPN therapy to detect early signs of complications. Glycosuria is to be expected during the first few days of therapy until the pancreas adjusts by secreting more insulin. A gradual weight gain is to be expected as the client's nutritional status improves. Some clients experience a decreased appetite during TPN therapy.

🔑 CN: Reduction of risk potential; CL: Analyze

62. 2. Too rapid infusion of a TPN solution can lead to circulatory overload. The client should be assessed carefully for indications of excessive fluid volume. A negative nitrogen balance occurs in nutritionally depleted individuals, not when TPN fluids are administered in excess. When TPN is administered too rapidly, the client is at risk for receiving an excess of dextrose and electrolytes. Therefore, the client is at risk for hyperglycemia and hyperkalemia.

🔑 CN: Pharmacological and parenteral therapies; CL: Analyze

The Client with Diverticular Disease

63. 1,2,4. Clients with diverticulosis are encouraged to follow a high-fiber diet. Bran, broccoli, and navy beans are foods high in fiber. Tomato juice and cheese are low-residue foods.

🔑 CN: Reduction of risk potential; CL: Apply

64. 3. The nurse should first assess the client for signs of peritonitis. Complications of diverticulitis include perforation with peritonitis, abscess, and fistula formation; bowel obstruction; ureteral obstruction; and bleeding. A computed tomography (CT) scan with oral contrast is the test of choice for diverticulitis. A client with acute diverticulitis does not receive a barium enema or colonoscopy because of the possibility of peritonitis and perforation. With acute diverticulitis, the goal of treatment is to allow the colon to rest and inflammation to subside. The client is kept on NPO status; parenteral fluid therapy is provided.

🔑 CN: Physiological adaptation; CL: Synthesize

65. 1. Barium enemas and colonoscopies are contraindicated in clients with acute diverticulitis

because they can lead to perforation of the colon and peritonitis. A barium enema may be prescribed after the client has been treated with antibiotic therapy and the inflammation has subsided. A barium enema is diagnostic in diverticulitis. A barium enema could increase the client's pain; however, that is not a reason for excluding this test. The client may be able to tolerate the procedure, but the concern is the potential for perforation of the intestine.

🔑 CN: Reduction of risk potential; CL: Apply

66. 4. Clients with diverticular disease should refrain from any activities, such as lifting, straining, or coughing, that increase intra-abdominal pressure and may precipitate an attack. Enemas are contraindicated because they increase intestinal pressure. Fluid intake should be increased, rather than decreased, to promote soft, formed stools. A low-fiber diet is used when inflammation is present.

🔑 CN: Reduction of risk potential; CL: Synthesize

67. 3,4,5. Clients who have diverticulosis should be instructed to maintain a diet high in fiber and, unless contraindicated, should increase their fluid intake to a minimum of 2,000 mL/day. Participating in a regular exercise program is also strongly encouraged. Diverticulosis can be controlled with treatment but cannot be cured. Clients should be instructed to avoid the regular use of cathartic laxatives. Bulk laxatives and stool softeners may be helpful to maintain regularity and decrease straining.

🔑 CN: Reduction of risk potential; CL: Evaluate

68. 1. Diverticular disease is treated with a high-fiber diet and bulk laxatives such as psyllium hydrophilic mucilloid. Fiber decreases the intraluminal pressure and makes it easier for stool to pass through the colon. Bulk laxatives do not manage diarrhea or relieve gas formation. The stool should remain soft and easy to expel.

🔑 CN: Pharmacological and parenteral therapies; CL: Evaluate

69. 1,2,3,5. Percussion will show resonance and tympany indicating paralytic ileus. Lack of liver dullness may indicate free air in the abdomen. The client with peritonitis will have fever, tachypnea, and tachycardia. The abdomen becomes rigid with rebound tenderness, and there will be absent bowel sounds. The client will not demonstrate excessive thirst but may have anorexia, nausea, and vomiting as peristalsis decreases.

🔑 CN: Physiological adaptation; CL: Analyze

The Client with Appendicitis

70. 4. The nurse should gently clean the area around the drain by moving in a circular motion away from the drain. Doing so prevents the introduction of microorganisms to the wound and drain site. The incision cannot be left open to air as long as the drain is intact. The nurse should note the amount and character of wound drainage, but the surgeon will determine when the drain should be removed. Surgical wound drains are not irrigated.

> CN: Safety and infection control;
> CL: Synthesize

71. 1. Appendicitis typically begins with periumbilical pain followed by anorexia, nausea, and vomiting. The pain is persistent and continuous, eventually shifting to the right lower quadrant and localizing at McBurney point (located halfway between the umbilicus and the right iliac crest). To relieve pain prior to surgery, the nurse assists the client to a comfortable position with the knees drawn to the chest and the head of the bed slightly elevated. The nurse may also administer analgesics and ice packs, if prescribed; heat is avoided as heat may precipitate rupture of the appendix. The abdomen is not palpated or massaged more than necessary to avoid increasing the pain. Distraction with music may be helpful, but positioning, using ice packs, and analgesics are most effective.

> CN: Physiological adaptation;
> CL: Synthesize

72. 2. Noting the client's first bowel movement after surgery is important because this indicates that normal peristalsis has returned. Sitz baths are used after rectal surgery, not appendectomy. Ambulation is started the day of surgery and is not confined to bathroom privileges. The abdomen should be auscultated for bowel sounds and palpated for softness, but there is no need to measure the girth every 2 hours.

> CN: Physiological adaptation;
> CL: Synthesize

73. 2. Drains are inserted postoperatively in appendectomies when an abscess was present or the appendix was perforated. The purpose is to promote drainage of exudate from the wound and facilitate healing. A drain is not used for irrigation of the wound. The drain will not minimize scar tissue development or decrease postoperative discomfort.

> CN: Reduction of risk potential;
> CL: Apply

The Client with an Inguinal Hernia

74. 3. The symptoms are indicative of a strangulated hernia. In a strangulated hernia, the hernia cannot be reduced back into the abdominal cavity. The intestinal lumen and the blood supply to the intestine are obstructed, causing an acute intestinal obstruction. Without immediate intervention, necrosis and gangrene may develop. Surgery is required to release the strangulation. Although many of these signs and symptoms are present with peritonitis or perforated bowel, abdominal rigidity, a cardinal sign of peritonitis and perforated bowel, is not mentioned. Therefore, the nurse would not immediately suspect these conditions. An incarcerated hernia refers to a hernia that is irreducible but has not necessarily resulted in an obstruction.

> CN: Physiological adaptation;
> CL: Analyze

75. 4. The client is instructed to avoid lifting items heavier than 5 lb for 4 to 6 weeks following hernia repair. The client continues to take deep breaths and expand the lungs but is instructed to avoid coughing. Ice, rather than heat, is used to reduce scrotal swelling. The client is instructed to sneeze with the mouth open to avoid sudden stress on the sutures.

> CN: Physiological adaptation; CL: Apply

76. 4. The most common complication after an inguinal hernia repair is the inability to void, especially in men. The nurse should evaluate the client carefully for urine retention. Hypostatic pneumonia, deep vein thrombosis, and paralytic ileus are potential postoperative problems with any surgical client but are not as likely to occur after an inguinal hernia repair as is urine retention.

> CN: Reduction of risk potential;
> CL: Analyze

Managing Care, Quality, and Safety of Clients with Lower Gastrointestinal Tract Health Problems

77. 2. The nurse administers the PRBCs using a separate infusion line and appropriate tubing, with normal saline as the priming solution. It is not necessary to discontinue the TPN infusion or wait until the TPN infusion is completed.

> CN: Safety and infection control;
> CL: Synthesize

78. 2,5. The nurse should consider client needs and scope of practice when assigning staff to provide care. The client who is recovering from inguinal hernia repair surgery and the client who is experiencing an exacerbation of ulcerative colitis are appropriate clients to assign to an **LPN/VN** 📖 as the care they require falls within the scope of practice for an LPN or a VN. It is not within the scope of practice for the LPN/VN to administer TPN, insert nasoenteric tubes, or provide client teaching related to medications.

🔑 CN: Management of care; CL: Synthesize

79. 2,4,5. The nurse can delegate the following basic care activities to the **UAP** 📖: providing skin care following bowel movements, maintaining intake and output records, and obtaining the client's weight. Assessing the client's bowel sounds and evaluating the client's response to medication are **registered nurse (RN)** 📖 activities that cannot be delegated.

🔑 CN: Management of care; CL: Synthesize

80. 3. This client has signs and symptoms of severe sepsis. Blood cultures should be drawn prior to administering the antibiotic (vancomycin); and the antibiotics should be administered within the first 45 minutes after recognition of these signs in order to try to prevent septic shock. Obtaining a chest x-ray and inserting a urinary catheter to accurately measure intake and output are also important actions but are not first priority for this client.

🔑 CN: Reduction of risk potential; CL: Synthesize

81. 4,5. *Clostridium difficile* is an organism that has developed very resistant and highly morbid strains. Universal precautions, most importantly handwashing, wearing personal protective gear, and modest use of antibiotics, are critical actions for stopping the spread. *C. difficile* is not spread via the respiratory tract; therefore, a mask is not needed. Alcohol-based hand sanitizers do not kill the spores of *C. difficile*; soap and water must be used. Sterile gloves are not needed to provide care; clean gloves may be worn.

🔑 CN: Safety and infection control; CL: Synthesize

82. 4. When TPN fluids are infused too rapidly or too slowly, the **HCP** 📖 should be notified. TPN solutions must be carefully and accurately infused. Rate adjustments should not be made without a written prescription from the HCP. Significant alterations in rate (10% increase or decrease) can result in fluctuations of blood glucose levels. Speeding up the solution can result in too much glucose entering the system.

🔑 CN: Management of care; CL: Synthesize

83. 3. The nurse should contact the pharmacy directly and request that a properly labeled medication be provided. The nurse should not administer any drug that is not properly labeled, even if the nurse or another nurse recognizes the medication. It is not necessary to notify the unit manager at this point because the client needs to receive the antibiotic as soon as possible.

🔑 CN: Safety and infection control; CL: Apply

84. 3. When dehiscence occurs, the nurse should immediately cover the wound with a sterile dressing moistened with normal saline. If the dehiscence is extensive, the incision must be resutured in surgery. Later, after the sutures are removed, additional support may be provided to the incision by applying strips of tape as directed by institutional policy or by the surgeon. An abdominal binder may also be utilized for additional support.

🔑 CN: Reduction of risk potential; CL: Synthesize

85. 2. Airborne precautions are required for clients with presumed or proven pulmonary tuberculosis (TB), chickenpox, or other airborne pathogens. Contact precautions are used for organisms that are spread by skin-to-skin contact, such as antibiotic-resistant organisms or *Clostridium difficile*. Droplet precautions are used for organisms such as influenza or *meningococcus* that can be transmitted by close respiratory or mucous membrane contact with respiratory secretions. The most important aspect of reducing the risk of bloodborne infection is avoidance of percutaneous injury. Extreme care is essential when needles, scalpels, and other sharp objects are handled.

🔑 CN: Safety and infection control; CL: Apply

86. 2,4. A black box warning for ciprofloxacin is that ciprofloxacin may increase the anticoagulant effects of warfarin. The nurse should instruct the client to report increased bleeding and to monitor the prothrombin time (PT) and the international normalized ratio (INR) closely. Although there is a drug-food interaction and taking ciprofloxacin may increase the stimulatory effect of caffeine, the client does not need to eliminate caffeine, but should report signs of stimulant effect. Ciprofloxacin may cause photosensitivity reactions; the nurse must advise the client to avoid excessive sunlight or artificial ultraviolet light during therapy. Clients must be advised not to crush, split, or chew the extended-release tablets. It is not necessary to increase the amount of fluids.

🔑 CN: Pharmacological and parenteral therapies; CL: Synthesize

The Client with Biliary Tract Disorders

- The Client with Cholecystitis
- The Client with Pancreatitis
- The Client with Viral Hepatitis
- The Client with Cirrhosis
- Managing Care, Quality, and Safety of Clients with Biliary Tract Disorders
- Answers, Rationales, and Test-Taking Strategies

The Client with Cholecystitis

1. A client has undergone a laparoscopic cholecystectomy. Which instruction should the nurse include in the discharge teaching?
- ☐ 1. Empty the bile bag daily.
- ☐ 2. Breathe deeply into a paper bag when nauseated.
- ☐ 3. Keep adhesive dressings in place for 6 weeks.
- ☐ 4. Report bile-colored drainage from any incision.

2. A 40-year-old client is admitted to the hospital with a diagnosis of acute cholecystitis. The nurse should contact the healthcare provider (HCP) to question which prescription?
- ☐ 1. IV fluid therapy of normal saline solution to be infused at 100 mL/h until further prescriptions.
- ☐ 2. Administer morphine sulfate 10 mg IM every 4 hours as needed for severe abdominal pain.
- ☐ 3. Nothing by mouth (NPO) until further prescriptions.
- ☐ 4. Insert a nasogastric tube, and connect to low intermittent suction.

3. A client is admitted to the hospital with a diagnosis of cholecystitis from cholelithiasis. The client has severe abdominal pain and nausea and has vomited 120 mL. Based on these data, which nursing action would have the **highest priority** at this time?
- ☐ 1. Manage anxiety.
- ☐ 2. Restore fluid loss.
- ☐ 3. Manage the pain.
- ☐ 4. Replace nutritional loss.

4. A client's stools are light gray in color. For what finding should the nurse assess the client? Select all that apply.
- ☐ 1. intolerance to fatty foods
- ☐ 2. fever
- ☐ 3. jaundice
- ☐ 4. respiratory distress
- ☐ 5. pain at McBurney's point
- ☐ 6. peptic ulcer disease

5. A client who has been scheduled to have a choledocholithotomy expresses anxiety about having surgery. Which nursing intervention would be the **most** appropriate to achieve the outcome of anxiety reduction?
- ☐ 1. providing the client with information about what to expect postoperatively
- ☐ 2. telling the client not to be afraid
- ☐ 3. reassuring the client by saying that surgery is a common procedure
- ☐ 4. stressing the importance of following the healthcare provider's (HCP's) instructions after surgery

6. A client has an open cholecystectomy with bile duct exploration. Following surgery, the client has a T tube. To evaluate the effectiveness of the T tube, the nurse should:
- ☐ 1. irrigate the tube with 20 mL of normal saline every 4 hours.
- ☐ 2. unclamp the T tube and empty the contents every day.
- ☐ 3. assess the color and amount of drainage every shift.
- ☐ 4. monitor the multiple incision sites for bile drainage.

7. At 0800, the nurse reviews the amount of T-tube drainage for a client who underwent an open cholecystectomy yesterday. After reviewing the output record (see chart), the nurse should:

Output Record

Time	T-Tube
1200	50 mL
1600	60 mL
2000	60 mL
0000	70 mL
0400	70 mL
0800	10 mL

☐ **1.** report the 24-hour drainage amount at 1200.
☐ **2.** clamp the T tube.
☐ **3.** evaluate the tube for patency.
☐ **4.** irrigate the T tube.

8. The nurse measures the amount of bile drainage from a T tube and records it by which method?
☐ **1.** adding it to the client's urine output
☐ **2.** charting it separately on the output record
☐ **3.** adding it to the amount of wound drainage
☐ **4.** subtracting it from the total intake for each day

9. The nurse is caring for a client who had an open cholecystectomy 24 hours ago. The client's vital signs have been stable over the last 24 hours, with most recent temperature 98.6°F (37°C), blood pressure (BP) 118/76 mm Hg, respiratory rate (RR) 16/minute, and heart rate (HR) 78 bpm, but are now changing. Which set of vital signs indicates that the nurse should contact the healthcare provider (HCP)?
☐ **1.** temperature 101.8°F (38.8°C), BP 140/86 mm Hg, HR 94 bpm, RR 24/min
☐ **2.** temperature 100.7°F (38.2°C), BP 118/68 mm Hg, HR 84 bpm, RR 20/min
☐ **3.** temperature 99.5°F (37.5°C), BP 126/80 mm Hg, HR 58 bpm, RR 16/min
☐ **4.** temperature 97.5°F (36.4°C), BP 98/64 mm Hg, HR 98 bpm, RR 18/min

10. After a cholecystectomy, the client is to follow a low-fat diet. Which food would be **most** appropriate to include in a low-fat diet?
☐ **1.** cheese omelet with onions
☐ **2.** peanut butter on wheat toast
☐ **3.** ham salad sandwich made with mayonnaise
☐ **4.** roast beef sandwich with lettuce and tomato

11. A client with cholecystitis continues to have severe right upper quadrant pain. The nurse obtains the following vital signs: temperature 101.1°F (38.4°C); pulse 114 bpm; respirations 22/min; blood pressure 142/90 mm Hg. Using the SBAR (Situation-Background-Assessment-Recommendation) technique for communication, the nurse recommends to the healthcare provider for the client to receive:
☐ **1.** hydromorphone IV.
☐ **2.** diltiazem PO.
☐ **3.** meperidine IM.
☐ **4.** promethazine IM.

12. The nurse prepares to administer promethazine 35 mg IM as prescribed PRN for a client with cholecystitis who has nausea. The ampule label reads that the medication is available in 25 mg/mL. How many milliliters should the nurse administer? Record your answer using one decimal place.

_____ ml.

13. A client undergoes a laparoscopic cholecystectomy. Which dietary instructions should the nurse give the client immediately after surgery?
☐ **1.** "You cannot eat or drink anything for 24 hours."
☐ **2.** "You may resume your normal diet the day after your surgery."
☐ **3.** "Drink liquids today and eat lightly for a few days."
☐ **4.** "You can progress from a liquid to a bland diet as tolerated."

14. Which discharge instruction would be appropriate for a client who has had a laparoscopic cholecystectomy and has sutures covered by a dressing?
☐ **1.** Avoid showering for 1 week after surgery.
☐ **2.** Return to work within 1 week.
☐ **3.** Leave dressing in place until you see the surgeon at the postoperative visit.
☐ **4.** Use acetaminophen to control any fever.

15. A client who has had a laparoscopic cholecystectomy has adhesive strips over the puncture sites. When preparing the client for discharge, which client statements indicate that the teaching has been successful? Select all that apply.
☐ **1.** "I can resume my normal diet when I want."
☐ **2.** "I need to avoid driving for about 4 weeks."
☐ **3.** "I may experience some pain in my right shoulder."
☐ **4.** "I should spend 2 to 3 days in bed before resuming activity."
☐ **5.** "I can take a shower 2 days later."

16. A client has been admitted to the medical surgical unit following an emergency cholecystectomy. There is a Jackson-Pratt drain with a portable suction unit attached. After 4 hours, the drainage unit is full. What should the nurse do?
☐ **1.** Notify the surgeon.
☐ **2.** Remove the drain and suction unit.
☐ **3.** Check the dressing for bleeding.
☐ **4.** Empty the drainage unit.

The Client with Pancreatitis

17. The client who has been hospitalized with pancreatitis does not drink alcohol because of religious convictions. The client comes upset when the healthcare provider (HCP) persists in asking about alcohol intake. The nurse should explain that the reason for these questions is that:
- ☐ **1.** there is a strong link between alcohol use and acute pancreatitis.
- ☐ **2.** alcohol intake can interfere with the tests used to diagnose pancreatitis.
- ☐ **3.** alcoholism is a major health problem, and all clients are questioned about alcohol intake.
- ☐ **4.** the HCP must obtain the pertinent facts, regardless of religious beliefs.

18. A client with acute pancreatitis has a blood pressure of 88/40 mm Hg, heart rate of 128 bpm, respirations of 28/min, and Grey Turner's sign. What prescription should the nurse implement **first**?
- ☐ **1.** Initiate intake/output record.
- ☐ **2.** Place an intravenous line.
- ☐ **3.** Position on the left side.
- ☐ **4.** Insert a nasogastric tube.

19. On 1/16 at 0800, the nurse is caring for a client with acute pancreatitis and reviewing progress notes as listed:

Nurses Progress Notes

Date	Time	Progress Notes
1/15	0800	Vital signs are: temperature 37.4°C; heart rate, 138; BP is 80/48; pain is 9 on a 10-point scale; client is restless. Robin Brown, RN
1/15	1000	Discussed following lab values with A. Smith, MD: hematocrit is 27.6%, hemoglobin is 7.6 g/dl, platelet count is 245,000 mm³, and INR is 0.8. Robin Brown, RN
1/15	1100	PRBCs infused; no adverse reactions. Robin Brown, RN

Which finding indicates that the desired outcome of the transfusion is obtained at this time?
- ☐ **1.** BP is 110/80 mm Hg.
- ☐ **2.** Pain is 4 on a 10-point scale.
- ☐ **3.** Hemoglobin is 12 g/dL.
- ☐ **4.** Platelet count is 144,000/mm³.

20. The nurse should question which prescription for medications for a client with acute pancreatitis?
- ☐ **1.** furosemide 20 mg IV push
- ☐ **2.** imipenem 500 mg IV
- ☐ **3.** morphine sulfate 2 mg IV push
- ☐ **4.** famotidine 20 mg IV push

21. The nurse should monitor the client with acute pancreatitis for which complication?
- ☐ **1.** heart failure
- ☐ **2.** duodenal ulcer
- ☐ **3.** cirrhosis
- ☐ **4.** pneumonia

22. When providing care for a client hospitalized with acute pancreatitis who has acute abdominal pain, which nursing intervention(s) would be **most** appropriate for this client? Select all that apply.
- ☐ **1.** Place the client in a side-lying position.
- ☐ **2.** Administer morphine sulfate for pain as needed.
- ☐ **3.** Maintain the client on a high-calorie, high-protein diet.
- ☐ **4.** Monitor the client's respiratory status.
- ☐ **5.** Obtain daily weights.

23. The nurse notes that a client with acute pancreatitis occasionally experiences muscle twitching and jerking. How should the nurse interpret the significance of these symptoms?
- ☐ **1.** The client may be developing hypocalcemia.
- ☐ **2.** The client is experiencing a reaction to meperidine.
- ☐ **3.** The client has a nutritional imbalance.
- ☐ **4.** The client needs a muscle relaxant to promote rest.

24. A client is receiving propantheline bromide in the management of acute pancreatitis. Which finding would indicate that the nurse should discuss withholding the medication with the healthcare provider (HCP)?
- ☐ **1.** absent bowel sounds
- ☐ **2.** increased urine output
- ☐ **3.** diarrhea
- ☐ **4.** decreased heart rate

25. Which dietary instruction would be appropriate for the nurse to give a client who is recovering from acute pancreatitis?
- ☐ **1.** Avoid crash dieting.
- ☐ **2.** Restrict carbohydrate intake.
- ☐ **3.** Eat six small meals a day.
- ☐ **4.** Decrease sodium in the diet.

26. Pancreatic enzyme replacements are prescribed for the client with chronic pancreatitis. When should the nurse instruct the client to take them to obtain the most therapeutic effect?
☐ 1. three times daily between meals
☐ 2. with each meal and snack
☐ 3. in the morning and at bedtime
☐ 4. every 4 hours, at specified times

27. The nurse should teach the client with chronic pancreatitis to monitor the effectiveness of pancreatic enzyme replacement therapy by:
☐ 1. recording daily fluid intake.
☐ 2. performing glucose fingerstick tests twice a day.
☐ 3. observing stools for steatorrhea.
☐ 4. testing urine for ketones.

28. The nurse is assessing a client with chronic hepatitis B who is receiving lamivudine. What information is **most** important to communicate to the healthcare provider (HCP)?
☐ 1. The client has had a 3-kg weight gain over 2 days.
☐ 2. The client has nausea.
☐ 3. The client now has a temperature of 99°F (37.2°C) orally.
☐ 4. The client has fatigue.

The Client with Viral Hepatitis

29. The nurse is assessing a client with hepatitis A and notices that the aspartate transaminase (AST) and alanine transaminase (ALT) lab values have increased. Which statement by the client indicates the need for further instruction by the nurse?
☐ 1. "I require increased periods of rest."
☐ 2. "I follow a low-fat, high-carbohydrate diet."
☐ 3. "I eat dry toast to relieve my nausea."
☐ 4. "I take acetaminophen for arthritis pain."

30. College freshmen are participating in a study abroad program. When teaching them about hepatitis B, the nurse should instruct the students on the need for:
☐ 1. water sanitation.
☐ 2. single dormitory rooms.
☐ 3. vaccination for hepatitis D.
☐ 4. safe sexual practices.

31. Which finding is normal for a client during the icteric phase of hepatitis A?
☐ 1. tarry stools
☐ 2. yellowed sclerae
☐ 3. shortness of breath
☐ 4. light, frothy urine

32. The nurse is teaching a client with hepatitis A about preventing transmission of the disease. The nurse should focus teaching on:
☐ 1. proper food handling.
☐ 2. insulin syringe disposal.
☐ 3. alpha-interferon.
☐ 4. use of condoms.

33. A client has a positive serologic test for anti-HCV (hepatitis C virus). The nurse should instruct the client:
☐ 1. how to self-administer alpha-interferon.
☐ 2. that the HCV will resolve in approximately 3 months.
☐ 3. that a follow-up appointment for HCV genotype testing is required.
☐ 4. to take alpha-interferon as prescribed.

34. A client with chronic hepatitis C is experiencing nausea, anorexia, and fatigue. During the health history, the client states that he is homosexual, drinks one to two glasses of wine with dinner, is taking St. John's wort for a "bit of depression," and takes acetaminophen for frequent headaches. What should the nurse do? Select all that apply.
☐ 1. Instruct the client that the wine with meals can be beneficial for cardiovascular health.
☐ 2. Instruct the client to ask the healthcare provider (HCP) about taking any other medications as they may interact with medications the client is currently taking.
☐ 3. Instruct the client to increase the protein in his diet and eat less frequently.
☐ 4. Advise the client of the need for additional testing for HIV.
☐ 5. Encourage the client to obtain sufficient rest.

35. A client who is recovering from hepatitis A has fatigue and malaise. The client asks the nurse, "When will my strength return?" Which response by the nurse is **most** appropriate?
☐ 1. "Your fatigue should be gone by now. We will evaluate you for a secondary infection."
☐ 2. "Your fatigue is an adverse effect of your drug therapy. It will disappear when your treatment regimen is complete."
☐ 3. "It is important for you to increase your activity level. That will help decrease your fatigue."
☐ 4. "It is normal for you to feel fatigued. The fatigue should go away in the next 2 to 4 months."

36. The nurse is caring for a client recently diagnosed with hepatitis C. In reviewing the client's history, what information will be **most** helpful as the nurse develops a teaching plan? The client:
- ☐ 1. has a history of exercise-induced asthma.
- ☐ 2. is a scientist and is frequently exposed to multiple chemicals.
- ☐ 3. traveled to Central America recently and ate uncooked vegetables.
- ☐ 4. has a known history of sexually transmitted disease.

37. A client recently diagnosed with hepatitis C states: "Now that you know what is wrong with me, you can just get me those new drugs to take care of it, right?" The nurse should tell the client:
- ☐ 1. "The treatment is complex. There are new antiviral drugs available that may make treatment more effective and help you tolerate it better."
- ☐ 2. "There are drugs to help with the symptoms, but once you have hepatitis C you will never be cured."
- ☐ 3. "The medicine currently used to treat hepatitis C is very expensive, and your insurance probably will not pay for it."
- ☐ 4. "If you continue to make the same lifestyle choices, the medicine will not make any difference."

38. The nurse is developing a plan of care for the client with viral hepatitis. The nurse should instruct the client to:
- ☐ 1. obtain adequate bed rest.
- ☐ 2. increase fluid intake.
- ☐ 3. take antibiotic therapy as prescribed.
- ☐ 4. drink 8 oz (240 mL) of an electrolyte solution every day.

39. When planning care for a client with hepatitis A, the nurse should review laboratory reports for which laboratory values?
- ☐ 1. prolonged prothrombin time
- ☐ 2. decreased blood glucose level
- ☐ 3. elevated serum potassium level
- ☐ 4. decreased serum calcium level

40. The nurse should teach the client with hepatitis A to:
- ☐ 1. limit caloric intake and reduce weight.
- ☐ 2. increase carbohydrates and protein in the diet.
- ☐ 3. avoid contact with others and sleep in a separate room.
- ☐ 4. intensify routine exercise and increase strength.

41. The nurse develops a teaching plan for the client about how to prevent the transmission of hepatitis A. Which discharge instruction is appropriate for the client?
- ☐ 1. Spray the house to eliminate infected insects.
- ☐ 2. Tell family members to try to stay away from the client.
- ☐ 3. Ask family members to wash their hands frequently.
- ☐ 4. Disinfect all clothing and eating utensils.

42. The client with hepatitis A is experiencing fatigue, weakness, and a general feeling of malaise. The client tires rapidly during morning care. The **most** appropriate goal for this client is to:
- ☐ 1. increase mobility.
- ☐ 2. learn new self-care skills.
- ☐ 3. adapt to new levels of energy.
- ☐ 4. gradually increase activity tolerance.

43. Interferon alfa-2b has been prescribed to treat a client with chronic hepatitis B. The nurse should assess the client for which common adverse effect?
- ☐ 1. retinopathy
- ☐ 2. constipation
- ☐ 3. flulike symptoms
- ☐ 4. hypoglycemia

44. The nurse is preparing a community education program about preventing hepatitis B infection. Which information should be incorporated into the teaching plan?
- ☐ 1. Hepatitis B is relatively uncommon among college students.
- ☐ 2. Frequent ingestion of alcohol can predispose an individual to development of hepatitis B.
- ☐ 3. Good personal hygiene habits are most effective at preventing the spread of hepatitis B.
- ☐ 4. The use of a condom is advised for sexual intercourse.

45. Which goal is appropriate for a client with hepatitis A? The client will:
- ☐ 1. demonstrate a decrease in fluid retention related to ascites.
- ☐ 2. verbalize the importance of reporting bleeding gums or bloody stools.
- ☐ 3. limit use of alcohol to two to three drinks per week.
- ☐ 4. restrict activity to within the home to prevent disease transmission.

The Client with Cirrhosis

46. A client had a liver biopsy 1 hour ago. The nurse should **first**:
☐ 1. auscultate lung sounds.
☐ 2. check for fever.
☐ 3. obtain a CBC.
☐ 4. apply packing to the biopsy site.

47. The nurse is assessing a client for ascites. Where does the nurse place the hands to percuss for the presence of fluid?

48. A client with cirrhosis is receiving lactulose. The nurse notes the client is more confused and has asterixis. The nurse should:
☐ 1. assess for gastrointestinal (GI) bleeding.
☐ 2. withhold the lactulose.
☐ 3. increase protein in the diet.
☐ 4. monitor serum bilirubin levels.

49. The nurse is assessing a client with cirrhosis who has developed hepatic encephalopathy. The nurse should notify the healthcare provider (HCP) of a decrease in which serum lab value that is a potential precipitating factor for hepatic encephalopathy?
☐ 1. aldosterone
☐ 2. creatinine
☐ 3. potassium
☐ 4. protein

50. A client has advanced cirrhosis of the liver. The client's spouse asks the nurse why his abdomen is swollen, making it very difficult for him to fasten his pants. How should the nurse respond to provide the **most** accurate explanation of the disease process?
☐ 1. "He must have been eating too many foods with salt in them. Salt pulls water with it."
☐ 2. "The swelling in his ankles must have moved up closer to his heart so the fluid circulates better."
☐ 3. "He must have forgotten to take his daily water pill."
☐ 4. "Blood is not able to flow readily through the liver now, and the liver cannot make protein to keep fluid inside the blood vessels."

51. A nurse is developing a care plan for a client with hepatic encephalopathy. Which are goals for the care for this client? Select all that apply.
☐ 1. Prevent constipation.
☐ 2. Administer lactulose to reduce blood ammonia levels.
☐ 3. Monitor coordination while walking.
☐ 4. Check the pupil reaction.
☐ 5. Provide food and fluids high in carbohydrate.
☐ 6. Encourage physical activity.

52. The nurse is assessing a client who is in the early stages of cirrhosis of the liver. Which focused assessment is appropriate?
☐ 1. peripheral edema
☐ 2. ascites
☐ 3. anorexia
☐ 4. jaundice

53. A client with cirrhosis begins to develop ascites. Spironolactone is prescribed to treat the ascites. The nurse should monitor the client closely for which drug-related adverse effect?
☐ 1. constipation
☐ 2. hyperkalemia
☐ 3. irregular pulse
☐ 4. dysuria

54. What diet should be implemented for a client who is in the early stages of cirrhosis?
☐ 1. high-calorie, high-carbohydrate
☐ 2. high-protein, low-fat
☐ 3. low-fat, low-protein
☐ 4. high-carbohydrate, low-sodium

55. A client with jaundice has pruritus and areas of irritation from scratching. What measures can the nurse suggest the client use to prevent skin breakdown? Select all that apply.
☐ 1. Avoid lotions containing calamine.
☐ 2. Add baking soda to the water in a tub bath.
☐ 3. Keep nails short and clean.
☐ 4. Rub the skin when it itches with knuckles instead of nails.
☐ 5. Massage skin with alcohol.
☐ 6. Increase sodium intake in diet.

56. Which health promotion activity should the nurse suggest that the client with cirrhosis add to the daily routine at home?
☐ 1. Supplement the diet with daily multivitamins.
☐ 2. Abstain from drinking alcohol.
☐ 3. Take a sleeping pill at bedtime.
☐ 4. Limit contact with other people whenever possible.

57. The nurse is reviewing the chart information for a client with increased ascites. The data include the following: temperature 98.9°F (37.2°C), heart rate 118 bpm, shallow respirations 26/min, blood pressure 128/76 mm Hg, and SpO$_2$ 89% on room air. The nurse should **first**:
- [ ] **1.** assess heart sounds.
- [ ] **2.** obtain a prescription for blood cultures.
- [ ] **3.** prepare for a paracentesis.
- [ ] **4.** raise the head of the bed.

58. Which position would be appropriate for a client with severe ascites?
- [ ] **1.** Fowler's
- [ ] **2.** side-lying
- [ ] **3.** reverse Trendelenburg
- [ ] **4.** Sims

59. The nurse is caring for a client with esophageal varices. The nurse should discuss which laboratory report finding with the healthcare provider (HCP)?
- [ ] **1.** normal serum albumin
- [ ] **2.** decreased ammonia
- [ ] **3.** slightly decreased levels of calcium
- [ ] **4.** elevated PT/INR

60. A client with cirrhosis who has ascites receives 100 mL of 25% serum albumin IV. Which finding would **best** indicate that the albumin is having its desired effect?
- [ ] **1.** reduced ascites
- [ ] **2.** increased serum albumin level
- [ ] **3.** decreased anorexia
- [ ] **4.** increased ease of breathing

61. A client with a Sengstaken-Blakemore tube has a sudden drop in SpO$_2$ and an increase in respiratory rate to 40 breaths/min. What should the nurse do in order from **first** to last? All options must be used.

1. Affirm airway obstruction by the tube.

2. Remove the tube.

3. Deflate the tube by cutting with bedside scissors.

4. Apply oxygen via face mask.

62. The healthcare provider (HCP) instructs a client with alcohol-induced cirrhosis to stop drinking alcohol. The expected outcome of this intervention is:
- [ ] **1.** absence of delirium tremens.
- [ ] **2.** having a balanced diet.
- [ ] **3.** improved liver function.
- [ ] **4.** reduced weight.

63. The nurse monitors a client with cirrhosis for the development of hepatic encephalopathy. Which would be an indication that hepatic encephalopathy is developing?
- [ ] **1.** decreased mental status
- [ ] **2.** elevated blood pressure
- [ ] **3.** decreased urine output
- [ ] **4.** labored respirations

64. A client's serum ammonia level is elevated, and the healthcare provider (HCP) prescribes 30 mL of lactulose. Which effect is common for this drug?
- [ ] **1.** increased urine output
- [ ] **2.** improved level of consciousness
- [ ] **3.** increased bowel movements
- [ ] **4.** nausea and vomiting

65. The nurse has a prescription to administer 2 oz of lactulose to a client who has cirrhosis. How many milliliters of lactulose should the nurse administer? Record your answer using a whole number.

_____ mL.

66. A client is to be discharged with a prescription for lactulose. The nurse teaches the client and the client's spouse how to administer this medication. Which statement would indicate that the client has understood the information?
- [ ] **1.** "I will take it with an antacid."
- [ ] **2.** "I will mix it with apple juice."
- [ ] **3.** "I will take it with a laxative."
- [ ] **4.** "I will mix the crushed tablets in some gelatin."

67. The nurse is providing discharge instructions for a client with cirrhosis. Which statement **best** indicates that the client has understood the teaching?
- [ ] **1.** "I should eat a high-protein, high-carbohydrate diet to provide energy."
- [ ] **2.** "It is safer for me to take acetaminophen for pain instead of aspirin."
- [ ] **3.** "I should avoid constipation to decrease chances of bleeding."
- [ ] **4.** "If I get enough rest and follow my diet, it is possible for my cirrhosis to be cured."

68. The nurse is preparing a client for a paracentesis. The nurse should:
- [ ] **1.** have the client void immediately before the procedure.
- [ ] **2.** place the client in a side-lying position.
- [ ] **3.** initiate an IV line to administer sedatives.
- [ ] **4.** place the client on nothing-by-mouth (NPO) status 6 hours before the procedure.

69. A client with ascites and peripheral edema is at risk for impaired skin integrity. To prevent skin breakdown, the nurse should:
- ☐ 1. institute range-of-motion (ROM) exercise every 4 hours.
- ☐ 2. massage the abdomen once a shift.
- ☐ 3. use an alternating air pressure mattress.
- ☐ 4. elevate the lower extremities.

Managing Care, Quality, and Safety of Clients with Biliary Tract Disorders

70. Which precautions should the healthcare team observe when caring for clients with hepatitis A?
- ☐ 1. gowning when entering a client's room
- ☐ 2. wearing a mask when providing care
- ☐ 3. assigning the client to a private room
- ☐ 4. wearing gloves when giving direct care

71. After completing assessment rounds, which client should the nurse discuss with the healthcare provider (HCP) **first**?
- ☐ 1. a client with cirrhosis who is depressed and has refused to eat for the past 2 days
- ☐ 2. a client with stable vital signs that has been receiving IV ciprofloxacin following a cholecystectomy for 1 day and has developed a rash on the chest and arms
- ☐ 3. a client with pancreatitis whose family requests to speak with the HCP regarding the treatment plan
- ☐ 4. a client with hepatitis whose pulse was 84 bpm and regular and is now 118 bpm and irregular

72. The nurse's assignment consists of four clients. From highest to lowest priority, in which order should the nurse assess the clients after receiving the morning report? All options must be used.

1. the client with cirrhosis who became confused and disoriented during the night

2. the client who is 1 day postoperative following a cholecystectomy and has a T tube inserted

3. the client with acute pancreatitis who is requesting pain medication

4. the client with hepatitis B who has questions about discharge instructions

73. The nurse should institute which measure to prevent transmission of the hepatitis C virus to healthcare personnel?
- ☐ 1. administering hepatitis C vaccine to all healthcare personnel
- ☐ 2. decreasing contact with blood and blood-contaminated fluids
- ☐ 3. wearing gloves when emptying the bed pan
- ☐ 4. wearing a gown and mask when providing direct care

74. The nurse is taking care of a client who has an IV infusion pump. The pump alarm rings. What should the nurse do in order from first to last? All options must be used.

1. Silence the pump alarm.

2. Determine if the infusion pump is plugged into an electrical outlet.

3. Assess the client's access site for infiltration or inflammation.

4. Assess the tubing for hindrances to flow of solution.

Answers, Rationales, and Test-Taking Strategies

*The answers and rationales for each question follow below, along with keys (🔑) to the client need (CN) and cognitive level (CL) for each question. In addition, you will also see a glossary icon (📖) highlighting specific terminology used on the licensing exam. As you check your answers, use the **Content Mastery and Test-Taking Skill Self-Analysis** worksheet (tear-out worksheet in back of book) to identify the reason(s) for not answering the questions correctly. For additional information about test-taking skills and strategies for answering questions, refer to pages 12–23 and pages 35–36 in Part 1 of this book.*

The Client with Cholecystitis

1. 4. There should be no bile-colored drainage coming from any of the incisions postoperatively. A laparoscopic cholecystectomy does not involve a bile bag. Breathing deeply into a paper bag will prevent a person from passing out due to hyperventilation; it does not alleviate nausea. If the adhesive dressings have not already fallen off, they are removed by the surgeon in 7 to 10 days, not 6 weeks.

CN: Management of care; CL: Create

2. 2. A nurse should question the prescription for morphine sulfate because it is believed to cause biliary spasm. Thus, the preferred opioid analgesic to treat cholecystitis is meperidine. Elderly clients should not be given meperidine because of the risk of acute confusion and seizures in this population. An alternative pain medication will be necessary. IV fluid therapy is used to maintain fluid and electrolyte balance that may result from NPO status and gastric suctioning. NPO status and gastric decompression prevent further gallbladder stimulation.

CN: Safety and infection control; CL: Synthesize

3. 3. The priority for nursing care at this time is to decrease the client's severe abdominal pain. The pain, which is frequently accompanied by nausea and vomiting, is caused by biliary spasm. Opioid analgesics are given to relieve the severe pain and spasm of cholecystitis. Relief of pain may decrease nausea and vomiting and thereby decrease the client's likelihood of developing further complications, such as severe fluid loss and inadequate nutrition. There are no data to suggest that the client is anxious.

CN: Physiological adaptation; CL: Analyze

4. 1,2,3. Bile is created in the liver, stored in the gallbladder, and released into the duodenum, giving stool its brown color. A bile duct obstruction can cause pale-colored stools. Other symptoms associated with cholelithiasis are right upper quadrant tenderness, fever from inflammation or infection, jaundice from elevated serum bilirubin levels, and nausea or right upper quadrant pain after a fatty meal. Pain at McBurney's point lies between the umbilicus and right iliac crest and is associated with appendicitis. A bleeding ulcer produces black, tarry stools. Respiratory distress is not a symptom of cholelithiasis.

CN: Physiological adaptation; CL: Analyze

5. 1. Providing information can help to answer the client's questions and decrease anxiety. Fear of the unknown can increase anxiety. Telling the client not to be afraid, that the procedure is common, or to follow the **HCP's** prescriptions will not necessarily decrease anxiety.

CN: Psychosocial adaptation; CL: Synthesize

6. 3. A T tube is inserted in the common bile duct to maintain patency when there is a likelihood of edema. The tube remains in place until edema from the duct exploration subsides. The bile color should be gold to dark green, and the amount of drainage should be closely monitored to ensure tube patency. Irrigation is not routinely done, unless prescribed using a smaller volume of fluid. The T tube is not clamped in the early post-op period to allow for continuous drainage. An open cholecystectomy has one right subcostal incision, whereas a laparoscopic cholecystectomy has multiple small incisions.

CN: Physiological adaptation; CL: Evaluate

7. 3. The T tube should drain approximately 300 to 500 mL in the first 24 hours, and after 3 to 4 days, the amount should decrease to <200 mL in 24 hours. With the sudden decrease in drainage at 0800, the nurse should immediately assess the tube for obstruction of flow that can be caused by kinks in the tube or the client lying on the tube. Drainage color must also be assessed for signs of bleeding. The tube should not be irrigated or clamped without a prescription.

CN: Physiological adaptation; CL: Synthesize

8. 2. T-tube bile drainage is recorded separately on the output record. Adding the T-tube drainage to the urine output or wound drainage makes it difficult to accurately determine the amounts of bile, urine, or drainage. The client's total intake will be incorrect if drainage is subtracted from it.

CN: Reduction of risk potential; CL: Apply

9. 1. This client is exhibiting three of four signs of systemic inflammatory response syndrome (SIRS): temperature >100.4°F (38°C) (or <96.8°F [36°C]), heart rate >90 bpm, and respiratory rate >20 breaths/min. The fourth indicator is an abnormal white blood cell count (>12,000 [12 × 10⁹/L], <4000 [4 × 10⁹/L], or >10% [0.1 × 10⁹/L] bands). At least two of these variables are required to define SIRS.

CN: Physiological integrity; CL: Evaluate

10. 4. Lean meats, such as beef, lamb, veal, and well-trimmed lean ham and pork, are low in fat. Rice, pasta, and vegetables are low in fat when not served with butter, cream, or sauces. Fruits are low in fat. The amount of fat allowed in a client's diet after a cholecystectomy will depend on the client's ability to tolerate fat. Typically, the client does not require a special diet but is encouraged to avoid excessive fat intake. A cheese omelet and peanut butter have high fat content. Ham salad is high in fat from the fat in a mayonnaise-based salad dressing.

CN: Basic care and comfort; CL: Apply

11. 1. Hydromorphone should be considered for pain management. It should be administered intravenously for rapid action to address the severe pain the client is experiencing. Intramuscular injections are painful and slower acting. Since meperidine's toxic metabolite can cause seizures, it is no longer the treatment choice for pain. Diltiazem, a calcium channel blocker, is not indicated. Elevation of heart rate and blood pressure is likely due to pain and fever. Promethazine is used to treat nausea.

   CN: Pharmacological and parenteral therapies; CL: Synthesize

12. 1.4 mL.
The following formula is used to calculate the correct dosage:

$$35 \text{ mg}/X \text{ mL} = 25\text{mg} /1 \text{ mL}$$
$$X = 1.4 \text{ mL}$$

   CN: Pharmacological and parenteral therapies; CL: Apply

13. 3. Immediately after surgery, the client will drink liquids. A light diet can be resumed the day after surgery. There is no need for the client to remain on nothing-by-mouth status after surgery because peristaltic bowel activity should not be affected. The client will probably not be able to tolerate a full meal comfortably the day after surgery. There is no need for the client to stay on a bland diet after a laparoscopic cholecystectomy. The client should, however, avoid excessive fats.

   CN: Physiological adaptation; CL: Synthesize

14. 3. After a laparoscopic cholecystectomy when there are sutures covered by a dressing, the client should not remove dressings from the puncture sites but should wait until visiting the surgeon. The client may shower 48 hours after surgery. A client can return to work within 1 week, but only if approved by the surgeon and no strenuous activity is involved. The client should report any fever, which could be an indication of a complication.

   CN: Reduction of risk potential; CL: Synthesize

15. 1,3,5. Following a laparoscopic cholecystectomy, the client can resume a normal diet as tolerated. The client may experience right shoulder pain from the gas that was used to inflate the abdomen during surgery. The client can take a shower 48 hours after the surgery. The adhesive strips will fall off in about 10 days. The client can resume driving within 3 to 4 days following surgery as long as the client is not taking pain medication. There is no need for the client to maintain bed rest in the days following surgery. Light exercise such as walking can be resumed immediately.

   CN: Physiological adaptation; CL: Evaluate

16. 4. Portable suction units should be emptied and drained every shift or when full. It is normal for the unit to fill within the first hours after surgery; the nurse does not need to contact the surgeon. There should not be bleeding on the dressing if the drainage system is emptied when full. The drain should not be removed until prescribed by the **healthcare provider (HCP)** 📖.

   CN: Management of care CL: Synthesize

The Client with Pancreatitis

17. 1. Alcoholism is a major cause of acute pancreatitis in the United States and Canada. Because some clients are reluctant to discuss alcohol use, staff may inquire about it in several ways. Generally, alcohol intake does not interfere with the tests used to diagnose pancreatitis. Recent ingestion of large amounts of alcohol, however, may cause an increased serum amylase level. Large amounts of ethyl and methyl alcohol may produce an elevated urinary amylase concentration. All clients are asked about alcohol and drug use on hospital admission, but this information is especially pertinent for clients with pancreatitis. **HCPs** 📖 do need to seek facts, but this can be done while respecting the client's religious beliefs. Respecting religious beliefs is important in providing holistic client care.

   CN: Health promotion and maintenance; CL: Apply

18. 2. Grey Turner's sign is a bluish discoloration in the flank area caused by retroperitoneal bleeding. The vital signs are showing hemodynamic instability. IV access should be obtained to provide immediate volume replacement. The urine output will provide information on the fluid status. A nasogastric tube is indicated for clients with uncontrolled nausea and vomiting or gastric distension. Repositioning the client may be considered for pain management once the client's vital signs are stable.

   CN: Physiological adaptation; CL: Synthesize

19. 3. PRBCs are ordered to improve the low hemoglobin level; therefore, the nurse assesses for an increase in hemoglobin. The PRBCs do not increase BP; colloid solutions are needed to increase the circulating blood volume and raise the BP. The client has acute pain and requires the use of analgesia to minimize the pain. The platelet count is within normal limits and is not affected by the infusion of PRBCs.

   CN: Physiological Adaptation; CL: Evaluate

20. 1. Furosemide can cause pancreatitis. Additionally, hypovolemia can develop with acute pancreatitis, and furosemide will further deplete fluid volume. Imipenem is indicated in the treatment of acute pancreatitis with necrosis and infection. Research no longer supports meperidine over other opiates. Morphine and hydromorphone are opiates of choice in acute pancreatitis to get pain under control. Famotidine is a histamine-2 receptor antagonist used to decrease acid secretion and prevent stress or peptic ulcers.

⚭ CN: Pharmacological and parenteral therapies; CL: Synthesize

21. 4. The client with acute pancreatitis is prone to complications associated with the respiratory system. Pneumonia, atelectasis, and pleural effusion are examples of respiratory complications that can develop as a result of pancreatic enzyme exudate. Pancreatitis does not cause heart failure, ulcer formation, or cirrhosis.

⚭ CN: Reduction of risk potential; CL: Analyze

22. 1,4,5. The client with acute pancreatitis usually experiences acute abdominal pain. Placing the client in a side-lying position relieves the tension on the abdominal area and promotes comfort. A semi-Fowler's position is also appropriate. The nurse should also monitor the client's respiratory status because clients with pancreatitis are prone to develop respiratory complications. Daily weights are obtained to monitor the client's nutritional and fluid volume status. While the client will likely need opioid analgesics to treat the pain, morphine sulfate is not appropriate as it stimulates spasm of the sphincter of Oddi, thus increasing the client's discomfort. During the acute phase of the illness while the client is experiencing pain, the pancreas is rested by withholding food and drink. When the diet is reintroduced, it is a high-carbohydrate, low-fat, bland diet.

⚭ CN: Physiological adaptation; CL: Synthesize

23. 1. Hypocalcemia develops in severe cases of acute pancreatitis. The exact cause is unknown. Signs and symptoms of hypocalcemia include jerking and muscle twitching, numbness of fingers and lips, and irritability. Meperidine may cause tremors or seizures as an adverse effect, but not muscle twitching. Muscle twitching is not caused by a nutritional deficit, nor does it indicate that the client needs a muscle relaxant.

⚭ CN: Reduction of risk potential; CL: Analyze

24. 1. Propantheline is an anticholinergic, antispasmodic medication that decreases vagal stimulation and pancreatic secretions. It is contraindicated in paralytic ileus; therefore, the nurse should be concerned with the absent bowel sounds. Side effects are urinary retention, constipation, and tachycardia.

⚭ CN: Pharmacological and parenteral therapies; CL: Analyze

25. 1. Crash dieting or bingeing may cause an acute attack of pancreatitis and should be avoided. Carbohydrate intake should be increased because carbohydrates are less stimulating to the pancreas. There is no need to maintain a dietary pattern of six meals a day; the client can eat whenever desired. There is no need to place the client on a sodium-restricted diet because pancreatitis does not promote fluid retention.

⚭ CN: Physiological adaptation; CL: Synthesize

26. 2. In chronic pancreatitis, destruction of pancreatic tissue requires pancreatic enzyme replacement. Pancreatic enzymes are prescribed to facilitate the digestion of proteins and fats and should be taken in conjunction with every meal and snack. Specified hours or limited times for administration are ineffective because the enzymes must be taken in conjunction with food ingestion.

⚭ CN: Pharmacological and parenteral therapies; CL: Apply

27. 3. If the dosage and administration of pancreatic enzymes are adequate, the client's stool will be relatively normal. Any increase in odor or fat content would indicate the need for dosage adjustment. Stable body weight would be another indirect indicator. Fluid intake does not affect enzyme replacement therapy. If diabetes has developed, the client will need to monitor glucose levels. However, glucose and ketone levels are not affected by pancreatic enzyme therapy and would not indicate effectiveness of the therapy.

⚭ CN: Pharmacological and parenteral therapies; CL: Evaluate

28. 1. The fluid weight gain is of concern since the drug should be used with caution with impaired renal function. Dosage adjustment may be needed with renal insufficiency since the drug is excreted in the urine. Nausea, mild temperature elevation, and fatigue are symptoms that should be monitored, but are associated with hepatitis.

⚭ CN: Pharmacological and parenteral therapies; CL: Synthesize

The Client with Viral Hepatitis

29. 4. Acetaminophen is toxic to the liver and should be avoided in a client with liver dysfunction. Increased periods of rest allow for liver regeneration. A low-fat, high-carbohydrate diet and dry toast to relieve nausea are appropriate.

⚭ CN: Health promotion and maintenance; CL: Evaluate

30. 4. Hepatitis B is considered a sexually transmitted disease, and students should observe safe sex practices. Poor sanitary conditions in underdeveloped countries relate to spread of hepatitis A and E. Focusing on routes of transmission and avoidance of infection can prevent the spread of hepatitis; isolation in single rooms is not required. There is no vaccine for hepatitis D.

⚷ CN: Reduction of risk potential;
CL: Synthesize

31. 2. Liver inflammation and obstruction block the normal flow of bile. Excess bilirubin turns the skin and sclerae yellow and the urine dark and frothy. Profound anorexia is also common. Tarry stools are indicative of gastrointestinal bleeding and would not be expected in hepatitis. Light- or clay-colored stools may occur in hepatitis owing to bile duct obstruction. Shortness of breath would be unexpected.

⚷ CN: Physiological adaptation;
CL: Analyze

32. 1. The main route of transmission for hepatitis A is the oral-fecal route, rarely parenteral. Good handwashing before eating or preparing food is essential to preventing spread of the disease. Percutaneous transmission is seen with hepatitis B, C, and D. Alpha-interferon is used for treatment of chronic hepatitis B and C.

⚷ CN: Safety and infection control;
CL: Synthesize

33. 3. Clients with hepatitis C should receive genotype testing to determine the most effective treatment approach, and it must be done prior to the start of drug treatment with alpha-interferon. There are six types of hepatitis C genotypes, and clients have different responses to drugs depending on their genotype. For example, clients with genotype 2 or 3 are three times more likely to respond to treatment than those with genotype 1. The recommended course of duration of treatment also depends on genotype. Clients with genotype 2 or 3 usually have a 24-week course of treatment, whereas a 48-week course is recommended for clients with genotype 1. HCV has a high possibility of converting to chronic HCV and will not resolve in 2 to 4 months.

⚷ CN: Physiologic adaptation; CL: Apply

34. 2,4,5. Clients with chronic hepatitis C should abstain from alcohol as it can speed cirrhosis and end-stage liver disease. Clients should also check with their **HCPs** 📖 before taking any nonprescription or prescription medications, or herbal supplements. It is also important that clients who are infected with HCV be tested for HIV, as clients who have both HIV and HCV have a more rapid progression of liver disease than do those who have HCV alone. Clients with HCV and nausea should be instructed to eat four to five times a day to help reduce anorexia and nausea. The client should obtain sufficient rest to manage the fatigue.

⚷ CN: Physiologic adaptation;
CL: Synthesize

35. 4. During the convalescent or posticteric stage of hepatitis, fatigue and malaise are the most common problems. These symptoms usually disappear within 2 to 4 months. Fatigue and malaise are not evidence of a secondary infection. Hepatitis A is not treated by drug therapy. It is important that the client continue to balance activity with periods of rest.

⚷ CN: Reduction of risk potential;
CL: Synthesize

36. 4. Although primarily bloodborne, unprotected sex with multiple partners and a history of sexually transmitted disease are risk factors for transmission of the hepatitis C virus. Other risk factors include blood transfusions, past treatment with chronic hemodialysis, being a child born to woman infected with hepatitis C virus, past/current illicit IV drug use, or needlestick injuries to healthcare workers. It is important for the nurse to be aware of the client's history in order to help determine the client's level of understanding of the disease, promote a healthy lifestyle, and discuss the role of viral transmission of the disease.

⚷ CN: Safety and infection control;
CL: Synthesize

37. 1. Current therapy includes a combination of IV interferon and ribavirin that often includes unpleasant side effects and requires frequent monitoring. The recent approval of oral, directly acting antiviral agents (telaprevir, boceprevir, sofosbuvir, simeprevir) is expected to decrease monitoring rates and increase cure rates, though these drugs are currently very expensive. Though answers 3 and 4 may be true, it is not appropriate for the nurse to make judgments about a client's health insurance or lifestyle choices.

⚷ CN: Pharmacological and parenteral
therapies; CL: Synthesize

38. 1. Treatment of hepatitis consists primarily of bed rest with bathroom privileges. Bed rest is maintained during the acute phase to reduce metabolic demands on the liver, thus increasing its blood supply and promoting liver cell regeneration. When activity is gradually resumed, the client should be taught to rest before becoming overly tired. Although adequate fluid intake is important, it is not necessary to force fluids to treat hepatitis. Antibiotics are not used to treat hepatitis. Electrolyte imbalances are not typical of hepatitis.

⚷ CN: Basic care and comfort;
CL: Synthesize

39. 1. The prothrombin time may be prolonged because of decreased absorption of vitamin K and decreased production of prothrombin by the liver. The client should be assessed carefully for bleeding tendencies. Blood glucose, serum potassium, and serum calcium levels are not affected by hepatitis.

CN: Reduction of risk potential; CL: Analyze

40. 2. Low-fat, high-protein, high-carbohydrate diet is encouraged for a client with hepatitis to promote liver rejuvenation. Nutrition intake is important because clients may be anorexic and experience weight loss. Activity should be modified and adequate rest obtained to promote recovery. Social isolation should be avoided, and education on preventing transmission should be provided; the client does not need to sleep in a separate room.

CN: Health promotion and maintenance; CL: Synthesize

41. 3. The hepatitis A virus is transmitted via the fecal-oral route. It spreads through contaminated hands, water, and food, especially shellfish growing in contaminated water. Certain animal handlers are at risk for hepatitis A, particularly those handling primates. Frequent handwashing is probably the single most important preventive action. Insects do not transmit hepatitis A. Family members do not need to stay away from the client with hepatitis. It is not necessary to disinfect food and clothing.

CN: Safety and infection control; CL: Synthesize

42. 4. The most appropriate goal for this client with hepatitis is to increase activity gradually as tolerated. Periods of alternating rest and activity should be included in the plan of care. There is no evidence that the client is physically immobile, is unable to provide self-care, or needs to adapt to new energy levels.

CN: Basic care and comfort; CL: Analyze

43. 3. Interferon alfa-2b most commonly causes flulike adverse effects, such as myalgia, arthralgia, headache, nausea, fever, and fatigue. Retinopathy is a potential adverse effect, but not a common one. Diarrhea may develop as an adverse effect. Clients are advised to administer the drug at bedtime and get adequate rest. Medications may be prescribed to treat the symptoms. The drug may also cause hematologic changes; therefore, laboratory tests such as a complete blood count and differential should be conducted monthly during drug therapy. Blood glucose laboratory values should be monitored for the development of hyperglycemia.

CN: Pharmacological and parenteral therapies; CL: Analyze

44. 4. Hepatitis B is spread through exposure to blood or blood products and through high-risk sexual activity. Hepatitis B is considered to be a sexually transmitted disease. High-risk sexual activities include sex with multiple partners, unprotected sex with an infected individual, male homosexual activity, and sexual activity with IV drug users. College students are at high risk for development of hepatitis B and are encouraged to be immunized. Alcohol intake by itself does not predispose an individual to hepatitis B, but it can lead to high-risk behaviors such as unprotected sex. Good personal hygiene alone will not prevent the transmission of hepatitis B.

CN: Safety and infection control; CL: Create

45. 2. The client should be able to verbalize the importance of reporting any bleeding tendencies that could be the result of a prolonged prothrombin time. Ascites is not typically a clinical manifestation of hepatitis; it is associated with cirrhosis. Alcohol use should be eliminated for at least 1 year after the diagnosis of hepatitis to allow the liver time to fully recover. There is no need for a client to be restricted to the home because hepatitis is not spread through casual contact between individuals.

CN: Physiological adaptation; CL: Evaluate

The Client with Cirrhosis

46. 1. Because the biopsy needle insertion site is close to the lung, there is a risk of lung puncture and pneumothorax; therefore, immediately after the procedure, the nurse should determine diminished or absent lung sounds in the right lung. Although fever indicates infection, a rise in temperature is not seen immediately. A CBC is warranted if the vital signs and client symptoms indicate potential hemorrhage. The needle insertion site is covered with a pressure dressing; there is no need for a dressing requiring packing.

CN: Safety and infection control; CL: Synthesize

47. The nurse places the client in supine position and percusses each flank for shifting dullness. If fluid is present, dullness is noted.

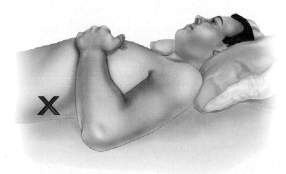

CN: Physiological Adaptation; CL: Apply

48. 1. Clients with cirrhosis can develop hepatic encephalopathy caused by increased ammonia levels. Asterixis, a flapping tremor, is a characteristic symptom of increased ammonia levels. Bacterial action on increased protein in the bowel will increase ammonia levels and cause the encephalopathy to worsen. GI bleeding and protein consumed in the diet increase protein in the intestine and can elevate ammonia levels. Lactulose is given to reduce ammonia formation in the intestine and should not be held since neurological symptoms are worsening. Bilirubin is associated with jaundice.

🔑 CN: Pharmacological and parenteral therapies; CL: Synthesize

49. 3. Hypokalemia is a precipitating factor in hepatic encephalopathy. A decrease in creatinine results from muscle atrophy; an increase in creatinine would indicate renal insufficiency. With liver dysfunction, increased aldosterone levels are seen. A decrease in serum protein will decrease colloid osmotic pressure and promote edema.

🔑 CN: Physiological adaptation; CL: Synthesize

50. 4. Portal hypertension and hypoalbuminemia as a result of cirrhosis cause a fluid shift into the peritoneal space causing ascites. In a cardiac or kidney problem, not cirrhosis, sodium can promote edema formation and subsequent decreased urine output. Edema does not migrate upward toward the heart to enhance its circulation. Although diuretics promote the excretion of excess fluid, occasionally forgetting or omitting a dose will not yield the ascites found in cirrhosis of the liver.

🔑 CN: Physiological adaptation; CL: Synthesize

51. 1,2,3,4,5. Constipation leads to increased ammonia production. Lactulose is a hyperosmotic laxative that reduces blood ammonia by acidifying the colon contents, which retards diffusion of nonionic ammonia from the colon to the blood while promoting its migration from the blood to the colon. Hepatic encephalopathy is considered a toxic or metabolic condition that causes cerebral edema; it affects a person's coordination and pupil reaction to light and accommodation. Food and fluids high in carbohydrates should be given because the liver is not synthesizing and storing glucose. Because exercise produces ammonia as a by-product of metabolism, physical activity should be limited, not encouraged.

🔑 CN: Management of care; CL: Create

52. 3. Early clinical manifestations of cirrhosis are subtle and usually include gastrointestinal symptoms, such as anorexia, nausea, vomiting, and changes in bowel patterns. These changes are caused by the liver's altered ability to metabolize carbohydrates, proteins, and fats. Peripheral edema, ascites, and jaundice are later signs of liver failure and portal hypertension.

🔑 CN: Physiological adaptation; CL: Analyze

53. 2. Spironolactone is a potassium-sparing diuretic; therefore, clients should be monitored closely for hyperkalemia. Other common adverse effects include abdominal cramping, diarrhea, dizziness, headache, and rash. Constipation and dysuria are not common adverse effects of spironolactone. An irregular pulse is not an adverse effect of spironolactone but could develop if serum potassium levels are not closely monitored.

🔑 CN: Pharmacological and parenteral therapies; CL: Analyze

54. 1. For clients who have cirrhosis without complications, a high-calorie, high-carbohydrate diet is preferred to provide an adequate supply of nutrients. In the early stages of cirrhosis, there is no need to restrict fat, protein, or sodium.

🔑 CN: Physiological adaptation; CL: Apply

55. 2,3,4. Baking soda baths can decrease pruritus. Keeping nails short and rubbing the area with knuckles can decrease breakdown when scratching. Calamine lotions help relieve itching. Alcohol will increase skin dryness. Sodium in the diet will increase edema and weaken skin integrity.

🔑 CN: Basic care and comfort; CL: Create

56. 2. General health promotion measures include maintaining good nutrition, avoiding infection, and abstaining from alcohol. It is not necessary to take multivitamins if the client is obtaining adequate nutrition. Rest and sleep are essential, but an impaired liver may not be able to detoxify sedatives and barbiturates. Such drugs must be used cautiously, if at all, by clients with cirrhosis. The client does not need to limit contact with others but should exercise caution to stay away from ill people.

🔑 CN: Health promotion and maintenance; CL: Synthesize

57. 4. Elevating the head of the bed will allow for increased lung expansion by decreasing the ascites pressing on the diaphragm. The client requires reassessment. A paracentesis is reserved for symptomatic clients with ascites with impaired respiration or abdominal pain not responding to other measures such as sodium restriction and diuretics. There is no indication for blood cultures. Heart sounds are assessed with the routine physical assessment.

🔑 CN: Physiological adaptation; CL: Synthesize

58. 1. Ascites can compromise the action of the diaphragm and increase the client's risk of respiratory problems. Ascites also greatly increases the risk of skin breakdown. Frequent position changes are important, but the preferred position is Fowler's. Placing the client in Fowler's position helps facilitate the client's breathing by relieving pressure on the diaphragm. The other positions do not relieve pressure on the diaphragm.

CN: Reduction of risk potential; **CL:** Synthesize

59. 4. The client with esophageal varices is at even higher risk for bleeding with elevated PT/INR. The nurse and **HCP** collaborate to prevent bleeding. The other laboratory findings are not as life threatening. A decreased serum albumin can cause fluid to move into the interstitial tissues. Increased ammonia levels are toxic to the brain. Calcium loss is more common to pancreatitis.

CN: Physiological Adaptation; **CL:** Synthesize

60. 1. Normal serum albumin is administered to reduce ascites. Hypoalbuminemia, a mechanism underlying ascites formation, results in decreased colloid osmotic pressure. Administering serum albumin increases the plasma colloid osmotic pressure, which causes fluid to flow from the tissue space into the plasma. Increased urine output is the best indication that the albumin is having the desired effect. An increased serum albumin level and increased ease of breathing may indirectly imply that the administration of albumin is effective in relieving the ascites. However, it is not as direct an indicator as increased urine output and reduced ascites. Anorexia is not affected by the administration of albumin.

CN: Pharmacological and parenteral therapies; **CL:** Evaluate

61. 1,3,2,4. The nurse should first assess the client to determine if the tube is obstructing the airway; assessment is done by assessing airflow. Once obstruction is established, the tube should be deflated and then quickly removed. A set of scissors should always be at the bedside to allow for emergency deflation of the balloon. Oxygen via face mask should then be applied once the tube is removed.

CN: Safety and infection control; **CL:** Synthesize

62. 3. The goal of abstinence from alcohol in clients with alcohol-induced cirrhosis is to improve the liver function; most clients have improved liver function when they abstain from alcohol. Clients with cirrhosis do not necessarily have delirium tremens. Abstaining from alcohol may allow the client to improve nutritional status, but additional dietary counseling may be needed to achieve that goal.

Clients with cirrhosis may have weight gain from ascites, but this is managed with diuretics.

CN: Pharmacological and parenteral therapies; **CL:** Evaluate

63. 1. The client should be monitored closely for changes in mental status. Ammonia has a toxic effect on central nervous system tissue and produces an altered level of consciousness, marked by drowsiness and irritability. If this process is unchecked, the client may lapse into coma. Increasing ammonia levels are not detected by changes in blood pressure, urine output, or respirations.

CN: Physiological adaptation; **CL:** Analyze

64. 3. Lactulose increases intestinal motility, thereby trapping and expelling ammonia in the feces. An increase in the number of bowel movements is expected as an adverse effect. Lactulose does not affect urine output. Any improvements in mental status would be the result of increased ammonia elimination, not an adverse effect of the drug. Nausea and vomiting are not common adverse effects of lactulose.

CN: Pharmacological and parenteral therapies; **CL:** Apply

65. 60 mL

$$30 \text{ mL} = 1 \text{ oz}$$

The following formula is used to calculate the correct dosage:

$$30 \text{ mL}/1 \text{ oz} = X \text{ mL}/2 \text{ oz}$$
$$X = 60 \text{ mL}.$$

CN: Pharmacological and parenteral therapies; **CL:** Apply

66. 2. The taste of lactulose is a problem for some clients. Mixing it with fruit juice, water, or milk can make it more palatable. Lactulose should not be given with antacids, which may inhibit its action. Lactulose should not be taken with a laxative because increased stooling is an adverse effect of the drug and would be potentiated by using a laxative. Lactulose comes in the form of syrup for oral or rectal administration.

CN: Pharmacological and parenteral therapies; **CL:** Evaluate

67. 3. Clients with cirrhosis should be instructed to avoid constipation and straining at stool to prevent hemorrhage. The client with cirrhosis has bleeding tendencies because of the liver's inability to produce clotting factors. A low-protein and high-carbohydrate diet is recommended. Clients with cirrhosis should not take acetaminophen, which is potentially hepatotoxic. Aspirin also should be avoided if esophageal varices are present. Cirrhosis is a chronic disease.

CN: Reduction of risk potential; **CL:** Evaluate

68. 1. Immediately before a paracentesis, the client should empty the bladder to prevent perforation. The client will be placed in a high Fowler's position or seated on the side of the bed for the procedure. IV sedatives are not usually administered. The client does not need to be NPO.

CN: Reduction of risk potential;
CL: Synthesize

69. 3. Edematous tissue is easily traumatized and must receive meticulous care. An alternating air pressure mattress will help decrease pressure on the edematous tissue. ROM exercises are important to maintain joint function, but they do not necessarily prevent skin breakdown. When abdominal skin is stretched taut due to ascites, it must be cleaned very carefully. The abdomen should not be massaged. Elevation of the lower extremities promotes venous return and decreases swelling.

CN: Reduction of risk potential;
CL: Synthesize

Managing Care, Quality, and Safety of Clients with Biliary Tract Disorders

70. 4. Contact precautions are recommended for clients with hepatitis A. This includes wearing gloves for direct care. A gown is not required unless substantial contact with the client is anticipated. It is not necessary to wear a mask. The client does not need a private room unless incontinent of stool.

CN: Safety and infection control;
CL: Create

71. 4. A change in a client's baseline vital signs should be brought to the **HCP's** 🔲 attention immediately. In this case, the client's heart rate has increased, and the rhythm appears to have changed; the HCP may prescribe an ECG to determine if treatment is necessary. The nurse should also have a complete set of current vital signs as well as a physical assessment before providing the HCP information using the SBAR format. The nutritional as well as psychological needs of a client must be addressed but are not first priority. A rash that develops after a new antibiotic is started must be brought to the HCP attention; however, this client is stable and is not the first priority. The nurse is responsible to facilitate discussion between the client, the client's family, and the HCP, but only after all of the immediate physical and psychological needs of all clients have been met.

CN: Reduction of risk potential;
CL: Synthesize

72. 1,3,2,4. The nurse should first assess the client with cirrhosis to ensure the client's safety and assess the client for the onset of hepatic encephalopathy. The nurse should then assess the client with acute pancreatitis who is requesting pain medication and administer the needed medication. The nurse should next assess the client who underwent a cholecystectomy and is 1 day postoperative to make sure that the T tube is draining and that the client is performing postoperative breathing exercises. This client's safety is not at risk, and the client is not reporting having pain. The nurse can speak last with the client with hepatitis B who has questions about discharge instructions because this client's issues are not urgent.

CN: Management of care; CL: Synthesize

73. 2. Hepatitis C is usually transmitted through blood exposure or needlesticks. A hepatitis C vaccine is currently under development, but it is not available for use. The first line of defense against hepatitis B is the hepatitis B vaccine. Hepatitis C is not transmitted through feces or urine. Wearing a gown and mask will not prevent transmission of the hepatitis C virus if the caregiver comes in contact with infected blood or needles.

CN: Safety and infection control;
CL: Apply

74. 1,3,4,2. Silencing the alarm will eliminate a stress to the client and allow the nurse to focus on the task at hand. The nurse should then assess the access site to note if the needle is inserted in the vein or if there is tissue trauma, infiltration, or inflammation. Next, the nurse should check for kinks in the tubing. Finally, the nurse can plug the pump into the wall to allow the battery to become recharged.

CN: Pharmacological and parenteral therapies; CL: Synthesize

The Client with Endocrine Health Problems

- The Client with Disorders of the Thyroid
- The Client with Diabetes Mellitus
- The Client with Pituitary Adenoma
- The Client with Addison's Disease
- The Client with Cushing's Disease
- Managing Care, Quality, and Safety of Clients with Endocrine Health Problems
- Answers, Rationales, and Test-Taking Strategies

The Client with Disorders of the Thyroid

1. The nurse is completing a health assessment of a 42-year-old female with suspected Graves' disease. The nurse should assess this client for:
- ☐ **1.** anorexia.
- ☐ **2.** tachycardia.
- ☐ **3.** weight gain.
- ☐ **4.** cold skin.

2. When conducting a health history with a female client with thyrotoxicosis, the nurse should ask about which changes in the menstrual cycle?
- ☐ **1.** dysmenorrhea
- ☐ **2.** metrorrhagia
- ☐ **3.** oligomenorrhea
- ☐ **4.** menorrhagia

3. A 34-year-old female is diagnosed with hypothyroidism. What should the nurse assess the client for? Select all that apply.
- ☐ **1.** rapid pulse
- ☐ **2.** decreased energy and fatigue
- ☐ **3.** weight gain of 10 lb (4.5 kg)
- ☐ **4.** fine, thin hair with hair loss
- ☐ **5.** constipation
- ☐ **6.** menorrhagia

4. Propylthiouracil (PTU) is prescribed for a client with Graves' disease. The nurse should teach the client to immediately report:
- ☐ **1.** sore throat.
- ☐ **2.** painful, excessive menstruation.
- ☐ **3.** constipation.
- ☐ **4.** increased urine output.

5. A client with thyrotoxicosis says to the nurse, "I am so irritable. I am having problems at work because I lose my temper very easily." Which response by the nurse would give the client the **most** accurate explanation of this behavior?
- ☐ **1.** "Your behavior is caused by temporary confusion brought on by your illness."
- ☐ **2.** "Your behavior is caused by the excess thyroid hormone in your system."
- ☐ **3.** "Your behavior is caused by your worrying about the seriousness of your illness."
- ☐ **4.** "Your behavior is caused by the stress of trying to manage a career and cope with illness."

6. The nurse is evaluating a client with hyperthyroidism who is taking propylthiouracil (PTU) 100 mg/day in three divided doses for maintenance therapy. Which statement from the client indicates the drug is effective?
- ☐ **1.** "I have excess energy throughout the day."
- ☐ **2.** "I am able to sleep and rest at night."
- ☐ **3.** "I have lost weight since taking this medication."
- ☐ **4.** "I do perspire throughout the entire day."

7. A client with hyperthyroidism is hospitalized to have a thyroidectomy. The healthcare provider (HCP) has prescribed propranolol. In reviewing the client's history, the nurse notes that the client has asthma. The nurse should **next**:
- ☐ **1.** take the client's pulse and withhold the propranolol if the pulse is <100 beats per minute.
- ☐ **2.** count the client's respirations and withhold the propranolol if the respirations are <20 breaths per minute.
- ☐ **3.** contact the HCP and discuss the prescription for propranolol because of the client's history of having asthma.
- ☐ **4.** instruct the client to make position changes slowly.

8. The nurse should teach the client with Graves' disease to prevent corneal irritation from mild exophthalmos by:

☐ 1. massaging the eyes at regular intervals.

☐ 2. instilling an ophthalmic anesthetic as prescribed.

☐ 3. wearing dark-colored glasses.

☐ 4. covering both eyes with moistened gauze pads.

9. After treatment with radioactive iodine (RAI, 1-131) I, the nurse should teach the client to:

☐ 1. monitor for signs and symptoms of hyperthyroidism.

☐ 2. rest for 1 week to prevent complications of the medication.

☐ 3. take thyroxine replacement for the remainder of the client's life.

☐ 4. assess for hypertension and tachycardia resulting from altered thyroid activity.

10. A client with a large goiter is scheduled for a subtotal thyroidectomy to treat thyrotoxicosis. Saturated solution of potassium iodide (SSKI) is prescribed preoperatively for the client. The expected outcome of using this drug is that it helps:

☐ 1. slow progression of exophthalmos.

☐ 2. reduce the vascularity of the thyroid gland.

☐ 3. decrease the body's ability to store thyroxine.

☐ 4. increase the body's ability to excrete thyroxine.

11. The nurse is administering a saturated solution of potassium iodide (SSKI). The nurse should:

☐ 1. pour the solution over ice chips.

☐ 2. mix the solution with an antacid.

☐ 3. dilute the solution with water, milk, or fruit juice and have the client drink it with a straw.

☐ 4. disguise the solution in a pureed fruit or vegetable.

12. Following a subtotal thyroidectomy, the nurse asks the client to speak immediately upon regaining consciousness. The nurse does this to monitor for signs of:

☐ 1. internal hemorrhage.

☐ 2. decreasing level of consciousness.

☐ 3. laryngeal nerve damage.

☐ 4. upper airway obstruction.

13. A client who has undergone a subtotal thyroidectomy is subject to complications in the first 48 hours after surgery. The nurse should obtain and keep at the bedside equipment to:

☐ 1. begin total parenteral nutrition.

☐ 2. initiate defibrillation.

☐ 3. administer tube feedings.

☐ 4. perform a tracheotomy.

14. One day following a subtotal thyroidectomy, a client begins to have tingling in the fingers and toes. The nurse should **first**:

☐ 1. encourage the client to flex and extend the fingers and toes.

☐ 2. notify the healthcare provider (HCP).

☐ 3. assess the client for thrombophlebitis.

☐ 4. ask the client to speak.

15. Which medication should be available to provide emergency treatment if a client develops tetany after a subtotal thyroidectomy?

☐ 1. sodium phosphate

☐ 2. calcium gluconate

☐ 3. echothiophate iodide

☐ 4. sodium bicarbonate

16. A 60-year-old female is diagnosed with hypothyroidism. The nurse should assess the client for:

☐ 1. tachycardia.

☐ 2. weight gain.

☐ 3. diarrhea.

☐ 4. nausea.

17. The nurse should assess a client with hypothyroidism for:

☐ 1. corneal abrasion due to inability to close the eyelids.

☐ 2. weight loss due to hypermetabolism.

☐ 3. fluid loss due to diarrhea.

☐ 4. decreased activity due to fatigue.

18. When discussing recent onset of feelings of sadness and depression in a client with hypothyroidism who has just started to take thyroid hormone replacement, the nurse should inform the client that these feelings are:

☐ 1. the effects of thyroid hormone replacement therapy and will diminish over time.

☐ 2. related to thyroid hormone replacement therapy and will not diminish over time.

☐ 3. a normal part of having a chronic illness.

☐ 4. most likely related to low thyroid hormone levels and will improve with treatment.

19. The nurse is instructing the client with hypothyroidism who takes levothyroxine 100 mcg, digoxin, and simvastatin. Teaching regarding the use of these medications is effective if the client will take:

☐ 1. the levothyroxine with breakfast and the other medications after breakfast.

☐ 2. the levothyroxine before breakfast and the other medications 4 hours later.

☐ 3. all medications together 1 hour after eating breakfast.

☐ 4. all medications before going to bed.

The Client with Diabetes Mellitus

20. The nurse is coaching a diabetic client using an empowerment approach. The nurse should initiate teaching by asking:
☐ 1. "How much does your family need to be involved in learning about your condition?"
☐ 2. "What is required for your family to manage your symptoms?"
☐ 3. "What activities are most important for you to be able to maintain control of your diabetes?"
☐ 4. "What do you know about your medications and condition?"

21. The nurse is obtaining a health history from a client with diabetes mellitus who has been taking insulin for 20 years. Currently, the client reports having periods of hypoglycemia followed by periods of hyperglycemia. The nurse should specifically ask if the client is:
☐ 1. eating snacks between meals.
☐ 2. initiating the use of the insulin pump.
☐ 3. injecting insulin at a site of lipodystrophy.
☐ 4. adjusting insulin according to blood glucose levels.

22. A nurse is participating in a diabetes screening program. Who are at risk for developing type 2 diabetes? Select all that apply.
☐ 1. a 32-year-old female who gave birth to a 9½-lb (4,300-g) infant.
☐ 2. a 44-year-old Native American (First Nations) who has a body mass index (BMI) of 32.
☐ 3. an 18-year-old immigrant from Mexico who jogs four times a week.
☐ 4. a 55-year-old Asian who has hypertension and two siblings with type 2 diabetes.
☐ 5. a 12-year-old who is overweight.

23. An adult with type 2 diabetes mellitus has been NPO since 2200 in preparation for having a nephrectomy the next day. At 0600 on the day of surgery, the nurse reviews the client's medical record and laboratory results. Which finding should the nurse report to the healthcare provider (HCP)?
☐ 1. urine output of 350 mL in 8 hours
☐ 2. urine specific gravity of 1.015
☐ 3. potassium of 4.0 mEq (4 mmol/L)
☐ 4. blood glucose of 140 mg/dL (7.8 mmol/L)

24. The nurse is checking the laboratory results of an adult client with type 1 diabetes (see chart). What laboratory result indicates a problem that should be managed?

Laboratory Results

Test	Result
Blood glucose	192 mg/dL (10.7 mmol/L)
Total cholesterol	250 mg/dL (6.5 mmol/L)
Hemoglobin	12.3 mg/dL (123 g/L)
Low-density lipoprotein cholesterol	125 mg/dL (3.2 mmol/L)

☐ 1. blood glucose
☐ 2. total cholesterol
☐ 3. hemoglobin
☐ 4. low-density lipoprotein (LDL) cholesterol

25. A client with type 1 diabetes mellitus has diabetic ketoacidosis. Which finding has the **greatest** effect on fluid loss?
☐ 1. hypotension
☐ 2. decreased serum potassium level
☐ 3. rapid, deep respirations
☐ 4. warm, dry skin

26. A client is to receive glargine insulin in addition to a dose of aspart. When the nurse checks the blood glucose level at the bedside, it is >200 mg/dL (11.1 mmol/L). How should the nurse administer the insulins?
☐ 1. Put air into the glargine insulin vial and then air into the aspart insulin vial, and draw up the correct dose of aspart insulin first.
☐ 2. Roll the glargine insulin vial, and then roll the aspart insulin vial. Draw up the longer-acting glargine insulin first.
☐ 3. Shake both vials of insulin before drawing up each dose in separate insulin syringes.
☐ 4. Put air into the glargine insulin vial, and draw up the correct dose in an insulin syringe; then with a different insulin syringe, put air into the aspart vial, and draw up the correct dose.

27. The client with type 2 insulin-requiring diabetes asks the nurse about having alcoholic beverages. Which is the **best** response by the nurse?
☐ 1. "You can have one or two drinks a day as long as you have something to eat with them."
☐ 2. "Alcohol is detoxified in the liver, so it is not a good idea for you to drink anything with alcohol."
☐ 3. "If you are going to have a drink, it is best to consume alcohol on an empty stomach."
☐ 4. "If you do have a drink, the blood glucose value may be elevated at bedtime, and you should skip having a snack."

50. A nurse is teaching a client with type 1 diabetes mellitus who jogs daily about the preferred sites for insulin absorption. What is the **most** appropriate site for a client who jogs?
- [ ] 1. arms
- [ ] 2. legs
- [ ] 3. abdomen
- [ ] 4. iliac crest

51. A client with diabetes is taking insulin lispro injections. The nurse should advise the client to eat:
- [ ] 1. within 10 to 15 minutes after the injection.
- [ ] 2. 1 hour after the injection.
- [ ] 3. at any time because timing of meals with lispro injections is unnecessary.
- [ ] 4. 2 hours before the injection.

52. The **best** indicator that the client has learned how to give an insulin self-injection correctly is when the client can:
- [ ] 1. perform the procedure safely and correctly.
- [ ] 2. critique the nurse's performance of the procedure.
- [ ] 3. explain all steps of the procedure correctly.
- [ ] 4. obtain 100% correct answers on a posttest.

53. The nurse is instructing the client on insulin administration. The client is performing a return demonstration for preparing the insulin. The client's morning dose of insulin is 10 units of regular and 22 units of NPH. The nurse checks the dose accuracy with the client. The nurse determines that the client has prepared the correct dose when the syringe reads how many units? Record your answer using a whole number.

_____ units.

54. Angiotensin-converting enzyme (ACE) inhibitors may be prescribed for the client with diabetes mellitus to reduce vascular changes and possibly prevent or delay development of:
- [ ] 1. chronic obstructive pulmonary disease (COPD).
- [ ] 2. pancreatic cancer.
- [ ] 3. renal failure.
- [ ] 4. cerebrovascular accident.

55. The nurse should teach the diabetic client that which symptom is **most** indicative of hypoglycemia?
- [ ] 1. nervousness
- [ ] 2. anorexia
- [ ] 3. Kussmaul's respirations
- [ ] 4. bradycardia

56. The nurse is assessing the client's understanding of the use of medications. Which medication may cause a complication with the treatment plan of a client with diabetes?
- [ ] 1. aspirin
- [ ] 2. steroids
- [ ] 3. sulfonylureas
- [ ] 4. angiotensin-converting enzyme (ACE) inhibitors

57. A client with type 1 diabetes mellitus has influenza. The nurse should instruct the client to:
- [ ] 1. increase the frequency of self-monitoring (blood glucose testing).
- [ ] 2. reduce food intake to diminish nausea.
- [ ] 3. discontinue that dose of insulin if unable to eat.
- [ ] 4. take half of the normal dose of insulin.

58. Which goal is a **priority** for the diabetic client who is taking insulin and has nausea and vomiting from a viral illness or influenza?
- [ ] 1. obtaining adequate food intake
- [ ] 2. managing own health
- [ ] 3. relieving pain
- [ ] 4. increasing activity

59. A client with diabetes begins to cry and says, "I just cannot stand the thought of having to give myself a shot every day." What would be the **best** response by the nurse?
- [ ] 1. "If you do not give yourself your insulin shots, you will be at greater risk for complications."
- [ ] 2. "We can teach a family member to give the shots so you will not have to do it."
- [ ] 3. "I can arrange to have a home care nurse give you the shots every day."
- [ ] 4. "What is it about giving yourself the insulin shots that bothers you?"

The Client with Pituitary Adenoma

60. A client is to have a transsphenoidal hypophysectomy to remove a large, invasive pituitary tumor. The nurse should instruct the client that the surgery will be performed through an incision in the:
- [ ] 1. back of the mouth.
- [ ] 2. nose.
- [ ] 3. sinus channel below the right eye.
- [ ] 4. upper gingival mucosa in the space between the upper gums and lip.

61. To minimize the risk of postoperative respiratory complications after a hypophysectomy, the nurse should instruct the client how to:
- [ ] 1. limit use of pain medications.
- [ ] 2. turn in bed.
- [ ] 3. take deep breaths.
- [ ] 4. clear the throat and cough.

62. Following a transsphenoidal hypophysectomy, the nurse should assess the client for:
- [ ] 1. cerebrospinal fluid (CSF) leak.
- [ ] 2. fluctuating blood glucose levels.
- [ ] 3. Cushing's syndrome.
- [ ] 4. cardiac arrhythmias.

63. A male client expresses concern about how a hypophysectomy will affect his sexual function. Which statement provides the **most** accurate information about the physiologic effects of hypophysectomy in a male?
- ☐ 1. Removing the source of excess hormone should restore the client's libido, erectile function, and fertility.
- ☐ 2. Potency will be restored, but the client will remain infertile.
- ☐ 3. Fertility will be restored, but impotence and decreased libido will persist.
- ☐ 4. Exogenous hormones will be needed to restore erectile function after the adenoma is removed.

64. Initial treatment for a cerebrospinal fluid (CSF) leak after transsphenoidal hypophysectomy would **most** likely involve:
- ☐ 1. repacking the nose with pressure dressings.
- ☐ 2. returning the client to surgery to close the leak.
- ☐ 3. maintaining bed rest with the head of the bed elevated to 30 degrees.
- ☐ 4. administering high-dose corticosteroid therapy.

65. To provide oral hygiene for a client recovering from transsphenoidal hypophysectomy, the nurse should instruct the client to:
- ☐ 1. rinse the mouth with saline.
- ☐ 2. perform frequent toothbrushing.
- ☐ 3. clean the teeth with an electric toothbrush.
- ☐ 4. floss the teeth thoroughly.

66. The nurse teaches the client to report signs and symptoms of which potential complication after hypophysectomy?
- ☐ 1. acromegaly
- ☐ 2. Cushing's disease
- ☐ 3. diabetes mellitus
- ☐ 4. hypopituitarism

67. After pituitary surgery, the nurse should assess the client for:
- ☐ 1. urine specific gravity <1.010.
- ☐ 2. urine output between 1 and 2 L/day.
- ☐ 3. blood glucose level higher than 300 mg/dL (16.7 mmol/L).
- ☐ 4. urine negative for glucose and ketones.

68. Vasopressin is administered to the client with diabetes insipidus because it:
- ☐ 1. decreases blood pressure.
- ☐ 2. increases tubular reabsorption of water.
- ☐ 3. increases release of insulin from the pancreas.
- ☐ 4. decreases glucose production within the liver.

69. Which indicates that the client with diabetes insipidus understands how to manage care?
- ☐ 1. The client will maintain normal fluid and electrolyte balance.
- ☐ 2. The client will select a diabetic diet correctly.
- ☐ 3. The client will state dietary restrictions.
- ☐ 4. The client will exhibit serum glucose level within normal range.

The Client with Addison's Disease

70. The nurse is instructing a college student with Addison's disease how to adjust the dose of glucocorticoids. The nurse should explain that the client may need an increased dosage of glucocorticoids in which situation?
- ☐ 1. completing the spring semester of school
- ☐ 2. gaining 4 lb (1.8 kg)
- ☐ 3. becoming engaged
- ☐ 4. having wisdom teeth extracted

71. Which goal is the **priority** for a client in addisonian crisis?
- ☐ 1. controlling hypertension
- ☐ 2. preventing irreversible shock
- ☐ 3. preventing infection
- ☐ 4. relieving anxiety

72. Which is an expected finding in a client with adrenal crisis (addisonian crisis)?
- ☐ 1. fluid retention
- ☐ 2. pain
- ☐ 3. peripheral edema
- ☐ 4. hunger

73. A client with Addison's disease is taking corticosteroid replacement therapy. The nurse should instruct the client about which side effects of corticosteroids? Select all that apply.
- ☐ 1. hyperkalemia
- ☐ 2. skeletal muscle weakness
- ☐ 3. mood changes
- ☐ 4. hypocalcemia
- ☐ 5. increased susceptibility to infection
- ☐ 6. hypotension

74. The client is receiving an IV infusion of 5% dextrose in normal saline running at 125 mL/h. When hanging a new bag of fluid, the nurse notes swelling and hardness at the infusion site. The nurse should **first**:
- ☐ 1. discontinue the infusion.
- ☐ 2. apply a warm soak to the site.
- ☐ 3. stop the flow of solution temporarily.
- ☐ 4. irrigate the needle with normal saline.

75. The client's wife asks the nurse whether the IV infusion is meeting her husband's nutritional needs because he has vomited several times. The nurse's response should be based on the knowledge that 1 L of 5% dextrose in normal saline delivers:
☐ 1. 170 cal.
☐ 2. 250 cal.
☐ 3. 340 cal.
☐ 4. 500 cal.

76. A client with Addison's disease has fluid and electrolyte loss due to inadequate fluid intake and to fluid loss secondary to inadequate adrenal hormone secretion. As the client's oral intake increases, which fluids would be **most** appropriate?
☐ 1. milk and diet soda
☐ 2. water and eggnog
☐ 3. chicken broth and juice
☐ 4. coffee and milkshakes

77. After stabilization of Addison's disease, the nurse teaches the client about stress management. The nurse should instruct the client to:
☐ 1. remove all sources of stress from daily life.
☐ 2. use relaxation techniques such as music.
☐ 3. take antianxiety drugs daily.
☐ 4. avoid discussing stressful experiences.

78. When teaching a client newly diagnosed with primary Addison's disease, the nurse should explain that the disease results from:
☐ 1. insufficient secretion of growth hormone (GH).
☐ 2. dysfunction of the hypothalamic pituitary.
☐ 3. idiopathic atrophy of the adrenal gland.
☐ 4. oversecretion of the adrenal medulla.

79. The nurse is conducting discharge education with a client newly diagnosed with Addison's disease. Which information should be included in the client and family teaching plan? Select all that apply.
☐ 1. Addison's disease will resolve over a few weeks, requiring no further treatment.
☐ 2. Avoiding stress and maintaining a balanced lifestyle will minimize risk for exacerbations.
☐ 3. Fatigue, weakness, dizziness, and mood changes need to be reported to the healthcare provider (HCP).
☐ 4. A medical identification bracelet should be worn.
☐ 5. Family members need to be informed about the warning signals of adrenal crisis.
☐ 6. Dental work or surgery will require adjustment of daily medication.

80. The nurse should assess a client with Addison's disease for:
☐ 1. weight gain.
☐ 2. hunger.
☐ 3. lethargy.
☐ 4. muscle spasms.

81. Which topic is **most** important to include in the teaching plan for a client newly diagnosed with Addison's disease who will be taking corticosteroids?
☐ 1. The importance of watching for signs of hyperglycemia
☐ 2. The need to adjust the steroid dose based on dietary intake and exercise
☐ 3. To notify the healthcare provider (HCP) when the blood pressure is suddenly high
☐ 4. How to decrease the dose of the corticosteroids when the client experiences stress

82. The client with Addison's disease is taking glucocorticoids at home. Which statement indicates that the client understands how to take the medication?
☐ 1. "Various circumstances increase the need for glucocorticoids, so I will need to adjust the dosage."
☐ 2. "My need for glucocorticoids will stabilize, and I will be able to take a predetermined dose once a day."
☐ 3. "Glucocorticoids are cumulative, so I will take a dose every third day."
☐ 4. "I must take a dose every 6 hours to ensure consistent blood levels of glucocorticoids."

83. Cortisone acetate and fludrocortisone acetate are prescribed as replacement therapy for a client with Addison's disease. What administration schedule should be followed for this therapy?
☐ 1. Take both drugs three times a day.
☐ 2. Take the entire dose of both drugs first thing in the morning.
☐ 3. Take all the fludrocortisone acetate and two-thirds of the cortisone acetate in the morning, and take the remaining cortisone acetate in the afternoon.
☐ 4. Take half of each drug in the morning and the remaining half of each drug at bedtime.

84. When teaching a client about taking oral glucocorticoids, how should the nurse instruct the client to take the medication?
☐ 1. with a full glass of water
☐ 2. on an empty stomach
☐ 3. at bedtime to increase absorption
☐ 4. with meals or with an antacid

85. Which indicator is **best** for determining whether a client with Addison's disease is receiving the correct amount of glucocorticoid replacement?
☐ 1. skin turgor
☐ 2. temperature
☐ 3. thirst
☐ 4. daily weight

86. Which outcome is a **priority** for the client with Addison's disease?
- ☐ **1.** maintenance of medication compliance
- ☐ **2.** avoidance of normal activities with stress
- ☐ **3.** adherence to a 2-g sodium diet
- ☐ **4.** prevention of hypertensive episodes

87. The client with Addison's disease should anticipate the need for increased glucocorticoid supplementation when:
- ☐ **1.** returning to work after a weekend.
- ☐ **2.** going on vacation.
- ☐ **3.** having oral surgery.
- ☐ **4.** having a routine medical checkup.

88. The nurse should teach the client with Addison's disease that the bronze-colored skin is thought to be caused by:
- ☐ **1.** hypersensitivity to sun exposure.
- ☐ **2.** increased serum bilirubin level.
- ☐ **3.** adverse effects of the glucocorticoid therapy.
- ☐ **4.** increased secretion of adrenocorticotropic hormone (ACTH).

The Client with Cushing's Disease

89. A client reports that she has gained weight and that her face and body are "rounder," while her legs and arms have become thinner. A tentative diagnosis of Cushing's disease is made. The nurse should further assess the client for:
- ☐ **1.** orthostatic hypotension.
- ☐ **2.** muscle hypertrophy in the extremities.
- ☐ **3.** bruised areas on the skin.
- ☐ **4.** decreased body hair.

90. A client diagnosed with Cushing's syndrome is admitted to the hospital and scheduled for a dexamethasone suppression test. During this test, the nurse should:
- ☐ **1.** collect a 24-hour urine specimen to measure serum cortisol levels.
- ☐ **2.** administer 1 mg of dexamethasone orally at night and obtain serum cortisol levels the next morning.
- ☐ **3.** draw blood samples before and after exercise to evaluate the effect of exercise on serum cortisol levels.
- ☐ **4.** administer an injection of adrenocorticotropic hormone (ACTH) 30 minutes before drawing blood to measure serum cortisol levels.

91. The nurse should monitor the client with Cushing's disease for which finding?
- ☐ **1.** postprandial hypoglycemia
- ☐ **2.** hypokalemia
- ☐ **3.** hyponatremia
- ☐ **4.** decreased urine calcium level

92. A client with Cushing's disease tells the nurse that the healthcare provider (HCP) said the morning serum cortisol level was within normal limits. The client asks, "How can that be? I am not imagining all these symptoms!" The nurse's response will be based on the fact that?
- ☐ **1.** Some clients are very sensitive to the effects of cortisol and develop symptoms even with normal levels.
- ☐ **2.** A single random blood test cannot provide reliable information about endocrine levels.
- ☐ **3.** The excessive cortisol levels seen in Cushing's disease commonly result from loss of the normal diurnal secretion pattern.
- ☐ **4.** Tumors tend to secrete hormones irregularly, and the hormones are generally not present in the blood.

93. The client with Cushing's disease needs to modify dietary intake to control symptoms. In addition to increasing protein, which strategy would be **most** appropriate?
- ☐ **1.** Increase calories.
- ☐ **2.** Restrict sodium.
- ☐ **3.** Restrict potassium.
- ☐ **4.** Reduce fat to 10%.

94. Bone resorption is a possible complication of Cushing's disease. To help the client prevent this complication, the nurse should recommend that the client:
- ☐ **1.** increase the amount of potassium in the diet.
- ☐ **2.** maintain a regular program of weight-bearing exercise.
- ☐ **3.** limit dietary vitamin D intake.
- ☐ **4.** perform isometric exercises.

95. A client has an adrenal tumor and is scheduled for a bilateral adrenalectomy. During preoperative teaching, the nurse teaches the client how to do deep-breathing exercises after surgery by telling the client to:
- ☐ **1.** "Sit in an upright position, and take a deep breath."
- ☐ **2.** "Hold your abdomen firmly with a pillow, and take several deep breaths."
- ☐ **3.** "Tighten your stomach muscles as you inhale, and breathe normally."
- ☐ **4.** "Raise your shoulders to expand your chest."

96. A **priority** in the first 24 hours after a bilateral adrenalectomy is:
- ☐ **1.** beginning oral nutrition.
- ☐ **2.** promoting self-care activities.
- ☐ **3.** preventing adrenal crisis.
- ☐ **4.** ambulating in the hallway.

97. A client undergoing a bilateral adrenalectomy has postoperative prescriptions for hydromorphone hydrochloride 2 mg to be administered subcutaneously every 4 hours PRN for pain. This drug is administered in relatively small doses **primarily** because it is:

☐ 1. less likely to cause dependency in small doses.

☐ 2. less irritating to subcutaneous tissues in small doses.

☐ 3. as potent as most other analgesics in larger doses.

☐ 4. excreted before accumulating in toxic amounts in the body.

98. The nurse is caring for a client who is scheduled for an adrenalectomy. Which drug may be included in the preoperative prescriptions to prevent Addison's crisis following surgery?

☐ 1. prednisone orally

☐ 2. fludrocortisones subcutaneously

☐ 3. spironolactone intramuscularly

☐ 4. methylprednisolone sodium succinate intravenously

99. Adrenal function is affected by the drug ketoconazole, an antifungal agent used to treat severe fungal infections. How is this effect manifested?

☐ 1. Ketoconazole suppresses adrenal steroid secretion.

☐ 2. Ketoconazole destroys adrenocortical cells, resulting in a "medical" adrenalectomy.

☐ 3. Ketoconazole increases adrenocorticotropic hormone (ACTH)-induced corticosteroid serum levels.

☐ 4. Ketoconazole decreases duration of adrenal suppression when administered with corticosteroids.

100. In the early postoperative period after a bilateral adrenalectomy, the client has an increased temperature. The nurse should assess the client specifically for signs of:

☐ 1. dehydration.

☐ 2. poor lung expansion.

☐ 3. wound infection.

☐ 4. urinary tract infection.

101. A client who is recovering from a bilateral adrenalectomy has a client-controlled analgesia (PCA) system with morphine sulfate. The nurse should:

☐ 1. observe the client at regular intervals for opioid addiction.

☐ 2. encourage the client to reduce analgesic use and tolerate the pain.

☐ 3. evaluate pain control at least every 2 hours.

☐ 4. increase the amount of morphine if the client does not administer the medication.

102. As the nurse assists the postoperative client out of bed, the client reports having gas pains in the abdomen. To reduce this discomfort, what should the nurse do?

☐ 1. Encourage the client to ambulate.

☐ 2. Insert a rectal tube.

☐ 3. Insert a nasogastric (NG) tube.

☐ 4. Encourage the client to drink carbonated liquids.

103. Because of steroid excess after a bilateral adrenalectomy, the nurse should assess the client for:

☐ 1. postoperative confusion.

☐ 2. delayed wound healing.

☐ 3. emboli.

☐ 4. malnutrition.

104. The client who has undergone a bilateral adrenalectomy is concerned about persistent body changes and unpredictable moods. The nurse should teach the client that:

☐ 1. the body changes are permanent and the client will not be the same as before this condition.

☐ 2. the body and mood will gradually return to normal.

☐ 3. the physical changes are permanent, but the mood swings will disappear.

☐ 4. the physical changes are temporary, but the mood swings are permanent.

105. After a bilateral adrenalectomy for Cushing's disease, the client will receive periodic testosterone injections. The expected outcome of these injections is:

☐ 1. balanced reproductive cycle.

☐ 2. restored sodium and potassium balance.

☐ 3. stimulated protein metabolism.

☐ 4. stabilized mood swings.

106. Which information should the nurse include in the teaching plan of a female client with bilateral adrenalectomy?

☐ 1. The client will need steroid replacement for the rest of her life.

☐ 2. The client must decrease the dose of steroid medication carefully to prevent crisis.

☐ 3. The client will require steroids only until her body can manufacture sufficient quantities.

☐ 4. The client will need to take steroids whenever her life involves physical or emotional stress.

Managing Care, Quality, and Safety of Clients with Endocrine Health Problems

107. The nurse is reviewing the postoperative prescriptions (see chart) just written by a healthcare provider (HCP) for a client with type 1 diabetes who has returned to the surgery floor from the recovery room following surgery for a left hip replacement. The client has pain of 5 on a scale of 1 to 10. The hand-off report from the nurse in the recovery room indicated that the vital signs have been stable for the last 30 minutes. After obtaining the client's glucose level, the nurse should **first**:

Prescriptions

Vital signs every 15 minutes for 4 hours, then every hour for 8 hours.
Oxygen 2 L/min per nasal canula.
1,000 mL NS every 8 hours.
10 mg morphine intramuscularly every 4 hours as needed.
10 U regular insulin stat.

☐ **1.** administer the morphine.
☐ **2.** contact the healthcare provider (HCP) to rewrite the insulin prescription.
☐ **3.** administer oxygen per nasal cannula at 2 L/min.
☐ **4.** take the vital signs.

108. The nurse is receiving results of a blood glucose level from the laboratory over the telephone. The nurse should:
☐ **1.** write down the results, read back the results to the caller from the laboratory, and receive confirmation from the caller.
☐ **2.** repeat the results to the caller from the laboratory, write the results on scrap paper, and then transfer the results to the medical record.
☐ **3.** indicate to the caller that the nurse cannot receive results from lab tests over the telephone and ask the lab to bring the written results to the nurses' station.
☐ **4.** request that the laboratory send the results by email to transfer to the client's medical record.

109. A client with type 1 diabetes is admitted to the emergency department with dehydration following the flu. The client has a blood glucose level of 325 mg/dL (18 mmol/L) and a serum potassium level of 3.5 mEq (3.5 mmol/L). The healthcare provider (HCP) has prescribed 1,000 mL 5% dextrose in water to be infused every 8 hours. Prior to implementing the HCP's prescriptions, the nurse should contact the HCP, explain the situation, provide background information, report the current assessment of the client, and:
☐ **1.** suggest adding potassium to the fluids.
☐ **2.** request an increase in the volume of intravenous fluids.
☐ **3.** verify the prescription for 5% dextrose in water.
☐ **4.** determine if the client should be placed in isolation.

110. Glulisine insulin is prescribed to be administered to a client before each meal. To assist the day-shift nurse who is receiving the report, the night-shift nurse gives the morning dose of glulisine. When the day-shift nurse goes to the room of the client who requires glulisine, the nurse finds that the client is not in the room. The client's roommate tells the nurse that the client "went for a test." What should the nurse do **next**?
☐ **1.** Bring a small glass of juice, and locate the client.
☐ **2.** Call the client's healthcare provider (HCP).
☐ **3.** Check the computerized care plan to determine what test was scheduled.
☐ **4.** Send the nurse's assistant to the x-ray department to bring the client back to his room.

111. A young adult client who has been diagnosed with type 1 diabetes has an insulin drip to aid in lowering the serum blood glucose level of 600 mg/dL (33.3 mmol/L). The client is also receiving ciprofloxacin IV. The healthcare provider (HCP) prescribes discontinuation of the insulin drip. What should the nurse do **next**?
☐ **1.** Discontinue the insulin drip, as prescribed.
☐ **2.** Hang the next IV dose of antibiotic before discontinuing the insulin drip.
☐ **3.** Inform the HCP that the client has not received any subcutaneous insulin yet.
☐ **4.** Add glargine to the insulin drip before discontinuing it.

112. The elderly client with type 2 diabetes has hyperglycemic hyperosmolar syndrome (HHS). The nurse should monitor the infusion for too rapid correction of the blood glucose in order to prevent:
☐ **1.** ketone body formation.
☐ **2.** a major vascular accident.
☐ **3.** fluid volume depletion.
☐ **4.** cerebral edema.

Answers, Rationales, and Test-Taking Strategies

The answers and rationales for each question follow below, along with keys (⚷) to the client need (CN) and cognitive level (CL) for each question. In addition, you will also see a

54. 3. Renal failure frequently results from the vascular changes associated with diabetes mellitus. ACE inhibitors increase renal blood flow and are effective in decreasing diabetic nephropathy. Chronic obstructive pulmonary disease is not a complication of diabetes nor is it prevented by ACE inhibitors. Pancreatic cancer is neither prevented by ACE inhibitors nor considered a complication of diabetes. Cerebrovascular accident is not directly prevented by ACE inhibitors, although management of hypertension will decrease vascular disease.

CN: Pharmacological and parenteral therapies; CL: Apply

55. 1. The four most commonly reported signs and symptoms of hypoglycemia are nervousness, weakness, perspiration, and confusion. Other signs and symptoms include hunger, incoherent speech, tachycardia, and blurred vision. Anorexia and Kussmaul's respirations are clinical manifestations of hyperglycemia or ketoacidosis. Bradycardia is not associated with hypoglycemia; tachycardia is.

CN: Reduction of risk potential; CL: Apply

56. 2. Steroids can cause hyperglycemia because of their effects on carbohydrate metabolism, making diabetic control more difficult. Aspirin is not known to affect glucose metabolism. Sulfonylureas are oral hypoglycemic agents used in the treatment of diabetes mellitus. ACE inhibitors are not known to affect glucose metabolism.

CN: Pharmacological and parenteral therapies; CL: Apply

57. 1. Colds and influenza present special challenges to the client with diabetes mellitus because the body's need for insulin increases during illness. Therefore, the client must take the prescribed insulin dose, increase the frequency of blood glucose testing, and maintain an adequate fluid intake to counteract the dehydrating effect of hyperglycemia. The nurse can encourage the client to drink clear fluids, juices, and electrolyte drinks. Not taking insulin when sick, or taking half the normal dose, may cause the client to develop ketoacidosis.

CN: Reduction of risk potential; CL: Synthesize

58. 1. The priority goal for the client with diabetes mellitus who is experiencing vomiting with influenza is to obtain adequate nutrition. The diabetic client should eat small, frequent meals of 50 g of carbohydrate or food equal to 200 cal. every 3 to 4 hours. If the client cannot eat the carbohydrates or take fluids, the **healthcare provider (HCP)** should be called, or the client should go to the emergency department. The diabetic client is in danger of complications with dehydration,

electrolyte imbalance, and ketoacidosis. Increasing the client's health management skills is important to lifestyle behaviors, but it is not a priority during this acute illness of influenza. Pain relief may be a need for this client, but it is not the priority at this time; neither is increasing activity during the illness.

CN: Basic care and comfort; CL: Analyze

59. 4. The best response is to allow the client to verbalize fears about performing self-injection. Tactics that increase fear such as threatening the client about complications are not effective in changing behavior. If possible, the client needs to be responsible for self-care, including giving self-injections. A nurse for home care visits is not justified if the client is capable of self-administration.

CN: Psychosocial integrity; CL: Synthesize

The Client with Pituitary Adenoma

60. 4. With transsphenoidal hypophysectomy, the sella turcica is entered from below, through the sphenoid sinus. There is no external incision; the incision is made between the upper lip and gums.

CN: Reduction of risk potential; CL: Apply

61. 3. Deep breathing is the best choice for helping prevent atelectasis. The client should be placed in the semi-Fowler's position (or as prescribed) and taught deep breathing, sighing, mouth breathing, and how to avoid coughing. The client should receive sufficient medication to control postoperative pain. Frequent position changes help loosen lung secretions, but deep breathing is most important in preventing atelectasis. Coughing is contraindicated because it increases intracranial pressure and can cause cerebrospinal fluid to leak from the point at which the sella turcica was entered.

CN: Reduction of risk potential; CL: Synthesize

62. 1. A major focus of nursing care after transsphenoidal hypophysectomy is the prevention of and monitoring for a CSF leak. CSF leakage can occur if the patch or incision is disrupted. The nurse should monitor for signs of infection, including elevated temperature, increased white blood cell count, rhinorrhea, nuchal rigidity, and persistent headache. Hypoglycemia and adrenocortical insufficiency may occur. Monitoring for fluctuating blood glucose levels is not related specifically to transsphenoidal hypophysectomy. The client will be given IV fluids postoperatively to supply carbohydrates. Cushing's disease results from adrenocortical excess, not insufficiency. Monitoring for cardiac arrhythmias is important, but arrhythmias are not anticipated following a transsphenoidal hypophysectomy.

🔑 CN: Reduction of risk potential; CL: Analyze

63. 1. The client's sexual problems are directly related to the excessive prolactin level. Removing the source of excessive hormone secretion should allow the client to return gradually to a normal physiologic pattern. Fertility will return, and erectile function and sexual desire will return to baseline as hormone levels return to normal.

🔑 CN: Physiological adaptation; CL: Apply

64. 3. If CSF leakage is suspected or confirmed, the client is treated initially with bed rest with the head of the bed elevated to decrease pressure on the graft site. Most leaks heal spontaneously, but occasionally, surgical repair of the site in the sella turcica is needed. Repacking the nose will not heal the leak at the graft site in the dura. The client will not be returned to surgery immediately because most leaks heal spontaneously. High-dose corticosteroid therapy is not effective in healing a CSF leak.

🔑 CN: Physiological adaptation; CL: Apply

65. 1. After transsphenoidal surgery, the client must be careful not to disturb the suture line while healing occurs. Frequent oral care should be provided with rinses of saline, and the teeth may be gently cleaned with oral swabs. Frequent or vigorous toothbrushing or flossing is contraindicated because it may disturb or cause tension on the suture line.

🔑 CN: Physiological adaptation; CL: Synthesize

66. 4. Most clients who undergo adenoma removal experience a gradual return of normal pituitary secretion and do not experience complications. However, hypopituitarism can cause growth hormone, gonadotropin, thyroid-stimulating hormone, and adrenocorticotropic hormone deficits. The client should be taught to monitor for change in mental status, energy level, muscle strength, and cognitive function. In adults, changes in sexual function, impotence, or decreased libido should be reported. Acromegaly and Cushing's disease are conditions of hypersecretion. Diabetes mellitus is related to the function of the pancreas and is not directly related to the function of the pituitary.

🔑 CN: Reduction of risk potential; CL: Analyze

67. 1. Pituitary diabetes insipidus is a potential complication after pituitary surgery because of possible interference with the production of antidiuretic hormone (ADH). One major manifestation of diabetes insipidus is polyuria because lack of ADH results in insufficient water reabsorption by the kidneys. The polyuria leads to a decreased urine specific gravity (between 1.001 and 1.010). The client may drink and excrete 5 to 40 L of fluid daily. Diabetes insipidus does not affect metabolism. A blood glucose level higher than 300 mg/dL (16.7 mmol/L) is associated with impaired glucose metabolism or diabetes mellitus. Urine negative for sugar and ketones is normal.

🔑 CN: Reduction of risk potential; CL: Analyze

68. 2. The major characteristic of diabetes insipidus is decreased tubular reabsorption of water due to insufficient amounts of antidiuretic hormone (ADH). Vasopressin is administered to the client with diabetes insipidus because it has pressor and ADH activities. Vasopressin works to increase the concentration of the urine by increasing tubular reabsorption, thus preserving up to 90% water. Vasopressin is administered to the client with diabetes insipidus because it is a synthetic ADH. The administration of vasopressin results in increased tubular reabsorption of water, and it is effective for emergency treatment or daily maintenance of mild diabetes insipidus. Vasopressin does not decrease blood pressure or affect insulin production or glucose metabolism nor is insulin production a factor in diabetes insipidus.

🔑 CN: Pharmacological and parenteral therapies; CL: Apply

69. 1. Because diabetes insipidus involves excretion of large amounts of fluid, maintaining normal fluid and electrolyte balance is a priority for this client. Special dietary programs or restrictions are not indicated in treatment of diabetes insipidus. Serum glucose levels are priorities in diabetes mellitus but not in diabetes insipidus.

🔑 CN: Physiological adaptation; CL: Evaluate

The Client with Addison's Disease

70. 4. Adrenal crisis can occur with physical stress, such as surgery, dental work, infection, flu, trauma, and pregnancy. In these situations, glucocorticoid and mineralocorticoid dosages are increased. Weight loss, not gain, occurs with adrenal insufficiency. Psychological stress has less effect on corticosteroid need than physical stress.

🔑 CN: Reduction of risk potential; CL: Synthesize

71. 2. Addison's disease is caused by a deficiency of adrenal corticosteroids and can result in severe hypotension and shock because of uncontrolled loss of sodium in the urine and impaired mineralocorticoid function. This results in loss of extracellular fluid and dangerously low blood volume. Glucocorticoids must be administered to reverse hypotension. Preventing infection is not an appropriate goal of care in this life-threatening situation. Relieving anxiety is appropriate when the client's condition is stabilized, but the calm, competent demeanor of the emergency department staff will be initially reassuring.

CN: Physiological adaptation; CL: Synthesize

72. 2. Adrenal hormone deficiency can cause profound physiologic changes. The client may experience severe pain (headache, abdominal pain, back pain, or pain in the extremities). Inhibited gluconeogenesis commonly produces hypoglycemia, and impaired sodium retention causes decreased, not increased, fluid volume. Edema would not be expected. Gastrointestinal disturbances, including nausea and vomiting, are expected findings in Addison's disease, not hunger.

CN: Physiological adaptation; CL: Analyze

73. 2,3,4,5. The long-term administration of corticosteroids in therapeutic doses often leads to serious complications or side effects. Corticosteroid therapy is not recommended for minor chronic conditions; the potential benefits of treatment must always be weighed against the risks. Hypokalemia may develop; corticosteroids act on the renal tubules to increase sodium reabsorption and enhance potassium and hydrogen excretion. Corticosteroids stimulate the breakdown of protein for gluconeogenesis, which can lead to skeletal muscle wasting. CNS adverse effects are euphoria, headache, insomnia, confusion, and psychosis. The nurse watches for changes in mood and behavior, emotional stability, sleep pattern, and psychomotor activity, especially with long-term therapy. Hypocalcemia related to anti–vitamin D effect may occur. Corticosteroids cause atrophy of the lymphoid tissue, suppress the cell-mediated immune responses, and decrease the production of antibodies. The nurse must be alert to the possibility of masked infection and delayed healing (anti-inflammatory and immunosuppressive actions). Retention of sodium (and subsequently water) increases blood volume and, therefore, blood pressure.

CN: Pharmacological parenteral therapies; CL: Apply

74. 1. Signs of infiltration include slowing of the infusion and swelling, pain, hardness, pallor, and coolness of the skin at the site. If these signs occur, the IV line should be discontinued and restarted at another infusion site. The new anatomic site, time, and type of cannula used should be documented. The nurse may apply a warm soak to the site, but only after the IV line is discontinued. Parenteral administration of fluids should not be stopped intermittently. Stopping the flow does not treat the problem nor does it address the client's needs for fluid replacement. Infiltrated IV sites should not be irrigated; doing so will only cause more swelling and pain.

CN: Pharmacological and parenteral therapies; CL: Synthesize

75. 1. Each liter of 5% dextrose in normal saline contains 170 cal. The nurse should consult with the **healthcare provider (HCP)** and dietitian when a client is on IV therapy or is on nothing-by-mouth status for an extended period because further electrolyte supplementation or alimentation therapy may be needed.

CN: Pharmacological and parenteral therapies; CL: Apply

76. 3. Electrolyte imbalances associated with Addison's disease include hypoglycemia, hyponatremia, and hyperkalemia. Regular salted (not low-salt) chicken or beef broth and fruit juices provide glucose and sodium to replenish these deficits. Diet soda does not contain sugar. Water could cause further sodium dilution. Coffee's diuretic effect would aggravate the fluid deficit. Milk contains potassium and sodium.

CN: Basic care and comfort; CL: Apply

77. 2. Finding alternative methods of dealing with stress, such as relaxation techniques, is a cornerstone of stress management. Removing all sources of stress from one's life is not possible. Antianxiety drugs are prescribed for temporary management during periods of major stress, and they are not an intervention in stress management classes. Avoiding discussion of stressful situations will not necessarily reduce stress.

CN: Psychosocial integrity; CL: Synthesize

78. 3. Primary Addison's disease refers to a problem in the gland itself that results from idiopathic atrophy of the glands. The process is believed to be autoimmune in nature. The most common causes of primary adrenocortical insufficiency are autoimmune destruction (70%) and tuberculosis (20%). Insufficient secretion of GH causes dwarfism or growth delay. Hyposecretion of glucocorticoids, aldosterone, and androgens occurs with Addison's disease. Pituitary dysfunction can cause Addison's disease, but this is not a primary disease process. Oversecretion of the adrenal medulla causes pheochromocytoma.

CN: Physiological adaptation; CL: Apply

79. 2,3,4,5,6. Addison's disease occurs when the client does not produce enough steroids from the adrenal cortex. Lifetime steroid replacement is needed. The client should be taught lifestyle management techniques to avoid stress and maintain rest periods. A medical identification bracelet should be worn, and the family should be taught signs and symptoms that indicate an impending adrenal crisis, such as fatigue, weakness, dizziness, or mood changes. Dental work, infections, and surgery commonly require an adjusted dosage of steroids.

CN: Physiological adaptation; CL: Create

80. 3. Although many of the disease signs and symptoms are vague and nonspecific, most clients experience lethargy and depression as early symptoms. Other early signs and symptoms include mood changes, emotional lability, irritability, weight loss, muscle weakness, fatigue, nausea, and vomiting. Most clients experience a loss of appetite. Muscles become weak, not spastic, because of adrenocortical insufficiency.

CN: Physiological adaptation; CL: Analyze

81. 1. Since Addison's disease can be life threatening, treatment often begins with administration of corticosteroids. Corticosteroids, such as prednisone, may be taken orally or intravenously, depending on the client. A serious adverse effect of corticosteroids is hyperglycemia. Clients do not adjust their steroid dose based on dietary intake and exercise; insulin is adjusted based on diet and exercise. Addisonian crisis can occur secondary to hypoadrenocorticism, resulting in a crisis situation of acute hypotension, not increased blood pressure. Addison's disease is a disease of inadequate adrenal hormone, and therefore, the client will have inadequate response to stress. If the client takes more medication than prescribed, there can be a potential increase in potassium depletion, fluid retention, and hyperglycemia. Taking less medication than was prescribed can trigger addisonian crisis state, which is a medical emergency manifested by signs of shock.

CN: Physiological adaptation; CL: Synthesize

82. 1. The need for glucocorticoids changes with circumstances. The basal dose is established when the client is discharged, but this dose covers only normal daily needs and does not provide for additional stressors. As the manager of the medication schedule, the client needs to know signs and symptoms of excessive and insufficient dosages. Glucocorticoid needs fluctuate. Glucocorticoids are not cumulative and must be taken daily. They must never be discontinued suddenly; in the absence of endogenous production, addisonian crisis could

result. Two-thirds of the daily dose should be taken at about 0800 and the remainder at about 1600. This schedule approximates the diurnal pattern of normal secretion, with highest levels between 0400 and 0600 and lowest levels in the evening.

CN: Pharmacological and parenteral therapies; CL: Evaluate

83. 3. Fludrocortisone acetate can be administered once a day, but cortisone acetate administration should follow the body's natural diurnal pattern of secretion, in which greater amounts of cortisol are secreted during the daytime to meet the increased demand of the body. To mimic this pattern, baseline administration of cortisone acetate is typically 25 mg in the morning and 12.5 mg in the afternoon. Taking it three times a day would result in an excessive dose. Taking the drug only in the morning would not meet the needs of the body later in the day and evening.

CN: Pharmacological and parenteral therapies; CL: Apply

84. 4. Oral steroids can cause gastric irritation and ulcers and should be administered with meals, if possible, or otherwise with an antacid. Only instructing the client to take the medication with a full glass of water will not help prevent gastric complications from steroids. Steroids should never be taken on an empty stomach. Glucocorticoids should be taken in the morning, not at bedtime.

CN: Pharmacological and parenteral therapies; CL: Apply

85. 4. Measuring daily weight is a reliable, objective way to monitor fluid balance. Rapid variations in weight reflect changes in fluid volume, which suggests insufficient control of the disease and the need for more glucocorticoids in the client with Addison's disease. Nurses should instruct clients taking oral steroids to weigh themselves daily and to report any unusual weight loss or gain. Skin turgor testing does supply information about fluid status, but daily weight monitoring is more reliable. Temperature is not a direct measurement of fluid balance. Thirst is a nonspecific and very late sign of weight loss.

CN: Pharmacological and parenteral therapies; CL: Evaluate

86. 1. Medication compliance is an essential part of the self-care required to manage Addison's disease. The client must learn to adjust the glucocorticoid dose in response to the normal and unexpected stresses of daily living. The nurse should instruct the client never to stop taking the drug without consulting the **healthcare provider (HCP)** ▢ to avoid an addisonian crisis. Regularity in daily habits makes adjustment easier, but the client should not be encouraged to withdraw from normal activities to avoid stress. The client does not need to restrict sodium. The client is at risk for hyponatremia. Hypotension, not hypertension, is more common with Addison's disease.

☞ CN: Reduction of risk potential; CL: Evaluate

87. 3. Illness or surgery places tremendous stress on the body, necessitating increased glucocorticoid dosage. Extreme psychological stress also necessitates dosage adjustment. Increased dosages are needed in times of stress to prevent drug-induced adrenal insufficiency. Returning to work after the weekend, a vacation, or a routine checkup usually will not alter glucocorticoid dosage needs.

☞ CN: Reduction of risk potential; CL: Synthesize

88. 4. Bronzing, or general deepening of skin pigmentation, is a classic sign of Addison's disease and is caused by melanocyte-stimulating hormone produced in response to increased ACTH secretion. The hyperpigmentation is typically found in the distal portion of extremities and in areas exposed to the sun. Additionally, areas that may not be exposed to the sun, such as the nipples, genitalia, tongue, and knuckles, become bronze colored. Treatment of Addison's disease usually reverses the hyperpigmentation. Bilirubin level is not related to the pathophysiology of Addison's disease. Hyperpigmentation is not related to the effects of the glucocorticoid therapy.

☞ CN: Physiological adaptation; CL: Apply

The Client with Cushing's Disease

89. 3. Skin bruising from increased skin and blood vessel fragility is a classic sign of Cushing's disease. Hyperpigmentation and bruising are caused by the hypersecretion of glucocorticoids. Fluid retention causes hypertension, not hypotension. Muscle wasting occurs in the extremities. Hair on the head thins, while body hair increases.

☞ CN: Physiological adaptation; CL: Analyze

90. 2. When Cushing's syndrome is suspected, a 24-hour urine collection for free cortisol is performed. Levels of 50 to 100 mcg/day (1,379 to 2,756 mmol/L) in adults indicate Cushing's syndrome. If these results are borderline, a high-dose dexamethasone suppression test is done. The dexamethasone is given at 2300 to suppress secretion of the corticotrophin-releasing hormone. A plasma cortisol sample is drawn at 0800. Normal cortisol level

<5 mcg/dL (140 mmol/L) indicates normal adrenal response.

☞ CN: Management of care; CL: Apply

91. 2. Sodium retention is typically accompanied by potassium depletion. Hypertension, hypokalemia, edema, and heart failure may result from the hypersecretion of aldosterone. The client with Cushing's disease exhibits postprandial or persistent hyperglycemia. Clients with Cushing's disease have hypernatremia, not hyponatremia. Bone resorption of calcium increases the urine calcium level.

☞ CN: Reduction of risk potential; CL: Analyze

92. 3. Cushing's disease is commonly caused by loss of the diurnal cortisol secretion pattern. The client's random morning cortisol level may be within normal limits, but secretion continues at that level throughout the entire day. Cortisol levels should normally decrease after the morning peak. Analysis of a 24-hour urine specimen is often useful in identifying the cumulative excess. Clients will not have symptoms with normal cortisol levels. Hormones are present in the blood.

☞ CN: Reduction of risk potential; CL: Apply

93. 2. A primary dietary intervention is to restrict sodium, thereby reducing fluid retention. Increased protein catabolism results in loss of muscle mass and necessitates supplemental protein intake. The client may be asked to restrict total calories to reduce weight. The client should be encouraged to eat potassium-rich foods because serum levels are typically depleted. Although reducing fat intake as part of an overall plan to restrict calories is appropriate, fat intake of <20% of total calories is not recommended.

☞ CN: Basic care and comfort; CL: Synthesize

94. 2. Osteoporosis is a serious outcome of prolonged cortisol excess because calcium is resorbed out of the bone. Regular daily weight-bearing exercise (e.g., brisk walking) is an effective way to drive calcium back into the bones. The client should also be instructed to have a dietary or supplemental intake of calcium of 1,500 mg daily. Potassium levels are not relevant to prevention of bone resorption. Vitamin D is needed to aid in the absorption of calcium. Isometric exercises condition muscle tone but do not build bones.

☞ CN: Reduction of risk potential; CL: Synthesize

95. 2. Effective splinting for a high incision reduces stress on the incision line, decreases pain, and increases the client's ability to deep breathe effectively. Deep breathing should be done hourly by the client after surgery. Sitting upright ignores the need to splint the incision to prevent pain. Tightening the stomach muscles is not an effective strategy for promoting deep breathing. Raising the shoulders is not a feature of deep-breathing exercises.

CN: Physiological adaptation; CL: Apply

96. 3. The priority in the first 24 hours after adrenalectomy is to identify and prevent adrenal crisis. Monitoring of vital signs is the most important evaluation measure. Hypotension, tachycardia, orthostatic hypotension, and arrhythmias can be indicators of pending vascular collapse and hypovolemic shock that can occur with adrenal crisis. Beginning oral nutrition is important, but not necessarily in the first 24 hours after surgery, and it is not more important than preventing adrenal crisis. Promoting self-care activities is not as important as preventing adrenal crisis. Ambulating in the hallway is not a priority in the first 24 hours after adrenalectomy.

CN: Physiological adaptation; CL: Synthesize

97. 3. Hydromorphone hydrochloride is about five times more potent than morphine sulfate, from which it is prepared. Therefore, it is administered only in small doses. Hydromorphone hydrochloride can cause dependency in any dose; however, fear of dependency developing in the postoperative period is unwarranted. The dose is determined by the client's need for pain relief. Hydromorphone hydrochloride is not irritating to subcutaneous tissues. As with opioid analgesics, excretion depends on normal liver function.

CN: Pharmacological and parenteral therapies; CL: Apply

98. 4. A glucocorticoid preparation will be administered intravenously or intramuscularly in the immediate preoperative period to a client scheduled for an adrenalectomy. Methylprednisolone sodium succinate protects the client from developing acute adrenal insufficiency (Addison's crisis) that occurs as a result of the adrenalectomy. Spironolactone is a potassium-sparing diuretic. Prednisone is an oral corticosteroid. Fludrocortisones is a mineral corticoid.

CN: Physiological integrity; CL: Apply

99. 1. Ketoconazole suppresses adrenal steroid secretion and may cause acute hypoadrenalism. The adverse effect should reverse when the drug is discontinued. Ketoconazole does not destroy adrenal cells; mitotane destroys the cells and may be used to obtain a medical adrenalectomy. Ketoconazole decreases, not increases, ACTH-induced serum corticosteroid levels. It increases the duration of adrenal suppression when given with steroids.

CN: Pharmacological and parenteral therapies; CL: Apply

100. 2. Poor lung expansion from bed rest, pain, and retained anesthesia is a common cause of slight postoperative temperature elevation. Nursing care includes turning the client and having the client cough and deep breathe every 1 to 2 hours or more frequently as prescribed. The client will have postoperative IV fluid replacement prescribed to prevent dehydration. Wound infections typically appear 4 to 7 days after surgery. Urinary tract infections would not be typical with this surgery.

CN: Physiological adaptation; CL: Analyze

101. 3. Pain control should be evaluated at least every 2 hours for the client with a PCA system. Addiction is not a common problem for the postoperative client. A client should not be encouraged to tolerate pain; in fact, other nursing actions besides PCA should be implemented to enhance the action of opioids. One of the purposes of PCA is for the client to determine frequency of administering the medication; the nurse should not interfere unless the client is not obtaining pain relief. The nurse should ensure that the client is instructed on the use of the PCA control button and that the button is always within reach.

CN: Pharmacological and parenteral therapies; CL: Synthesize

102. 1. Decreased mobility is one of the most common causes of abdominal distention related to retained gas in the intestines. Peristalsis has been inhibited by general anesthesia, analgesics, and inactivity during the immediate postoperative period. Ambulation increases peristaltic activity and helps move gas. Walking can prevent the need for a rectal tube, which is a more invasive procedure. An NG tube is also a more invasive procedure and requires a prescription. It is not a preferred treatment for gas postoperatively. Walking should prevent the need for further interventions. Carbonated liquids can increase gas formation.

CN: Reduction of risk potential; CL: Synthesize

103. 2. Persistent cortisol excess undermines the collagen matrix of the skin, impairing wound healing. It also carries an increased risk of infection and of bleeding. The wound should be observed and documentation performed regarding the status of healing. Confusion and emboli are not expected complications after adrenalectomy. Malnutrition also is not an expected complication after adrenalectomy. Nutritional status should be regained postoperatively.

CN: Reduction of risk potential; CL: Analyze

104. 2. As the body readjusts to normal cortisol levels, mood and physical changes will gradually return to a normal state. The body changes are not permanent, and the mood swings should level off.

🔑 CN: Physiological adaptation;
CL: Synthesize

105. 3. Testosterone is an androgen hormone that is responsible for protein metabolism as well as maintenance of secondary sexual characteristics; therefore, it is needed by both males and females. Removal of both adrenal glands necessitates replacement of glucocorticoids and androgens. Testosterone does not balance the reproductive cycle, stabilize mood swings, or restore sodium and potassium balance.

🔑 CN: Physiological adaptation; CL: Apply

106. 1. Bilateral adrenalectomy requires lifelong adrenal hormone replacement therapy. If unilateral surgery is performed, most clients gradually reestablish a normal secretion pattern. The client and family will require extensive teaching and support to maintain self-care management at home. Information on dosing, adverse effects, what to do if a dose is missed, and follow-up examinations is needed in the teaching plan. Although steroids are tapered when given for an intermittent or onetime problem, they are not discontinued when given to clients who have undergone bilateral adrenalectomy because the clients will not regain the ability to manufacture steroids. Steroids must be taken on a daily basis, not just during periods of physical or emotional stress.

🔑 CN: Physiological adaptation;
CL: Synthesize

Managing Care, Quality, and Safety of Clients with Endocrine Health Problems

107. 2. Insulin is on the list of error-prone medications, and the nurse should ask the **HCP** 📖 to rewrite the prescription to spell out the word "units" and to indicate the route by which the drug is to be administered. The nurse should contact the HCP immediately as the nurse is to administer the insulin now. The nurse can then also report the most current glucose level. While waiting for the insulin prescription to be rewritten, the nurse can administer the pain medication if needed, start the oxygen, and check the client's vital signs.

🔑 CN: Safety and infection control;
CL: Synthesize

108. 1. To assure client safety, the nurse first writes the results on the chart, then reads them back to the caller, and waits for the caller to confirm that the nurse has understood the results. The nurse may receive results by telephone; and although electronic transfer to the client's **medical record** 📖 is appropriate, the nurse can also accept the telephone results if the laboratory has called the results to the nurses' station.

🔑 CN: Management of Care; CL: Apply

109. 3. The client needs fluid volume replacement due to the dehydration. However, the nurse should verify the prescription for IV dextrose with the **HCP** 📖 due to the risk of hyperglycemia that dextrose would present when administered to a client with diabetes. The potassium level is within normal limits. The client does not have restrictions on oral fluids, and the nurse can encourage the client to drink fluids. The client does not need to be placed in isolation at this time.

🔑 CN: Management of care; CL: Synthesize

110. 3. Glulisine is a rapid-acting insulin with an action onset of 15 minutes. The client could experience hypoglycemia with the insulin in the bloodstream and no breakfast. It is not necessary to call the client's **HCP** 📖; the nurse should determine what test was scheduled and then locate the client and provide either breakfast or 4 oz (120 mL) of fruit juice. To bring the client back to the room would be wasting valuable time needed to prevent or correct hypoglycemia.

🔑 CN: Management of care; CL: Synthesize

111. 3. Because subcutaneous administration of insulin has a slower rate of absorption than IV insulin, there must be an adequate level of insulin in the bloodstream before discontinuing the insulin drip; otherwise, the glucose level will rise. Adding an IV antibiotic has no influence on the insulin drip; it should not be piggy-backed into the insulin drip. Glargine cannot be administered IV and should not be mixed with other insulins or solutions.

🔑 CN: Management of care; CL: Synthesize

112. 4. HHS can be caused by acute illness, such as an infection like pneumonia or sepsis. In HHS, there is a residual amount of insulin that suppresses ketosis but cannot control hyperglycemia. This leads to severe dehydration and impaired renal function. Ketone bodies are usually absent in HHS, and they do not form as a result of too rapid correction of blood glucose. The nurse should assess the client for a major vascular accident in the elderly as an etiology for a hyperglycemic crisis. Volume depletion must be treated first in HHS. Cerebral edema is a risk with too rapid correction of blood glucose.

🔑 CN: Reduction of risk potential;
CL: Apply

TEST 9

The Client with Urinary Tract Health Problems

- The Client with Cancer of the Bladder
- The Client with Renal Calculi
- The Client with Acute Renal Failure
- The Client with Urinary Tract Infection
- The Client with Pyelonephritis
- The Client with Chronic Renal Failure
- The Client with Urinary Incontinence
- Managing Care, Quality, and Safety of Clients with Urinary Tract Health Problems
- Answers, Rationales, and Test-Taking Strategies

The Client with Cancer of the Bladder

1. A client has undergone a cystectomy and an ileal conduit diversion. What should the nurse include in the discharge instructions? Select all that apply.
- ☐ 1. Drink at least 3,000 mL of fluid each day.
- ☐ 2. Minimize daily activities.
- ☐ 3. Keep urine alkaline to prevent urinary tract infections.
- ☐ 4. Avoid odor-producing foods, such as onions, fish, eggs, and cheese.
- ☐ 5. Wear snug clothing over the stoma to encourage urine flow into the drainage bag.

2. A nurse is caring for a client with an ileal conduit. When assessing the stoma, which outcomes are not desirable? Select all that apply.
- ☐ 1. dermatitis
- ☐ 2. bleeding
- ☐ 3. fungal infection
- ☐ 4. use of adhesive solvent on the skin around the stoma
- ☐ 5. placing skin cement on the faceplate of the collection bag

3. A client is admitted to the recovery room after cystoscopy with biopsy. Before the nurse can discharge the client, the nurse should be sure the client:
- ☐ 1. has a bowel movement.
- ☐ 2. has received the first dose of pain medication.
- ☐ 3. has voided.
- ☐ 4. has no blood in the urine.

4. The nurse should conduct a focused assessment for the client with suspected bladder cancer for which common sign of the disease?
- ☐ 1. suprapubic pain
- ☐ 2. dysuria
- ☐ 3. painless hematuria
- ☐ 4. urine retention

5. Which symptom indicates that a client has developed a complication after a cystoscopy?
- ☐ 1. dizziness
- ☐ 2. chills
- ☐ 3. pink-tinged urine
- ☐ 4. bladder spasms

6. If the client develops lower abdominal pain after a cystoscopy, what should the nurse instruct the client to do?
- ☐ 1. Apply an ice pack to the pubic area.
- ☐ 2. Massage the abdomen gently.
- ☐ 3. Ambulate as much as possible.
- ☐ 4. Sit in a tub of warm water.

7. A client who has been diagnosed with bladder cancer is scheduled for an ileal conduit. Preoperatively, the nurse reinforces the client's understanding of the surgical procedure by explaining that an ileal conduit:
- ☐ 1. is a temporary procedure that can be reversed later.
- ☐ 2. diverts urine into the sigmoid colon, where it is expelled through the rectum.
- ☐ 3. conveys urine from the ureters to a stoma opening on the abdomen.
- ☐ 4. creates an opening in the bladder that allows urine to drain into an external pouch.

8. After surgery for an ileal conduit, the nurse should closely assess the client for the occurrence of which complication specifically related to this pelvic surgery?
- ☐ 1. peritonitis
- ☐ 2. thrombophlebitis
- ☐ 3. ascites
- ☐ 4. inguinal hernia

9. The nurse is assessing the urine of a client who has had an ileal conduit and notes that there is a moderate amount of mucus in the urine. The nurse should:
- ☐ 1. change the appliance bag.
- ☐ 2. notify the healthcare provider (HCP).
- ☐ 3. obtain a urine specimen for culture.
- ☐ 4. encourage a high fluid intake.

10. When teaching the client to care for an ileal conduit, the nurse instructs the client to empty the appliance frequently. Which outcome indicates that the client is following instructions?
- ☐ 1. The skin around the stoma is red.
- ☐ 2. The urine is a deep yellow.
- ☐ 3. There is no odor present.
- ☐ 4. The seal around the stoma is intact.

11. The nurse should teach the client with an ileal conduit to prevent urine leakage when changing the appliance by:
- ☐ 1. inserting a gauze wick into the stoma.
- ☐ 2. closing the opening temporarily with a cellophane seal.
- ☐ 3. suctioning the stoma before changing the appliance.
- ☐ 4. avoiding oral fluids for several hours before changing the appliance.

12. The client with an ileal conduit will be using a reusable appliance at home. The nurse should teach the client to clean the appliance routinely with which product?
- ☐ 1. baking soda
- ☐ 2. soap
- ☐ 3. hydrogen peroxide
- ☐ 4. alcohol

13. The nurse is evaluating the discharge teaching for a client who has an ileal conduit. Which statements indicate that the client has correctly understood the teaching? Select all that apply.
- ☐ 1. "If I limit my fluid intake, I will not have to empty my ostomy pouch as often."
- ☐ 2. "I can place an aspirin tablet in my pouch to decrease odor."
- ☐ 3. "I can usually keep my ostomy pouch on for 3 to 7 days before changing it."
- ☐ 4. "I must use a skin barrier to protect my skin from urine."
- ☐ 5. "I should empty my ostomy pouch of urine when it is full."

14. A client has an ileal conduit. Which solutions will be useful to help control odor in the urine collecting bag after it has been cleaned?
- ☐ 1. salt water
- ☐ 2. vinegar
- ☐ 3. ammonia
- ☐ 4. bleach

15. A female client who has a urinary diversion tells the nurse, "This urinary pouch is embarrassing. Everyone will know that I am not normal. I do not see how I can go out in public anymore." The **most** appropriate goal for this client is to:
- ☐ 1. manage her anxiety about her health.
- ☐ 2. learn how to care for the urinary diversion.
- ☐ 3. overcome feelings of worthlessness.
- ☐ 4. express fears about the urinary diversion.

16. The nurse teaches the client with a urinary diversion to attach the appliance to a standard urine collection bag at night. The **most** important reason for doing this is to prevent:
- ☐ 1. urine reflux into the stoma.
- ☐ 2. appliance separation.
- ☐ 3. urine leakage.
- ☐ 4. the need to restrict fluids.

17. The nurse is teaching the client with an ileal conduit how to prevent a urinary tract infection. Which measure would be **most** effective?
- ☐ 1. Avoid people with respiratory tract infections.
- ☐ 2. Maintain a daily fluid intake of 2,000 to 3,000 mL.
- ☐ 3. Use sterile technique to change the appliance.
- ☐ 4. Irrigate the stoma daily.

18. The nurse evaluates the effectiveness of the client's postoperative plan of care. Which outcome is expected for a client with an ileal conduit?
- ☐ 1. The client verbalizes the understanding that physical activity must be curtailed.
- ☐ 2. The client will place an aspirin in the drainage pouch to help control odor.
- ☐ 3. The client demonstrates how to catheterize the stoma.
- ☐ 4. The client will empty the drainage pouch frequently throughout the day.

19. A client is scheduled to undergo weekly intravesical chemotherapy for bladder cancer for the next 8 weeks. Which statement indicates that the client understands how to manage the urine as a biohazard? The client will:
- ☐ 1. void into a bedpan and then empty the urine into the toilet.
- ☐ 2. disinfect the urine and toilet with bleach for 6 hours following a treatment.
- ☐ 3. clean the bathroom daily with disinfectant wipes.
- ☐ 4. use a separate bathroom from the rest of the family for the next 8 weeks.

20. A nurse is planning care for a client who underwent a percutaneous needle biopsy of the kidney. What should the nurse plan to do immediately after the biopsy? Select all that apply.
- [ ] 1. Assess the biopsy site.
- [ ] 2. Take vital signs every hour.
- [ ] 3. Assess urine for hematuria.
- [ ] 4. Place the client in a prone position.
- [ ] 5. Assess the client for chest pain.

The Client with Renal Calculi

21. A client had a lithotripsy to treat renal calculi. The client is having ureteral spasms and hematuria. What should the nurse do? Select all that apply.
- [ ] 1. Strain all urine.
- [ ] 2. Apply a heating pad to the lower back area.
- [ ] 3. Contact the healthcare provider (HCP) to report hematuria.
- [ ] 4. Encourage fluid intake of 1,000 mL/day.
- [ ] 5. Assess pain level.

22. A client has renal colic due to renal lithiasis. What is the nurse's **first** priority in managing care for this client?
- [ ] 1. Do not allow the client to ingest fluids.
- [ ] 2. Encourage the client to drink at least 500 mL of water each hour.
- [ ] 3. Request the central supply department to send supplies for straining urine.
- [ ] 4. Administer an opioid analgesic as prescribed.

23. A client is admitted to the hospital with a diagnosis of renal calculi. The client is experiencing severe flank pain and nausea; the temperature is 100.6°F (38.1°C). Which outcome is a **priority** for this client?
- [ ] 1. prevention of urinary tract complications
- [ ] 2. alleviation of nausea
- [ ] 3. alleviation of pain
- [ ] 4. maintenance of fluid and electrolyte balance

24. The client is scheduled to have a kidney, ureter, and bladder (KUB) radiograph. To prepare the client for this procedure, the nurse should explain to the client that:
- [ ] 1. fluid and food will be withheld the morning of the examination.
- [ ] 2. a tranquilizer will be given before the examination.
- [ ] 3. an enema will be given before the examination.
- [ ] 4. no special preparation is required for the examination.

25. In addition to nausea and severe flank pain, a female client with renal calculi has pain in the groin and bladder. The nurse should assess the client further for signs of:
- [ ] 1. nephritis.
- [ ] 2. referred pain.
- [ ] 3. urine retention.
- [ ] 4. additional stone formation.

26. Which is likely to provide the **most** relief from the pain associated with renal colic?
- [ ] 1. applying moist heat to the flank area
- [ ] 2. administering meperidine
- [ ] 3. encouraging high fluid intake
- [ ] 4. maintaining complete bed rest

27. A client who has been diagnosed with renal calculi reports that the pain is intermittent and less colicky. Which nursing action is **most** important at this time?
- [ ] 1. Report hematuria to the healthcare provider (HCP).
- [ ] 2. Strain the urine carefully.
- [ ] 3. Administer meperidine every 3 hours.
- [ ] 4. Apply warm compresses to the flank area.

28. The client is scheduled for an intravenous pyelogram (IVP) to determine the location of the renal calculi. Which action would be **most** important for the nurse to include in pretest preparation?
- [ ] 1. Ensure adequate fluid intake on the day of the test.
- [ ] 2. Prepare the client for the possibility of bladder spasms during the test.
- [ ] 3. Check the client's history for allergy to iodine.
- [ ] 4. Determine when the client last had a bowel movement.

29. After an intravenous pyelogram (IVP), the nurse should include which measure in the client's plan of care?
- [ ] 1. Maintain bed rest.
- [ ] 2. Encourage adequate fluid intake.
- [ ] 3. Assess for hematuria.
- [ ] 4. Administer a laxative.

30. A client has a ureteral catheter in place after renal surgery. A **priority** nursing action for care of the ureteral catheter is to:
- [ ] 1. irrigate the catheter with 30 mL of normal saline every 8 hours.
- [ ] 2. ensure that the catheter is draining freely.
- [ ] 3. clamp the catheter every 2 hours for 30 minutes.
- [ ] 4. ensure that the catheter drains at least 30 mL/h.

31. Which would be the **most** appropriate measure for preventing the development of a paralytic ileus in a client who has undergone renal surgery?
☐ 1. Encourage the client to ambulate every 2 to 4 hours.
☐ 2. Offer 3 to 4 oz (90 to 120 mL) of a carbonated beverage periodically.
☐ 3. Encourage use of a stool softener.
☐ 4. Continue IV fluid therapy.

32. The nurse is conducting a postoperative assessment of a client on the first day after renal surgery. The nurse should report which finding to the healthcare provider (HCP)?
☐ 1. temperature, 99.8°F (37.7°C)
☐ 2. urine output, 20 mL/h
☐ 3. absence of bowel sounds
☐ 4. a 2″ × 2″ (5 cm × 5 cm) area of serosanguineous drainage on the flank dressing

33. A client with a history of renal calculi formation is being discharged after surgery to remove the calculus. What instruction should the nurse include in the client's discharge teaching plan?
☐ 1. Increase daily fluid intake to at least 2 to 3 L.
☐ 2. Strain urine at home regularly.
☐ 3. Eliminate dairy products from the diet.
☐ 4. Follow measures to alkalinize the urine.

34. Because a client's renal stone was found to be composed of uric acid, a low-purine, alkaline-ash diet was prescribed. Incorporation of which food items into the home diet would indicate that the client understands the necessary diet modifications?
☐ 1. milk, apples, tomatoes, and corn
☐ 2. eggs, spinach, dried peas, and gravy
☐ 3. salmon, chicken, caviar, and asparagus
☐ 4. grapes, corn, cereals, and liver

35. Allopurinol, 200 mg/day, is prescribed for the client with renal calculi to take at home. The nurse should teach the client about which adverse effect of this medication?
☐ 1. retinopathy
☐ 2. maculopapular rash
☐ 3. nasal congestion
☐ 4. dizziness

36. A client has been prescribed allopurinol for renal calculi that are caused by high uric acid levels. Which symptoms indicate the client is experiencing adverse effects of this drug? Select all that apply.
☐ 1. nausea
☐ 2. rash
☐ 3. constipation
☐ 4. flushed skin
☐ 5. bone marrow depression

37. The nurse is reviewing laboratory reports for a client who is taking allopurinol. Which finding indicates that the drug has had a therapeutic effect?
☐ 1. decreased urine alkaline phosphatase level
☐ 2. increased urine calcium excretion
☐ 3. increased serum calcium level
☐ 4. decreased serum uric acid level

The Client with Acute Renal Failure

38. A client is to receive peritoneal dialysis. To prepare for the procedure, the nurse should:
☐ 1. assess the dialysis access for a bruit and thrill.
☐ 2. insert an indwelling urinary catheter and drain all urine from the bladder.
☐ 3. ask the client to turn toward the left side.
☐ 4. warm the dialysis solution in the warmer.

39. A client has been admitted with acute renal failure. What should the nurse do? Select all that apply.
☐ 1. Elevate the head of the bed 30 to 45 degrees.
☐ 2. Take vital signs.
☐ 3. Establish an IV access site.
☐ 4. Call the admitting healthcare provider (HCP) for prescriptions.
☐ 5. Contact the hemodialysis unit.

40. Which initial manifestation of acute renal failure is the **most** common?
☐ 1. dysuria
☐ 2. anuria
☐ 3. hematuria
☐ 4. oliguria

41. A client developed cardiogenic shock after a severe myocardial infarction and has now developed acute renal failure. The client's family asks the nurse why the client has developed acute renal failure. The nurse should base the response on the knowledge that there was:
☐ 1. a decrease in the blood flow through the kidneys.
☐ 2. an obstruction of urine flow from the kidneys.
☐ 3. a blood clot formed in the kidneys.
☐ 4. structural damage to the kidney resulting in acute tubular necrosis.

42. The client who is in acute renal failure has an elevated blood urea nitrogen (BUN). What is the **likely** cause of this finding?
☐ 1. fluid retention
☐ 2. hemolysis of red blood cells
☐ 3. below-normal metabolic rate
☐ 4. reduced renal blood flow

43. The client's serum potassium level is elevated in acute renal failure, and the nurse administers sodium polystyrene sulfonate. The mechanism of action for this drug is to:
- ☐ 1. increase potassium excretion from the colon.
- ☐ 2. release hydrogen ions for sodium ions.
- ☐ 3. increase calcium absorption in the colon.
- ☐ 4. exchange sodium for potassium ions in the colon.

44. A client with acute renal failure has an increase in the serum potassium level. The nurse should monitor the client for:
- ☐ 1. cardiac arrest.
- ☐ 2. pulmonary edema.
- ☐ 3. circulatory collapse.
- ☐ 4. hemorrhage.

45. A high-carbohydrate, low-protein diet is prescribed for the client with acute renal failure. The intended outcome of this diet is to:
- ☐ 1. act as a diuretic.
- ☐ 2. reduce demands on the liver.
- ☐ 3. help maintain urine acidity.
- ☐ 4. prevent the development of ketosis.

46. The client with acute renal failure asks the nurse for a snack. Because the client's potassium level is elevated, which snack is **most** appropriate?
- ☐ 1. a gelatin dessert
- ☐ 2. yogurt
- ☐ 3. an orange
- ☐ 4. peanuts

47. In the oliguric phase of acute renal failure, the nurse should assess the client for:
- ☐ 1. pulmonary edema.
- ☐ 2. metabolic alkalosis.
- ☐ 3. hypotension.
- ☐ 4. hypokalemia.

48. The client in acute renal failure has an external cannula inserted in the forearm for hemodialysis. Which nursing measure is appropriate for the care of this client?
- ☐ 1. Use the unaffected arm for blood pressure measurements.
- ☐ 2. Draw blood from the cannula for routine laboratory work.
- ☐ 3. Percuss the cannula for bruits each shift.
- ☐ 4. Inject heparin into the cannula each shift.

49. During dialysis, the client has disequilibrium syndrome. The nurse should **first**:
- ☐ 1. administer oxygen per nasal cannula.
- ☐ 2. slow the rate of dialysis.
- ☐ 3. reassure the client that the symptoms are normal.
- ☐ 4. place the client in Trendelenburg's position.

50. Which abnormal blood value would not be improved by dialysis treatment?
- ☐ 1. elevated serum creatinine level
- ☐ 2. hyperkalemia
- ☐ 3. decreased hemoglobin concentration
- ☐ 4. hypernatremia

51. The nurse teaches the client how to recognize infection in the shunt by telling the client to assess the shunt each day for:
- ☐ 1. absence of a bruit.
- ☐ 2. sluggish capillary refill time.
- ☐ 3. coolness of the involved extremity.
- ☐ 4. swelling at the shunt site.

52. The client with acute renal failure is recovering and asks the nurse, "Will my kidneys ever function normally again?" The nurse's response is based on knowledge that the client's renal status will **most** likely:
- ☐ 1. continue to improve over a period of weeks.
- ☐ 2. result in the need for permanent hemodialysis.
- ☐ 3. improve only if the client receives a renal transplant.
- ☐ 4. result in end-stage renal failure.

The Client with Urinary Tract Infection

53. The nurse is teaching an older adult with a urinary tract infection about the importance of increasing fluids in the diet. What puts this client at a risk for not obtaining sufficient fluids?
- ☐ 1. diminished liver function
- ☐ 2. increased production of antidiuretic hormone
- ☐ 3. decreased production of aldosterone
- ☐ 4. decreased ability to detect thirst

54. A client with a urinary tract infection is to take nitrofurantoin four times each day. The client asks the nurse, "What should I do if I forget a dose?" What should the nurse tell the client?
- ☐ 1. "You can wait and take the next dose when it is due."
- ☐ 2. "Double the amount prescribed with your next dose."
- ☐ 3. "Take the prescribed dose as soon as you remember it, and if it is very close to the time for the next dose, delay that next dose."
- ☐ 4. "Take a lot of water with a double amount of your prescribed dose."

55. What should the nurse do to prevent catheter-associated urinary tract infection (CAUTI)? Select all that apply.
- ☐ 1. Change the catheter daily.
- ☐ 2. Provide perineal care several times a day.
- ☐ 3. Monitor the temperature as an indicator of the infection.
- ☐ 4. Encourage the client to drink 3,000 mL fluids daily.
- ☐ 5. Recommend the healthcare provider (HCP) prescribe antibiotics.

56. A nurse is assessing a client with a urinary tract infection who takes an antihypertensive drug. The nurse reviews the client's urinalysis results (see chart). The nurse should:

Laboratory Results

Test	Result
pH	6.8
Red blood cells	3 per high power field
Color	Yellow
Specific gravity	1.030

☐ 1. encourage the client to increase fluid intake.
☐ 2. withhold the next dose of antihypertensive medication.
☐ 3. restrict the client's sodium intake.
☐ 4. encourage the client to eat at least half of a banana per day.

57. A client has nephropathy. The healthcare provider (HCP) prescribes a 24-hour urine collection for creatinine clearance. Which action is necessary to ensure proper collection of the specimen?
☐ 1. Collect the urine in a preservative-free container and keep it on ice.
☐ 2. Inform the client to discard the last voided specimen at the conclusion of urine collection.
☐ 3. Obtain a self-report of the client's weight before beginning the collection of urine.
☐ 4. Request a prescription for insertion of an indwelling urinary catheter.

58. A client who weighs 207 lb (94.1 kg) is to receive 1.5 mg/kg of gentamicin sulfate IV three times each day. How many milligrams of medication should the nurse administer for each dose? Round to the nearest whole number.

_____ mg.

59. A 24-year-old female client comes to an ambulatory care clinic in moderate distress with a probable diagnosis of acute cystitis. When obtaining the client's history, the nurse should ask the client if she has had:
☐ 1. fever and chills.
☐ 2. frequency and burning on urination.
☐ 3. flank pain and nausea.
☐ 4. hematuria.

60. The client asks the nurse, "How did I get this urinary tract infection?" The nurse should explain that in **most** instances, cystitis is caused by:
☐ 1. congenital strictures in the urethra.
☐ 2. an infection elsewhere in the body.
☐ 3. urinary stasis in the urinary bladder.
☐ 4. an ascending infection from the urethra.

61. The client, who is a newlywed, is afraid to discuss her diagnosis of cystitis with her husband. Which approach would be **best**?
☐ 1. Arrange a meeting with the client, her husband, the healthcare provider (HCP), and the nurse.
☐ 2. Insist that the client talk with her husband because good communication is necessary for a successful marriage.
☐ 3. Talk first with the husband alone and then with both of them together to share the husband's reactions.
☐ 4. Spend time with the client addressing her concerns and then, if the client requests, stay with her while she talks with her husband.

62. The nurse teaches a female client who has cystitis methods to relieve her discomfort until the antibiotic takes effect. Which response by the client would indicate that she understands the nurse's instructions?
☐ 1. "I will place ice packs on my perineum."
☐ 2. "I will take hot tub baths."
☐ 3. "I will drink a cup of warm tea every hour."
☐ 4. "I will void every 5 to 6 hours."

63. The client with first-time bacterial cystitis is being treated with an antibiotic to be taken for 7 days. The nurse should instruct the client to:
☐ 1. limit fluids to 1,000 mL/day.
☐ 2. notify the healthcare provider (HCP) when the urine is clear.
☐ 3. take the entire prescription as ordered.
☐ 4. use condoms if having sex.

64. When teaching the client with a urinary tract infection about taking a prescribed antibiotic for 7 days, the nurse should tell the client to report which symptoms to the healthcare provider (HCP)? Select all that apply.
☐ 1. cloudy urine for the first few days
☐ 2. blood in the urine
☐ 3. rash
☐ 4. mild nausea
☐ 5. fever above 100°F (37.8°C)
☐ 6. urinating every 3 to 4 hours

65. A client has been prescribed nitrofurantoin for treatment of a lower urinary tract infection. Which instructions should the nurse include when teaching the client about this medication? Select all that apply.
☐ 1. "Take the medication on an empty stomach."
☐ 2. "Your urine may become brown in color."
☐ 3. "Increase your fluid intake."
☐ 4. "Take the medication until your symptoms subside."
☐ 5. "Take the medication with an antacid to decrease gastrointestinal distress."

66. Nitrofurantoin, 75 mg four times per day, has been prescribed for a client with a lower urinary tract infection. The medication comes in an oral suspension of 25 mg/5 mL. How many milliliters should the nurse administer for each dose? Record your answer using a whole number.

_____ mL.

67. Which statements by a female client would indicate that she is at high risk for a recurrence of cystitis?
- ☐ **1.** "I can usually go 8 to 10 hours without needing to empty my bladder."
- ☐ **2.** "I take a tub bath every evening."
- ☐ **3.** "I wipe from front to back after voiding."
- ☐ **4.** "I work out by lifting weights three times a week."

68. To prevent recurrence of cystitis, the nurse should plan to encourage the female client to include which measure in her daily routine?
- ☐ **1.** wearing cotton underpants
- ☐ **2.** increasing citrus juice intake
- ☐ **3.** douching regularly with 0.25% acetic acid
- ☐ **4.** using vaginal sprays

69. The nurse explains to the client the importance of drinking large quantities of fluid to prevent cystitis. The nurse should tell the client to drink:
- ☐ **1.** twice as much fluid as usual.
- ☐ **2.** at least 1,000 mL more than usual.
- ☐ **3.** as much water or juice, as possible.
- ☐ **4.** at least 3,000 mL of fluids daily.

The Client with Pyelonephritis

70. A client is at risk for acute pyelonephritis. The nurse should instruct the client about which health promotion behaviors that will be **most** effective in preventing pyelonephritis?
- ☐ **1.** Wash the perineum with warm water and soap, cleaning from front to back.
- ☐ **2.** Treat fungal infections such as athlete's foot immediately.
- ☐ **3.** Have a pneumonia immunization to prevent streptococcal infection.
- ☐ **4.** Treat skin lesions with antibiotics, and cover any open lesions.

71. A client is diagnosed with acute pyelonephritis. What should the nurse instruct the client to do?
- ☐ **1.** Urinate frequently.
- ☐ **2.** Take bubble baths instead of showers.
- ☐ **3.** Take antibiotics for the rest of the client's life.
- ☐ **4.** Decrease fluid intake.

72. Which factor would put the client at increased risk for pyelonephritis?
- ☐ **1.** history of hypertension
- ☐ **2.** intake of large quantities of cranberry juice
- ☐ **3.** fluid intake of 2,000 mL/day
- ☐ **4.** history of diabetes mellitus

73. The client with pyelonephritis asks the nurse, "How will I know whether the antibiotics are effectively treating my infection?" What should the nurse tell the client?
- ☐ **1.** "After you take the antibiotics for 2 weeks, you will not have any infection."
- ☐ **2.** "Your healthcare provider can tell by the color and odor of your urine."
- ☐ **3.** "Your healthcare provider will take a urine culture."
- ☐ **4.** "When your symptoms disappear, you will know that your infection is gone."

74. The nurse is to administer 1,200 mg of an antibiotic. The drug is prepared with 6 g of the drug in 2 mL of solution. The nurse should administer how many milliliters of the drug? Record your answer using one decimal point.

_____ mL.

75. The client with acute pyelonephritis wants to know the possibility of developing chronic pyelonephritis. The nurse's response is based on knowledge of which disorder that **most** commonly leads to chronic pyelonephritis?
- ☐ **1.** acute pyelonephritis
- ☐ **2.** recurrent urinary tract infections
- ☐ **3.** acute renal failure
- ☐ **4.** glomerulonephritis

76. A client is diagnosed with pyelonephritis. Which nursing action is a **priority** for care now?
- ☐ **1.** Monitor hemoglobin levels.
- ☐ **2.** Insert a urinary catheter.
- ☐ **3.** Stress importance of use of long-term antibiotics.
- ☐ **4.** Ensure sufficient hydration.

The Client with Chronic Renal Failure

77. A client with end-stage renal failure has an internal arteriovenous fistula in the left arm for vascular access during hemodialysis. What should the nurse instruct the client to do? Select all that apply.
- ☐ **1.** Remind healthcare providers (HCPs) to draw blood from veins on the left side.
- ☐ **2.** Avoid sleeping on the left arm.
- ☐ **3.** Wear wristwatch on the right arm.
- ☐ **4.** Assess fingers on the left arm for warmth.
- ☐ **5.** Obtain BP from the left arm.

78. A client with end-stage chronic renal failure is admitted to the hospital with a serum potassium level of 7 mEq/L. In what order of priority from first to last does the nurse perform the prescriptions? All options must be used.

| **1.** Administer calcium gluconate. |
| **2.** Start an IV access site. |
| **3.** Administer sodium polystyrene sulfonate. |
| **4.** Attach the client to a cardiac monitor. |

| |
| |
| |
| |

79. A client with chronic renal failure is receiving hemodialysis three times a week. In order to protect the fistula, the nurse should:
☐ **1.** take the blood pressure in the arm with the fistula.
☐ **2.** report the loss of a thrill or bruit on the arm with the fistula.
☐ **3.** maintain a pressure dressing on the shunt.
☐ **4.** start a second IV in the arm with the fistula.

80. A client with chronic renal failure who receives hemodialysis three times a week is experiencing severe nausea. What should the nurse advise the client to do to manage the nausea? Select all that apply.
☐ **1.** Drink fluids before eating solid foods.
☐ **2.** Have limited amounts of fluids only when thirsty.
☐ **3.** Limit activity.
☐ **4.** Keep all dialysis appointments.
☐ **5.** Eat smaller, more frequent meals.

81. The dialysis solution is warmed before use in peritoneal dialysis **primarily** to:
☐ **1.** encourage the removal of serum urea.
☐ **2.** force potassium back into the cells.
☐ **3.** add extra warmth to the body.
☐ **4.** promote abdominal muscle relaxation.

82. A client is receiving peritoneal dialysis. While the dialysis solution is dwelling in the client's abdomen, the nurse should:
☐ **1.** assess for urticaria.
☐ **2.** observe respiratory status.
☐ **3.** check capillary refill time.
☐ **4.** monitor electrolyte status.

83. During the peritoneal dialysis, the nurse observes that the solution draining from the client's abdomen is consistently blood tinged. The client has a permanent peritoneal catheter in place. The nurse should recognize that the bleeding:
☐ **1.** is expected with a permanent peritoneal catheter.
☐ **2.** indicates abdominal blood vessel damage.
☐ **3.** can indicate kidney damage.
☐ **4.** is caused by too-rapid infusion of the dialysate.

84. During peritoneal dialysis, the nurse observes that the flow of dialysate stops before all the solution has drained out. The nurse should:
☐ **1.** have the client sit in a chair.
☐ **2.** turn the client from side to side.
☐ **3.** reposition the peritoneal catheter.
☐ **4.** have the client walk.

85. A client undergoing long-term peritoneal dialysis at home is currently experiencing a reduced outflow from the dialysis catheter. To determine if the catheter is obstructed, the nurse should inquire whether the client has:
☐ **1.** diarrhea.
☐ **2.** vomiting.
☐ **3.** flatulence.
☐ **4.** constipation.

86. Which should be included in the client's plan of care during dialysis therapy?
☐ **1.** Limit the client's visitors.
☐ **2.** Monitor the client's blood pressure.
☐ **3.** Pad the side rails of the bed.
☐ **4.** Keep the client on nothing-by-mouth (NPO) status.

87. The client performs self peritoneal dialysis. What should the nurse teach the client about preventing peritonitis? Select all that apply.
☐ **1.** Broad-spectrum antibiotics may be administered to prevent infection.
☐ **2.** Antibiotics may be added to the dialysate to treat peritonitis.
☐ **3.** Clean technique is permissible for prevention of peritonitis.
☐ **4.** Peritonitis is characterized by cloudy dialysate drainage and abdominal discomfort.
☐ **5.** Peritonitis is the most common and serious complication of peritoneal dialysis.

88. After completion of peritoneal dialysis, the nurse should assess the client for:
☐ **1.** hematuria.
☐ **2.** weight loss.
☐ **3.** hypertension.
☐ **4.** increased urine output.

89. Aluminum hydroxide gel is prescribed for the client with chronic renal failure to take at home. What is the expected outcome of giving this drug?
- ☐ 1. relieving the pain of gastric hyperacidity
- ☐ 2. preventing Curling's stress ulcers
- ☐ 3. binding phosphate in the intestine
- ☐ 4. reversing metabolic acidosis

90. The nurse teaches the client with chronic renal failure when to take aluminum hydroxide gel. Which statement indicates that the client understands the teaching?
- ☐ 1. "I will take it every 4 hours around the clock."
- ☐ 2. "I will take it between meals and at bedtime."
- ☐ 3. "I will take it when I have an upset stomach."
- ☐ 4. "I will take it with meals and bedtime snacks."

91. Which teaching approach for the client with chronic renal failure who has difficulty concentrating due to high uremia levels would be **most** appropriate?
- ☐ 1. Provide all needed teaching in one extended session.
- ☐ 2. Validate the client's understanding of the material frequently.
- ☐ 3. Conduct a one-on-one session with the client.
- ☐ 4. Use video clips to reinforce the material as needed.

92. The nurse is instructing the client with chronic renal failure to maintain adequate nutritional intake. Which diet would be **most** appropriate?
- ☐ 1. high-carbohydrate, high-protein
- ☐ 2. high-calcium, high-potassium, high-protein
- ☐ 3. low-protein, low-sodium, low-potassium
- ☐ 4. low-protein, high-potassium

93. The nurse is discussing concerns about sexual activity with a client with chronic renal failure. Which strategy would be **most** useful?
- ☐ 1. Help the client to accept that sexual activity will be decreased.
- ☐ 2. Suggest using alternative forms of sexual expression and intimacy.
- ☐ 3. Tell the client to plan rest periods after sexual activity.
- ☐ 4. Refer the client to a counselor.

94. A client with chronic renal failure has asked to be evaluated for a home continuous ambulatory peritoneal dialysis (CAPD) program. The nurse should explain that the major advantage of this approach is that it:
- ☐ 1. is relatively low in cost.
- ☐ 2. allows the client to be more independent.
- ☐ 3. is faster and more efficient than standard peritoneal dialysis.
- ☐ 4. has fewer potential complications than does standard peritoneal dialysis.

95. The client asks about diet changes when using continuous ambulatory peritoneal dialysis (CAPD). Which response by the nurse would be **best**?
- ☐ 1. "Diet restrictions are more rigid with CAPD because standard peritoneal dialysis is a more effective technique."
- ☐ 2. "Diet restrictions are the same for both CAPD and standard peritoneal dialysis."
- ☐ 3. "Diet restrictions with CAPD are fewer than with standard peritoneal dialysis because dialysis is constant."
- ☐ 4. "Diet restrictions with CAPD are fewer than with standard peritoneal dialysis because CAPD works more quickly."

96. A client is receiving continuous ambulatory peritoneal dialysis (CAPD). The nurse should assess the client for which sign of peritoneal infection?
- ☐ 1. cloudy dialysate fluid
- ☐ 2. swelling in the legs
- ☐ 3. poor drainage of the dialysate fluid
- ☐ 4. redness at the catheter insertion site

The Client with Urinary Incontinence

97. A client who is 70 years of age and lives alone has stress incontinence. To prevent incontinence, the nurse advises the client to:
- ☐ 1. ask someone else to lift heavy objects.
- ☐ 2. wear disposable protective underwear.
- ☐ 3. perform perineal muscle exercises (i.e., Kegel exercises).
- ☐ 4. apply estrogen vaginal cream to the urinary meatus after each intentional voiding.

98. What should the nurse teach the client to do to prevent stress incontinence? Select all that apply.
- ☐ 1. Use techniques that strengthen the sphincter and structural supports of the bladder, such as Kegel exercises.
- ☐ 2. Avoid natural diuretics such as caffeine or alcoholic beverages.
- ☐ 3. Carry an extra incontinence pad when away from home.
- ☐ 4. Maintain a fluid intake of 500 mL/day.
- ☐ 5. Refrain from coughing or laughing.

99. A client has stress incontinence. Which data from the client's history contribute to the client's incontinence?
- ☐ 1. the client's intake of 2 to 3 L of fluid per day
- ☐ 2. the client's history of three full-term pregnancies
- ☐ 3. the client's age of 45 years
- ☐ 4. the client's history of competitive swimming

100. The **primary** goal of nursing care for a client with stress incontinence is to:
- ☐ 1. help the client adjust to the frequent episodes of incontinence.
- ☐ 2. eliminate all episodes of incontinence.
- ☐ 3. prevent the development of urinary tract infections.
- ☐ 4. decrease the number of incontinence episodes.

101. The nurse is developing a teaching plan for a client with stress incontinence. Which instruction should be included?
- ☐ 1. Avoid activities that are stressful and upsetting.
- ☐ 2. Avoid caffeine and alcohol.
- ☐ 3. Do not wear a girdle.
- ☐ 4. Limit physical exertion.

102. A client has urge incontinence. When obtaining the health history, the nurse should ask if the client has:
- ☐ 1. inability to empty the bladder.
- ☐ 2. loss of urine when coughing.
- ☐ 3. involuntary urination with minimal warning.
- ☐ 4. frequent dribbling of urine.

103. Which nursing action is **most** appropriate for a client who has urge incontinence?
- ☐ 1. Have the client urinate on a timed schedule.
- ☐ 2. Provide a bedside commode.
- ☐ 3. Administer prophylactic antibiotics.
- ☐ 4. Teach the client intermittent self-catheterization technique.

Managing Care, Quality, and Safety of Clients with Urinary Tract Health Problems

104. Which hospitalized client is at **highest** risk for catheter-associated urinary tract infection (CAUTI)?
- ☐ 1. client with diabetes mellitus
- ☐ 2. client who had one course of antibiotic therapy
- ☐ 3. client with a family history of UTIs
- ☐ 4. client with a urinary calculus

105. A client is scheduled for an intravenous pyelogram (IVP). The evening before the procedure, the nurse learns that the client has a sensitivity to shellfish. The nurse should:
- ☐ 1. administer a cathartic to the client to empty the colon.
- ☐ 2. administer an antiflatulent to the client to relieve gas.
- ☐ 3. keep the client on nothing-by-mouth (NPO) status.
- ☐ 4. cancel the IVP and notify the healthcare provider (HCP).

106. The nurse finds a container with the client's urine specimen sitting on a counter in the bathroom. The client states that the specimen has been sitting in the bathroom for at least 2 hours. The nurse should:
- ☐ 1. discard the urine and obtain a new specimen.
- ☐ 2. send the urine to the laboratory as quickly as possible.
- ☐ 3. add fresh urine to the collected specimen and send the specimen to the laboratory.
- ☐ 4. refrigerate the specimen until it can be transported to the laboratory.

107. A client with early acute renal failure has anemia, tachycardia, hypotension, and shortness of breath. The healthcare provider (HCP) has prescribed 2 units of packed red blood cells (RBCs). What should the nurse determine prior to initiating the blood transfusion? Select all that apply.
- ☐ 1. There is an IV access with the appropriate tubing and normal saline as the priming solution.
- ☐ 2. There is a signed informed consent for transfusion therapy.
- ☐ 3. Blood typing and cross-matching are documented in the medical record.
- ☐ 4. The vital signs have been taken and documented in accordance with facility policy and procedure.
- ☐ 5. There is the second unit of blood in the medication room.
- ☐ 6. The client has an identification bracelet.

108. The nurse is instructing the unlicensed assistive personnel (UAP) about the correct technique for obtaining a clean-catch urine culture from a female client. Which statement indicates that the UAP has understood the instructions?
- ☐ 1. "I will have the client completely empty her bladder into the specimen cup."
- ☐ 2. "I will need to catheterize the client to get the urine specimen."
- ☐ 3. "I will ask the client to clean her labia, void into the toilet, and then into the specimen cup."
- ☐ 4. "I will obtain the specimen in the afternoon after the client has had plenty of fluids."

109. An elderly client admitted with new-onset confusion, headache, poor skin turgor, bounding pulse, and urinary incontinence has been drinking copious amounts of water. Upon reviewing the lab results, the nurse discovers a sodium level of 122 mEq/L (122 mmol/L). A report to the healthcare provider (HCP) should include what recommendations? Select all that apply.
- ☐ 1. fluid restriction
- ☐ 2. encourage fluids
- ☐ 3. vital signs every 4 hours instead of every shift
- ☐ 4. bed alarm
- ☐ 5. Foley catheter
- ☐ 6. strict intake and output
- ☐ 7. repeat electrolytes, urine for sodium and specific gravity in the morning
- ☐ 8. 2-g sodium diet

110. Which of the responsibilities related to the care of a client with a Foley catheter are appropriate for the nurse to delegate to the unlicensed assistive personnel (UAP)? Select all that apply.

☐ 1. Flush the catheter as needed to ensure patency.

☐ 2. Empty drainage bag, and record output at specified times.

☐ 3. Apply catheter-securing device to client's leg.

☐ 4. Perform bladder irrigation as prescribed.

☐ 5. Provide Foley catheter and perineal care each shift.

☐ 6. Ensure the urine drainage bag is below the level of the bladder at all times.

111. The client is to receive antibiotic intravenous (IV) therapy in the home. The nurse should develop a teaching plan to ensure that the client and family can manage the IV fluid and infusion correctly and avoid complications. What should the nurse instruct the client to do? Select all that apply.

☐ 1. Report signs of redness or inflammation at the site.

☐ 2. Wear sterile gloves to change the fluids.

☐ 3. Call the healthcare provider (HCP) for a temperature above 100°F (37.8°C).

☐ 4. Cleanse the port with alcohol wipes.

☐ 5. Place the IV bag on a table level with the client's arm.

112. Prior to discharging a client with end-stage cancer of the bladder from the hospital, what should the nurse do? Select all that apply.

☐ 1. Determine if the client is likely to become suicidal.

☐ 2. Give a list of the client's medications to the client before discharge.

☐ 3. Instruct the client to update information when medications are discontinued, doses are changed, or new medications are added.

☐ 4. Explain the need to carry medication information with the client at all times.

☐ 5. Instruct the client that the use of over-the-counter products need not be reported to the healthcare provider (HCP).

Answers, Rationales, and Test-Taking Strategies

*The answers and rationales for each question follow below, along with keys (🔑) to the client need (CN) and cognitive level (CL) for each question. In addition, you will also see a glossary icon (📖) highlighting specific terminology used on the licensing exam. As you check your answers, use the **Content Mastery and Test-Taking Skill Self-Analysis** worksheet (tear-out worksheet in back of book) to identify the*

reason(s) for not answering the questions correctly. For additional information about test-taking skills and strategies for answering questions, refer to pages 12–23 and pages 35–36 in Part 1 of this book.

The Client with Cancer of the Bladder

1. 1,4. An adequate fluid intake aids in the prevention of urinary calculi and infection. Odor-producing foods can produce offensive odors that may impact the client's lifestyle and relationships. Lack of activity leads to urinary stasis, which promotes urinary calculi development and infection. Acidic urine helps prevent urinary tract infections. Tight clothing over the stoma obstructs blood circulation and urine flow.

🔑 CN: Reduction of risk potential; CL: Synthesize

2. 1,2,3. Dermatitis with alkaline encrustations may occur when alkaline urine comes in contact with exposed skin. Yeast infections (or fungal infections) are another common peristomal skin problem. If the stoma is irritated from rubbing, there will be bleeding. The nurse and client should avoid irritating the stoma. Adhesive solvent should be used on a gauze pad to remove old adhesive and should, therefore, not contact the stoma directly. Only a minimal amount of skin cement is applied to the faceplate of the collection bag and skin to secure the appliance over the stoma, so obstruction of the stoma by the cement would not be possible if correct technique is followed.

🔑 CN: Physiological adaptation; CL: Evaluate

3. 3. The nurse should verify that the client has voided prior to discharge in order to evaluate bladder function. Bowel function is not expected to be affected by this procedure. There may not be a need for pain medication immediately postprocedure and before discharge, but the nurse should assess the client's pain status and inform the client about the use and side effects of the medication. It is normal for the client to have hematuria because of the procedure.

🔑 CN: Management of care; CL: Synthesize

4. 3. Painless hematuria is the most common clinical finding in bladder cancer. Other symptoms include urinary frequency, dysuria, and urinary urgency, but these are not as common as hematuria. Suprapubic pain and urine retention do not occur in bladder cancer.

🔑 CN: Physiological adaptation; CL: Analyze

5. 2. Chills could indicate the onset of acute infection that can progress to septic shock. Dizziness would not be an anticipated symptom after a cystoscopy. Pink-tinged urine and bladder spasms are common after cystoscopy.

🔑 CN: Reduction of risk potential;
CL: Analyze

6. 4. Lower abdominal pain after a cystoscopy is frequently caused by bladder spasms. Warm water can help relax muscles. Ice is not effective in relieving spasms. Massage and ambulation may increase bladder irritability.

🔑 CN: Basic care and comfort;
CL: Synthesize

7. 3. An ileal conduit is a permanent urinary diversion in which a portion of the ileum is surgically resected and one end of the segment is closed. The ureters are surgically attached to this segment of the ileum, and the open end of the ileum is brought to the skin surface on the abdomen to form the stoma. The client must wear a pouch to collect the urine that continually flows through the conduit. The bladder is removed during the surgical procedure, and the ileal conduit is not reversible. Diversion of urine to the sigmoid colon is called a *ureteroileosigmoidostomy*. An opening in the bladder that allows urine to drain externally is called a *cystostomy*.

🔑 CN: Reduction of risk potential;
CL: Apply

8. 2. After pelvic surgery, there is an increased chance of thrombophlebitis owing to the pelvic manipulation that can interfere with circulation and promote venous stasis. Peritonitis is a potential complication of any abdominal surgery, not just pelvic surgery. Ascites is most frequently an indication of liver disease. Inguinal hernia may be caused by an increase in intra-abdominal pressure or a congenital weakness of the abdominal wall; ventral hernia occurs at the site of a previous abdominal incision.

🔑 CN: Reduction of risk potential;
CL: Analyze

9. 4. Mucus is secreted by the intestinal segment used to create the conduit and is a normal occurrence. The client should be encouraged to maintain a large fluid intake to help flush the mucus out of the conduit. Because mucus in the urine is expected, it is not necessary to change the appliance bag or to notify the **HCP** 📖. The mucus is not an indication of an infection, so a urine culture is not necessary.

🔑 CN: Reduction of risk potential;
CL: Synthesize

10. 4. If the appliance becomes too full, it is likely to pull away from the skin completely or to leak urine onto the skin; thus, if the seal is intact, the client is emptying the appliance regularly. The skin around the seal should not be red or irritated, which could indicate a leak. There will likely be an odor from the urine. Deep yellow urine indicates that the client should be increasing fluid intake.

🔑 CN: Physiological adaptation;
CL: Evaluate

11. 1. Inserting a gauze wick into the stoma helps prevent urine leakage when changing the appliance. The stoma should not be sealed or suctioned. Oral fluids do not need to be avoided.

🔑 CN: Physiological adaptation;
CL: Synthesize

12. 2. A reusable appliance should be routinely cleaned with soap and water. Other products are not necessary and may damage the appliance or be caustic to the client's skin.

🔑 CN: Physiological adaptation; CL: Apply

13. 3,4. The client with an ileal conduit must learn self-care activities related to care of the stoma and ostomy appliances. The client should be taught to increase fluid intake to about 3,000 mL/day and should not limit intake. Adequate fluid intake helps to flush mucus from the ileal conduit. The ostomy appliance should be changed approximately every 3 to 7 days and whenever a leak develops. A skin barrier is essential to protecting the skin from the irritation of the urine. An aspirin should not be used as a method of odor control because it can be an irritant to the stoma and lead to ulceration. The ostomy pouch should be emptied when it is one-third to one-half full to prevent the weight of the urine from pulling the appliance away from the skin.

🔑 CN: Reduction of risk potential;
CL: Evaluate

14. 2. A distilled vinegar solution acts as a good deodorizing agent after an appliance has been cleaned well with soap and water. If the client prefers, a commercial deodorizer may be used. Salt solution does not deodorize. Ammonia and bleaching agents may damage the appliance.

🔑 CN: Basic care and comfort; CL: Apply

15. 4. It is normal for clients to express fears and concerns about the body changes associated with a urinary diversion. Allowing the client time to verbalize concerns in a supportive environment and suggesting that she discuss these concerns with people who have successfully adjusted to ostomy surgery can help her begin coping with these changes in a positive manner. Although the client may be anxious about this situation and may be feeling worthless, the underlying problem is a disturbance in body image. There are no data to indicate that the client does not know how to care for the urinary diversion.

CN: Psychosocial integrity; CL: Analyze

16. 1. The most important reason for attaching the appliance to a standard urine collection bag at night is to prevent urine reflux into the stoma and ureters, which can result in infection. Use of a standard collection bag also keeps the appliance from separating from the skin and helps prevent urine leakage from an overly full bag, but the primary purpose is to prevent reflux of urine. A client with a urinary diversion should drink 2,000 to 3,000 mL of fluid each day; it would be inappropriate to suggest decreasing fluid intake.

CN: Physiological adaptation; CL: Apply

17. 2. Maintaining a fluid intake of 2,000 to 3,000 mL/day is likely to be most effective in preventing urinary tract infection. A high fluid intake results in high urine output, which prevents urinary stasis and bacterial growth. Avoiding people with respiratory tract infections will not prevent urinary tract infections. Clean, not sterile, technique is used to change the appliance. An ileal conduit stoma is not irrigated.

CN: Physiological adaptation; CL: Synthesize

18. 4. It is important that the client empty the drainage pouch throughout the day to decrease the risk of leakage. The client does not normally need to curtail physical activity. Aspirin should never be placed in a pouch because aspirin can irritate or ulcerate the stoma. The client does not catheterize an ileal conduit stoma.

CN: Physiological adaptation; CL: Evaluate

19. 2. After intravesical chemotherapy, the client must treat the urine as a biohazard; this involves disinfecting the urine and the toilet with household bleach for 6 hours following a treatment. It is not necessary to use a bedpan and then empty the urine in the toilet; the client can use the toilet, but must disinfect the urine with bleach. The bathroom does not need to be cleaned daily with disinfectant wipes. The client does not need to use a separate bathroom as long as the client's urine is disinfected with bleach.

CN: Physiological integrity; CL: Evaluate

20. 1,3,4. The nurse should assess the biopsy site for bleeding and hematoma formation. The client should remain prone for 8 to 24 hours after the biopsy. A pressure dressing will aid in blood coagulation. Vital signs assessment should be taken every 5 to 15 minutes for the first hour and then less often if the client is stable. The urine does not need to be collected and kept on ice. The nurse should collect serial urine specimens to assess for hematuria. A renal biopsy does not put the client at increased risk for chest pain.

CN: Reduction of risk potential; CL: Synthesize

The Client with Renal Calculi

21. 1,2,5. Following lithotripsy, the nurse strains all urine to collect and identify stone composition. Providing heat to the flank area may be helpful to relieve muscle spasms when renal colic is present; the nurse assesses the client's pain level and administers analgesics as needed. Hematuria is common after lithotripsy, and it is not necessary to notify the HCP. The nurse should promote a fluid intake of at least 2,000 mL/day to flush stones and clots through the urinary tract.

CN: Physiological adaptation; CL: Synthesize

22. 4. If infection or blockage caused by calculi is present, a client can experience sudden severe pain in the flank area, known as *renal colic*. Pain from a kidney stone is considered an emergency situation and requires analgesic intervention. Withholding fluids will make urine more concentrated and stones more difficult to pass naturally. Forcing large quantities of fluid may cause hydronephrosis if urine is prevented from flowing past calculi. Straining urine for small stones is important, but does not take priority over pain management.

CN: Management of care; CL: Synthesize

23. 3. The priority nursing goal for this client is to alleviate the pain, which can be excruciating. Prevention of urinary tract complications and alleviation of nausea are appropriate throughout the client's hospitalization, but relief of the severe pain is a priority. The client is at little risk for fluid and electrolyte imbalance.

CN: Physiological adaptation; CL: Synthesize

24. 4. A KUB radiographic examination ordinarily requires no preparation. It is usually done while the client lies supine and does not involve the use of radiopaque substances. It is not necessary for the client to withhold fluids; the client will not need to take a tranquilizer; an enema is not included in the preparation.

CN: Reduction of risk potential; CL: Apply

25. 2. The pain associated with renal colic due to calculi is commonly referred to the groin and bladder in female clients and to the testicles in male clients. Nausea, vomiting, abdominal cramping, and diarrhea may also be present. Nephritis or urine retention is an unlikely cause of the referred pain. The type of pain described in this situation is unlikely to be caused by additional stone formation.

⚷━ CN: Physiological adaptation;
CL: Analyze

26. 2. During episodes of renal colic, the pain is excruciating. It is necessary to administer opioid analgesics to control the pain. Application of heat, encouraging high fluid intake, and limitation of activity are important interventions, but they will not relieve the renal colic pain.

⚷━ CN: Reduction of risk potential;
CL: Synthesize

27. 2. Intermittent pain that is less colicky indicates that the calculi may be moving along the urinary tract. Fluids should be encouraged to promote movement, and the urine should be strained to detect passage of the stone. Hematuria is to be expected from the irritation of the stone. Analgesics should be administered when the client needs them, not routinely. Moist heat to the flank area is helpful when renal colic occurs, but it is less necessary as pain is lessened.

⚷━ CN: Physiological adaptation;
CL: Synthesize

28. 3. A client scheduled for an IVP should be assessed for allergies to iodine and shellfish. Clients with such allergies may be allergic to the IVP dye and be at risk for an anaphylactic reaction. Adequate fluid intake is important after the examination. Bladder spasms are not common during an IVP. Bowel preparation is important before an IVP to allow visualization of the ureters and bladder, but checking for allergies is most important.

⚷━ CN: Reduction of risk potential;
CL: Synthesize

29. 2. After an IVP, the nurse should encourage fluids to decrease the risk of renal complications caused by the contrast agent. There is no need to place the client on bed rest or administer a laxative. An IVP would not cause hematuria.

⚷━ CN: Reduction of risk potential;
CL: Synthesize

30. 2. The ureteral catheter should drain freely without bleeding at the site. The catheter is rarely irrigated, and any irrigation would be done by the **healthcare provider (HCP)** 📖. The catheter is never clamped. The client's total urine output (ureteral catheter plus voiding or indwelling urinary catheter output) should be at least 30 mL/h.

⚷━ CN: Reduction of risk potential;
CL: Synthesize

31. 1. Ambulation stimulates peristalsis. A client with paralytic ileus is kept on nothing-by-mouth status until peristalsis returns. Carbonated beverages will increase gas and distention but will not stimulate peristalsis. A stool softener will not stimulate peristalsis. IV fluid infusion is a routine postoperative prescription that does not have any effect on preventing paralytic ileus.

⚷━ CN: Physiological adaptation;
CL: Synthesize

32. 2. The decrease in urine output may reflect inadequate renal perfusion and should be reported immediately. Urine output of 30 mL/h or greater is considered acceptable. A slight elevation in temperature is expected after surgery. Peristalsis returns gradually, usually the second or third day after surgery. Bowel sounds will be absent until then. A small amount of serosanguineous drainage is to be expected.

⚷━ CN: Physiological adaptation;
CL: Analyze

33. 1. A high daily fluid intake is essential for all clients who are at risk for calculi formation because it prevents urinary stasis and concentration, which can cause crystallization. Depending on the composition of the stone, the client also may be instructed to institute specific dietary measures aimed at preventing stone formation. Clients may need to limit purine, calcium, or oxalate. Urine may need to be either alkaline or acid. There is no need to strain urine regularly.

⚷━ CN: Basic care and comfort;
CL: Synthesize

34. 1. Because a high-purine diet contributes to the formation of uric acid, a low-purine diet is advocated. An alkaline-ash diet is also advocated because uric acid crystals are more likely to develop in acid urine. Foods that may be eaten as desired in a low-purine diet include milk, all fruits, tomatoes, cereals, and corn. Foods allowed on an alkaline-ash diet include milk, fruits (except cranberries, plums, and prunes), and vegetables (especially legumes and green vegetables). Gravy, which can be made with organ meats such as liver, chicken, and liver are high in purine. In the absence of specific information from the **healthcare provider (HCP)** 📖 or dietician about limiting calcium, the client can include dairy products in this diet.

⚷━ CN: Basic care and comfort; CL: Evaluate

35. 2. Allopurinol is used to treat renal calculi composed of uric acid. Adverse effects of allopurinol include drowsiness, maculopapular rash, anemia, abdominal pain, nausea, vomiting, and bone marrow depression. Clients should be instructed to report rashes and unusual bleeding or bruising.

Retinopathy, nasal congestion, and dizziness are not adverse effects of allopurinol.

   CN: Pharmacological and parenteral therapies; CL: Synthesize

36. 1,2,5. Common adverse effects of allopurinol include gastrointestinal distress, such as anorexia, nausea, vomiting, and diarrhea. A rash is another potential adverse effect. A potentially life-threatening adverse effect is bone marrow depression. Constipation and flushed skin are not associated with this drug.

   CN: Pharmacological and parenteral therapies; CL: Analyze

37. 4. By inhibiting uric acid synthesis, allopurinol decreases its excretion. The drug's effectiveness is assessed by evaluating for a decreased serum uric acid concentration. Allopurinol does not alter the level of alkaline phosphatase, nor does it affect urine calcium excretion or the serum calcium level.

   CN: Pharmacological and parenteral therapies; CL: Evaluate

The Client with Acute Renal Failure

38. 4. Solution for peritoneal dialysis should be warmed to body temperature in a warmer or with a heating pad; do not use the microwave. Cold dialysate increases discomfort. Assessment for a bruit and thrill is necessary with hemodialysis when the client has a fistula, graft, or shunt. An indwelling urinary catheter is not required for this procedure. The nurse should position the client in a supine or low Fowler's position.

   CN: Reduction of risk potential; CL: Synthesize

39. 1,2,3,4. Elevation of the head of the bed will promote ease of breathing. Respiratory manifestations of acute renal failure include shortness of breath, orthopnea, crackles, and the potential for pulmonary edema. Therefore, priority is placed on facilitation of respiration. The nurse should assess the vital signs because the pulse and respirations will be elevated. Establishing a site for IV therapy will become important because fluids will be administered IV in addition to orally. The **HCP** will need to be contacted for further prescriptions; there is no need to contact the hemodialysis unit.

   CN: Physiological adaptation; CL: Synthesize

40. 4. Oliguria is the most common initial symptom of acute renal failure. Anuria is rarely the initial symptom. Dysuria and hematuria are not associated with acute renal failure.

   CN: Physiological adaptation; CL: Analyze

41. 1. There are three categories of acute renal failure: prerenal, intrarenal, and postrenal. Causes of prerenal failure occur outside the kidney and include poor perfusion and decreased circulating volume resulting from such factors as trauma, septic shock, impaired cardiac function, and dehydration. In this case of severe myocardial infarction, there was a decrease in perfusion of the kidneys caused by impaired cardiac function. An obstruction within the urinary tract, such as from kidney stones, tumors, or benign prostatic hypertrophy, is called *postrenal failure*. Structural damage to the kidney resulting from acute tubular necrosis is called *intrarenal failure*. It is caused by such conditions as hypersensitivity (allergic disorders), renal vessel obstruction, and nephrotoxic agents.

   CN: Physiological adaptation; CL: Apply

42. 4. Urea, an end product of protein metabolism, is excreted by the kidneys. Impairment in renal function caused by reduced renal blood flow results in an increase in the plasma urea level. Fluid retention, hemolysis of red blood cells, and lowered metabolic rate do not cause an elevated BUN value.

   CN: Reduction of risk potential; CL: Analyze

43. 4. Polystyrene sulfonate, a cation-exchange resin, causes the body to excrete potassium through the gastrointestinal tract. In the intestines, particularly the colon, the sodium of the resin is partially replaced by potassium. The potassium is then eliminated when the resin is eliminated with feces. Although the result is to increase potassium excretion, the specific method of action is the exchange of sodium ions for potassium ions. Polystyrene sulfonate does not release hydrogen ions or increase calcium absorption.

   CN: Pharmacological and parenteral therapies; CL: Apply

44. 1. Hyperkalemia places the client at risk for serious cardiac arrhythmias and cardiac arrest. Therefore, the nurse should carefully monitor the client for cardiac arrhythmias and be prepared to treat cardiac arrest when caring for a client with hyperkalemia. Increased potassium levels do not result in pulmonary edema, circulatory collapse, or hemorrhage.

   CN: Pharmacological and parenteral therapies; CL: Analyze

45. 4. High-carbohydrate foods meet the body's caloric needs during acute renal failure. Protein is limited because its breakdown may result in accumulation of toxic waste products. The main goal of nutritional therapy in acute renal failure is to decrease protein catabolism. Protein catabolism causes increased levels of urea, phosphate, and potassium. Carbohydrates provide energy and decrease the need for protein breakdown. They do not have a diuretic effect. Some specific carbohydrates influence urine pH, but this is not the reason for encouraging a high-carbohydrate, low-protein diet. There is no need to reduce demands on the liver through dietary manipulation in acute renal failure.

CN: Basic care and comfort; CL: Apply

46. 1. Gelatin desserts contain little or no potassium and can be served to a client on a potassium-restricted diet. Foods high in potassium include bran and whole grains; most dried, raw, and frozen fruits and vegetables; most milk and milk products; and chocolate, nuts, raisins, coconut, and strong brewed coffee.

CN: Basic care and comfort; CL: Apply

47. 1. Pulmonary edema can develop during the oliguric phase of acute renal failure because of decreased urine output and fluid retention. Metabolic acidosis develops because the kidneys cannot excrete hydrogen ions, and bicarbonate is used to buffer the hydrogen. Hypertension may develop as a result of fluid retention. Hyperkalemia develops as the kidneys lose the ability to excrete potassium.

CN: Physiological adaptation; CL: Analyze

48. 1. The unaffected arm should be used for blood pressure measurement. The external cannula must be handled carefully and protected from damage and disruption. In addition, a tourniquet or clamps should be kept at the bedside because dislodgment of the cannula would cause arterial hemorrhage. The arm with the cannula is not used for blood pressure measurement, IV therapy, or venipuncture. Patency is assessed by auscultating for bruits every shift. Heparin is not injected into the cannula to maintain patency. Because it is part of the general circulation, the cannula cannot be heparinized.

CN: Reduction of risk potential; CL: Synthesize

49. 2. If disequilibrium syndrome occurs during dialysis, the most appropriate intervention is to slow the rate of dialysis. The syndrome is believed to result from too-rapid removal of urea and excess electrolytes from the blood; this causes transient cerebral edema, which produces the symptoms. Administration of oxygen and position changes do not affect the symptoms. It would not be appropriate to reassure the client that the symptoms are normal.

CN: Reduction of risk potential; CL: Synthesize

50. 3. Dialysis has no effect on hemoglobin levels because some red blood cells are injured during the procedure; dialysis aggravates a low hemoglobin concentration and may contribute to anemia. Dialysis will clear metabolic waste products from the body and correct electrolyte imbalances, correct electrolyte imbalances such as creatinine, potassium and sodium levels.

CN: Reduction of risk potential; CL: Apply

51. 4. Signs and symptoms of an external access shunt infection include redness, tenderness, swelling, and drainage from around the shunt site. The absence of a bruit indicates closing of the shunt. Sluggish capillary refill time and coolness of the extremity indicate decreased blood flow to the extremity.

CN: Reduction of risk potential; CL: Analyze

52. 1. The kidneys have a remarkable ability to recover from serious insult. Recovery may take 3 to 12 months. The client should be taught how to recognize the signs and symptoms of decreasing renal function and to notify the **healthcare provider (HCP)** if such problems occur. In a client who is recovering from acute renal failure, there is no need for renal transplantation or permanent hemodialysis. Chronic renal failure develops before end-stage renal failure.

CN: Physiological adaptation; CL: Apply

The Client with Urinary Tract Infection

53. 4. The sensation of thirst diminishes in those greater than 60 years of age; hence, fluid intake is decreased, and dissolved particles in the extracellular fluid compartment become more concentrated. There is no change in liver function in older adults, nor is there a reduction of ADH and aldosterone as a normal part of aging.

CN: Physiological adaptation; CL: Apply

54. 3. Antibiotics have the maximum effect when the level of the medication in the blood is maintained. However, because nitrofurantoin is readily absorbed from the gastrointestinal tract and is primarily excreted in urine, toxicity may develop by doubling the dose. The client should not skip a dose, if one dose is missed. Additional fluids, especially water, should be encouraged, but not forced, to promote elimination of the antibiotic from the body. Adequate fluid intake aids in the prevention of urinary tract infections, in addition to an acidic urine.

CN: Pharmacological and parenteral therapies; CL: Synthesize

55. 2,3,4. Catheter-associated urinary tract infection is the most frequent type of healthcare-acquired infection (HAI) and represents as much as 80% of HAIs in hospitals. The nurse should provide meticulous perineal care, encourage the client to obtain an adequate fluid intake, and assess the client for signs of infection such as an elevated temperature. It is not necessary to change the catheter daily. It is recommended that long-term use of an indwelling urinary catheter be evaluated carefully and other methods considered if the catheter will be in place longer than 2 weeks. It is not necessary to request a prescription for antibiotics as the client does not currently have an infection.

CN: Safety and infection control; CL: Synthesize

56. 1. The client's urine specific gravity is elevated. Specific gravity is a reflection of the concentrating ability of the kidneys. This level indicates that the urine is concentrated. By increasing fluid intake, the urine will become more dilute. Antihypertensives do not make urine more concentrated unless there is a diuretic component within them. The nurse should not hold a dose of antihypertensive medication. Sodium tends to pull water with it; by restricting sodium, less water, not more, will be present. Bananas do not aid in the dilution of urine.

CN: Reduction of risk potential; CL: Synthesize

57. 1. All urine for creatinine clearance determination must be saved in a container with no preservatives and refrigerated or kept on ice. The first urine voided at the beginning of the collection is discarded, not the last. A self-report of weight may not be accurate. It is not necessary to have an indwelling urinary catheter inserted for urine collection.

CN: Reduction of risk potential; CL: Apply

58. 141 mg

$$1.5\,mg \times 94.1 = 141.15 = 141\,mg$$

CN: Pharmacological and parenteral therapies; CL: Apply

59. 2. The classic symptoms of cystitis are severe burning on urination, urgency, and frequent urination. Systemic symptoms, such as fever and nausea and vomiting, are more likely to accompany pyelonephritis than cystitis. Hematuria may occur, but it is not as common as frequency and burning.

CN: Physiological adaptation; CL: Analyze

60. 4. Although various conditions may result in cystitis, the most common cause is an ascending infection from the urethra. Strictures and urine retention can lead to infections, but these are not the most common cause. Systemic infections are rarely causes of cystitis.

CN: Physiological adaptation; CL: Apply

61. 4. As newlyweds, the client and her husband need to develop a strong communication base. The nurse can facilitate communication by preparing and supporting the client. Given the situation, an interdisciplinary conference is inappropriate and would not promote intimacy for the client and her husband. Insisting that the client talk with her husband is not addressing her fears. Being present allows the nurse to facilitate the discussion of a difficult topic. Having the nurse speak first with the husband alone shifts responsibility away from the couple.

CN: Psychosocial integrity; CL: Synthesize

62. 2. Hot tub baths promote relaxation and help relieve urgency, discomfort, and spasm. Applying heat to the perineum is more helpful than cold because heat reduces inflammation. Although liberal fluid intake should be encouraged, caffeinated beverages, such as tea, coffee, and cola, can be irritating to the bladder and should be avoided. Voiding at least every 2 to 3 hours should be encouraged because it reduces urinary stasis.

CN: Basic care and comfort; CL: Evaluate

63. 3. The client should take the prescription as ordered. The client should increase fluid intake to 3,000 mL/day to increase urination. Even though the urine may become clear in a short period, it is not necessary to notify the **HCP**. The client should continue to take the entire prescription of antibiotics. Cystitis is not sexually transmitted, so protection by using a condom is not necessary.

CN: Pharmacological and parenteral therapies; CL: Synthesize

64. 2,3,5. The nurse should instruct the client to report signs of adverse reaction to the antibiotic or indications that the urinary tract infection is not clearing. Blood in the urine is not an expected outcome, rash is an adverse response to the antibiotic, and an elevated temperature indicates a persistent infection. These signs should be reported to the **HCP**. Cloudy urine can be expected during the first few days of antibiotic treatment. Mild nausea is a side effect of antibiotic therapy, but it can be managed with eating small, frequent meals. Urinating every 3 to 4 hours or more is expected, particularly if the client is increasing the fluid intake as directed.

CN: Pharmacological and parenteral therapies; CL: Synthesis

65. **2,3.** Clients who are taking nitrofurantoin should be instructed to take the medication with meals and to increase their fluid intake to minimize gastrointestinal distress. The urine may become brown in color. Although this change is harmless, clients need to be prepared for this color change. The client should be instructed to take the full prescription and not to stop taking the drug because symptoms have subsided. The medication should not be taken with antacids as this may interfere with the drug's absorption.

⚷— CN: Pharmacological and parenteral therapies; CL: Synthesize

66. **15 mL**
The following formula is used to calculate the correct dosage:

$$25\,mg\,/\,5\,mL = 75\,mg\,/\,X\,mL$$
$$X = 15\,mL.$$

⚷— CN: Pharmacological and parenteral therapies; CL: Apply

67. **1.** Stasis of urine in the bladder is one of the chief causes of bladder infection, and a client who voids infrequently is at greater risk for reinfection. A tub bath does not promote urinary tract infections as long as the client avoids harsh soaps and bubble baths. Scrupulous hygiene and liberal fluid intake (unless contraindicated) are excellent preventive measures, but the client also should be taught to void every 2 to 3 hours during the day. Lifting weights is not a risk factor for cystitis.

⚷— CN: Reduction of risk potential; CL: Analyze

68. **1.** A woman can adopt several health promotion measures to prevent the recurrence of cystitis, including avoiding too-tight pants, non-cotton underpants, and irritating substances, such as bubble baths and vaginal soaps and sprays. Increasing citrus juice intake can be a bladder irritant. Regular douching is not recommended; it can alter the pH of the vagina, increasing the risk of infection.

⚷— CN: Health promotion and maintenance; CL: Synthesize

69. **4.** Instructions should be as specific as possible, and the nurse should avoid general statements such as "a lot." A specific goal is most useful. A mix of fluids will increase the likelihood of client compliance. It may not be sufficient to tell the client to drink twice as much as or 1 quart (950 mL) more than she usually drinks if her intake was inadequate to begin with.

⚷— CN: Basic care and comfort; CL: Apply

The Client with Pyelonephritis

70. **1.** Acute pyelonephritis usually begins with a bacterial infection of the lower urinary tract via the ascending urethral route; most infections are due to gram-negative bacilli, such as *Escherichia coli*, normally found in the GI tract. Thorough perineal care using soap and warm water, and cleansing from front to back, decreases the likelihood that organisms will be introduced into the urinary tract and ascend upward toward the kidneys. Although preventing and treating all infections are appropriate, fungal infections from the feet and bacterial infections in the throat or skin are less likely to be immediate sources of infection causing pyelonephritis.

⚷— CN: Health promotion and maintenance; CL: Synthesize

71. **1.** Pyelonephritis usually begins with colonization and infection of the lower urinary tract via the ascending urethral route, and the client should have an adequate intake of fluids to promote the flushing action of urination. Bubble baths and limiting fluid intake increase the risk of developing a urinary tract infection. Antibiotics should be used on a short-term basis because the risk of antibiotic resistance may lead to breakthrough infections with increasingly virulent pathogens.

⚷— CN: Health promotion and maintenance; CL: Synthesize

72. **4.** A client with a history of diabetes mellitus, urinary tract infections, or renal calculi is at increased risk for pyelonephritis. Others at high risk include pregnant women and people with structural alterations of the urinary tract. A history of hypertension may put the client at risk for kidney damage, but not kidney infection. Intake of large quantities of cranberry juice and a fluid intake of 2,000 mL/day are not risk factors for pyelonephritis.

⚷— CN: Reduction of risk potential; CL: Analyze

73. **3.** Antibiotics are usually prescribed for a 2- to 4-week period. A urine culture is needed to evaluate the effectiveness of antibiotic therapy. Urine must be examined microscopically to adequately determine the presence of bacteria; looking at the color of the urine or checking the odor is not sufficient. Symptoms usually disappear 48 to 72 hours after antibiotic therapy is started, but antibiotics may need to continue for up to 4 weeks.

⚷— CN: Pharmacological and parenteral therapies; CL: Evaluate

74. **0.4 mL**

⚷— CN: Pharmacologic and parenteral therapy; CL: Apply

75. 2. Chronic pyelonephritis is most commonly the result of recurrent urinary tract infections. Chronic pyelonephritis can lead to chronic renal failure. Single cases of acute pyelonephritis rarely cause chronic pyelonephritis. Acute renal failure is not a cause of chronic pyelonephritis. Glomerulonephritis is an immunologic disorder, not an infectious disorder.

🔑 CN: Physiological adaptation; CL: Apply

76. 4. The nurse should ensure the client has adequate hydration. A urinary catheter is discouraged because of the risk of urinary tract infection. Monitoring of the hemoglobin level is not necessary for clients with pyelonephritis. Although antibiotics may be prescribed for long-term management and for chronic pyelonephritis, at this time the nurse should focus on helping the client maintain hydration.

🔑 CN: Physiologic adaptation; CL: Analyze

The Client with Chronic Renal Failure

77. 2,3,4. The nurse instructs the client to protect the site of the fistula. The client should avoid pressure on the involved arm such as sleeping on it, wearing tight jewelry, or obtaining BP. The client is also advised to assess the area distal to the fistula for adequate circulation, such as warmth and color. When the client is hospitalized, the nurse posts a sign on the client's bed not to draw blood or obtain BP on the left side; the client is also instructed to be sure that none of the healthcare team members do so.

🔑 CN: Physiological adaptation; CL: Synthesize

78. 2,4,1,3. The nurse first assures an IV access site in case the client has respiratory or cardiac arrest. Next, the nurse monitors the client's heart rate and rhythm: Cardiovascular signs of elevated serum potassium levels are irregular, slow heart rate; decreased BP; narrow, peaked T waves; widened QRS complexes, prolonged PR intervals, and flattened D waves; frequent ectopy; ventricular fibrillation; and ventricular standstill. The nurse then administers calcium gluconate, which has an immediate action to antagonize the effect of hyperkalemia on cardiac muscle. Last, the nurse administers polystyrene sulfonate, which is a cation-exchange resin that removes potassium from the body by exchanging sodium ion for potassium; potassium-containing resin is then excreted; onset is in several hours to days.

🔑 CN: Physiological adaptation; CL: Synthesize

79. 2. The nurse must always auscultate for a bruit and palpate for a thrill in the arm with the fistula and promptly report the absence of either a thrill or bruit to the **healthcare provider (HCP)** 📖 as it indicates an occlusion. The client should not have a pressure dressing on the shunt and should avoid wearing tight clothing or carrying heavy items such as purse over the area of the shunt to avoid restricting blood flow in the shunt. No procedures such as IV access, blood pressure measurements, or blood draws are done on an arm with a fistula as they could damage the fistula.

🔑 CN: Physiological adaptation; CL: Synthesize

80. 2,4,5. To manage nausea, the nurse can advise the client to drink limited amounts of fluid only when thirsty and eat food before drinking fluids to alleviate dry mouth, and encourage strict follow-up for blood work, dialysis, and **healthcare provider (HCP)** 📖 visits. Smaller, more frequent meals may help to reduce nausea and facilitate medication taking. The client should be as active as possible to avoid immobilization because it increases bone demineralization. The client should also maintain the dialysis schedule because the dialysis will remove wastes that can contribute to nausea.

🔑 CN: Physiological adaptation; CL: Synthesize

81. 1. The main reason for warming the peritoneal dialysis solution is that the warm solution helps dilate peritoneal vessels, which increases urea clearance. Warmed dialyzing solution also contributes to client comfort by preventing chilly sensations, but this is a secondary reason for warming the solution. The warmed solution does not force potassium into the cells or promote abdominal muscle relaxation.

🔑 CN: Reduction of risk potential; CL: Apply

82. 2. During dwell time, the dialysis solution is allowed to remain in the peritoneal cavity for the time prescribed by the **healthcare provider (HCP)** 📖 (usually 20 to 45 minutes). During this time, the nurse should monitor the client's respiratory status because the pressure of the dialysis solution on the diaphragm can create respiratory distress. The dialysis solution would not cause urticaria or affect circulation to the fingers. The client's laboratory values are obtained before beginning treatment and are monitored every 4 to 8 hours during the treatment, not just during the dwell time.

🔑 CN: Reduction of risk potential; CL: Analyze

83. 2. Because the client has a permanent catheter in place, blood-tinged drainage should not occur. Persistent blood-tinged drainage could indicate damage to the abdominal vessels, and the **health-care provider (HCP)** 📖 should be notified. The bleeding is originating in the peritoneal cavity, not the kidneys. Too-rapid infusion of the dialysate can cause pain, not blood-tinged drainage.

🔑 CN: Reduction of risk potential;
CL: Analyze

84. 2. Fluid return with peritoneal dialysis is accomplished by gravity flow. Actions that enhance gravity flow include turning the client from side to side, raising the head of the bed, and gently massaging the abdomen. The client is usually confined to a recumbent position during the dialysis. The nurse should not attempt to reposition the catheter.

🔑 CN: Reduction of risk potential;
CL: Synthesize

85. 4. Constipation may contribute to reduced urine outflow in part because peristalsis facilitates drainage outflow. For this reason, bisacodyl suppositories can be used prophylactically, even without a history of constipation. Diarrhea, vomiting, and flatulence typically do not cause decreased outflow in a peritoneal dialysis catheter.

🔑 CN: Physiological integrity; CL: Analyze

86. 2. Because hypotension is a complication associated with peritoneal dialysis, the nurse records intake and output, monitors vital signs, and observes the client's behavior. The nurse also encourages visiting and other diversional activities. A client on peritoneal dialysis does not need to be placed in a bed with padded side rails or kept on NPO status.

🔑 CN: Reduction of risk potential;
CL: Synthesize

87. 1,2,4,5. Broad-spectrum antibiotics may be administered to prevent infection when a peritoneal catheter is inserted for peritoneal dialysis. If peritonitis is present, antibiotics may be added to the dialysate. Aseptic technique is imperative. Peritonitis, the most common and serious complication of peritoneal dialysis, is characterized by cloudy dialysate drainage, diffuse abdominal pain, and rebound tenderness.

🔑 CN: Safety and infection control;
CL: Synthesize

88. 2. Weight loss is expected because of the removal of fluid. The client's weight before and after dialysis is one measure of the effectiveness of treatment. Blood pressure usually decreases because of the removal of fluid. Hematuria would not occur after completion of peritoneal dialysis. Dialysis only minimally affects the damaged kidneys' ability to manufacture urine.

🔑 CN: Reduction of risk potential;
CL: Evaluate

89. 3. A client in renal failure develops hyperphosphatemia that causes a corresponding excretion of the body's calcium stores, leading to renal osteodystrophy. To decrease this loss, aluminum hydroxide gel is prescribed to bind phosphates in the intestine and facilitate their excretion. Gastric hyperacidity is not necessarily a problem associated with chronic renal failure. Antacids will not prevent Curling's stress ulcers and do not affect metabolic acidosis.

🔑 CN: Pharmacological and parenteral therapies; CL: Evaluate

90. 4. Aluminum hydroxide gel is administered to bind the phosphates in ingested foods and must be given with or immediately after meals and snacks. There is no need for the client to take it on a 24-hour schedule. It is not administered to treat an upset stomach caused by hyperacidity in clients with chronic renal failure and therefore is not prescribed between meals.

🔑 CN: Pharmacological and parenteral therapies; CL: Evaluate

91. 2. Uremia can cause decreased alertness, so the nurse needs to validate the client's comprehension frequently. Because the client's ability to concentrate is limited, short lessons are most effective. If family members are present at the sessions, they can reinforce the material. Written materials that the client can review are superior to videos because the client may not be able to maintain alertness during the viewing of the videotape.

🔑 CN: Physiological adaptation;
CL: Synthesize

92. 3. Dietary management for clients with chronic renal failure is usually designed to restrict protein, sodium, and potassium intake. Protein intake is reduced because the kidney can no longer excrete the by-products of protein metabolism. The degree of dietary restriction depends on the degree of renal impairment. The client should also receive a high-carbohydrate diet along with appropriate vitamin and mineral supplements. Calcium requirements remain 1,000 to 2,000 mg/day.

🔑 CN: Basic care and comfort;
CL: Synthesize

93. 2. Altered sexual functioning commonly occurs in chronic renal failure and can stress marriages and relationships. Altered sexual functioning can be caused by decreased hormone levels, anemia, peripheral neuropathy, or medication.

The client should not decrease or avoid sexual activity but instead should modify it. The client should rest before sexual activity. Unless the client provides additional information, it is not necessary to refer the client to counseling at this time.

CN: Psychosocial integrity;
CL: Synthesize

94. 2. The major benefit of CAPD is that it frees the client from daily dependence on dialysis centers, healthcare personnel, and machines for life-sustaining treatment. This independence is a valuable outcome for some people. CAPD is costly and must be done daily. Adverse effects and complications are similar to those of standard peritoneal dialysis. Peritoneal dialysis usually takes less time but cannot be done at home.

CN: Reduction of risk potential;
CL: Apply

95. 3. Dietary restrictions with CAPD are fewer than those with standard peritoneal dialysis because dialysis is constant, not intermittent. The constant slow diffusion of CAPD helps prevent accumulation of toxins and allows for a more liberal diet. CAPD does not work more quickly, but more consistently. Both types of peritoneal dialysis are effective.

CN: Basic care and comfort;
CL: Synthesize

96. 1. Cloudy drainage indicates bacterial activity in the peritoneum. Other signs and symptoms of infection are fever, hyperactive bowel sounds, and abdominal pain. Swollen legs may indicate heart failure. Poor drainage of dialysate fluid is probably the result of a kinked catheter. Redness at the insertion site indicates local infection, not peritonitis. However, a local infection that is left untreated can progress to the peritoneum.

CN: Reduction of risk potential;
CL: Analyze

The Client with Urinary Incontinence

97. 3. Perineal muscle exercises (Kegel exercises) increase the tone of the urethral sphincters; the nurse teaches the client to perform the exercises in sets of at least 10 contractions, four to five times per day. Asking someone else to lift heavy loads may not always be practical. Wearing disposable protective underwear is only a temporary measure because long-term use discourages continence and can lead to skin problems. Applying estrogen vaginal cream to the urinary meatus after each intentional voiding can lead to UTIs. Drug therapy has a very limited role in the management of stress urinary incontinence.

CN: Health promotion and maintenance;
CL: Synthesize

98. 1,2. Kegel exercises strengthen the sphincter and structural supports of the bladder, and the nurse should be sure the client knows how to do these exercises. Establishing a voiding schedule is more effective than carrying incontinence pads in preventing stress incontinence. In nonrestricted clients, a fluid intake of at least 2 to 3 L/day is encouraged; clients with stress incontinence may reduce their fluid intake to avoid incontinence at the risk of developing dehydration and urinary tract infections. Natural diuretics, such as caffeine and alcoholic beverages, may increase stress incontinence. It is unlikely that the client can prevent laughing or coughing or other activities that might put stress on the sphincter.

CN: Health promotion and maintenance;
CL: Synthesize

99. 2. The history of three pregnancies is most likely the cause of the client's current episodes of stress incontinence. The client's fluid intake, age, or history of swimming would not create an increase in intra-abdominal pressure.

CN: Reduction of risk potential;
CL: Analyze

100. 4. The primary goal of nursing care is to decrease the number of incontinence episodes and the amount of urine expressed in an episode. Behavioral interventions (e.g., diet and exercise) and medications are the nonsurgical management methods used to treat stress incontinence. Without surgical intervention, it may not be possible to eliminate all episodes of incontinence. Helping the client adjust to the incontinence is not treating the problem. Clients with stress incontinence are not prone to the development of urinary tract infection.

CN: Physiological adaptation;
CL: Synthesize

101. 2. Clients with stress incontinence are encouraged to avoid substances that are bladder irritants, such as caffeine and alcohol. Emotional stressors do not cause stress incontinence. It is most commonly caused by relaxed pelvic musculature. Wearing girdles is not contraindicated. Although clients may want to limit physical exertion to avoid incontinence episodes, they should be encouraged to seek treatment instead of limiting their activities.

CN: Reduction of risk potential; CL: Create

102. 3. A characteristic of urge incontinence is involuntary urination with little or no warning. The inability to empty the bladder is urine retention. Loss of urine when coughing occurs with stress incontinence. Frequent dribbling of urine is common in male clients after some types of prostate surgery or may occur in women after the development of a vesicovaginal or urethrovaginal fistula.

CN: Physiological adaptation; CL: Analyze

103. 1. Instructing the client to void at regularly scheduled intervals can help decrease the frequency of incontinence episodes. Providing a bedside commode does not decrease the number of incontinence episodes and does not help the client who leads an active lifestyle. Infections are not a common cause of urge incontinence, so antibiotics are not an appropriate treatment. Intermittent self-catheterization is appropriate for overflow or reflux incontinence but not urge incontinence, because it does not treat the underlying cause.

CN: Physiological adaptation; CL: Synthesize

Managing Care, Quality, and Safety of Clients with Urinary Tract Health Problems

104. 1. Clients who are immunosuppressed, have diabetes mellitus, or have undergone multiple courses of antibiotic therapy are prone to bacterial, fungal, and parasitic infections. Taking one course of antibiotic therapy or having a family history of UTIs does not make a client at high risk for development of a UTI. A predisposing factor for a UTI is ongoing problems of urinary calculi; one calculus would not place a client at high risk.

CN: Management of care; CL: Analyze

105. 4. Sensitivity to shellfish or iodine may cause an anaphylactic reaction to the contrast material, which contains iodine. Administering a cathartic or antiflatulent will not prevent an anaphylactic reaction to the contrast material. Keeping a client on NPO status for 8 hours before the procedure is part of the usual preparation for such a procedure to prevent aspiration of food or fluids if the client vomits when lying on the x-ray table.

CN: Reduction of risk potential; CL: Synthesize

106. 1. The appropriate action would be to discard the specimen and obtain a new one. Urine that is allowed to stand at room temperature will become alkaline, with multiplying bacteria. The specimen should be examined within 1 hour after urination.

CN: Reduction of risk potential; CL: Synthesize

107. 1,2,3,4,6. Before prescribing and administering packed RBCs, the nurse should assess the IV site to make sure it has an 18G to 20G infusion set. The nurse should also ensure that normal saline solution is used to prime the tubing to prevent RBCs from adhering to the tubing. The client must

indicate **informed consent** for the procedure by signing the consent form. The client's blood must be typed to determine ABO blood typing and Rh factor and ensure that the client receives compatible blood. Cross-matching is done to detect the presence of recipient antibodies to the donor's minor antigens. Vital signs provide a baseline reference for continuous monitoring throughout the transfusion. An identification bracelet and red blood band are essential for client identification per facility policy. Two nurses must double-check the client's identification with the client listed on the unit of RBCs. The transfusion should be started within 30 minutes of the time that the RBC unit is checked out of the blood bank. Thus, no blood should be kept in the medication room before transfusion.

CN: Safety and infection control; CL: Synthesize

108. 3. The correct technique for a clean-catch urine culture specimen is to have the female client clean the labia from front to back, void into the toilet, and then void into the cup. The client does not need to fully empty her bladder into the cup. It is not necessary to catheterize the client to obtain the specimen. The **first** voided specimen of the day has the highest bacterial counts.

CN: Basic care and comfort; CL: Evaluate

109. 1,3,4,5,6,7. The client is hyponatremic; the nurse will closely monitor vital signs, restrict fluids, accurately record intake and output with the aid of a Foley catheter, prescribe labs for morning, and ensure client safety with use of a bed alarm. Encouraging fluids and restricting dietary sodium to 2 g may further exacerbate the hyponatremia. The nurse will also monitor for neurological changes and inform the **HCP** immediately of any change or if the client becomes unable to take food/fluids by mouth.

CN: Management of care; CL: Synthesize

110. 2,3,5,6. While the scope of practice for a **UAP** may vary by state, province, or territory, as well as by place of employment, general duties include recording input and output, including emptying and recording urine output from a Foley catheter. A UAP with proper training may apply a securing device to maintain safety, provide regular Foley catheter and perineal care, and ambulate a client with a catheter, continually monitoring that the collection bag remains below the level of the bladder to help prevent infection. Activities such as irrigating or flushing a catheter should not be assigned to a UAP as these activities involve nursing assessment skills.

CN: Management of care; CL: Evaluate

111. 1,3,4. When intravenous (IV) therapy must be administered in the home setting, teaching is essential. Written instructions as well as demonstration and return demonstration help reinforce key points. The client and/or caregiver is responsible for adhering to the established plan of care that includes the treatment plan, monitoring plan, potential for complications, expected outcome/outcomes, potential adverse effects, and plan for communicating with the **HCP** 📖. Periodic laboratory testing may be necessary to assess the effects of IV therapy and the client's progress. The client should report signs of redness or inflammation that could indicate infection, and also report an elevated temperature. Prior to changing the fluids, the caregiver should cleanse the port with alcohol wipes. It is not necessary to use sterile gloves; the IV bag should be elevated to promote gravity flow.

🔑 CN: Reduction of risk potential; CL: Create

112. 1,2,3,4. To ensure client safety, the nurse should assess clients that might be at risk for suicide, such as those with end-stage cancer. The nurse should also communicate accurate medication information by explaining the importance of managing medication information to the client when he/she is discharged from the hospital or at the end of an outpatient encounter. Examples include instructing the client to give a list of medications to his/her **HCP** 📖; to update the information when medications are discontinued, doses are changed, or new medications including over-the-counter products are added; and to carry medication information at all times in the event of emergency situations.

🔑 CN: Safety and infection control; CL: Application

The Client with Reproductive Health Problems

The Client with a Vaginal Infection

1. A nurse is reviewing a client's medical record and notes the Papanicolaou smear laboratory report indicates visualization of clue cells and a vaginal pH of 3.8. What should the nurse teach this client? Select all that apply.
- ☐ **1.** Seek care if the vaginal discharge has a fishy odor.
- ☐ **2.** Seek care if experiencing white, adherent vaginal discharge.
- ☐ **3.** All vaginal infections are sexually transmitted infections.
- ☐ **4.** Do not douche unless instructed by a health-care provider (HCP).
- ☐ **5.** Usually, vaginal infections can be treated with over-the-counter preparations.

2. A nurse is teaching a client how to prevent a vaginal infection. Which activity puts the client at risk for altering the normal pH of her vagina?
- ☐ **1.** consuming over four cups of coffee per day
- ☐ **2.** having sexual intercourse during the menstrual cycle
- ☐ **3.** douching unless instructed to do so by the healthcare provider (HCP)
- ☐ **4.** using tampons during the menstrual cycle

3. A client is prescribed oral metronidazole for treatment of bacterial vaginosis. What should the nurse instruct the client to avoid during treatment and for 24 hours thereafter?
- ☐ **1.** douching
- ☐ **2.** sexual intercourse
- ☐ **3.** hot tub baths
- ☐ **4.** alcohol consumption

4. A female client with which condition would be at risk for increased severity of vulvovaginal candidiasis? Select all that apply.
- ☐ **1.** uncontrolled diabetes
- ☐ **2.** immunosuppression due to cancer
- ☐ **3.** human immunodeficiency virus (HIV) infection
- ☐ **4.** hypertension
- ☐ **5.** asthma

5. A client taking oral contraceptives is placed on a 10-day course of antibiotics for an infection. Which instruction should the nurse include in the teaching plan?
- ☐ **1.** "Use a barrier method of birth control for the rest of your cycle."
- ☐ **2.** "You should stop taking the oral contraceptives while taking the antibiotic."
- ☐ **3.** "Call your healthcare provider for increased hunger or fluid retention."
- ☐ **4.** "Take the antibiotics 2 hours after the oral contraceptive."

6. A client is asking for information about using an intrauterine device (IUD). Which question when asked by the nurse would provide pertinent information on whether or not a client is a candidate for an IUD?
- ☐ **1.** "Do you smoke?"
- ☐ **2.** "Do you have hypertension?"
- ☐ **3.** "How often do you have sex?"
- ☐ **4.** "Are you in a monogamous relationship?"

7. A nurse is caring for a hospitalized 22-year-old female client with type 1 diabetes mellitus and toxic shock syndrome (TSS). Which action should the nurse perform **first**?
- ☐ **1.** Administer 5% dextrose in half-normal saline solution at 150 mL/h IV.
- ☐ **2.** Administer 50 mg of meperidine IM every 4 hours as needed for pain.
- ☐ **3.** Teach the client to use pads at night instead of tampons during her menstrual period.
- ☐ **4.** Administer 400 mg of ciprofloxacin IV every 12 hours infused over 1 hour.

The Client with Uterine Fibroids

8. A 39-year-old female client has been experiencing intermittent vaginal bleeding for several months. Her healthcare provider (HCP) tells her that she has uterine fibroids and recommends an abdominal hysterectomy. When the client expresses fear about the surgery, the nurse should:
- ☐ **1.** reassure the client of her HCP's competence.
- ☐ **2.** give the client opportunities to express her fears.
- ☐ **3.** teach the client that fear impedes recovery.
- ☐ **4.** change the topic of conversation.

9. A female with uterine fibroids has dysmenorrhea and menorrhagia. After reviewing the laboratory reports, the nurse should report which results to the healthcare provider (HCP)? Select all that apply.
- ☐ **1.** hemoglobin, 9.0 g/dL (90 g/L)
- ☐ **2.** hematocrit, 27.1% (0.27)
- ☐ **3.** white blood cell count, 10,000 cells/mm³ (10 × 10⁹/L)
- ☐ **4.** potassium, 4.0 mEq/L (4.0 mmol/L)
- ☐ **5.** normocytic red blood cells

10. The client will have an abdominal hysterectomy tomorrow. Which information will be **most** important for the nurse to give to the client prior to admission to the hospital?
- ☐ **1.** what to wear to the hospital
- ☐ **2.** what she can eat and drink before admission
- ☐ **3.** the type of pain medication that will be prescribed postoperatively
- ☐ **4.** the amount of activity she can have after surgery

11. The nurse is witnessing the client's signature on the informed surgical consent for an abdominal hysterectomy. It is important to ascertain that the client understands that with this surgical procedure she will have:
- ☐ **1.** decreased libido.
- ☐ **2.** infertility.
- ☐ **3.** depression.
- ☐ **4.** weight gain.

12. Which is the correct order, from first to last, for proper placement of a urinary catheter? All options must be used.

1. Lubricate the catheter adequately with a water-soluble lubricant.
2. Ensure free flow of urine.
3. Insert the catheter far enough into the bladder to prevent trauma to the urethral tissue.
4. Prepare a sterile field.

13. Which physical sensation will the client who has had an abdominal hysterectomy **most** likely experience if she hyperventilates while performing deep-breathing exercises?
- ☐ **1.** dyspnea
- ☐ **2.** dizziness
- ☐ **3.** blurred vision
- ☐ **4.** mental confusion

14. Which nursing measure would **most** likely relieve postoperative gas pains after abdominal hysterectomy?
- ☐ **1.** offering the client a hot beverage
- ☐ **2.** providing extra warmth
- ☐ **3.** applying a snugly fitting abdominal binder
- ☐ **4.** helping the client walk

15. On the second postoperative day after an abdominal hysterectomy, the client develops a temperature of 100.4°F (38°C). The nurse's **first** action should be to:
☐ 1. increase the number of wound dressing changes to minimize infection.
☐ 2. obtain a culture and sensitivity study of the urine to determine the source of infection.
☐ 3. ensure that the client takes at least 10 deep breaths every hour.
☐ 4. change the site of the client's IV fluid catheter to reduce the risk of infection.

16. The nurse is changing the dressing of a client after an abdominal hysterectomy. If the dressing adheres to the client's incisional area, what should the nurse do?
☐ 1. Pull off the dressing quickly, and then apply slight pressure over the area.
☐ 2. Lift an easily moved portion of the dressing, and then remove it slowly.
☐ 3. Moisten the dressing with sterile normal saline solution, and then remove it.
☐ 4. Remove part of the dressing, and then remove the remainder gradually over a period of several minutes.

17. The client with an abdominal hysterectomy is being prepared for discharge in the morning. The client has a handicapped adult son whom she cares for at home. The nurse should discuss with the healthcare provider (HCP) the need for referral to:
☐ 1. home health care.
☐ 2. social work.
☐ 3. pastoral care.
☐ 4. volunteer services.

18. When preparing discharge instructions for a client after an abdominal hysterectomy, the nurse should **first**:
☐ 1. have the client watch an educational video.
☐ 2. assess the client's available social supports.
☐ 3. call the social worker to evaluate the client.
☐ 4. read the discharge instructions to the client.

19. A client who had a hysterectomy 2 hours ago is returning to the postsurgical unit from the recovery room. The nurse is assessing the client. The vital signs are as follows: temperature 99°F (32°C), pulse 98 bmp, respirations 20 breaths/min, and BP 100/65 mm Hg. The urinary catheter is draining freely, and the client wants to try voiding without the catheter. The IV is infusing at 60 gtt/min. The perineal pad is saturated with bright red blood. The nurse reviews the progress notes from the recovery room (see notes).

Nurses Progress Notes

Date	Time	Progress Notes
5/24	1145	Client ready for transfer to room. Vital signs T = 37°C, P = 78; R = 14, BP = 114/70, O₂ Sat of 95% per pulse oximetry; catheter to straight drainage; IV in left cephalic vein infusing at keep open rate; client awake and oriented x3. Peri pad changed; moderately saturated. Bonnie Slater, RN

What should the nurse do **first**?
☐ 1. Change the perineal pad.
☐ 2. Contact the surgeon.
☐ 3. Increase the IV fluids.
☐ 4. Remove the urinary catheter.

20. When preparing a client for discharge 2 days after an abdominal hysterectomy, the nurse should instruct the client to avoid which activity until recovery is complete?
☐ 1. swimming in a pool treated with chlorine for 6 weeks after surgery
☐ 2. walking at a leisurely pace for 30 minutes at least once a day
☐ 3. driving until the client can push the brake pedal without pain
☐ 4. lifting >2 lb (0.9 kg) until the abdominal incision has healed

21. A client returned to the recovery room after a dilatation and curettage has the postoperative medication prescriptions shown in the medical record. What should the nurse do **next**?

> **Prescriptions**
>
> Rx   Meperidine 50 mg I.M. every 4 hours for severe pain
> Acetaminophen P.O. every 4 hours for pain
> Ibuprofen 800 mg P.O. every 4 hours for pain.

☐ 1. Ask the client to rate the intensity of her pain on a scale of 1 to 10, and administer the analgesia according to the intensity of the pain.
☐ 2. Administer the meperidine first because the client had surgery today.
☐ 3. Administer the acetaminophen first, and if it does not relieve the pain in 2 hours, administer the meperidine.
☐ 4. Administer the ibuprofen first, and if it does not relieve the pain, administer the meperidine.

22. On the second day following an abdominal hysterectomy, a client reports she has had three brown, loose stools in moderate amount. The morning medications include a prescription for 100 mg of docusate sodium daily or as needed. What should the nurse do **next**?
☐ 1. Administer the docusate sodium according to the prescription.
☐ 2. Ask the client if she is having gas pains or hunger.
☐ 3. Withhold the medication, and document the client's report of loose stools.
☐ 4. Administer the docusate sodium, and instruct the client to avoid high-fiber foods.

23. Which information should the nurse include when teaching a 55-year-old woman in the beginning of menopause? Select all that apply.
☐ 1. The average age of onset for menopause is 50 to 52 years.
☐ 2. Vaginal infections will increase.
☐ 3. Depression is very common as a result of menopause.
☐ 4. Hot flashes, especially at night, can occur in about 80% of women.
☐ 5. When periods become irregular, contraception is unnecessary.

The Client with Breast Cancer

24. A nurse is palpating a female client's breast while assessing for breast disease. In the illustration, indicate the area of the breast in which tumors are **most** commonly found.

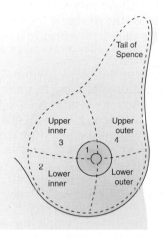

25. The client states that she has noticed that her bra fits more snugly at certain times of the month. She asks the nurse if this is a sign of breast disease. The nurse should base the reply to this client on the knowledge that:
☐ 1. benign cysts tend to cause the breasts to vary in size.
☐ 2. it is normal for the breasts to increase in size before menstruation begins.
☐ 3. a change in breast size warrants further investigation.
☐ 4. differences in breast size are related to normal growth and development.

26. A 70-year-old client asks the nurse if she needs to have a mammogram. Which is the nurse's **best** response?
☐ 1. "Having a mammogram when you are older is less painful."
☐ 2. "The incidence of breast cancer increases with age."
☐ 3. "We need to consider your family history of breast cancer first."
☐ 4. "It will be sufficient if you perform breast examinations monthly."

27. Prior to surgery for a modified radical mastectomy, the client is extremely anxious and asks many questions. Which approach offers the **best** guide for the nurse to answer these questions?
☐ 1. Tell the client as much as she wants to know and is able to understand.
☐ 2. Delay discussing the client's questions with her until she is convalescing.
☐ 3. Delay discussing the client's questions with her until her apprehension subsides.
☐ 4. Explain to the client that she should discuss her questions first with the healthcare provider (HCP).

28. Following a simple mastectomy, the nurse is totaling the amount of drainage in 24 hours from a suction drain in the incision. The nurse notes there is 200 ml of serosanguineous drainage for the first 24 hours. The nurse should:
☐ **1.** document the findings.
☐ **2.** notify the surgeon.
☐ **3.** remove the drain.
☐ **4.** place the client's arm in a dependent position.

29. Atropine sulfate is included in the preoperative prescriptions for a client undergoing a modified radical mastectomy. The expected outcome is to:
☐ **1.** promote general muscular relaxation.
☐ **2.** decrease pulse and respiratory rates.
☐ **3.** decrease nausea.
☐ **4.** inhibit oral and respiratory secretions.

30. During the postoperative period after a modified radical mastectomy, the client confides in the nurse that she thinks she got breast cancer because she had an abortion and she did not tell her husband. What is the **best** response by the nurse?
☐ **1.** "Cancer is not a punishment; it is a disease."
☐ **2.** "You might feel better if you confided in your husband."
☐ **3.** "Tell me more about your feelings about this."
☐ **4.** "I can have the social worker talk to you if you would like."

31. Following a modified radical mastectomy, a client has an incisional drainage tube attached to Hemovac suction. The nurse determines the suction is effective when:
☐ **1.** the intrathoracic pressure is decreased and the client breathes easier.
☐ **2.** there is an increased collateral lymphatic flow toward the operative area.
☐ **3.** accumulated serum and blood in the operative area are removed.
☐ **4.** no adhesions are formed between the skin and chest wall in the operative area.

32. Which position would be **best** for a client's right arm when she returns to her room after a right modified radical mastectomy with multiple lymph node excisions?
☐ **1.** across her chest wall
☐ **2.** at her side at the same level as her body
☐ **3.** in the position that affords her the greatest comfort without placing pressure on the incision
☐ **4.** on pillows, with her hand higher than her elbow and her elbow higher than her shoulder

33. A client develops lymphedema after a left mastectomy with lymph node dissection. The nurse should include which points in the discharge teaching plan? Select all that apply.
☐ **1.** Do not allow blood pressures or blood draws in the affected arm.
☐ **2.** Avoid application of sunscreen on the left arm.
☐ **3.** Use an electric razor for shaving.
☐ **4.** Immobilize the left arm.
☐ **5.** Elevate the left arm.
☐ **6.** Perform hand pump exercises.

34. The client with breast cancer is prescribed tamoxifen 20 mg daily. The client states she does not like taking medicine and asks the nurse if the tamoxifen is really worth taking. The nurse should tell the client:
☐ **1.** "This drug is part of your chemotherapy program."
☐ **2.** "This drug has been found to decrease metastatic breast cancer."
☐ **3.** "This drug will act as an estrogen in your breast tissue."
☐ **4.** "This drug will prevent hot flashes since you cannot take hormone replacement."

35. A client undergoing chemotherapy after a modified radical mastectomy asks the nurse questions about breast prosthesis and wigs. After answering the questions directly, the nurse should also:
☐ **1.** provide a list of resources, including the local breast cancer support group.
☐ **2.** offer a referral to the social worker.
☐ **3.** call the home healthcare agency.
☐ **4.** contact the plastic surgeon.

36. A client is to have radiation therapy after a modified radical mastectomy. The nurse should teach the client to care for the skin at the site of therapy by:
☐ **1.** washing the area with water.
☐ **2.** exposing the area to dry heat.
☐ **3.** applying an ointment to the area.
☐ **4.** using talcum powder on the area.

37. The nurse should teach a client that a normal local tissue response to radiation following surgery for breast cancer is:
☐ **1.** atrophy of the skin.
☐ **2.** scattered pustule formation.
☐ **3.** redness of the surface tissue.
☐ **4.** sloughing of two layers of skin.

38. The nurse is providing discharge instructions about preventing infection to a client who had a modified radical mastectomy and will be pruning flowers when she returns to work. To prevent infection, what should the nurse instruct the client to do?
- ☐ 1. Wear protective gloves when gardening.
- ☐ 2. Avoid crowded areas.
- ☐ 3. Keep cuticles cut.
- ☐ 4. Remove underarm hair with a sharp razor.

The Client with Benign Prostatic Hypertrophy

39. An adult male client has been unable to void for the past 12 hours. The **best** method for the nurse to use when assessing for bladder distention in a male client is to check for:
- ☐ 1. a rounded swelling above the pubis.
- ☐ 2. dullness in the lower left quadrant.
- ☐ 3. rebound tenderness below the symphysis.
- ☐ 4. urine discharge from the urethral meatus.

40. When emptying the client's bladder during a urinary catheterization, the nurse should allow the urine to drain from the bladder slowly to prevent:
- ☐ 1. renal failure.
- ☐ 2. abdominal cramping.
- ☐ 3. possible shock.
- ☐ 4. atrophy of bladder musculature.

41. The **primary** reason for lubricating the urinary catheter generously before inserting the catheter into a male client is that this technique helps reduce:
- ☐ 1. spasms at the orifice of the bladder.
- ☐ 2. friction along the urethra when the catheter is being inserted.
- ☐ 3. the number of organisms gaining entrance to the bladder.
- ☐ 4. the formation of encrustations that may occur at the end of the catheter.

42. The **primary** reason for taping an indwelling catheter laterally to the thigh of a male client is to:
- ☐ 1. eliminate pressure at the penoscrotal angle.
- ☐ 2. prevent the catheter from kinking in the urethra.
- ☐ 3. prevent accidental catheter removal.
- ☐ 4. allow the client to turn without kinking the catheter.

43. The nurse is providing preoperative instructions to a client who is having a transurethral resection of the prostate. The nurse should tell the client:
- ☐ 1. "You will have a central venous access inserted just prior to the procedure."
- ☐ 2. "Plan on being in the hospital anywhere from 5 to 7 days following the procedure."
- ☐ 3. "You will be taught care of the incision and suture line prior to your discharge home."
- ☐ 4. "Expect blood in your urine in the first couple of days following the procedure."

44. When providing client teaching about continuous bladder irrigation following prostate surgery, the nurse should tell the client:
- ☐ 1. "The catheter is disconnected from the drainage tubing one time per shift to enable manual irrigation of the bladder."
- ☐ 2. "The purpose of the irrigation is to keep bladder drainage clear and to prevent the formation of blood clots in the bladder."
- ☐ 3. "The fluid drips into the bladder at a slow rate to prevent the effects of overhydration and hyponatremia."
- ☐ 4. "The catheter is clamped off approximately 4 hours after returning to the nursing unit."

45. When caring for a client with a history of benign prostatic hypertrophy (BPH), what should the nurse do? Select all that apply.
- ☐ 1. Provide privacy and time for the client to void.
- ☐ 2. Monitor intake and output.
- ☐ 3. Catheterize the client for postvoid residual urine.
- ☐ 4. Ask the client if he has urinary retention.
- ☐ 5. Test the urine for hematuria.

46. The nurse should specifically assess a client with prostatic hypertrophy for:
- ☐ 1. voiding at less frequent intervals.
- ☐ 2. difficulty starting the flow of urine.
- ☐ 3. painful urination.
- ☐ 4. increased force of the urine stream.

47. The nurse is reviewing the medication history of a client with benign prostatic hypertrophy (BPH). Which medication will likely aggravate BPH?
- ☐ 1. metformin
- ☐ 2. buspirone
- ☐ 3. inhaled ipratropium
- ☐ 4. ophthalmic timolol

48. A client is scheduled to undergo transurethral resection of the prostate. The procedure is to be done under spinal anesthesia. Postoperatively, the nurse should assess the client for:
- ☐ 1. seizures.
- ☐ 2. cardiac arrest.
- ☐ 3. renal shutdown.
- ☐ 4. respiratory paralysis.

49. A client with benign prostatic hypertrophy (BPH) is being treated with terazosin 2 mg at bedtime. The nurse should monitor the client's:
- ☐ 1. urine nitrites.
- ☐ 2. white blood cell count.
- ☐ 3. blood pressure.
- ☐ 4. pulse.

50. A client, who had a transurethral resection of the prostate (TURP), has a three-way indwelling urinary catheter with continuous bladder irrigation. In which circumstance should the nurse increase the flow rate of the continuous bladder irrigation?
- ☐ 1. when drainage is continuous but slow
- ☐ 2. when drainage appears cloudy and dark yellow
- ☐ 3. when drainage becomes bright red
- ☐ 4. when there is no drainage of urine and irrigating solution

51. A client is to receive belladonna and opium suppositories, as needed, postoperatively after transurethral resection of the prostate (TURP). The nurse should give the client these drugs when he demonstrates signs of:
- ☐ 1. a urinary tract infection.
- ☐ 2. urine retention.
- ☐ 3. frequent urination.
- ☐ 4. pain from bladder spasms.

52. An unlicensed assistive personnel (UAP) tells the nurse, "I think the client is confused. He keeps telling me he has to void, but that is not possible because he has a catheter in place that is draining well." The nurse should tell the UAP:
- ☐ 1. "His catheter is probably plugged. I will irrigate it."
- ☐ 2. "That is a common problem after prostate surgery. The client only imagines the urge to void."
- ☐ 3. "The urge to void is usually created by the large catheter, and he may be having some bladder spasms."
- ☐ 4. "I think he may be somewhat confused."

53. A healthcare provider (HCP) has prescribed amoxicillin 100 PO two times a day. What should the nurse instruct the client to do? Select all that apply.
- ☐ 1. Drink 300 to 500 mL of fluids daily.
- ☐ 2. Void frequently, at least every 2 to 3 hours.
- ☐ 3. Take time to empty the bladder completely.
- ☐ 4. Take the last dose of the antibiotic for the day at bedtime.
- ☐ 5. Take the antibiotic with or without food.

54. In discussing home care with a client after transurethral resection of the prostate (TURP), the nurse should teach the male client that dribbling of urine:
- ☐ 1. can be a chronic problem.
- ☐ 2. can persist for several months.
- ☐ 3. is an abnormal sign that requires intervention.
- ☐ 4. is a sign of healing within the prostate.

55. A client is being discharged to home 3 days after transurethral resection of the prostate (TURP). What should the nurse instruct the client to do? Select all that apply.
- ☐ 1. Drink at least 3,000 mL water per day.
- ☐ 2. Increase calorie intake by eating six small meals a day.
- ☐ 3. Report bright red bleeding to the healthcare provider (HCP).
- ☐ 4. Take deep breaths and cough every 2 hours.
- ☐ 5. Report a temperature over 99°F (37.2°C).

56. A client with benign prostatic hypertrophy (BPH) has an elevated prostate-specific antigen (PSA) level. The nurse should:
- ☐ 1. instruct the client to request having a colonoscopy before coming to conclusions about the PSA results.
- ☐ 2. instruct the client that a urologist will monitor the PSA level biannually when elevated.
- ☐ 3. determine if the prostatic palpation was done before or after the blood sample was drawn.
- ☐ 4. ask the client if he emptied his bladder before the blood sample was obtained.

The Client with a Sexually Transmitted Disease

57. What is **most** important information for the nurse to teach a client newly diagnosed with genital herpes?
- ☐ 1. Use condoms at all times during sexual intercourse.
- ☐ 2. A urologist should be seen only when lesions occur.
- ☐ 3. Oral sex is permissible without a barrier.
- ☐ 4. Determine if your partner has received a vaccine against herpes.

58. A nurse is planning care for a 25-year-old female client who has just been diagnosed with human immunodeficiency virus (HIV) infection. The client asks the nurse, "How could this have happened?" The nurse responds to the question based on the **most** frequent mode of HIV transmission, which is:
- ☐ 1. hugging an HIV-positive sexual partner without using barrier precautions.
- ☐ 2. inhaling cocaine.
- ☐ 3. sharing food utensils with an HIV-positive person without proper cleaning of the utensils.
- ☐ 4. having sexual intercourse with an HIV-positive person without using a condom.

59. A client with human immunodeficiency virus (HIV) infection is taking zidovudine (AZT). The expected outcome of AZT is to:
- ☐ 1. destroy the virus.
- ☐ 2. enhance the body's antibody production.
- ☐ 3. slow replication of the virus.
- ☐ 4. neutralize toxins produced by the virus.

60. Women who have human papillomavirus (HPV) are at risk for development of:
- ☐ **1.** sterility.
- ☐ **2.** cervical cancer.
- ☐ **3.** uterine fibroid tumors.
- ☐ **4.** irregular menses.

61. The **primary** reason that a herpes simplex virus (HSV) infection is a serious concern to a client with human immunodeficiency virus (HIV) infection is that it:
- ☐ **1.** is an acquired immunodeficiency virus (AIDS)–defining illness.
- ☐ **2.** is curable only after 1 year of antiviral therapy.
- ☐ **3.** leads to cervical cancer.
- ☐ **4.** causes severe electrolyte imbalances.

62. When teaching a client about human immunodeficiency virus (HIV), the nurse should take into account the fact that the **most** effective method known to control the spread of HIV infection is:
- ☐ **1.** premarital serologic screening.
- ☐ **2.** prophylactic treatment of exposed people.
- ☐ **3.** laboratory screening of pregnant women.
- ☐ **4.** ongoing sex education about preventive behaviors.

63. A male client with human immunodeficiency virus (HIV) infection becomes depressed and tells the nurse: "I have nothing worth living for now." Which statement would be the **best** response by the nurse?
- ☐ **1.** "You are a young person and have a great deal to live for."
- ☐ **2.** "You should not be too depressed; we are close to finding a cure for AIDS."
- ☐ **3.** "You are right; it is very depressing to have HIV."
- ☐ **4.** "Tell me more about how you are feeling about being HIV positive."

64. The typical chancre of syphilis appears as:
- ☐ **1.** a grouping of small, tender pimples.
- ☐ **2.** an elevated wart.
- ☐ **3.** a painless, moist ulcer.
- ☐ **4.** an itching, crusted area.

65. The nurse is interviewing a client with newly diagnosed syphilis. In order to prevent the spread of the disease, the nurse should focus the interview by:
- ☐ **1.** motivating the client to undergo treatment.
- ☐ **2.** obtaining a list of the client's sexual contacts.
- ☐ **3.** increasing the client's knowledge of the disease.
- ☐ **4.** reassuring the client that medical records are confidential.

66. Benzathine penicillin G, 2.4 million units IM, is prescribed as treatment for an adult client with primary syphilis. The nurse should administer the injection in the:
- ☐ **1.** deltoid.
- ☐ **2.** upper outer quadrant of the buttock.
- ☐ **3.** quadriceps lateralis of the thigh.
- ☐ **4.** midlateral aspect of the thigh.

67. An 18-year-old female is to have a pelvic exam. Which response by the nurse would be **best** when the client says that she is nervous about the upcoming pelvic examination?
- ☐ **1.** "Can you tell me more about how you are feeling?"
- ☐ **2.** "You are not alone. Most women feel uncomfortable about this examination."
- ☐ **3.** "Do not worry about Dr. Smith. He is a specialist in female problems."
- ☐ **4.** "We will do everything we can to avoid embarrassing you."

68. When educating a female client with gonorrhea, the nurse should emphasize that for women, gonorrhea:
- ☐ **1.** is often marked by symptoms of dysuria or vaginal bleeding.
- ☐ **2.** does not lead to serious complications.
- ☐ **3.** can be treated but not cured.
- ☐ **4.** may not cause symptoms until serious complications occur.

69. Which group has experienced the **greatest** rise in the incidence of sexually transmitted diseases (STDs) over the past two decades?
- ☐ **1.** teenagers
- ☐ **2.** divorced people
- ☐ **3.** young married couples
- ☐ **4.** older adults

70. A sexually active male client has burning on urination and a milky discharge from the urethral meatus. What documentation should be included on the client's medical record? Select all that apply.
- ☐ **1.** history of unprotected sex (sex without a condom)
- ☐ **2.** length of time since symptoms presented
- ☐ **3.** history of fever or chills
- ☐ **4.** presence of any enlarged lymph nodes on examination
- ☐ **5.** names and phone numbers of all sexual contacts
- ☐ **6.** allergies to any medications

71. A male client is diagnosed with a chlamydial infection. Azithromycin 1 g is prescribed. The supply of azithromycin is in 250-mg tablets. How many tablets should the nurse administer? Record your answer using a whole number.
_____ tablets.

72. A female client with gonorrhea informs the nurse that she has had sexual intercourse with her boyfriend and asks the nurse, "Would he have any symptoms?" The nurse responds that in men, the symptoms of gonorrhea include:
- ☐ **1.** impotence.
- ☐ **2.** scrotal swelling.
- ☐ **3.** urine retention.
- ☐ **4.** dysuria.

73. The nurse assesses the mouth and oral cavity of a client with human immunodeficiency virus (HIV) infection because the **most** common opportunistic infection initially presents as:
- ☐ 1. herpes simplex virus (HSV) lesions on the lips.
- ☐ 2. oral candidiasis.
- ☐ 3. cytomegalovirus (CMV) infection.
- ☐ 4. aphthae on the gingiva.

74. The nurse is administering didanosine to a client with HIV. Before administering this medication, the nurse should check which lab test results? Select all that apply.
- ☐ 1. elevated serum creatinine
- ☐ 2. elevated blood urea nitrogen (BUN)
- ☐ 3. elevated aspartate aminotransferase (AST)
- ☐ 4. elevated alanine aminotransferase (ALT)
- ☐ 5. elevated serum amylase

75. The nurse is caring for a client from Southeast Asia who has HIV/AIDS. The client does not speak or comprehend the English language. What should the nurse do?
- ☐ 1. Contact the hospital's chaplain.
- ☐ 2. Do an Internet search for the Joint United Nations Programme on HIV/AIDS.
- ☐ 3. Utilize language-appropriate interpreters.
- ☐ 4. Ask a family member to obtain informed consent.

The Client with Cancer of the Cervix

76. The nurse is preparing a 45-year-old female for a vaginal examination. The nurse should place the client in which position?
- ☐ 1. Sims' position
- ☐ 2. lithotomy position
- ☐ 3. genupectoral position
- ☐ 4. dorsal recumbent position

77. A client asks the nurse to explain the meaning of her abnormal Papanicolaou (Pap) smear result of atypical squamous cells. The nurse should tell the client that an atypical Pap smear means that:
- ☐ 1. abnormal viral cells were found in the smear.
- ☐ 2. cancer cells were found in the smear.
- ☐ 3. the Pap smear alone is not very important diagnostically because there are many false-positive results.
- ☐ 4. the cells could cause various conditions and help identify a problem early.

78. Which is a risk factor for cervical cancer?
- ☐ 1. sexual experiences with one partner
- ☐ 2. sedentary lifestyle
- ☐ 3. obesity
- ☐ 4. adolescent pregnancy

79. A woman tells the nurse, "There has been a lot of cancer in my family." The nurse should instruct the client to report which possible sign of cervical cancer?
- ☐ 1. pain
- ☐ 2. leg edema
- ☐ 3. urinary and rectal symptoms
- ☐ 4. light bleeding or watery vaginal discharge

80. A 30-year-old female client asks the nurse about douching. What information should the nurse include in the teaching plan?
- ☐ 1. Douching during menstruation is safe.
- ☐ 2. Daily douching will decrease vaginal odor.
- ☐ 3. Perfumed douches are recommended to decrease odors.
- ☐ 4. Douching removes natural mucus and changes the balance of normal vaginal flora.

81. A young woman will receive 6 months of chemotherapy for cervical cancer. She is a single parent of two young children and can no longer work. The nurse contacts a social worker to help plan continuing care. The client states, "I feel overwhelmed. How can the social worker help me?" Which responses by the nurse about the role of the social worker are appropriate? Select all that apply.
- ☐ 1. "The social worker is a part of a multidisciplinary team that provides care for clients with cancer."
- ☐ 2. "The social worker can assist in locating resources and programs to assist you during your treatment."
- ☐ 3. "Based on your financial situation and need to care for your children, the social worker can help you identify needed resources at this time."
- ☐ 4. "Your entire family will be included in the treatment plan. Your needs and those of your children will be assessed and determined so that referrals can be made to appropriate resources."
- ☐ 5. "The social worker can authorize temporary funds to help you with child care and to pay your bills while you are sick."

82. The husband of a client with cervical cancer says to the nurse, "The doctor told my wife that her cancer is curable. Is he just trying to make us feel better?" Which would be the nurse's **most** accurate response?
- ☐ 1. "When cervical cancer is detected early and treated aggressively, the cure rate is almost 100%."
- ☐ 2. "The 5-year survival rate is about 75%, which makes the odds pretty good."
- ☐ 3. "Saying a cancer is curable means that 50% of all women with the cancer survive at least 5 years."
- ☐ 4. "Cancers of the female reproductive tract tend to be slow growing and respond well to treatment."

83. A client with suspected cervical cancer is undergoing a colposcopy with conization. The nurse gives instructions to the client about her menstrual periods, emphasizing that:
- ☐ 1. her periods will return to normal after 6 months.
- ☐ 2. her next two or three periods may be heavier and more prolonged than usual.
- ☐ 3. her next two or three periods will be lighter than normal.
- ☐ 4. she may skip her next two periods.

84. A client with cervical cancer is undergoing internal radium implant therapy. A lead-lined container and a pair of long forceps are kept in the client's hospital room for:
- ☐ 1. disposal of emesis or other bodily secretions.
- ☐ 2. handling of a dislodged radiation source.
- ☐ 3. disposal of the client's eating utensils.
- ☐ 4. storage of the radiation dose.

85. The mother of a client who has a radium implant asks why so many nurses are involved in her daughter's care. She states, "The doctor said I can be in the room for up to 2 hours each day, but the nurses say they are restricted to 30 minutes." The nurse explains that this variation is based on the fact that nurses:
- ☐ 1. touch the client, which increases their exposure to radiation.
- ☐ 2. work with many clients and could carry infection to a client receiving radiation therapy, if exposure is prolonged.
- ☐ 3. work with radiation on an ongoing basis, while visitors have infrequent exposure to radiation.
- ☐ 4. are at greater risk from the radiation because they are younger than the mother.

86. A client with human papillomavirus (HPV) infection is being treated by a colposcopy. The client asks the nurse if this procedure is really necessary. The nurse explains that the procedure to treat the warts is important because HPV can lead to:
- ☐ 1. infertility.
- ☐ 2. cervical cancer.
- ☐ 3. pelvic inflammatory disease.
- ☐ 4. rectal cancer.

87. Which action should be included in the nursing care for a client with cervical cancer who has an internal radium implant in place?
- ☐ 1. Offer the bed pan every 2 hours.
- ☐ 2. Provide perineal care twice daily.
- ☐ 3. Check the position of the applicator hourly.
- ☐ 4. Offer a low-residue diet.

88. The nurse should carefully observe a client with internal radium implants for typical adverse effects associated with radiation therapy to the cervix. These effects include:
- ☐ 1. severe vaginal itching.
- ☐ 2. confusion.
- ☐ 3. high fever in the afternoon or evening.
- ☐ 4. nausea and a foul vaginal discharge.

The Client with Cancer of the Ovaries

89. When teaching a client about ovarian cancer, the nurse should include which information? Select all that apply.
- ☐ 1. details about the prognosis
- ☐ 2. staging and grading of ovarian cancer
- ☐ 3. need for routine colonoscopy beginning at age 30
- ☐ 4. procedures for diagnosis if there is a pelvic mass
- ☐ 5. symptoms occurring early in the disease process

90. Interprofessional management of ovarian cancer includes which measures? Select all that apply.
- ☐ 1. combination chemotherapy to cure the cancer
- ☐ 2. bilateral salpingo-oophorectomy to remove diseased organs
- ☐ 3. radiation therapy to eliminate all cancer cells
- ☐ 4. referral to social services for supportive care
- ☐ 5. nutrition therapy for parenteral lipids

91. A client with ovarian cancer asks the nurse, "What is the cause of this cancer?" Which is the **most** accurate response by the nurse?
- ☐ 1. Use of oral contraceptives increases the risk of ovarian cancer.
- ☐ 2. Women who have had at least two live births are protected from ovarian cancer.
- ☐ 3. There is less chance of developing ovarian cancer when one lives in an industrialized country.
- ☐ 4. The risk of developing ovarian cancer is related to environmental, endocrine, and genetic factors.

92. The nurse is planning a presentation about ovarian cancer to a group of women. Which topic should receive **priority** attention in the lesson plan?
- ☐ 1. Ovarian cancer signs and symptoms are often vague until late in development.
- ☐ 2. Ovarian cancer should be considered in any woman older than 30 years of age.
- ☐ 3. A rigid board-like abdomen is the most common sign.
- ☐ 4. Methods for early detection have made a dramatic reduction in the mortality rate due to ovarian cancer.

The Client with Testicular Disease

93. A 28-year-old male is diagnosed with acute epididymitis. The nurse should assess the client for:
☐ 1. burning and pain on urination.
☐ 2. severe tenderness and swelling in the scrotum.
☐ 3. foul-smelling ejaculate.
☐ 4. foul-smelling urine.

94. A 30-year-old client is being treated for epididymitis. Teaching for this client should include the fact that epididymitis is commonly a result of a:
☐ 1. virus.
☐ 2. parasite.
☐ 3. sexually transmitted infection.
☐ 4. protozoon.

95. When teaching a client to perform testicular self-examination, the nurse explains that the examination should be performed:
☐ 1. after intercourse.
☐ 2. at the end of the day.
☐ 3. after a warm bath or shower.
☐ 4. after exercise.

96. The nurse is assessing a client's testes. Which finding indicates the testes are normal?
☐ 1. soft
☐ 2. egg-shaped
☐ 3. spongy
☐ 4. lumpy

97. A client has a testicular nodule that is highly suspicious for testicular cancer. A laboratory test that supports this diagnosis is:
☐ 1. decreased alpha fetoprotein (AFP).
☐ 2. decreased beta–human chorionic gonadotropin (hCG).
☐ 3. increased testosterone.
☐ 4. increased AFP.

98. Although the cause of testicular cancer is unknown, it is associated with a history of:
☐ 1. undescended testes.
☐ 2. sexual relations at an early age.
☐ 3. seminal vesiculitis.
☐ 4. epididymitis.

99. Risk factors associated with testicular malignancies include:
☐ 1. African race.
☐ 2. residing in a rural area.
☐ 3. lower socioeconomic status.
☐ 4. age older than 40 years.

100. A client with a testicular malignancy undergoes a radical orchiectomy. In the immediate postoperative period, the nurse should particularly assess the client for:
☐ 1. bladder spasms.
☐ 2. urine output.
☐ 3. pain.
☐ 4. nausea.

101. A right orchiectomy is performed on a client with a testicular malignancy. The client expresses concerns regarding his sexuality. The nurse should base the response on the knowledge that the client:
☐ 1. is not a candidate for sperm banking.
☐ 2. should retain normal sexual drive and function.
☐ 3. will be impotent.
☐ 4. will have a change in secondary sexual characteristics.

102. A client diagnosed with seminomatous testicular cancer expresses fear and questions the nurse about his prognosis. The nurse should base the response on the knowledge that:
☐ 1. testicular cancer can be cured.
☐ 2. testicular cancer has a cure rate of 90% when diagnosed early.
☐ 3. surgery is the treatment of choice for testicular cancer.
☐ 4. testicular cancer has a 50% cure rate when diagnosed early.

The Client with Cancer of the Prostate

103. The nurse is developing an educational program about prostate cancer. The nurse should provide information about which topic?
☐ 1. The prostate-specific antigen (PSA) test is reliable for detecting the presence of prostate cancer.
☐ 2. For all men, age 50 and older, the American and Canadian Cancer Societies recommend an annual rectal examination.
☐ 3. Not lifting more than 20 lb (9.1 kg) aids in prevention of prostate cancer.
☐ 4. Regular sexual activity promotes health of the prostate gland to prevent cancer.

104. The nurse is caring for a client who will have a bilateral orchiectomy. The client asks what is involved with this procedure. Which statement is the nurse's **most** appropriate response? "The surgery:
☐ 1. removes the entire prostate gland, prostatic capsule, and seminal vesicles."
☐ 2. tends to cause urinary incontinence and impotence."
☐ 3. freezes prostate tissue, killing cells."
☐ 4. results in reduction of the major circulating androgen, testosterone."

105. The nurse is teaching a client about prostate cancer. Which points should be included in the instruction? Select all that apply.
☐ 1. Prostate cancer is usually multifocal and slow growing.
☐ 2. Most prostate cancers are adenocarcinoma.
☐ 3. The incidence of prostate cancer is higher in men of African descent, and the onset is earlier.
☐ 4. A prostate-specific antigen (PSA) lab test >4 ng/mg will need to be monitored.
☐ 5. Cancer cells are detectable in the urine.

106. What should the nurse do for a client who is receiving hormone replacement for prostate cancer? Select all that apply.
- ☐ 1. Inform the client that increased libido is expected with hormone therapy.
- ☐ 2. Reassure the client that erectile dysfunction will not occur as a consequence of hormone therapy.
- ☐ 3. Provide the client the opportunity to communicate concerns and needs.
- ☐ 4. Utilize communication strategies that enable the client to gain some feeling of control.
- ☐ 5. Suggest that an appointment be made to see a psychiatrist.

107. A client asks the nurse why the prostate-specific antigen (PSA) level is determined before the digital rectal examination. The nurse's **best** response is:
- ☐ 1. "It is easier for the client."
- ☐ 2. "A prostate examination can possibly decrease the PSA."
- ☐ 3. "A prostate examination can possibly increase the PSA."
- ☐ 4. "If the PSA is normal, the client will not have to undergo the rectal examination."

108. The nurse is performing a digital rectal examination. Which finding is a **key** sign for prostate cancer?
- ☐ 1. a hard prostate, localized or diffuse
- ☐ 2. abdominal pain
- ☐ 3. a boggy, tender prostate
- ☐ 4. a nonindurated prostate

109. A client is undergoing a total prostatectomy for prostate cancer. The client asks questions about his sexual function. The **best** response by the nurse is "Loss of the prostate gland means that:
- ☐ 1. you will be impotent."
- ☐ 2. you will be infertile and there will be no ejaculation. You can still experience the sensations of orgasm."
- ☐ 3. you will have no loss of sexual function and drive."
- ☐ 4. your erectile capability will return immediately after surgery."

110. A 65-year-old client has been told by the healthcare provider (HCP) that his prostate cancer was graded at stage IIB. The client inquires if this means he is going to die soon. What is the **best** response by the nurse?
- ☐ 1. "Prostate cancer at this stage is very slow growing."
- ☐ 2. "Prostate cancer at this stage is very fast growing."
- ☐ 3. "Prostate cancer at this stage has spread to the bone."
- ☐ 4. "Prostate cancer at this stage is difficult to predict."

111. A client with prostate cancer is treated with a luteinizing hormone-releasing hormone agonist and antagonist goserelin. The nurse should instruct the client to expect to have:
- ☐ 1. tenderness of the scrotum.
- ☐ 2. flushing.
- ☐ 3. loss of pubic hair.
- ☐ 4. decreased blood pressure.

The Client with Erectile Dysfunction

112. The client is taking sildenafil orally for erectile dysfunction. What instruction should the nurse give the client?
- ☐ 1. Sildenafil may be taken more than one time per day.
- ☐ 2. The healthcare provider (HCP) should be notified promptly if the client experiences sudden or diminished vision.
- ☐ 3. Sildenafil offers protection against some sexually transmitted diseases (STDs).
- ☐ 4. Sildenafil does not require sexual stimulation to work.

113. A male client reports having impotence. The nurse examines the client's medication regimen and determines that a contributing factor to impotence could be:
- ☐ 1. aspirin.
- ☐ 2. antihypertensives.
- ☐ 3. nonsteroidal anti-inflammatory drugs.
- ☐ 4. anticoagulants.

114. A 65-year-old male client with erectile dysfunction (ED) asks the nurse, "Is all this just in my head? Am I crazy?" The **best** response by the nurse is based on the knowledge that:
- ☐ 1. ED is believed to be psychogenic in most cases.
- ☐ 2. more than 50% of the cases are attributed to organic causes.
- ☐ 3. evaluation of nocturnal erections does not help differentiate psychogenic or organic causes.
- ☐ 4. ED is an uncommon problem among men older than age 65.

115. The nurse should teach the client with erectile dysfunction (ED) to alter his lifestyle to:
- ☐ 1. avoid alcohol.
- ☐ 2. follow a low-salt diet.
- ☐ 3. decrease smoking.
- ☐ 4. increase attempts at sexual intercourse.

Managing Care, Quality, and Safety of Clients with Reproductive Health Problems

116. The nurse is assigning tasks to the unlicensed assistive personnel (UAP) for a client with an abdominal hysterectomy on the first postoperative day. Which task **cannot** be delegated to the UAP?
- [ ] 1. taking vital signs
- [ ] 2. recording intake and output
- [ ] 3. giving perineal care
- [ ] 4. assessing the incision site

117. The nurse-manager on a gynecologic surgical unit is addressing reports from clients that they have to wait too long on the night shift for their pain medication. Which course of action should the nurse-manager take **first**?
- [ ] 1. Change the staffing schedule on nights to include a medication nurse.
- [ ] 2. Consult the nursing supervisor.
- [ ] 3. Consult the nurses on the evening shift about their evaluation of the night nurses regarding these reports from the clients.
- [ ] 4. Complete a quality improvement study with the night nurses to document the waiting times for pain medication and other data, including staffing and client acuity.

118. A nurse is reviewing the healthcare provider's (HCP's) admitting prescriptions for a 52-year-old client scheduled for a dilatation and curettage. The nurse is unable to decipher the handwriting but thinks the medication prescription reads either metoprolol or topiramate. What should the nurse do **next**?
- [ ] 1. Ask the client if she has hypertension.
- [ ] 2. Ask the client if she has migraines.
- [ ] 3. Call the HCP to clarify the prescription.
- [ ] 4. Ask the pharmacist to interpret the prescription.

119. The unlicensed assistive personnel (UAP) reports to the nurse that the client with an abdominal hysterectomy who returned from the recovery room 1 hour earlier has saturated the blue pad with bright red blood. What should the nurse do?
- [ ] 1. Call the surgeon to report the bleeding.
- [ ] 2. Ask the UAP to obtain vital signs while the nurse calls the surgeon.
- [ ] 3. Ask the UAP to increase the flow of IV fluids to prevent shock.
- [ ] 4. Assess the client again in 15 minutes before the nurse takes any further action.

120. A nurse on the gynecologic surgery unit observes a respiratory therapist (RT) take a medication cup with pills that was sitting in the medication room. What course of action should the nurse take?
- [ ] 1. Report the situation to the supervisor of respiratory therapy.
- [ ] 2. Tell the RT that you saw her take the pills from the medication room.
- [ ] 3. Report the situation to the nursing supervisor.
- [ ] 4. Tell the nurse who was administering medications not to leave pills out.

Answers, Rationales, and Test-Taking Strategies

*The answers and rationales for each question follow below, along with keys (🔑) to the client need (CN) and cognitive level (CL) for each question. In addition, you will also see a glossary icon (📖) highlighting specific terminology used on the licensing exam. As you check your answers, use the **Content Mastery and Test-Taking Skill Self-Analysis** worksheet (tear-out worksheet in back of book) to identify the reason(s) for not answering the questions correctly. For additional information about test-taking skills and strategies for answering questions, refer to pages 12–23 and pages 35–36 in Part 1 of this book.*

The Client with a Vaginal Infection

1. 1,2,4. Bacterial vaginosis is a clinical syndrome resulting from the replacement of the normal vaginal *Lactobacillus* species with overgrowth of anaerobic bacteria that cause a cluster of symptoms. Presence of a thick, white, adherent vaginal discharge with a fishy odor is evidence for bacterial vaginosis, and the client should seek treatment. The client should not douche unless under medical prescriptions because douching can cause bacteria to ascend into the uterus. Bacterial vaginosis is not sexually transmitted, and it does not require treatment of the partner. Vaginal infections commonly require an examination and diagnostic assessment.

🔑 CN: Reduction of risk potential; CL: Synthesize

2. 3. Douching may disrupt the normal flora of the vaginal lactobacilli and change the pH, which could result in overgrowth of other bacteria. Coffee, intercourse during menses, and tampons are not related to changes in vaginal pH or the incidence of bacterial vaginosis.

🔑 CN: Health promotion and maintenance; CL: Apply

3. 4. Metronidazole interacts with alcohol and can cause a serious disulfiram-type reaction, with severe, prolonged vomiting. The client should not douche unless following a medical prescription, but douching does not interact with metronidazole. Sexual intercourse and hot tub baths are not known to affect the incidence or treatment of bacterial vaginosis.

🔑 CN: Pharmacological and parenteral therapies; CL: Synthesize

4. 1,2,3. Women with underlying medical conditions, such as uncontrolled diabetes and HIV infection or cancer-causing immunosuppression, correlate with an increasing severity of candidiasis. Hypertension and asthma are not related to immunosuppression or complicated candidiasis.

🔑 CN: Health promotion and maintenance; CL: Analyze

5. 1. Antibiotics may decrease the effectiveness of oral contraceptives. The client should be instructed to continue the contraceptives and use a barrier method as a backup method of birth control until the next menstrual cycle. The client should not stop taking her oral contraceptives, and there is no indication for or benefit to taking the antibiotic 2 hours after the contraceptive. There is no incidence of the adverse effects of increased hunger and fluid retention with the interaction of antibiotic therapy and oral contraceptives.

🔑 CN: Pharmacological and parenteral therapies; CL: Create

6. 4. Due to the increased risk of pelvic inflammatory disease, candidates for the IUD should be in a monogamous relationship. Smoking and hypertension are not contraindications for an IUD. The frequency of sexual relations will not affect IUD use.

🔑 CN: Pharmacological and parenteral therapies; CL: Analyze

7. 1. Fluid losses can occur from vomiting, diarrhea, and fever and can lead to hypovolemic shock. The first nursing action is to treat the hypovolemic shock that accompanies toxic shock, so the IV fluids must be administered immediately. The fluid replacement is critical to avoid circulatory collapse. Pain medication and teaching can be implemented later. Antibiotics will be given because TSS is caused by a staphylococcal infection; however, fluid replacement is initiated **first** to treat life-threatening hypovolemic shock.

🔑 CN: Reduction of risk potential; CL: Synthesize

The Client with Uterine Fibroids

8. 2. The best approach for a client who is fearful about having surgery is to allow the client opportunities to express her fears. Open-ended questions should elicit the client's individual and specific fears. This then gives the nurse the opportunity to provide clarification, information, and support and possibly to offer other resources. The other actions are not supportive and deny the client the opportunity to express her feelings.

🔑 CN: Psychosocial adaptation; CL: Synthesize

9. 1,2. A woman with uterine fibroids and dysmenorrhea is at risk for iron deficiency anemia. The hemoglobin and hematocrit indicate the likelihood that the fibroids causing heavy menstrual blood loss have resulted in anemia. A hemoglobin of <12 g/dL (120 g/L) in women is considered low. The white blood cell count and potassium levels are within normal parameters, and normocytic red blood cells are normal.

🔑 CN: Management of care; CL: Synthesize

10. 2. It is a priority that the client knows she will not be able to eat or drink for 8 hours before admission. A client who consumes food and fluid before receiving a general anesthetic is at risk for aspiration, which can lead to aspiration pneumonia, respiratory arrest, and even death. The clothing she should wear to the hospital and the type of medication she will receive are important, but not the priority. Information on exercise and resumption of normal activities can be included in the discharge teaching.

🔑 CN: Basic care and comfort; CL: Synthesize

11. 2. The client needs to understand that with removal of the uterus, she will no longer be able to bear children or have menstrual periods. The surgical procedure should not change her libido or sexual functioning. Research does not support the idea that hysterectomy contributes to depression or weight gain. Research demonstrates that women who have managed health problems for some time before the hysterectomy may actually have a more positive effect, with less worry about their health condition, contraception, or pregnancy.

🔑 CN: Management of care; CL: Apply

12. 4,1,3,2. After gathering appropriate supplies, the nurse should prepare a sterile field. After lubricating the catheter adequately with a water-soluble lubricant to minimize trauma to the urethra, the nurse should insert the catheter far enough into the bladder so the retention balloon does not traumatize urethral tissues. Ensuring a free flow of urine prevents infection; improper drainage occurs when tubing is kinked or twisted.

🔑 CN: Safety and infection control; CL: Apply

13. 2. Hyperventilation occurs when the client breathes so rapidly and deeply that she exhales excessive amounts of carbon dioxide. A characteristic symptom of hyperventilation is dizziness. To avoid hyperventilation, the nurse should assist the client in the practice of slow, deep breathing in a regular breathing pattern. Dyspnea, blurred vision, and mental confusion are not associated with hyperventilation.

🔑 CN: Physiological adaptation; CL: Apply

14. 4. The discomfort associated with gas pains is likely to be relieved when the client ambulates. The gas will be more easily expelled with exercise. The anesthesia, analgesics, and immobility have altered normal peristalsis. Peristalsis will be stimulated by exercise. Offering a hot beverage, providing extra warmth, and applying an abdominal binder are not recommended and could aggravate the discomfort of postoperative gas pains.

CN: Physiological adaptation; CL: Synthesize

15. 3. Elevated temperature on the second postoperative day is suggestive of a respiratory tract infection. Respiratory infections most often occur during the first 48 hours after surgery. The nurse should encourage the client to take deep breaths frequently. The nurse should also monitor the client's vital signs and report significant changes to the surgeon. Signs of infection, if present in the wound or urinary tract, are likely to occur later in the postoperative period. There is no indication that the IV catheter is the source of infection.

CN: Physiological adaptation; CL: Synthesize

16. 3. When a dressing sticks to a wound, it is best to moisten the dressing with sterile normal saline solution and then remove it carefully. Trying to remove a dry dressing is likely to irritate the skin and wound. This may contribute to tension or tearing along the suture line.

CN: Management of care; CL: Apply

17. 2. The social worker will be able to coordinate respite care for the son and other community resources for this family. Home health care would provide care for the client herself, but respite care for the son is the priority need for this family. Pastoral care provides spiritual care. The volunteer department would not be responsible for coordination of care at the client's home.

CN: Management of care; CL: Apply

18. 2. Assessment is the first step in planning client education. Assessing social support resources is a key aspect of discharge planning that begins when the client is admitted to the hospital. It is imperative to know what assistance and support the client has at home. Assessment includes obtaining data about any family or home responsibilities the client is concerned with during the recovery period. It is within the scope of nursing practice to provide discharge instructions. A social worker is not needed at this time. The nurse should assess the client's needs before determining whether using a video or reading instructions to the client is appropriate.

CN: Health promotion and maintenance; CL: Create

19. 2. The nurse's first action is to notify the surgeon as the amount of bleeding on the perineal pad is not normal. Excessive bleeding is also indicated by elevated heart rate and decreased BP. Urinary catheters are not removed until the second or third postoperative day. The surgeon may prescribe an increase in the rate of the IV fluids. The nurse changes the perineal pad and offers comfort measures once the client is stable.

CN: Physiological adaptation; CL: Synthesize

20. 3. The client should be prepared for what to expect after surgery. The client should not drive until she can use the brake pedal without abdominal pain. The nurse should teach the client to avoid activities that may increase pelvic congestion, such as dancing or brisk walking, for several months, whereas activities, such as swimming and leisurely walking, may be both physically and mentally helpful. Heavy lifting should be avoided for 2 months, but the client can lift up to 10 lb (4.5 kg) as long as there is no tension on the abdomen or abdominal pain.

CN: Physiological adaptation; CL: Synthesize

21. 1. The nurse must first assess the intensity of the client's pain before selecting the correct analgesia. A high score would necessitate administering the meperidine. If the intensity rating is low, an oral analgesic would be appropriate. If acetaminophen is given without assessing the intensity of the client's pain, the nurse must then wait 4 hours before administering another analgesic.

CN: Pharmacological and parenteral therapies; CL: Synthesize

22. 3. The nurse should withhold administering docusate sodium, a stool softener, and document that the woman has had loose stools. The nurse is responsible for assessing contraindications and adverse effects of medications, and administering the medication when the client already has loose stools is unsafe. The assessment should also include auscultation of bowel sounds and inquiry about gas pains, but the stool softener should still be withheld.

CN: Pharmacological and parenteral therapies; CL: Synthesize

23. 1,4. The average age of menopause is 50 to 52 years, although some variation exists. Vaginal infections do not necessarily increase during menopause. Hot flashes occur in about 80% of women; they can range from mild to very debilitating with disruption of sleep patterns. Depression is not usual during menopause; if symptoms of depression do occur, the nurse should refer the woman to her **healthcare provider (HCP)** 📖. Contraception should be used until menses has ceased for a full year.

CN: Physiological adaptation; CL: Create

The Client with Breast Cancer

24. The upper outer quadrant is the area of the breast in which most breast tumors are found. This area should be palpated thoroughly. Although breast tumors can be found in any area of the breast, including the nipple, the tumors are most often in the upper outer quadrant.

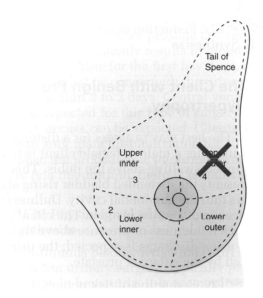

CN: Health promotion and maintenance; CL: Apply

25. 2. The breasts may vary in size before menstruation because of breast engorgement caused by hormonal changes. A woman may then note that her bra fits more tightly than usual. Benign cysts do not cause variation in breast size. A change in breast size that does not follow hormonal changes could warrant further assessment. The breasts normally are about the same size, although some women have one breast slightly larger than the other.

CN: Health promotion and maintenance; CL: Apply

26. 2. The nurse should explain that the incidence of breast cancer increases with age and current guidelines recommend women have a mammogram every 2 years until age 74. While mammograms are less painful as breast tissue becomes softer, the nurse should advise the woman to have the mammogram. Family history is important, but only about 5% of breast cancers are genetic. Several breast cancer screening guidelines recommend against breast self-examinations for women.

CN: Health promotion and maintenance; CL: Synthesize

27. 1. An important nursing responsibility is preoperative teaching, and the most frequently recommended guide for teaching is to tell the client as much as she wants to know and is able to understand. Delaying discussion of issues about which the client has concerns is likely to aggravate the situation and cause the client to feel distrust. As a general guide, the client would not ask the question if she were not ready to discuss her situation. The nurse is available to answer the client's questions and concerns and should not delay discussing these with the client.

CN: Psychosocial adaptation; CL: Synthesize

28. 1. The nurse documents serosanguineous drainage of 100 to 200 ml because this is normal during the first 24 hours after surgery. The nurse notifies the surgeon only if there is excessive or very bloody drainage. The surgeon removes the drain within 24 to 48 hours. The client is instructed to keep her arm on the affected side and supported in an adducted position.

CN: Physiological adaptation; CL: Synthesize

29. 4. Atropine sulfate, a cholinergic blocking agent, is given preoperatively to reduce secretions in the mouth and respiratory tract, which assists in maintaining the integrity of the respiratory system during general anesthesia. Atropine is not used to promote muscle relaxation, decrease nausea and vomiting, or decrease pulse and respiratory rates. It causes the pulse to increase.

CN: Pharmacological and parenteral therapies; CL: Evaluate

30. 3. The nurse should respond with an open-ended statement that elicits further exploration of the client's feelings. Women with cancer may feel guilt or shame. Previous life decisions, sexuality, and religious beliefs may influence a client's adjustment to a diagnosis of cancer. The nurse should not contradict the client's feelings of punishment or offer advice such as confiding in the husband. A social worker referral may be beneficial in the future, but it is not the first response needed to elicit exploration of the client's feelings.

CN: Psychosocial adaptation; CL: Synthesize

31. 3. A drainage tube is placed in the wound after a modified radical mastectomy to help remove accumulated blood and fluid in the area. Removal of the drainage fluids assists in wound healing and is intended to decrease the incidence of hematoma, abscess formation, and infection. Drainage tubes placed in a wound do not decrease intrathoracic pressure, increase collateral lymphatic flow, or prevent adhesion formation.

CN: Reduction of risk potential; CL: Evaluate

90. 2,4. Ovarian cancer is a malignant tumor of the ovary. Ovarian cancer is the fourth most common gynecologic cancer, but the most lethal. It is usually found in advanced stages because it is asymptomatic in early stages. Interdisciplinary management may involve chemotherapy, radiation therapy, surgery, and supportive services. Chemotherapy may be used to achieve remission of the disease; it is not, however, curative. Surgery is the treatment of choice, usually involving total hysterectomy with bilateral salpingo-oophorectomy and removal of the omentum. Radiation therapy may be performed for palliative purposes only. The nurse should provide referral to home health services, financial assistance, psychological counseling, clergy, and other social services, as appropriate. Nutrition therapy for parenteral lipids is not part of management of ovarian cancer.

🔑 CN: Health promotion and maintenance; CL: Create

91. 4. A definitive cause of carcinoma of the ovary is unknown, and the disease is multifactorial. The risk of developing ovarian cancer is related to environmental, endocrine, and genetic factors. The highest incidence is in industrialized Western countries. Endocrine risk factors for ovarian cancer include women who are nulliparous. Use of oral contraceptives does not increase the risk for developing ovarian cancer but may actually be protective.

🔑 CN: Health promotion and maintenance; CL: Apply

92. 1. Ovarian cancer is rarely diagnosed early. Methods for mass screening and early detection have not been successful. Signs and symptoms are often vague until late in development. Ovarian cancer should be considered in any woman older than 40 years of age who has vague abdominal and/or pelvic discomfort or enlargement, a sense of bloating, or flatulence. Enlargement of the abdomen due to the accumulation of fluid is the most common sign.

🔑 CN: Health promotion and maintenance; CL: Synthesize

The Client with Testicular Disease

93. 2. Epididymitis causes acute tenderness and pronounced swelling of the scrotum. Gradual onset of unilateral scrotal pain, urethral discharge, and fever are other key signs. Epididymitis is occasionally, but not routinely, associated with urinary tract infection. Burning and pain on urination and foul-smelling ejaculate or urine are not classic symptoms of epididymitis.

🔑 CN: Physiological adaptation; CL: Analyze

94. 3. Among men younger than age 35, epididymitis is most frequently caused by a sexually transmitted infection. Causative organisms are usually chlamydia or *Neisseria gonorrhoeae*. The other major form of epididymitis is bacterial, caused by the *Escherichia coli* or *Pseudomonas* organisms. The nurse should always include safe sex teaching for a client with epididymitis. The client should also be advised against anogenital intercourse because this is a mode of transmission of gram-negative rods to the epididymis.

🔑 CN: Reduction of risk potential; CL: Apply

95. 3. After a warm bath or shower, the testes hang lower and are both relaxed and in the ideal position for manual evaluation and palpation. The testes are not relaxed or in the best position after intercourse, at the end of the day, or after exercise.

🔑 CN: Health promotion and maintenance; CL: Apply

96. 2. Normal testes feel smooth, egg-shaped, and firm to the touch, without lumps. The surface should feel smooth and rubbery. The testes should not be soft or spongy to the touch. Testicular malignancies are usually nontender, nonpainful hard lumps. Lumps, swelling, nodules, or signs of inflammation should be reported to the **healthcare provider (HCP)** 📖.

🔑 CN: Health promotion and maintenance; CL: Analyze

97. 4. AFP and hCG are considered markers that indicate the presence of testicular disease. Elevated AFP and hCG and decreased testosterone are markers for testicular disease. Measurements of AFP, hCG, and testosterone are also obtained throughout the course of therapy to help measure the effectiveness of treatment.

🔑 CN: Physiological adaptation; CL: Apply

98. 1. Cryptorchidism (undescended testes) carries a greatly increased risk for testicular cancer. Undescended testes occur in about 3% of male infants, with an increased incidence in premature infants. Other possible causes of malignancy include chemical carcinogens, trauma, orchitis, and environmental factors. Testicular cancer is not associated with early sexual relations in men, even though cervical cancer is associated with early sexual relations in women. Testicular cancer is not associated with seminal vesiculitis or epididymitis.

🔑 CN: Health promotion and maintenance; CL: Apply

99. 2. The incidence of testicular cancer is higher in men who live in rural rather than suburban areas. Testicular cancer is more common in white than black men. Men with higher socioeconomic status seem to have a greater incidence of testicular cancer. The exact cause of testicular cancer is unknown. Cancer of the testes is the leading cause of death from cancer in the 15- to 35-year-old age group.

🔑 CN: Health promotion and maintenance; CL: Analyze

100. 3. Because of the location of the incision in the high inguinal area, pain is a major problem during the immediate postoperative period. The incisional area and discomfort caused by movement contribute to increased pain. Bladder spasms and elimination problems are more commonly associated with prostate surgery. Nausea is not a priority problem.

🔑 CN: Physiological adaptation; CL: Synthesize

101. 2. Unilateral orchiectomy alone does not result in impotence if the other testis is normal. The other testis should produce enough testosterone to maintain normal sexual drive, functioning, and characteristics. Sperm banking before treatment is commonly recommended because radiation or chemotherapy can affect fertility.

🔑 CN: Psychosocial adaptation; CL: Synthesize

102. 2. When diagnosed early and treated aggressively, testicular cancer has a cure rate of about 90%. Treatment of testicular cancer is based on tumor type, and seminoma cancer has the best prognosis. Modes of treatment include combinations of orchiectomy, radiation therapy, and chemotherapy. The chemotherapeutic regimen used currently is responsible for the successful treatment of testicular cancer. The nurse should not indicate to the client that the cancer will be cured, even though cure rates are high.

🔑 CN: Physiological adaptation; CL: Apply

The Client with Cancer of the Prostate

103. 2. Most cases of prostate cancer are adenocarcinomas. An adenocarcinoma is palpable on rectal examination because it arises from the posterior portion of the gland. Although the prostate-specific antigen (PSA) is not a perfect screening test, the American Cancer Society and the Canadian Cancer Society recommend an annual rectal examination and blood PSA level for all men age 50 years and older, or starting at age 40 years if the client is of African descent, or if there is family history of prostate cancer. Avoiding heavy lifting does not prevent cancer, nor does having regular sexual activity.

🔑 CN: Health promotion and maintenance; CL: Synthesize

104. 4. Bilateral orchiectomy (removal of testes) results in reduction of the major circulating androgen, testosterone, as a palliative measure to reduce symptoms and progression of prostate cancer. A radical prostatectomy (removal of entire prostate gland, prostatic capsule, and seminal vesicles) may include pelvic lymphadenectomy. Complications include urinary incontinence, impotence, and rectal injury with the radical prostatectomy. Cryosurgery freezes prostate tissue, killing tumor cells without prostatectomy.

🔑 CN: Health promotion and maintenance; CL: Apply

105. 1,2,3. Cancer of the prostate gland is the second leading cause of cancer death among American and Canadian men and is the most common carcinoma in men older than age 65. Incidence of prostate cancer is higher in men of African descent, and onset is earlier. Most prostate cancers are adenocarcinoma. Prostate cancer is usually multifocal and slow growing and can spread by local extension, by lymphatics, or through the bloodstream. Prostate-specific antigen (PSA) >4 ng/mg is diagnostic; a free PSA level can help stratify the risk of elevated PSA levels. Metastatic workup may include skeletal x-ray, bone scan, and computed tomography or magnetic resonance imaging to detect local extension, bone, and lymph node involvement. The urine does not have prostate cancer cells.

🔑 CN: Health promotion and maintenance; CL: Create

106. 3,4. Hormone manipulation deprives tumor cells of androgens or their by-products and, thereby, alleviates symptoms and retards disease progression. Complications of hormonal manipulation include hot flashes, nausea and vomiting, gynecomastia, and sexual dysfunction. As part of supportive care, provide explanations of diagnostic tests and treatment options and help the client gain some feeling of control over his disease and decisions related to it. To help achieve optimal sexual function, give the client the opportunity to communicate his concerns and sexual needs. Inform the client that decreased libido is expected after hormonal manipulation therapy and that impotence may result from some surgical procedures and radiation. A psychiatrist is not needed.

🔑 CN: Psychosocial adaptation; CL: Synthesize

107. 3. Manipulation of the prostate during the digital rectal examination may falsely increase the PSA levels. The PSA determination and the digital rectal examination are no longer recommended as screening tools for prostate cancer. Prostate cancer is the most common cancer in men and the second leading killer from cancer among men in the United States and Canada. Incidence increases sharply with age, and the disease is predominant in the 60- to 70-year-old age group.

🗝 CN: Health promotion and maintenance; CL: Apply

108. 1. On digital rectal examination, key signs of prostate cancer are a hard prostate, induration of the prostate, and an irregular, hard nodule. Accompanying symptoms of prostate cancer can include constipation, weight loss, and lymphadenopathy. Abdominal pain usually does not accompany prostate cancer. A boggy, tender prostate is found with infection (e.g., acute or chronic prostatitis).

🗝 CN: Health promotion and maintenance; CL: Analyze

109. 2. Loss of the prostate gland interrupts the flow of semen, so there will be no ejaculation fluid. The sensations of orgasm remain intact. The client needs to be advised that return of erectile capability is often disrupted after surgery, but within 1 year, 95% of men have returned to normal erectile function with sexual intercourse.

🗝 CN: Physiological adaptation; CL: Synthesize

110. 1. Clients who have stage IA or IIB prostate cancer have an excellent survival rate. Prostate cancer is usually slow growing, and many men who have prostate cancer do not die from it. A stage I or II tumor is confined to the prostate gland and has not spread to the extrapelvic region or bone.

🗝 CN: Physiological adaptation; CL: Synthesize

111. 2. Goserelin is used to decrease testosterone production in men to slow or stop the production of cancer cells. A common side effect is flushing or hot flashes. Changes in blood pressure, tenderness of the scrotum, and dramatic changes in secondary sexual characteristics should not occur.

🗝 CN: Pharmacological and parenteral therapies; CL: Apply

The Client with Erectile Dysfunction

112. 2. The client should notify his **HCP** 📖 promptly if he experiences sudden or decreased vision loss in one or both eyes. Sildenafil should not be taken more than once per day. Sildenafil offers no protection against sexually transmitted diseases. Sildenafil has no effect in the absence of sexual stimulation.

🗝 CN: Pharmacological and parenteral therapies; CL: Synthesize

113. 2. Antihypertensives, especially beta-blockers such as propranolol, can cause impotence. When a male client has impotence, the nurse should always examine his medication regimen as a potential contributing factor. Aspirin, nonsteroidal anti-inflammatory drugs, and anticoagulants do not cause erectile dysfunction.

🗝 CN: Pharmacological and parenteral therapies; CL: Synthesize

114. 2. ED is multifactorial in origin, and more than 50% of the cases can be attributed to organic causes, which include alteration in vascular supply, hormonal changes, neurologic dysfunction, medications, and associated systemic diseases, such as diabetes mellitus or alcoholism. The presence of nocturnal erections is the first evaluation to differentiate between organic and psychogenic causes. ED is a common problem among men older than age 65.

🗝 CN: Psychosocial adaptation; CL: Apply

115. 1. Avoidance of alcohol can improve the outcome of therapy. Alcohol and smoking can affect a man's ability to have and maintain an erection. The client should be encouraged to follow a healthy diet, but no specific diet is associated with improvement of sexual function. The client should cease smoking, not just decrease smoking. Increasing attempts at intercourse without treatment will not facilitate improvement. The client should be reassured that ED is a common problem and that help is available.

🗝 CN: Reduction of risk potential; CL: Synthesize

Managing Care, Quality, and Safety of Clients with Reproductive Health Problems

116. 4. The **registered nurse (RN)** 📖 is responsible for monitoring the surgical site for condition of the dressing, status of the incision, and signs and symptoms of complications. **UAP** 📖 who have been trained to report abnormalities to the RN supervising the care may take vital signs, record intake and output, and give perineal care.

🗝 CN: Management of care; CL: Synthesize

117. 4. To determine the cause of this problem, a quality improvement study should be conducted. Before implementing solutions to a problem, the precise issues in the hospital system must be observed and documented. Consulting with the evening nurses may result in biased observations because the evening nurses are not conducting care under the same environment as the night nurses. Including a medication nurse is not the first step in understanding the problem and may be an unrealistic or expensive solution. The supervisor is not directly involved with the problem and should only be consulted if the problem cannot be solved by those involved.

CN: Management of care; CL: Synthesize

118. 3. The nurse must clarify this prescription with the admitting **HCP** 📖 to ensure medication accuracy and client safety. In healthcare settings without computerized medical records or computer prescribing, misinterpretation of handwriting remains a leading cause of medication errors. It is not safe practice to question the client regarding a diagnosis and assume the medication is correctly prescribed. The pharmacist will need clarification of the prescription as well. It is not the role of the pharmacist to interpret the prescription.

CN: Pharmacological and parenteral therapies; CL: Synthesize

119. 2. The surgeon should be notified when a client who has had an abdominal hysterectomy develops vaginal bleeding that saturates a blue pad in 1 hour, and care should be managed so that other personnel can obtain vital signs while the nurse contacts the surgeon. The client may need to have IV fluids increased, but the surgeon needs to be notified first. Waiting 15 minutes while the client is having bright red bleeding is an unsafe nursing action; the client may lose a large amount of blood.

CN: Management of care; CL: Synthesize

120. 3. The nurse should follow the line of authority or chain of command by reporting the observation immediately to the nursing supervisor. The nurse should not confront the person or the medication nurse because the line of authority for reporting incidents should be followed. The RT supervisor may subsequently be involved in the incident, but the nursing supervisor should initiate and follow the policy and procedure.

CN: Management of care; CL: Synthesize

The Client with Neurologic Health Problems

- The Client with a Head Injury
- The Client with Seizures
- The Client with a Stroke
- The Client with Parkinson's Disease
- The Client with Multiple Sclerosis
- The Client with Myasthenia Gravis
- The Unconscious Client
- The Client in Pain
- Managing Care, Quality, and Safety of Clients with Neurologic Health Problems
- Answers, Rationales, and Test-Taking Strategies

The Client with a Head Injury

1. The nurse has established a goal to maintain intracranial pressure (ICP) within the normal range for a client who had a craniotomy 12 hours ago. What should the nurse do? Select all that apply.

☐ 1. Encourage the client to cough to expectorate secretions.

☐ 2. Elevate the head of the bed 15 to 20 degrees.

☐ 3. Contact the healthcare provider (HCP) if ICP is >15 mm Hg.

☐ 4. Monitor neurologic status using the Glasgow Coma Scale.

☐ 5. Stimulate the client with active range-of-motion exercises.

2. The nurse is monitoring a client with increased intracranial pressure (ICP). What indicators are the **most** critical for the nurse to monitor? Select all that apply.

☐ 1. systolic blood pressure

☐ 2. urine output

☐ 3. breath sounds

☐ 4. cerebral perfusion pressure

☐ 5. level of pain

3. A nurse is assessing a client with increasing intracranial pressure. What is a client's mean arterial pressure (MAP) in mm Hg when blood pressure (BP) is 120/60 mm Hg?

_____ mm Hg.

4. A client with a contusion has been admitted for observation following a motor vehicle accident when he was driving his pregnant wife to the hospital. The next morning, instead of asking about his wife and baby, he asked to see the football game on television that he thinks is starting in 5 minutes. He is agitated because the nurse will not turn on the television. What should the nurse do **next**? Select all that apply.

☐ 1. Find a television so the client can view the football game.

☐ 2. Determine if the client's pupils are equal and react to light.

☐ 3. Ask the client if he has a headache.

☐ 4. Arrange for the client to be with his wife and baby.

☐ 5. Administer a sedative.

5. The nurse is assessing the level of consciousness in a client with a head injury who has been unresponsive for the last 8 hours. Using the Glasgow Coma Scale, the nurse notes that the client opens the eyes only as a response to pain, responds with sounds that are not understandable, and has abnormal extension of the extremities. What should the nurse do?

Glasgow Coma Scale

Parameter	Finding	Score
Eye opening	Spontaneously	4
	To speech	3
	To pain	2
	Do not open	1
Best verbal response	Oriented	5
	Confused	4
	Inappropriate speech	3
	Incomprehensible sounds	2
	No verbalization	1
Best motor response	Obeys command	6
	Localizes pain	5
	Withdraws from pain	4
	Abnormal flexio	3
	Abnormal extension	2
	No motor response	1

Interpretation: Best score = 15; worst score = 3; 7 or less generally indicates coma; changes from baseline are most important.

☐ 1. Attempt to arouse the client.
☐ 2. Reposition the client with the extremities in normal alignment.
☐ 3. Chart the client's level of consciousness as coma.
☐ 4. Notify the healthcare provider (HCP).

6. An unconscious client with multiple injuries to the head and neck arrives in the emergency department. What should the nurse do **first**?
☐ 1. Establish an airway.
☐ 2. Determine the identity of the client.
☐ 3. Stop bleeding from open wounds.
☐ 4. Check for a neck fracture.

7. A client has delirium following a head injury. The client is disoriented and agitated. In which order from first to last should the nurse initiate care for this client? All options must be used.

| 1. Request a prescription for haloperidol. |
| 2. Maintain a quiet environment. |
| 3. Assure the client's safety. |
| 4. Approach the client using short sentences. |

| |
| |
| |
| |

8. A client is at risk for increased intracranial pressure (ICP). Which finding is the **priority** for the nurse to monitor?
☐ 1. unequal pupil size
☐ 2. decreasing systolic blood pressure
☐ 3. tachycardia
☐ 4. decreasing body temperature

9. What should the nurse do **first** when a client with a head injury begins to have clear drainage from the nose?
☐ 1. Compress the nares.
☐ 2. Tilt the head back.
☐ 3. Collect the drainage.
☐ 4. Administer an antihistamine for postnasal drip.

10. Which respiratory pattern indicates increasing intracranial pressure in the brain stem?
☐ 1. slow, irregular respirations
☐ 2. rapid, shallow respirations
☐ 3. asymmetric chest excursion
☐ 4. nasal flaring

11. A client has an increased intracranial pressure (ICP) of 20 mm Hg. The nurse should:
☐ 1. give the client a warming blanket.
☐ 2. administer low-dose barbiturates.
☐ 3. encourage the client to take deep breaths to hyperventilate.
☐ 4. restrict fluids.

12. The nurse is assessing a client with increasing intracranial pressure (ICP). The nurse should notify the healthcare provider (HCP) about which early change in the client's condition?
☐ 1. widening pulse pressure
☐ 2. decrease in the pulse rate
☐ 3. dilated, fixed pupils
☐ 4. decrease in level of consciousness (LOC)

13. The client has a sustained increased intracranial pressure (ICP) of 20 mm Hg. Which client position would be **most** appropriate?
☐ 1. the head of the bed elevated 15 to 20 degrees
☐ 2. Trendelenburg's position
☐ 3. left Sims' position
☐ 4. the head elevated on two pillows

14. The nurse administers mannitol to the client with increased intracranial pressure. Which parameter requires close monitoring?
☐ 1. muscle relaxation
☐ 2. intake and output
☐ 3. widening of the pulse pressure
☐ 4. pupil dilation

15. The nurse is assessing a client for movement after halo traction placement for a C8 fracture. The nurse should document that:
☐ 1. the client's shoulders shrug against downward pressure of the examiner's hands.
☐ 2. the client's arm pulls up from a resting position against resistance.
☐ 3. the client's arm straightens out from a flexed position against resistance.
☐ 4. the client's hand-grasp strength is equal.

16. A client who is regaining consciousness after a craniotomy becomes restless and attempts to pull out the IV line. Which nursing intervention protects the client without increasing the intracranial pressure (ICP)?
☐ 1. Place the client in a jacket restraint.
☐ 2. Wrap the hands in soft "mitten" restraints.
☐ 3. Tuck the arms and hands under the sheet.
☐ 4. Apply a wrist restraint to each arm.

17. Which activity should the nurse encourage the client to avoid when there is a risk for increased intracranial pressure (ICP)?
☐ 1. deep breathing
☐ 2. turning
☐ 3. coughing
☐ 4. passive range-of-motion (ROM) exercises

18. A client who had a serious head injury with increased intracranial pressure is to be discharged to a rehabilitation facility. Which outcome of rehabilitation would be appropriate for the client? The client will:
☐ 1. exhibit no further episodes of short-term memory loss.
☐ 2. be able to return to his construction job in 3 weeks.
☐ 3. actively participate in the rehabilitation process as appropriate.
☐ 4. be emotionally stable and display preinjury personality traits.

19. The nurse is assessing a client for decerebrate posturing. The nurse should assess the client for:
☐ 1. internal rotation and adduction of arms with flexion of elbows, wrists, and fingers.
☐ 2. back hunched over and rigid flexion of all four extremities with supination of arms and plantar flexion of feet.
☐ 3. supination of arms and dorsiflexion of the feet.
☐ 4. back arched and rigid extension of all four extremities.

20. A client receiving continuous mandatory ventilation begins to experience cluster breathing after recent intracranial occipital bleeding. What should the nurse do?
☐ 1. Count the rate to be sure that ventilations are deep enough to be sufficient.
☐ 2. Notify the healthcare provider (HCP) of the client's breathing pattern.
☐ 3. Increase the rate of ventilations.
☐ 4. Increase the tidal volume on the ventilator.

21. The nurse is planning the care for a client who has had a posterior fossa (infratentorial) craniotomy. What should the nurse **avoid** when positioning the client?
☐ 1. keeping the client flat on one side or the other
☐ 2. elevating the head of the bed to 30 degrees
☐ 3. logrolling or turning as a unit when turning
☐ 4. keeping the neck in a neutral position

22. A young adult is admitted to the hospital with a head injury and possible temporal skull fracture sustained in a motorcycle accident. On admission, the client was conscious but lethargic; vital signs included temperature 99°F (37°C), pulse 100 bpm, respirations 18 breaths/min, and BP 140/70 mm Hg. The nurse should report which changes should they occur to the healthcare provider (HCP)? Select all that apply.
☐ 1. decreasing urinary output
☐ 2. decreasing systolic BP
☐ 3. bradycardia
☐ 4. widening pulse pressure
☐ 5. tachycardia
☐ 6. increasing diastolic BP

23. A client with a head injury regains consciousness after several days. When the client **first** awakes, what should the nurse say to the client?
☐ 1. "I will get your family."
☐ 2. "Can you tell me your name and where you live?"
☐ 3. "I will bet you are a little confused right now."
☐ 4. "You are in the hospital. You were in an accident and unconscious."

The Client with Seizures

24. The nurse sees a client walking in the hallway who begins to have a seizure. What should the nurse do in order of priority from first to last? All options must be used.

| 1. Maintain a patent airway. |
| 2. Record the seizure activity observed. |
| 3. Ease the client to the floor. |
| 4. Obtain vital signs. |

| |
| |
| |
| |

25. Which finding will the nurse observe in the client in the ictal phase of a generalized tonic-clonic seizure?
- [ ] 1. jerking in one extremity that spreads gradually to adjacent areas
- [ ] 2. vacant staring and abruptly ceasing all activity
- [ ] 3. facial grimaces, patting motions, and lip smacking
- [ ] 4. loss of consciousness, body stiffening, and violent muscle contractions

26. It is the night before a client is to have a computed tomography (CT) scan of the head without contrast. The nurse should tell the client:
- [ ] 1. "You must shampoo your hair tonight to remove all oil and dirt."
- [ ] 2. "You may drink fluids until midnight, but after that, drink nothing until the scan is completed."
- [ ] 3. "You will have some hair shaved to attach the small electrode to your scalp."
- [ ] 4. "You will need to hold your head very still during the examination."

27. The client will have an electroencephalogram (EEG) in the morning. The nurse should instruct the client to have which foods/fluids for breakfast?
- [ ] 1. no food or fluids
- [ ] 2. only coffee or tea if needed
- [ ] 3. a full breakfast as desired without coffee, tea, or energy drinks
- [ ] 4. a liquid breakfast of fruit juice, oatmeal, or smoothie

28. The client is scheduled to receive phenytoin through a nasogastric tube (NGT) and has a tube-feeding supplement running continuously. The head of the bed is elevated to 30 degrees. Prior to administering the medication, the nurse should:
- [ ] 1. elevate the head of the bed to 60 degrees.
- [ ] 2. draw blood to determine the phenytoin level after giving the morning dose in order to determine if the client has toxic blood level.
- [ ] 3. stop the tube feeding 1 hour before giving phenytoin and hold tube feeding for 1 hour after giving the medication.
- [ ] 4. flush the NGT with 150 mL of water before and after giving the phenytoin.

29. Which instruction should the nurse include in the teaching plan for a client with seizures who is going home with a prescription for gabapentin?
- [ ] 1. Take all the medication until it is gone.
- [ ] 2. Notify the healthcare provider (HCP) if vision changes occur.
- [ ] 3. Store gabapentin in the refrigerator.
- [ ] 4. Take gabapentin with an antacid to protect against ulcers.

30. What is the **priority** nursing intervention in the postictal phase of a seizure?
- [ ] 1. Reorient the client to time, person, and place.
- [ ] 2. Determine the client's level of sleepiness.
- [ ] 3. Assess the client's breathing pattern.
- [ ] 4. Position the client comfortably.

31. Which intervention is **most** effective in minimizing the risk of seizure activity in a client who is undergoing diagnostic studies after having experienced several episodes of seizures?
- [ ] 1. Maintain the client on bed rest.
- [ ] 2. Administer butabarbital sodium 30 mg PO, three times per day.
- [ ] 3. Close the door to the room to minimize stimulation.
- [ ] 4. Administer carbamazepine 200 mg PO, twice per day.

32. What nursing assessments should be documented at the beginning of the ictal phase of a seizure?
- [ ] 1. heart rate, respirations, pulse oximeter, and blood pressure
- [ ] 2. last dose of anticonvulsant and circumstances at the time
- [ ] 3. type of visual, auditory, and olfactory aura the client experienced
- [ ] 4. movement of the head and eyes and muscle rigidity

33. The nurse is assessing a client in the postictal phase of generalized tonic-clonic seizure. The nurse should determine if the client has:
- [ ] 1. drowsiness.
- [ ] 2. inability to move.
- [ ] 3. paresthesia.
- [ ] 4. hypotension.

34. When preparing to teach a client about phenytoin sodium therapy, the nurse should urge the client not to stop the drug suddenly because:
- ☐ 1. physical dependency on the drug develops over time.
- ☐ 2. status epilepticus may develop.
- ☐ 3. a hypoglycemic reaction develops.
- ☐ 4. heart block is likely to develop.

35. The nurse is teaching a client to recognize an aura. The nurse should instruct the client to note:
- ☐ 1. a postictal state of amnesia.
- ☐ 2. a hallucination that occurs during a seizure.
- ☐ 3. a symptom that occurs just before a seizure.
- ☐ 4. a feeling of relaxation as the seizure begins to subside.

36. Which statement by a client with a seizure disorder who has been prescribed topiramate indicates the client has understood the nurse's instruction about this drug?
- ☐ 1. "I will take the medicine before going to bed."
- ☐ 2. "I will drink six to eight glasses of water a day."
- ☐ 3. "I will eat plenty of fresh fruits."
- ☐ 4. "I will take the medicine with a meal or snack."

37. Which clinical manifestation is a typical reaction to long-term phenytoin sodium therapy?
- ☐ 1. weight gain
- ☐ 2. insomnia
- ☐ 3. excessive growth of gum tissue
- ☐ 4. deteriorating eyesight

38. A 21-year-old female client takes clonazepam. What should the nurse ask this client about? Select all that apply.
- ☐ 1. seizure activity
- ☐ 2. pregnancy status
- ☐ 3. alcohol use
- ☐ 4. cigarette smoking
- ☐ 5. intake of caffeine and sugary drinks

The Client with a Stroke

39. Which outcomes indicate effective management of a conscious client who is being treated with recombinant tissue plasminogen therapy during the initial phase of an ischemic cerebral vascular accident (CVA)? Select all that apply.
- ☐ 1. headache reduced
- ☐ 2. dysphagia improved
- ☐ 3. visual disturbances improved
- ☐ 4. responds to comfort measures
- ☐ 5. no signs or symptoms of bleeding

40. Following a stroke, a client has dysphagia and left-sided facial paralysis. Which feeding technique will be **most** helpful at this time?
- ☐ 1. Encourage sipping diluted liquid meal supplements from a straw.
- ☐ 2. Position the client with the bed at a 30-degree angle.
- ☐ 3. Offer solid foods from the unaffected side of the mouth.
- ☐ 4. Feed the client a soft diet from a spoon into the left side of the mouth.

41. A client is being monitored for transient ischemic attacks. The client is oriented, can open the eyes spontaneously, and follows commands. What is the Glasgow Coma Scale score?
_____ points.

42. The nurse is teaching a client about taking prophylactic warfarin sodium. Which statement indicates that the client understands how to take the drug? Select all that apply.
- ☐ 1. "The drug's action peaks in 2 hours."
- ☐ 2. "Maximum dosage is not achieved until 3 to 4 days after starting the medication."
- ☐ 3. "Effects of the drug continue for 4 to 5 days after discontinuing the medication."
- ☐ 4. "Protamine sulfate is the antidote for warfarin."
- ☐ 5. "I should have my blood levels tested periodically."

43. Which action is **not** appropriate when providing oral hygiene for a client who has had a stroke?
- ☐ 1. placing the client on the back with a small pillow under the head
- ☐ 2. keeping portable suctioning equipment at the bedside
- ☐ 3. opening the client's mouth with a padded tongue blade
- ☐ 4. cleaning the client's mouth and teeth with a toothbrush

44. A client arrives in the emergency department with an ischemic stroke. Because the healthcare team is considering administering tissue plasminogen activator (t-PA) administration, the nurse should **first**:
- ☐ 1. ask what medications the client is taking.
- ☐ 2. complete a history and health assessment.
- ☐ 3. identify the time of onset of the stroke.
- ☐ 4. determine if the client is scheduled for any surgical procedures.

45. During the **first** 24 hours after thrombolytic treatment for an ischemic stroke, the **primary** goal is to control the client's:
- ☐ 1. pulse.
- ☐ 2. respirations.
- ☐ 3. blood pressure.
- ☐ 4. temperature.

46. What is a **priority** nursing assessment in the **first** 24 hours after admission of the client with a thrombotic stroke?
- ☐ **1.** cholesterol level
- ☐ **2.** pupil size and pupillary response
- ☐ **3.** bowel sounds
- ☐ **4.** echocardiogram

47. A client with a hemorrhagic stroke is slightly agitated, heart rate is 118 bpm, respirations are 22 breaths/min, bilateral rhonchi are auscultated, SpO_2 is 94%, blood pressure is 144/88 mm Hg, and oral secretions are noted. What order of interventions from first to last should the nurse follow when suctioning the client to prevent increased intracranial pressure (ICP) and maintain adequate cerebral perfusion? All options must be used.

1. Suction the airway.

2. Hyperoxygenate.

3. Suction the mouth.

4. Provide sedation.

48. In planning care for the client who has had a stroke, the nurse should obtain a history of the client's functional status before the stroke because:
- ☐ **1.** the rehabilitation plan will be guided by it.
- ☐ **2.** functional status before the stroke will help predict outcomes.
- ☐ **3.** it will help the client recognize physical limitations.
- ☐ **4.** the client can be expected to regain most functional status.

49. Which positioning technique is **not** appropriate when the nurse changes a client's position in bed if the client has hemiparalysis?
- ☐ **1.** rolling the client onto the side
- ☐ **2.** sliding the client to move up in bed
- ☐ **3.** lifting the client when moving the client up in bed
- ☐ **4.** having the client help lift off the bed using a trapeze

50. The nurse is caring for a client who is paraplegic as the result of a stroke. At home, the client uses a wheelchair for mobility and can transfer independently. The client is now being treated with IV antibiotics for a sacral wound via a peripherally inserted central catheter. The client is alert and oriented and has no previous history of falling. Using the Morse Fall Scale (see exhibit), what is this client's total score?

Morse Fall Risk/Scale

Item	Scale		Scoring
1. History of falling; immediate or within 3 months	No	0	
	Yes	25	
2. Secondary diagnosis	No	0	
	Yes	15	
3. Ambulatory aid			
Bed rest/nurse assist		0	
Crutches/cane/walker		15	
Furniture		30	
4. IV/Heparin Lock	No	0	
	Yes	20	
5. Gait/Transferring			
Normal/bedrest/immobile		0	
Weak		10	
Impaired		20	
6. Mental status			
Oriented to own ability		0	
Forgets limitations		15	

_____ fall risk score.

51. Which is the **most** effective means of preventing plantar flexion in a client who has had a stroke with residual paralysis?
- ☐ **1.** Place the client's feet against a firm footboard.
- ☐ **2.** Reposition the client every 2 hours.
- ☐ **3.** Have the client wear ankle-high tennis shoes at intervals throughout the day.
- ☐ **4.** Massage the client's feet and ankles regularly.

52. The nurse is planning the care of a hemiplegic client to prevent joint deformities of the arm and hand. Which position is appropriate? Select all that apply.
- ☐ **1.** placing a pillow in the axilla so the arm is away from the body
- ☐ **2.** inserting a pillow under the slightly flexed arm so the hand is higher than the elbow
- ☐ **3.** immobilizing the extremity in a sling
- ☐ **4.** positioning a hand cone in the hand so the fingers are barely flexed
- ☐ **5.** keeping the arm at the side using a pillow

53. For the client who is experiencing expressive aphasia, which nursing intervention is **most** helpful in promoting communication?
- ☐ 1. speaking loudly and slowly
- ☐ 2. using a "picture board" for the client to point to pictures
- ☐ 3. writing directions so the client can read them
- ☐ 4. speaking in short sentences

54. The nurse is teaching the family of a client with dysphagia about decreasing the risk of aspiration while eating. Which strategies should the nurse include in the teaching plan? Select all that apply.
- ☐ 1. maintaining an upright position while eating
- ☐ 2. restricting the diet to liquids until swallowing improves
- ☐ 3. introducing foods on the unaffected side of the mouth
- ☐ 4. keeping distractions to a minimum
- ☐ 5. cutting food into large pieces of finger food

55. The nurse is assisting a client with a stroke who has homonymous hemianopia. The nurse should understand that the client will:
- ☐ 1. have a preference for foods high in salt.
- ☐ 2. eat food on only half of the plate.
- ☐ 3. forget the names of foods.
- ☐ 4. not be able to swallow liquids.

56. A nurse is teaching a client who had a stroke about ways to adapt to a visual disability. Which does the nurse identify as the **primary** safety precaution to use?
- ☐ 1. Wear a patch over one eye.
- ☐ 2. Place personal items on the sighted side.
- ☐ 3. Lie in bed with the unaffected side toward the door.
- ☐ 4. Turn the head from side to side when walking.

57. A client is experiencing mood swings after a stroke and often has episodes of tearfulness that are distressing to the family. Which is the **best** technique for the nurse to instruct family members to try when the client experiences a crying episode?
- ☐ 1. Sit quietly with the client until the episode is over.
- ☐ 2. Ignore the behavior.
- ☐ 3. Attempt to divert the client's attention.
- ☐ 4. Tell the client that this behavior is unacceptable.

58. When communicating with a client who has aphasia, which approaches are helpful? Select all that apply.
- ☐ 1. Present one thought at a time.
- ☐ 2. Avoid writing messages.
- ☐ 3. Speak with normal volume.
- ☐ 4. Make use of gestures.
- ☐ 5. Encourage pointing to the needed object.

59. What is the expected outcome of thrombolytic drug therapy for stroke?
- ☐ 1. increased vascular permeability
- ☐ 2. vasoconstriction
- ☐ 3. dissolved emboli
- ☐ 4. prevention of hemorrhage

The Client with Parkinson's Disease

60. Which nursing approach is **most** helpful to a client with Parkinson's disease who is experiencing a freezing of gait with difficulty initiating movement?
- ☐ 1. Pull the client forward to initiate walking.
- ☐ 2. Instruct the client to use a wheelchair.
- ☐ 3. Have the client remain still.
- ☐ 4. Tell the client to march in place.

61. A healthcare provider (HCP) has prescribed carbidopa-levodopa four times per day for a client with Parkinson's disease. The client wants "to end it all now that the Parkinson's disease has progressed." What should the nurse do? Select all that apply.
- ☐ 1. Explain that the new prescription for carbidopa-levodopa will treat the depression.
- ☐ 2. Encourage the client to discuss feelings as the carbidopa-levodopa is being administered.
- ☐ 3. Contact the HCP before administering the carbidopa-levodopa.
- ☐ 4. Determine if the client is on antidepressants or monoamine oxidase (MAO) inhibitors.
- ☐ 5. Determine if the client is at risk for suicide.

62. Which is an initial sign of Parkinson's disease?
- ☐ 1. rigidity
- ☐ 2. tremor
- ☐ 3. bradykinesia
- ☐ 4. akinesia

63. The nurse develops a teaching plan for a client newly diagnosed with Parkinson's disease. Which topic is **most** important to include in the plan?
- ☐ 1. maintaining a balanced nutritional diet
- ☐ 2. enhancing the immune system
- ☐ 3. maintaining a safe environment
- ☐ 4. engaging in diversional activity

64. The nurse observes that a when a client with Parkinson's disease unbuttons the shirt, the upper arm tremors disappear. Which statement **best** guides the nurse's analysis of this observation about the client's tremors?
- ☐ 1. The tremors are probably psychological and can be controlled at will.
- ☐ 2. The tremors sometimes disappear with purposeful and voluntary movements.
- ☐ 3. The tremors disappear when the client's attention is diverted by some activity.
- ☐ 4. There is no explanation for the observation; it is a chance occurrence.

65. At what time of day should the nurse encourage a client with Parkinson's disease to schedule the most demanding physical activities to minimize the effects of hypokinesia?
- ☐ **1.** early in the morning, when the client's energy level is high
- ☐ **2.** to coincide with the peak action of drug therapy
- ☐ **3.** immediately after a rest period
- ☐ **4.** when family members will be available

66. Which goal is the **most** realistic for a client diagnosed with Parkinson's disease?
- ☐ **1.** to cure the disease
- ☐ **2.** to stop progression of the disease
- ☐ **3.** to begin preparations for terminal care
- ☐ **4.** to maintain optimal body function

67. Which of the goals is collaboratively established by the client with Parkinson's disease, nurse, and physical therapist?
- ☐ **1.** to maintain joint flexibility
- ☐ **2.** to build muscle strength
- ☐ **3.** to improve muscle endurance
- ☐ **4.** to reduce ataxia

68. A client with Parkinson's disease is prescribed levodopa (L-dopa) therapy. Improvement in which area indicates effective therapy?
- ☐ **1.** mood
- ☐ **2.** muscle rigidity
- ☐ **3.** appetite
- ☐ **4.** alertness

69. A client is being switched from levodopa (L-dopa) to carbidopa-levodopa. The nurse should monitor for which possible complication during medication changes and dosage adjustment?
- ☐ **1.** euphoria
- ☐ **2.** jaundice
- ☐ **3.** vital sign fluctuation
- ☐ **4.** signs and symptoms of diabetes

70. A client with Parkinson's disease needs a long time to complete morning care but becomes annoyed when the nurse offers assistance and refuses all help. Which action is the nurse's **best** initial response in this situation?
- ☐ **1.** Tell the client firmly that he or she needs assistance and help with the morning care.
- ☐ **2.** Praise the client for the desire to be independent and give extra time and encouragement.
- ☐ **3.** Tell the client that he or she is being unrealistic about the abilities and must accept the fact that he or she needs help.
- ☐ **4.** Suggest to the client to at least modify the morning care routine if he or she insists on self-care.

71. Which is an expected outcome for a client with Parkinson's disease who has had a pallidotomy?
- ☐ **1.** improved functional ability
- ☐ **2.** reduced emotional stress
- ☐ **3.** increased alertness
- ☐ **4.** better appetite

The Client with Multiple Sclerosis

72. When assessing the client with multiple sclerosis for potential complications of the disease, the nurse should asses the client for which of the following? Select all that apply.
- ☐ **1.** dehydration
- ☐ **2.** falls
- ☐ **3.** seizures
- ☐ **4.** skin breakdown
- ☐ **5.** fatigue

73. The nurse is teaching a client with bladder dysfunction from multiple sclerosis (MS) about bladder training at home. Which instructions should the nurse include in the teaching plan? Select all that apply.
- ☐ **1.** Restrict fluids to 1,000 mL/24 hours.
- ☐ **2.** Drink 400 to 500 mL with each meal.
- ☐ **3.** Drink fluids midmorning, midafternoon, and late afternoon.
- ☐ **4.** Attempt to void at least every 2 hours.
- ☐ **5.** Use intermittent catheterization as needed.

74. Which is **not** a typical clinical manifestation of multiple sclerosis (MS)?
- ☐ **1.** double vision
- ☐ **2.** sudden bursts of energy
- ☐ **3.** weakness in the extremities
- ☐ **4.** muscle tremors

75. A client with multiple sclerosis (MS) is receiving baclofen. The nurse determines that the drug is effective when it:
- ☐ **1.** induces sleep.
- ☐ **2.** stimulates the client's appetite.
- ☐ **3.** relieves muscular spasticity.
- ☐ **4.** reduces the urine bacterial count.

76. A client has had multiple sclerosis (MS) for 15 years and has received various drug therapies. What is the **primary** reason why the nurse has found it difficult to evaluate the effectiveness of the drugs that the client has used?
- ☐ **1.** The client exhibits intolerance to many drugs.
- ☐ **2.** The client experiences spontaneous remissions from time to time.
- ☐ **3.** The client requires multiple drugs simultaneously.
- ☐ **4.** The client endures long periods of exacerbation before the illness responds to a particular drug.

77. When the nurse talks with a client with multiple sclerosis who has slurred speech, which nursing intervention is **contraindicated**?
☐ 1. encouraging the client to speak slowly
☐ 2. encouraging the client to speak distinctly
☐ 3. asking the client to repeat indistinguishable words
☐ 4. asking the client to speak louder when tired

78. The right hand of a client with multiple sclerosis trembles severely whenever she attempts a voluntary action. She spills her coffee twice at lunch and cannot get her dress fastened securely. Which is the **best** legal documentation in nurses' notes of the medical record for this client assessment?
☐ 1. "Has an intention tremor of the right hand."
☐ 2. "Right-hand tremor worsens with purposeful acts."
☐ 3. "Needs assistance with dressing and eating due to severe trembling and clumsiness."
☐ 4. "Slight shaking of right hand increases to severe tremor when client tries to button her clothes or drink from a cup."

79. A client with multiple sclerosis (MS) is experiencing bowel incontinence and is starting a bowel retraining program. Which strategy is **not** appropriate?
☐ 1. eating a diet high in fiber
☐ 2. setting a regular time for elimination
☐ 3. using an elevated toilet seat
☐ 4. limiting fluid intake to 1,000 mL/day

80. Which outcome is **not** realistic to establish with a client who has multiple sclerosis (MS)? The client will develop:
☐ 1. increased joint mobility.
☐ 2. improved muscle strength.
☐ 3. clearer thinking.
☐ 4. mood elevation.

81. The nurse is preparing a client with multiple sclerosis (MS) for discharge from the hospital to home. The nurse should tell the client:
☐ 1. "You will need to accept the necessity for a quiet and inactive lifestyle."
☐ 2. "Keep active, use stress reduction strategies, and avoid fatigue."
☐ 3. "Follow good health habits to change the course of the disease."
☐ 4. "Practice using the mechanical aids that you will need when future disabilities arise."

82. Which information should the nurse include in the discharge plan for a client with multiple sclerosis who has an impaired peripheral sensation? Select all that apply.
☐ 1. Carefully test the temperature of bath water.
☐ 2. Avoid kitchen activities because of the risk of injury.
☐ 3. Avoid hot water bottles and heating pads.
☐ 4. Inspect the skin daily for injury or pressure points.
☐ 5. Wear warm clothing when outside in cold temperatures.

83. Which intervention should the nurse suggest to help a client with multiple sclerosis avoid episodes of urinary incontinence?
☐ 1. Limit fluid intake to 1,000 mL/day.
☐ 2. Insert an indwelling urinary catheter.
☐ 3. Establish a regular voiding schedule.
☐ 4. Administer prophylactic antibiotics, as prescribed.

84. A client with multiple sclerosis (MS) lives with her daughter and 3-year-old granddaughter. The daughter asks the nurse what she can do at home to help her mother. Which measure would be **most** beneficial?
☐ 1. psychotherapy
☐ 2. regular exercise
☐ 3. day care for the granddaughter
☐ 4. weekly visits by another person with MS

The Client with Myasthenia Gravis

85. When planning care for a client with myasthenia gravis, the nurse understands that the client is at highest risk for:
☐ 1. aspiration.
☐ 2. bladder dysfunction.
☐ 3. hypertension.
☐ 4. sensory loss.

86. The nurse is discussing discharge instructions with a client with myasthenia gravis who is taking pyridostigmine. The nurse should tell the client to:
☐ 1. administer artificial tears.
☐ 2. avoid contact with crowds.
☐ 3. take pyridostigmine in the afternoon.
☐ 4. decrease protein in the diet.

87. After teaching a client about myasthenia gravis, the nurse would judge that the client has formed a realistic concept of her health problem when she says that by taking her medication and pacing her activities:
☐ 1. she will live longer, but ultimately the disease will cause her death.
☐ 2. her symptoms will be controlled, and eventually the disease will be cured.
☐ 3. she should be able to control the disease and enjoy a healthy lifestyle.
☐ 4. her fatigue will be relieved, but she should expect occasional periods of muscle weakness.

The Unconscious Client

88. A client is brought to the emergency department unconscious. An empty bottle of aspirin was found in the car, and a drug overdose is suspected. Which medication should the nurse have available for further emergency treatment?
- [ ] 1. vitamin K
- [ ] 2. dextrose 50%
- [ ] 3. activated charcoal powder
- [ ] 4. sodium thiosulfate

89. Which clinical manifestations should the nurse expect to assess in a client diagnosed with an overdose of a cholinergic agent? Select all that apply.
- [ ] 1. dry mucous membranes
- [ ] 2. urinary incontinence
- [ ] 3. central nervous system (CNS) depression
- [ ] 4. seizures
- [ ] 5. skin rash

90. The nurse is caring for a client who is unconscious following an attempted suicide by drug overdose. When speaking with the client's distraught wife, what should the nurse do **first**?
- [ ] 1. Explain that because the client was found on hospital property, he was probably asking for help and did not intentionally overdose.
- [ ] 2. Ask the wife if she would like to speak to a member of the clergy.
- [ ] 3. Encourage the wife to express her feelings and concerns, and listen carefully.
- [ ] 4. Allow the wife to help care for the client by rubbing his back when he is turned.

91. Which nursing action is a **priority** during the **first** 24 hours of hospitalization for a comatose client with suspected drug overdose?
- [ ] 1. Educate regarding drug abuse.
- [ ] 2. Minimize pain.
- [ ] 3. Maintain intact skin.
- [ ] 4. Increase caloric intake.

92. The nurse is caring for an unconscious intubated client with normal intracranial pressure. The nurse should:
- [ ] 1. monitor the oral temperature, keep the room temperature at 70° F (21.1° C), and place the client on a cooling blanket if the client's temperature is higher than 101° F (38.3° C).
- [ ] 2. clean the mouth carefully, apply a thin coat of a water-based lubricant, and move the endotracheal tube to the opposite side daily.
- [ ] 3. position the client in the supine position with the head to the side and slightly elevated on two pillows.
- [ ] 4. turn the client with a drawsheet, and place a pillow behind the back and one between the legs.

93. The unconscious client is to be placed in a right side-lying position. The nurse should intervene when observing a client in which position?
- [ ] 1. The head is placed on a small pillow.
- [ ] 2. The right leg is extended without pillow support.
- [ ] 3. The left arm is rested on the mattress with the elbow flexed.
- [ ] 4. The left leg is supported on a pillow with the knee flexed.

94. Which indicates that performing passive range-of-motion (ROM) exercises on an unconscious client has been successful?
- [ ] 1. preservation of muscle mass
- [ ] 2. prevention of bone demineralization
- [ ] 3. increase in muscle tone
- [ ] 4. maintenance of joint mobility

95. When the nurse performs oral hygiene for an unconscious client, which nursing intervention is the **priority**?
- [ ] 1. Keep a suction machine available.
- [ ] 2. Place the client in a prone position.
- [ ] 3. Wear sterile gloves while brushing the client's teeth.
- [ ] 4. Use gauze wrapped around the fingers to clean the client's gums.

96. The nurse observes that the right eye of an unconscious client does not close completely. Which nursing intervention is **most** appropriate?
- [ ] 1. Have the client wear eyeglasses at all times.
- [ ] 2. Lightly tape the eyelid shut.
- [ ] 3. Instill artificial tears once every shift.
- [ ] 4. Clean the eyelid with a washcloth every shift.

97. Which sign is an early indicator of hypoxia in the unconscious client?
- [ ] 1. cyanosis
- [ ] 2. decreased respirations
- [ ] 3. restlessness
- [ ] 4. hypotension

98. When administering intermittent enteral feeding to an unconscious client, the nurse should:
- [ ] 1. heat the formula in a microwave.
- [ ] 2. place the client in a semi-Fowler's position.
- [ ] 3. obtain a sterile gavage bag and tubing.
- [ ] 4. weigh the client before administering the feeding.

99. The unconscious client is to receive 200 mL of tube feeding every 4 hours. The nurse checks for the client's gastric residual before administering the next scheduled feeding and obtains 40 mL of gastric residual. The nurse should:
- [ ] 1. withhold the tube feeding and notify the healthcare provider (HCP).
- [ ] 2. dispose of the residual and continue with the feeding.
- [ ] 3. delay feeding the client for 1 hour and then recheck the residual.
- [ ] 4. readminister the residual to the client and continue with the feeding.

The Client in Pain

100. The healthcare provider (HCP) prescribes morphine sulfate 2 to 4 mg IV push every 2 hours PRN pain for a client who has postoperative pain following abdominal surgery. Prior to performing an abdominal dressing change with packing at 1000, the nurse assesses the client's pain level as 1 on a scale of 0 = no pain to 10 = the worst pain. The client is awake and oriented, and vital signs are within normal limits. The nurse reviews the pain medication record (see chart). What should the nurse do?

Medication Record

Time	Pain Level	Intervention
0700	8	Morphine 4 mg IV
0900	4	Morphine 2 mg IV
1000	1	

- [ ] 1. Perform the dressing change.
- [ ] 2. Administer morphine 2 mg IV before the dressing change.
- [ ] 3. Administer morphine 4 mg IV after the dressing change.
- [ ] 4. Call the HCP for a new medication prescription.

101. The nurse finds it difficult to relieve a client's pain satisfactorily. Which measure should the nurse take **next** when continuing efforts to promote comfort?
- [ ] 1. Increase the client's confidence in the nurse.
- [ ] 2. Enlist the help of the client's family.
- [ ] 3. Allow the client additional time to work through his or her own responses to pain.
- [ ] 4. Arrange to have the client share a room with a client who has little pain.

102. The client's healthcare provider (HCP) changes the analgesia medication from meperidine hydrochloride 75 mg IM every 4 hours as needed to meperidine hydrochloride by the oral route. What dosage of oral meperidine is required to provide an equivalent analgesic dose?
- [ ] 1. 25 to 50 mg
- [ ] 2. 75 to 100 mg
- [ ] 3. 125 to 150 mg
- [ ] 4. 250 to 300 mg

103. After administering meperidine hydrochloride, the nurse determines its effectiveness as an analgesic was related to its ability to:
- [ ] 1. reduce the perception of pain.
- [ ] 2. decrease the sensitivity of pain receptors.
- [ ] 3. interfere with pain impulses traveling along sensory nerve fibers.
- [ ] 4. block the conduction of pain impulses along the central nervous system.

104. A client is arousing from a coma and keeps saying, "Just stop the pain." The nurse responds based on the knowledge that the client's **first** response to pain will be to:
- [ ] 1. tolerate the pain.
- [ ] 2. decrease the perception of pain.
- [ ] 3. escape the source of pain.
- [ ] 4. divert attention from the source of pain.

105. Ergotamine tartrate is prescribed for a client's migraine headaches. Which is an expected outcome of the use of this drug?
- [ ] 1. prevention of the migraine
- [ ] 2. aborting of the developing migraine
- [ ] 3. relief from the sleeplessness experienced in the past after a migraine
- [ ] 4. relief from the vision problems experienced in the past after a migraine

106. The purpose of biofeedback is to enable a client to exert control over physiologic processes by:
- [ ] 1. regulating the body processes through electrical control.
- [ ] 2. shocking the client when an undesirable response is elicited.
- [ ] 3. monitoring the body processes for the therapist to interpret.
- [ ] 4. translating the signals of body processes into observable forms.

107. The nurse explains to the client that the **main** reason a back rub is used as therapy to relieve pain is because the massage:
- [ ] 1. blocks pain impulses from the spinal cord to the brain.
- [ ] 2. blocks pain impulses from the brain to the spinal cord.
- [ ] 3. stimulates the release of endorphins.
- [ ] 4. distracts the client's focus on the source of the pain.

108. Nursing responsibilities for the client with a patient-controlled analgesia (PCA) system include:
- [ ] 1. reassuring the client that pain will be relieved.
- [ ] 2. documenting the client's response to pain medication.
- [ ] 3. instructing the client to continue pressing the system's button whenever pain occurs.
- [ ] 4. titrating the client's pain medication until the client is free from pain.

109. A client has a patient-controlled analgesia (PCA) infusion to manage postoperative pain. In spite of receiving a dose of pain medication, the client rates the pain at 8 on a 0 to 10 pain scale. What should the nurse do **first**?
- [ ] 1. Check the patient-controlled analgesia (PCA) pump function.
- [ ] 2. Inspect the infusion site.
- [ ] 3. Assess vital signs.
- [ ] 4. Notify the healthcare provider (HCP).

110. The nurse using healing touch affects a client's pain **primarily** through:
- ☐ 1. directing the flow of energy fields.
- ☐ 2. lightly touching the client skin.
- ☐ 3. massaging the client's muscles.
- ☐ 4. increasing endorphin production.

111. When a nurse is assessing a client for pain, what finding is **most** significant? The client:
- ☐ 1. protects a specific area of the body.
- ☐ 2. tells the nurse about experiencing pain.
- ☐ 3. has a change in vital signs.
- ☐ 4. appears to be uncomfortable.

112. A client who is 89 years of age is in traction for a broken hip. At 1100 on 3/26, the client is experiencing pain. Prescriptions include morphine sulfate 2 to 4 mg intravenous push every 2 to 4 hours for pain. The client rates the pain as an 8 on the visual analog scale (0 to 10). Prior to intervening to manage the pain, the nurse reviews the progress notes (see exhibit).

Nurse Progress Notes

Date	Time	Progress Notes
3/26	0900	Client is alert and oriented. Vital signs: pulse 80, respirations 14, BP 100/80, and oxygen saturation by pulse oximeter 92%. Received Morphine Sulfate 2 mg by intravenous push (IVP). Fred Lewis, RN
3/26	1000	Client has pain of 4 on the Visual Analog Scale (0-10). Respirations are 10. Fred Lewis, RN

At 1100 on 3/26, the nurse should:
- ☐ 1. reposition the client for comfort and administer pain medication in another 2 hours.
- ☐ 2. administer 2 mg morphine sulfate IVP now and reassess in 10 to 15 minutes.
- ☐ 3. call the healthcare provider (HCP) for supplemental medication to relax the client and promote sedation.
- ☐ 4. administer 2 mg morphine sulfate IVP in 2 hours if the respirations are above 12 breaths per minute.

Managing Care, Quality, and Safety of Clients with Neurologic Health Problems

113. When caring for a client with Guillain-Barre syndrome, the nurse can delegate which activity to the unlicensed assistive personnel (UAP)?
- ☐ 1. Assess weakness with range-of-motion exercises.
- ☐ 2. Reposition client every 2 hours.
- ☐ 3. Suction the endotracheal tube.
- ☐ 4. Show the client how to do deep-breathing exercises.

114. An unlicensed assistive personnel (UAP) is providing care to a client with left-sided paralysis. Which action by the UAP requires the nurse to provide further instruction?
- ☐ 1. providing passive range-of-motion exercises to the left extremities during the bed bath
- ☐ 2. elevating the foot of the bed to reduce edema
- ☐ 3. pulling up the client under the left shoulder when getting the client out of bed to a chair
- ☐ 4. putting high top tennis shoes on the client after bathing

115. The nurse notices that a client with Parkinson's disease is coughing frequently when eating. Which intervention should the nurse consider?
- ☐ 1. Have the client hyperextend the neck when swallowing.
- ☐ 2. Tell the client to place the chin firmly against the chest when eating.
- ☐ 3. Thicken all liquids before offering to the client.
- ☐ 4. Place the client on a clear liquid diet.

116. After receiving a change-of-shift report at 0700, the nurse should assess which client **first**?
- ☐ 1. a 23-year-old with a migraine headache who has severe nausea associated with retching
- ☐ 2. a 45-year-old who is scheduled for a craniotomy in 30 minutes and needs preoperative teaching
- ☐ 3. a 59-year-old with Parkinson's disease who will need a swallowing assessment before breakfast
- ☐ 4. a 63-year-old with multiple sclerosis who has an oral temperature of 101.8° F (38.8° C) and flank pain.

117. The nurse has asked the unlicensed assistive personnel (UAP) to ambulate a client with Parkinson's disease. The nurse observes the UAP pulling on the client's arms to get the client to walk forward. The nurse should:
- ☐ 1. have the UAP keep a steady pull on the client to promote forward ambulation.
- ☐ 2. explain how to overcome a freezing gait by telling the client to march in place.
- ☐ 3. assist the UAP with getting the client back in bed.
- ☐ 4. give the client a muscle relaxant.

118. Which pressure point areas should the nurse monitor for an unconscious client positioned on the left side? (See figure.) Select all that apply.

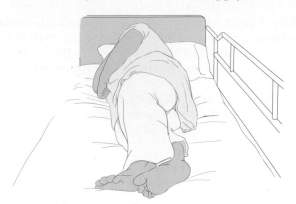

☐ **1.** ankles
☐ **2.** ear
☐ **3.** greater trochanter
☐ **4.** heels
☐ **5.** occiput
☐ **6.** sacrum
☐ **7.** shoulder

119. The nurse ascertains that there is a discrepancy in the records of use of a controlled substance for a client who is taking large doses of narcotic pain medication. What should the nurse do **next**?
☐ **1.** Notify the police.
☐ **2.** Contact the hospital's administration or legal department.
☐ **3.** Notify the pharmacy technician who delivered the controlled substance.
☐ **4.** Notify the nursing supervisor of the clinical unit.

120. The nurse is caring for a client who is confused about time and place. The client has intravenous fluid infusing. The nurse attempts to reorient the client, but the client remains unable to demonstrate appropriate use of the call light. In order to maintain client safety, what should the nurse do **first**?
☐ **1.** Ask the family to stay with the client.
☐ **2.** Contact the healthcare provider (HCP), and request a prescription for soft wrist restraints.
☐ **3.** Increase the frequency of client observation.
☐ **4.** Administer a sedative.

121. The nurse finds a confused client with soft wrist restraints in place (see figure). The nurse should **first**:

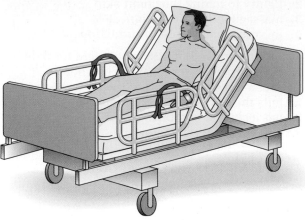

☐ **1.** assess and document the condition of the client's skin beneath the restraint.
☐ **2.** untie the restraint and resecure to the bed frame using a quick-release knot.
☐ **3.** release the restraint and perform passive range of motion.
☐ **4.** ask if the client needs to use the restroom.

Answers, Rationales, and Test-Taking Strategies

*The answers and rationales for each question follow below, along with keys (⚷) to the client need (CN) and cognitive level (CL) for each question. In addition, you will also see a glossary icon (📖) highlighting specific terminology used on the licensing exam. As you check your answers, use the **Content Mastery and Test-Taking Skill Self-Analysis** worksheet (tear-out worksheet in back of book) to identify the reason(s) for not answering the questions correctly. For additional information about test-taking skills and strategies for answering questions, refer to pages 12–23 and pages 35–36 in Part 1 of this book.*

The Client with a Head Injury

1. **2,3,4.** The nurse should maintain ICP by elevating the head of the bed 15 to 20 degrees and monitoring neurologic status. An ICP >15 mm Hg with 20 to 25 mm Hg as upper limits of normal indicates increased ICP, and the nurse should notify the **HCP** 📖. Coughing and range-of-motion exercises will increase ICP and should be avoided in the early postoperative stage.

⚷ CN: Physiological adaptation;
CL: Synthesize

2. 1,4. The nurse must monitor the systolic and diastolic blood pressure to obtain the mean arterial pressure (MAP), which represents the pressure needed for each cardiac cycle to perfuse the brain. The nurse must also monitor the cerebral perfusion pressure (CPP), which is obtained from the ICP and the MAP. The nurse should also monitor urine output, respirations, and pain; however, crucial measurements needed to maintain CPP are ICP and MAP. When ICP equals MAP, there is no CPP.

🔑 CN: Management of care; CL: Analyze

3. 80 mm Hg
To obtain the MAP, use this formula:

$$MAP = [systolic\ BP + (2 \times diastolic\ BP)] \div 3$$
$$MAP = [120 + (2 \times 60)] \div 3$$
$$MAP = 240 \div 3 = 80.$$

🔑 CN: Management of care; CL: Apply

4. 2,3. The nurse should determine if the client's pupils are equal and react to light, and ask the client if he has a headache. Confusion, agitation, and restlessness are subtle clinical manifestations of increased intracranial pressure (ICP). At this time, it is not appropriate for the nurse to find a television or arrange for the client to see his wife and baby. Administering a sedative at this time will obscure assessment of increased ICP.

🔑 CN: Management of care; CL: Synthesize

5. 3. The client has a score of 6 (eye opening to pain = 2; verbal response, incomprehensible sounds = 2; best motor response, abnormal extension = 2); a score <7 is indicative of coma. While the nurse should continue to speak to the client, at this time the client will not be able to be aroused. The nurse should continue to provide skin care and appropriate alignment, but the client will continue to have a motor response of limb extension. It is not necessary to notify the **HCP** 📖 as this assessment does not represent a significant change in neurological status.

🔑 CN: Physiological adaptation; CL: Analyze

6. 1. The highest priority for a client with multiple head and neck injuries is to establish an open airway for effective ventilation and oxygenation. Unless the client has a patent airway, other care measures will be futile. Determining the client's identity, blood loss, stopping bleeding from open wounds, and checking for a neck fracture are important nursing interventions to be completed after the airway and ventilation are established.

🔑 CN: Safety and infection control; CL: Synthesize

7. 4,3,2,1. The first step in providing care for a client with delirium is to approach the client calmly, introduce oneself, and use short sentences when explaining the care given. The nurse should also assure the client's safety by protecting the client from injury. Maintaining a quiet and calm environment by removing extraneous noises will prevent overstimulation. Pharmacologic intervention is used only when other plans for care are not effective. When the underlying problems related to the head injury are resolved, the delirium likely will improve.

🔑 CN: Physiological adaptation; CL: Synthesize

8. 1. Increasing ICP causes unequal pupils as a result of pressure on the third cranial nerve. Increasing ICP causes an increase in the systolic pressure, which reflects the additional pressure needed to perfuse the brain. It increases the pressure on the vagus nerve, which produces bradycardia, and it causes an increase in body temperature from hypothalamic damage.

🔑 CN: Reduction of risk potential; CL: Analyze

9. 3. The clear drainage must be analyzed to determine whether it is nasal drainage or cerebrospinal fluid (CSF). The nurse should not give the client tissues because it is important to know how much leakage of CSF is occurring. Compressing the nares will obstruct the drainage flow. It is inappropriate to tilt the head back, which would allow the fluid to drain down the throat and not be collected for a sample. It is inappropriate to administer an antihistamine because the drainage may not be from postnasal drip.

🔑 CN: Reduction of risk potential; CL: Synthesize

10. 1. Neural control of respiration takes place in the brain stem. Deterioration and pressure produce slow and irregular respirations. Rapid and shallow respirations, asymmetric chest movements, and nasal flaring are more characteristic of respiratory distress or hypoxia.

🔑 CN: Physiological adaptation; CL: Apply

11. 3. Normal ICP is 15 mm Hg or less for 15 to 30 seconds or longer. Hyperventilation causes vasoconstriction, which reduces cerebrospinal fluid and blood volume, two important factors for reducing a sustained ICP of 20 mm Hg. A cooling blanket is used to control the elevation of temperature because a fever increases the metabolic rate, which in turn increases ICP. High doses of barbiturates may be used to reduce the increased cellular metabolic demands. Fluid volume and inotropic drugs are used to maintain cerebral perfusion by supporting the cardiac output and keeping the cerebral perfusion pressure >80 mm Hg.

🔑 CN: Physiological adaptation;
CL: Synthesize

12. 4. A decrease in the client's LOC is an early indicator of deterioration of the client's neurologic status. Changes in LOC, such as restlessness and irritability, may be subtle. Widening of the pulse pressure, decrease in the pulse rate, and dilated, fixed pupils occur later if the increased ICP is not treated.

🔑 CN: Physiological adaptation;
CL: Analyze

13. 1. The client's ICP is elevated, and the client should be positioned to avoid extreme neck flexion or extension. The head of the bed is usually elevated 15 to 20 degrees to drain the venous sinuses and thus decrease the ICP. Trendelenburg's position places the client's head lower than the body, which would increase ICP. Sims' position (side lying) and elevating the head on two pillows may extend or flex the neck, which increases ICP.

🔑 CN: Reduction of risk potential;
CL: Synthesize

14. 2. After administering mannitol, the nurse closely monitors intake and output because mannitol promotes diuresis and is given primarily to pull water from the extracellular fluid of the edematous brain. Mannitol can cause hypokalemia and may lead to muscle contractions, not muscle relaxation. Signs and symptoms, such as widening pulse pressure and pupil dilation, should not occur because mannitol serves to decrease ICP.

🔑 CN: Pharmacological and parenteral therapies; CL: Analyze

15. 4. The correct motor function test for C8 is a hand-grasp check. The motor function check for C4 to C5 is shoulders shrugging against downward pressure of the examiner's hands. The motor function check for C5 to C6 is an arm pulling up from a resting position against resistance. The motor function check for C7 is an arm straightening out from a flexed position against resistance.

🔑 CN: Management of care; CL: Analyze

16. 2. It is best for the client to wear mitts, which help prevent the client from pulling on the IV without causing additional agitation. Using a jacket or wrist restraint or tucking the client's arms and hands under the sheet restricts movement and adds to feelings of being confined, all of which would add to the agitation and increase ICP.

🔑 CN: Physiological adaptation;
CL: Synthesize

17. 3. Coughing is contraindicated for a client at risk for increased ICP because coughing increases ICP. Deep breathing can be continued. Turning and passive ROM exercises can be continued with care not to extend or flex the neck.

🔑 CN: Reduction of risk potential;
CL: Synthesize

18. 3. Recovery from a serious head injury is a long-term process that may continue for months or years. Depending on the extent of the injury, clients who are transferred to rehabilitation facilities most likely will continue to exhibit cognitive and mobility impairments as well as behavior and personality changes. The client would be expected to participate in the rehabilitation efforts to the extent he is capable. Family members and significant others will need long-term support to help them cope with the changes that have occurred in the client.

🔑 CN: Physiological adaptation; CL: Evaluate

19. 4. Decerebrate posturing occurs in clients with damage to the upper brain stem, midbrain, or pons and is demonstrated clinically by arching of the back, rigid extension of the extremities, pronation of the arms, and plantar flexion of the feet. Internal rotation and adduction of arms with flexion of elbows, wrists, and fingers describes decorticate posturing, which indicates damage to corticospinal tracts and cerebral hemispheres.

🔑 CN: Physiological adaptation; CL: Apply

20. 2. Cluster breathing consists of clusters of irregular breaths followed by periods of apnea on an irregular basis. A lesion in the upper medulla or lower pons is usually the cause of cluster breathing. Because the client had a bleed in the occipital lobe, which is just superior and posterior to the pons and medulla, clinical manifestations that indicate a new lesion are monitored very closely in case another bleed ensues. The nurse should notify the HCP 📖 immediately so that treatment can begin before respirations cease. The client is not obtaining sufficient oxygen, and the depth of breathing is assisted by the ventilator. The HCP will determine changes in the ventilator settings.

🔑 CN: Physiological adaptation;
CL: Synthesize

21. 2. Elevating the head of the bed to 30 degrees is contraindicated for infratentorial craniotomies because it could cause herniation of the brain down onto the brain stem and spinal cord, resulting in sudden death. Elevation of the head of the bed to 30 degrees with the head turned to the side opposite the incision, if not contraindicated by the increased intracranial pressure, is used for supratentorial craniotomies.

🔑 CN: Physiological adaptation;
CL: Synthesize

22. 3,4. The nurse should immediately report changes that indicate increasing intracranial pressure (ICP): bradycardia, increasing systolic pressure, and widening pulse pressure. As ICP increases and the brain becomes more compressed, respirations become rapid, BP decreases, and the pulse slows further; these are very ominous signs. Decreased arterial BP and tachycardia can indicate bleeding elsewhere in the body. Decreasing urinary output indicates decreased tissue perfusion. The nurse monitors changes and notifies the **HCP** 📖 if trends continue.

🔑 CN: Physiological adaptation; CL: Synthesize

23. 4. It is important to first explain where a client is to orient him or her to time, person, and place. Offering to get the family and asking questions to determine orientation are important, but the first comments should let the client know where he or she is and what has happened. It is useful to be empathetic to the client, but making a comment such as "I will bet you are a little confused" is not helpful and may cause anxiety.

🔑 CN: Psychosocial adaptation; CL: Synthesize

The Client with Seizures

24. 3,1,4,2. To protect the client from falling, the nurse first should ease the client to the floor. It is important to protect the head and maintain a patent airway since altered breathing and excessive salivation can occur. The assessment of the postictal period should include level of consciousness and vital signs. The nurse should record details of the seizure once the client is stable. The events preceding the seizure, timing with descriptions of each phase, body parts affected and sequence of involvement, and autonomic signs should be recorded.

🔑 CN: Safety and infection control; CL: Synthesize

25. 4. A generalized tonic-clonic seizure involves both a tonic phase and a clonic phase. The tonic phase consists of loss of consciousness, dilated pupils, and muscular stiffening or contraction, which lasts about 20 to 30 seconds. The clonic phase involves repetitive movements. The seizure ends with confusion, drowsiness, and resumption of respiration. A partial seizure starts in one region of the cortex and may stay focused or spread (e.g., jerking in the extremity spreading to other areas of the body). An absence seizure usually occurs in children and involves a vacant stare with a brief loss of consciousness that often goes unnoticed. A complex partial seizure involves facial grimacing with patting and smacking.

🔑 CN: Physiological adaptation; CL: Analyze

26. 4. The client will be asked to hold the head very still during the examination, which lasts about 30 to 60 minutes. In some instances, food and fluids may be withheld for 4 to 6 hours before the procedure if a contrast medium is used because the radiopaque substance sometimes causes nausea. There is no special preparation for a CT scan, so a shampoo the night before is not required. The client may drink fluids until 4 hours before the scan is scheduled. Electrodes are not used for a CT scan, nor is the head shaved.

🔑 CN: Physiological adaptation; CL: Synthesize

27. 3. Beverages containing caffeine, such as coffee, tea, cola, and energy drinks, are withheld before an EEG because of the stimulating effects of the caffeine on the brain waves. A meal should not be omitted before an EEG because low blood sugar could alter brain wave patterns; the client can have the entire meal except for the coffee. The client does not need to be on a liquid diet or NPO.

🔑 CN: Physiological adaptation; CL: Synthesize

28. 3. In order for phenytoin to be properly absorbed and provide maximum benefit to the client, nutritional supplements must be stopped before and after delivery. The head of the bed is elevated 30 degrees since this client has a tube feeding infusing; it is not necessary to elevate the bed any further. Blood levels are usually drawn before giving a dose of phenytoin, not after. It is not necessary to flush with such a large amount of water (150 mL) before and after administering phenytoin.

🔑 CN: Pharmacological and parenteral therapies; CL: Synthesize

29. 2. Gabapentin may impair vision. Changes in vision, concentration, or coordination should be reported to the **HCP** 📖. Gabapentin should not be stopped abruptly because of the potential for status epilepticus; this is a medication that must be tapered off. Gabapentin is to be stored at room temperature and out of direct light. It should not be taken with antacids.

🔑 CN: Pharmacological and parenteral therapies; CL: Synthesize

30. 3. A priority for the client in the postictal phase (after a seizure) is to assess the client's breathing pattern for effective rate, rhythm, and depth. The nurse should apply oxygen and ventilation to the client as appropriate. Other interventions, to be completed after the airway has been established, include reorientation of the client to time, person, and place. Determining the client's level of sleepiness is useful, but it is not a priority.

Positioning the client comfortably promotes rest but is of less importance than ascertaining that the airway is patent.

🔑 CN: Reduction of risk potential; CL: Synthesize

31. 4. Carbamazepine is an anticonvulsant that helps prevent further seizures and is the most effective intervention for preventing seizure risk while the client is undergoing diagnostic tests for seizures. Bed rest, sedation (phenobarbital), and providing privacy do not minimize the risk of seizures.

🔑 CN: Pharmacological and parenteral therapies; CL: Synthesize

32. 4. During a seizure, the nurse should note movement of the client's head and eyes and muscle rigidity, especially when the seizure first begins, to obtain clues about the location of the trigger focus in the brain. Other important assessments would include noting the progression and duration of the seizure, respiratory status, loss of consciousness, pupil size, and incontinence of urine and stool. It is typically not possible to assess the client's pulse and blood pressure during a tonic-clonic seizure because the muscle contractions make assessment difficult to impossible. The last dose of anticonvulsant medication can be evaluated later. The nurse should focus on maintaining an open airway, preventing injury to the client, and assessing the onset and progression of the seizure to determine the type of brain activity involved. The type of aura should be assessed in the preictal phase of the seizure.

🔑 CN: Physiological adaptation; CL: Analyze

33. 1. The nurse should expect a client in the postictal phase to experience drowsiness to somnolence because exhaustion results from the abnormal spontaneous neuron firing and tonic-clonic motor response. An inability to move a muscle part is not expected after a tonic-clonic seizure because a lack of motor function would be related to a complication, such as a lesion, tumor, or stroke, in the correlating brain tissue. A change in sensation would not be expected because this would indicate a complication such as an injury to the peripheral nerve pathway to the corresponding part from the central nervous system. Hypotension is not typically a problem after a seizure.

🔑 CN: Physiological adaptation; CL: Analyze

34. 2. Anticonvulsant drug therapy should never be stopped suddenly; doing so can lead to life-threatening status epilepticus. Phenytoin sodium does not carry a risk of physical dependency or lead to hypoglycemia. Phenytoin has antiarrhythmic properties, and discontinuation does not cause heart block.

🔑 CN: Pharmacological and parenteral therapies; CL: Apply

35. 3. An aura is a premonition of an impending seizure. Auras usually are of a sensory nature (e.g., an olfactory, visual, gustatory, or auditory sensation); some may be of a psychic nature. Evaluating an aura may help identify the area of the brain from which the seizure originates. Auras occur before a seizure, not during or after (postictal). They are not similar to hallucinations or amnesia or related to relaxation.

🔑 CN: Physiological adaptation; CL: Synthesize

36. 2. Toxic effects of topiramate include nephrolithiasis, and clients are encouraged to drink six to eight glasses of water a day to dilute the urine and flush the renal tubules to avoid stone formation. Topiramate is taken in divided doses because it produces drowsiness. Although eating fresh fruits is desirable from a nutritional standpoint, this is not related to the topiramate. The drug does not have to be taken with meals.

🔑 CN: Pharmacological and parenteral therapies; CL: Evaluate

37. 3. A common adverse effect of long-term phenytoin therapy is an overgrowth of gingival tissues. Problems may be minimized with good oral hygiene, but in some cases, overgrown tissues must be removed surgically. Phenytoin does not cause weight gain, insomnia, or deteriorating eyesight.

🔑 CN: Pharmacological and parenteral therapies; CL: Evaluate

38. 1,2,3. The nurse should assess the number and type of seizures the client has experienced since starting clonazepam monotherapy for seizure control. The nurse should also determine if the client might be pregnant because clonazepam crosses the placental barrier. The nurse should also ask about the client's use of alcohol because alcohol potentiates the action of clonazepam. Although the nurse may want to check on the client's diet or use of cigarettes for health maintenance and promotion, such information is not specifically related to clonazepam therapy.

🔑 CN: Pharmacological and parenteral therapies; CL: Evaluate

The Client with a Stroke

39. 1,4,5. A headache (which is treated with analgesics) is commonly associated with an ischemic CVA. A conscious client responds to comfort measures. Bleeding is a side effect of recombinant tissue plasminogen (t-PA) therapy to dissolve the clots; absence of bleeding is a desired outcome. Reduction of dysphagia and visual disturbances is unpredictable and less likely to occur during this phase.

🔑 CN: Pharmacological and parenteral therapies; CL: Evaluate

40. 3. Following a stroke, it is easiest for clients with dysphagia (difficulty swallowing) to swallow solid foods; the nurse introduces foods on the unaffected side. Liquid foods are difficult to swallow, and the client with facial paralysis will have difficulty sipping using a straw. The head of the bed is elevated to 90 degrees, or the client is instructed to sit up, if possible, while eating to prevent choking and aspiration.

CN: Physiological adaptation; CL: Apply

41. 15 points
The Glasgow Coma Scale provides three objective neurologic assessments: spontaneity of eye opening, best motor response, and best verbal response on a scale of 3 to 15. The client who scores the best on all three assessments scores 15 points.

CN: Management of care; CL: Apply

42. 2,3,5. The maximum dosage of warfarin sodium is not achieved until 3 to 4 days after starting the medication, and the effects of the drug continue for 4 to 5 days after discontinuing the medication. The client should have blood levels tested periodically to make sure that the desired level is maintained. Warfarin has a peak action of 9 hours. Vitamin K is the antidote for warfarin; protamine sulfate is the antidote for heparin.

CN: Pharmacological and parenteral therapies; CL: Evaluate

43. 1. A helpless client should be positioned on the side, not on the back, with the head on a small pillow. A lateral position helps secretions escape from the throat and mouth, minimizing the risk of aspiration. It may be necessary to suction the client if he aspirates. Suction equipment should be nearby. It is safe to use a padded tongue blade, and the client should receive oral care, including brushing with a toothbrush.

CN: Reduction of risk potential; CL: Synthesize

44. 3. Studies show that clients who receive recombinant t-PA treatment within 3 hours after the onset of a stroke have better outcomes. The time from the onset of a stroke to t-PA treatment is critical. A complete health assessment and history is not possible when a client is receiving emergency care. Upcoming surgical procedures may need to be delayed because of the administration of t-PA, which is a priority in the immediate treatment of the current stroke. While the nurse should identify which medications the client is taking, it is more important to know the time of the onset of the stroke to determine the course of action for administering t-PA.

CN: Pharmacological and parenteral therapies; CL: Synthesize

45. 3. Control of blood pressure is critical during the first 24 hours after treatment because an intracerebral hemorrhage is the major adverse effect of thrombolytic therapy. Vital signs are monitored, and blood pressure is maintained as identified by the **healthcare provider (HCP)** 📖 and specific to the client's ischemic tissue needs and risk of bleeding from treatment. The other vital signs are important, but the priority is to monitor blood pressure.

CN: Reduction of risk potential; CL: Synthesize

46. 2. It is crucial to monitor the pupil size and pupillary response to indicate changes around the cranial nerves. The cholesterol level is not a priority assessment, although it may be an assessment to be addressed for long-term healthy lifestyle rehabilitation. Bowel sounds need to be assessed because an ileus or constipation can develop, but this is not a priority in the first 24 hours, when the primary concerns are cerebral hemorrhage and increased intracranial pressure. An echocardiogram is not needed for the client with a thrombotic stroke without heart problems.

CN: Physiological adaptation; CL: Analyze

47. 4,2,1,3. Increased agitation with suctioning will increase ICP; therefore, sedation should be provided first. The client should be hyperoxygenated before and after suctioning to prevent hypoxia since hypoxia causes vasodilation of the cerebral vessels and increases ICP. The airway should then be suctioned for no more than 10 seconds. The mouth can be suctioned once the airway is clear to remove oral secretions. Once the mouth is suctioned, the suction catheter should be discarded.

CN: Physiological adaptation; CL: Synthesize

48. 1. The primary reason for the nursing assessment of a client's functional status before and after a stroke is to guide the plan. The assessment does not help to predict how far the rehabilitation team can help the client to recover from the residual effects of the stroke, only what plans can help a client who has moved from one functional level to another. The nursing assessment of the client's functional status is not a motivating factor.

CN: Physiological adaptation; CL: Apply

49. 2. Sliding a client on a sheet causes friction and is to be avoided. Friction injures skin and predisposes to pressure ulcer formation. Rolling the client is an acceptable method to use when changing positions as long as the client is maintained in anatomically neutral positions and the limbs are properly supported. The client may be lifted as long as the nurse has assistance and uses proper body mechanics to avoid injury to himself or herself or the client. Having the client help lift off the bed with a trapeze is an acceptable means to move a client without causing friction burns or skin breakdown.

CN: Reduction of risk potential;
CL: Synthesize

50. 35. This client has a fall risk score of 35 and is at medium fall risk due to the client's secondary diagnosis (15) and IV access (20). Though paraplegic, this does not affect the client's fall risk assessment as the client will be either in bed or in a wheelchair; the client therefore is not assessed points on the fall risk for "ambulatory aid" or "gait."

CN: Safety and infection control;
CL: Evaluate

51. 3. The use of ankle-high tennis shoes has been found to be most effective in preventing plantar flexion (footdrop) because they add support to the foot and keep it in the correct anatomic position. Footboards stimulate spasms and are not routinely recommended. Regular repositioning and range-of-motion exercises are important interventions, but the client's foot needs to be in the correct anatomic position to prevent overextension of the muscle and tendon. Massaging does not prevent plantar flexion and, if rigorous, could release emboli.

CN: Reduction of risk potential;
CL: Synthesize

52. 1,2,4. Placing a pillow in the axilla so the arm is away from the body keeps the arm abducted and prevents skin from touching skin to avoid skin breakdown. Placing a pillow under the slightly flexed arm so the hand is higher than the elbow prevents dependent edema. Positioning a hand cone (not a rolled washcloth) in the hand prevents hand contractures. Immobilization of the extremity may cause a painful shoulder-hand syndrome. Flexion contractures of the hand, wrist, and elbow can result from immobility of the weak or paralyzed extremity. It is better to extend the arms to prevent contractures.

CN: Reduction of risk potential;
CL: Synthesize

53. 2. Expressive aphasia is a condition in which the client understands what is heard or written but cannot say what he or she wants to say. A communication or picture board helps the client communicate with others in that the client can point to objects or activities that he or she desires. Receptive aphasia is a condition in which the client does not comprehend what is being said. For this client it is helpful to speak clearly using short sentences or writing out directions.

CN: Physiological adaptation;
CL: Synthesize

54. 1,3,4. A client with dysphagia (difficulty swallowing) commonly has the most difficulty ingesting thin liquids, which are easily aspirated. Liquids should be thickened to avoid aspiration. Maintaining an upright position while eating is appropriate because it minimizes the risk of aspiration. Introducing foods on the unaffected side allows the client to have better control over the food bolus. The client should concentrate on chewing and swallowing; therefore, distractions should be avoided. Large pieces of food could cause choking; the food should be cut into bite-sized pieces.

CN: Safety and infection control;
CL: Synthesize

55. 2. Homonymous hemianopia is blindness in half of the visual field; therefore, the client would see only half of the plate. Eating only the food on half of the plate results from an inability to coordinate visual images and spatial relationships. There may be an increased preference for foods high in salt after a stroke, but this would not be related to homonymous hemianopia. Forgetting the names of foods is a sign of aphasia, which involves a cerebral cortex lesion. Being unable to swallow liquids is dysphagia, which involves motor pathways of cranial nerves IX and X, including the lower brain stem.

CN: Physiological adaptation;
CL: Analyze

56. 4. To expand the visual field, the partially sighted client should be taught to turn the head from side to side when walking. Neglecting to do so may result in accidents. This technique helps maximize the use of remaining sight. Covering an eye with a patch will limit the field of vision. Personal items can be placed within sight and reach, but most accidents occur from tripping over items that cannot be seen. It may help the client to see the door, but walking presents the primary safety hazard.

CN: Reduction of risk potential;
CL: Synthesize

57. 3. A client who has brain damage may be emotionally labile and may cry or laugh for no explainable reason. Crying is best dealt with by attempting to divert the client's attention. Ignoring the behavior will not affect the mood swing or the crying and may increase the client's sense of isolation. Telling the client to stop is inappropriate.

CN: Psychosocial adaptation;
CL: Synthesize

58. 1,3,4,5. The goal of communicating with a client with aphasia is to minimize frustration and exhaustion. The nurse should encourage the client to write messages or use alternative forms of communication to avoid frustration. Presenting one thought at a time decreases stimuli that may distract the client, as does speaking in a normal volume and tone. The nurse should ask the client to point to objects and encourage the use of gestures to assist in communicating.

🔑 CN: Psychosocial adaptation; CL: Synthesize

59. 3. Thrombolytic enzyme agents are used for clients with a thrombotic stroke to dissolve emboli, thus reestablishing cerebral perfusion. They do not increase vascular permeability, cause vasoconstriction, or prevent further hemorrhage.

🔑 CN: Pharmacological and parenteral therapies; CL: Evaluate

The Client with Parkinson's Disease

60. 4. When a freezing gait occurs, having the client march in place or step over actual lines, imaginary lines, or objects on the floor can promote walking. Instructing the client to take one step backward and two steps forward may also stimulate walking. Pulling the client forward can cause imbalance. The nurse does not instruct the client to use a wheelchair. The client obtains much exercise as possible; having the client remain still does not help the client obtain the momentum needed to walk.

🔑 CN: Physiological adaptation; CL: Apply

61. 3,4,5. The nurse should contact the **HCP** 📖 before administering carbidopa-levodopa because this medication can cause further symptoms of depression. Suicide threats in clients with chronic illness should be taken seriously. The nurse should also determine if the client is on an MAO inhibitor because concurrent use with carbidopa-levodopa can cause a hypertensive crisis. Carbidopa-levodopa is not a treatment for depression. Having the client discuss feelings is appropriate when the prescription is finalized.

🔑 CN: Pharmacological and parenteral therapies; CL: Synthesize

62. 2. The first sign of Parkinson's disease is usually tremors. The client commonly is the first to notice this sign because the tremors may be minimal at first. Rigidity is the second sign, and bradykinesia is the third sign. Akinesia is a later stage of bradykinesia.

🔑 CN: Physiological adaptation; CL: Analyze

63. 3. The primary focus is on maintaining a safe environment because the client with Parkinson's disease usually has a propulsive gait, characterized by a tendency to take increasingly quicker steps while walking. This type of gait commonly causes

the client to fall or to have trouble stopping. The client should maintain a balanced diet, enhance the immune system, and enjoy diversional activities; however, safety is the primary concern.

🔑 CN: Reduction of risk potential; CL: Synthesize

64. 2. Voluntary and purposeful movements often temporarily decrease or stop the tremors associated with Parkinson's disease. In some clients, however, tremors may increase with voluntary effort. Tremors associated with Parkinson's disease are not psychogenic but are related to an imbalance between dopamine and acetylcholine. Tremors cannot be reduced by distracting the client.

🔑 CN: Physiological adaptation; CL: Analyze

65. 2. Demanding physical activity should be performed during the peak action of drug therapy. Clients should be encouraged to maintain independence in self-care activities to the greatest extent possible. Although some clients may have more energy in the morning or after rest, tremors are managed with drug therapy.

🔑 CN: Physiological adaptation; CL: Synthesize

66. 4. Helping the client function at his or her best is most appropriate and realistic. There is no known cure for Parkinson's disease. Parkinson's disease progresses in severity, and there is no known way to stop its progression. However, many clients live for years with the disease, and it would not be appropriate to start planning terminal care at this time.

🔑 CN: Physiological adaptation; CL: Synthesize

67. 1. The primary goal of physical therapy and nursing interventions is to maintain joint flexibility and muscle strength. Parkinson's disease involves a degeneration of dopamine-producing neurons; therefore, it would be an unrealistic goal to attempt to build muscles or increase endurance. The decrease in dopamine neurotransmitters results in ataxia secondary to extrapyramidal motor system effects. Attempts to reduce ataxia through physical therapy would not be effective.

🔑 CN: Physiological adaptation; CL: Synthesize

68. 2. Levodopa is prescribed to decrease severe muscle rigidity. Levodopa does not improve mood, appetite, or alertness in a client with Parkinson's disease.

🔑 CN: Pharmacological and parenteral therapies; CL: Evaluate

69. 3. Vital signs should be monitored, especially during periods of adjustment. Changes, such as orthostatic hypotension, cardiac irregularities, palpitations, and light-headedness, should be reported immediately. The client may actually experience suicidal or paranoid ideation instead of euphoria. The nurse should monitor the client for elevated liver enzyme levels, such as lactate dehydrogenase, aspartate aminotransferase, alanine aminotransferase, blood urea nitrogen, and alkaline phosphatase, but the client should not be jaundiced. The client should not experience signs and symptoms of diabetes or a low serum glucose level, but the nurse should check the hemoglobin and hematocrit levels.

🔑 CN: Pharmacological and parenteral therapies; CL: Analyze

70. 2. Ongoing self-care is a major focus for clients with Parkinson's disease. The client should be given additional time as needed and praised for efforts to remain independent. Firmly telling the client that he or she needs assistance will undermine self-esteem and defeat efforts to be independent. Telling the client that perception of the situation is unrealistic does not foster hope in the ability to perform self-care measures. Suggesting that the client modify the morning routine seems to put the hospital or the nurse's time schedule before the client's needs. This will only decrease the client's self-esteem and the desire to try to continue self-care, which is obviously important to the client.

🔑 CN: Psychosocial adaptation; CL: Synthesize

71. 1. The goal of a pallidotomy is to improve functional ability for the client with Parkinson's disease. This is a priority. The pallidotomy creates lesions in the globus pallidus to control extrapyramidal disorders that affect control of movement and gait. If functional ability is improved by the pallidotomy, the client may experience a secondary response of an improved emotional response, but this is not the primary goal of the surgical procedure. The procedure will not improve alertness or appetite.

🔑 CN: Basic care and comfort; CL: Apply

The Client with Multiple Sclerosis

72. 2,4,5. The client with multiple sclerosis is at risk for falls due to muscle weakness, skin breakdown due to bowel and bladder incontinence, and fatigue. The client is not at risk for dehydration; seizures are not associated with myelin destruction.

🔑 CN: Physiological integrity; CL: Analyze

73. 2,3,4,5. Maintaining urinary function in a client with neurogenic bladder dysfunction from MS is an important goal. The client should ideally drink 400 to 500 mL with each meal; drink 200 mL midmorning, midafternoon, and late afternoon; and attempt to void at least every 2 hours to prevent infection and stone formation. The client may need to catheterize herself to drain residual urine in the bladder. Restricting fluids during the day will not produce sufficient urine. However, in bladder training for nighttime continence, the client may restrict fluids for 1 to 2 hours before going to bed. The client should drink at least 2,000 mL every 24 hours.

🔑 CN: Physiological adaptation; CL: Create

74. 2. With MS, hyperexcitability and euphoria may occur, but because of muscle weakness, sudden bursts of energy are unlikely. Visual disturbances, weakness in the extremities, and loss of muscle tone and tremors are common symptoms of MS.

🔑 CN: Physiological adaptation; CL: Analyze

75. 3. Baclofen is a centrally acting skeletal muscle relaxant that helps relieve the muscle spasms common in MS. Drowsiness is an adverse effect, and driving should be avoided if the medication produces a sedative effect. Baclofen does not stimulate the appetite or reduce bacteria in the urine.

🔑 CN: Pharmacological and parenteral therapies; CL: Evaluate

76. 2. Evaluating drug effectiveness is difficult because a high percentage of clients with MS exhibit unpredictable episodes of remission, exacerbation, and steady progress without apparent cause. Clients with MS do not necessarily have increased intolerance to drugs, nor do they endure long periods of exacerbation before the illness responds to a particular drug. Multiple drug use is not what makes evaluation of drug effectiveness difficult.

🔑 CN: Physiological adaptation; CL: Analyze

77. 4. Asking a client to speak louder even when tired may aggravate the problem. Asking the client to speak slowly and distinctly and to repeat hard-to-understand words helps the client to communicate effectively.

🔑 CN: Psychosocial adaptation; CL: Synthesize

78. 4. The nurses' notes should be concise, objective, clearly stated, and relevant. This client trembles when she attempts voluntary actions, such as drinking a beverage or fastening clothing. This activity should be described exactly as it occurs so that others reading the note will have no doubt about the nurse's observation of the client's behavior.

Identifying the "intentional" activity of daily living will help the interdisciplinary team individualize the client's plan of care. Clarifying what is meant by "worsening" with a purposeful act will facilitate the interrater reliability of the team. It is better to state what the client did than to give vague nursing orders in the nurses' notes.

CN: Management of care; CL: Apply

79. 4. Limiting fluid intake is likely to aggravate rather than relieve symptoms when a bowel retraining program is being implemented. Furthermore, water imbalance, as well as electrolyte imbalance, tends to aggravate the signs and symptoms of MS. A diet high in fiber helps keep bowel movements regular. Setting a regular time each day for elimination helps train the body to maintain a schedule. Using an elevated toilet seat facilitates transfer of the client from the wheelchair to the toilet or from a standing to a sitting position.

CN: Physiological adaptation;
CL: Synthesize

80. 3. MS is a progressive, chronic neurologic disease characterized by patchy demyelination throughout the central nervous system. This interferes with the transmission of electrical impulses from one nerve cell to the next. MS affects speech, coordination, and vision, but not cognition. Care for the client with MS is directed toward maintaining joint mobility, preventing deformities, maintaining muscle strength, rehabilitation, preventing and treating depression, and providing client motivation.

CN: Reduction of risk potential;
CL: Synthesize

81. 2. The nurse's most positive approach is to encourage a client with MS to keep active, use stress reduction strategies, and avoid fatigue because it is important to support the immune system while remaining active. A quiet, inactive lifestyle is not necessarily indicated. Good health habits are not likely to alter the course of the disease, although they may help minimize complications. Practicing using aids that will be needed for future disabilities may be helpful but also can be discouraging.

CN: Physiological adaptation;
CL: Synthesize

82. 1,3,4,5. A client with impaired peripheral sensation does not feel pain as readily as does someone whose sensation is unimpaired; therefore, water temperatures should be tested carefully. The client should be advised to avoid using hot water bottles or heating pads and to protect against cold temperatures. Because the client cannot rely on minor pain as an indicator of damaged skin or sore spots, the client should carefully inspect the skin daily to visualize any injuries that he or she cannot feel. The client should not be instructed to avoid

kitchen activities out of fear of injury; independence and self-care are also important. However, the client should meet with an occupational therapist to learn about assistive devices and techniques that can reduce injuries, such as burns and cuts that are common in kitchen activities.

CN: Reduction of risk potential;
CL: Create

83. 3. Maintaining a regular voiding pattern is the most appropriate measure to help the client avoid urinary incontinence. Fluid intake is not related to incontinence. Incontinence is related to the strength of the detrusor and urethral sphincter muscles. Inserting an indwelling catheter would be a treatment of last resort because of the increased risk of infection. If catheterization is required, intermittent self-catheterization is preferred because of its lower risk of infection. Antibiotics do not influence urinary incontinence.

CN: Physiological adaptation;
CL: Synthesize

84. 2. An individualized regular exercise program helps the client to relieve muscle spasms. The client can be trained to use unaffected muscles to promote coordination because MS is a progressive, debilitating condition. The data do not indicate that the client needs psychotherapy, day care for the granddaughter, or visits from other clients.

CN: Physiological adaptation;
CL: Synthesize

The Client with Myasthenia Gravis

85. 1. Loss of motor function to the face and throat can cause dysphagia and places the client at risk for aspiration. Bladder dysfunction and hypertension are not associated with myasthenia gravis. Myasthenia affects nerve impulses at the neuromuscular junction, causing loss of motor function; there is no sensory deficit.

CN: Reduction of risk potential;
CL: Synthesize

86. 1. The nurse instructs the client regarding use of artificial tears because eyelid and extraocular muscles are frequently affected by myasthenia gravis and there is a risk of corneal abrasion if the eyelids do not close completely. The client is encouraged to maintain social contacts and prevent social isolation by staying at home. Medication is taken in the morning, prior to activities, so the client is able to complete them. A nutritious diet is encouraged, and there is no indication to limit protein.

CN: Reduction of risk potential;
CL: Synthesize

87. 3. With a well-managed regimen, a client with myasthenia gravis should be able to control symptoms, maintain a normal lifestyle, and achieve a normal life expectancy. Myasthenia gravis can be controlled and need not be a fatal disease. Myasthenia gravis can be controlled, not cured. Episodes of increased muscle weakness should not occur if treatment is well managed.

CN: Physiological adaptation;
CL: Evaluate

The Unconscious Client

88. 3. Activated charcoal powder is administered to absorb remaining particles of salicylate. Vitamin K is an antidote for warfarin sodium. Dextrose 50% is used to treat hypoglycemia. Sodium thiosulfate is an antidote for cyanide.

CN: Pharmacological and parenteral therapies; CL: Synthesize

89. 2,3,4. An excess of cholinergic agents produces urinary and fecal incontinence, increased salivation, diarrhea, and diaphoresis. In a severe overdose, CNS depression, seizures and muscle fasciculations, bradycardia or tachycardia, weakness, and respiratory arrest due to respiratory muscle paralysis occur. Anticholinergics produce dry mucous membranes. Skin rash is not a sign of overdose with a cholinergic agent.

CN: Pharmacological and parenteral therapies; CL: Analyze

90. 3. The wife's initial response to this crisis is high anxiety. Anxiety must dissipate before a person can deal with the actual situation. Allowing the wife to express her feelings can help diffuse their anxiety. The reasons for the client's actions are unknown; assumptions must be validated before they become facts. The nurse should first listen to the wife's needs before recommending meeting with clergy. Asking the wife to help with the client's care is appropriate at a later time.

CN: Psychosocial adaptation;
CL: Synthesize

91. 3. Maintaining intact skin is a priority for the unconscious client. Unconscious clients need to be turned every hour to prevent complications of immobility, which include pressure ulcers and stasis pneumonia. The unconscious client cannot be educated at this time. Pain is not a concern. During the first 24 hours, the unconscious client will mostly likely be on nothing-by-mouth status.

CN: Reduction of risk potential;
CL: Synthesize

92. 2. The nurse must clean the unconscious client's mouth carefully, apply a thin coat of petroleum jelly, and move the endotracheal tube to the opposite side daily to prevent dryness, crusting, inflammation, and parotiditis. The unconscious client's temperature should be monitored by a route other than the oral (e.g., rectal, tympanic) because oral temperatures will be inaccurate. The client should be positioned in a lateral or semiprone position, not a supine position, to allow for drainage of secretions and for the jaw and tongue to fall forward. The client should not be dragged when turned, as may happen when a drawsheet is used. Care should be taken to lift the client's heels, buttocks, arms, and head off of the sheets when turning. Trochanter rolls, splints, foam boot aids, specialty beds, and so on—not just two pillows—should be used to keep the client in correct body position and to decrease pressure on bony prominences.

CN: Reduction of risk potential;
CL: Synthesize

93. 3. The client is not in proper body alignment if, when in the right side-lying position, the client's left arm rests on the mattress with the elbow flexed. This positioning of the arm pulls the left shoulder out of good alignment, restricting respiratory movements. The arm should be supported on a pillow. The client's head also should be placed on a small pillow to keep it in alignment with the body. The right leg should be extended on the mattress without a pillow to avoid hyperrotation of the hip. A pillow should be placed between the left and right legs with the left knee flexed so that on no parts of the legs is skin touching skin.

CN: Physiological adaptation;
CL: Synthesize

94. 4. The goal of performing passive ROM exercises is to maintain joint mobility. Active exercise is needed to preserve bone and muscle mass. Passive ROM movements do not prevent bone demineralization or have a positive effect on the client's muscle tone.

CN: Physiological adaptation;
CL: Evaluate

95. 1. Maintaining a patent airway is the priority. Therefore, the nurse should keep suction equipment available to remove secretions. The client should be placed in a side-lying, not prone, position. Performing oral hygiene is a clean procedure; therefore, the nurse wears clean gloves, not sterile gloves. The nurse should never place any fingers in an unconscious client's mouth; the client may bite down. Padded tongue blades, swabs, or a toothbrush should be used instead; but maintaining the airway is the priority.

CN: Physiological adaptation;
CL: Synthesize

96. 2. When the blink reflex is absent or the eyes do not close completely, the cornea may become dry and irritated. Corneal abrasion can occur. Taping the eye closed will prevent injury. Having the client wear eyeglasses or cleaning the eyelid will not protect the cornea from dryness or irritation. Artificial tears instilled once per shift are not frequent enough for preventing dryness.

   CN: Reduction of risk potential; CL: Synthesize

97. 3. Restlessness is an early indicator of hypoxia. The nurse should suspect hypoxia in the unconscious client who becomes restless. The most accurate method for determining the presence of hypoxia is to evaluate the pulse oximeter value or arterial blood gas values. Cyanosis and decreased respirations are late indicators of hypoxia. Hypertension, not hypotension, is a sign of hypoxia.

   CN: Physiological adaptation; CL: Apply

98. 2. The client should be placed in a semi-Fowler's position to reduce the risk of aspiration. The formula should be at room temperature, not heated. Administering enteral tube feedings is a clean procedure, not a sterile one; therefore, sterile supplies are not required. Clients receiving enteral feedings should be weighed regularly, but not necessarily before each feeding.

   CN: Reduction of risk potential; CL: Synthesize

99. 4. Gastric residuals are checked before administration of enteral feedings to determine whether gastric emptying is delayed. A residual of <50% of the previous feeding volume is usually considered acceptable. In this case, the amount is not excessive and the nurse should reinstill the aspirate through the tube and then administer the feeding. If the amount of gastric residual is excessive, the nurse should notify the **HCP** and withhold the feeding. Disposing of the residual can cause electrolyte and fluid losses.

   CN: Reduction of risk potential; CL: Synthesize

The Client in Pain

100. 2. Morphine 2 mg was given 1 hour ago, and the client can have up to 4 mg every 2 hours. Although the pain level is at 1, the nurse should give medication prior to the dressing change with packing that is likely to cause discomfort. A 4-mg dose of morphine would exceed the 2-hour limit and, if given after the dressing change, would not manage pain during the procedure. The client has been responding to the pain medication dosing, and a new prescription is not required at this time.

   CN: Management of care; CL: Synthesize

101. 1. Experience has demonstrated that clients who feel confidence in the persons who are caring for them do not require as much therapy for pain relief as do those who have less confidence. Without the client's confidence, developed in an effective nurse-client relationship, other interventions may be less effective. The client's family can be an important source of support, but it is the nurse who plans strategies for pain relief. The client may require time to adjust to the pain, but the nurse and client can collaborate to try to evaluate a variety of pain relief strategies. Arranging for the client to share a room with another client who has little pain may have negative effects on the client who has pain that is difficult to relieve.

   CN: Basic care and comfort; CL: Synthesize

102. 4. Although meperidine hydrochloride can be given orally, it is more effective when given intramuscularly. The equianalgesic dose of oral meperidine is up to four times the IM dose (75 × 4 = 300).

   CN: Pharmacological and parenteral therapies; CL: Apply

103. 1. Opioid analgesics relieve pain by reducing or altering the perception of pain. Meperidine hydrochloride does not decrease the sensitivity of pain receptors, interfere with pain impulses traveling along sensory nerve fibers, or block the conduction of pain impulses in the central nervous system.

   CN: Pharmacological and parenteral therapies; CL: Evaluate

104. 3. The client's innate responses to pain are directed initially toward escaping from the source of pain. Variations in tolerance and perception of pain are apparent only in conscious clients, and only conscious clients can employ distraction to help relieve pain.

   CN: Physiological adaptation; CL: Apply

105. 2. Ergotamine tartrate is used to help abort a migraine attack. It should be taken as soon as prodromal symptoms appear. Reduced migraine severity and relief from sleeplessness and vision problems address symptoms that occur after the migraine has occurred and are not effects of ergotamine.

   CN: Pharmacological and parenteral therapies; CL: Evaluate

106. 4. Biofeedback translates body processes into observable signs so that the client can develop some control over certain body processes. Biofeedback does not involve electrical stimulation. Use of unpleasant stimuli such as electrical shock is a form of aversion therapy. Biofeedback does not involve monitoring body processes for the therapist to interpret; rather, it is a self-directed, self-care activity that reinforces learning because the client can see the results of his or her actions.

CN: Psychosocial adaptation; CL: Apply

107. 1. A back rub stimulates the large-diameter cutaneous fibers, which block transmission of pain impulses from the spinal cord to the brain. It does not block the transmission of pain impulses or stimulate the release of endorphins. A back rub may distract the client, but the physiologic process of fiber stimulation is the main reason a back rub is used as therapy for pain relief.

CN: Basic care and comfort; CL: Apply

108. 2. It is essential that the nurse document the client's response to pain medication on a routine, systematic basis. Reassuring the client that pain will be relieved is often not realistic. A client who continually presses the PCA button may not be getting adequate pain relief, but through careful assessment and documentation, the effectiveness of pain relief interventions can be evaluated and modified. Pain medication is not titrated until the client is free from pain but rather until an acceptable level of pain management is reached.

CN: Pharmacological and parenteral therapies; CL: Synthesize

109. 2. The nurse should first check the infusion site to be sure the site has not infiltrated. Next, the nurse should check the PCA pump to determine if it is functioning properly. Assessing vital signs would be important to provide additional data about the possible cause of pain, but is not the first action at this time. It is not necessary to notify the **healthcare provider (HCP)** 📖 unless the infusion site or pump is malfunctioning and other methods of managing the pain are required.

CN: Pharmacological and parenteral therapies; CL: Synthesize

110. 1. The nurse using healing touch affects a client's pain primarily through assessing and directing the flow of energy fields. Healing touch removes energy congestion so energy channels can facilitate integration of the body, mind, and soul to promote healing. Healing touch can involve touching, but it does not have to involve body contact. Massage is not involved with healing touch. The goal of healing touch is not to increase the production of endorphins.

CN: Physiological adaptation; CL: Apply

111. 2. Pain is whatever the client perceives it is; using a pain scale is the best way to have the client quantify the amount of pain. The fact that the client is protecting an area of the body, the client's vital signs, and the client's appearance of discomfort are objective rather than subjective findings; the nurse should confirm the meaning of these changes before assuming the client has pain.

CN: Basic care and comfort; CL Analyze

112. 2. The nurse administers between 2 and 4 mg of morphine sulfate IVP every 2 to 4 hours according to the prescription for pain management. Even though the client received pain medication 2 hours ago, the client is still experiencing pain of the intensity of 8 on a scale of 0 to 10. Elderly clients may have slowed pain perception, but not diminished pain intensity. The nurse starts out conservatively, administering 2 mg of morphine sulfate IVP and reassessing in 15 minutes to determine the effectiveness of pain management and respiratory effort. If pain is still not relieved, the titration of morphine sulfate upward to 4 mg is optional. The single provision of nonpharmacologic interventions such as repositioning is not sufficient pain management when a client rates pain at 8 on a scale of 0 to 10. Requesting a prescription for sedation only causes the client to be unable to express her pain and does not treat the pain. Although the nurse continues to monitor the client's respirations, the respirations are not dangerously depressed, and waiting another 2 hours to administer pain medication does not address the client's need for pain relief.

CN: Pharmacological parenteral therapies; CL: Synthesize

Managing Care, Quality, and Safety of Clients with Neurologic Health Problems

113. 2. Assessments, teaching, and suctioning are roles of the nurse. Basic care with frequent positioning is the most appropriate to delegate to the UAP 📖.

CN: Management of care; CL: Apply

114. 3. Pulling the client up under the arm can cause shoulder displacement. A belt around the waist should be used to move the client. Passive range-of-motion exercises prevent contractures and atrophy. Raising the foot of the bed assists in venous return to reduce edema. High top tennis shoes are used to prevent foot drop.

CN: Management of care; CL: Synthesize

115. 3. Clients with Parkinson's disease can experience dysphagia. Thickening liquids assists with swallowing, preventing aspiration. Hyperextending the neck opens the airway and can increase risk of aspiration. Pressing the chin firmly on the chest makes swallowing more difficult. The chin should be slightly tucked to promote swallowing. The nurse should suggest a speech therapy consult for evaluation of the client's ability to swallow.

CN: Safety and infection control; CL: Synthesize

116. 4. Urinary tract infections are a frequent complication in clients with multiple sclerosis because of the effect on bladder function; therefore, that client should been seen first by the nurse. The elevated temperature and flank pain suggest that this client may have pyelonephritis. The client should be notified immediately so that antibiotic therapy can be started quickly. The other clients should be assessed soon but do not have needs as urgent as this client.

CN: Management of care; CL: Synthesize

117. 2. Clients with Parkinson's disease may experience a freezing gait when they are unable to move forward. Instructing the client to march in place, step over lines in the flooring, or visualize stepping over a log allows them to move forward. It is important to ambulate the client and not keep him or her on bed rest. A muscle relaxant is not indicated.

CN: Management of care; CL: Synthesize

118. 1,2,3,7. Pressure points in the side-lying position include the ears, shoulders, ribs, greater trochanter, medial or lateral condyles, and ankles. The sacrum, occiput, and heels are pressure point areas affected in the supine position.

CN: Safety and infection control; CL: Analyze

119. 4. All healthcare facilities in which controlled medications are stored for dispensing and/or administration to clients are required to follow procedures for the proper maintenance of narcotic inventory. Narcotic inventory maintenance includes, but is not limited to, thorough and appropriate documentation of any discrepancy with accompanying reasons (i.e., tablet/amp/vial breakage, additional medication volume, etc.), timely resolution of inventory discrepancies, and timely notification of persons in oversight areas (i.e., pharmacy, security, nursing house supervisor). In the event of a significant incident, the proper external authorities will be notified by the Quality and Risk Management/Legal Department.

CN: Pharmacological and parenteral therapies; CL: Synthesize

120. 3. The first intervention for a confused client is to increase the frequency of observation, moving the client closer to the nurses' station if possible and/or delegating the **unlicensed assistive personnel (UAP)** to check on the client more frequently. If the family is able to stay with the client, that is an option, but it is the nurse's responsibility, not the family's, to keep the client safe. Wrist restraints are not used simply because a client is confused; there is no mention of this client pulling at intravenous lines, which is one of the main reasons to use wrist restraints. Administering a sedative simply because a client is confused is not appropriate nursing care and may actually potentiate the problem.

CN: Safety and infection control; CL: Synthesize

121. 2. To ensure the client's safety when using restraints, the restraint must be secured to the bed frame (not the side rail) using a quick-release slip knot (not a square knot). Assessing and documenting skin should be done regularly when restraints are in use, but safety is first priority. Regularly releasing restraints and performing range of motion is essential but not priority in this case. Providing for the client's basic needs while in restraints (i.e., toileting) is important but not first priority.

CN: Safety and infection control; CL: Synthesize

The Client with Musculoskeletal Health Problems

- The Client with Rheumatoid Arthritis
- The Client with Osteoarthritis
- The Client with a Hip Fracture
- The Client Having Hip Replacement Surgery
- The Client Having Knee Replacement Surgery
- The Client with a Herniated Disk
- The Client with an Amputation due to Peripheral Vascular Disease
- The Client with Fractures
- The Client with a Femoral Fracture
- The Client with a Spinal Cord Injury
- Managing Care, Quality, and Safety of Clients with Musculoskeletal Health Problems
- Answers, Rationales, and Test-Taking Strategies

The Client with Rheumatoid Arthritis

1. On a visit to the clinic, a client reports the onset of early symptoms of rheumatoid arthritis. The nurse should conduct a focused assessment for:
- ☐ **1.** limited motion of joints.
- ☐ **2.** deformed joints of the hands.
- ☐ **3.** early morning stiffness.
- ☐ **4.** rheumatoid nodules.

2. A client with rheumatoid arthritis states, "I cannot do my household chores without becoming tired. My knees hurt whenever I walk." Which goal for this client should take **priority**?
- ☐ **1.** Conserve energy.
- ☐ **2.** Adapt self-care skills.
- ☐ **3.** Develop coping skills.
- ☐ **4.** Employ a housekeeping service.

3. Of the clients listed below, who is at risk for developing rheumatoid arthritis (RA)? Select all that apply.
- ☐ **1.** adults between the ages of 20 and 50 years
- ☐ **2.** adults who have had an infectious disease with the Epstein-Barr virus
- ☐ **3.** adults who are of the male gender
- ☐ **4.** adults who possess the genetic link, specifically HLA-DR4
- ☐ **5.** adults who also have osteoarthritis

4. A client is in the acute phase of rheumatoid arthritis. In which order of priority from first to last should the nurse establish the goals? All options must be used.

1. Relieve pain.

2. Preserve joint function.

3. Maintain usual ways of accomplishing tasks.

4. Prevent joint deformity.

5. The nurse teaches a client about heat and cold treatments to manage arthritis pain. Which statement indicates that the client still has a knowledge deficit?
- [ ] 1. "I can use heat and cold as often as I want."
- [ ] 2. "With heat, I should apply it for no longer than 20 minutes at a time."
- [ ] 3. "Heat-producing liniments can be used with other heat devices."
- [ ] 4. "Ten to fifteen minutes per application is the maximum time for cold applications."

6. The client with rheumatoid arthritis tells the nurse, "I have a friend who took gold shots and had a wonderful response. Why did my healthcare provider not let me try that?" Which response by the nurse would be **most** appropriate?
- [ ] 1. "It is the healthcare provider's prerogative to decide how to treat you. The healthcare provider has chosen what is best for your situation."
- [ ] 2. "Tell me more about your friend's arthritic condition. Maybe I can answer that question for you."
- [ ] 3. "That drug is used for cases that are more advanced than yours. You are not eligible for this treatment now."
- [ ] 4. "Every person is different. What works for one client may not always be effective for another."

7. The teaching plan for the client with rheumatoid arthritis includes rest promotion. What position of the involved joints should the nurse tell the client to **avoid** when at rest?
- [ ] 1. keeping all joints aligned
- [ ] 2. elevating the affected joints
- [ ] 3. lying in a prone position
- [ ] 4. maintaining the joints in a flexed position

8. After teaching the client with rheumatoid arthritis about measures to conserve energy in activities of daily living involving the small joints, which activity observed by the nurse indicates the need for additional teaching?
- [ ] 1. pushing with palms when rising from a chair
- [ ] 2. holding packages close to the body
- [ ] 3. sliding objects
- [ ] 4. carrying a laundry basket with clinched fingers and fists

9. After teaching the client with severe rheumatoid arthritis about prescribed methotrexate, which statement indicates the need for further teaching?
- [ ] 1. "I will take my vitamins while I am on this drug."
- [ ] 2. "I must not drink any alcohol while I am taking this drug."
- [ ] 3. "I should brush my teeth after every meal."
- [ ] 4. "I will continue taking my birth control pills."

10. A 25-year-old client taking hydroxychloroquine for rheumatoid arthritis reports difficulty seeing out of the left eye. What does this finding indicate?
- [ ] 1. development of a cataract
- [ ] 2. possible retinal degeneration
- [ ] 3. part of the disease process
- [ ] 4. a coincidental occurrence

11. A client with rheumatoid arthritis is taking high doses of nonsteroidal anti-inflammatory medications. The nurse should instruct the client to:
- [ ] 1. take prescribed medication with food to lessen the likelihood of an upset stomach.
- [ ] 2. not stop taking the medication suddenly; the dose needs to be decreased gradually.
- [ ] 3. use mouthwash to rinse the mouth after taking this medication.
- [ ] 4. not drive if dizziness occurs.

12. A client with rheumatoid arthritis tells the nurse, "I know it is important to exercise my joints so that I will not lose mobility, but my joints are so stiff and painful that exercising is difficult." Which response by the nurse would be **most** appropriate?
- [ ] 1. "You are probably exercising too much. Decrease your exercise to every other day."
- [ ] 2. "Tell the healthcare provider about your symptoms. Maybe your analgesic medication can be increased."
- [ ] 3. "Stiffness and pain are part of the disease. Learn to cope by focusing on activities you enjoy."
- [ ] 4. "Take a warm tub bath or shower before exercising. This may help with your discomfort."

13. Which information should the nurse include in the teaching session when preparing a client for arthrocentesis? Select all that apply.
- [ ] 1. "A local anesthetic agent may be injected into the joint site for your comfort."
- [ ] 2. "A syringe and needle will be used to withdraw fluid from your joint."
- [ ] 3. "The procedure, although not painful, will provide immediate relief."
- [ ] 4. "We will want you to keep your joint active after the procedure to increase blood flow."
- [ ] 5. "You will need to wear a compression bandage for several days after the procedure."

The Client with Osteoarthritis

14. A client with osteoarthritis will undergo an arthrocentesis on a painful, edematous knee. What information should be included in the nursing plan of care? Select all that apply.
- [ ] 1. Explain the procedure.
- [ ] 2. Administer preoperative medication 1 hour before surgery.
- [ ] 3. Instruct the client to immobilize the knee for 2 days after the surgery.
- [ ] 4. Assess the site for bleeding.
- [ ] 5. Offer pain medication.

15. A postmenopausal client is scheduled for a bone density scan. The nurse should instruct the client to:
☐ 1. remove all metal objects on the day of the scan.
☐ 2. consume foods and beverages with a high content of calcium for 2 days before the test.
☐ 3. ingest 600 mg of calcium gluconate by mouth for 2 weeks before the test.
☐ 4. report any significant pain to the healthcare provider (HCP) at least 2 days before the test.

16. A healthcare provider (HCP) prescribes a lengthy x-ray examination for a client with osteoarthritis. Which action by the nurse would demonstrate client advocacy?
☐ 1. Contact the x-ray department, and ask the technician if the lengthy session can be divided into shorter sessions.
☐ 2. Contact the HCP to determine if an alternative examination could be scheduled.
☐ 3. Request a prescription for acetaminophen prior to the examination.
☐ 4. Request padding for the hard x-ray table.

17. Which condition should the nurse assess when completing the history and physical examination of a client diagnosed with osteoarthritis?
☐ 1. anemia
☐ 2. osteoporosis
☐ 3. weight loss
☐ 4. local joint pain

18. Which information should be included in the teaching plan for a client with osteoporosis? Select all that apply.
☐ 1. Maintain a diet with adequate amounts of vitamin D, as found in fortified milk and cereals.
☐ 2. Choose good calcium sources, such as figs, broccoli, and almonds.
☐ 3. Use alcohol in moderation because a moderate intake has no known negative effects.
☐ 4. Try swimming as a good exercise to maintain bone mass.
☐ 5. Avoid high-fat foods, such as avocados, salad dressings, and fried foods.

19. Which statement indicates that the client with osteoarthritis understands the effects of capsaicin cream?
☐ 1. "I always wash my hands right after I apply the cream."
☐ 2. "After I apply the cream, I wrap my knee with an elastic bandage."
☐ 3. "I keep the cream in the cabinet above the stove in the kitchen."
☐ 4. "I also use the same cream when I get a cut or a burn."

20. At which time should the nurse instruct the client to take ibuprofen, prescribed for left hip pain secondary to osteoarthritis, to minimize gastric mucosal irritation?
☐ 1. at bedtime
☐ 2. on arising
☐ 3. immediately after a meal
☐ 4. on an empty stomach

21. The client diagnosed with osteoarthritis tells the nurse, "My friend takes steroid pills for her rheumatoid arthritis. Should I be taking steroids, too?" What should the nurse explain to the client?
☐ 1. Intra-articular corticosteroid injections are used to treat osteoarthritis.
☐ 2. Oral corticosteroids can be used in osteoarthritis.
☐ 3. A systemic effect is needed in osteoarthritis.
☐ 4. Rheumatoid arthritis and osteoarthritis are two similar diseases.

22. After teaching a client with osteoarthritis about the importance of regular exercise, which statement indicates the client has understood the teaching?
☐ 1. "Performing range-of-motion exercises will increase my joint mobility."
☐ 2. "Exercise helps to drive synovial fluid through the cartilage."
☐ 3. "Joint swelling should determine when to stop exercising."
☐ 4. "Exercising in the outdoors year-round promotes joint relaxation."

The Client with a Hip Fracture

23. A client in a double hip spica cast is constipated. The surgeon cuts a window into the front of the cast. Which outcome is intended?
☐ 1. The window will allow the nurse to palpate the superior mesenteric artery.
☐ 2. The window will allow the surgeon to manipulate the fracture site.
☐ 3. The window will allow the nurses to reposition the client.
☐ 4. The window will provide some relief from pressure due to abdominal distention as a result of constipation.

24. A client has an intracapsular hip fracture. The nurse should conduct a focused assessment to detect:
☐ 1. internal rotation.
☐ 2. muscle flaccidity.
☐ 3. shortening of the affected leg.
☐ 4. absence of pain in the fracture area.

25. When teaching a client with an extracapsular hip fracture scheduled for surgical internal fixation with the insertion of a pin, the nurse bases the teaching on the understanding that this surgical repair is the treatment of choice because:
☐ **1.** hemorrhage at the fracture site is prevented.
☐ **2.** neurovascular impairment risk is decreased.
☐ **3.** the risk of infection at the site is lessened.
☐ **4.** the client is able to be mobilized sooner.

26. A client with an extracapsular hip fracture returns to the nursing unit after internal fixation and pin insertion with a drainage tube at the incision site. Her husband asks, "Why does she have this tube inserted in her hip?" Which response would be **best**?
☐ **1.** "The tube helps us to detect a wound infection early on."
☐ **2.** "This way we will not have to irrigate the wound."
☐ **3.** "Fluid will not be allowed to accumulate at the site."
☐ **4.** "We have a way to administer antibiotics into the wound."

27. A client with a hip fracture has undergone surgery for insertion of a femoral head prosthesis. Which activity should the nurse instruct the client to avoid?
☐ **1.** crossing the legs while sitting down
☐ **2.** sitting on a raised commode seat
☐ **3.** using an abductor splint while lying on the side
☐ **4.** rising straight from a chair to a standing position

28. The nurse is caring for an older adult male who had open reduction internal fixation (ORIF) of the right hip 24 hours ago. The client is now experiencing shortness of breath and reports having "tightness in my chest." The nurse reviews the recent lab results. The nurse should report which lab results to the healthcare provider (HCP)?
☐ **1.** hematocrit (Hct): 40% (0.4)
☐ **2.** serum glucose: 120 mg/dL (6.7 mmol/L)
☐ **3.** troponin: 1.4 mcg/L (1.4 µg/L)
☐ **4.** erythrocyte sedimentation rate (ESR): 22 mm/h

29. The nurse advises the client who has had a femoral head prosthesis placement on the type of chair to sit in during the first 6 to 8 weeks after surgery. Which chair would be the correct type to recommend?
☐ **1.** a desk-type swivel chair
☐ **2.** a padded upholstered chair
☐ **3.** a high-backed chair with armrests
☐ **4.** a recliner with an attached footrest

30. The nurse is to apply a sequential compression device (intermittent pneumatic compression). Identify the area of the compression device that is placed on the client's calf.

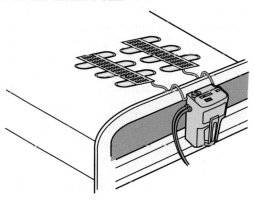

31. The nurse is assessing the home environment of an elderly client who is using crutches during the postoperative recovery phase after hip pinning. Which poses the **greatest** hazard to the client as a risk for falling at home?
☐ **1.** a 4-year-old cocker spaniel
☐ **2.** scatter rugs
☐ **3.** snack tables
☐ **4.** rocking chairs

The Client Having Hip Replacement Surgery

32. A frail elderly client with a hip fracture is to use an alternating air pressure mattress at home to prevent pressure ulcers while recovering from surgery. The nurse is assisting the client's family to place the mattress (see below). What should the nurse instruct the family to do?

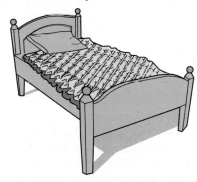

☐ **1.** Turn the mattress over so the air cells face the mattress of the bed, and cover the mattress with a bedsheet.
☐ **2.** Put a thick pad over the pressure mattress to prevent soiling, and place the bedsheet on top of the pad.
☐ **3.** Make the bed with the bedsheet on top of the pressure mattress.
☐ **4.** Make the bed, and then remove the pillow to allow full use of the mattress on the neck.

33. A client had a posterolateral total hip replacement 2 days ago. What information should the nurse include in the client's plan of care? Select all that apply.
- ☐ 1. When using a walker, encourage the client to keep the toes pointing inward.
- ☐ 2. Position a pillow between the legs to maintain abduction.
- ☐ 3. Allow the client to be in the supine position or in the lateral position on the unoperated side.
- ☐ 4. Do not allow the client to bend down to tie or slip on shoes.
- ☐ 5. Place ice on the incision after physical therapy.

34. Which information should the nurse include when performing discharge teaching with a client who had an anterolateral approach for a total hip replacement? Select all that apply.
- ☐ 1. Avoid turning the toes or knee outward.
- ☐ 2. Use an abduction pillow between the legs when in bed.
- ☐ 3. Use an elevated toilet seat and shower chair.
- ☐ 4. Do not extend the operative leg backward.
- ☐ 5. Restrict motion for 2 weeks after surgery.

35. The nurse is assessing a client for neurologic impairment after a total hip replacement. Which finding indicates impairment in the affected extremity?
- ☐ 1. decreased distal pulse
- ☐ 2. inability to move
- ☐ 3. diminished capillary refill
- ☐ 4. coolness to the touch

36. The nurse is instructing a client who will have a total hip replacement tomorrow. Which information is **most** important to include in the teaching plan at this time?
- ☐ 1. Teach how to prevent hip flexion.
- ☐ 2. Demonstrate coughing and deep-breathing techniques.
- ☐ 3. Show the client what an actual hip prosthesis looks like.
- ☐ 4. Assess the client's fears about the procedure.

37. After surgery and insertion of a total hip prosthesis, a client develops severe sudden pain and an inability to move the extremity. The nurse interprets these findings as indicating:
- ☐ 1. a developing infection.
- ☐ 2. bleeding in the operative site.
- ☐ 3. joint dislocation.
- ☐ 4. glue seepage into soft tissue.

38. A client who had a total hip replacement 2 days ago has developed an infection with a fever and profuse diaphoresis. The nurse establishes a goal to reduce the fluid deficit. Which outcome is the **most** appropriate?
- ☐ 1. The client drinks 2,000 mL of fluid per day.
- ☐ 2. The client understands how to manage the incision.
- ☐ 3. The client's bed linens are changed as needed.
- ☐ 4. The client's skin remains cool throughout hospitalization.

39. Following a total hip replacement, the nurse should position the client by:
- ☐ 1. placing weights alongside the affected extremity to keep the extremity from rotating.
- ☐ 2. elevating both feet on two pillows.
- ☐ 3. keeping the lower extremities adducted by use of an immobilization binder around both legs.
- ☐ 4. maintaining the extremity in slight abduction using an abduction splint or pillows placed between the thighs.

40. Following a client's total hip replacement, what should the nurse do? Select all that apply.
- ☐ 1. With the aid of a coworker, turn the client from the supine to the prone position every 2 hours.
- ☐ 2. Encourage the client to use the overhead trapeze to assist with position changes.
- ☐ 3. For meals, elevate the head of the bed to 90 degrees.
- ☐ 4. Use a fracture bedpan when needed by the client.
- ☐ 5. When the client is in bed, prevent thromboembolism by encouraging the client to do toe-pointing exercises.

41. A client is to have a total hip replacement. What nursing actions should the preoperative plan include? Select all that apply.
- ☐ 1. Administer antibiotics as prescribed to ensure therapeutic blood levels.
- ☐ 2. Apply leg compression device.
- ☐ 3. Request a trapeze be added to the bed.
- ☐ 4. Teach isometric exercises of quadriceps and gluteal muscles.
- ☐ 5. Demonstrate crutch walking with a three-point gait.
- ☐ 6. Place Buck's traction on the bed.

42. The nurse is teaching the client to administer enoxaparin following a total hip replacement. What should the nurse instruct the client to do? Select all that apply.
- ☐ 1. Report promptly any difficulty breathing, rash, or itching.
- ☐ 2. Notify the healthcare provider (HCP) of unusual bruising.
- ☐ 3. Avoid all aspirin-containing medications.
- ☐ 4. Wear or carry medical identification.
- ☐ 5. Expel the air bubble from the syringe before the injection.
- ☐ 6. Remove the needle immediately after the medication is injected.

43. A client who had a total hip replacement 4 days ago is worried about dislocation of the prosthesis. The nurse should respond by saying:
- ☐ 1. "Do not worry. Your new hip is very strong."
- ☐ 2. "Use of a cushioned toilet seat helps to prevent dislocation."
- ☐ 3. "Activities that tend to cause adduction of the hip tend to cause dislocation, so try to avoid them."
- ☐ 4. "Decreasing use of the abductor pillow will strengthen the muscles to prevent dislocation."

44. The nurse is assessing a client who had a left hip replacement 36 hours ago. Which findings indicate the prosthesis is dislocated? Select all that apply.
- ☐ 1. The client reported a "popping" sensation in the hip.
- ☐ 2. The left leg is shorter than the right leg.
- ☐ 3. The client has sharp pain in the groin.
- ☐ 4. The client cannot move the right leg.
- ☐ 5. The client cannot wiggle the toes on the left leg.

45. A client who has had a total hip replacement has a dislocated hip prosthesis. The nurse should **first**:
- ☐ 1. stabilize the leg with Buck's traction.
- ☐ 2. apply an ice pack to the affected hip.
- ☐ 3. position the client toward the opposite side of the hip.
- ☐ 4. notify the orthopedic surgeon.

46. The nurse has established a goal with a client to improve mobility following hip replacement. Which outcome is realistic at the time of discharge from the surgical unit?
- ☐ 1. The client can walk throughout the entire hospital with a walker.
- ☐ 2. The client can walk the length of a hospital hallway with minimal pain.
- ☐ 3. The client has increased independence in transfers from bed to chair.
- ☐ 4. The client can raise the affected leg 6 inches (15.2 cm) with assistance.

47. Following a total joint replacement, which complication has the **greatest** likelihood of occurring?
- ☐ 1. deep vein thrombosis (DVT)
- ☐ 2. polyuria
- ☐ 3. displacement of the new joint
- ☐ 4. wound evisceration

The Client Having Knee Replacement Surgery

48. In preparation for total knee surgery, a 200-lb (90.7-kg) client with osteoarthritis must lose weight. Which exercise should the nurse recommend as **best** if the client has no contraindications?
- ☐ 1. weight lifting
- ☐ 2. walking
- ☐ 3. aquatic exercise
- ☐ 4. tai chi exercise

49. The client has just had a total knee replacement for severe osteoarthritis. When assessing the client, which finding should lead the nurse to suspect possible nerve damage?
- ☐ 1. numbness
- ☐ 2. bleeding
- ☐ 3. dislocation
- ☐ 4. pinkness

50. After knee arthroplasty, the client has a sequential compression device (SCD). What should the nurse do?
- ☐ 1. Elevate the SCD on two pillows.
- ☐ 2. Change the settings on the SCD to make the client more comfortable.
- ☐ 3. Stop the SCD to remove dressings, and bathe the leg.
- ☐ 4. Discontinue the SCD when the client is ambulatory.

51. A client returns from the first session of scheduled physical therapy following total knee replacement surgery. The nurse assesses that the client's knee is swollen, slightly erythematous, and painful. The client rates the pain as 7 out of 10 and has not had any scheduled or PRN pain medication today. What should the nurse do? Select all that apply.
- ☐ 1. Gently massage the area to increase circulation to reduce pain.
- ☐ 2. Administer pain medication as prescribed.
- ☐ 3. Elevate the leg and apply a cold pack.
- ☐ 4. Notify the healthcare provider (HCP).
- ☐ 5. Call physical therapy to cancel the next treatment.

52. The nurse is preparing a client who has had a knee replacement with a metal joint to go home. What should the nurse instruct the client to do? Select all that apply.
- ☐ 1. Notify healthcare provider (HCP) about the joint prior to invasive procedures.
- ☐ 2. Inform healthcare provider (HCP) prior to having magnetic resonance imaging (MRI) scans.
- ☐ 3. Notify airport security that the joint may set off alarms on metal detectors.
- ☐ 4. Refrain from carrying items weighing more than 5 lb (2.3 kg).
- ☐ 5. Limit fluid intake to 1,000 mL/day.

53. The laboratory notifies the nurse that a client who had a total knee replacement 3 days ago and is receiving heparin has an activated partial thromboplastin time (aPTT) of 95 seconds. After verifying the values, the nurse calls the healthcare provider (HCP). The nurse should discuss with the HCP giving the client a prescription for:
- ☐ 1. protamine sulfate.
- ☐ 2. vitamin K.
- ☐ 3. warfarin.
- ☐ 4. packed red blood cells.

54. The nurse is assessing a client's left leg for neurovascular changes following a total left knee replacement. Which are expected normal findings? Select all that apply.
- ☐ 1. moderate edema of the left knee
- ☐ 2. skin warm to touch
- ☐ 3. capillary refill response of <3 seconds
- ☐ 4. moves toes
- ☐ 5. pain absent
- ☐ 6. pulse on left leg weaker than right leg

55. On the evening of surgery for total knee replacement, a client wants to get out of bed. To safely assist the client, the nurse should:
- ☐ 1. encourage the client to apply full weight bearing.
- ☐ 2. prescribe a walker for the client.
- ☐ 3. place a straight-backed chair at the foot of the bed.
- ☐ 4. apply a knee immobilizer.

56. When preparing a client for discharge from the hospital after a total knee replacement, the nurse should include which information in the discharge plan? Select all that apply.
- ☐ 1. Report signs of infection to healthcare provider (HCP).
- ☐ 2. Keep the affected leg and foot on the floor when sitting in a chair.
- ☐ 3. Remove antiembolism stockings when sleeping.
- ☐ 4. The physical therapist will encourage progressive ambulation with use of assistive devices.
- ☐ 5. Change the dressing daily.

The Client with a Herniated Disk

57. The nurse is observing a client who is recovering from back strain lift a box as shown below. What should the nurse do?
- ☐ 1. Praise the client for using correct body mechanics.
- ☐ 2. Suggest to the client to put both knees on the floor before attempting to lift the box.
- ☐ 3. Advise the client to bend from the waist rather than stretching the back in this position.
- ☐ 4. Instruct the client to keep the back straight by squatting with both knees parallel.

58. The nurse should instruct the client with low back pain to **avoid**:
- ☐ 1. keeping light objects below the level of the elbows when lifting.
- ☐ 2. leaning forward while bending the knees.
- ☐ 3. exceeding the prescribed exercise program.
- ☐ 4. sleeping on the side with legs flexed.

59. A client is discharged with the following prescription for severe back pain from a herniated intravertebral disc: hydrocodone 5 mg, acetaminophen 500 mg, one-half to one tablet by mouth each 8 to 12 hours as needed. The nurse should instruct the client to:
- ☐ 1. start with one-half tablet and take one every 12 hours.
- ☐ 2. start with one-half tablet and take one every 8 hours.
- ☐ 3. start with one tablet and then take one tablet every 8 hours.
- ☐ 4. start with one tablet and then take one tablet every 12 hours.

60. A client attempting to get out of bed stops midway because of low back pain radiating down to the right heel and lateral foot. What should the nurse do in order of priority from first to last? All options must be used.

| 1. Apply a warm compress to the client's back. |

| 2. Notify the healthcare provider (HCP). |

| 3. Assist the client to lie down. |

| 4. Administer the prescribed celecoxib. |

| |

| |

| |

| |

61. A client with a ruptured intervertebral disc at L4–L5 stands with a flattened spine slightly tilted forward and slightly flexed to the affected side. The nurse interprets this finding as indicating:
- ☐ **1.** motor changes.
- ☐ **2.** postural deformity.
- ☐ **3.** alteration of reflexes.
- ☐ **4.** sensory changes.

62. Which position would be **most** comfortable for a client with a ruptured disc at L5–S1 right?
- ☐ **1.** prone
- ☐ **2.** supine with the legs flexed
- ☐ **3.** high Fowler's
- ☐ **4.** right Sims'

63. Which action would **not** be appropriate to include when preparing a client for magnetic resonance imaging (MRI) to evaluate a ruptured disc?
- ☐ **1.** informing the client that the procedure is painless
- ☐ **2.** taking a thorough history of past surgeries
- ☐ **3.** checking for previous claustrophobia
- ☐ **4.** starting an IV line at keep-open rate

64. A client tells the nurse about having numbness from the back of the left buttock to the dorsum of the foot and big toe. The client is scheduled to undergo a laminectomy, and the operative consent form states "a left lumbar laminectomy of L3–L4." What should the nurse do **next**?
- ☐ **1.** Have the client sign the consent form.
- ☐ **2.** Call the surgeon.
- ☐ **3.** Change the consent form.
- ☐ **4.** Review the client's history.

65. Immediately after a lumbar laminectomy, the nurse administers ondansetron hydrochloride to the client as prescribed. The nurse determines that the drug is effective when which sign is controlled?
- ☐ **1.** muscle spasms
- ☐ **2.** nausea
- ☐ **3.** shivering
- ☐ **4.** dry mouth

66. After a laminectomy, the client states, "The doctor said that I can do anything I want to." Which activity that the client intends to do indicates the need for further teaching?
- ☐ **1.** drying the dishes
- ☐ **2.** sitting outside on firm cushions
- ☐ **3.** making the bed walking from side to side
- ☐ **4.** sweeping the front porch

67. The nurse is developing the discharge teaching plan for a client after a lumbar laminectomy L4–L5. What action should the nurse encourage the client to **avoid** when returning to work in 6 weeks?
- ☐ **1.** placing one foot on a step stool during prolonged standing
- ☐ **2.** sleeping on the back with support under the knees
- ☐ **3.** maintaining average body weight for height
- ☐ **4.** sitting whenever possible

68. A male client underwent a lumbar spinal fusion yesterday. Which nursing assessment should alert the nurse to the development of a possible complication?
- ☐ **1.** lateral rotation of the head and neck
- ☐ **2.** clear yellowish fluid on the dressing
- ☐ **3.** use of the standing position to void
- ☐ **4.** nonproductive cough

69. After the nurse teaches a client about wearing a back brace after a spinal fusion, which statement indicates effective teaching?
- ☐ **1.** "I will apply lotion before putting on the brace."
- ☐ **2.** "I will be sure to pad the area around my iliac crest."
- ☐ **3.** "I can use baby powder under the brace to absorb perspiration."
- ☐ **4.** "I should wear a thin cotton undershirt under the brace."

70. The nurse develops a teaching plan for a client scheduled for a spinal fusion. What should the nurse tell the client?
- ☐ **1.** The client will typically experience more pain at the donor site than at the fusion site.
- ☐ **2.** The surgeon will apply a simple gauze dressing to the donor site.
- ☐ **3.** Neurovascular checks are unnecessary if the fibula is the donor site.
- ☐ **4.** The client's level of activity restriction is determined by the amount of pain.

71. A client who has had a lumbar laminectomy with a spinal fusion is sitting in a chair. Which is the correct position for this client?
☐ 1. with the feet flat on the floor
☐ 2. on a low footstool
☐ 3. in any comfortable position with legs uncrossed
☐ 4. on a high footstool so the feet are level with the chair seat

72. The nurse develops a plan of care for a client in the initial postoperative period following a lumbar laminectomy. Which activity is **contraindicated**?
☐ 1. assisting with daily hygiene activities
☐ 2. lying flat in bed
☐ 3. walking in the hall
☐ 4. sitting all afternoon in her room

73. Which exercise should the nurse advise the client to **avoid** after a lumbar laminectomy?
☐ 1. knee-to-chest lifts
☐ 2. hip tilts
☐ 3. sit-ups
☐ 4. pelvic tilts

The Client with an Amputation due to Peripheral Vascular Disease

74. Which factor contributes to a risk for amputation in a client with peripheral vascular disease? Select all that apply.
☐ 1. uncontrolled diabetes mellitus for 15 years
☐ 2. a 20-pack-year history of cigarette smoking
☐ 3. current age of 39 years
☐ 4. a serum cholesterol concentration of 275 mg/dL (15.3 mmol/L)
☐ 5. work that requires prolonged standing

75. A client has severe arterial occlusive disease and gangrene of the left great toe. Which finding is expected?
☐ 1. edema around the ankle
☐ 2. loss of hair on the lower leg
☐ 3. thin, soft toenails
☐ 4. warmth in the foot

76. A client with absent peripheral pulses and pain at rest is scheduled for an arterial Doppler study of the affected extremity. When preparing the client for this test, the nurse should:
☐ 1. have the client sign an informed consent form for the procedure.
☐ 2. administer a pretest sedative as appropriate.
☐ 3. keep the client tobacco free for 30 minutes before the test.
☐ 4. wrap the client's affected foot with a blanket.

77. Which action is **most** helpful to promote circulation for the client with peripheral arterial disease?
☐ 1. resting with the legs elevated above the level of the heart
☐ 2. walking slowly but steadily for 30 minutes twice a day
☐ 3. minimizing activity as much and as often as possible
☐ 4. wearing antiembolism stockings at all times when out of bed

78. What information should the nurse include in the teaching plan for a client with arterial insufficiency to the feet that is being managed conservatively?
☐ 1. Lubricate the feet daily.
☐ 2. Soak the feet in warm water.
☐ 3. Apply antiembolism stockings.
☐ 4. Wear firm, supportive leather shoes.

79. A client says, "I hate the idea of being an invalid after they cut off my leg." Which response by the nurse would be the **most** therapeutic?
☐ 1. "At least you will still have one good leg to use."
☐ 2. "Tell me more about how you are feeling."
☐ 3. "Let us finish the preoperative teaching."
☐ 4. "You are lucky to have a wife to care for you."

80. The client asks the nurse, "Why will the healthcare provider not tell me exactly how much of my leg he is going to take off? Do you not think I should know that?" On which information should the nurse base the response?
☐ 1. the need to remove as much of the leg as possible
☐ 2. the adequacy of the blood supply to the tissues
☐ 3. the ease with which a prosthesis can be fitted
☐ 4. the client's ability to walk with a prosthesis

81. A client who has had an above-the-knee amputation develops a dime-sized bright red spot on the dressing after 45 minutes in the postanesthesia recovery unit. The nurse should **first**:
☐ 1. elevate the stump.
☐ 2. reinforce the dressing.
☐ 3. call the surgeon.
☐ 4. draw a mark around the site.

82. A client in the postanesthesia care unit with a left below-the-knee amputation has pain in the left big toe. What should the nurse do **first**?
☐ 1. Tell the client it is impossible to feel the pain.
☐ 2. Show the client that the toes are not there.
☐ 3. Explain to the client that the pain is real.
☐ 4. Give the client the prescribed opioid analgesic.

83. The client with an above-the-knee amputation is to use crutches while the prosthesis is being adjusted. Which exercises will **best** prepare the client for using crutches?
- ☐ 1. abdominal exercises
- ☐ 2. isometric shoulder exercises
- ☐ 3. quadriceps setting exercises
- ☐ 4. triceps strengthening exercises

84. The nurse teaches a client about using crutches, instructing the client to support the weight **primarily** on the:
- ☐ 1. axillae.
- ☐ 2. elbows.
- ☐ 3. upper arms.
- ☐ 4. hands.

85. The client is to be discharged on a low-fat, low-cholesterol, low-sodium diet. When coaching the client about the diet, the nurse should **first**:
- ☐ 1. determine the client's knowledge level about cholesterol.
- ☐ 2. ask the client to name foods that are high in fat, cholesterol, and salt.
- ☐ 3. explain the importance of complying with the diet.
- ☐ 4. assess the client's and family's typical food preferences.

The Client with Fractures

86. A client has a leg immobilized in traction. Which observation by the nurse indicates that the client understands actions to take to prevent muscle atrophy?
- ☐ 1. The client adducts the affected leg every 2 hours.
- ☐ 2. The client rolls the affected leg away from the body's midline twice per day.
- ☐ 3. The client performs isometric exercises to the affected extremity three times per day.
- ☐ 4. The client asks the nurse to add a 5-lb (2.3-kg) weight to the traction for 30 min/day.

87. The client with a fractured tibia has been taking methocarbamol. Which finding indicates that the drug is having the intended effect?
- ☐ 1. lack of infection
- ☐ 2. reduction in itching
- ☐ 3. relief of muscle spasms
- ☐ 4. decrease in nervousness

88. When developing a teaching plan for a client who is prescribed acetaminophen for muscle pain, which information should the nurse expect to include? Select all that apply.
- ☐ 1. The drug can be used if the person is allergic to aspirin.
- ☐ 2. Acetaminophen does not affect platelet aggregation.
- ☐ 3. This drug causes little or no gastric distress.
- ☐ 4. Acetaminophen exerts a strong anti-inflammatory effect.
- ☐ 5. The client should have the international normalized ratio (INR) checked regularly.

89. A client who has been taking hydrocodone with acetaminophen at home for 6 weeks following a fractured tibia is admitted with a blood pressure of 80/50 mm Hg, a pulse rate of 115 bpm, and respirations of 8 breaths/min and shallow. The nurse interprets these findings as indicating:
- ☐ 1. expected common adverse effects of the hydrocodone.
- ☐ 2. hypersensitivity reaction to the acetaminophen.
- ☐ 3. possible habituating effect of the long-term drug use.
- ☐ 4. hemorrhage from gastrointestinal irritation associated with the pain medication.

90. The nurse is caring for a client who is 30 years of age with a fracture of the right femur and left tibia. Both legs have casts. The nurse assesses the following: respirations are 30 per minute and are rapid and shallow; there is presence of faint expiratory wheeze; and coughing produces thin pink sputum. The client is yelling at the nurse and wants to be released from the hospital; this is behavior unlike that previously reported. The last pain medication was administered 3 hours ago. The nurse should **first**:
- ☐ 1. cut slits in the top of the casts.
- ☐ 2. administer pain medication.
- ☐ 3. notify the healthcare provider (HCP).
- ☐ 4. obtain a chest x-ray.

91. A client is being discharged following an open reduction and internal fixation of the left ankle and is to wear a non–weight-bearing cast for 2 weeks. What should the nurse teach the client to do when using crutches?
- ☐ 1. Use a four-point gait.
- ☐ 2. Maintain two to three finger widths between the axillary fold and underarm piece grip.
- ☐ 3. Keep leg dependent when sitting.
- ☐ 4. Maintain balance by supporting body's weight on the axillae.

92. The nurse is caring for an adult with a grade III compound fracture of the right femur; the client has been placed in skeletal traction. The intended outcome of the traction is to:
☐ 1. prevent skin breakdown.
☐ 2. prevent movement in the bed.
☐ 3. preserve normal length of the leg.
☐ 4. reduce and immobilize the fracture.

93. An older adult is admitted with a fracture of the femur. The nurse should **first** assess:
☐ 1. ability to change positions.
☐ 2. type of pain.
☐ 3. mechanism of injury.
☐ 4. extent of anxiety.

94. When admitting a client with a fractured extremity, the nurse should **first** assess:
☐ 1. the area proximal to the fracture.
☐ 2. the actual fracture site.
☐ 3. the area distal to the fracture.
☐ 4. the opposite extremity for baseline comparison.

95. Which client statement identifies a knowledge deficit about cast care?
☐ 1. "I will elevate the cast above my heart initially."
☐ 2. "I will exercise my joints above and below the cast."
☐ 3. "I can pull out cast padding to scratch inside the cast."
☐ 4. "I will apply ice for 10 minutes to control edema for the first 24 hours."

96. Which nursing action would be **least** appropriate for a client who is in a double hip spica cast?
☐ 1. encouraging the intake of cranberry juice
☐ 2. advising the client to eat large amounts of cheese
☐ 3. establishing regular times for elimination
☐ 4. having the client dangle at the bedside

97. The nurse is preparing a teaching plan for a client about crutch walking using a two-point gait pattern. What information should the nurse include?
☐ 1. Advance a crutch on one side, and then advance the opposite foot; repeat on the opposite side.
☐ 2. Advance a crutch on one side, and simultaneously advance and bear weight on the opposite foot; repeat on the opposite side.
☐ 3. Advance both crutches together, and then follow by lifting both lower extremities to the level of the crutches.
☐ 4. Advance both crutches together, and then follow by lifting both lower extremities past the level of the crutches.

98. A client returned from surgery with a debrided open tibial fracture and has a three-way drainage system. The client's vital signs are within normal limits. What should the nurse do **next**?
☐ 1. Review the results of culture and sensitivity testing of the wound.
☐ 2. Look for the presence of a pressure dressing over the wound.
☐ 3. Determine if the client has increased pain from exposed nerve endings.
☐ 4. Check laboratory results for electrolyte imbalances.

99. A client has a left tibial fracture that required casting. Approximately 5 hours later, the client has increasing pain distal to the fracture despite the morphine injection administered 30 minutes previously. Which area should be the nurse's **next** assessment?
☐ 1. distal pulses
☐ 2. pain with a pain rating scale
☐ 3. vital sign changes
☐ 4. potential for drug tolerance

100. A client with a fracture develops compartment syndrome. Which sign should alert the nurse to impending organ failure?
☐ 1. crackles
☐ 2. jaundice
☐ 3. generalized edema
☐ 4. dark, scanty urine

The Client with a Femoral Fracture

101. A client with a fractured right femur has not had any immunizations since childhood. Which biologic products should the nurse administer to provide the client with passive immunity for tetanus?
☐ 1. tetanus toxoid
☐ 2. tetanus antigen
☐ 3. tetanus vaccine
☐ 4. tetanus antitoxin

102. After teaching the client about the use of skeletal traction which statement about the purpose of the traction indicates the client needs additional teaching?
☐ 1. to align injured bones.
☐ 2. to provide long-term pull.
☐ 3. to apply 25 lb (11.3 kg) of traction.
☐ 4. to pull weight with a boot.

103. The nurse is planning care for the client with a femoral fracture who is in balanced suspension traction. Which nursing action is **least** likely to be included in the plan of care?
- [ ] 1. use of a fracture bedpan
- [ ] 2. checks for redness over the ischial tuberosity
- [ ] 3. elevation of the head of bed no more than 25 degrees
- [ ] 4. personal hygiene with a complete bed bath

104. The client in balanced suspension traction is transported to surgery for closed reduction and internal fixation of a fractured femur. What should the nurse do when transporting the client to the operating room?
- [ ] 1. Transfer the client to a cart with manually suspended traction.
- [ ] 2. Call the surgeon to request a prescription to temporarily remove the traction.
- [ ] 3. Send the client on the bed with extra help to stabilize the traction.
- [ ] 4. Remove the traction and send the client on a cart.

105. A client has a Pearson attachment on the traction setup. What is the purpose of this attachment?
- [ ] 1. to support the lower portion of the leg
- [ ] 2. to support the thigh and upper leg
- [ ] 3. to allow attachment of the skeletal pin
- [ ] 4. to prevent flexion deformities in the ankle and foot

106. Which sign indicates that a client with a fracture of the right femur may be developing a fat embolus?
- [ ] 1. acute respiratory distress syndrome
- [ ] 2. migraine-like headaches
- [ ] 3. numbness in the right leg
- [ ] 4. muscle spasms in the right thigh

107. Which goal is the **priority** for a client with a fractured femur who is in traction at this time?
- [ ] 1. Prevent effects of immobility while in traction.
- [ ] 2. Develop skills to cope with prolonged immobility.
- [ ] 3. Choose appropriate diversional activities during the prolonged recovery.
- [ ] 4. Adapt to inactivity from the impaired mobility.

108. The client in traction for a fractured femur is having difficulty managing self-care activities. Which outcome indicates a successful completion of a goal of promoting independence for this client?
- [ ] 1. The client assists as much as possible in care, demonstrating increased participation over time.
- [ ] 2. The client allows the nurse to complete care in an efficient manner without interfering.
- [ ] 3. The client allows the spouse to assume total responsibility for care.
- [ ] 4. The client accepts that self-care is not possible while in traction.

109. The client with an open femoral fracture was discharged to home and reports having a fever, night sweats, chills, restlessness, and restrictive movement of the fractured leg. The nurse should interpret these findings as the client may be experiencing:
- [ ] 1. a pulmonary embolus.
- [ ] 2. osteomyelitis.
- [ ] 3. a fat embolus.
- [ ] 4. a urinary tract infection.

110. The nurse is planning care for a client with osteomyelitis. The client is taking an antibiotic, but the infection has not resolved. The nurse should advise the client to:
- [ ] 1. use herbal supplements.
- [ ] 2. eat a diet high in protein and vitamins C and D.
- [ ] 3. ask the healthcare provider (HCP) for a change of antibiotics.
- [ ] 4. encourage frequent passive range of motion to the affected extremity.

The Client with a Spinal Cord Injury

111. When planning to move a person with a possible spinal cord injury, the nurse should direct the team to:
- [ ] 1. limit movement of the arms by wrapping them next to the body.
- [ ] 2. move the person gently to help reduce pain.
- [ ] 3. immobilize the head and neck to prevent further injury.
- [ ] 4. cushion the back with pillows to ensure comfort.

112. The nurse is caring for a client with a spinal cord injury. The client is experiencing blurred vision and has a blood pressure of 204/102 mm Hg. What should the nurse do **first**?
- [ ] 1. Position the client on the left side.
- [ ] 2. Control the environment by turning the lights off and decreasing stimulation for the client.
- [ ] 3. Check the client's bladder for distention.
- [ ] 4. Administer pain medications.

113. The nurse is taking care of a client with a spinal cord injury. The extent of the client's injury is shown below. Which finding is expected when assessing this client?
☐ 1. inability to move the arms
☐ 2. loss of sensation in the hands and fingers
☐ 3. dysfunction of bowel and bladder
☐ 4. difficulty breathing

114. When the client has a cord transection at T4, the nurse should focus the assessment on:
☐ 1. renal status.
☐ 2. vascular status.
☐ 3. gastrointestinal function.
☐ 4. biliary function.

115. When assessing the client with a cord transection above T5 for possible complications, which complication is **least** likely to occur?
☐ 1. diarrhea
☐ 2. paralytic ileus
☐ 3. stress ulcers
☐ 4. intra-abdominal bleeding

116. Which is the **best** method to assess for the development of deep vein thrombosis in a client with a spinal cord injury?
☐ 1. Homans' sign
☐ 2. pain
☐ 3. tenderness
☐ 4. leg girth

117. During the period of spinal shock, the nurse should expect the client's bladder function to be:
☐ 1. spastic.
☐ 2. normal.
☐ 3. atonic.
☐ 4. uncontrolled.

118. After 1 month of therapy, the client in spinal shock begins to experience muscle spasms in the legs and calls the nurse in excitement to report the leg movement. Which response by the nurse would be the **most** accurate?
☐ 1. "These movements indicate that the damaged nerves are healing."
☐ 2. "This is a good sign. Keep trying to move all the affected muscles."
☐ 3. "The return of movement means that eventually you should be able to walk again."
☐ 4. "The movements occur from muscle reflexes that cannot be initiated or controlled by the brain."

119. The client with a spinal cord injury asks the nurse why the dietitian has recommended to decrease the total daily intake of calcium. Which response by the nurse would provide the **most** accurate information?
☐ 1. "Excessive intake of dairy products makes constipation more common."
☐ 2. "Immobility increases calcium absorption from the intestine."
☐ 3. "Lack of weight bearing causes demineralization of the long bones."
☐ 4. "Dairy products likely will contribute to weight gain."

120. As a first step in teaching a woman with a spinal cord injury and quadriplegia about her sexual health, the nurse assesses her understanding of her current sexual functioning. Which statement by the client indicates she understands her current ability?
☐ 1. "I will not be able to have sexual intercourse until the urinary catheter is removed."
☐ 2. "I can participate in sexual activity but might not experience orgasm."
☐ 3. "I cannot have sexual intercourse because it causes hypertension, but other sexual activity is okay."
☐ 4. "I should be able to participate in sexual activity, but I will be infertile."

121. A client with a spinal cord injury who has been active in sports and outdoor activities talks almost obsessively about his past activities. In tears, one day he asks the nurse, "Why am I unable to stop talking about these things? I know those days are gone forever." Which response by the nurse conveys the **best** understanding of the client's behavior?
☐ 1. "Be patient. It takes time to adjust to such a massive loss."
☐ 2. "Talking about the past is a form of denial. We have to help you focus on today."
☐ 3. "Reviewing your losses is a way to help you work through your grief and loss."
☐ 4. "It is a simple escape mechanism to go back and live again in happier times."

Managing Care, Quality, and Safety of Clients with Musculoskeletal Health Problems

122. The nurse should asses which clients for risk for falling? Select all that apply.
☐ 1. client who is 45 years of age, in hospice with terminal cancer, and receiving morphine every 2 hours
☐ 2. client who is 70 years of age, hospitalized for lung biopsy, and receiving no medications
☐ 3. client who is 62 years of age, recovering from breast biopsy in outpatient surgery, and has a fear of falling
☐ 4. client who is 80 years of age and in a locked facility for clients with cognitive impairment
☐ 5. client who is 75 years of age and recovering at home from hip replacement surgery on the left hip

123. Four days after surgery for internal fixation of a C3–C4 fracture, a nurse is moving a client from the bed to the wheelchair. The nurse is checking the wheelchair for correct features for this client. Which features of the wheelchair are appropriate for the needs of this client? Select all that apply.
☐ 1. back at the level of the client's scapula
☐ 2. back and head that are high
☐ 3. seat that is lower than normal
☐ 4. seat with firm cushions
☐ 5. chair controlled by the client's breath

124. The nurse is planning care for a group of clients who have had total hip replacement. Of the clients listed below, who is at **highest** risk for infection and should be assessed **first**?
☐ 1. a 55-year-old client who is 6 feet (180 cm) tall and weighs 180 lb (81.7 kg)
☐ 2. a 90-year-old who lives alone
☐ 3. a 74-year-old who has periodontal disease with periodontitis
☐ 4. a 75-year-old who has asthma and uses an inhaler

125. The nurse is documenting care of a client who is restrained in bed with bilateral wrist restraints. Following assessment of the restraints, what should the nurse's documentation include? Select all that apply.
☐ 1. nutrition and hydration needs
☐ 2. capillary refill
☐ 3. continued need for restraints
☐ 4. need for medication
☐ 5. skin integrity

126. The nurse is instituting a falls prevention program. Which personnel should be involved in the program? Select all that apply.
☐ 1. registered nurses (RNs)
☐ 2. insurance providers
☐ 3. unlicensed assistive personnel (UAP)
☐ 4. housekeeping services
☐ 5. family members
☐ 6. client

127. The nurse unit manager is making rounds on a team of clients and notices a client who is wearing red slipper socks and a color-coded armband that indicates the client is at risk for falling walking down the hall unassisted. The client is already at the end of the hallway farthest from the client's room, but is not tired. What should the nurse do **first**?
☐ 1. Obtain a wheel chair, and take the client back to the room.
☐ 2. Walk with the client back to the room, and assist the client to get in bed.
☐ 3. Locate an unlicensed nursing personnel (UAP) to walk with the client back to the room.
☐ 4. Instruct the client to walk only in the room at this time.

128. The healthcare provider has prescribed 5 mg warfarin orally for a hospitalized client. In planning care for this client, the nurse should verify that which services have been contacted? Check all that apply.
☐ 1. pharmacy
☐ 2. dietary
☐ 3. laboratory
☐ 4. discharge planning
☐ 5. chaplain

129. Unlicensed assistive personnel (UAP) are helping a client who has had knee surgery 2 days ago get into bed. As the nurse makes rounds, which information requires the nurse to intervene?
☐ 1. The call light is pinned to the head of the bed in the client's reach.
☐ 2. The night light is dimmed, giving low-level lighting to the room.
☐ 3. There is a clear path to the bathroom.
☐ 4. The side rails on the head and foot of the bed are in the up position.

130. The nurse on the orthopedic unit is going to lunch and is conducting a "hand-off" to the charge nurse. The goal of the "hand-off" communication is:
☐ 1. to ensure the charge nurse understands that the nurse is going to lunch.
☐ 2. to be sure the charge nurse assigns someone else to take care of the client.
☐ 3. to provide accurate information about client's care to the next caregiver.
☐ 4. to provide in-depth information about the client's history.

131. The client has been diagnosed with septic arthritis in a hip joint. Which outcomes are desired from a client-focused teaching plan? Select all that apply.

☐ 1. Report pain that is severe enough to limit activities.

☐ 2. Discuss how to take prescribed medications.

☐ 3. Describe how the application of a heating pad set on "high" readily resolves edema.

☐ 4. Describe the septic arthritis physiologic process.

☐ 5. Explain the importance of supporting the affected joint.

☐ 6. Describe how to use ambulatory aids and assistive devices.

132. The nurse should perform passive range-of-motion (ROM) exercises on which clients? Select all that apply.

☐ 1. a client who has septic joints

☐ 2. a client who has temporary loss of sensation

☐ 3. a client who is unconsciousness

☐ 4. a client who has plantar flexion of the foot

☐ 5. a client who has supination of the hand

Answers, Rationales, and Test-Taking Strategies

*The answers and rationales for each question follow below, along with keys (🔑) to the client need (CN) and cognitive level (CL) for each question. In addition, you will also see a glossary icon (📖) highlighting specific terminology used on the licensing exam. As you check your answers, use the **Content Mastery and Test-Taking Skill Self-Analysis** worksheet (tear-out worksheet in back of book) to identify the reason(s) for not answering the questions correctly. For additional information about test-taking skills and strategies for answering questions, refer to pages 12–23 and pages 35–36 in Part 1 of this book.*

The Client with Rheumatoid Arthritis

1. 3. Initially, most clients with early symptoms of rheumatoid arthritis report early morning stiffness or stiffness after sitting still for a while. Later symptoms of rheumatoid arthritis include limited joint range of motion; deformed joints, especially of the hand; and rheumatoid nodules.

🔑 CN: Physiological adaptation; CL: Analyze

2. 1. Based on the information from the client, the nurse should develop a plan with the client that will conserve energy and decrease episodes of fatigue. Although the client may develop a self-care deficit related to the increasing joint pain, the client is voicing concerns about household chores and difficulty around the house and yard, not self-care issues. Over time, the client may have difficulty coping, but that is not the current concern. Employing cleaning services may not be within the client's budget, and the client should first try a plan that balances rest and activity.

🔑 CN: Basic care and comfort; CL: Analyze

3. 1,2,4. RA affects women three times more often than men between the ages of 20 and 55 years. Research has determined that RA occurs in clients who have had infectious disease, such as the Epstein-Barr virus. The genetic link, specifically HLA-DR4, has been found in 65% of clients with RA. People with osteoarthritis are not necessarily at risk for developing RA.

🔑 CN: Reduction of risk potential; CL: Analyze

4. 1,2,4,3. Pain relief is the highest priority during the acute phase because pain is typically severe and interferes with the client's ability to function. Preserving joint function is the next goal to set, followed by preventing joint deformity during the acute phase to promote an optimal level of functioning and reduce the risk of contractures. Maintaining usual ways of accomplishing tasks is the goal with the lowest priority during the acute phase. Rather, the focus is on developing less stressful ways of accomplishing routine tasks.

🔑 CN: Physiological adaptation; CL: Synthesize

5. 3. Heat-producing liniment can produce a burn if used with other heat devices that could intensify the response to the heat. Heat and cold can be used as often as the client desires. However, each application of heat should not exceed 20 minutes, and each application of cold should not exceed 10 to 15 minutes. Application for longer periods results in the opposite of the intended effect: vasoconstriction instead of vasodilation with heat, and vasodilation instead of vasoconstriction with cold.

🔑 CN: Reduction of risk potential; CL: Evaluate

6. 4. The nurse's most appropriate response is one that is therapeutic. The basic principle of therapeutic communication and a therapeutic relationship is honesty. Therefore, the nurse needs to explain truthfully that each client is different and that there are various forms of arthritis and arthritis treatment. To state that it is the **HCP's** 📖 prerogative to decide how to treat the client implies that the client is not a member of his or her own healthcare team and is not a participant in his or her care. The statement also is defensive, which serves to block any further communication or questions. Asking the client to tell more about the friend presumes that the client knows correct and complete information, which is not a valid assumption to make. The nurse does not know about the client's friend and should not make statements about another client's condition. Stating that the drug is for advanced disease demonstrates that the nurse is making assumptions that are not necessarily valid or appropriate. Also, telling the client that he or she is not eligible for the drug now is not within the scope of the nurse's practice.

🗝️ CN: Psychosocial adaptation; CL: Synthesize

7. 4. Positions of flexion should be avoided to prevent loss of functional ability of affected joints. Proper body alignment during rest periods is encouraged to maintain correct muscle and joint placement. Lying in the prone position is encouraged to avoid further curvature of the spine and internal rotation of the shoulders.

🗝️ CN: Physiological adaptation; CL: Synthesize

8. 4. Carrying a laundry basket with clinched fingers and fists is not an example of conserving energy of small joints. The laundry basket should be held with both hands opened as wide as possible and with outstretched arms so that pressure is not placed on the small joints of the fingers. When rising from a chair, the palms should be used instead of the fingers so as to distribute weight over the larger area of the palms. Holding packages close to the body provides greater support to the shoulder, elbow, and wrist joints because muscles of the arms and hands are used to stabilize the weight against the body. This decreases the stress and weight or pull on small joints such as the fingers. Objects can be slid with the palm of the hand, which distributes weight over the larger area of the palms instead of stressing the small joints of the fingers to pick up the weight of the object to move it to another place.

🗝️ CN: Basic care and comfort; CL: Evaluate

9. 1. Because some over-the-counter vitamin supplements contain folic acid, the client should avoid self-medication with vitamins while taking methotrexate, a folic acid antagonist. Because methotrexate is hepatotoxic, the client should avoid the intake of alcohol, which could increase the risk for hepatotoxicity. Methotrexate can cause bone marrow depression, placing the client at risk for infection. Therefore, meticulous mouth care is essential to minimize the risk of infection. Contraception should be used during methotrexate therapy and for 8 weeks after the therapy has been discontinued because of its effect on mitosis. Methotrexate is considered teratogenic.

🗝️ CN: Pharmacological and parenteral therapies; CL: Evaluate

10. 2. Difficulty seeing out of one eye, when evaluated in conjunction with the client's medication therapy regimen, leads to the suspicion of possible retinal degeneration. The possibility of an irreversible retinal degeneration caused by deposits of hydroxychloroquine in the layers of the retina requires an ophthalmologic examination before therapy is begun and at 6-month intervals. Although cataracts may develop in young adults, they are less likely, and damage from the hydroxychloroquine is the most obvious at-risk factor. Eyesight is not affected by the disease process of rheumatoid arthritis.

🗝️ CN: Pharmacological and parenteral therapies; CL: Analyze

11. 1. Gastric upset is a side effect of nonsteroidal anti-inflammatory medications; taking medication with food minimizes this effect. Corticosteroids affect adrenal gland function and are discontinued by lowering the dose gradually, but this is not true of nonsteroidal anti-inflammatory medications. It is not necessary to rinse the mouth, as stomatitis is not a usual side effect. Dizziness is not an effect of this drug.

🗝️ CN: Pharmacological and parenteral therapies; CL: Synthesize

12. 4. Superficial heat applications, such as tub baths, showers, and warm compresses, can be helpful in relieving pain and stiffness. Exercises can be performed more comfortably and more effectively after heat applications. The client with rheumatoid arthritis must balance rest with exercise every day, not every other day. Typically, large doses of analgesics, which can lead to hepatotoxic effects, are not necessary. Learning to cope with the pain by refocusing is inappropriate.

🗝️ CN: Basic care and comfort; CL: Synthesize

13. 1,2,5. An arthrocentesis is performed to aspirate excess synovial fluid, pus, or blood from a joint cavity to relieve pain or to diagnose inflammatory diseases such as rheumatoid arthritis. A local agent may be used to decrease the pain of the needle insertion through the skin and into the joint cavity. Aspiration of the fluid into the syringe can be very painful because of the size and inflammation of the joint. Usually, a steroid medication is injected locally to alleviate the inflammation; a compression bandage is applied to help decrease swelling; and the client is asked to rest the joint for up to 24 hours afterward to help relieve the pain and promote rest to the inflamed joint. The client may experience pain during this time until the inflammation begins to resolve and swelling decreases.

🔑 CN: Reduction of risk potential; CL: Create

The Client with Osteoarthritis

14. 1,4,5. To prepare a client for an arthrocentesis, the nurse should tell the client that a local anesthetic administered by the **healthcare provider (HCP)** 📖 will decrease discomfort. There may be bleeding after the procedure, so the nurse should check the dressing. The client may experience pain. The nurse should offer pain medication and evaluate outcomes for pain relief. Because a local anesthetic is used, the client will not require preoperative medication. The client will rest the knee for 24 hours and then should begin range-of-motion and muscle-strengthening exercises.

🔑 CN: Management of care; CL: Create

15. 1. Metal will interfere with the test. Metallic objects within the examination field, such as jewelry, earrings, and dental amalgams, may inhibit organ visualization and can produce unclear images. Ingesting foods and beverages days before the test will not affect bone mineral status. Short-term calcium gluconate intake will also not influence bone mineral status. The client may already have had chronic pain as a result of a bone fracture or from osteoporosis.

🔑 CN: Management of care; CL: Synthesize

16. 1. Shorter sessions will allow the client to rest between the sessions. Changing the **HCP's** 📖 prescription to a different examination will not provide the information needed for this client's treatment. Acetaminophen is a nonopioid analgesic and an antipyretic, not an anti-inflammatory agent; thus, it would not help this client avoid the adverse effects of a lengthy x-ray examination. Although the x-ray table is hard, it is not possible to provide padding and obtain the needed diagnostic x-rays.

🔑 CN: Management of care; CL: Synthesize

17. 4. Osteoarthritis is a degenerative joint disease with local manifestations such as local joint pain. Rheumatoid arthritis has systemic manifestation such as anemia and osteoporosis. Weight loss occurs in rheumatoid arthritis, whereas most clients with osteoarthritis are overweight.

🔑 CN: Physiological adaptation; CL: Analyze

18. 1,2,3. A diet with adequate amounts of vitamin D aids in the regulation, absorption, and subsequent utilization of calcium and phosphorus, which are necessary for the normal calcification of bone. Figs, broccoli, and almonds are very good sources of calcium. Moderate intake of alcohol has no known negative effects on bone density, but excessive alcohol intake does reduce bone density. Swimming, biking, and other non–weight-bearing exercises do not maintain bone mass. Walking and running, which are weight-bearing exercises, do maintain bone mass. The client should eat a balanced diet but does not need to avoid high-fat foods.

🔑 CN: Reduction of risk potential; CL: Create

19. 1. Capsaicin cream, which produces analgesia by preventing the reaccumulation of substance P in the peripheral sensory neurons, is made from the active ingredients of hot peppers. Therefore, clients should wash their hands immediately after applying capsaicin cream if they do not wear gloves, to avoid possible contact between the cream and mucous membranes. Clients are instructed to avoid wearing tight bandages over areas where capsaicin cream has been applied because swelling may occur from inflammation of the arthritis in the joint and lead to constriction on the peripheral neurovascular system. Capsaicin cream should be stored in areas between 59°F and 86°F (15°C and 30°C). The cabinet over the stove in the kitchen would be too warm. Capsaicin cream should not come in contact with irritated and broken skin, mucous membranes, or eyes. Therefore, it should not be used on cuts or burns.

🔑 CN: Pharmacological and parenteral therapies; CL: Evaluate

20. 3. Drugs that cause gastric irritation, such as ibuprofen, are best taken after or with a meal, when stomach contents help minimize the local irritation. Taking the medication on an empty stomach at any time during the day will lead to gastric irritation. Taking the drug at bedtime with food may cause the client to gain weight, possibly aggravating the osteoarthritis. When the client arises, he or she is stiff from immobility and should use warmth and stretching until he or she gets food in the stomach.

🔑 CN: Pharmacological and parenteral therapies; CL: Synthesize

21. 1. Corticosteroids are used for clients with osteoarthritis to obtain a local effect. Therefore, they are given only via intra-articular injection. Oral corticosteroids are avoided because they can cause an acceleration of osteoarthritis. Rheumatoid arthritis and osteoarthritis are two different diseases.

⊶ CN: Pharmacological and parenteral therapies; CL: Synthesize

22. 2. Weight-bearing exercise plays a very important role in stimulating regeneration of cartilage, which lacks blood vessels, by driving synovial fluid through the joint cartilage. Joint mobility is increased by weight-bearing exercises, not range-of-motion exercises, because surrounding muscles, ligaments, and tendons are strengthened. Pain is an early sign of degenerative joint bone problems. Swelling may not occur for some time after pain, if at all. Osteoarthritic pain is worsened in cold, damp weather; therefore, exercising outdoors is not recommended year round in all settings.

⊶ CN: Health promotion and maintenance; CL: Evaluate

The Client with a Hip Fracture

23. 4. The hip spica cast is used for treatment of femoral fractures; it immobilizes the affected extremity and the trunk securely. It extends from above the nipple line to the base of the foot of both extremities in a double hip spica. Constipation, possible due to lack of mobility, can cause abdominal distention or bloating. When the spica cast becomes too tight due to distention, the cast will compress the superior mesenteric artery against the duodenum. The compression produces abdominal pain, abdominal pressure, nausea, and vomiting. To relieve the compression, the surgeon can cut a "window" in the cast. The nurse should assess the abdomen for decreased bowel sounds, not the superior mesenteric artery. The surgeon cannot manipulate a fracture through a small window in a double hip spica cast. The nurse cannot use the window to aid in repositioning because the window opening can break and negate the effect of the cast.

⊶ CN: Reduction of risk potential; CL: Evaluate

24. 3. With an intracapsular hip fracture, the affected leg is shorter than the unaffected leg because of the muscle spasms and external rotation. The client also experiences severe pain in the region of the fracture.

⊶ CN: Physiological adaptation; CL: Analyze

25. 4. Insertion of a pin for the internal fixation of an extracapsular fractured hip provides good fixation of the fracture. The fracture site is stabilized, and fractured bone ends are well approximated. As a result, the client is able to be mobilized sooner, thus reducing the risks of complications related to immobility. Internal fixation with a pin insertion does not prevent hemorrhage or decrease the risk of neurovascular impairment, which are potential complications associated with any joint or bone surgery. It does not lessen the client's risk of infection at the site.

⊶ CN: Reduction of risk potential; CL: Apply

26. 3. The primary purpose of the drainage tube is to prevent fluid accumulation in the wound. Fluid, when it accumulates, creates dead space. Elimination of the dead space by keeping the wound free of fluid greatly enhances wound healing and helps prevent abscess formation. Although the characteristics of the drainage from the tube, such as a change in color or appearance, may suggest a possible infection, this is not the tube's primary purpose. The drainage tube does not eliminate the need for wound irrigation or provide a way to instill antibiotics into the wound.

⊶ CN: Reduction of risk potential; CL: Apply

27. 1. Any activity or position that causes flexion, adduction, or internal rotation of >90 degrees should be avoided until the soft tissue surrounding the prosthesis has stabilized, at approximately 6 weeks. Crossing the legs while sitting down causes internal rotation and can lead to dislocation of the femoral head from the hip socket. Sitting on a raised commode seat prevents hip flexion and adduction. Using an abductor splint while side-lying keeps the hip joint in abduction, thus preventing adduction and possible dislocation. Rising straight from a chair to a standing position is acceptable for this client because this action avoids hip flexion, adduction, and internal rotation of >90 degrees.

⊶ CN: Reduction of risk potential; CL: Synthesize

28. 3. Troponin is a cardiac biomarker and is normally almost undetectable in the blood. A level of 1.4 means there has likely been some damage to the heart muscle. Though serum glucose (normal 60 to 100 mg/dL [3.3 to 5.5 mmol/L]) and ESR (normal is <20 for males >50 years old) are slightly elevated, this could be explained by normal stress and inflammatory response to surgery. The hematocrit is low (normal 40 to 45 [0.4 to 0.5] for men) but also not unexpected for a client following surgery.

⊶ CN: Physiological adaption; CL: Synthesize

29. 3. A high-backed straight chair with arm-rests is recommended to help keep the client in the best possible alignment after surgery for a femoral head prosthesis placement. Use of this type of chair helps to prevent dislocation of the prosthesis from the socket. A desk-type swivel chair, padded uphol-stered chair, or recliner should be avoided because it does not provide for good body alignment and can cause the overly flexed femoral head to dislocate.

🔑 CN: Reduction of risk potential;
CL: Synthesize

30. The air cell should be centered on the back of the client's calf.

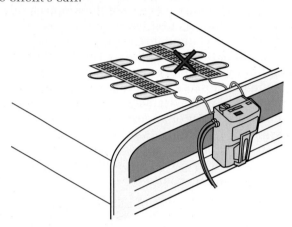

🔑 CN: Safety and infection control;
CL: Apply

31. 2. Although pets and furniture, such as snack tables and rocking chairs, may pose a problem, scatter rugs are the single greatest hazard in the home, especially for elderly people who are unsure and unsteady with walking. Falls have been found to account for almost half the accidental deaths that occur in the home. The risk of falls is further com-pounded by the client's need for crutches.

🔑 CN: Safety and infection control;
CL: Synthesize

The Client Having Hip Replacement Surgery

32. 3. To obtain best results, one sheet should be used to cover the mattress. The air cells should be facing up as shown. Thick pads should not be used; if the client is incontinent, a "breathable" inconti-nent pad can be added. The client can use a pillow as needed.

33. 2,3,4,5. A client who has had a posterolateral total hip replacement should not adduct the hip joint, which would lead to dislocation of the ball out of the socket; therefore, the client should be encour-aged to keep the toes pointed slightly outward when using a walker. An abduction pillow should be kept between the legs to keep the hip joint in an abducted position. The client should rotate between lying supine and lateral on the unoperated side, but not on the operated side. Ice is used to reduce swell-ing on the operative side. The client should not flex the operated hip beyond a 90-degree angle, such as when bending down to tie or slip on shoes. Doing so could lead to joint dislocation.

🔑 CN: Reduction of risk potential;
CL: Create

34. 1,3,4. A client who has had a total hip replacement via an anterolateral approach has almost the opposite precautions as those for a client who has had a total hip replacement through the posterolateral approach. The hip joint should not be actively abducted. The client should avoid turning the toes or knee outward. The client should keep the legs side by side without a pillow or wedge. The client should use an elevated toilet seat and shower chair and should not extend the operative leg back-ward. The client should perform range-of-motion exercises as directed by the physical therapist.

🔑 CN: Reduction of risk potential;
CL: Create

35. 2. Being unable to move the affected leg sug-gests neurologic impairment. A decrease in the dis-tal pulse, diminished capillary refill, and coolness to touch of the affected extremity suggest vascular compromise.

🔑 CN: Reduction of risk potential;
CL: Analyze

36. 4. The nurse should first identify and discuss the client's fears about the procedure. Only then can the client begin to hear what the nurse has to share about the individualized teaching plan designed to meet the client's needs. In the preoperative period, the client needs to learn how to correctly prevent hip flexion and to demonstrate coughing and deep breathing. However, this teaching can be effective only after the client's fears have been assessed and addressed. Although the client may appreciate see-ing what a hip prosthesis looks like, so as to under-stand the new body part, this is not a necessity.

🔑 CN: Psychosocial adaptation;
CL: Synthesize

37. 3. The joint has dislocated when the client with a total joint prosthesis develops severe sudden pain and an inability to move the extremity. Clinical manifestations of an infection would include inflammation, redness, erythema, and possibly drainage and separation of the wound. Bleeding could be external (e.g., blood visible from the wound or on the dressing) or internal and manifested by signs of shock (e.g., pallor, coolness, hypotension, tachycardia). The seepage of glue into soft tissue would have occurred in the operating room, when the glue is still in the liquid form. The glue dries into the hard, fixed form before the wound is closed.

⚷ CN: Reduction of risk potential;
CL: Analyze

38. 1. An average adult requires approximately 1,100 to 1,400 mL of fluids per day. In some instances, such as when a person has an increase in body temperature or has increased perspiration, additional water may be necessary. With an increase in body temperature, there is also an increase in insensible fluid loss. The increased loss of fluid causes an increased need for fluid replacement. If the loss is significant and/or goes untreated, an individual's intake will not be balanced with output. Managing the incision, changing the bed linens, or keeping the client's skin cool are not outcomes indicative of resolution of a fluid volume deficit.

⚷ CN: Physiological adaptation;
CL: Synthesize

39. 4. After total hip replacement, proper positioning by the nurse prevents dislocation of the prosthesis. The nurse should place the client in a supine position and keep the affected extremity in slight abduction using an abduction splint or pillows or Buck's extension traction. The client must not abduct or flex the operated hip because this may produce dislocation.

⚷ CN: Reduction of risk potential;
CL: Synthesize

40. 2,4,5. Following total hip replacement, the client should use the overhead trapeze to assist with position changes. The head of the bed should not be elevated more than 45 degrees; any height >45 degrees puts a strain on the hip joint and may cause dislocation. To use a fracture bedpan, instruct the client to flex the unoperated hip and knee to lift the buttocks onto the pan. Toe-pointing exercises stimulate circulation in the lower extremities to prevent the formation of thrombi and potential emboli. The prone position is avoided shortly after a total hip replacement.

⚷ CN: Reduction of risk potential;
CL: Synthesize

41. 1,3,4. Administration of antibiotics as prescribed will aid in the acquisition of therapeutic blood levels during and immediately after surgery to prevent osteomyelitis. The nurse can request that a trapeze be added to the bed so the client can assist with lifting and turning. The nurse should also demonstrate and have the client practice isometric exercises (muscle setting) of quadriceps and gluteal muscles. The client will not use crutches after surgery; a physical therapy assistant will initially assist the client with walking by using a walker. The client will not use Buck's traction. The client will require antiembolism stockings and use of a leg compression device to minimize the risk of thrombus formation and potential emboli; the leg compression device is applied during surgery and maintained per prescription.

⚷ CN: Physiological adaptation; CL: Create

42. 1,2,3,4. Client/family teaching should include advising the client to report any symptoms of unusual bleeding or bruising, dizziness, itching, rash, fever, swelling, or difficulty breathing to **HCP** 📖 immediately. Instruct the client not to take aspirin or nonsteroidal anti-inflammatory drugs without consulting the HCP while on therapy. A low-molecular-weight heparin is considered to be a high-risk medication, and the client should wear or carry medical identification. The air bubble should not be expelled from the syringe because the bubble ensures the client receives the full dose of the medication. The client should allow 5 seconds to pass before withdrawing the needle to prevent seepage of the medication out of the site.

⚷ CN: Pharmacological and parenteral therapies; CL: Create

43. 3. Dislocation precautions include the following: avoid extremes of internal rotation, adduction, and 90-degree flexion of affected hip for at least 4 to 6 weeks after the procedure. Use of an abduction pillow prevents adduction. Decreasing use of the abductor pillow does not strengthen the muscles to prevent dislocation. Informing a client to "not worry" is not therapeutic. A cushioned toilet seat does not prevent hip dislocation.

⚷ CN: Psychosocial adaptation;
CL: Synthesize

44. 1,2,3. Dislocation of a hip prosthesis may occur with positioning that exceeds the limits of the prosthesis. The nurse must recognize dislocation of the prosthesis. Signs of prosthesis dislocation include acute groin pain in the affected hip, shortening of the affected leg, restricted ability or inability to move the affected leg, and reported "popping" sensation in the hip. Toe wiggling is not a test for potential hip dislocation.

⚷ CN: Reduction of risk potential;
CL: Analyze

45. 4. If a prosthesis becomes dislocated, the nurse should immediately notify the surgeon. This is done so the hip can be reduced and stabilized promptly to prevent nerve damage and to maintain circulation. After closed reduction, the hip may be stabilized with Buck's traction or a brace to prevent recurrent dislocation. If prescribed by the surgeon, an ice pack may be applied postreduction to limit edema, although caution must be utilized due to potential muscle spasms. Some orthopedic surgeons may prescribe the client be turned toward the side of the reduced hip, but that is not the nurse's first response.

☞ CN: Reduction of risk potential;
CL: Synthesize

46. 3. Expected outcomes at the time of discharge from the surgical unit after a hip replacement include the following: increased independence in transfers, participates in progressive ambulation without pain or assistance, and raises the affected leg without assistance. The client will not be able to walk throughout the hospital, walk for a distance without some postoperative pain, or raise the affected leg more than several inches. The client may be referred to a rehabilitation unit in order to achieve the additional independence, strength, and pain relief.

☞ CN: Physiological adaptation;
CL: Evaluate

47. 1. DVT is a complication of total joint replacement and may occur during hospitalization or develop later when the client is home. Clients who are obese or have previous history of a deep vein thrombosis or pulmonary embolism are at high risk. Immobility produces venous stasis, increasing the client's chance to develop a venous thromboembolism. Signs of a DVT include unilateral calf tenderness, warmth, redness, and edema (increased calf circumference). Findings should be reported promptly to the **healthcare provider (HCP)** 📖 for definitive evaluation and therapy. Polyuria may be indicative of diabetes mellitus. Displacement of the new joint is unlikely. Wound evisceration is more likely to occur after abdominal surgeries.

☞ CN: Reduction of risk potential;
CL: Analyze

The Client Having Knee Replacement Surgery

48. 3. When combined with a weight loss program, aquatic exercise would be best because it cushions the joints and allows the client to burn off calories. Aquatic exercise promotes circulation, muscle toning, and lung expansion, which promote healthy preoperative conditioning. Weight lifting and walking are too stressful to the joints, possibly exacerbating the client's osteoarthritis. Although tai chi exercise is designed for stretching and coordination, it would not be the best exercise for this client to help with weight loss.

☞ CN: Physiological adaptation;
CL: Synthesize

49. 1. The nurse should suspect nerve damage if numbness is present. However, whether the damage is short term and related to edema or long term and related to permanent nerve damage would not be clear at this point. The nurse needs to continue to assess the client's neurovascular status, including pain, pallor, pulselessness, paresthesia, and paralysis (the five Ps). Bleeding would suggest vascular damage or hemorrhage. Dislocation would suggest malalignment. Pink color would suggest adequate circulation to the area. Numbness would suggest neurologic damage.

☞ CN: Reduction of risk potential;
CL: Analyze

50. 4. After knee arthroplasty, the knee will be extended and immobilized with a firm compression dressing and an adjustable soft extension splint in place. An SCD will be applied. The SCD can be discontinued when the client is ambulatory, but while the client is in bed the SCD needs to be maintained to prevent thromboembolism. The SCD should be positioned on the bed, but not on two pillows. Settings for the SCD are prescribed by the orthopedic surgeon. Initial dressing changes are completed by the orthopedic surgeon and changed as needed per prescription.

☞ CN: Reduction of risk potential;
CL: Synthesize

51. 2,3. It is anticipated that there might be some swelling, redness, and discomfort immediately after activity, including physical therapy. Ideally, pain medication could be offered or given prior to therapy to reduce posttreatment pain but should be administered now. Elevation and cold packs can also reduce swelling and decrease pain. It is not appropriate to notify the **HCP** 📖 as pain and swelling are normal after therapy. It is also not appropriate to massage the area. This will increase circulation and therefore increase swelling and pain.

☞ CN: Management of care; CL: Synthesize

52. 1,2,3. The nurse should instruct the client to notify the dentist and other **HCPs** of the need to take prophylactic antibiotics if undergoing any procedure (e.g., tooth extraction) due to the potential of bacteremia. The nurse should also advise the client that the metal components of the joint may set off the metal-detector alarms in airports. The client should also report having the metal joint prior to having MRI studies because, depending on the type of joint replacement, the implanted metal components could be pulled toward the large magnet core of the MRI. Any weight bearing that is permitted is prescribed by the orthopedic surgeon and is usually not limited to 5 lb (2.3 kg). Postsurgery, the client can resume a normal diet with regular fluid intake.

CN: Health promotion and maintenance; CL: Create

53. 1. The aPTT is at a critical value, and the client should receive protamine sulfate as the antidote for heparin. Vitamin K is the antidote for warfarin. Packed red blood cells are administered to increase the hematocrit.

CN: Pharmacological and parenteral therapies; CL: Apply

54. 1,2,3,4. Postoperatively, the knee in a total knee replacement is dressed with a compression bandage, and ice may be applied to control edema and bleeding. Recurrent assessment by the nurse for neurovascular changes can prevent loss of limb. Normal neurovascular findings include color normal, extremity warm, capillary refill <3 seconds, moderate edema, tissue not palpably tense, pain controllable, normal sensations, no paresthesia, normal motor abilities, no paresis or paralysis, and pulses strong and equal.

CN: Reduction of risk potential; CL: Analyze

55. 4. The knee is usually protected with a knee immobilizer (splint, cast, or brace) and is elevated when the client sits in a chair. Pre- and postsurgery, the **healthcare provider (HCP)** prescribes weight-bearing limits and use of assistive devices for progressive ambulation. Positioning a straight-backed chair at the foot of the bed is not an action conducive to getting the client out of bed on the evening of surgery for a total knee replacement.

CN: Reduction of risk potential; CL: Synthesize

56. 1,4. After a total knee replacement, efforts are directed at preventing complications, such as thromboembolism, infection, limited range of motion, and peroneal nerve palsy. The nurse should instruct the client to report signs of infection, such as an increased temperature. To prevent edema, the affected leg must remain elevated when the client sits in a chair. The client will wear antiembolism stockings at all times, including when sleeping. After discharge, the client may undergo physical therapy on an outpatient basis per **HCP** prescription. The client should leave the dressing in place until the follow-up visit with the surgeon.

CN: Reduction of risk potential; CL: Create

The Client with a Herniated Disk

57. 1. The client is using correct body mechanics for lifting because she is keeping her back as straight as possible and is holding the box close to her body. She is using her large leg muscles to lift the box. She is using a broad base of support by placing her feet as wide apart as possible. The other suggestions would cause the client to put a strain on her back.

CN: Reduction of risk potential; CL: Synthesize

58. 3. The client with low back pain should not exceed the prescribed exercises even though the client may think, "If this will make me well, double will make me well quicker." When exceeding prescribed exercise programs, the client's muscle may be unconditioned and easily tired, leading to injury and increased pain. To use proper body mechanics when lifting light objects, the client should bring the item close to the center of gravity, which occurs when the object is kept below the level of the elbows. Leaning forward while bending the knees allows for the muscles of the thigh to be used instead of those of the lower back. Sleeping on the side with the legs flexed is appropriate because the spine is kept in a neutral position without twisting or pulling on muscles.

CN: Reduction of risk potential; CL: Synthesize

59. 1. The nurse instructs the client to start the prescription by taking the least amount of the medication. The client is advised to monitor pain level and adjust the dosage according to the amount of pain relief.

CN: Pharmacological and parenteral therapies; CL: Synthesize

60. 3,4,1,2. When the client is not entirely able to get out of bed, the nurse should first assist the client to lie down for comfort/safety before administering the prescribed celecoxib. Applying a warm compress will further promote relaxation of skeletal muscles. The **HCP** should be kept informed of the client's status and nursing actions already taken.

CN: Basic care and comfort; CL: Synthesize

61. 2. Standing with a flattened spine slightly tilted forward and slightly flexed to the affected side indicates a postural deformity. Motor changes would include findings such as hypotonia or muscle weakness. Absent or diminished reflexes related to the level of herniation would indicate alteration in reflexes. Sensory changes would include findings such as paresthesia and numbness related to the specific tract of the herniation.

8━ CN: Physiological adaptation; CL: Analyze

62. 2. A supine position with the client's legs flexed is the most comfortable position because it allows for the disc to recess off of the nerve, thus alleviating the pressure and pain. The prone position causes hyperextension of the spine and increased pressure of the disc on the nerve root on the right. A ruptured disc at L5–S1 right identifies a ruptured disc compressing the right nerve root exiting the L5–S1 spinous process; terms such as this are commonly used in the analysis of a magnetic resonance image, myelogram, or history and physical examination. If the ruptured area of the disc were in the central area of the spinous process, the prone position and hyperextension might relieve the disc pressure on the nerve. A high Fowler's or sitting position increases the pressure of the disc on the nerve root because of gravity, as does a right Sims' position.

8━ CN: Physiological adaptation; CL: Synthesize

63. 4. An IV line is not required for an MRI. If a client has an IV line, it is usually converted to an intermittent infusion device, such as a saline lock, to avoid infiltration during transport of the client and completion of the procedure. When a contrast agent is used, the client is moved out of the cylinder, the contrast material is injected, and the client is moved back in. An MRI scan is painless. Typically, the staff positions the client with pillows, blankets, earplugs, and music, to ensure client comfort, before the procedure is started. A history of past surgeries is important, especially if the surgery involved implantation of any metallic devices (e.g., implants, clips, pacemakers). Additionally, the nurse needs to assess for hearing aids, electronic devices, shrapnel, bra hooks, necklaces, jewelry, credit cards, zippers, or any type of metal that the magnet of the MRI unit would attract. Although open MRI units are now available, they are not in widespread use. Therefore, the nurse needs to determine whether the client is claustrophobic because the unit is a closed cylinder in which the client hears pops of noise. A number of clients develop claustrophobia that causes the procedure to be canceled. If the client is claustrophobic, the procedure may need to be rescheduled after an open MRI unit is located or made available.

8━ CN: Reduction of risk potential; CL: Synthesize

64. 2. Based on the client's comments, the nurse should call the surgeon to verify the location of the surgery. The client's comments indicate radiculopathy of L4–L5, but the **informed consent** 📖 form states L3–L4. Radiculopathy of L3–L4 involves pain radiating from the back to the buttocks to the posterior thigh to the inner calf. The nurse must act as a client advocate and not ask the client to sign the consent until the correct procedure is identified and confirmed on the consent. The nurse has no legal authority or responsibility to change the consent. The history is a source of information, but when the client is coherent and the history is contradictory, the **healthcare provider (HCP)** 📖 should be contacted to clarify the situation. Ultimately, it is the surgeon's responsibility to identify the site of surgery specified on the surgical consent form.

8━ CN: Management of care; CL: Synthesize

65. 2. Ondansetron hydrochloride is a selective serotonin receptor antagonist that acts centrally to control the client's nausea in the postoperative phase. It does not control muscle spasms, shivering, or dry mouth.

8━ CN: Pharmacological and parenteral therapies; CL: Evaluate

66. 4. Sweeping causes a twisting motion, which should be avoided because twisting can cause undue stress on the recently ruptured disc site, muscle spasms, and a potential recurrent disc rupture. Although the client should not bend at the waist, such as when washing dishes at the sink, the client can dry dishes because no bending is necessary. The client can sit in a firm chair that keeps the back anatomically aligned. The client should not twist and pull, so when making the bed, the client should pull the covers up on one side and then walk around to the other side before trying to pull the covers up there.

8━ CN: Physiological adaptation; CL: Evaluate

67. 4. After a lumbar laminectomy L4–L5, a client who is returning to work should avoid sitting whenever possible. If the client must sit, he or she should sit only in chairs that allow the knees to be higher than the hips and support the arms to maintain correct body alignment and reduce undue stress on the spine. Maintaining good body postures is most important after a lumbar laminectomy L4–L5. By 6 weeks after the surgery, the client should have regained stamina. To maintain correct body posture, the client should also place one foot on a step stool during prolonged standing. Sleeping on the back with a support under the knees is effective in maintaining correct body posture. Maintaining an average weight for height is important in maintaining a healthy back because carrying extra weight causes undue stress on back muscles.

8━ CN: Physiological adaptation; CL: Synthesize

68. 2. Clear yellowish fluid on the dressing may be cerebrospinal fluid (CSF). This fluid must be tested for glucose to determine whether it is CSF. If so, the client is at great risk for an infection of the central nervous system, which has a high mortality rate. The client should be able to laterally rotate the head and neck, which is above the surgical site in the spinal column. During the nursing postoperative neuromuscular-vascular assessment of movement of the head and neck, the nurse should find results consistent with the preoperative baseline status. Using the standing position to void is normal for a male client. Coughing is the body's defense mechanism to help clear the lungs of the anesthetic agents and to ventilate the lungs in response to a sustained deep inspiration for ventilation of the lower lobes of the lungs. A frequent cough could place a strain on the incision site and should be avoided. Also, a productive cough of thick, yellow sputum would indicate the complication of a respiratory infection.

⚷ CN: Reduction of risk potential;
CL: Analyze

69. 4. The client should wear a thin cotton undershirt under the brace to prevent the brace from abrading directly against the skin. The cotton material also aids in absorbing any moisture, such as perspiration, that could lead to skin irritation and breakdown. Applying lotion is not recommended before applying the brace because further skin breakdown can result (related to the collection of moisture where microorganisms can grow). Applying extra padding (e.g., to the iliac crests) is not recommended because the padding can become wrinkled, producing more pressure sites and skin breakdown. Use of baby or talcum powder and lotion is not recommended because they can cause irritation and skin breakdown.

⚷ CN: Reduction of risk potential;
CL: Evaluate

70. 1. Typically, the donor site causes more pain than the fused site does because inflammation, swelling, and venous oozing around the nerve endings in the donor site, where the subcutaneous tissue was removed, occur during the first 24 to 48 hours postoperatively. After surgery, the surgeon applies a pressure dressing to the donor site to compress the veins that were transected for the removal of subcutaneous tissue but that did not stop oozing blood after surgical cauterization. Pressure on a transected vein, which is low pressure, stops the oozing and loss of blood from the venous site. When the donor site is the fibula, neurovascular checks must be performed every hour to ensure adequate neurologic function of and circulation to the area. The surgeon, not the degree or amount of pain, specifies activity restrictions.

⚷ CN: Physiological adaptation;
CL: Synthesize

71. 1. A client who has had back surgery should place his feet flat on the floor to avoid strain on the incision. Placing the feet on a low or high footstool or in any other position of comfort with the legs uncrossed increases the pressure on the suture line and increases the inflammation around the involved nerve root, thereby increasing the risk of possible rerupture of the disc site.

⚷ CN: Reduction of risk potential;
CL: Evaluate

72. 4. After a lumbar laminectomy, a client should not sit for prolonged periods in a chair because of the increased pressure against the nerve root and incision site. Assisting with daily hygiene is an appropriate activity during the initial postoperative period because, as with any surgical procedure, the client needs to return to an optimal level of functioning as soon as possible. There is no limitation on the client's participation in daily hygiene activities except for individual responses of pain, nausea, vomiting, or weakness. Lying flat in bed is appropriate because it does not cause stress on the spinal column where the laminectomy was performed and the disc tissue was removed. Positions that should be avoided are those that would cause twisting and flexion of the spine. Walking in the hall is an acceptable activity. It promotes good postoperative ventilation, circulation, and return of peristalsis, which are needed for all surgical clients. In addition, walking provides the postoperative lumbar laminectomy client an opportunity to build up endurance and muscle strength and to promote circulation to the operative and incision sites for healing without twisting or stressing them.

⚷ CN: Physiological adaptation;
CL: Synthesize

73. 3. Sit-ups are not recommended for the client who has had a lumbar laminectomy because these exercises place too great a stress on the back. Knee-to-chest lifts, hip tilts, and pelvic tilt exercises are recommended to strengthen back and abdominal muscles.

⚷ CN: Reduction of risk potential;
CL: Synthesize

The Client with an Amputation due to Peripheral Vascular Disease

74. **1,2,4.** Uncontrolled diabetes mellitus is considered a risk factor for peripheral vascular disease because of the macroangiopathic and microangiopathic changes that result from poor blood glucose control. Cigarette smoking is a known risk factor for peripheral vascular disease; nicotine is a potent vasoconstrictor. Serum cholesterol levels >200 mg/dL (11.1 mmol/L) are considered a risk factor for peripheral vascular disease. Typically, peripheral vascular disease is considered to be a disorder affecting older adults. Therefore, an age of 39 years would not be considered as a risk factor contributing to the development of peripheral vascular disease. Prolonged standing is a risk factor for venous stasis and varicose veins.

⚷ CN: Health promotion and maintenance; CL: Analyze

75. **2.** The client with severe arterial occlusive disease and gangrene of the left great toe would have lost the hair on the leg due to decreased circulation to the skin. Edema around the ankle and lower leg would indicate venous insufficiency of the lower extremity. Thin, soft toenails (i.e., not thickened and brittle) are a normal finding. Warmth in the foot indicates adequate circulation to the extremity. Typically, the foot would be cool to cold if a severe arterial occlusion were present.

⚷ CN: Physiological adaptation; CL: Analyze

76. **3.** The client should be tobacco free for 30 minutes before the test to avoid false readings related to the vasoconstrictive effects of smoking on the arteries. Because this test is noninvasive, the client does not need to sign an **informed consent** 📖 form. The client should receive an opioid analgesic, not a sedative, to control the pain as the blood pressure cuffs are inflated during the Doppler studies to determine the ankle-to-brachial pressure index. The client's ankle should not be covered with a blanket because the weight of the blanket on the ischemic foot will cause pain. A bed cradle should be used to keep even the weight of a sheet off the affected foot.

⚷ CN: Reduction of risk potential; CL: Synthesize

77. **2.** Slow, steady walking is a recommended activity for the client with peripheral arterial disease because it stimulates the development of collateral circulation needed to ensure adequate tissue oxygenation. The client with peripheral arterial disease should not minimize activity. Activity is necessary to foster the development of collateral circulation. Elevating the legs above the heart is an appropriate strategy for reducing venous congestion. Wearing antiembolism stockings promotes the return of venous circulation, which is important for clients with venous insufficiency. However, their use in clients with peripheral arterial disease may cause the disease to worsen.

⚷ CN: Physiological adaptation; CL: Evaluate

78. **1.** Daily lubrication, inspection, cleaning, and patting dry of the feet should be performed to prevent cracking of the skin and possible infection. Soaking the feet in warm water should be avoided because soaking can lead to maceration and subsequent skin breakdown. Additionally, the client with arterial insufficiency typically experiences sensory changes, so the client may be unable to detect water that is too warm, thus placing the client at risk for burns. Antiembolism stockings, appropriate for clients with venous insufficiency, are inappropriate for clients with arterial insufficiency and could lead to a worsening of the condition. Footwear should be roomy, soft, and protective and allow air to circulate. Therefore, firm, supportive leather shoes would be inappropriate.

⚷ CN: Reduction of risk potential; CL: Synthesize

79. **2.** Encouraging the client who will be undergoing amputation to verbalize his feelings is the most therapeutic response. Asking the client to tell more about how he is feeling helps to elicit information, providing insight into his view of the situation and also providing the nurse with ideas to help him cope. The nurse should avoid value-laden responses, such as, "At least you will still have one good leg to use," that may make the client feel guilty or hostile, thereby blocking further communication. Furthermore, stating that the client still has one good leg ignores his expressed concerns. The client has verbalized feelings of helplessness by using the term "invalid." The nurse needs to focus on this concern and not try to complete the teaching first before discussing what is on the client's mind. The client's needs, not the nurse's needs, must be met first. It is inappropriate for the nurse to assume to know the relationship between the client and his wife or the roles they now must assume as dependent client and caregiver. Additionally, the response about the client's wife caring for him may reinforce the client's feelings of helplessness as an invalid.

⚷ CN: Psychosocial adaptation; CL: Synthesize

80. 2. The level of amputation often cannot be accurately determined until during surgery, when the surgeon can directly assess the adequacy of the circulation of the residual limb. From a moral, ethical, and legal viewpoint, the surgeon attempts to remove as little of the leg as possible. Although a longer residual limb facilitates prosthesis fitting, unless the stump is receiving a good blood supply, the prosthesis will not function properly because tissue necrosis will occur. Although the client's ability to walk with a prosthesis is important, it is not a determining factor in the decision about the level of amputation required. Blood supply to the tissue is the primary determinant.

CN: Physiological adaptation;
CL: Synthesize

81. 4. The priority action is to draw a mark around the site of bleeding to determine the rate of bleeding. Once the area is marked, the nurse can determine whether the bleeding is increasing or decreasing by the size of the area marked. Because the spot is bright red, the bleeding is most likely arterial in origin. Once the rate and source of bleeding are identified, the surgeon should be notified. The stump is not elevated because adhesions may occur, interfering with the ability to fit a prosthesis. The dressing would be reinforced if the bleeding is determined to be of venous origin, characterized by slow oozing of darker blood that ceases with the application of a pressure dressing. Typically, operative dressings are not changed for 24 hours. Therefore, the dressing is reinforced to prevent organisms from penetrating through the blood-soaked areas of the initial postoperative dressing.

CN: Physiological adaptation;
CL: Synthesize

82. 4. The nurse's first action should be to administer the prescribed opioid analgesic to the client because this phenomenon is phantom sensation and interventions should be provided to relieve it. Pain relief is the priority. Phantom sensation is a real sensation. It is incorrect and inappropriate to tell a client that it is impossible to feel the pain. Although it does relieve the client's apprehensions to be told that phantom sensations are a real phenomenon, the client needs prompt treatment to relieve the pain sensation. Usually, phantom sensation will go away. However, showing the client that the toes are not there does nothing to provide the client with relief.

CN: Physiological adaptation;
CL: Synthesize

83. 4. Use of crutches requires significant strength from the triceps muscles. Therefore, efforts are focused on strengthening these muscles in anticipation of crutch walking. Bed and wheelchair push-ups are excellent exercises targeted at the triceps muscles. Abdominal exercises, range-of-motion and isometric exercises of the shoulders, and quadriceps and gluteal setting exercises are not helpful in preparing for crutch walking.

CN: Reduction of risk potential;
CL: Synthesize

84. 4. When using crutches, the client is taught to support weight primarily on the hands. Supporting body weight on the axillae, elbows, or upper arms must be avoided to prevent nerve damage from excessive pressure.

CN: Reduction of risk potential;
CL: Synthesize

85. 4. Before beginning dietary instructions and interventions, the nurse must first assess the client's and family's food preferences, such as pattern of food intake, lifestyle, food preferences, and ethnic, cultural, and financial influences. Once this information is obtained, the nurse can begin teaching based on the client's current knowledge level and then building on this knowledge base.

CN: Physiological adaptation;
CL: Synthesize

The Client with Fractures

86. 3. Isometric contractions increase the tension within a muscle but do not produce movement. Repeated isometric contractions make muscles grow larger and stronger. Adduction of the leg puts work onto the hip joint as well as altering the pull of traction. Rolling the leg, or *external rotation*, alters the pull of traction. Additional weight should not be added to traction unless prescribed by the **health-care provider (HCP)** ; it will not prevent muscle atrophy.

CN: Reduction of risk potential;
CL: Evaluate

87. 3. Methocarbamol is a muscle relaxant and acts primarily to relieve muscle spasms. It has no effect on microorganisms, does not reduce itching, and has no effect on nervousness.

CN: Pharmacological and parenteral therapies; CL: Evaluate

88. 1,2,3. Acetaminophen is an alternative for a client who is allergic to aspirin. It does not affect platelet aggregation, and the client does not need to have coagulation studies (such as INR). Acetaminophen causes little or no gastric distress. Acetaminophen exerts no anti-inflammatory effects.

CN: Pharmacological and parenteral therapies; CL: Create

89. 3. Hypotension and depressed respirations are signs of high levels of ingestion of hydrocodone, and the client may be developing a habit of taking this drug for a prolonged period. Expected common adverse effects of hydrocodone and acetaminophen would include drowsiness, confusion, blurred vision, and constipation. Hemorrhage from gastrointestinal irritation is not associated with this drug. Hypersensitivity reactions would be manifested by pruritus and rashes.

⚱ CN: Pharmacological and parenteral therapies; CL: Evaluate

90. 3. The nurse's first action is to notify the **HCP** 📖 because the client is likely experiencing a fat embolus. Fat emboli are associated with embolization of marrow or tissue fat or platelets and free fatty acids to the pulmonary capillaries, producing rapid onset of symptoms. Multiple fractures and fractures of the long bones or pelvis increase a client's risk for developing a fat embolus; in addition, young adults between 20 and 30 years of age are at a higher risk for fat emboli with fractures. When fat emboli do occur, hypoxia results; therefore, it is most important the nurse assess changes in level of consciousness and observe changes in behavior such as restlessness and irritability. The nurse does not cut the cast; there is no indication that the casts are obstructing circulation. ABGs are used to confirm the diagnosis, not a chest x-ray. The client's behavior is a result of hypoxemia, not pain.

⚱ CN: Reduction of risk potential; CL: Synthesize

91. 2. The nurse instructs the client to maintain two finger widths between the axillary fold and the underarm piece grip of the crutches to prevent pressure on the brachial plexus. The client is advised to use the three-point gait; in the four-point and two-point gait, there is partial weight bearing of both feet. The client is also advised to keep the affected leg elevated when sitting to prevent swelling and to use the arms, not the axillae, to maintain balance and support.

⚱ CN: Reduction of risk potential; CL: Apply

92. 4. Skeletal traction is often used to regain normal length of the bone, but in this situation, the main purpose of the traction is to reduce and immobilize the fracture. This type of traction allows the client to move in bed without dislocating the fracture. This client has an open fracture, but skeletal traction will not prevent further skin breakdown.

⚱ CN: Physiological adaptation; CL: Evaluate

93. 3. The nurse first assesses the mechanism of injury to help determine related injuries, tests needed, and potential treatment options. The next step is to assess the location, type, quality, and intensity of the pain. Neurovascular stasis of the injured site is assessed after pain; therefore, the nurse checks for functional ability or changing positions. Although the nurse can also determine the extent of anxiety while assessing the injury and can use communication strategies to minimize anxiety, it is not the first priority for assessing this client.

⚱ CN: Physiological adaptation; CL: Synthesize

94. 3. The nursing assessment is first focused on the region distal to the fracture for neurovascular injury or compromise. When a nerve or blood vessel is severed or obstructed at the actual fracture site, innervation to the nerve or blood flow to the vessel is disrupted below the site; therefore, the area distal to the fracture site is the area of compromised neurologic input or vascular flow and return, not the area above the fracture site or the fracture site itself. The nurse may assess the opposite extremity at the area proximal to the fracture site for a baseline comparison of pulse quality, color, temperature, size, and so on, but the comparison would be made after the initial neurovascular assessment.

⚱ CN: Physiological adaptation; CL: Analyze

95. 3. Clients should not pull out cast padding to scratch inside the cast because of the hazard of skin breakdown and subsequent potential for infection. Clients are encouraged to elevate the casted extremity above the level of the heart to reduce edema and to exercise or move the joints above and below the cast to promote and maintain flexibility and muscle strength. Applying ice for 10 minutes during the first 24 hours helps to reduce edema.

⚱ CN: Reduction of risk potential; CL: Evaluate

96. 2. The client in a double hip spica cast should avoid eating foods that can be constipating, such as cheese. Rather, fresh fruits and vegetables should be encouraged, and the client should be encouraged to drink at least 2,500 mL/day. Drinking cranberry juice, which helps keep urine acidic, thereby avoiding the development of renal calculi, is encouraged. The client should be encouraged to establish regular times for elimination to promote regularity in bowel and bladder habits. The client will develop orthostatic hypotension unless the circulatory system is reconditioned slowly through dangling and standing exercises.

⚱ CN: Physiological adaptation; CL: Synthesize

97. 2. A two-point gait involves partial weight bearing on each foot, with each crutch advancing simultaneously with the opposing leg. Advancing a crutch on one side and then advancing the opposite foot, and repeating on the opposite side, illustrates the four-point gait. When the client advances both crutches together and follows by lifting both lower extremities to the same level as the crutches, the gait is called a "swing-to" gait. When the client advances both crutches together and follows by lifting both lower extremities past the level of the crutches, the gait is called a "swing-through" gait. The "swing-through" gait is often used by paraplegic clients because it allows them to place weight on their legs while the crutches are moved one stride ahead.

CN: Reduction of risk potential; CL: Synthesize

98. 1. The wound was left open with a three-way drainage system in place to irrigate the debrided wound with normal saline or an antibiotic. Before the debridement, a sample of the wound would be taken for culture and sensitivity testing so that an organism-specific antibiotic could be administered to prevent possible serious sequelae of osteomyelitis. Therefore, the nurse should review the results of the culture and sensitivity report before initiating care. A pressure dressing would not be applied to an open wound. Rather, a wet-to-dry dressing most likely would be used. There should not be increased pain related to the exposure of nerve endings in the subcutaneous tissue of the wound that was left open to the environment. The first priority is to determine if there is an infection as this is the biggest risk to the client; the nurse can check other lab values later.

CN: Physiological adaptation; CL: Synthesize

99. 1. The nurse should assess the client's ability to move the toes and for the presence of distal pulses, including a neurovascular assessment of the area below the cast. Increasing pain unrelieved by usual analgesics and occurring 4 to 12 hours after the onset of casting or trauma may be the first sign of compartment syndrome, which can lead to permanent damage to nerves and muscles. Although the nurse can use a pain rating scale or assess for changes in vital signs to objectively assess the client's pain, the client's comments suggest early and important signs of compartment syndrome requiring immediate intervention. The nurse should not confuse these signs with the potential for drug tolerance. This assessment might be appropriate once the suspicion of compartment syndrome has been ruled out.

CN: Physiological adaptation; CL: Analyze

100. 4. The client with compartment syndrome may release myoglobin from damaged muscle cells into the circulation. This becomes trapped in the renal tubules, resulting in dark, scanty urine, possibly leading to acute renal failure. Crackles may suggest respiratory complications; jaundice suggests liver failure; and generalized edema may suggest heart failure. However, these are not associated with compartment syndrome.

CN: Reduction of risk potential; CL: Analyze

The Client with a Femoral Fracture

101. 4. Passive immunity for tetanus is provided in the form of tetanus antitoxin or tetanus immune globulin. An antitoxin is an antibody to the toxin of an organism. Administering tetanus toxoid, antigen, or vaccine would provide active immunity by stimulating the body to produce its own antibodies.

CN: Pharmacological and parenteral therapies; CL: Apply

102. 4. Skeletal traction is NOT used to pull weight with a boot, and the nurse should explain to the client that skeletal traction involves the insertion of a wire or a pin into the bone to maintain a pull of 5 to 45 lb (2.3 to 20.4 kg) on the area which will align the injured bones by providing a long-term pull to realign the fracture.

CN: Reduction of risk potential; CL: Evaluate

103. 4. The client with a femoral fracture in balanced suspension traction should not be given a complete bed bath. Rather, the client is encouraged to participate in self-care and movement in bed, such as with a trapeze triangle. Use of a fracture bedpan is appropriate. A fracture bedpan is lower, and it is easier for the client to move on and off the bedpan without altering the line of traction. Checking for areas of redness or pressure over all areas in contact with the traction or bed, including the ischial tuberosity, is important to prevent possible skin breakdown. The client should be positioned so that the feet do not press against the footboard. Therefore, elevating the head of the bed no more than 25 degrees is recommended to keep the client from moving down in the bed.

CN: Reduction of risk potential; CL: Synthesize

104. 3. The nurse should send the client to the operating room on the bed with extra help to keep the traction from moving to maintain the femur in the proper alignment before surgery. Transferring the client to a cart with manually suspended traction is inappropriate because doing so places the client at risk for additional trauma to the surrounding neurovascular and soft tissues, as would removing the traction. The surgeon need not be called because the decision about transferring the client is an independent nursing action.

⚷ CN: Reduction of risk potential;
CL: Synthesize

105. 1. The Pearson attachment supports the lower leg and provides increased stability in the overall traction setup. It also makes it easier to maintain correct alignment. It does not support the thigh and the upper leg or prevent flexion deformities in the ankle and foot. It is not attached to the skeletal pin.

⚷ CN: Reduction of risk potential;
CL: Apply

106. 1. Fat emboli usually result in symptoms of acute respiratory distress syndrome, such as apprehension, chest pain, cyanosis, dyspnea, tachypnea, tachycardia, and decreased partial pressure of arterial oxygen resulting from poor oxygen exchange. Migraine-like headaches are not a symptom of a fat embolism, but mental confusion, memory loss, and a headache from poor oxygen exchange may be seen with central nervous system involvement. Numbness in the right leg is a peripheral neurovascular response that most likely is related to the femoral fracture. Muscle spasms in the right thigh are a symptom of a neuromuscular response affecting the local muscle around the femoral fracture site.

⚷ CN: Reduction of risk potential;
CL: Analyze

107. 1. The priority for this client is to prevent the effects of prolonged immobility, such as by preventing skin breakdown and encouraging the client to take deep breaths, and use active range-of-motion exercises for the joints that are not immobilized. Although not the priority, the nurse also should seek ways to help the client adjust to and cope with the present state of immobility. Emphasis should be placed on what the client can do, such as participating in daily care and exercises to maintain muscle strength. Finding diversional activities is not a **priority** at this moment. Although the client must adapt to the inactivity, helping the client develop coping skills is the priority at this time.

⚷ CN: Psychosocial adaptation;
CL: Analyze

108. 1. The client's assisting as much as possible in self-care and increasing participation over time indicate that the client has accomplished self-care by gaining a sense of control. If the client lets the nurse complete the care without interfering, the behavior would indicate passivity, possibly from denial or depression. If the client allows the spouse to assume total responsibility, a successful outcome has not been reached. The client is able to accomplish self-care activities within the limits of immobilization from the traction.

⚷ CN: Basic care and comfort; CL: Evaluate

109. 2. Fever, night sweats, chills, restlessness, and restrictive movement of the fractured leg are clinical manifestations of osteomyelitis, which is a pyogenic bone infection caused by bacteria (usually staphylococci), a virus, or a fungus. The bone is inaccessible to macrophages and antibodies for protection against infections, so an infection in this site can become serious quickly. The client with a pulmonary or fat embolus would develop symptoms of pulmonary compromise, such as shortness of breath, chest pain, angina, and mental confusion. Signs and symptoms of urinary tract infection would include pain over the suprapubic, groin, or back region with fever and chills, with no restrictive movement of the leg.

⚷ CN: Reduction of risk potential;
CL: Analyze

110. 2. The goal of care for this client is healing and tissue growth while the client continues on long-term antibiotic therapy to clear the infection. A diet high in protein and vitamins C and D promotes healing. Herbal supplements may potentiate bleeding (e.g., ginkgo, ginger, tumeric, chamomile, kelp, horse chestnut, garlic, and dong quai) and have not been proven through research to promote healing. Frequent passive motion will increase circulation but may also aggravate localized bone pain. It is not appropriate to advise the client to change antibiotics as treatment may take time.

⚷ CN: Physiological adaptation;
CL: Synthesize

The Client with a Spinal Cord Injury

111. 3. The priority concern is to immobilize the head and neck to prevent further trauma when a fractured vertebra is unstable and easily displaced. Although wrapping and supporting the extremities is important, it does not take priority over immobilizing the head and neck. Pain usually is not a significant consideration with this type of injury. Cushioning is contraindicated. The neck should be kept in a neutral position and immobilized. Flexion of the neck is avoided.

⚷ CN: Safety and infection control;
CL: Synthesize

112. 3. The client is experiencing autonomic dysreflexia, which is a medical emergency. The nurse should immediately evaluate the client for bladder distention and be prepared to catheterize the client. Positioning the client on the left side, reducing environmental stimuli, and administering pain medications are not used to treat autonomic hyperreflexia.

⚷ CN: Physiological adaptation;
CL: Synthesize

113. 3. This client has a spinal cord injury of the sacral region of the spinal cord and will have bladder and bowel dysfunction, as well as loss of sensation and muscle control below the injury. The other options are true of a client who has quadriplegia.

⚷ CN: Physiological adaptation;
CL: Analyze

114. 2. Although assessment of renal status, gastrointestinal function, and biliary function is important, with the spinal cord transection at T4 the client's vascular status is the primary focus of the nursing assessment because the sympathetic feedback system is lost and the client is at risk for hypotension and bradycardia.

⚷ CN: Physiological adaptation;
CL: Analyze

115. 1. The client with a spinal cord transection above T5 is least likely to develop diarrhea. Rather, constipation due to atonia would be possible. The client with a spinal cord transection above T5 is at risk for development of a paralytic ileus because the sympathetic nerve innervation to the vagus nerve, which dominates all the vessels and organs below T5 (e.g., the intestinal tract), has been disrupted and, therefore, so has movement or peristalsis. The client is at risk for development of stress ulcers because the sympathetic nerve innervation to the stomach has been disrupted, which results in an excessive release of hydrochloric acid in the stomach, allowing contact of hydrochloric acid with the stomach mucosa. The client does not feel subjective signs of stress ulcers (e.g., pain, guarding, tenderness) and therefore is at increased risk for bleeding because complications of an ulcer can develop before early diagnosis.

⚷ CN: Reduction of risk potential;
CL: Synthesize

116. 4. Measuring the leg girth is the most appropriate method because the usual signs, such as a positive Homans' sign, pain, and tenderness, are not present. Other means of assessing for deep vein thrombosis in a client with a spinal cord injury are through a Doppler examination and impedance plethysmography.

⚷ CN: Reduction of risk potential;
CL: Analyze

117. 3. During the period of spinal shock, the bladder is completely atonic and will continue to fill passively unless the client is catheterized. The bladder will not go into spasms or cause uncontrolled urination. Bladder function will not be normal during the period of spinal shock.

⚷ CN: Reduction of risk potential;
CL: Analyze

118. 4. The movements occur from muscle reflexes and cannot be initiated or controlled by the brain. After the period of spinal shock, the muscles gradually become spastic owing to an increased sensitivity of the lower motor neurons. It is an expected occurrence and does not indicate that healing is taking place or that the client will walk again. The movement is not voluntary and cannot be brought under voluntary control.

⚷ CN: Physiological adaptation;
CL: Synthesize

119. 3. Long-bone demineralization is a serious consequence of the loss of weight bearing. An excessive calcium load is brought to the kidneys, and precipitation may occur, predisposing to stone formation. Excessive intake of dairy products may promote constipation. However, this is not the most accurate reason for decreasing calcium intake. Immobility does not increase calcium absorption from the intestine. Dairy products do not necessarily contribute to weight gain.

⚷ CN: Basic care and comfort;
CL: Synthesize

120. 2. The woman with spinal cord injury can participate in sexual activity but might not experience orgasm. Cessation in the nerve pathway may occur in spinal cord injury, but this does not negate the client's mental and emotional needs to creatively participate with her partner in a sexual relationship and to reach orgasm. An indwelling urinary catheter may be left in place during intercourse and need not be removed because the indwelling urinary catheter is placed in the urethra, which is not the channel used for sexual intercourse. There are no contraindications, such as hypertension, to sexual activity in a woman with spinal cord injury. Sexual intercourse is allowed, and hypertension should be manageable. Because a spinal cord injury does not affect fertility, the client should have access to family planning information so that an unplanned pregnancy can be avoided.

⚷ CN: Basic care and comfort; CL: Evaluate

121. **3.** Spinal cord injury represents a physical loss; grief is the normal response to this loss. Working through grief entails reviewing memories and eventually letting go of them. The process may take as long as 2 years. Telling the client to be patient and that adjustment takes time is a clichéd type of response, one that is not empathetic or responsive to the client's needs. Telling the client to focus on today does not allow time for the grief process, which is necessary for the client to work through and adjust to the loss. The client is not escaping but is reminiscing on what is lost, to work through the grieving process.

🔑 CN: Psychosocial adaptation; CL: Synthesize

Managing Care, Quality, and Safety of Clients with Musculoskeletal Health Problems

122. **1,3,4,5.** Clients who are at risk for falling include the client taking narcotics, the client with a known fear of falling, the client with cognitive impairment, and the client with gait problems. Age and setting are not necessarily risks for fallings.

🔑 CN: Management of care; CL: Synthesize

123. **2,3,5.** The client with a C3–C4 fracture has neck control but may tire easily using sore muscles around the incision area to hold up the head. Therefore, the head and neck of the wheelchair should be high. The seat of the wheelchair should be lower than normal to facilitate transfer from the bed to the wheelchair. When a client can use the hands and arms to move the wheelchair, the placement of the back to the client's scapula is necessary. This client cannot use the arms and will need an electric chair with breath, chin, or voice control to manipulate movement of the chair. A firm or hard cushion adds pressure to bony prominences; the cushion should instead be padded to reduce the risk of pressure ulcers.

🔑 CN: Basic care and comfort; CL: Synthesize

124. **3.** Infection is a serious complication of total hip replacement and may necessitate removal of the implant. Clients who are obese, poorly nourished, or elderly and those who have poorly controlled diabetes, rheumatoid arthritis, or concurrent infections (e.g., dental, urinary tract) are at high risk for infection. Clients who are of normal weight and have well-controlled chronic diseases are not at risk for infection. Living alone is not a risk factor for infection.

🔑 CN: Reduction of risk potential; CL: Synthesize

125. **1,2,3,5.** A restraint is a method of involuntary physical restriction of a client's freedom of movement, physical activity, or normal access to his/her body. The nurse must monitor and provide care to optimize the physical and psychological well-being of the client including, but not limited to, respiratory and circulatory status, skin integrity, and vital signs. With each assessment, the nurse needs to ascertain that restraints are still required for client safety. The least restrictive intervention based on an individualized assessment of the client's medical or behavioral status or condition is needed.

🔑 CN: Safety and infection control; CL: Analyze

126. **1,3,4,5,6.** Client safety is a priority for the client, the client's family, and all of the personnel working on this unit. All of these persons must be engaged in using strategies to prevent falls. The insurance provider does not need to be involved in developing a falls program.

🔑 CN: Safety and infection control; CL: Create

127. **2.** The client is identified as being at risk for falling, and a staff member or family member should accompany the client when walking. The nurse should first accompany the client back the room. Because the client is not fatigued, the client does not need a wheelchair, but must have assistance. The nurse can delegate the task of ambulating the client to the **UAP** 📖, but it may take a while to locate one that it available at this time. Walking only in the room will not provide an opportunity for the client to gain strength and improve ambulation, but the nurse should remind the client to have assistance.

🔑 CN: Reduction of risk potential; CL: Synthesize

128. **1,2,3.** To assure client safety when using anticoagulants, the nurse should coordinate care at this time with the pharmacist, dietitian, and laboratory. The pharmacist will collaborate in teaching the client about using the drug; dietary services will plan a diet that limits foods that have high amounts of vitamin K (spinach, cabbage, blueberries) that will interfere with anticoagulation; and the laboratory will draw daily INR levels to assure accurate dosing. Although the nurse coordinates discharge planning at the time of admission to the hospital, at this point it is too soon for discharge planning services to be involved because it is not known if the client will continue to take the warfarin when discharged. There is no indication a chaplain is needed at this time.

🔑 CN: Management of care; CL: Synthesize

129. 4. Side rails are considered restraints and are not used at both the head and foot of the bed. Using side rails at the head of the bed will aid the client in sitting up and are safe, but using side rails at both the head and the foot of the bed presents risks for a client who might become wedged between the rail and the bed or attempt to climb over them. The nurse discusses side rail use with the **UAP** 📖 and lowers the side rail at the foot of the bed. The nurse assures the bed is placed in low position. The accessible call light, dim lighting, and clear path to the bathroom are factors that contribute to fall prevention.

🗝 CN: Management of care: CL: Synthesize

130. 3. Hand-off communication is an interactive communication allowing the opportunity for questioning between the giver and receiver of client information, including up-to-date information regarding the client's care, treatment, and services, as well as the client's current condition and any recent or anticipated changes. "Hand-off" communication does occur when a nurse is leaving the nursing unit, but the purpose is not to let the charge nurse know that the nurse is going to lunch or to have someone else assigned to care for the client. "Hand-off" communication focuses on current information, not the client's history.

🗝 CN: Management of care; CL: Synthesize

131. 1,2,4,5,6. The nurse should determine that a client with rheumatoid arthritis can describe the septic arthritis physiologic process and knows how to relieve pain using pharmacologic and nonpharmacologic interventions. Prolonged immobility and limited activity may promote formation of a deep vein thrombosis and possibly subsequent pulmonary emboli. The client should also understand the importance of supporting the affected joint, weight-bearing and activity restrictions, and how to use ambulatory aids and assistive devices safely to promote recovery of normal function. The local application of heat and cold to an injured body part can provide therapeutic benefits; however, "high" heat may cause a thermal injury and further promote edema formation. The client should inform the **healthcare provider (HCP)** 📖 about pain that is not relieved by the current management plan.

🗝 CN: Management of care; CL: Evaluate

132. 2,3. Passive ROM exercises are used to move the client's joints through as full a ROM as possible. Passive ROM exercises improve or maintain joint mobility and help prevent contractures. These exercises are indicated for the client with temporary or permanent loss of mobility, sensation, or consciousness. Exercises help with joint mobility, strength, and endurance. Plantar flexion of the foot and supination of the hand may be normal joint movements if the client can do active ROM. Septic joints have infection that may be spread either hematogenously or through trauma.

🗝 CN: Reduction of risk potential; CL: Apply

The Client with Cancer

The Client at Risk for Cancer

1. Which client is at **highest** risk for colorectal cancer?
- ☐ 1. the client who smokes
- ☐ 2. the client who eats a vegetarian diet
- ☐ 3. the client who has been treated for Crohn's disease for 20 years
- ☐ 4. the client who has a family history of lung cancer

2. A nurse is conducting a cancer risk screening program. Which client is at **greatest** risk for skin cancer?
- ☐ 1. a 45-year-old healthcare worker
- ☐ 2. a 15-year-old high school student
- ☐ 3. a 30-year-old butcher
- ☐ 4. a 60-year-old mountain biker

3. A client diagnosed with testicular cancer expresses concerns about fertility. The client and his spouse desire to eventually have a family, and the nurse discusses the option of sperm banking. The nurse should inform the couple that sperm banking would need to be performed:
- ☐ 1. before treatment is started.
- ☐ 2. once the client is tolerating the treatment.
- ☐ 3. upon completion of treatment.
- ☐ 4. when tumor markers drop to normal levels.

4. Cancer prevalence is defined as:
- ☐ 1. the likelihood cancer will occur in a lifetime.
- ☐ 2. the number of persons with cancer at a given point in time.
- ☐ 3. the number of new cancers in a year.
- ☐ 4. all cancer cases more than 5 years old.

5. A nurse is planning an educational program about cancer prevention and detection. Which group would benefit **most** from education regarding potential risk factors for melanoma?
- ☐ 1. adults older than age 35
- ☐ 2. senior citizens who have been repeatedly exposed to the effects of ultraviolet A and ultraviolet B rays
- ☐ 3. parents with children
- ☐ 4. employees of a chemical factory

6. A nurse is providing education in a community setting about general measures to avoid excessive sun exposure. Which recommendation is appropriate?
- ☐ 1. Apply sunscreen only after going into the water.
- ☐ 2. Avoid peak exposure hours from 0900 to 1300.
- ☐ 3. Wear loosely woven clothing for added ventilation.
- ☐ 4. Apply sunscreen with a sun protection factor (SPF) of 15 or more before sun exposure.

7. A 29-year-old woman is concerned about her personal risk factors for malignant melanoma. She is upset because her 49-year-old sister was recently diagnosed with the disease. After gathering information about the client's history of sun exposure, the nurse's **best** response would be to explain that:
- ☐ 1. some melanomas have a familial component, and she should seek medical advice.
- ☐ 2. her personal risk is low because most melanomas occur at age 60 or later.
- ☐ 3. her personal risk is low because melanoma does not have a familial component.
- ☐ 4. she should not worry because she did not experience severe sunburn as a child.

8. A client with a family history of cancer asks the nurse what the single most important risk factor is for cancer. Which risk factor should the nurse discuss?
- ☐ **1.** family history
- ☐ **2.** lifestyle choices
- ☐ **3.** age
- ☐ **4.** menopause or hormonal events

9. A 42-year-old female highway construction worker is concerned about her cancer risks. She has been married for 18 years, has two children, smokes one pack of cigarettes per day, and occasionally drinks one to two beers. She is 30 lb (13.6 kg) overweight, eats fried fast food often, and rarely eats fresh fruits and vegetables. Her mother was diagnosed with breast cancer 2 years ago. Her father and an aunt both died of lung cancer. She had a basal cell carcinoma removed from her cheek 3 years earlier. What behavioral changes should the nurse coach this client to make to decrease her risk of cancer? Select all that apply.
- ☐ **1.** Improve nutrition.
- ☐ **2.** Decrease alcohol consumption.
- ☐ **3.** Use sunscreen.
- ☐ **4.** Stop smoking.
- ☐ **5.** Lose weight.
- ☐ **6.** Change her job to work inside.

10. The incidence and risk of cancer increase when smoking is combined with:
- ☐ **1.** asbestos exposure and alcohol consumption.
- ☐ **2.** ultraviolet radiation exposure and alcohol consumption.
- ☐ **3.** asbestos exposure and ultraviolet radiation exposure.
- ☐ **4.** alcohol consumption and human papillomavirus (HPV) infection.

11. The nurse is assessing a 60-year-old who has hoarseness and a chronic sore throat. What should the nurse determine while conducting a focused assessment? Select all that apply.
- ☐ **1.** use of acetaminophen
- ☐ **2.** exposure to sun
- ☐ **3.** consumption of a high-fat diet
- ☐ **4.** history of tobacco use
- ☐ **5.** amount of alcohol consumption

12. A 42-year-old is interested in making dietary changes to reduce the risk of colon cancer. What dietary selections should the nurse suggest?
- ☐ **1.** croissant, granola and peanut butter squares, whole milk
- ☐ **2.** bran muffin, skim milk, stir-fried broccoli
- ☐ **3.** granola, bagel with cream cheese, cauliflower salad
- ☐ **4.** oatmeal raisin cookies, baked potato with sour cream, turkey sandwich

13. The nurse is conducting a cancer risk assessment for a middle-aged client. Which environmental factor increases the risk of cancer?
- ☐ **1.** gender
- ☐ **2.** nutrition
- ☐ **3.** immunologic status
- ☐ **4.** age

14. A client at risk for lung cancer asks about the reason for having a computed tomography (CT) scan as part of the initial exam. What is the nurse's **best** response? "A CT scan is:
- ☐ **1.** far superior to magnetic resonance imaging for evaluating lymph node metastasis."
- ☐ **2.** noninvasive and readily available."
- ☐ **3.** useful for distinguishing small differences in tissue density and detecting nodal involvement."
- ☐ **4.** used to distinguish a malignant from a non-malignant adenopathy."

15. Lifestyle influences that are considered risk factors for colorectal cancer include:
- ☐ **1.** a diet low in vitamin C.
- ☐ **2.** a high dietary intake of artificial sweeteners.
- ☐ **3.** a high-fat, low-fiber diet.
- ☐ **4.** multiple sex partners.

16. When planning a culturally sensitive health education program, the nurse should:
- ☐ **1.** locate the program at a facility that will not charge for use.
- ☐ **2.** integrate folk beliefs and traditions of the target population into the content.
- ☐ **3.** prepare materials in the primary language of the program sponsor.
- ☐ **4.** exclude community leaders from the dominant culture from initial planning efforts.

The Client with Pain

17. A client in a hospice program has increasing pain. The nurse and client collaborate to schedule analgesics to provide:
- ☐ **1.** doses of analgesic when pain is a 5 on a scale of 1 to 10.
- ☐ **2.** enough analgesia to keep the client semisomnolent.
- ☐ **3.** an analgesia-free period so that the client can carry out daily hygienic activities.
- ☐ **4.** around-the-clock routine administration of analgesics for continuous pain relief.

18. A client with pancreatic cancer has been receiving morphine via a subcutaneous pump for 2 weeks. The client is requiring an increased dose of the morphine to manage the pain. The nurse should document that the client is:
☐ 1. tolerating the medication well.
☐ 2. showing addiction to morphine.
☐ 3. developing a tolerance for the medication.
☐ 4. experiencing physical dependence.

19. A client with advanced ovarian cancer takes 150 mg of long-acting morphine orally every 12 hours for abdominal pain. When the client develops a small bowel obstruction, the healthcare provider (HCP) discontinues the oral morphine and prescribes morphine 6 mg/h IV. After calculating the equianalgesic conversion from oral to intravenous morphine, the nurse should:
☐ 1. continue the oral morphine for one more dose after the IV morphine is started.
☐ 2. contact the HCP to suggest a higher equianalgesic dose of IV morphine.
☐ 3. administer the morphine IV as prescribed.
☐ 4. clarify the prescription to recommend the initial morphine dose of 4 mg/h.

20. A client had a craniotomy for removal of a malignant brain tumor in the occipital region. The nurse should question a prescription for which of these drugs?
☐ 1. ibuprofen
☐ 2. naproxen
☐ 3. morphine sulfate
☐ 4. acetaminophen

21. A 62-year-old female is taking long-acting morphine 120 mg every 12 hours for pain from metastatic breast cancer. She can have 20 mg of immediate-release morphine every 3 to 4 hours as needed for breakthrough pain. The healthcare provider (HCP) should be notified if the client uses **more** than how many breakthrough doses of morphine in 24 hours?
☐ 1. seven
☐ 2. four
☐ 3. two
☐ 4. one

22. Assessment of a client taking a nonsteroidal anti-inflammatory drug (NSAID) for pain management should include specific questions regarding which body system?
☐ 1. gastrointestinal
☐ 2. renal
☐ 3. pulmonary
☐ 4. cardiac

23. The nurse is assessing a client with chronic pain. What findings are expected for a client in chronic pain? Select all that apply.
☐ 1. facial grimacing
☐ 2. normal vital signs
☐ 3. physical inactivity
☐ 4. moaning
☐ 5. depression

24. A client with lung cancer is being cared for by his wife at home. His pain is increasing in severity. The nurse recognizes that teaching has been effective when the wife: (Select all that apply.)
☐ 1. gives her husband a long-acting or sustained-release oral pain medication regularly around the clock.
☐ 2. uses an immediate-release medication (oxycodone) for breakthrough pain.
☐ 3. avoids long-acting opioids due to her concern about addiction.
☐ 4. uses music for distraction as well as heat or cold in combination with medications.
☐ 5. substitutes acetaminophen to avoid tolerance to the medications.
☐ 6. has her husband use a pain rating scale to measure the effectiveness at reaching his individual pain goal.

25. A 52-year-old male was discharged from the hospital for cancer-related pain. His pain appeared to be well controlled on the IV morphine. He was switched to oral morphine when discharged 2 days ago. He now reports his pain as an 8 on a 10-point scale and wants the IV morphine. Which explanation is the **most** likely for the client's reports of inadequate pain control?
☐ 1. He is addicted to the IV morphine.
☐ 2. He is going through withdrawal from the IV opioid.
☐ 3. He is physically dependent on the IV morphine.
☐ 4. He is undermedicated on the oral opioid.

26. A nurse is assessing a client with bone cancer pain. Which part of a thorough pain assessment is **most** significant for this client?
☐ 1. intensity
☐ 2. cause
☐ 3. aggravating factors
☐ 4. location

27. A client with chronic cancer pain has been receiving opiates for 4 months. She rated the pain as an 8 on a 10-point scale before starting the opioid medication. Following a thorough examination, there is no new evidence of increased disease, yet the pain is close to 8 again. The **most** likely explanation for the increasing pain is:
☐ 1. development of an addiction to the opioids.
☐ 2. tolerance to the opioid.
☐ 3. withdrawal from the opioid.
☐ 4. placebo effect has decreased.

28. The nurse teaches the client with chronic cancer pain about optimal pain control. Which recommendation is **most** effective for pain control?
- ☐ 1. Get used to some pain, and use a little less medication than needed to keep from being addicted.
- ☐ 2. Take prescribed analgesics on an around-the-clock schedule to prevent recurrent pain.
- ☐ 3. Take analgesics only when pain returns.
- ☐ 4. Take enough analgesics around the clock so that you can sleep 12 to 16 hours a day to block the pain.

The Client Who Is Receiving Chemotherapy

29. When preparing to administer a chemotherapeutic agent to a client, the nurse should:
- ☐ 1. recap all needles used to prepare agents.
- ☐ 2. dispose of chemotherapy wastes in the client's bedside trash.
- ☐ 3. use gloves and disposable long-sleeved gowns when handling agents.
- ☐ 4. administer only prepackaged agents from the manufacturer.

30. A client who is receiving chemotherapy develops stomatitis. What should the nurse instruct the client to do?
- ☐ 1. Rinse the mouth with full-strength hydrogen peroxide every 4 hours.
- ☐ 2. Use a soft-bristled toothbrush after each meal.
- ☐ 3. Drink hot tea with honey to soothe the painful oral mucosa.
- ☐ 4. Avoid using dental floss until the stomatitis is resolved.

31. Doxorubicin is prescribed for a female client with breast cancer. The client is distressed about hair loss. What should the nurse do?
- ☐ 1. Have the client wash and massage the scalp daily to stimulate hair growth.
- ☐ 2. Explain that hair loss is temporary and will quickly grow back to its original appearance.
- ☐ 3. Provide resources for a wig selection before hair loss begins.
- ☐ 4. Recommend that the client limit social contacts until hair regrows.

32. A client is receiving chemotherapy for the diagnosis of brain cancer. When teaching the client about contamination from excretion of the chemotherapy drugs within 48 hours, the nurse should instruct the client that:
- ☐ 1. a bathroom can be shared with an adult who is not pregnant.
- ☐ 2. urinary and bowel excretions are not considered contaminated.
- ☐ 3. disposable plates and plastic utensils must be used during the entire course of chemotherapy.
- ☐ 4. any contaminated linens should be washed separately and then washed a second time, if necessary.

33. A client is receiving vincristine. Client teaching by the nurse should include instructions on:
- ☐ 1. use of loperamide.
- ☐ 2. fluid restriction.
- ☐ 3. low-fiber, bland diet.
- ☐ 4. bowel regimen.

34. The client who is receiving chemotherapy is not eating well but otherwise feels healthy. What should the nurse suggest the client eat?
- ☐ 1. cereal with milk and strawberries
- ☐ 2. toast, gelatin dessert, and cookies
- ☐ 3. broiled chicken, green beans, and cottage cheese
- ☐ 4. steak and french fries

35. A nurse is assessing a woman who is receiving the second administration of chemotherapy for breast cancer. When obtaining this client's health history, the nurse should ask the client which question?
- ☐ 1. "Has your hair been falling out in clumps?"
- ☐ 2. "Have you had nausea or vomiting?"
- ☐ 3. "Have you been sleeping at night?"
- ☐ 4. "Do you have your usual energy level?"

36. A client is receiving monthly doses of chemotherapy for treatment of stage III colon cancer. Which laboratory results should the nurse report to the oncologist before the **next** dose of chemotherapy is administered? Select all that apply.
- ☐ 1. hemoglobin of 14.5 g/dL (145 g/L)
- ☐ 2. platelet count of 40,000/mm³ (40 × 10⁹/L)
- ☐ 3. blood urea nitrogen (BUN) level of 12 mg/dL (4.3 mmol/L)
- ☐ 4. white blood cell count of 2,300/mm³ (2.3 × 10⁹/L)
- ☐ 5. temperature of 101.2°F (38.4°C)
- ☐ 6. urine specific gravity of 1.020

37. A nurse is checking the laboratory results of a client with colon cancer admitted for further chemotherapy. The client has lost 30 lb (13.6 kg) since initiation of the treatment. Which laboratory result should be reported to the healthcare provider (HCP)?
- ☐ 1. blood glucose level of 95 mg/dL (5.3 mmol/L)
- ☐ 2. total cholesterol level of 182 mg/dL (4.71 mmol/L)
- ☐ 3. hemoglobin level of 12.3 mg/dL (123 g/L)
- ☐ 4. albumin level of 2.8 g/dL (28 g/L)

38. The **most** reliable early indicator of infection in a client who is neutropenic is:
- ☐ 1. fever.
- ☐ 2. chills.
- ☐ 3. tachycardia.
- ☐ 4. dyspnea.

39. A nurse is caring for a client who is undergoing chemotherapy. Current laboratory values are noted on the medical record. Which action would be **most** appropriate for the nurse to implement?

Laboratory Results

Test	Result
Hemoglobin	12.0 g/dL (120 g/L)
Platelet count	108,000/mm^3 (108 × 10^9/L)
WBC count	1,600/mm^3 (1.6 × 10^9/L)
ANC	< 1,000/mm^3 (1 × 10^9/L)

☐ 1. wearing a protective gown and particulate respiratory mask when completing treatments
☐ 2. washing hands before and after entering the room
☐ 3. restricting visitors
☐ 4. contacting the healthcare provider (HCP) for a prescription for hematopoietic factors such as erythropoietin

40. A client is using an herbal therapy while receiving chemotherapy. The nurse should:
☐ 1. determine what substances the client is using, and make sure that the healthcare provider (HCP) is aware of all therapies the client is using.
☐ 2. guide the client in the decision-making process to select either Western or alternative medicine.
☐ 3. encourage the client to seek alternative modalities that do not require the ingestion of substances.
☐ 4. recommend that the client stop using the alternative medicines immediately.

41. A client diagnosed with cancer is receiving chemotherapy. The nurses should assess which diagnostic value while the client is receiving chemotherapy?
☐ 1. bone marrow cells
☐ 2. liver tissues
☐ 3. heart tissues
☐ 4. pancreatic enzymes

42. A client is receiving chemotherapy that has the potential to cause pulmonary toxicity. Which signs or symptoms indicate a toxic response to the chemotherapy?
☐ 1. decrease in appetite
☐ 2. drowsiness
☐ 3. spasms of the diaphragm
☐ 4. cough and shortness of breath

43. A client is to start chemotherapy to treat lung cancer. A venous access device has been placed to permit administration of chemotherapeutic medications. Three days later at the scheduled appointment to receive chemotherapy, the nurse assesses that the client is dyspneic and the skin is warm and pale. The vital signs are blood pressure 80/30 mm Hg, pulse 132 bpm, respirations 28 breaths/min, temperature 103°F (39.4°C), and oxygen saturation 84%. The central line insertion site is inflamed. After calling the rapid response team, what should the nurse do **next**?
☐ 1. Place cold, wet compresses on the client's head.
☐ 2. Obtain a portable ECG monitor.
☐ 3. Administer a prescribed antipyretic.
☐ 4. Insert a peripheral intravenous fluid line and infuse normal saline.

44. A client receiving chemotherapy for cancer has an elevated serum creatinine level. The nurse should **next**:
☐ 1. cancel the next scheduled chemotherapy.
☐ 2. administer the scheduled dose of chemotherapy.
☐ 3. notify the HCP.
☐ 4. obtain a urine specimen.

The Client Who Is Receiving Radiation Therapy

45. The nurse is instructing a client about skin care while receiving radiation therapy to the chest. What should the nurse instruct the client to do?
☐ 1. Apply lotion if the skin becomes dry.
☐ 2. Shave the chest to prevent contamination from chest hair.
☐ 3. Wash the area with tepid water and mild soap.
☐ 4. Keep the area covered with a nonadherent dressing between treatments.

46. A client with cancer who is receiving radiation therapy develops thrombocytopenia. The **priority** nursing goal is to prevent:
☐ 1. pain related to spontaneous bleeding episodes.
☐ 2. altered nutrition related to anemia.
☐ 3. injury related to the decreased platelet count.
☐ 4. skin breakdown related to decreased tissue perfusion.

47. A client is beginning external beam radiation therapy to the right axilla after a lumpectomy for breast cancer. Which information should the nurse include in client teaching?
☐ 1. Use a heating pad under the right arm.
☐ 2. Immobilize the right arm.
☐ 3. Place ice on the area after each treatment.
☐ 4. Apply deodorant only under the left arm.

48. A client receiving radiation therapy for lung cancer is having difficulty sleeping. The nurse should:
- [ ] 1. suggest the client stop watching television before bed.
- [ ] 2. assess the client's usual sleep patterns, amount of sleep, and bedtime rituals.
- [ ] 3. tell the client sleeplessness is expected with radiation therapy.
- [ ] 4. suggest that the client stop drinking coffee until the therapy is completed.

49. A 56-year-old female client is currently receiving radiation therapy to the chest wall for recurrent breast cancer. She has pain while swallowing and burning and tightness in her chest. The nurse should further assess the client for indications of:
- [ ] 1. hiatal hernia.
- [ ] 2. stomatitis.
- [ ] 3. radiation enteritis.
- [ ] 4. esophagitis.

50. A 36-year-old female is scheduled to receive external radiation therapy and a cesium implant for cancer of the cervix and is asking about the effects of the radiation on sexual relations. The nurse should inform the client about which potential effects of radiation therapy on sexuality?
- [ ] 1. "You can have sexual intercourse while the implant is in place."
- [ ] 2. "You may notice some vaginal dryness after treatment is completed."
- [ ] 3. "You may notice some vaginal relaxation after treatment is completed."
- [ ] 4. "You will continue to have normal menstrual periods during treatment."

51. The nurse caring for a client who is receiving external beam radiation therapy for treatment of lung cancer should assess the client for:
- [ ] 1. diarrhea.
- [ ] 2. improved energy level.
- [ ] 3. dysphagia.
- [ ] 4. normal white blood cell count.

The Client Who Requires Symptom Management

52. A client receiving radiation to the head and neck is experiencing stomatitis. The nurse should recommend:
- [ ] 1. evaluation by a dentist.
- [ ] 2. alcohol-based mouthwash rinses.
- [ ] 3. artificial saliva.
- [ ] 4. vigorous brushing of teeth after each meal.

53. A client undergoing chemotherapy has a white blood cell count of 2,300/mm³ (2.3 × 10⁹/L), hemoglobin of 9.8 g/dL (98 g/L), platelet count of 80,000/mm³ (80 × 10⁹/L), and potassium of 3.8. Which finding should take **priority**?
- [ ] 1. blood pressure 136/88 mm Hg
- [ ] 2. emesis of 90 mL
- [ ] 3. temperature 101°F (38.3°C)
- [ ] 4. urine output 40 mL/h

54. A client with bladder cancer has gross hematuria. The client's hemoglobin is 8.0 g/dL (80 g/L), and the healthcare provider (HCP) prescribes a unit of packed blood cells. The client has an existing intravenous infusion of normal saline using a 19-gauge needle. To administer the packed red blood cells, the nurse should:
- [ ] 1. attach the packed cells to the existing 19-gauge IV of normal saline solution using Y tubing.
- [ ] 2. start an additional 22-gauge IV site because the packed blood cells must be given in a separate line.
- [ ] 3. attach the packed blood cells to the existing 22-gauge IV of 5% dextrose using Y tubing.
- [ ] 4. start an additional IV access device with a 22-gauge intravenous cannulation device.

55. A nurse is caring for a client 24 hours after an abdominal-perineal resection for a bowel tumor. The client's wife asks if she can bring him some of his favorite home-cooked Italian minestrone soup. What should the nurse do **first**?
- [ ] 1. Auscultate for bowel sounds.
- [ ] 2. Ask the client if he feels hunger or gas pains.
- [ ] 3. Consult the dietician.
- [ ] 4. Encourage the wife to bring the soup.

56. Which nursing intervention would be **most** helpful in improving the respiratory effort of a client with metastatic lung cancer?
- [ ] 1. teaching the client diaphragmatic breathing techniques
- [ ] 2. administering cough suppressants as prescribed
- [ ] 3. teaching and encouraging pursed-lip breathing
- [ ] 4. placing the client in a low semi-Fowler's position

57. Which information should be included in the teaching plan for a client with cancer who is experiencing thrombocytopenia? Select all that apply.
- [ ] 1. Use an electric razor.
- [ ] 2. Use a soft-bristle toothbrush.
- [ ] 3. Avoid frequent flossing for oral care.
- [ ] 4. Include an over-the-counter nonsteroidal anti-inflammatory (NSAID) daily for pain control.
- [ ] 5. Monitor temperature daily.
- [ ] 6. Report bleeding, such as nosebleed, petechiae, or melena, to a healthcare provider (HCP).

58. A client with cancer is afraid of experiencing a febrile reaction associated with blood transfusions. The nurse should explain to the client that:

☐ 1. "Febrile reactions are caused when antibodies on the surface of blood cells in the transfusion are directed against antigens of the recipient."

☐ 2. "Febrile reactions can usually be prevented by administering antipyretics and antihistamines before the start of the transfusion."

☐ 3. "Febrile reactions are rarely immune-mediated reactions and can be a sign of hemolytic transfusion."

☐ 4. "Febrile reactions primarily occur within 15 minutes after initiation of the transfusion and can occur during the blood transfusion."

59. An adult who recently had a right pneumonectomy for lung cancer is admitted to the oncology unit with dyspnea and fever. The nurse should:

☐ 1. place the client on the left side.

☐ 2. position the client for postural drainage.

☐ 3. provide education on deep-breathing exercises.

☐ 4. instruct the client to maintain bed rest with bathroom privileges.

60. A client undergoing chemotherapy tells the nurse, "I do not want to get out of bed in the morning, because I am so tired." The nursing plan of care should include:

☐ 1. education on the use of filgrastim.

☐ 2. individually tailored exercise program.

☐ 3. weight lifting when not experiencing fatigue.

☐ 4. bed rest until chemotherapy is completed.

61. A nurse is reviewing the medical record of an adult male with cancer. The healthcare provider (HCP) has prescribed filgrastim 400 mcg, subcutaneously once daily. The nurse reviews the laboratory report and determines treatment has been effective when:

Laboratory Results

Hemoglobin: 16 g/dL (160 g/L)

White blood cell (WBC) count: 3,500/mm³ (3.5 × 10⁹/L)

Platelet count: 200,000/mm³ (200 × 10⁹/L)

Red blood cell (RBC) count: 4.3 million/mm³ (4.3 × 10¹²/L)

☐ 1. hemoglobin is 16 g/dL (160 g/L).

☐ 2. WBC count is 3,500/mm³ (3.5 × 10⁹/L).

☐ 3. platelet count is 200,000/mm³ (200 × 10⁹/L).

☐ 4. RBC count is 4.3 million/mm³ (4.3 × 10¹²/L).

62. The nurse is teaching the client who is receiving chemotherapy and the family how to manage possible nausea and vomiting at home. The nurse should include information about:

☐ 1. eating frequent, small meals throughout the day.

☐ 2. eating three normal meals a day.

☐ 3. eating only cold foods with no odor.

☐ 4. limiting the amount of fluid intake.

63. A terminally ill client in hospice care is experiencing nausea and vomiting because of a partial bowel obstruction. To respect the client's wishes for palliative care, the nurse should recommend the use of:

☐ 1. a nasogastric (NG) suction tube.

☐ 2. IV antiemetics.

☐ 3. osmotic laxatives.

☐ 4. a clear liquid diet.

64. An adult is dying from metastatic lung cancer, and all treatments have been discontinued. The client's breathing pattern is labored, with gurgling sounds. The client's spouse asks the nurse, "Can you do something to help with the breathing?" Which is the nurse's **best** response in this situation?

☐ 1. Direct the unlicensed assistive personnel (UAP) to assess the client's vital signs and provide oral care.

☐ 2. Suction the client so that the client's spouse knows all interventions were performed.

☐ 3. Reposition the client, elevate the head of the bed, and provide a cool compress.

☐ 4. Explain to the spouse that it is standard practice not to suction clients when treatments have been discontinued.

65. A 65-year-old client with brown hair is concerned about losing the hair on the head as a result of chemotherapy. The nurse should tell the client:

☐ 1. "The new growth of hair will be gray."

☐ 2. "The hair loss is temporary."

☐ 3. "New hair growth will be the same texture and color as it was before chemotherapy."

☐ 4. "The client should avoid use of wigs when possible."

66. An adult with a history of chronic obstructive pulmonary disease (COPD) and metastatic carcinoma of the lung has not responded to radiation therapy and is being admitted to the hospice program. The nurse should conduct a focused client assessment for:

☐ 1. ascites.

☐ 2. pleural friction rub.

☐ 3. dyspnea.

☐ 4. peripheral edema.

67. The nurse is planning with a client who has cancer to improve the client's independence in activities of daily living after radiation therapy. What should the nurse do?
☐ 1. Refer the client to a community support group after discharge from the rehabilitation unit.
☐ 2. Make certain that a family member is present for the rehabilitation sessions.
☐ 3. Provide positive reinforcement for skills achieved.
☐ 4. Inform the client of rehabilitation plans made by the rehabilitation team.

68. When teaching about prevention of infection to a client with a long-term venous catheter, the nurse determines that the client has understood discharge instructions when the client states:
☐ 1. "I will not remove the dressing until I return to the clinic next week."
☐ 2. "My husband will change the dressing three times a week, using sterile technique."
☐ 3. "I will monitor my temperature every other day."
☐ 4. "I know it is very important to wash my hands after irrigating the catheter."

69. When caring for a client with a central venous line, which nursing actions should be implemented in the plan of care for chemotherapy administration? Select all that apply.
☐ 1. Verify patency of the line by the presence of a blood return at regular intervals.
☐ 2. Inspect the insertion site for swelling, erythema, or drainage.
☐ 3. Administer a cytotoxic agent to keep the regimen on schedule even if blood return is not present.
☐ 4. If unable to aspirate blood, reposition the client and encourage the client to cough.
☐ 5. Contact the healthcare provider (HCP) about verifying placement if the status is questionable.

70. Indicate on the illustration the area that correctly identifies the position of the distal tip of a central line that is inserted into the subclavian vein.

71. A client with pancreatic cancer, who has been bed-bound for 3 weeks, has just returned from having a left subclavian, long-term, tunneled catheter inserted for administration of analgesics. The nurse has not yet received radiographic results for confirmation of placement. The client becomes restless and dyspneic and has chest pain radiating to the middle of the back. Physical assessment reveals tachycardia and absent breath sounds in the left lung. The nurse should further assess the client for:
☐ 1. an air embolus.
☐ 2. a pneumothorax.
☐ 3. a pulmonary embolus.
☐ 4. a myocardial infarction.

72. In setting goals for a client with advanced liver cancer who has poor nutrition, which is a desired outcome for the client? The client will:
☐ 1. have normalized albumin levels.
☐ 2. return to ideal body weight.
☐ 3. gain 1 lb (0.5 kg) every 2 weeks.
☐ 4. maintain current weight.

73. The nurse administers a bolus tube feeding to a client with cancer. To decrease the risk of aspiration, the nurse should:
☐ 1. place the client on bed rest with the head of the bed elevated to 60 degrees for 2 hours.
☐ 2. turn the client on the left side with the head of the bed at 45 degrees for 15 minutes.
☐ 3. assist the client out of bed to sit upright in a chair for 1 hour.
☐ 4. ask the client to rest in bed with the head of the bed elevated to 30 degrees for 20 minutes.

74. A client with colon cancer had a left hemicolectomy 3 weeks ago. The client is still having difficulty maintaining an adequate oral intake to meet metabolic needs for optimal healing. The nurse should recommend to the healthcare provider (HCP) which nutritional support to maintain the nutritional needs of the client?
☐ 1. total parenteral nutrition through a central catheter
☐ 2. IV infusion of dextrose
☐ 3. nasogastric feeding tube with protein supplement
☐ 4. jejunostomy for high-caloric feedings

75. A client with colon cancer undergoes surgical removal of a segment of colon and creation of a sigmoid colostomy. What assessments by the nurse indicate the client is developing complications within the first 24 hours? Select all that apply.
☐ 1. coarse breath sounds auscultated bilaterally at the bases
☐ 2. dusky appearance of the stoma
☐ 3. no drainage in the ostomy appliance
☐ 4. temperature >101.2°F (38.4°C)
☐ 5. decreased bowel sounds

76. A client receiving chemotherapy for metastatic colon cancer is admitted to the hospital because of prolonged vomiting. Assessment findings include irregular pulse of 120 bpm, blood pressure of 88/48 mm Hg, respiratory rate of 14 breaths/min, serum potassium of 2.9 mEq/L (2.9 mmol/L), and arterial blood gas—pH 7.46, PCO_2 45 mm Hg (6.0 kPA), PO_2 95 mm Hg (12.6 kPA), and bicarbonate level 29 mEq/L (29 mmol/L). The nurse should implement which prescription **first**?
- ☐ **1.** oxygen at 4 L per nasal cannula
- ☐ **2.** repeat lab work in 4 hours
- ☐ **3.** 5% dextrose in 0.45% normal saline with KCl 40 mEq/L at 125 mL/h
- ☐ **4.** 12-lead ECG

77. One week after a left mastectomy, the client reports her appetite is still not good, she is not getting much sleep, and her husband is avoiding her. She is eager to get back to work. What should the nurse do **first**?
- ☐ **1.** Call the healthcare provider (HCP) to discuss allowing the client to return to work earlier.
- ☐ **2.** Suggest that the client learn relaxation techniques for help with insomnia.
- ☐ **3.** Perform a nutritional assessment to assess for anorexia.
- ☐ **4.** Ask open-ended questions about sexuality issues related to her mastectomy.

78. The nurse is making a follow-up telephone call to a 52-year-old client with lung cancer. The client now has a low-grade fever (100.6°F [38.1°C]), nonproductive cough, and increasing fatigue. The client completed the radiation therapy to the mass in the right lung and mediastinum 10 weeks ago and has a follow-up appointment to see the healthcare provider in 2 weeks. The nurse should advise the client:
- ☐ **1.** to take two acetaminophen tablets every 4 to 6 hours for 2 days and call the healthcare provider (HCP) if the temperature increases to 101°F (38.3°C) or greater.
- ☐ **2.** that this is an expected side effect of the radiation therapy and to keep his appointment in 2 weeks.
- ☐ **3.** to contact the healthcare provider (HCP) for an appointment today.
- ☐ **4.** to go to the nearest emergency department.

79. A client with malignant pleural effusions has dyspnea and chest pain. In which order of priority from first to last should the nurse manage the client's care? All options must be used.

1. Administer morphine sulfate 2 mg IV.

2. Apply oxygen at 2 L via nasal cannula.

3. Educate the client in anticipation of a thoracentesis.

4. Coach the client on deep-breathing exercise.

80. What instructions should the nurse provide to a client who develops cellulitis in the right arm after a right modified radical mastectomy?
- ☐ **1.** Antibiotics will need to be taken for 1 to 2 weeks.
- ☐ **2.** Arm exercises will get rid of the cellulitis.
- ☐ **3.** Ice packs should be applied to the affected area for 20-minute periods to reduce swelling.
- ☐ **4.** The right extremity should be lowered to improve blood flow to the forearm.

81. An adult has just had a sclerosing agent instilled after chest tube drainage of a pleural effusion. The nurse should instruct the client to:
- ☐ **1.** lie still to prevent a pneumothorax.
- ☐ **2.** sit upright with arms on an overhead table to promote lung expansion.
- ☐ **3.** change position frequently to distribute the agent.
- ☐ **4.** lie on the side where the thoracentesis was done to hold pressure on the chest tube site.

82. After surgery for head and neck cancer, a client has a permanent tracheostomy. Which is the **most** important point for the nurse to include in the teaching plan for the client and family?
- ☐ **1.** providing tracheostomy site care
- ☐ **2.** addressing the psychosocial issues related to tracheostomy
- ☐ **3.** observing for early signs and symptoms of skin breakdown around the tracheostomy site
- ☐ **4.** using humidifiers to prevent thick, tenacious secretions

83. A client has malignant pleural effusions. The nurse should conduct a focused assessment to determine if the client has which signs and symptoms? Select all that apply.
☐ 1. hiccups
☐ 2. weight gain
☐ 3. peripheral edema
☐ 4. chest pain
☐ 5. dyspnea
☐ 6. cough

84. A client with suspected lung cancer is undergoing a thoracentesis. Which outcomes of the procedure are expected? Select all that apply.
☐ 1. treatment of recurrent malignant effusion
☐ 2. diagnosis of underlying disease
☐ 3. palliation of symptoms
☐ 4. relief of acute respiratory distress
☐ 5. removal of the cancer cells

85. The nurse is assessing a client with anemia. In order to plan nursing care, the nurse should focus the assessment on which signs and symptoms?
☐ 1. decreased salivation
☐ 2. bradycardia
☐ 3. cold intolerance
☐ 4. nausea

86. A nurse is assessing an adult who has been receiving chemotherapy. The client has a platelet count of 22,000 cells/mm³ (22 × 10⁹/L) and has petechiae on the lower extremities. The nurse should advise the client to:
☐ 1. increase the amount of iron in the client's diet.
☐ 2. apply lotion to the lower extremities.
☐ 3. elevate the legs.
☐ 4. consult the healthcare provider (HCP).

87. A nurse is teaching an older adult who has had a left modified radical mastectomy with axillary node dissection about lymphedema. The nurse should tell the client that lymphedema occurs:
☐ 1. if all cancer cells are not removed.
☐ 2. in older women.
☐ 3. at any time after surgery.
☐ 4. only with radical mastectomy.

88. A middle-aged female with a history of breast-conserving surgery, axillary node dissection, and radiation therapy reports that her arm is red, warm to touch, and slightly swollen. Which action should the nurse suggest?
☐ 1. Apply warm compresses to the affected arm.
☐ 2. Elevate the arm on two pillows.
☐ 3. See the healthcare provider (HCP) immediately.
☐ 4. Schedule an appointment within 2 to 3 weeks.

89. The nurse is assessing a middle-aged client with cancer who has lost 1 lb (0.5 kg) in 4 weeks. The client is taking ondansetron for nausea and now has a temperature of 101°F (38.3°C). The fever is indicative of:
☐ 1. inadequate nutrition.
☐ 2. new resistance to current antiemetic therapy.
☐ 3. expected response to chemotherapy treatment.
☐ 4. infection.

90. A nurse is assessing a client with lymphoma who reports distress 9 days after chemotherapy. Because of the risk for septic shock, the nurse should assess the client for which cluster of symptoms?
☐ 1. flushing, decreased oxygen saturation, mild hypotension
☐ 2. low-grade fever, chills, tachycardia
☐ 3. elevated temperature, oliguria, hypotension
☐ 4. high-grade fever, normal blood pressure, increased respirations

91. An appropriate nursing intervention for a client with fatigue related to cancer treatment includes teaching the client to:
☐ 1. increase fluid intake.
☐ 2. minimize naps or periods of rest during day.
☐ 3. conserve energy by prioritizing activities.
☐ 4. limit dietary intake of high-fiber foods.

92. The **most** common issue associated with sleep disturbances in the hospitalized client with cancer is:
☐ 1. social.
☐ 2. nutritional.
☐ 3. cultural.
☐ 4. psychological.

93. Which is the **most** appropriate nursing intervention for a hospitalized client with pruritus caused by medications used to treat cancer?
☐ 1. administration of antihistamines
☐ 2. steroids
☐ 3. silk sheets
☐ 4. medicated cool baths

94. A client receiving chemotherapy has pruritus. In order to develop a care plan, the nurse should ask if the client has been:
☐ 1. wearing clothes made from 100% cotton.
☐ 2. sleeping in a cool, humidified room.
☐ 3. increasing fluid intake to at least 3,000 mL/day.
☐ 4. taking daily baths with a deodorant soap.

95. Which factor is **most** important to assess when determining the impact of the cancer diagnosis and treatment modalities on a long-term survivor's quality of life?
☐ 1. occupation and employability
☐ 2. functional status
☐ 3. evidence of disease
☐ 4. individual values and beliefs

96. A client with breast cancer has abdominal bloating and cramping with no bowel movement for 5 days. She says she usually has a bowel movement every day after her morning coffee. Bowel sounds are present in all four quadrants. She received 80 mg of doxorubicin hydrochloride 10 days ago. The nurse should contact the healthcare provider (HCP) to request a prescription for:
- [ ] 1. a ready-to-use enema to stimulate peristalsis.
- [ ] 2. a soapsuds enema until clear.
- [ ] 3. an oral cathartic until the client has a bowel movement; then evaluate the need for daily stool softeners.
- [ ] 4. a daily stool softener for constipation and a mild opioid for abdominal discomfort.

97. A client with cancer has diarrhea and inflamed areas of skin around the rectum. What actions should the nurse take? Select all that apply.
- [ ] 1. Use sitz baths.
- [ ] 2. Apply zinc oxide ointment to the rectal area after each bowel movement.
- [ ] 3. Apply a skin barrier dressing daily to the rectal area.
- [ ] 4. Clean the rectal area with unscented soap and water after each bowel movement, rinse well, and pat dry.
- [ ] 5. Increase fluid intake.

98. When explaining the long-term toxic effects of cancer treatments on the immune system, what should the nurse tell the client?
- [ ] 1. Clients with persistent immunologic abnormalities after treatment are at a much greater risk for infection than clients with a history of splenectomy.
- [ ] 2. The use of radiation and combination chemotherapy can result in more frequent and more severe immune system impairment.
- [ ] 3. Long-term immunologic effects have been studied only in clients with breast and lung cancer.
- [ ] 4. The helper T cells recover more rapidly than do the suppressor T cells, which results in positive helper cell balance that can last 5 years.

The Client Who Is Coping with Loss, Grief, Bereavement, and Spiritual Distress

99. A client is newly diagnosed with cancer and is beginning a treatment plan. Which action by the nurse will be **most** effective in helping the client cope?
- [ ] 1. Assume decision making for the client until treatment is completed.
- [ ] 2. Encourage the client to observe strict compliance with all treatment regimens.
- [ ] 3. Inform the client of all possible adverse treatment effects.
- [ ] 4. Identify available resources for the client and family.

100. A daughter is concerned that her mother is in denial because when they discuss the diagnosis of breast cancer, the mother says that breast cancer is not that serious and then changes the subject. The nurse can tell the daughter that denial can be a healthy defense mechanism if it is used:
- [ ] 1. to permit her mother to seek unconventional treatments.
- [ ] 2. when making decisions about her care.
- [ ] 3. alone and not in combination with other defense mechanisms.
- [ ] 4. to allow her mother to continue in her role as a mother.

101. A 45-year-old single mother of three teenaged boys has metastatic breast cancer. Her parents live 750 miles (1,200 km) away and have only been able to visit twice since her initial diagnosis 14 months ago. The progression of her disease has forced the client to consider high-dose chemotherapy. She is concerned about her children's welfare during the treatment. When assessing the client's present support systems, the nurse will be **most** concerned about the potential problems with:
- [ ] 1. denial as a primary coping mechanism.
- [ ] 2. support systems and coping strategies.
- [ ] 3. decision-making abilities.
- [ ] 4. transportation and money for the boys.

102. Which characteristic displayed by the wife of a 36-year-old man with pancreatic cancer suggests that she may be at risk for negative bereavement outcomes?
- [ ] 1. She is preparing for her husband's death.
- [ ] 2. She has a high socioeconomic status.
- [ ] 3. She has strong family support.
- [ ] 4. She blames herself for her husband's cancer.

103. The nurse is counseling the family of an older adult who died today. Which factor facilitates attainment of a positive bereavement outcome?
- [ ] 1. being a teenager
- [ ] 2. having a history of anxiety
- [ ] 3. being a spouse
- [ ] 4. possessing adequate financial resources

104. Which nursing intervention will be **most** effective when caring for a client who is experiencing powerlessness?
- [ ] 1. Make certain that all staff members focus only on the client's capabilities.
- [ ] 2. Encourage family members to become more responsible for the client's care.
- [ ] 3. Request a referral to a psychologist.
- [ ] 4. Include the client in decision making whenever possible.

105. During the initial stage of adaptation to the diagnosis of cancer and its treatment, the nurse can facilitate the client's adaptation by:
- [ ] 1. encouraging the client to maintain her usual role.
- [ ] 2. facilitating family-related disagreements and conflicts.
- [ ] 3. supporting the client in her use of denial as a coping strategy.
- [ ] 4. arranging transportation and child care on treatment days.

106. When explaining hospice care to a client, the nurse should tell the client:
- [ ] 1. "Hospice care uses a team approach to direct hospice activity."
- [ ] 2. "Clients and their families are the focus of care."
- [ ] 3. "Your healthcare provider coordinates all the care."
- [ ] 4. "All hospice clients will die at home."

107. A client's husband expresses concern that his dying wife keeps saying, "I have to go to the store." Which statement by the nurse will be **most** effective in assisting the husband to understand the dying process?
- [ ] 1. "Many dying clients are restless and can be treated with sedatives."
- [ ] 2. "The client may be fighting death, and you should leave her alone."
- [ ] 3. "Comments related to going somewhere or leaving on a trip are common in dying clients."
- [ ] 4. "You can tell your wife that you will take her to the store."

108. The wife of a terminally ill client asks the nurse, "Why is my husband having frequent bowel movements if he is not eating?" The nurse should tell the wife:
- [ ] 1. "I know he is having frequent loose stools and it is distressing for you, but that is just the way it is."
- [ ] 2. "I do not know when the bowels will shut down, but they will eventually."
- [ ] 3. "The pain medication will eventually help to slow the process of bowel function."
- [ ] 4. "The intestines still produce some waste products even when a person is not eating."

109. The client who is in end stages of cancer is requesting spiritual support. The nurse should:
- [ ] 1. inform the family and ask for their suggestions.
- [ ] 2. call a chaplain and set up an appointment for spiritual guidance.
- [ ] 3. help the client reflect on past accomplishments.
- [ ] 4. ask the client what spiritual activities would be most helpful.

110. An older adult with end-stage cancer needs assistance with arranging the finances for end-of-life home care. The nurse should refer the client to:
- [ ] 1. the business manager of the healthcare agency.
- [ ] 2. a social worker.
- [ ] 3. the healthcare provider (HCP).
- [ ] 4. the executor of the client's will.

111. The family members of a client who is near death from colon cancer ask the nurse what to expect if the client becomes dehydrated. What should the nurse tell them?
- [ ] 1. The healthcare provider (HCP) will make the decision regarding hydration therapy.
- [ ] 2. Dehydration may prolong the dying process.
- [ ] 3. Hydration is used only in extreme situations of dehydration.
- [ ] 4. Dehydration is expected during the dying process.

112. When caring for a client who is experiencing spiritual distress, what should the nurse do **first**?
- [ ] 1. Make a referral to a member of the clergy.
- [ ] 2. Explain the major beliefs of different religions.
- [ ] 3. Suggest reading material.
- [ ] 4. Help the client explore his or her own values and beliefs.

113. A nurse is caring for a client who is receiving hospice care at home. The client's neighbors have been calling the nurse to inquire about the client's condition. The nurse should tell the callers:
- [ ] 1. "Please call the oncologist."
- [ ] 2. "The client is in a coma now."
- [ ] 3. "Please call the client's sister."
- [ ] 4. "The client is not expected to live much longer."

114. A 42-year-old client with breast cancer is concerned that her husband is depressed by her diagnosis. Which change in her husband's behavior may confirm her fears?
- [ ] 1. increased decisiveness
- [ ] 2. problem-focused coping style
- [ ] 3. increase in social interactions
- [ ] 4. disturbance in his sleep patterns

115. The **most** cost-effective suggestion for bereavement support for the hospice nurse to give a woman whose husband died 3 months ago and her three young children would be to:
- [ ] 1. seek group counseling support for the three children.
- [ ] 2. request individual counseling and medication to manage depression.
- [ ] 3. remind her gently that bereavement care before death minimizes grieving.
- [ ] 4. continue bereavement support offered through hospice.

116. Which strategy will be **most** effective in improving transcultural communications with clients with cancer and their families?
☐ 1. Use touch to show concern and caring for the client.
☐ 2. Focus attention on verbal communication skills only.
☐ 3. Establish a rapport and listen to their concerns.
☐ 4. Maintain eye contact at all times.

117. Which outcome is expected of a nursing referral to a cancer support group? The client can:
☐ 1. choose the best treatment options.
☐ 2. find financial help.
☐ 3. obtain home health care.
☐ 4. cope with cancer.

118. A cancer survivor feels guilty when attending a cancer support group meeting. The nurse can help the client manage feelings of guilt by pointing out that:
☐ 1. these actually are feelings of anger at the terminally ill clients in the group.
☐ 2. it is an unexpected response to volatile emotions.
☐ 3. this is a spiritual response to the client's own illness.
☐ 4. this is a normal reaction when surviving a life-threatening experience.

119. The 65-year-old widower whose only son is 500 miles (800 km) away is at higher risk for psychosocial distress because the client:
☐ 1. has been successful in dealing with stress all his life.
☐ 2. does not have to deal with other stressors right now.
☐ 3. is able to use denial as a coping mechanism.
☐ 4. perceives he has minimal social support.

120. A client with a diagnosis of cancer is frequently disruptive and challenges the nurse. This behavior may be caused by:
☐ 1. uncertainty and an underlying fear of recurrence.
☐ 2. the usual trajectory of a short-term illness.
☐ 3. a history of a behavioral illness.
☐ 4. the one-time crisis from learning of the diagnosis.

121. A 42-year-old husband and father of a 7-year-old girl and a 10-year-old boy is concerned about what he should tell his children regarding his wife's impending death from aggressive breast cancer. The nurse should **first**:
☐ 1. refer the family to pastoral care services.
☐ 2. encourage the husband to come to terms with his own grief.
☐ 3. suggest that the healthcare provider (HCP) tell the children about the seriousness of their mother's illness.
☐ 4. begin education about strategies for communication with his children.

122. While talking to her husband, who is caring for their children, a middle-aged woman who has stage 4 breast cancer slams the phone down. She begins to cry and states that she is feeling guilty for being hospitalized. Which nursing action will **best** support the client emotionally?
☐ 1. Ask the client if she would like to speak with a grief counselor.
☐ 2. Call the healthcare provider (HCP), and request an antidepressant.
☐ 3. Sit with the client, and help her acknowledge and discuss her feelings.
☐ 4. Suggest the client call her husband when she is calmer.

123. A middle-aged woman who is receiving radiation therapy tells the nurse that she feels inadequate as a wife and mother because she can no longer carry out her usual duties with the same energy as before. What recommendations should the nurse make to help the client cope with this situation?
☐ 1. Suggest that she reassign all household chores to other members of the family.
☐ 2. Suggest that she prioritize her activities and ask for help from friends and family.
☐ 3. Suggest that she ignore the household chores during the crisis period.
☐ 4. Tell her not to worry so much because everyone gets a little tired at this phase of the therapy.

124. An older adult woman who is usually meticulous about her appearance and dress arrives today for her 23rd day of radiation therapy. She appears disheveled and emotionally labile, and her responses to the usual questions are a little inappropriate. Her heart rate is 124 bpm, her respirations are 32 breaths/min, and her skin is cold and clammy. These findings would suggest that the nurse should further assess the client for:
☐ 1. schizophrenia.
☐ 2. panic disorder.
☐ 3. depression.
☐ 4. delirium.

125. The nurse is planning future care with a middle-aged woman who has undergone surgical resection for lung cancer. Which plan will **best** promote adaptation and rehabilitation?
☐ 1. arranging a visit from a client who has recovered from a similar surgery
☐ 2. planning a progressive activity regimen
☐ 3. teaching about dressing care
☐ 4. requesting house cleaning services for 3 months

126. Which activity indicates that the client with cancer is adapting well to body image changes?
☐ 1. The client names his brother as the person to call if he is experiencing suicidal ideation.
☐ 2. The client continuously looks at the incision.
☐ 3. The client discusses a date to return to work.
☐ 4. The client serves as a volunteer in a client-to-client visitation program.

The Client Who Is Experiencing Problems with Sexuality

127. A 36-year-old female has increased vaginal dryness during sexual intercourse. She has received chemotherapy in the past and has menopausal symptoms due to ovarian suppression. The nurse should instruct the client on the use of:
☐ **1.** vaginal dilators.
☐ **2.** douching with a soothing solution.
☐ **3.** water-soluble vaginal lubricants.
☐ **4.** relaxation techniques.

128. A 49-year-old male with a tracheostomy tube confides to the nurse that he is beginning to avoid sexual activity because of the increased tracheostomy secretions. Which statement by the nurse will be **most** helpful to the client?
☐ **1.** "Use a scopolamine patch to decrease secretions."
☐ **2.** "Avoid fluid intake 2 hours before sexual activity."
☐ **3.** "Place a thin piece of gauze over the tracheostomy."
☐ **4.** "Wash the tracheostomy area with deodorizing antibacterial soap before sexual activity."

129. A 52-year-old client is scheduled for a total abdominal hysterectomy for cervical cancer. When discussing the potential impact of this procedure on the client's sexuality, the nurse should respond by saying:
☐ **1.** "All women experience sexual problems with this surgical procedure. Do you have any questions?"
☐ **2.** "When can I schedule an appointment with you and your partner to discuss any issues either of you may have regarding sexuality?"
☐ **3.** "Do you anticipate any problems with sex related to your scheduled hysterectomy?"
☐ **4.** "Most women have concerns about their sexuality after this type of surgery. Do you have any concerns or questions?"

130. A young man with early-stage testicular cancer is scheduled for a unilateral orchiectomy. The client confides to the nurse that he is concerned about what effects the surgery will have on his sexual performance. Which response by the nurse provides accurate information about sexual performance after an orchiectomy?
☐ **1.** "Most impotence resolves in a couple of months."
☐ **2.** "You could have early ejaculation with this type of surgery."
☐ **3.** "We will refer you to a sex therapist because you will probably notice erectile dysfunction."
☐ **4.** "Because your surgery does not involve other organs or tissues, you will likely not notice much change in your sexual performance."

131. A young female client is receiving chemotherapy and mentions to the nurse that she and her husband are using a diaphragm for birth control. Which information is **most** important for the nurse to discuss?
☐ **1.** inconvenience of the diaphragm
☐ **2.** transmission of sexually transmitted diseases
☐ **3.** body changes related to hormones
☐ **4.** infection control

132. To promote comfort and optimal respiratory expansion for a client with chronic obstructive pulmonary disease during sexual intimacy, the nurse can suggest that the couple:
☐ **1.** use a foam mattress.
☐ **2.** use pillows to raise the affected partner's head and upper torso.
☐ **3.** have the affected partner assume a dependent position.
☐ **4.** limit the duration of the sexual activity.

Ethical and Legal Issues Related to Clients with Cancer

133. A hospitalized client with end-stage heart failure does not want to be resuscitated. The healthcare provider (HCP) has written the do-not-resuscitate (DNR) prescription on the client's record. The client has a cardiac arrest, and the wife tells the nurse she wants the client to be resuscitated and asks the nurse to "do something." The nurse should:
☐ **1.** begin CPR.
☐ **2.** call a "code."
☐ **3.** page the healthcare provider (HCP).
☐ **4.** discuss the DNR prescription with the wife.

134. A registered nurse (RN) is assigning care on the oncology unit and assigns the client with Kaposi's sarcoma and human immunodeficiency virus (HIV) infection to the unlicensed assistive personnel (UAP). This person does not want to care for this client. How should the nurse respond?
☐ **1.** "I will assign this client to another nurse."
☐ **2.** "I will help you take care of this client so you are confident with the care."
☐ **3.** "You seem worried about this assignment."
☐ **4.** "I will review blood and body fluid precautions with you."

135. A woman employed full-time wants to request a leave of absence to care for her father who is being treated for colon cancer 300 miles (480 km) away. What should the nurse advise the client to do **first**?
- ☐ 1. Contact her employee resources department about policies guiding leaves of absence.
- ☐ 2. Make a plan to see how long she can be out of work without financial concerns.
- ☐ 3. Find someone to do her work while she is away.
- ☐ 4. Ask her father if he can afford a caregiver.

136. The nurse is developing a care plan for a client with cancer receiving hospice home care. Which would be the **most** appropriate action for managing the client's chronic pain?
- ☐ 1. Administer analgesics regularly and additionally as needed for breakthrough pain.
- ☐ 2. Sedate the client with tranquilizers.
- ☐ 3. Avoid intravenous pain medication until the client is terminal.
- ☐ 4. Administer analgesics when vital signs indicate increased pain severity.

137. A client and nurse have established a goal for the client to be more autonomous in decision making. Which situation indicates that the goal has been met?
- ☐ 1. The healthcare provider (HCP) directs the client's care.
- ☐ 2. The nurse provides the client with the facts and then allows the client to reach an unassisted decision.
- ☐ 3. The nurse respects a client's choice not to know particular information.
- ☐ 4. The healthcare team makes health and treatment decisions.

End-of-Life Care

138. A client who is near death is receiving hospice care to manage severe pain. The client is receiving a narcotic pain medication intravenously per a patient-controlled analgesia (PCA) pump. The client is lethargic and is sleeping much of the time, and has not had any pain for the last 12 hours. The nurse plans care based on the fact that the client:
- ☐ 1. Received too much medication through an overdose of medication administered through the PCA pump.
- ☐ 2. May be nearing death as specific dosages and time intervals for self-administration of the analgesic is programmed into the PCA pump to prevent overdose.
- ☐ 3. Has obtained sufficient pain relief because of not having pain in the last 12 hours.
- ☐ 4. Has an IV that has infiltrated and the analgesic has been injected into the subcutaneous tissues, thereby being absorbed faster than prescribed.

139. The family of a hospitalized client demonstrates understanding of the teaching about legal documents related to end-of-life care such as "advance directive" and "power of attorney" when they make which statements? Select all that apply.
- ☐ 1. "Advance directives give instructions about future medical care and treatment."
- ☐ 2. "If people are not capable of communicating their wishes, healthcare providers and family together can agree on measures or actions that will be taken."
- ☐ 3. "Ethics experts agree that the family is the sole deciding factor when the client is competent."
- ☐ 4. "Medical power of attorney gives primarily financial access to the designee."
- ☐ 5. "Medical power of attorney or durable power of attorney for health care is a document that lists who can make healthcare decisions should a person be unable to make an informed decision for himself or herself."
- ☐ 6. "Advance directives give details about the client's past medical history."

140. The nurse can be an important advocate for the client who is considering an alternative method of cancer treatment. Which statement **best** demonstrates the nurse as client advocate? The nurse will:
- ☐ 1. provide the information about standard therapies.
- ☐ 2. monitor blood tests as indicated by the alternative therapy.
- ☐ 3. document the client's desire to try an alternative therapy.
- ☐ 4. allow the client to make healthcare choices but will assist in ensuring the client is fully informed when making those decisions.

141. After completing the nursing assessment for a client and family entering the palliative care program, the nurse should develop a teaching plan that includes an understanding of which outcome? Select all that apply.
- ☐ 1. alteration in the family's usual coping strategies
- ☐ 2. achievement of a dignified and respectful death
- ☐ 3. improvement in the client's quality of life
- ☐ 4. provision of comfort during the dying process
- ☐ 5. provision of support for client and family
- ☐ 6. advocation for prolonging life while curing the disease

142. When a client and family receive the initial diagnosis of colon cancer, the nurse can act as an advocate by:
- ☐ 1. helping them maintain a sense of optimism and hopefulness.
- ☐ 2. determining their understanding of the results of the diagnostic testing.
- ☐ 3. listening carefully to their perceptions of what their needs are.
- ☐ 4. providing them with written materials about the cancer site and its treatment.

143. A client who is dying of acquired immunodeficiency syndrome (AIDS) is admitted to the inpatient psychiatric unit because he attempted suicide. His close friend recently died of AIDS. The client begins to talk about his feelings related to his illness and the loss of his friend. He begins to cry. Which response by the nurse would be **most** appropriate?
- [ ] 1. Give the client some tissues, and tell him it is okay to cry.
- [ ] 2. Tell the client to stop crying and that everything will be okay.
- [ ] 3. Sort the client's mail to distract the client.
- [ ] 4. Change the subject.

144. The wife of an older adult who has been admitted to the hospital with kidney failure tells the nurse, "I know he does not want to die in a hospital, but it is so hard for me to take care of him at home. He said he does not want any more treatment, but I am not ready to let him go. We have so many arrangements to decide before he dies." Which statement by the nurse to the client's wife would be **most** appropriate? Select all that apply.
- [ ] 1. "He is not going to die that soon judging by his current symptoms."
- [ ] 2. "What are your fears about your husband dying?"
- [ ] 3. "I can imagine that it is hard for you to care for him at home."
- [ ] 4. "What do you and your husband know about advance directives?"
- [ ] 5. "We can discuss types of hospice and home care available."
- [ ] 6. "What kind of arrangements do you think need to be made before he dies?"

145. A terminally ill client's husband tells the nurse, "I wish we had taken that trip to Europe last year. We just kept putting it off, and now I am furious that we did not go." The nurse interprets the husband's statement as indicating which stage of adaptation to dying?
- [ ] 1. anger
- [ ] 2. denial
- [ ] 3. bargaining
- [ ] 4. depression

146. Which philosophy should the nurse integrate into the plan of care for a client and family to help them **best** cope during the final stages of the client's illness?
- [ ] 1. living each day as it comes as fully as possible
- [ ] 2. reliving the pleasant memories of days gone by
- [ ] 3. expecting the worst and being grateful when it does not happen
- [ ] 4. planning ahead for the remaining good times that will be spent together

147. A client who is in the end stages of cancer is increasingly upset about receiving chemotherapy. Which approach by the nurse would likely be **most** helpful in gaining the client's cooperation?
- [ ] 1. Tell the client how the treatment can be expected to help.
- [ ] 2. Describe the probable effect that missing a treatment would have.
- [ ] 3. Explain that being upset makes the treatment more difficult.
- [ ] 4. Suggest having a massage during the treatment.

148. A client suspects that he will not live. However, others talk about only pleasant matters with him and maintain a persistently cheerful facade around him. The nurse plans care for this client by recognizing that these behaviors will **most** likely cause the client to feel:
- [ ] 1. relief.
- [ ] 2. isolated.
- [ ] 3. hopeful.
- [ ] 4. independent.

149. The young sister of a young adult client with leukemia asks, "Can you check my blood? When my sister got pneumonia, so did I. And I think I have this, too." How should the nurse respond? Select all that apply.
- [ ] 1. Ask the client's healthcare provider (HCP) to take a sample of the sister's blood.
- [ ] 2. Explain to the sister that leukemia is not a communicable disease.
- [ ] 3. Discuss the sister's concern with her parents.
- [ ] 4. Tell the sister's parents about a group for siblings of clients with terminal illness.
- [ ] 5. Ask the sister about her concerns.

150. When talking with the nurse, the brother of a client with leukemia says, "We used to play pretty rough games together. Maybe some of the bruises he got when I tackled him caused this." Which statement is the nurse's **best** response?
- [ ] 1. "Do not feel guilty. You did not cause your brother's illness."
- [ ] 2. "I can see you are worried. Let us talk about how people get leukemia."
- [ ] 3. "Here is some information about leukemia for you to read."
- [ ] 4. "Lots of people worry about things like this. It is not your fault."

Managing Care, Quality, and Safety of Clients with Cancer

151. A nurse is making follow-up phone calls to clients being treated for cancer. In which order of priority from first to last should the nurse return the calls? All options must be used.

1. the client receiving chemotherapy who has a loss of appetite

2. the client who underwent a mastectomy 2 weeks ago who called for information on the Reach for Recovery program

3. the client receiving spinal radiation for bone cancer metastases who has urinary incontinence

4. the client with colon cancer who has questions about a high-fiber diet

152. The nurse is making client rounds following shift report. Which client should the nurse assess **first**?
- ☐ 1. a 38-year-old woman receiving internal radiation therapy for cervical cancer
- ☐ 2. a 27-year-old man with leukemia hospitalized for induction of high-dose chemotherapy
- ☐ 3. a 75-year-old man with metastatic prostate cancer with a pathologic fracture of the femur who is in pain
- ☐ 4. a 23-year-old woman undergoing surgery for placement of a central venous catheter

153. The RN is administering intravenous chemotherapy to a client with cancer. Which precautions are necessary when administering chemotherapy? Select all that apply.
- ☐ 1. taping all IV tubing connections
- ☐ 2. wearing gloves when handling the client's urine
- ☐ 3. disposing of chemotherapy waste as hazardous material
- ☐ 4. wearing a long-sleeved gown when administering chemotherapy
- ☐ 5. disposing of sharps in a specifically labeled container.

154. During the intravenous administration of a chemotherapeutic vesicant drug, the nurse observes that there is a lack of blood return from the intravenous catheter. The nurse should **first**:
- ☐ 1. stop the administration of the drug.
- ☐ 2. reposition the client's arm and continue with administration of the drug.
- ☐ 3. irrigate the catheter with normal saline.
- ☐ 4. continue to administer the drug and assess for edema at the IV site.

155. The nurse is caring for a client with end-stage cancer whose health status is declining. A prescription is written by the attending healthcare provider (HCP) to withhold all fluid, but the healthcare team cannot locate a family member or guardian. The nurse requests an ethics consultation. Which information is true of an ethics consultation? Select all that apply.
- ☐ 1. Persons requesting an ethics consultation may do so without intimidation or fear of reprisal.
- ☐ 2. Ethics consultations may prevent poor outcomes in cases involving ethical problems.
- ☐ 3. The recommendations of ethics consultants are advisory only.
- ☐ 4. Requests for ethics consultations may only be made by the HCP or nurse.
- ☐ 5. Ethics consultation is intended to provide legal advice on client care.

156. The nurse-manager on the oncology unit wants to address the issue of correct documentation of the effectiveness of analgesia medication within 30 minutes after administration. What should the nurse-manager do **first**?
- ☐ 1. Change the policy of documentation to 45 minutes.
- ☐ 2. Consult the pharmacist.
- ☐ 3. Consult the nurses on the evening shift where documentation of analgesia is the greatest problem.
- ☐ 4. Complete a brief quality improvement study and chart audit to document the rate of adherence to the policy and the pattern of documentation over shifts.

157. A registered nurse (RN) instructs the unlicensed assistive personnel (UAP) to check the urine intake and output (I&O) on clients on the oncology unit at the end of the 8-hour shift. It is important for the nurse to instruct the UAP to do what?
- ☐ 1. Ask the clients if they are thirsty when calculating the I&O.
- ☐ 2. Report back to the nurse immediately if any client has an output <240 mL.
- ☐ 3. Document the I&O results on the medical records.
- ☐ 4. Write the I&O results down for the nurse to give report to the next shift.

158. An alert and oriented older adult female with metastatic lung cancer is admitted to the medical-surgical unit for treatment of heart failure. She was given 80 mg of furosemide in the emergency department. Although the client is ambulatory, the unlicensed assistive personnel (UAP) are concerned about urinary incontinence because the client is frail and in a strange environment. The nurse should instruct the UAP to assist with implementing the nursing plan of care by:
- ☐ 1. prescribing adult diapers for the client so she will not have to worry about incontinence.
- ☐ 2. requesting an indwelling urinary catheter to avoid incontinence.
- ☐ 3. padding the bed with extra absorbent linens.
- ☐ 4. placing a commode at the bedside and instructing the client in its use.

159. The nursing team on an oncology unit consists of a registered nurse (RN), a licensed practical/vocational nurse (LPN/VN), and one unlicensed assistive personnel (UAP). Which client should be assigned to the RN?
- ☐ 1. a 52-year-old client with lung cancer admitted for acute dyspnea
- ☐ 2. a 45-year-old client receiving tube feedings
- ☐ 3. a 28-year-old client being evaluated for a bone marrow transplant
- ☐ 4. a 65-year-old client diagnosed with endometrial cancer who underwent an abdominal hysterectomy 3 days ago

160. The nurse is to wear personal protective equipment (PPE) to administer a chemotherapeutic agent to the client. What guidelines should the nurse use for PPE use and care? Select all that apply.
- ☐ 1. Understand the proper use and limitations of PPE.
- ☐ 2. Use care in removing all items to reduce contamination.
- ☐ 3. Ensure that PPE is made of materials that allow for air ventilation.
- ☐ 4. Cleanse hands with alcohol-based solution before putting gloves on and after removing gloves.
- ☐ 5. Discard the PPE in containers for contaminated waste.

161. The nurse should ensure that which item is placed when the client is to receive intravascular therapy for more than 6 days?
- ☐ 1. short peripheral catheter
- ☐ 2. central venous access in the femoral vein
- ☐ 3. intravenous catheter insertion device
- ☐ 4. peripherally inserted central catheter (PICC)

Answers, Rationales, and Test-Taking Strategies

*The answers and rationales for each question follow below, along with keys (🔑) to the client need (CN) and cognitive level (CL) for each question. In addition, you will also see a glossary icon (📖) highlighting specific terminology used on the licensing exam. As you check your answers, use the **Content Mastery and Test-Taking Skill Self-Analysis** worksheet (tear-out worksheet in back of book) to identify the reason(s) for not answering the questions correctly. For additional information about test-taking skills and strategies for answering questions, refer to pages 12–23 and pages 35–36 in Part 1 of this book.*

The Client at Risk for Cancer

1. 3. Clients over age 50 who have a history of inflammatory bowel disease are at risk for colon cancer. The client who smokes is at high risk for lung cancer. While the exact cause is not always known, other risk factors for colon cancer are a diet high in animal fats, including a large amount of red meat and fatty foods with low fiber, and the presence of colon cancer in a first-generation relative.

🔑 CN: Reduction of risk potential; CL: Analyze

2. 4. Basal cell carcinoma occurs most commonly in sun-exposed areas of the body. The incidence of skin cancer is highest in older people who live in the mountains or spend outdoor leisure time at higher altitudes.

🔑 CN: Health promotion and maintenance; CL: Analyze

3. 1. Because of the high risk of infertility with chemotherapy, pelvic irradiation, and retroperitoneal lymph node dissection that may follow an orchiectomy, cryopreservation of sperm is completed before treatment is started and should be discussed with the client.

🔑 CN: Physiological adaptation; CL: Apply

4. 2. The word *prevalence* in a statistical setting is defined as the number of cases of a disease present in a specified population at a given time.

🔑 CN: Health promotion and maintenance; CL: Apply

5. 3. Sun damage is a cumulative process. Parents should be taught to apply sunscreen and teach their children to use sunscreen at an early age. Although preventive education is always valuable, serious sunburns in childhood are associated with an increased risk of melanoma. Adults and senior citizens have already been exposed to the harmful effects of the sun and, although they, too, should use sunscreen, they are not the group that will most benefit from intervention. Exposure to chemicals is not a risk factor for melanoma.

CN: Health promotion and maintenance; CL: Analyze

6. 4. A sunscreen with an SPF of 15 or higher should be worn on all sun-exposed skin surfaces. It should be applied before sun exposure and reapplied after being in the water. Peak sun exposure usually occurs from 0010 to 1400. Tightly woven clothing, protective hats, and sunglasses are recommended to decrease sun exposure. Sun tanning parlors should be avoided.

CN: Health promotion and maintenance; CL: Synthesize

7. 1. Malignant melanoma may have a familial basis, especially in families with dysplastic nevi syndrome. First-degree relatives should be monitored closely. Malignant melanoma occurs most often in the 20- to 45-year-old age group. Severe sunburn as a child does increase the risk; however, this client is at increased risk because of her family history.

CN: Health promotion and maintenance; CL: Apply

8. 3. Because more than 50% of the cancers occur in people who are older than age 65, the single most important factor in determining risk would be age.

CN: Health promotion and maintenance; CL: Apply

9. 1,3,4,5. The client is at increased risk for development of lung, skin, or breast cancer. Consequently, the client should improve nutrition (e.g., eating food with lower animal fat content, increasing fiber, adding fruits and vegetables to the diet), stop smoking, use sunscreen, and lose weight. The client's alcohol consumption is not excessive and not a risk. It is not necessary and would be difficult for the client to change jobs to work inside as long as the client uses protection from the sun.

CN: Health promotion and maintenance; CL: Synthesize

10. 1. Asbestos and alcohol, when combined with smoking, produce a synergistic effect and result in increased cancer risk and incidence.

Ultraviolet radiation exposure is associated with skin cancer. HPV exposure is associated with cervical cancer. However, the risks of contracting these types of cancer are not markedly increased when combined with smoking.

CN: Health promotion and maintenance; CL: Apply

11. 4,5. Hoarseness and chronic sore throat are indicative of cancer of head and neck cancers, particularly cancer of the pharynx. Tobacco use and heavy consumption of alcohol are risk factors for these cancers and may have a synergistic effect. Heavy use of acetaminophen is not a risk factor for head and neck cancer, but is related to liver failure. Exposure to the sun increases the risk of skin cancers, but not cancers of the head and neck. Consuming a high-fat diet is not related to head and neck cancer, but may be a risk factor for other cancers and heart disease. Exposure to wood dust and other inhaled particles is associated with lung cancer.

CN: Health promotion and maintenance; CL: Analyze

12. 2. High-fiber, low-fat diets are recommended to reduce the risk of colon cancer. Stir-frying, poaching, steaming, and broiling are all low-fat methods to prepare foods. Croissants are made of refined flour. They are also high in fat, as are peanut butter squares and whole milk, granola, cream cheese, and sour cream.

CN: Health promotion and maintenance; CL: Apply

13. 2. Environmental factors include place of residence, nutrition, occupation, personal habits, iatrogenic factors, and physical environment. Gender, immunologic status, and age are individual factors.

CN: Health promotion and maintenance; CL: Apply

14. 3. CT scanning is the standard noninvasive method used in a workup for lung cancer because it can distinguish small differences in tissue density and can detect nodal involvement. CT is comparable to magnetic resonance imaging in evaluating lymph node metastasis. CT is noninvasive and usually available, but these are not the main reasons for its use. CT can distinguish malignancy in some situations only.

CN: Physiological adaptation; CL: Synthesize

15. 3. A high-fat, low-fiber diet is a risk factor for colorectal cancer. A diet low in vitamin C, use of artificial sweeteners, and multiple sex partners are not considered risk factors for colorectal cancer.

CN: Health promotion and maintenance; CL: Analyze

16. 2. Strategies to reach clients in all cultures should include incorporating the folk beliefs and traditions of the target population into the program. Identification of a centrally located building with available access by the target population, use of materials in the native or primary language of the target population, and involvement by all community leaders will also help the program succeed.

🗝 CN: Health promotion and maintenance; CL: Synthesize

The Client with Pain

17. 4. The desired outcome for management of pain is that the client's or family's subjective report of pain is acceptable and documented using a pain scale; the goal is that behavioral and physiologic indicators of pain are absent around the clock. The nurse and client/family should develop a systematic approach to pain management using information gathered from history and a hierarchy of pain measurement. Pain should be assessed at frequent intervals. The client should not wait to receive medication until the pain is midpoint on the pain scale, nor should the client receive so much pain medication that he or she is not alert. Continuous pain relief is the goal, not just during particular periods during the day.

🗝 CN: Basic care and comfort; CL: Synthesize

18. 3. Tolerance develops from taking opioids over an extended period. It is characterized by the need for an increased dose to achieve the same degree of analgesia. Addiction is characterized by a drive to take the medication for the psychic effect rather than the therapeutic effect. Physical dependence is a response to ongoing exposure to a medication manifested by withdrawal symptoms when discontinued abruptly.

🗝 CN: Pharmacological and parenteral therapies; CL: Analyze

19. 4. The conversion ratio for morphine is 10 mg IV equals 30 mg oral, or 1:3. The client is receiving 300 mg orally per 24 hours, which is equivalent to 100 mg of IV morphine. Morphine 100 mg IV/24 hours = approximately 4 mg/h IV. The effect of the IV morphine is quick, and the oral morphine should be discontinued prior to starting the IV morphine. Administering too much morphine can cause untoward side effects.

🗝 CN: Pharmacological and parenteral therapies; CL: Synthesize

20. 3. Administration of morphine sulfate is contraindicated because morphine causes respiratory depression. It may also increase intracranial pressure if the client is not ventilating properly, which could result in an accumulation of CO_2, a potent vasodilator. Ibuprofen, naproxen, and acetaminophen are not likely to mask symptoms of increased intracranial pressure or impact respiratory status.

🗝 CN: Pharmacological and parenteral therapies; CL: Synthesize

21. 1. If the maximum dose specified by the prescription is required every 3 to 4 hours for breakthrough pain, the **HCP** 📖 should be notified to increase the long-acting medication or rotate to another type of opioid. Around-the-clock dosing is mandatory to achieve a steady state of analgesia. The rescue dose for breakthrough pain is administered over and above the regularly scheduled medication. If three to four analgesic doses are required every 24 hours, the sustained-release around-the-clock dose should be increased to include the amount used for previous breakthrough pain while maintaining a dose for future breakthrough pain.

🗝 CN: Pharmacological and parenteral therapies; CL: Synthesize

22. 1. The most common toxicities from NSAIDs are gastrointestinal disorders (nausea, epigastric pain, ulcers, bleeding, diarrhea, and constipation). Renal dysfunction, pulmonary complications, and cardiovascular complications from NSAIDs are much less common.

🗝 CN: Pharmacological and parenteral therapies; CL: Analyze

23. 2,3. In the client with chronic pain, physiologic adaptation results in minimal changes in behavior and vital signs; clients have normal vital signs and are generally physically inactive. Clients with chronic pain are not necessarily depressed. Elevated vital signs, grimacing, and moaning are characteristic responses to acute pain.

🗝 CN: Basic care and comfort; CL: Analyze

24. 1,2,4,6. Scheduled use of long-acting opioids and an around-the-clock dosing are necessary to achieve a steady level of analgesia. Whatever the route or frequency, a prescription should be available for "breakthrough" pain medication to be administered in addition to the regularly scheduled medication. Oral drug administration is the route of choice for economy, safety, and ease of use. Even severe pain requiring high doses of opioids can be managed orally as long as the client can swallow medication and has a functioning gastrointestinal system. Tolerance occurs due to the need for increasing doses to achieve the same pain relief and will not be avoided with the use of acetaminophen. Addiction is a complex condition in which the drug is used for psychological effect and not analgesia. Nurses need to educate families about the appropriate use of opioids and assure them that addiction is not a concern when managing cancer pain. Non-pharmacologic methods are useful as an adjunct to assist in pain control. Self-report is the best assessment of pain and is an individual response.

> 🔑 CN: Pharmacological and parenteral therapies; CL: Evaluate

25. 4. Most clients with cancer who are experiencing inadequate pain control while taking an oral opioid after being switched from IV administration have been undermedicated. Equianalgesic conversions should be made to provide estimates of the equivalent dose needed for the same level of relief as provided by the IV dose. There is research to suggest that cancer clients do not become addicted to opioids when dosed adequately. There is no evidence to suggest that the client is physically addicted or is having withdrawal symptoms.

> 🔑 CN: Pharmacological and parenteral therapies; CL: Analyze

26. 1. Intensity is indicative of the severity of pain and is important for evaluating the efficacy of pain management. The cause and location of the pain cannot be managed, but the intensity of the pain can be controlled. The nurse and client can collaborate to reduce aggravating factors; however, the goal will ultimately be to reduce the intensity of the pain.

> 🔑 CN: Basic care and comfort; CL: Analyze

27. 2. Tolerance to an opioid occurs when a larger dose of the analgesic is needed to provide the same level of pain control. The risk of addiction is low with opioids to treat cancer pain. There are no data to support that this client is experiencing withdrawal. Although the client may have experienced a placebo effect at one time, placebo effects tend to diminish over time, especially in regard to chronic cancer pain.

> 🔑 CN: Pharmacological and parenteral therapies; CL: Analyze

28. 2. The regular administration of analgesics provides a consistent serum level of medication, which can help prevent breakthrough pain. Therefore, taking the prescribed analgesics on a regular schedule is the best way to manage chronic cancer-related pain. There is little risk for the client with cancer-related pain to become addicted. Sleeping 12 to 16 hours a day would not allow the client to participate in usual daily activities or preferred activities.

> 🔑 CN: Pharmacological and parenteral therapies; CL: Synthesize

The Client Who Is Receiving Chemotherapy

29. 3. Chemotherapeutic agents are very toxic; therefore, precautions are taken such as the use of gloves and long-sleeved gowns when handling agents to prevent incidental contact with skin. Recapping needles is against universal precaution standards, and chemotherapy waste is disposed of in biohazard containers according to institution policy. Prepackaged agents can still be hazardous if not handled properly.

> 🔑 CN: Pharmacological and parenteral therapies; CL: Synthesize

30. 2. Stomatitis is an inflammation of the mucous membranes of the mouth resulting from chemotherapy. Using a soft-bristled toothbrush prevents further bleeding and irritation to the already irritated gums and mucous membranes. Hydrogen peroxide can further irritate the mouth. Fluids need to be lukewarm instead of hot; dental floss can be used if it is done gently.

> 🔑 CN: Basic care and comfort; CL: Synthesize

31. 3. Resources should be provided for acquiring a wig since it is easier to match hairstyle and color before hair loss begins. The client has expressed negative feelings of self-image with hair loss. Excessive shampooing and manipulation of hair will increase hair loss. Hair usually grows back in 3 to 4 weeks after the chemotherapy is finished; however, new hair may have a new color or texture. A wig, hairpiece, hat, scarf, or turban can be used to conceal hair loss. Social isolation should be avoided, and the client should be encouraged to socialize with others.

> 🔑 CN: Pharmacological and parenteral therapies; CL: Synthesize

32. 4. The client may excrete the chemotherapeutic agent for 48 hours or more after administration. Blood, emesis, and excretions may be considered contaminated during this time, and the client should not share a bathroom with children or pregnant women. Any contaminated linens or clothing should be washed separately and then washed a second time, if necessary. All contaminated disposable items should be sealed in plastic bags and disposed of as hazardous waste.

> 🔑 CN: Physiological integrity; CL: Synthesize

33. 4. A side effect of vincristine is constipation, and a bowel protocol should be considered. Loperamide is used to treat diarrhea. Fluids should be encouraged, along with high-fiber foods to prevent constipation.

> 🔑 CN: Pharmacological and parenteral therapies; CL: Synthesize

34. 3. Carbohydrates are the first substance used by the body for energy. Proteins are needed to maintain muscle mass, repair tissue, and maintain osmotic pressure in the vascular system. Fats, in a small amount, are needed for energy production. Chicken, green beans, and cottage cheese are the best selection to provide a nutritionally well-balanced diet of carbohydrate, protein, and a small amount of fat. Cereal with milk and strawberries as well as toast, gelatin dessert, and cookies have a large amount of carbohydrates and not enough protein. Steak and french fries provide some carbohydrates and a good deal of protein; however, they also provide a large amount of fat.

🗝 CN: Health promotion and maintenance; CL: Synthesize

35. 2. Chemotherapy agents typically cause nausea and vomiting when not controlled by antiemetic drugs. Antineoplastic drugs attack rapidly growing normal cells, such as in the gastrointestinal tract. These drugs also stimulate the vomiting center in the brain. Hair loss, loss of energy, and sleep are important aspects of the health history, but are not as critical as the potential for dehydration and electrolyte imbalance caused by nausea and vomiting.

🗝 CN: Pharmacological and parenteral therapies; CL: Analyze

36. 2,4,5. Chemotherapy causes bone marrow suppression and risk of infection. A platelet count of 40,000/mm³ (40 × 10⁹/L) and a white blood cell count of 2,300/mm³ (2.3 × 10⁹/L) are low. A temperature of 101.2°F (38.4°C) is high and could indicate an infection. Further assessment and examination should be performed to rule out infection. The BUN, hemoglobin, and specific gravity values are normal.

🗝 CN: Reduction of risk potential; CL: Analyze

37. 4. The nurse must recognize that an albumin level of 2.8 g/dL (28 g/L) indicates catabolism and potential for malnutrition. Normal albumin is 3.5 to 5.0 g/dL (35 to 50 g/L); <3.5 (35 g/L) indicates malnutrition. The other laboratory results are normal.

🗝 CN: Reduction of risk potential; CL: Analyze

38. 1. Fever is an early sign requiring clinical intervention to identify potential causes. Chills and dyspnea may or may not be observed. Tachycardia can be an indicator in a variety of clinical situations when associated with infection; it usually occurs in response to an elevated temperature or change in cardiac function.

🗝 CN: Reduction of risk potential; CL: Analyze

39. 2. Chemotherapy causes myelosuppression with a decrease in red blood cells (RBCs), WBCs, and platelets. This client's data demonstrate neutropenia, placing the client at risk for infection. An ANC of 500 to 1,000/mm³ (0.5 to 1 × 10⁹/L) indicates a moderate risk of infection; <500/mm³ (0.5 × 10⁹/L) indicates severe neutropenia and a high risk of infection. When the WBC count is low and immature WBCs are present, normal phagocytosis is impaired. Precautions to protect the client from life-threatening infections may be instituted when ANC is <1,000/mm³ (1 × 10⁹/L). Handwashing is the best way to avoid the spread of infection. It is not necessary to wear a gown and mask to take care of this client. It is also not necessary to restrict visitors; however, visitors should be screened to avoid exposing the client to possible infections. Erythropoietin is used for stimulating RBCs, not WBCs. Granulocyte colony-stimulating factors or granulocyte macrophage colony-stimulating factors are useful for treating neutropenia.

🗝 CN: Safety and infection control; CL: Synthesize

40. 1. The role of the nurse is to assess what substances or medications the client is using and to document and inform other members of the health-care team. It is very important to encourage the client to keep the **HCP** 📖 informed of all therapeutic agents, medications, and supplements he or she is using, to avoid adverse interactions. It is not appropriate for the nurse to suggest that the client choose either Western or alternative therapies or to discourage the client's use of alternative therapies. The nurse should remain objective about the client's treatment choices and respect the client's autonomy.

🗝 CN: Reduction of risk potential; CL: Synthesize

41. 1. The fast-growing, normal cells most likely to be affected by certain cancer treatments are blood-forming cells in the bone marrow, as well as cells in the digestive track, reproductive system, and hair follicles. Fortunately, most normal cells recover quickly when treatment is over. Bone marrow suppression (a decreased ability of the bone marrow to manufacture blood cells) is a common side effect of chemotherapy. A low white blood cell count (neutropenia) increases the risk of infection during chemotherapy, but other blood cells made in the bone marrow can be affected as well. Most cancer agents do not affect tissues and organs, such as heart, liver, and pancreas.

🗝 CN: Physiologic adaptation; CL: Apply

42. 4. Cough and shortness of breath are significant symptoms because they may indicate decreasing pulmonary function secondary to drug toxicity.

Decrease in appetite, difficulty in thinking clearly, and spasms of the diaphragm may occur as a result of chemotherapy; however, they are not indicative of pulmonary toxicity.

CN: Physiological adaptation; **CL:** Evaluate

43. 4. The client is experiencing severe sepsis, and it is essential to increase circulating fluid volume to restore the blood pressure and cardiac output. The wet compress, administering the antipyretic, and monitoring the client's cardiac status may be beneficial for this client, but they are not the highest priority action at this time. These three interventions may require the nurse to leave the client, which is not advisable at this time.

CN: Physiological adaptation; **CL:** Synthesize

44. 3. Nephrotoxicity caused by chemotherapy is assessed by monitoring serum creatinine. Creatinine is the most sensitive indicator of proper kidney function. In this case, the client is experiencing decreased kidney function, most likely due to the chemotherapy. The nurse consults the **HCP** 📖 for guidance. Administering the next dose of chemotherapy could potentially cause further kidney damage. It is inappropriate to cancel the chemotherapy without checking with the HCP or to tell the client that the cancer is spreading. A urine specimen will not provide other helpful information.

CN: Pharmacological and parenteral therapies; **CL:** Synthesize

The Client Who Is Receiving Radiation Therapy

45. 3. Clients receiving radiation experience dryness or redness in the area of the radiation. The nurse instructs the client to wash the area with soap and water and keep the area dry. The client does not apply lotion, shave, or cover the area.

CN: Basic care and comfort; **CL:** Apply

46. 3. This client is at high risk for bleeding because of the decreased platelet count. The priority nursing goal is to prevent injury to this client by preventing bleeding occurrences. Spontaneous bleeding may cause pain but is not the priority. The client has a low platelet count, but not a low hemoglobin count such as exists in anemia. Skin integrity is a risk but not a priority.

CN: Reduction of risk potential; **CL:** Synthesize

47. 4. The nurse should instruct the client to avoid applying chemicals (such as a deodorant) or heat or cold (such as with a heating pad or ice pack) to the area being treated. The client should be encouraged to use the extremity to prevent muscle atrophy and contractures.

CN: Health promotion and maintenance; **CL:** Synthesize

48. 2. Since sleeplessness is often an adverse effect of radiation therapy, the nurse should first assess the client's usual sleep patterns, hours of sleep required before treatment, and usual bedtime routine. Refraining from watching television before bedtime and avoiding caffeine intake are helpful suggestions. Determining the client's usual sleep pattern is essential before telling the client that sleeplessness is expected and making suggestions for improving sleep patterns.

CN: Health promotion and maintenance; **CL:** Synthesize

49. 4. Difficulty in swallowing, pain, and tightness in the chest are signs of esophagitis, which is a common complication of radiation therapy of the chest wall. Hiatal hernia is a herniation of a portion of the stomach into the esophagus. The client could experience burning and tightness in the chest secondary to a hiatal hernia, but not pain when swallowing. Also, hiatal hernia is not a complication of radiation therapy. Stomatitis is an inflammation of the oral cavity characterized by pain, burning, and ulcerations. The client with stomatitis may experience pain with swallowing, but not burning and tightness in the chest. Radiation enteritis is a disorder of the large and small bowel that occurs during or after radiation therapy to the abdomen, pelvis, or rectum. Nausea, vomiting, abdominal cramping, the frequent urge to have a bowel movement, and watery diarrhea are the signs and symptoms.

CN: Physiological adaptation; **CL:** Analyze

50. 2. Radiation fields that include the ovaries usually result in premature menopause. Vaginal dryness will occur without estrogen replacement. There should be no sexual intercourse while the implant is in place. Cesium is a radioactive isotope used for therapeutic irradiation of cancerous tissue. There is no documentation to support vaginal relaxation after treatment. Because the client will have premature menopause, she will not have normal menstrual periods.

CN: Physiological adaptation; **CL:** Synthesize

51. 3. Radiation-induced esophagitis with dysphagia is particularly common in clients who receive radiation to the chest. The anatomic location of the esophagus is posterior to the mediastinum and is within the field of primary treatment. Diarrhea may occur with radiation to the abdomen. Decreased energy level and decreased white blood cell count are potential complications of radiation therapy.

CN: Reduction of risk potential; **CL:** Analyze

The Client Who Requires Symptom Management

52. 3. Head and neck radiation can cause the complication of stomatitis and decreased salivary flow. A saliva substitute will assist with dryness, moistening food, and swallowing. Meticulous mouth care is needed; however, alcohol and vigorous brushing will increase irritation. Evaluation by a dentist to perform necessary dental work is done prior to initiation of therapy.

CN: Physiological adaptation;
CL: Synthesize

53. 3. The client has a low white blood cell count from the chemotherapy and has a temperature. Signs and symptoms of infection may be diminished in a client receiving chemotherapy; therefore, the temperature elevation is significant. Early detection of the source of infection facilitates early intervention. Surveillance for bleeding is important with the low hemoglobin and platelet count; however, the high blood pressure does not indicate bleeding. Vomiting is a side effect of chemotherapy and should be treated. The urine output and potassium are within normal limits.

CN: Physiological adaptation;
CL: Synthesize

54. 1. The packed cells should be administered using a central catheter or 19-gauge needle. Y tubing and the normal saline solution are used to keep the vein open when the blood transfusion is complete. Blood is not compatible with dextrose because dextrose may cause blood coagulation. Blood products should be given with normal saline solution. A blood filter must be used for all blood products to filter out sediment from stored blood products. It is not necessary to add another IV access.

CN: Pharmacological and parenteral therapies; CL: Synthesize

55. 1. The nurse should perform a thorough assessment of the abdomen and auscultate for bowel sounds in all four quadrants. Clients who have gastrointestinal surgery may have decreased peristalsis for several days after surgery. The nurse should check the abdomen for distention and check with the client and the **medical record** 📖 regarding the passage of flatus or stool. Consulting a dietician would be inappropriate because the client must be kept on nothing-by-mouth status until bowel sounds are present. The nurse should explain to the wife that it is too soon after surgery for her husband to eat.

CN: Reduction of risk potential;
CL: Synthesize

56. 3. For clients with obstructive versus restrictive disorders, extending exhalation through pursed-lip breathing will make the respiratory effort more efficient. The usual position of choice for this client is the upright position, leaning slightly forward to allow greater lung expansion. Teaching diaphragmatic breathing techniques will be more helpful to the client with a restrictive disorder. Administering cough suppressants will not help respiratory effort. A low semi-Fowler's position does not encourage lung expansion. Lung expansion is enhanced in the upright position.

CN: Basic care and comfort;
CL: Synthesize

57. 1,2,3,6. Thrombocytopenia places the client at risk for bleeding. Therefore, electric razors will reduce the potential for skin nicks and bleeding. Oral hygiene should be provided with a soft toothbrush and with minimal friction to gently clean without trauma. Clients should be instructed to read labels on all over-the-counter medications and avoid medications such as aspirin or NSAIDs due to their effect on platelet adhesiveness. Clients should evaluate mucous membranes, skin, stools, or other sources of potential bleeding. Monitoring temperature may be an important part of assessment but is focused on neutropenia instead of the problem of thrombocytopenia.

CN: Reduction of risk potential;
CL: Create

58. 2. The administration of antipyretics and antihistamines before initiation of the transfusion in the frequently transfused client can decrease the incidence of febrile reactions. Febrile reactions are immune mediated and are caused by antibodies in the recipient that are directed against antigens present on the granulocytes, platelets, and lymphocytes in the transfused component. They are the most common transfusion reactions and may occur with onset, during transfusion, or hours after transfusion is completed.

CN: Pharmacological and parenteral therapies; CL: Synthesize

59. 3. The fever and dyspnea suggest a respiratory infection. Education on deep-breathing exercises or incentive spirometry, elevating the head of the bed, and getting out of bed to a chair are necessary to promote lung expansion. When in bed, positioning the client with good lung down should be avoided, since this impedes expansion of the only lung. Postural drainage positioning will lower the head of bed and increase dyspnea.

CN: Physiological adaptation;
CL: Synthesize

60. 2. An individualized exercise program will increase stamina and endurance. Weight lifting may be too vigorous. Filgrastim is used to increase white blood cells and is not applicable in this situation. Decreased hemoglobin and hematocrit predisposes the client to fatigue due to decreased oxygen availability. Bed rest causes muscle atrophy, adding to fatigue, and can contribute to deep vein thrombosis (DVT).

CN: Health promotion and maintenance; CL: Synthesize

61. 1. Chemotherapy may cause suppression of the immune system, resulting in a reduction in the WBC count and placing the client at risk for infection. This client has a normal white blood cell count indicating that the filgrastim has been effective. Decreased hemoglobin (Hgb) indicates anemia. The Hgb is within normal limits for an adult male. A decreased platelet count would indicate thrombocytopenia, and platelets would be prescribed. The platelet count is within normal limits for an adult male. Epoetin alfa is used to treat low red blood cell counts (anemia) caused by chemotherapy.

CN: Pharmacologic and parenteral therapy; CL: Evaluate

62. 1. Dietary suggestions to reduce adverse effects of cancer and cancer therapies include a soft, bland diet low in fat and sugar. Frequent, small meals are usually better tolerated. It is not necessary to restrict the diet to cold foods. Fluid intake should be encouraged to avoid dehydration.

CN: Basic care and comfort; CL: Synthesize

63. 4. The use of diet modification is a conservative approach to treat the terminally ill or hospice clients who have nausea and vomiting related to bowel obstruction. Osmotic laxatives would be harder for the client to tolerate. An NG tube is more aggressive and invasive. IV antiemetics are also invasive. The hospice philosophy involves comfort and palliative care for the terminally ill.

CN: Basic care and comfort; CL: Synthesize

64. 3. Repositioning the client, elevating the head of the bed, and providing a cool compress are comfort interventions consistent with the concept of palliative care of the dying. Directing the UAP to assess vital signs focuses on the dying process, not the client. Suctioning may not benefit the client and is considered invasive and uncomfortable. Telling the spouse an intervention is not needed discounts the spouse's judgment and concerns.

CN: Basic care and comfort; CL: Synthesize

65. 2. Alopecia from chemotherapy is temporary. The new hair will not be necessarily gray, but the texture and color of new hair growth may be different. Clients who will be receiving chemotherapy should be encouraged to purchase a wig while they still have hair so that they can match the color and texture of their hair. Loss of hair, or alopecia, is a serious threat to self-esteem and should be addressed quickly before treatment.

CN: Pharmacological and parenteral therapies; CL: Apply

66. 3. Dyspnea is a distressing symptom in clients with advanced cancer including metastatic carcinoma of the lung, previous radiation therapy, and coexisting COPD. Ascites does occur in clients with metastatic carcinoma; however, in the client with COPD and lung cancer, dyspnea is a more common finding. A pleural friction rub is usually associated with pneumonia, pleurisy, or pulmonary infarct.

CN: Physiological adaptation; CL: Analyze

67. 3. The positive reinforcement builds confidence and facilitates achievement of rehabilitation goals. Community support may or may not be applicable after discharge. Although family support is an important component of rehabilitation, reinforcing the skills the client has acquired is of greater importance when regaining independence. Rehabilitation plans should include the client, family, or both.

CN: Psychosocial integrity; CL: Synthesize

68. 2. The most important intervention for infection control is to continue meticulous catheter site care. Dressings are to be changed two to three times per week depending on institutional policies. Temperature should be monitored at least once a day in someone with a vascular access device. Handwashing before and after irrigation or any manipulation of the site is a must for infection prevention.

CN: Safety and infection control; CL: Evaluate

69. 1,2,4,5. A major concern with IV administration of cytotoxic agents is vessel irritation or extravasation. The Oncology Nursing Society and hospital guidelines require frequent reevaluation of blood return when administering vesicant or nonvesicant chemotherapy due to the risk of extravasation. These guidelines apply to peripheral and central venous lines. The nurse should also assess the insertion site for signs of infiltration, such as swelling and redness. In addition, central venous lines may be long-term venous access devices. Thus, difficulty drawing or aspirating blood may indicate the line is against the vessel wall or may indicate the line has occlusion. Having the client cough or move position may change the status of the line if it is temporarily against a vessel wall. Occlusion warrants more thorough evaluation via x-ray study to verify placement if the status is questionable and may require a declotting regimen. The nurse should not administer any drug if the IV line is not open or does not have an adequate blood return.

CN: Pharmacological and parenteral therapies; CL: Create

70. The distal tip of a central line should be placed in the subclavian vein.

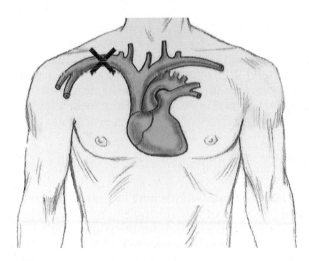

CN: Pharmacological and parenteral therapies; CL: Apply

71. 2. The client is exhibiting signs and symptoms of a pneumothorax from the insertion of the subclavian venous catheter. Although it is possible that the client suffered an air embolus during the procedure, and the client is at risk for pulmonary emboli because of his immobility, absent breath sounds immediately after insertion of a subclavian line are strongly suggestive of a pneumothorax. Unilateral absent breath sounds are not associated with a myocardial infarction.

CN: Physiological adaptation; CL: Analyze

72. 4. An appropriate and realistic outcome would be for the client to maintain current weight or not lose weight. It is unrealistic to expect that the client with advanced liver cancer will have normal albumin levels or will be able to gain weight.

CN: Basic care and comfort; CL: Synthesize

73. 3. As long as the client is able to get out of bed, the preferred position and time frame for preventing aspiration after a bolus tube feeding is sitting upright out of bed in a chair for 30 to 60 minutes. The client should have the head of the bed elevated more than 60 degrees; it is not necessary to remain in an upright position for more than an hour after the feeding. Placing the client on the right, not the left, side may facilitate gastric emptying, but this is not the preferred position. Elevating the bed 30 degrees decreases the risk of aspiration, but this elevation must be maintained for at least 45 to 60 minutes.

CN: Basic care and comfort; CL: Synthesize

74. 1. Total parenteral nutrition solutions supply the body with sufficient amounts of dextrose, amino acids, fats, vitamins, and minerals to meet metabolic needs. Clients who are unable to tolerate adequate quantities of foods and fluids and those who have had extensive bowel surgery may not be candidates for enteral feedings. The nurse would anticipate total parenteral nutrition via central catheter to promote wound healing. IV dextrose does not supply all the nutrients required to promote wound healing.

CN: Pharmacological and parenteral therapies; CL: Synthesize

75. 1,2,4. Elevated temperature in the first 24 hours along with coarse breath sounds may indicate a respiratory complication or the result of general anesthesia. Use of incentive spirometry and increasing activity would be key interventions. A healthy stoma will be beefy red. A dusky appearance of the stoma indicates decreased blood supply and is of concern. It is not uncommon to have decreased bowel sounds initially after gastrointestinal surgery. In addition, it usually will take time for the ostomy to function.

CN: Reduction of risk potential; CL: Analyze

76. 3. The vital signs suggest that the client is dehydrated from the vomiting, and the nurse should first infuse the IV fluids with the addition of potassium. There is no indication that the client needs oxygen at this time since the PO_2 is 95 (12.6 kPa). Although the client has a rapid and irregular pulse, the infusion of fluids may cause the heart rate to return to normal, and the 12-lead ECG can be prescribed after starting the intravenous fluids.

CN: Physiological adaptation; CL: Synthesize

77. 4. The content of the client's comments suggests that she is concerned about her husband avoiding her. Addressing sexuality issues is appropriate for a client who has undergone a mastectomy. Rushing her return to work may add to her exhaustion. Suggesting that she learn relaxation techniques for help with her insomnia is appropriate; however, the nurse must first address the psychosocial and sexual issues. A nutritional assessment may be useful, but there is no indication that she has anorexia.

CN: Psychosocial integrity; CL: Synthesize

78. 3. The client is exhibiting early symptoms of pulmonary toxicity as a result of the radiation therapy. These are not expected adverse effects of radiation. The client should be examined to differentiate between an infection and radiation pneumonitis. Suggesting that the client take acetaminophen and call back in 2 days is inappropriate. These signs and symptoms are not indicative of a true emergency, but the client should be seen by an **HCP** 📖 before the next appointment.

🔑 CN: Reduction of risk potential;
CL: Synthesize

79. 2,1,4,3. The client is short of breath. The head of the bed should be elevated to enable breathing, and oxygen should be applied. Morphine should be administered for pain prior to initiating deep-breathing exercises. Deep-breathing exercises improve lung expansion and decrease dyspnea. Education can be provided on the thoracentesis that is anticipated once the symptoms are managed.

🔑 CN: Physiological adaptation;
CL: Synthesize

80. 1. Treatment for cellulitis includes oral or intravenous antibiotics for 1 to 2 weeks, elevation of the affected extremity, and application of warm, moist packs to the site. Arm exercises help to reduce swelling, but do not treat the infection.

🔑 CN: Physiological adaptation;
CL: Synthesize

81. 3. Changing positions frequently aids in distributing the agent to the pleura for sealing. The majority of the pleural fluid is drained, and the lung should already be reexpanded before instillation of the sclerosing agent. A pressure dressing is applied to the chest tube exit site, and it is not necessary to lie on that side to hold pressure on the area.

🔑 CN: Reduction of risk potential;
CL: Synthesize

82. 4. Providing adequate humidification for the client with a tracheostomy is essential. The client no longer has the functions of the nose for warming, moistening, or filtering the air when breathing through the tracheostomy site. Providing tracheostomy site care, addressing the psychosocial issues, and observing for early signs and symptoms of skin breakdown around the tracheostomy site are also important; however, using humidifiers to prevent thick, tenacious secretions is the most important recommendation for long-term management and the prevention of pulmonary infection.

🔑 CN: Reduction of risk potential;
CL: Synthesize

83. 4,5. A malignant pleural effusion is an accumulation of excessive fluid within the pleural space that occurs when cancer cells irritate the pleural membrane. Dyspnea can result from the increased pressure, which may contribute to increased anxiety and fear of suffocation. Pain is a consequence of the pleural irritation. Cough is related to the atelectasis of the bronchi and inability to clear the airways. Hiccups are usually associated with pericardial effusions. Weight gain and peripheral edema may occur with peritoneal effusion.

🔑 CN: Physiological adaptation;
CL: Analyze

84. 2,3,4. Thoracentesis is usually successful for diagnosis of underlying disease, palliation of symptoms, and treating the acute respiratory distress; alleviation of the symptoms and distress is usually short term. The thoracentesis is not used as a treatment for recurrent pleural effusion because the fluid accumulates rapidly. Thoracentesis does not remove cancer cells.

🔑 CN: Reduction of risk potential;
CL: Evaluate

85. 3. Cold intolerance may be associated with anemia because of the diminished oxygen supply to the peripheral circulation. Decreased salivation is not associated with anemia. Tachycardia may be expected in severe anemia. Clients with anemia are usually not nauseated.

🔑 CN: Physiological adaptation;
CL: Analyze

86. 4. Petechiae are tiny, purplish, hemorrhagic spots visible under the skin. Petechiae usually appear when platelets are depleted. Bleeding gums or oozing of blood may accompany the petechiae, and the client should seek medical assistance immediately. Increasing iron in the diet will not improve the platelet count. Lotion will not treat the petechiae. Elevating the legs will not cause the petechiae to disappear.

🔑 CN: Physiological adaptation;
CL: Synthesize

87. 3. Lymphedema after breast cancer surgery is the accumulation of lymph tissue in the tissues of the upper extremity extending down from the upper arm. It may occur at any time after surgery in women of any age. It is caused by the interruption or removal of lymph channels and nodes after axillary node dissection. Removal results in less efficient filtration of lymph fluid and a pooling of lymph fluid in the tissues on the affected side. Treatments or interventions should be instituted as soon as lymphedema is noted to prevent or reduce further progression. Range-of-motion exercises, elevation, and avoidance of injury in the affected arm are important when completing client teaching. The **healthcare provider (HCP)** 📖 may also prescribe a compression sleeve. Lymphoma is not caused by failure to remove all cancer cells. Lymphedema can occur after any surgery that disrupts lymph flow, not just radical mastectomy.

🔑 CN: Reduction of risk potential;
CL: Synthesize

88. 3. Redness, warmth, and swelling are all signs of infection. Treatment with antibiotics is usually indicated. Infection usually increases fluid accumulation and could worsen the lymphedema. Warm compresses could also increase fluid accumulation. Elevation will not treat the infection. It is critical that the client not delay treatment.

🔑 CN: Reduction of risk potential;
CL: Synthesize

89. 4. Fever is most commonly related to infection. In a neutropenic client, fever frequently occurs in the absence of the usual clinical signs and symptoms of infection. Inadequate nutrition or antiemetic therapy resistance would not result in fever. Fever is not usually expected with most chemotherapy drugs.

🔑 CN: Physiological adaptation;
CL: Analyze

90. 2. Nine days after chemotherapy, it is expected for the client to be immunocompromised. The clinical signs and symptoms of shock reflect changes in cardiac function, vascular resistance, cellular metabolism, and capillary permeability. Low-grade fever, tachycardia, and chills may be early signs of shock. The client with signs and symptoms of impending septic shock may not have decreased oxygen saturation levels. Oliguria and hypotension are late signs of shock. Urine output can be initially normal or increased.

🔑 CN: Pharmacological and parenteral therapies; CL: Analyze

91. 3. Prioritizing physical activities helps to conserve energy, which promotes adaptation to fatigue. The client should learn to take short naps or short rest periods during the day for additional energy conversation. Increased fluid intake is important but may interrupt rest periods by causing frequent urination. Limiting intake of high-fiber foods can add to constipation, which may be a problem because of inactivity in fatigued clients.

🔑 CN: Basic care and comfort;
CL: Synthesize

92. 4. Most hospitalized persons are at risk for sleep disturbances. Psychological issues (such as anxiety and depression) and pain are related to sleep deprivation. Social, nutritional, and cultural issues are not necessarily associated with sleep disturbances.

🔑 CN: Psychosocial integrity; CL: Apply

93. 4. Nursing interventions to decrease the discomfort of pruritus include those that prevent vasodilation, decrease anxiety, and maintain skin integrity and hydration. Medicated baths with salicylic acid or colloidal oatmeal can be soothing as a temporary relief. The use of antihistamines or topical steroids depends on the cause of the pruritus, and these agents should be used with caution. Using silk sheets is not a practical intervention for the hospitalized client with pruritus.

🔑 CN: Basic care and comfort; CL: Apply

94. 4. Use of deodorant or fragrant soaps is drying to the skin. Cotton clothing gives the least irritation to skin. A cool, humidified environment adds to the client's comfort as well as providing hydration for skin comfort. Fluid intake of 3,000 mL/day is recommended for adequate hydration.

🔑 CN: Basic care and comfort; CL: Analyze

95. 4. Individuals with cancer have various cultural values and beliefs that help them cope with the cancer experience. Quality of life cannot be evaluated solely by quantifiable factors such as employability, functional status, or evidence of disease. It must be evaluated by the survivors within the context of their subjective and individual values and beliefs.

🔑 CN: Psychosocial integrity; CL: Analyze

96. 3. Constipation lasting 3 days or longer is unusual in this client and warrants immediate action. However, because the client had chemotherapy with doxorubicin 10 days ago, she is susceptible to infection and should avoid rectal medications and treatments. Abdominal discomfort secondary to constipation will be relieved after the client has a bowel movement; an opioid would contribute to the constipation.

🔑 CN: Pharmacological and parenteral therapies; CL: Synthesize

97. 1,4,5. The rectal area needs to be cleaned and gently dried after each bowel movement to prevent skin breakdown and inhibit growth of bacteria. Sitz baths are appropriate because they promote comfort. The client should increase fluid consumption to prevent dehydration. Zinc oxide ointment does form a protective skin barrier, but it makes it difficult to thoroughly clean the perirectal area of feces and increases the risk of infection, as do skin barrier dressings.

🔑 CN: Safety and infection control;
CL: Synthesize

98. 2. Studies of long-term immunologic effects in clients treated for leukemia, Hodgkin's disease, and breast cancer reveal that combination treatments of chemotherapy and radiation can cause overall bone marrow suppression, decreased leukocyte counts, and profound immunosuppression. Persistent and severe immunologic impairment may follow radiation and chemotherapy (especially multiagent therapy). There is no evidence of greater risk of infection in clients with persistent immunologic abnormalities. Suppressor T cells recover more rapidly than do the helper T cells.

🔑 CN: Pharmacological and parenteral therapies; CL: Apply

The Client Who Is Coping with Loss, Grief, Bereavement, and Spiritual Distress

99. 4. Identifying available resources for the client and family represents a respectful effort to make options available and encourages the client to become involved in treatment decisions. Assuming decision making for the client may foster dependence. Encouraging strict compliance with all treatment regimens may increase anxiety and limit the client's options and treatment choices. Informing the client of all possible adverse treatment effects may increase anxiety and fear by focusing on adverse outcomes too soon.

🔑 CN: Psychosocial integrity; CL: Synthesize

100. 4. Denial is a defense mechanism used to shut out a situation that is too frightening or threatening to tolerate. In this case, denial allows the client to vacillate between acceptance of the illness and its treatment and denial of the actual or potential seriousness of the disease. This may allow the client more psychological freedom to maintain her current roles in the family and elsewhere. Denial can be harmful if the client ignores standard medical therapies in favor of unconventional treatments. Denial is not helpful when it interferes with a client's willingness to seek treatment or make decisions about care. Using any one defense mechanism exclusively usually reflects maladaptive coping. Other defense mechanisms that may be used include regression, humor, and sublimation.

🔑 CN: Psychosocial integrity; CL: Apply

101. 2. The client's resources for coping with the emotional and practical needs of herself and her family need to be assessed because usual coping strategies and support systems are often inadequate in especially stressful situations. The nurse may be concerned with the client's use of denial,

decision-making abilities, and ability to pay for transportation; however, the client's support systems will be of more importance in this situation.

🔑 CN: Psychosocial integrity; CL: Analyze

102. 4. Variables that are most predictive of negative bereavement outcomes include anger and self-reproach, low socioeconomic status, lack of preparation for death, and lack of family support. Making preparations suggests that she is coping with her husband's approaching death.

🔑 CN: Psychosocial integrity; CL: Analyze

103. 4. Having adequate financial resources facilitates bereavement. Younger people are at higher risk for negative bereavement outcomes. Having a history of depressive illness or anxiety is a risk factor for negative bereavement outcomes. Being a spouse does not make grieving easier.

🔑 CN: Psychosocial integrity; CL: Analyze

104. 4. Focusing on the client's physical capabilities is important, but powerlessness reflects a perceived lack of control over the current situation and the belief that one's actions will not affect the outcome. Participation in decision making is key to getting the client involved and feeling more in control of his or her own care. Apathy and dependence on others are characteristics of powerlessness. Encouraging others to take responsibility for the client's care will increase the client's feelings of powerlessness. A referral to a psychologist is not necessarily indicated. The nurse should implement strategies to involve the client in decisions about the client's care and evaluate the response to this intervention before suggesting a referral.

🔑 CN: Psychosocial integrity; CL: Synthesize

105. 1. Maintaining role function has been found to be a supportive source of normalcy and positive self-esteem for the client and family during the cancer experience. Facilitating family-related disagreements and conflicts is not the nurse's role. Supporting the client in her use of denial as a coping strategy will not help facilitate the client's adaptation to the diagnosis. Arranging transportation and child care on treatment days may be helpful but does not necessarily facilitate adaptation to the diagnosis.

🔑 CN: Psychosocial integrity; CL: Synthesize

106. 2. The most important central component of hospice care is focus of care on the client as well as the family or significant other. The team approach and the **HCP's** 📖 coordination of the hospice team are important, but they are not the focus. Not all hospice clients want to die at home.

🔑 CN: Basic care and comfort; CL: Apply

107. 3. Mental changes and decreased level of consciousness are common in the dying process, and the client may talk about travel, trips, or going somewhere. Suggesting that the client be sedated ignores the husband's question about what his wife is experiencing. Suggesting that the client is fighting death and that the husband should leave her alone is inappropriate and denies the husband time to spend with his wife. The husband should not make misleading statements to his wife.

CN: Psychosocial integrity; CL: Synthesize

108. 4. It is important to give factual information to answer a loved one's questions and concerns. Stating "That is just the way it is" is unprofessional and uncaring. Saying "I do not know when the bowels will shut down, but they will eventually" projects an uncaring attitude and does not address the wife's concern for her husband or her need for information. Although it may be true that the pain medication will slow bowel function, this does not provide the wife with the information she is seeking.

CN: Psychosocial integrity; CL: Apply

109. 4. It is important to allow the client to choose his or her own form of spiritual support, and the nurse can begin by asking the client what would be most supportive now. The client must be consulted before referral to a chaplain is made. Reflection on past accomplishments may be comforting to the client, but it does not directly address spiritual concerns. The client is able to communicate with the nurse, and discussing the conversation with the family does not respect the client's right to privacy.

CN: Psychosocial integrity; CL: Synthesize

110. 2. A social worker can provide information for supportive services and can help the client determine which resources are necessary at this time. The business office of the healthcare agency does not provide advice about managing finances. The **HCP** 📖 will be part of the team, but will focus on managing the client's health and end-of-life care. The client may or may not have a will; it is not the role of an executor to make financial decisions about health care.

CN: Psychosocial integrity; CL: Synthesize

111. 4. Dehydration is an expected event within the dying process. Hydration may be used in any situation of dehydration as long as it is within the client and family's wishes. Rehydrating the client may actually prolong the dying process. Decisions about treatment are made with the family.

CN: Basic care and comfort; CL: Apply

112. 4. The nurse must first allow the client to explore his or her own beliefs and values before making referrals, explaining various religious beliefs, or suggesting appropriate reading material.

CN: Psychosocial integrity; CL: Synthesize

113. 3. The family is in the best position to give the information they elect to disclose to friends and community members. The hospice nurse and the oncologist must maintain client confidentiality and follow privacy guidelines for release of confidential information. Therefore, disclosing any information about the client's condition would be inappropriate.

CN: Management of care; CL: Synthesize

114. 4. Depression can be a mixture of affective responses (feelings of worthlessness, hopelessness, sadness), behavioral responses (appetite changes, withdrawal, sleep disturbances, lethargy), and cognitive responses (decreased ability to concentrate, indecisiveness, suicidal ideation). Increased decisiveness, problem-solving ability, and increased social interactions are reflective of adaptive coping.

CN: Psychosocial integrity; CL: Analyze

115. 4. Bereavement support after death usually continues for about 1 year or as needed at little or no cost to the remaining family. Mutual support groups by nonprofessionals are usually free or inexpensive but are not necessarily appropriate for young children. Professional individual counseling and medication are expensive, and medication may not be appropriate for young children. To remind someone of what she should have done before the death is not helpful at this time.

CN: Psychosocial integrity; CL: Synthesize

116. 3. It is important to establish rapport with the client and family by listening to verbal and nonverbal concern and showing respect for cultural differences. The use of touch or eye contact is culture-specific and cannot be generalized as an intervention for all individuals with cancer. Miscommunication between individuals of different cultures is often caused by language differences, rules of communication, age, and gender.

CN: Psychosocial integrity; CL: Synthesize

117. 4. Support groups are designed to educate clients and their families experiencing cancer about the disease and methods of coping positively with it. These are self-help and support groups monitored by professionals and cancer survivors who have undergone a training course that helps them to facilitate small groups.

CN: Psychosocial integrity; CL: Apply

118. 4. Many cancer survivors question why they are doing so well and others are not. Often, they express feeling guilty when they hear that others are not doing well. Suggesting that the client does not know how to describe his own emotions is inappropriate and may discourage him from expressing his feelings. Although the client may be experiencing volatile emotions, this is not the likely source of his feelings of guilt. Guilt about doing well after cancer treatment is not a spiritual response to illness.

🔑 CN: Psychosocial integrity; CL: Synthesize

119. 4. The person who has minimal social support, has not been successful in dealing with stressors, and has multiple other stressors is at greater risk for psychosocial distress. Being successful in dealing with stress all his life would decrease the client's risk for psychosocial distress. Not having to deal with other stressors would be helpful in managing the current stressful situation. The denial coping mechanism, if used for short periods, can decrease the risk for psychosocial distress.

🔑 CN: Psychosocial integrity; CL: Analyze

120. 1. Clients with cancer report that the lifelong fear of recurrence is one of the most disruptive aspects of the disease. The trajectory of the disease is unpredictable and can be intertwined with many short- and long-term illnesses related to cancer and the treatment modalities. A diagnosis of cancer challenges the individual and the family with a series of crises rather than a time-limited episode. There are no data to indicate that the client has an underlying behavioral disorder.

🔑 CN: Psychosocial integrity; CL: Analyze

121. 4. Without clear, consistent communication, the parent-child relationship may become strained during the illness and subsequent death of a parent. A great number of parents do not know how to communicate with their children, especially about difficult emotional topics at a time when they are also under great emotional stress. The nurse should begin by providing information and developmentally appropriate books about the grieving process for children. Referral to pastoral care services may be appropriate; however, the nurse's direct intervention of beginning education about strategies for communication will be of immediate and long-term benefit. The grieving process cannot be rushed for the husband, nor should an opportunity for the father and children to communicate and grieve together be delayed. Excluding children from participating in the grieving ritual does not shield them from the sorrow and sadness, and having the **HCP** 🖵 tell the children does not promote healthy communication between the father and the children.

🔑 CN: Psychosocial integrity;
CL: Synthesize

122. 3. Acknowledgment and discussion of the client's feelings begin the establishment of a therapeutic relationship between nurse and client. It also acknowledges the seriousness of the current situation and validates the client's feelings. Grief counseling antidepressant medication may be options if the depression is severe and prolonged. The client is not ready at this point to continue the conversation with her husband.

🔑 CN: Psychosocial integrity;
CL: Synthesize

123. 2. Individuals who are experiencing fatigue need to prioritize their activities and ask for assistance from others. It is best not to take away all of the client's activities because her role as wife and mother is obviously important to her and to her sense of self-worth. Suggesting that she ignore the household chores or telling her not to worry because everyone gets tired disregards the client's feelings and is not appropriate.

🔑 CN: Basic care and comfort; CL: Synthesize

124. 4. Tachycardia, tachypnea, moist or clammy skin, and disorientation are classic symptoms of delirium. Clients with panic disorder do not exhibit disorientation. Clients with depression exhibit a flat affect, apathy, and sleep disturbances. Clients with schizophrenia have thought disorders such as hallucinations or delusions.

🔑 CN: Physiological adaptation;
CL: Analyze

125. 2. A progressive activity regimen may be prescribed to increase pulmonary function after surgical lung resection. Rehabilitation should include walking and some stair climbing as tolerated. It is not necessary at this point for the client to speak with someone who has had similar surgery. Depending on the surgeon's preference, there may not be a dressing to change. There is no indication that the client would not be able to manage cleaning the house as her energy increases.

🔑 CN: Psychosocial integrity;
CL: Synthesize

126. 4. Serving as a volunteer in a client-to-client program represents reintegration with constructive channeling of energies, which indicates a higher level of adaptation than attention to safety, knowledge, or planned activity. Discussing suicide is an indication the client is not adapting to the changes in health status. Continuing to look at the incision indicates the client is still concerned about the changes to the body. While looking forward to returning to work is a positive sign, being able to help others demonstrates an integration of the experience into the client's life.

🔑 CN: Psychosocial integrity; CL: Evaluate

The Client Who Is Experiencing Problems with Sexuality

127. 3. Water-soluble lubricants used during sexual intercourse can augment reduced natural vaginal lubrication caused by ovarian dysfunction and decreased circulating estrogen related to chemotherapy. The use of vaginal dilators, relaxation techniques, or nightly douches would not increase vaginal lubrication. Frequent douching can disrupt the normal vaginal environment.

⚷ CN: Health promotion and maintenance; CL: Synthesize

128. 3. Placing a thin piece of gauze over the tracheostomy during sexual activity will help to contain the secretions and yet allow ventilation. Although a scopolamine patch may depress the salivary and bronchial secretions, it is not recommended for long-term use and would not be indicated in this situation. Avoiding fluids before sexual activity is not recommended to decrease secretions. Washing the tracheostomy area with any deodorizing soap may cause skin irritation and place the client at risk for infection.

⚷ CN: Health promotion and maintenance; CL: Synthesize

129. 4. This question introduces some basic information and allows for support for the client who may be experiencing some sexuality concerns. Not all women experience sexual problems after undergoing a hysterectomy. Assuming that the client will want to schedule an appointment with her partner is inappropriate and may embarrass her. Simply asking the client whether she expects to have problems with sex is too abrupt and does not provide any information.

⚷ CN: Psychosocial integrity; CL: Synthesize

130. 4. Although there may not be a big change in sexual function with a unilateral orchiectomy, the loss of a gonad and testosterone may result in decreased libido and sterility. Sperm banking may be an option worth exploring if the number and motility of the sperm are adequate. The population most affected by testicular cancer is generally young men aged 15 to 34, and in this crucial stage of life, sexual anxieties may be a large concern. Since there will likely not be a big change in sexual function, it is not appropriate to tell the client he will experience impotence, have early ejaculation, or require a referral to a sex therapist.

⚷ CN: Psychosocial integrity; CL: Synthesize

131. 4. The risk of becoming neutropenic during chemotherapy is very high. Therefore, an inserted foreign object such as a diaphragm may be a nidus for infection. Although the nurse may wish to inform the client about the ease with which various contraceptive modalities may be used, the focus of this discussion should be on preventing an infection, which can be fatal for the neutropenic client. There are no data to suggest the client is at risk for acquiring a sexually transmitted disease. The client will not be experiencing body changes directly related to hormonal changes.

⚷ CN: Safety and infection control; CL: Synthesize

132. 2. Raising the upper torso for the affected partner facilitates respiratory function. The use of a foam mattress is not necessary and will not help promote respiratory expansion. A dependent position may compromise respiratory expansion, even though energy may be conserved. Duration of sexual activity is not necessarily related to exertion.

⚷ CN: Health promotion and maintenance; CL: Synthesize

Ethical and Legal Issues Related to Clients with Cancer

133. 4. The nurse must respect the wishes of the client who has indicated that he does not wish to be resuscitated and not to initiate CPR. Nurses who resuscitate clients who have directed otherwise may be considered to be battering the client. In this situation, the **HCP** 📖 has written the DNR prescription, and it is not necessary for the nurse to page the HCP. The nurse can be most helpful by explaining the client's decision to the wife and helping her understand her husband's wishes and manage her own grief.

⚷ CN: Management of care; CL: Synthesize

134. 3. The **RN** 📖 assigning care should first give the UAP the opportunity to explore concerns and fears about caring for a client with HIV infection. Reassigning care for this client, assisting with care, and reviewing precautions do not address the present concern or create an environment that will generate useful knowledge regarding future assignments for client care.

⚷ CN: Management of care; CL: Synthesize

135. 1. The nurse should advise the client to check with her employer to determine the policies and legislation followed there regarding leaves of absence. While the client can consider the other options, the first step is to obtain information from her employer.

⚷ CN: Management of care; CL: Apply

136. 1. Maintaining a steady blood level of analgesics is beneficial for the client with chronic cancer pain. Administering analgesics regularly helps control pain more efficiently. Additional doses of medication may be necessary as ordered for breakthrough pain. Keeping the client overly sedated may not help to control pain. Intravenous analgesics are more effective than oral medications at controlling pain because their distribution is more predictable. Vital signs are not a reliable indicator of how much pain the client is experiencing.

CN: Management of care; CL: Apply

137. 3. The goal of client autonomy is to respect the client's choice not to know particular information. The client's best interests should be determined by the client after he or she receives all the necessary information and in conjunction with other people of the client's choice, including family, **HCP** 📖, and other healthcare personnel. The client's best interests are not totally directed by the HCP or the healthcare team.

CN: Management of care; CL: Evaluate

End-of-Life Care

138. 2. The client is likely becoming more comatose and is not self-administering the pain medication. The client is not receiving too much medication because the PCA pump has controls to prevent overdose. The client is likely having pain, but is not able to recognize it. There is no indication that the IV has infiltrated.

CN: Pharmacological and parenteral therapies CL: Analyze

139. 1,2,5. Advance directives are written statements of person's wishes related to health care if they are unable to decide for themselves. Power of attorney is a written authorization to represent or act on another's behalf in private affairs, business, or some other legal matter. These documents relate to current or future health care and not past medical history. Competent adults are responsible for their own healthcare decisions and their own right to accept or refuse treatment. Advance directives are used when the person cannot make the decision. Medical power of attorney is a term used to describe the person who makes healthcare decisions should someone be unable to make informed decisions for himself or herself. The focus is not primarily financial access.

CN: Management of care; CL: Evaluate

140. 4. The advocacy role of the nurse implies that the nurse will ensure that the client's wishes are being respected and the client is making informed decisions. Therefore, the nurse will assist in ensuring that the client is fully informed. The other interventions are appropriate for the nurse but are not related to client advocacy. The client may not understand or have all the necessary information for standard therapy. A client who is taking an alternative therapy should be monitored for adverse effects. If a client is taking an alternative therapy, it is essential for the **healthcare provider (HCP)** 📖 to know so that the therapy can be incorporated into the client's treatment plan and to ensure that there are no incompatibilities with other therapies or medications.

CN: Management of care; CL: Evaluate

141. 2,3,4,5. End-of-life care is the term currently used for issues related to death and dying. End-of-life care focuses on physical and psychosocial needs at the end of life for the client and client's family. Palliative care is health care aimed at symptom management rather than curative treatment for diseases. Goals would include providing comfort and support for the client and family and improving the client's quality of life. Grief counseling is a component, and efforts would be to enhance the coping of all involved and not to alter usual coping methods.

CN: Management of care; CL: Create

142. 3. The best nursing advocacy intervention is listening carefully to the client's and family's perceptions of their needs. Studies have demonstrated that these needs are not necessarily what the nurse thinks they are. Intervening without listening carefully may result in a lack of responsiveness to the real needs. Helping the client and family maintain a sense of optimism and hopefulness is appropriate but is not necessarily advocacy. Determining the client's and family's understanding of the results of the diagnostic testing and providing written materials about the cancer site and its treatment are examples of the nurse's role as educator.

CN: Psychosocial integrity; CL: Synthesize

143. 1. The nurse would give the client a tissue and indicate that it is okay to cry to convey acceptance and empathy. He needs to know that it is natural to have tremendous feelings of loss and sadness. Telling the client to stop crying, busying oneself in the client's room, and changing the subject are not helpful to the client because they ignore his needs and inhibit the expression of emotion.

CN: Psychosocial integrity; CL: Synthesize

144. 2,3,4,5,6. With serious, chronic, and terminal illnesses, it is important to help clients and families address fears, difficulties with home care, advance directives, hospice and home care options, and final arrangements. Predicting the length of life for this client is not appropriate at admission.

🔑 CN: Psychosocial integrity;
CL: Synthesize

145. 1. The client's husband is experiencing anger, much of which stems from feelings of guilt about not taking the trip. During the stage of denial, the husband is more likely to deny the client's diagnosis and prognosis. During the stage of bargaining, the husband would offer to do certain things in exchange for more time before the client dies. In the stage of depression, the husband is likely to make few or no comments and to act dejected.

🔑 CN: Psychosocial integrity;
CL: Analyze

146. 1. When supporting the friends or family of a terminally ill client, it is best to focus on the present. This can be accomplished by living each day to its fullest. Friends and families also want to know what to expect and want someone to listen to them as they express grief over the approaching death. Focusing on the past can interfere with enjoying the present. Expecting the worst interferes with focusing on day-to-day positive experiences. Planning ahead is inappropriate because of uncertainty when the length of life is unknown.

🔑 CN: Psychosocial integrity;
CL: Synthesize

147. 1. The best course of action when the client has outbursts concerning treatments is to explain how the treatment is expected to help. Describing the effect if the client misses a treatment is a negative approach and may be threatening to the client. Explaining the effects of being upset does not deal with the client's feelings. Offering to arrange for a massage during the chemotherapy may be helpful, but does not deal with the client's immediate feelings.

🔑 CN: Psychosocial integrity;
CL: Synthesize

148. 2. Clients tend to experience isolation and loneliness when those around them are trying to hide or mask the truth. They are then left to face the realities of death alone. Clients do not experience relief or hopefulness when others are falsely cheerful. Independence is promoted by offering realistic choices about care at the end of life.

🔑 CN: Health promotion and maintenance;
CL: Analyze

149. 3,4,5. Taking a blood sample is an unnecessary, invasive procedure that would not directly address the sister's fear. Leukemia is not considered a communicable disease. The nurse should first determine the sister's concerns, and then alert the parents to the sister's concerns and also tell the parents about resources that are available to assist siblings to cope with a terminal illness in the family.

🔑 CN: Psychosocial integrity;
CL: Synthesize

150. 2. A response that acknowledges the brother's concern and provides him with information is most helpful. Therefore, telling the brother that the nurse sees that he is worried and then following this up with a discussion about leukemia is most appropriate. Providing reassurance or information without acknowledging the expressed concern is not as helpful as acknowledging the concern and providing the information. Although acknowledging his worry is appropriate, more importantly, the brother needs factual information about the disease.

🔑 CN: Psychosocial integrity;
CL: Synthesize

Managing Care, Quality, and Safety of Clients with Cancer

151. 3,1,4,2. Using Maslow's hierarchy of needs to set priorities, the nurse should first call the client with bone cancer metastases to the spine because this client is at risk for compression, damage, or severing of the spinal cord. The nurse should evaluate the client immediately for urinary incontinence, paralysis, difficulty ambulating, and possible weakness or loss of motor function. The nurse should next call the client with loss of appetite to assess weight loss and suggest ways to increase the appetite. The client with colon cancer requires assistance with diet planning, also a physiologic need, but this client is not at high risk for weight loss. Lastly, the nurse should obtain information on Reach to Recovery and return the call to the client with a mastectomy. The needs of this client are the least urgent.

🔑 CN: Reduction of risk potential;
CL: Synthesize

152. 3. The nurse should first assess the 75-year-old man with prostate cancer because of the client's age, need for pain management, extended bed rest, and the potential for preexisting nutritional deficits. The nurse should plan to spend a focused but short time with the woman receiving internal radiation. The client who will receive chemotherapy will require more observation after receiving the medication. The nurse can assess the client who will have a central venous catheter after assuring the older client is comfortable.

🔑 CN: Management of care; CL: Synthesize

153. 2,3,4,5. Nurses preparing and administering chemotherapy wear gloves and a disposable, long-sleeved gown. Antineoplastic agents are disposed of as hazardous material, and gloves are always worn when handling the excretions of clients who have received chemotherapy. Sharps must be disposed of in a sharps container labeled "chemotherapy items". It is not appropriate to tape IV tubing connections; antineoplastic agents are administered using Luer-Lok fittings on all intravenous tubing to minimize the risk of exposure from needlestick injury.

🔑 CN: Pharmacological and parenteral therapies; CL: Synthesize

154. 1. An intravenous catheter with no blood return is most likely occluded and not patent. A chemotherapeutic vesicant drug extravasates into the surrounding skin tissue and causes tissue necrosis. The nurse stops administration of the drug immediately. Repositioning the arm does not improve patency. Irrigating the catheter may cause the medication to enter tissue. It is inappropriate to wait and see if the arm becomes edematous because of the vesicant action of the drug.

🔑 CN: Pharmacological and parenteral therapies; CL: Synthesize

155. 1,2,3. Ethics consultation seeks to facilitate communication and shared decision making in client care. Ethics consultations also tend to increase knowledge of clinical ethics, improve client care, and prevent poor outcomes in cases involving ethical problems. Requests for ethics consultations can be made by any member of the healthcare team and by clients, family members, guardians, students, or others with a legitimate interest in the client. The recommendations of ethics consultants are advisory only; the ethics consultation process is intended to supplement and support existing departmental and institutional mechanisms for making decisions and resolving conflict in clinical practice. Clinicians are encouraged to seek an ethics consultation when the client is incapacitated and when no family member/s or guardian/s exist or can be found or when the client's family members disagree about the ethically appropriate action to be taken. Ethics consultation is not intended or authorized to provide legal advice on client care. Persons requesting an ethics consultation may do so without intimidation or fear of reprisal.

🔑 CN: Management of care; CL: Synthesize

156. 4. To determine the cause of this problem, a quality improvement study should be conducted along with a chart audit. Before implementing solutions to a problem, the precise issues in the hospital system must be observed and documented. Changing the time to chart from 30 to 45 minutes does not solve the problem. It is not the pharmacist's role to provide consultation about documentation of drugs administered by nurses. Consulting the evening nurses may be helpful, but this is a systems issue of the entire unit and involves every **registered nurse (RN)** 📖 administering analgesia.

🔑 CN: Management of care; CL: Create

157. 2. The **RN** 📖 is responsible for describing to the **UAP** 📖 when to report to the RN a result that indicates a potential client problem with dehydration. The RN must assess and interpret results, but must give concrete feedback to the UAP on what is an expected situation or a specific result to report back to the RN. Urine output should be at least 30 mL/h, or 240 mL, over the 8-hour shift. Dehydrated clients may be thirsty, and the UAP can ask if the client is thirsty and offer water if permitted. However, because urine output is the critical indicator of dehydration, the UAP should document I&O and give results outside the normal range to the nurse. The nurse is specifically assessing dehydration and should request to receive this information from the UAP before it is charted and reported to the next shift.

🔑 CN: Management of care; CL: Synthesize

158. 4. A bedside commode should be near the client for easy, safe access. Measurement of urine output is also important in a client with heart failure. Putting diapers on an alert and oriented individual would be demeaning and inappropriate. Indwelling catheters are associated with increased risk of infection and are not a solution to possible incontinence. There is no reason to think that the client would not be able to use the bedside commode.

🔑 CN: Safety and infection control; CL: Synthesize

159. 1. Ongoing assessment by the **RN** 📖 is required to evaluate the client with dyspnea to monitor for potential deterioration of the respiratory status. If the RN is the care provider, the RN will have greater interaction with the individual client. The RN is responsible for assessment of all the clients. The other clients would not be considered unstable, and maintaining a patent airway is always the priority in providing care. Care for the other clients could be assigned safely, according to the abilities of the **LPN/VN** 📖 and **UAP** 📖.

🔑 CN: Management of care; CL: Synthesize

160. 1,2,5. Employers should provide appropriate PPE to protect workers who handle hazardous drugs in the workplace. The following general guidelines apply to PPE use and care: select specific respirators and protective clothing based on an assessment of the potential exposure to hazardous drugs; understand proper use and limitations of any selected PPE to ensure that it functions properly; and use care in donning and removing all items to prevent damage to PPE and to reduce the spread of contamination. The PPE must be constructed of materials that are appropriate for hazardous drug exposure. Hands must be thoroughly washed with soap and water both before donning and after removing gloves. Consider all PPE worn when handling hazardous drugs as being contaminated; contain and dispose of such PPE as contaminated waste.

CN: Safety and infection control; CL: Synthesize

161. 4. When the duration of intravascular therapy is likely to be more than 6 days, a midline catheter or peripherally inserted central catheter (PICC) is preferred to a short peripheral catheter. In adult clients, use of the femoral vein for central venous access should be avoided. Steel needles should be avoided when administering fluids and medications that might cause tissue necrosis if extravasation occurs.

CN: Reduction of risk potential; CL: Apply

The Client Having Surgery

■ The Client Who Is Preparing for Surgery

■ The Client Who Is Receiving or Recovering from Anesthesia

■ The Client Who Has Had Surgery

■ Legal and Ethical Issues Associated with Surgery

■ Managing Care, Quality, and Safety of Clients Having Surgery

■ Answers, Rationales, and Test-Taking Strategies

The Client Who Is Preparing for Surgery

1. A client tells the nurse on admission that she is uneasy about having to leave her children with a relative while being in the hospital for surgery. What should the nurse do?

☐ **1.** Reassure the client that her children will be fine and she should stop worrying.

☐ **2.** Contact the relative to determine his/her capacity to be an adequate care provider.

☐ **3.** Encourage the client to call the children to make sure they are doing well.

☐ **4.** Gather more information about the client's feelings about the childcare arrangements.

2. The client has a latex allergy. What should the nurse teach the client to do before having surgery? Select all that apply.

☐ **1.** Determine that there will be a latex-safe environment for surgery.

☐ **2.** Report symptoms experienced with the latex allergy (e.g., rhinitis, conjunctivitis, flushing).

☐ **3.** Notify the healthcare providers (HCPs) at the surgery center.

☐ **4.** Wear a stainless steel medical alert bracelet into the surgical suite.

☐ **5.** Ask to have the surgery at a hospital.

3. When the nurse asks the client who is having abdominal surgery today if the client understands the procedure, the client replies, "No, not really; I talked about several different things with my surgeon, and I am just not sure." The nurse should:

☐ **1.** teach the client all the details of the planned procedure.

☐ **2.** utilize a second witness when the client signs for consent.

☐ **3.** notify the surgeon of the client's expressed lack of understanding.

☐ **4.** administer the prescribed preoperative narcotics and/or sedatives.

4. During preadmission testing for same-day surgery, a client states that she has added two cloves of garlic each day to her diet to help control her blood pressure. The nurse should further inquire about:

☐ **1.** the type of surgery the client is having.

☐ **2.** what her blood pressure has been running.

☐ **3.** the amount of garlic she is eating.

☐ **4.** her preference for the type of anesthesia.

5. When removing protective covering, what action should this nurse (see figure) take to avoid spreading nosocomial infections?

☐ **1.** Remove the face mask.

☐ **2.** Place the face mask over the mouth and nose before removing the hair covering.

☐ **3.** Wash hands before tying the strings on the mask.

☐ **4.** Tie the dangling strings of the mask around the neck.

6. The client is to have surgery on the fourth metatarsal. Identify the place on the illustration below where the client should confirm the operative site to the healthcare provider (HCP).

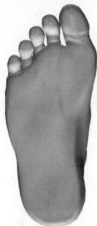

7. The nurse is reviewing the medical record of a 55-year-old male client who is scheduled for a lumbar laminectomy. The nurse should report which finding to the surgeon?
☐ **1.** pimple on the lower back
☐ **2.** abnormal electrocardiogram (ECG)
☐ **3.** hearing aid
☐ **4.** allergy to iodine

8. Prior to going to surgery, the client tells the nurse that she cannot hear without her hearing aid and asks to wear it to surgery and recovery. What is the nurse's **best** response?
☐ **1.** Explain to the client that it is policy not to take personal items to surgery because they may be lost or broken.
☐ **2.** Tell the client that a nurse will bring the hearing aid to the postanesthesia care unit so that she can have it as soon as she wakes up.
☐ **3.** Explain to the client that she will have a pre-medication that will make her sleepy before she goes to surgery and she will not need to hear.
☐ **4.** Call the surgery unit to explain the client's concern, and ask if she can wear her hearing aid to surgery.

9. The adult daughters of an elderly male client inform the nurse that they fully expect their father to be combative after surgery. Preoperatively, they request that the nurse put all four side rails up and use restraints to keep him safe. The nurse should tell the daughters:
☐ **1.** "Certainly; we will want to be sure to keep your father safe too."
☐ **2.** "We will call the healthcare provider (HCP) to get a prescription right away."
☐ **3.** "We will first try to keep him safe without restraint."
☐ **4.** "Restraint use is prohibited at our hospital at all times."

10. The client is to take nothing by mouth after 0400. The nurse recognizes that the client has deficient knowledge when he states that he:
☐ **1.** ate a gelatin dessert at 0330.
☐ **2.** brushed his teeth at 0400 but did not swallow.
☐ **3.** held a cold washcloth against his lips.
☐ **4.** smoked a cigarette at 0600.

11. The surgeon prescribes cefazolin 1 g to be given IV at 0730 when the client's surgery is scheduled at 0800. What is the **primary** reason to start the antibiotic exactly at 0730?
☐ **1.** Legally the medication has to be given at the prescribed time.
☐ **2.** The antibiotic is most effective in preventing infection if it is given 30 to 60 minutes before the operative incision is made.
☐ **3.** The postoperative dose of cefazolin needs to be started exactly 8 hours after the preoperative dose of cefazolin.
☐ **4.** The peak and titer levels are needed for antibiotic therapy.

12. Which approach is the **best** way for the nurse to begin the preoperative interview?
☐ **1.** Walk in the client's room and ask, "Are you Mrs. Smith?"
☐ **2.** Walk in the client's room, sit down, and take the client's blood pressure.
☐ **3.** Walk in the client's room, sit down, maintain eye contact, and make an introduction.
☐ **4.** Walk in the client's room, and ask the client's name.

13. A client who is to receive general anesthesia has a serum potassium level of 5.8 mEq/L (5.8 mmol/L). What should be the nurse's **first** response?
☐ **1.** Call the operating room to cancel the surgery.
☐ **2.** Send the client to surgery.
☐ **3.** Make a note on the client's record.
☐ **4.** Notify the anesthesiologist.

14. Prior to being transported to the surgery suite, the nurse asks the client whether the client has any allergies. The client responds, "Does anyone communicate with anyone? I have been asked that question over and over!" What is the nurse's **best** response?
☐ **1.** "I am sorry! I just have to ask that question for the record."
☐ **2.** "It is an important question, and we just have to check."
☐ **3.** "You will hear it again and again as you go through surgery."
☐ **4.** "This question is asked for verification and safety with each new phase of treatment."

15. On the day of surgery, a client with diabetes who takes insulin on a sliding scale is to have nothing by mouth and all medications withheld. The client's 0600 glucose level is 300 mg/dL (16.7 mmol/L). What should the nurse do?
- [ ] 1. Withhold all medications.
- [ ] 2. Administer the insulin dose dictated by the sliding scale.
- [ ] 3. Call the healthcare provider (HCP) for specific prescriptions based on the glucose level.
- [ ] 4. Notify the surgery department.

16. The nurse is preparing a preoperative teaching plan for a client who is undergoing a bilateral breast reduction. Which aspect of the plan is the **priority**?
- [ ] 1. reduction of risk potential
- [ ] 2. physiologic adaptation
- [ ] 3. psychosocial integrity
- [ ] 4. health promotion and maintenance

17. A client is scheduled to have an elective mandibular osteotomy to correct a mandibular fracture sustained in an accident 6 months earlier. Which statement by the client indicates to the nurse the client is having difficulty coping?
- [ ] 1. "I will be glad to have my jaw fixed because my wife thinks I do not look like myself."
- [ ] 2. "I am somewhat afraid to have the surgery but feel OK about it."
- [ ] 3. "My wife will help me, but I do not think I will need that much help."
- [ ] 4. "I am ready to get this over with."

18. The nurse is assessing a client's nutritional status before surgery. Which observation would indicate poor nutrition in a 5-foot 7-inch female (170 cm) client who is 21 years of age?
- [ ] 1. poor posture
- [ ] 2. brittle nails
- [ ] 3. dull expression
- [ ] 4. weight of 128 lb (58.1 kg)

19. A 92-year-old is being discharged following a repair of an inguinal hernia. The client is independent and lives alone, and the client's family lives 60 miles from the client's house. When at home, the client is to cleanse and inspect the incision for signs of infection. The client and family are able to read and understand written instructions. When giving discharge instructions, what should the nurse do? Select all that apply.
- [ ] 1. Explain the instructions to the client.
- [ ] 2. Ask the client to demonstrate the procedure.
- [ ] 3. Explain the instructions to a family member.
- [ ] 4. Provide written instructions for the client.
- [ ] 5. Give the family a link to a video showing the procedure.

20. A client is admitted for an arthroscopy of the right shoulder through same-day surgery. Which nurse is responsible for starting the client's discharge planning?
- [ ] 1. preadmission nurse
- [ ] 2. preoperative nurse
- [ ] 3. intraoperative nurse
- [ ] 4. postoperative nurse

21. The nurse is preparing to administer a preoperative medication that includes a sedative to a client who is having abdominal surgery. The nurse should **first**:
- [ ] 1. have the family present.
- [ ] 2. ensure that the operative area has been shaved.
- [ ] 3. have the client empty the bladder.
- [ ] 4. make sure the client is covered with a warm blanket.

22. Before surgery, a client expresses a fear of surgery because 10 years ago the client's sister died in surgery related to complications of anesthesia. What should the nurse do?
- [ ] 1. Reassure the client that technology has changed over the last 10 years.
- [ ] 2. Encourage the client to further express concerns.
- [ ] 3. Explain to the client that it is normal to be afraid.
- [ ] 4. Ask the client if anyone else in the family has had trouble when they had surgery.

23. The nurse is preparing to start an intravenous infusion and has raised the head of the client's bed. After the nurse applies gloves to insert an IV catheter, the client begins to rub the eyes and wipe away nasal drainage. What should the nurse do **first**?
- [ ] 1. Distract the client's attention.
- [ ] 2. Assess the client for pain.
- [ ] 3. Remove the gloves and assess the client's vital signs.
- [ ] 4. Lower the head of the client's bed.

24. When evaluating a client's preoperative cognitive-perceptual pattern, which question should the nurse ask the client?
- [ ] 1. "Do you have difficulty swallowing?"
- [ ] 2. "Do you need special equipment to walk?"
- [ ] 3. "Do you smoke?"
- [ ] 4. "Do you wear glasses?"

25. When attempting to check the pupils of a client scheduled to receive general anesthesia, the nurse notices that the client has trouble tilting the head back. What is the **primary** concern related to this finding?
- [ ] 1. The client has limited movement of his neck.
- [ ] 2. The client is at risk for postoperative neck pain.
- [ ] 3. The client is at risk for difficult intubation.
- [ ] 4. The ability to assess the client's pupils is limited.

26. A client is to have a below-the-knee amputation. Prior to the surgery, the circulating nurse in the operating room should:
- ☐ **1.** insert a Foley catheter.
- ☐ **2.** start an intravenous infusion.
- ☐ **3.** initiate a time-out.
- ☐ **4.** verify that the surgeon possesses the degree of expertise needed.

27. The nurse is developing a plan to teach a client deep-breathing exercises to expand collapsed alveoli and prevent postoperative atelectasis and pneumonia. Which steps should be included? Select all that apply.
- ☐ **1.** Splint or support the incision to promote maximal comfort.
- ☐ **2.** Inhale slowly through the nostrils; exhale through pursed lips.
- ☐ **3.** Hold the breath for about 5 seconds to expand the alveoli.
- ☐ **4.** Repeat this breathing method 5 to 10 times hourly.
- ☐ **5.** Close one nostril while inhaling.

28. The nurse receives the preoperative blood work report for a client who is scheduled to undergo surgery. Which laboratory finding should be reported to the surgeon and anesthesiologist?
- ☐ **1.** red blood cells, 4.5 million/mm³ (4.5×10^{12}/L)
- ☐ **2.** creatinine, 2.6 mg/dL (198 µmol/L).
- ☐ **3.** hemoglobin, 12.2 g/dL (122 g/L)
- ☐ **4.** blood urea nitrogen, 15 mg/dL (5.4 mmol/L)

29. A client will receive IV midazolam hydrochloride during surgery. Which finding indicates a therapeutic effect?
- ☐ **1.** amnesia
- ☐ **2.** nausea
- ☐ **3.** mild agitation
- ☐ **4.** blurred vision

30. As the client receives IV midazolam hydrochloride, the nurse should:
- ☐ **1.** assess the blood pressure.
- ☐ **2.** monitor the pulse oximeter.
- ☐ **3.** encourage slow, deep breaths.
- ☐ **4.** explain relaxation techniques.

31. When the nurse administers IV midazolam hydrochloride, the client demonstrates signs of an overdose. The nurse should **next** collaborate with the surgical team to:
- ☐ **1.** ventilate with an oxygenated bag-valve mask.
- ☐ **2.** shock the client with ECG paddles.
- ☐ **3.** administer 0.5 mL 1:1,000 epinephrine.
- ☐ **4.** titrate flumazenil.

32. Metoclopramide is prescribed as a premedication for a client about to undergo a gastroduodenoscopy. The expected therapeutic effect is:
- ☐ **1.** increased gastric pH.
- ☐ **2.** increased gastric emptying.
- ☐ **3.** reduced anxiety.
- ☐ **4.** inhibited respiratory secretions.

33. What therapeutic outcome does the nurse expect for a client who has received a premedication of glycopyrrolate?
- ☐ **1.** increased heart rate
- ☐ **2.** increased respiratory rate
- ☐ **3.** decreased secretions
- ☐ **4.** decreased amnesia

34. Atropine sulfate is contraindicated as a preoperative medication for which clients? Select all that apply.
- ☐ **1.** a client with diabetes
- ☐ **2.** a client with glaucoma
- ☐ **3.** a client with urine retention
- ☐ **4.** a client with bowel obstruction

35. After the nurse has administered droperidol, care is taken to move the client slowly based on the knowledge of droperidol's effect on the:
- ☐ **1.** central nervous system.
- ☐ **2.** respiratory system.
- ☐ **3.** cardiovascular system.
- ☐ **4.** psychoneurologic system.

36. A client is to receive enoxaparin 6 hours before the scheduled time of laparoscopically assisted vaginal hysterectomy. Which effect does the nurse recognize as an intended therapeutic action of the enoxaparin?
- ☐ **1.** increase in red blood cell production
- ☐ **2.** reduction of postoperative thrombi
- ☐ **3.** decrease in postoperative bleeding
- ☐ **4.** promotion of tissue healing

37. During the preoperative interview, the nurse obtains information about the client's medication history. Which information is **not** necessary to record about the client?
- ☐ **1.** current use of medications, herbs, and vitamins
- ☐ **2.** over-the-counter medication use in the last 6 weeks
- ☐ **3.** steroid use in the last year
- ☐ **4.** all drugs taken in the last 18 months

38. When the nurse is conducting a preoperative interview with a client who is having a vaginal hysterectomy, the client states that she forgot to tell her surgeon that she had a total hip replacement 3 years ago. The nurse communicates this information to the perioperative nurse because:
- ☐ **1.** the prosthesis may cause a problem with the electrosurgical unit used to control bleeding.
- ☐ **2.** the client should not have her hip externally rotated when she is positioned for the procedure.
- ☐ **3.** the perioperative nurse can inform the rest of the team about the total hip replacement.
- ☐ **4.** there is not enough time to notify the surgeon and note this finding on the history and physical information before the procedure.

39. The nurse learns that a client who is scheduled for a tonsillectomy has been taking 40 mg of oral prednisone daily for the last week for poison ivy on the leg. What should the nurse do **first**?
☐ 1. Document the prednisone with current medications.
☐ 2. Notify the surgeon of the poison ivy.
☐ 3. Notify the anesthesiologist of the prednisone administration.
☐ 4. Send the client to surgery.

40. A client who is scheduled for an open cholecystectomy has been smoking a pack of cigarettes a day for 20 years. For which postoperative complication is the client **most** at risk?
☐ 1. deep vein thrombosis
☐ 2. atelectasis
☐ 3. delayed wound healing
☐ 4. prolonged immobility

41. The family cannot go with the client past the doors that separate the public from the restricted area of the operating room suite. These measures are designed to:
☐ 1. protect the privacy of clients.
☐ 2. prevent electrical sparks that could ignite the anesthetic gases.
☐ 3. separate the family from the surgical team while they are operating on the client.
☐ 4. provide for an aseptic environment to prevent infection.

42. Which client is **most** at risk for potential hazards from the surgical experience?
☐ 1. an 80-year-old client
☐ 2. a 50-year-old client
☐ 3. a 30-year-old client
☐ 4. a 15-year-old client

43. In which client is an autotransfusion possible?
☐ 1. the client who has cancer
☐ 2. the client who is in danger of cardiac arrest
☐ 3. the client with a contaminated wound
☐ 4. the client with a ruptured bowel

44. The nurse teaches a client who had cystoscopy about the urge to void when the procedure is over. What other teaching should be included?
☐ 1. Ignore the urge to void.
☐ 2. Increase intake of fluids.
☐ 3. Ask for the bedpan.
☐ 4. Ring for assistance to go to the bathroom.

45. Which nursing intervention is **most** important in preventing postoperative complications?
☐ 1. progressive diet planning
☐ 2. pain management
☐ 3. bowel and elimination monitoring
☐ 4. early ambulation

46. When preparing a teaching plan for an adult client about general anesthesia induction, which explanation would be **most** appropriate?
☐ 1. "Your premedication will put you to sleep."
☐ 2. "You will breathe in an inhalant anesthetic mixed with oxygen through a facial mask and receive intravenous medication to make you sleepy."
☐ 3. "You will receive intravenous medication to make you sleepy."
☐ 4. "You will breathe in medication through a facial mask to make you sleepy."

The Client Who Is Receiving or Recovering from Anesthesia

47. A client who had a gastrectomy has been in the postanesthesia recovery room for 30 minutes when the vital signs suddenly change. The nurse checks the recovery room record (see chart). In addition to notifying the healthcare provider (HCP), what other action should the nurse take immediately?

Vital Signs			
Date	06/30	06/30	06/30
Time	1345	1400	1415
Pulse	70	82	90
Respiration	12	14	20
Blood pressure	100/60	110/70	140/90
Temperature	98°F	99°F	102°F
	(36.7°C)	(37.2°C)	(38.9°C)

☐ 1. Administer dantrolene.
☐ 2. Elevate the head of the bed 30 degrees.
☐ 3. Administer a bolus of IV fluids.
☐ 4. Insert an indwelling urinary catheter.

48. To decrease a female client's anxiety about being placed in the lithotomy position for surgery, the nurse should:
☐ 1. explain in detail what will occur in the operating room.
☐ 2. determine what the client is concerned about.
☐ 3. pad the stirrups for comfort.
☐ 4. reassure the client that an all-female surgical team will be present.

49. A client is to receive medication by a continuous nerve block route. Prior to insertion of the catheter by the anesthesiologist, what information must the nurse document? Select all that apply.
☐ 1. vital signs
☐ 2. weakness/numbness
☐ 3. location of pain
☐ 4. results of laboratory tests
☐ 5. allergies

50. Prior to placement of an epidural/intrathecal catheter, what should the nurse instruct the client to do? Select all that apply.
☐ 1. Take showers instead of baths while the catheter is in place.
☐ 2. Tell the nurse about having nausea or vomiting.
☐ 3. Call for assistance with turning or repositioning while in bed.
☐ 4. Inform the nurse of numbness or weakness in the legs.
☐ 5. Take shallow breaths to prevent dislodging the catheter.
☐ 6. Call the nurse if the catheter becomes dislodged.

51. A client arrives from surgery to the postanesthesia care unit. Which respiratory assessment should the nurse complete **first**?
☐ 1. oxygen saturation
☐ 2. respiratory rate
☐ 3. breath sounds
☐ 4. airway flow

52. The nurse assesses vital signs on a client who had epidural anesthesia 4 hours ago. The nurse should assess the client **first** for:
☐ 1. bladder distention.
☐ 2. headache.
☐ 3. postoperative pain.
☐ 4. ability to move the legs.

53. When assessing a client who has had spinal anesthesia, which finding is expected?
☐ 1. The client feels pain before moving the legs.
☐ 2. The blood pressure is significantly increased.
☐ 3. Sensation returns to the toes first and then progresses to the perineal area.
☐ 4. The client has a headache while in the lying position.

54. The nurse in the postanesthesia care unit notes that one of the client's pupils is larger than the other. The nurse should:
☐ 1. rate the client on the Glasgow Coma Scale.
☐ 2. administer oxygen.
☐ 3. check the client's baseline data.
☐ 4. call the surgeon.

55. A client is admitted to the postanesthesia care unit following a left hip replacement. The initial nursing assessment is as follows: temperature, 96.6°F (35.9°C); pulse, 90 bpm; respiration rate, 14 breaths/min; and blood pressure, 128/80 mm Hg. The client only responds with moaning when spoken to. What should the nurse do **first**?
☐ 1. Observe the surgical dressing.
☐ 2. Position the client on the right side.
☐ 3. Remove the oral airway remaining from surgery.
☐ 4. Administer sedation reversal agent such as flumazenil.

56. The surgical floor receives a client from the postanesthesia care unit. Ten minutes ago, the final assessment in the postanesthesia care unit indicated that the client had a patent airway and stable vital signs. The client's pain level was 2. The nurse should **next**:
☐ 1. check the dressing for signs of bleeding.
☐ 2. empty any peri-incisional drains.
☐ 3. reassess the client's pain level.
☐ 4. determine if the client has a full bladder.

57. A client with impaired cardiac functioning is at risk during anesthesia induction with thiopental sodium because this drug causes:
☐ 1. bradycardia.
☐ 2. complete muscle relaxation.
☐ 3. hypotension.
☐ 4. tachypnea.

58. The nurse anticipates that a client who has received propofol as the induction and maintenance agent for general anesthesia will **most** likely experience:
☐ 1. minimal nausea and vomiting.
☐ 2. hypotension.
☐ 3. slow induction of anesthesia.
☐ 4. small tremors of the skeletal muscles.

59. What is the **main** reason desflurane and sevoflurane, volatile liquid anesthesia agents, are used for surgical clients who go home the day of surgery?
☐ 1. These agents are better tolerated.
☐ 2. These agents are predictable in their cardiovascular effects.
☐ 3. These agents are nonirritating to the respiratory tract.
☐ 4. These agents are rapidly eliminated.

60. A 250-lb (113-kg) male client recovering from general anesthesia has the following assessment findings: pulse, 150 bpm; blood pressure, 90/50 mm Hg; respiratory rate, 28 breaths/min; tympanic temperature, 99.8°F (37.7°C); and rigid muscles. The nurse determines that the client is:
☐ 1. recovering as expected from the anesthesia and continues monitoring him.
☐ 2. exhibiting the effects of excessive blood loss experienced in the operating room and increases the rate of his IV infusion.
☐ 3. in the early stages of malignant hyperthermia and obtains emergency medications and notifies the anesthesiologist.
☐ 4. in pain and offers him pain medication.

61. The nurse is assessing a client recovering from anesthesia. Which is an early indicator of hypoxemia?
☐ 1. somnolence
☐ 2. restlessness
☐ 3. chills
☐ 4. urgency

62. When administering flumazenil intravenously for reversal of sedation, what should the nurse do? Select all that apply.
☐ 1. Administer the medication as a 2-mg bolus.
☐ 2. Give the medication undiluted in incremental doses.
☐ 3. Be alert for shivering and hypotension.
☐ 4. Use only a free-flowing IV line in a large vein.
☐ 5. Monitor the client's level of consciousness.

63. An 80-year-old client had spinal anesthesia for a transurethral resection of the prostate and received 4,000 mL of room temperature isotonic bladder irrigation. He now has continuous irrigation through a three-way indwelling urinary catheter. Which postoperative nursing intervention is **most** important to include in his plan of care?
☐ 1. Empty the catheter drainage bag.
☐ 2. Cover the client with warm blankets.
☐ 3. Hang new bags of irrigation.
☐ 4. Turn the client.

64. Which client is expected to retain anesthetic agents longest?
☐ 1. a client who is 6 feet 2 inches tall (188 cm) and weighs 250 lb (113 kg)
☐ 2. a client who is 5 feet 4 inches (163 cm) tall and weighs 110 lb (49.9 kg)
☐ 3. a client who is 5 feet 1 inches (155 cm) tall and weighs 200 lb (90.7 kg)
☐ 4. a client who is 5 feet 7 inches (170 cm) tall and weighs 145 lb (65.8 kg)

65. An awake postoperative client received an intravenous regional nerve block (Bier block) in the arm that is now casted and elevated on a pillow. What action should the nurse encourage the client to avoid until sensation returns?
☐ 1. holding the operated arm close to the face
☐ 2. holding the operated arm with the unoperated arm
☐ 3. using the unoperated arm
☐ 4. using pain medication

66. The healthcare provider (HCP) prescribed intravenous naloxone to reverse the respiratory depression from morphine administration. After administration of the naloxone, the nurse should:
☐ 1. check respirations in 5 minutes because naloxone is immediately effective in relieving respiratory depression.
☐ 2. check respirations in 30 minutes because the effects of morphine will have worn off by then.
☐ 3. monitor respirations frequently for 4 to 6 hours because the client may need repeated doses of naloxone.
☐ 4. monitor respirations each time the client receives morphine sulfate 10 mg IM.

67. When administering naloxone, the nurse should monitor the surgical client closely for which clinical manifestation?
☐ 1. dizziness
☐ 2. biliary colic
☐ 3. bleeding
☐ 4. urine retention

68. The nurse anticipates that the client who has received epidural anesthesia is at decreased risk for a spinal headache because:
☐ 1. a 17-gauge needle is used.
☐ 2. a subarachnoid injection is made.
☐ 3. a noncutting needle is used.
☐ 4. a faster onset occurs.

69. Which body system is **not** blocked by spinal anesthesia?
☐ 1. the sympathetic nervous system
☐ 2. the sensory system
☐ 3. the parasympathetic nervous system
☐ 4. the motor system

70. The nurse is to administer midazolam 2.5 mg. The medication is available in a 5-mg/mL vial. How many mL should the nurse administer? Record your answer using one decimal point.

_____ mL.

The Client Who Has Had Surgery

71. On the first day after abdominal surgery, the nurse auscultates a client's abdomen for bowel sounds; there are none. The nurse should:
- ☐ **1.** notify the healthcare provider (HCP).
- ☐ **2.** ask another nurse to validate the absence of bowel sounds.
- ☐ **3.** encourage the client to take more ice chips.
- ☐ **4.** document assessment findings in the client's medical record.

72. Three days after a cholecystectomy, a client states, "I feel like my stomach is going to burst." The client is taking a regular diet. After determining that vital signs are stable, in which order of priority from first to last does the nurse assist the client? All options must be used.

1. Position the client on the right side.

2. Offer 120 mL of hot liquids.

3. Auscultate for bowel sounds.

4. Encourage ambulation.

73. The nurse assesses that a client is restless in the immediate postoperative period. The nurse should **first**:
- ☐ **1.** administer a sedative.
- ☐ **2.** offer ice chips.
- ☐ **3.** administer oxygen.
- ☐ **4.** apply wrist restraints.

74. A client requests a narcotic analgesic shortly after the oncoming nurse receives change-of-shift report. The nurse who is leaving reported that the client had received morphine 10 mg (IM) within the past hour. In what order from first to last should the oncoming registered nurse (RN) perform the actions? All options must be used.

1. Validate with the outgoing RN that morphine 10 mg (IM) had been administered.

2. Assess the client for manifestations of pain.

3. Check the medication documentation as to when morphine 10 mg (IM) was dispensed and to whom.

4. Check to ascertain if any discrepancy had been documented with accompanying reason(s).

75. On the day of surgery, a client has been breathing room air. The vital signs are normal, and the O_2 saturation is 89%. The nurse should **first**:
- ☐ **1.** lower the head of the bed.
- ☐ **2.** notify the healthcare provider (HCP).
- ☐ **3.** assist the client to take several deep breaths and cough.
- ☐ **4.** administer oxygen by nasal cannula as prescribed at 2 L/min.

76. A client has been unable to void since having abdominal surgery 7 hours ago. The nurse should **first**:
- ☐ **1.** encourage the client to increase oral fluid intake.
- ☐ **2.** insert an intermittent urinary catheter.
- ☐ **3.** notify the healthcare provider (HCP).
- ☐ **4.** assist the client up to the toilet to attempt to void.

77. Following abdominal surgery, a client refuses to deep breathe and cough every 2 hours as prescribed. What should the nurse do **first**?
- ☐ **1.** Ask the client's wife to insist that the client take the deep breaths every 2 hours.
- ☐ **2.** Respect the client's wishes, and turn the client from side to side more frequently.
- ☐ **3.** Suggest that the client increase the daily fluid intake to at least 2,500 mL.
- ☐ **4.** Explain the risks of not expanding the lungs and why the exercise is important.

78. Eight hours after laparoscopic abdominal surgery, a client has a distended bladder and is unable to void in bed using a urinal. The client can be out of bed as tolerated, but has not done so yet. The nurse should **first**:

☐ 1. Assist the client to stand at the bedside to use the urinal.

☐ 2. Pour running water over perineum to stimulate emptying of the bladder.

☐ 3. Encourage the client to ambulate to prevent further bladder distention.

☐ 4. Notify the healthcare provider (HCP) to request a prescription for catheterization.

79. The nurse is assessing the level of consciousness for a client who just had open heart surgery. When asked, the client can give his name but is not sure about where he is or the time of day. What should the nurse do?

☐ 1. Notify the surgeon.

☐ 2. Rub the client's sternum to arouse the client.

☐ 3. Encourage the client's wife to orient the client.

☐ 4. Tell the client where he is and the time of day.

80. Following surgery, a client is receiving 1,000 mL normal saline (IV) with 40 mEq (40 mmol/L) KCl, which has been prescribed to be infused at 125 mL/h. The client states, "My IV hurts." What should the nurse do **first**?

☐ 1. Contact the client's healthcare provider (HCP) for a different IV prescription.

☐ 2. Slow down the infusion to a keep-open rate (20 to 50 mL/h).

☐ 3. Assess the IV site for signs of phlebitis, extravasation, or IV-related infection.

☐ 4. Check the hanging parenteral fluid and administration set for documentation as to when they were last changed.

81. A nurse is assessing a client when she returns from same-day surgery for a dilatation and curettage. The nurse checks preoperative vital signs at 0830 to compare them with the current vital signs at 2230 (see chart). What should the nurse do **first**?

Vital Signs		
	0830	2230
Pulse	80	90
Respirations	16	20
Blood pressure	90/60	100/80
Temperature	99.5 (37.5)	97 (36.1)

☐ 1. Call the healthcare provider (HCP) for pain medication.

☐ 2. Cover the client with warmed blankets.

☐ 3. Administer oxygen at 4 L/min.

☐ 4. Increase the IV fluid rate.

82. The nurse is caring for a client receiving morphine in an intravenous infusion using a patient-controlled anesthesia pump (PCA) for relief of postoperative pain. On assessment, the client's vital signs are as follows: heart rate, 84 bpm; respirations, 8 breaths/min; blood pressure, 104/56 mm Hg; and oxygen saturation of 88% on room air. What should the nurse do **first**?

☐ 1. Contact the healthcare provider (HCP) to request a prescription for naloxone.

☐ 2. Stop the infusion of morphine.

☐ 3. Assist the client to sit and stimulate coughing/deep breathing.

☐ 4. Call the rapid response team.

83. A client had a colectomy 8½ hours ago and has received 1,500 mL of dextrose 5% in water with normal saline solution. The client has just used a patient-controlled analgesia pump to administer morphine for pain, has been repositioned for comfort, and has stable pulse rate, respirations, and blood pressure. What should the nurse do **next**?

☐ 1. Check that the family is comfortable.

☐ 2. Assess vital signs following the use of morphine.

☐ 3. Dim the lights in the room.

☐ 4. Increase nasal oxygen from 2 to 3 L.

84. A client who had an esophageal hernia repair 4 hours ago has a pulse rate of 90 bpm; respiration rate of 16 breaths/min; blood pressure of 130/80 mm Hg; pulse oximeter of 91%, on room air; and a temperature of 100.4°F (38°C). What should the nurse do **first**?

☐ 1. Obtain a culture of the incision.

☐ 2. Notify the surgeon to obtain an antibiotic prescription.

☐ 3. Offer pain medication.

☐ 4. Assist the client to a sitting position to take deep breaths.

85. After completing client teaching on the use of patient-controlled analgesia (PCA), the nurse determines that the client understands the use of the PCA when the client states:

☐ 1. "It is OK for my family to press the button for me if I am too tired to do it myself."

☐ 2. "I should wait until the pain is really bad before I push the button to get more pain medicine."

☐ 3. "The machine will only give me the prescribed amount of pain medication even if I push the button too soon."

☐ 4. "I have to be careful about pushing the button too many times or I will overdose myself."

86. A client had a total abdominal hysterectomy and bilateral oophorectomy for ovarian carcinoma yesterday. She received 2 mg of morphine sulfate IV by patient-controlled analgesia (PCA) 10 minutes ago. The nurse was assisting her from the bed to a chair when the client felt dizzy and fell into the chair. The nurse should:
- ☐ 1. discontinue the PCA pump.
- ☐ 2. administer oxygen.
- ☐ 3. take the client's blood pressure.
- ☐ 4. assist the client back to bed.

87. Immediately following pelvic surgery, a client has an indwelling urinary catheter. Which nursing action would be **most** helpful to prevent a catheter-related urinary tract infection?
- ☐ 1. Provide catheter and perineal care twice daily.
- ☐ 2. Monitor the color, clarity, and amount of urine output.
- ☐ 3. Advocate for limited use of and duration of indwelling urinary catheters.
- ☐ 4. Palpate for lower abdominal distension once per shift.

88. A nurse is instructing a client who had abdominal surgery that day to do deep-breathing exercises. In which order from first to last should the nurse teach the client to perform diaphragmatic breathing and coughing? All options must be used.

1. Inhale through the nose.

2. Cough deeply from the lungs.

3. Exhale through pursed lips.

4. Splint the incisional site.

89. The postoperative nursing assessment of a client's ability to swallow fluids before providing oral fluids is based on the type of anesthesia given. Which client would **not** have delayed fluid restrictions?
- ☐ 1. the client who has undergone a bronchoscopy under local anesthesia
- ☐ 2. the client who has undergone a transurethral resection of a bladder tumor under general anesthesia
- ☐ 3. the client who has undergone a repair of carpal tunnel syndrome under local anesthesia
- ☐ 4. the client who has undergone an inguinal herniorrhaphy with spinal and intravenous conscious sedation

90. The client has just returned to bed following the first ambulation since abdominal surgery. The client's heart rate and blood pressure are slightly elevated; oxygen saturation is 91% on room air. The client reports being "a little short of breath," but does not have dizziness or pain. The nurse should **first**:
- ☐ 1. Obtain a 12-lead ECG.
- ☐ 2. Administer pain medication.
- ☐ 3. Allow the client to rest for a few minutes, then reassess.
- ☐ 4. Request new activity prescriptions from the healthcare provider (HCP).

91. Eight hours following bowel surgery, the nurse observes that the client's urine output has decreased from 50 to 20 mL/h. The nurse should assess the client further for:
- ☐ 1. bowel obstruction.
- ☐ 2. adverse effect of opioid analgesics.
- ☐ 3. hemorrhage.
- ☐ 4. hypertension.

92. A client who had a left thoracoscopy sustained an injury secondary to the surgery position. The nurse should assess the client for:
- ☐ 1. foot drop.
- ☐ 2. knee swelling and pain.
- ☐ 3. tingling in the arm.
- ☐ 4. absence of the Achilles reflex.

93. The nurse is evaluating a client who is using a flow incentive spirometer (see figure) following abdominal surgery 1 day ago. The client is performing the procedure correctly when the client: Select all that apply.

- ☐ 1. inhales before using the spirometer.
- ☐ 2. inhales for 3 seconds following fully expanding the lungs.
- ☐ 3. coughs after using the spirometer.
- ☐ 4. uses the spirometer once every 8 hours.
- ☐ 5. exhales passively before using the spirometer.
- ☐ 6. is sitting upright.

94. The nurse is teaching a client how to take care of an incision at home. The nurse should tell the client:
- ☐ 1. "Do not touch your incision before your next appointment."
- ☐ 2. "Clean your incision three times a day with hydrogen peroxide and water."
- ☐ 3. "Do not be concerned about uneven lumps under the suture lines."
- ☐ 4. "If the staples do not come out by themselves before your next appointment, the surgeon will remove them."

95. The nurse is removing the client's staples from an abdominal incision when the client sneezes and the incision splits open, exposing the intestines. What should the nurse do **first**?
- ☐ 1. Press the emergency alarm to call the resuscitation team.
- ☐ 2. Cover the abdominal organs with sterile dressings moistened with sterile normal saline.
- ☐ 3. Have all visitors and family leave the room.
- ☐ 4. Call the surgeon to come to the client's room immediately.

96. On the fourth day after surgery, a client's incision is red and inflamed. There is moderate drainage from the incision. The client has a temperature of 102°F (38.9°C). The total white blood count (WBC) 10,000/mm³ (10 × 109/L). The nurse should **first**:
- ☐ 1. encourage the client to increase the fluid intake.
- ☐ 2. cleanse the incision site with soap and water.
- ☐ 3. ask the client about the level of pain.
- ☐ 4. notify the healthcare provider (HCP).

97. The nurse is making rounds and observes the client receiving oxygen (see figure). The nurse should:

O₂ line
Reservoir bag

- ☐ 1. position the mask lower on the client's nose.
- ☐ 2. verify that the reservoir bag remains deflated.
- ☐ 3. confirm that the flow rate is set to deliver oxygen at 6 to 10 L/min.
- ☐ 4. loosen the elastic band on the client's face.

98. When changing a wet-to-dry dressing covering a surgical wound, what should the nurse do?
- ☐ 1. Place a dry dressing in the wound.
- ☐ 2. Use an aqueous solution of aluminum acetate (Burow's solution) to wet the dressing.
- ☐ 3. Pack the wet dressing tightly into the wound.
- ☐ 4. Cover the wet packing with a dry sterile dressing.

99. Two days following abdominal surgery, a client is refusing to take a narcotic pain medication, even though the pain rating is an 8 on a 0 to 10 scale. The client tells the nurse, "I do not want to get dependent on that stuff." Which response from the nurse is the **most** appropriate?
- ☐ 1. "You will recover more quickly and more effectively if you take pain medication now."
- ☐ 2. "Newer pain medications do not cause dependence or addiction."
- ☐ 3. "It is your right to not take pain medication."
- ☐ 4. "You do not need to worry about becoming addicted so soon."

100. The nurse empties a Jackson-Pratt drainage bulb. Which nursing action ensures correct functioning of the drain?
- ☐ 1. irrigating it with normal saline
- ☐ 2. connecting it to low intermittent suction
- ☐ 3. compressing it and then plugging it to establish suction
- ☐ 4. connecting it to a drainage bag and clamping it off

101. To prevent pulmonary emboli in a client who has had abdominal surgery, the nurse should:
- ☐ 1. have the client perform leg exercises every hour while awake.
- ☐ 2. encourage the client to cough and deep breathe.
- ☐ 3. massage the client's calves.
- ☐ 4. have the client wear antiembolism stockings when out of bed.

102. The nurse assesses a client who has just received morphine sulfate. The client's blood pressure is 90/50 mm Hg; pulse rate, 58 bpm; and respiration rate, 4 breaths/min. The nurse should check the client's record for a prescription to administer:
- ☐ 1. flumazenil.
- ☐ 2. naloxone hydrochloride.
- ☐ 3. doxacurium.
- ☐ 4. remifentanil.

103. The nurse observes the client with an intermittent compression device in place after abdominal surgery (see figure). The nurse should:

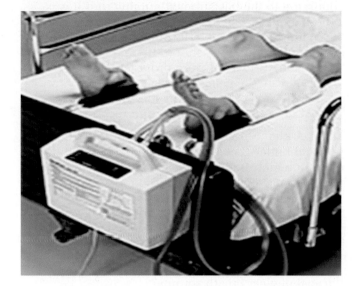

☐ **1.** elevate the client's legs.
☐ **2.** apply thromboembolic stockings to be worn under the device.
☐ **3.** instruct the client not to move while the device is inflated.
☐ **4.** make sure the client is comfortable.

104. A client is being discharged from same-day surgery. Which statement indicates that the client does not understand postoperative instructions about transportation to home?
☐ **1.** "My husband is taking the day off from work to drive me home."
☐ **2.** "I can drive myself home after surgery."
☐ **3.** "I am taking a taxi home, and my daughter will meet me at home."
☐ **4.** "My son will be here at noon to take me home."

105. The initial postoperative assessment is completed on a client who had an arthroscopy of the knee. Which information is **not** necessary to obtain every 15 minutes during the first postoperative hour?
☐ **1.** vital signs including pulse oximeter
☐ **2.** pain rating of the operative site
☐ **3.** urine output
☐ **4.** neurovascular check distal to the operative site

106. After surgery, a client was treated for postoperative nausea and vomiting and now is experiencing hypotension and tachycardia. The nurse should review the medication record to determine if the client has received which medication?
☐ **1.** ondansetron hydrochloride
☐ **2.** droperidol
☐ **3.** prochlorperazine
☐ **4.** promethazine

107. When an epidural catheter is used for postoperative pain management, the nurse should:
☐ **1.** assess but not disturb the epidural dressing.
☐ **2.** change the epidural dressing daily.
☐ **3.** change the epidural dressing daily only if it is wet.
☐ **4.** use strict aseptic technique when handling the epidural catheter.

108. The nurse understands that the client who has epidural pain management postoperatively can ambulate because:
☐ **1.** the analgesia is periodically administered through the epidural catheter.
☐ **2.** a low concentration of analgesia is used with the catheter.
☐ **3.** the analgesia from the epidural catheter bathes the spinal fluid.
☐ **4.** the epidural medication affects the sympathetic and motor function.

109. The nurse is caring for a client who is using a portable wound suction unit (see figure). Six hours following surgery, the drainage unit is full. What should the nurse do?

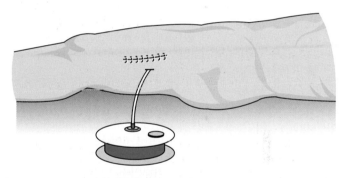

☐ **1.** Remove the drain from the incision.
☐ **2.** Notify the surgeon.
☐ **3.** Empty drainage.
☐ **4.** Record the amount in the unit as output on the client's medical record.

110. Three days after surgery, a client continues to take hydrocodone 7.5 mg and acetaminophen 500 mg for postoperative pain. What should the nurse ask the client before administering the pain medication?
☐ **1.** "When did you last have a bowel movement?"
☐ **2.** "Have you emptied your bladder?"
☐ **3.** "How long has it been since your last dose?"
☐ **4.** "Is your pain better than before you had surgery?"

111. Upon waking up in the postanesthesia care unit and seeing a drain with bright red fluid in it exiting from his total hip incision, a client asks the nurse, "Is this the way it is supposed to be?" The nurse should tell the client:
☐ 1. "The drainage is blood and fluid that must be drained out for healing."
☐ 2. "Do not worry about it. I will explain it when you are more awake."
☐ 3. "This blood is being kept sterile and will be given back to you."
☐ 4. "I will give you something to make you sleep so you will not worry."

112. A client has a Jackson-Pratt drainage tube in place the first day after surgical repair of a ruptured diverticulum. The client asks the nurse the purpose of the drain. What is the nurse's **best** response? "The drainage tube is used to prevent:
☐ 1. infection in the peritoneal cavity."
☐ 2. bleeding into the peritoneal cavity."
☐ 3. pressure on the bladder."
☐ 4. pressure on the gallbladder."

113. A client who had a cholecystectomy has a biliary drainage tube in place. What color of the drainage is expected?
☐ 1. pinkish red
☐ 2. dark yellow-orange
☐ 3. clear
☐ 4. green

114. A client is to be discharged from same-day surgery 7 hours after his inguinal hernia repair. Which nursing observation indicates this client is ready to be discharged?
☐ 1. The client voids 500 mL of urine.
☐ 2. The client tolerates eating a hamburger.
☐ 3. The client is pain free.
☐ 4. The client walks in the hallway unassisted.

115. A client is eligible for patient-controlled analgesia (PCA) when:
☐ 1. a family member is able to assist with self-dosing.
☐ 2. there are advanced directives in place.
☐ 3. the client has the ability to self-administer.
☐ 4. there is a nurse to assist with self-administration.

116. How often should the client's temperature be assessed during the first 24 hours after surgery?
☐ 1. every 2 hours
☐ 2. every 4 hours
☐ 3. every 6 hours
☐ 4. every 8 hours

117. A nurse is assessing a client's blood pressure 8 hours after surgery. The client's blood pressure before surgery was 120/80 mm Hg, and on admission to the postsurgical nursing unit it was 110/80 mm Hg. The client's blood pressure is now 90/70 mm Hg. After determining that other vital signs are normal, what should the nurse do **first**?
☐ 1. Notify the healthcare provider (HCP).
☐ 2. Elevate the head of the bed.
☐ 3. Administer pain medication.
☐ 4. Check the intake and output record.

118. A client has been positioned in the lithotomy position under general anesthesia for a pelvic procedure. In which anatomic area may the client expect to experience postoperative discomfort?
☐ 1. shoulders
☐ 2. thighs
☐ 3. legs
☐ 4. feet

119. Which nursing action does **not** aid in meeting the goal of clear breath sounds?
☐ 1. offering pain relief before having the client cough
☐ 2. providing a minimum of 1,000 mL of fluid per day
☐ 3. using an incentive spirometer
☐ 4. assisting with early ambulation

120. The nurse is teaching the client about deep-breathing techniques. Which statement from the client indicates the need for additional education?
☐ 1. "I will use my incentive spirometer every hour while I am awake."
☐ 2. "I should place my hands lightly over my lower ribs and upper abdomen."
☐ 3. "I should get into a comfortable position before doing my breathing exercises."
☐ 4. "I should take four deep breaths and then cough deeply from the lungs."

121. A client has had a nasogastric tube connected to low intermittent suction. The client is at risk for:
☐ 1. confusion.
☐ 2. muscle cramping.
☐ 3. edema.
☐ 4. tremors.

Legal and Ethical Issues Associated with Surgery

122. On admission to same-day surgery, the nurse reviews the medical record to verify the client's identification documentation. Which information is **most** important?
☐ 1. admitting record
☐ 2. preprinted labels
☐ 3. identification bracelet
☐ 4. location of family

123. A 15-year-old client needs lifesaving emergency surgery, but the relatives live an hour away from the hospital and cannot sign the consent form. What is the nurse's **best** response?
- ☐ 1. Send the client to surgery without the consent.
- ☐ 2. Call the family for a consent over the telephone, and have another nurse listen as a witness.
- ☐ 3. No action is necessary in this case because consent is not needed.
- ☐ 4. Have the family sign the consent form as soon as they arrive.

124. A client who has type 1 diabetes is being prepared to have a craniotomy for a brain tumor. As a client advocate, the nurse is evaluating the client's understanding of the informed consent before witnessing the client's signature on the operative consent form. Which statement from the client indicates that the nurse needs to contact the surgeon for further communication with the client?
- ☐ 1. "We talked about the effect of my diabetes on healing."
- ☐ 2. "The surgeon explained how the craniotomy was done."
- ☐ 3. "There are no major risks from this surgery."
- ☐ 4. "I will die if the tumor is not removed from my brain."

125. The nurse is helping to prepare a client for nonemergency surgery. The nurse should:
- ☐ 1. obtain informed consent from the client.
- ☐ 2. explain the surgical procedure in detail.
- ☐ 3. verify that the client understands the informed consent form.
- ☐ 4. inform the client about the risks of the surgery to be performed.

126. When a client cannot read or write but is of sound mind, the nurse should read the informed consent to the client in the presence of two witnesses and:
- ☐ 1. have the client's next of kin sign the informed consent.
- ☐ 2. have the client put an "X" on the signature line.
- ☐ 3. have a court appoint a guardian for the client.
- ☐ 4. have a hospital quality management coordinator sign for the client.

Managing Care, Quality, and Safety of Clients Having Surgery

127. The nurse should review the glucose level of which clients who are going to surgery today? Select all that apply.
- ☐ 1. a client with diabetes mellitus controlled by diet
- ☐ 2. a client with a high stress response to surgery
- ☐ 3. a client receiving corticosteroids for the past 3 months
- ☐ 4. a client with a family history of diabetes receiving dextrose 5% in lactated Ringer's solution (D_5LR) IV fluids
- ☐ 5. a client who consumes a high-carbohydrate diet

128. Which client has the **greatest** risk for latex allergies?
- ☐ 1. a woman who is admitted for her seventh surgery
- ☐ 2. a man who works as a sales clerk
- ☐ 3. a man with well-controlled type 2 diabetes
- ☐ 4. a woman who is having laser surgery

129. A client is admitted on the day of surgery for an arthroscopy of the left knee. Which nursing activities should be completed prior to administering anesthesia to the client to avoid wrong-site surgery? Select all that apply.
- ☐ 1. Verify that the surgeon has marked with a permanent marker the correct knee for the surgical site.
- ☐ 2. Verbally ask the client to state his or her name, surgical site, and procedure.
- ☐ 3. Verify the correct client with the correct operative site from medical records and diagnostic reports.
- ☐ 4. Call a "time-out" in the operating room to have the surgeon verify the correct knee before making the incision.
- ☐ 5. Show the client an anatomic model of the surgery site.

130. The nurse is planning care for a client with severe postoperative pain. There is a prescription for morphine written as "10 mg MSO_4" on the medical record. What should the nurse do **first**?
- ☐ 1. Obtain an intravenous infusion system.
- ☐ 2. Prepare the medication for administration.
- ☐ 3. Contact the pharmacy department.
- ☐ 4. Contact the healthcare provider (HCP) who prescribed the medication.

131. The client has returned to the surgery unit from the postanesthesia care unit (PACU). The client's respirations are rapid and shallow, the pulse is 120 bpm, and the blood pressure is 88/52 mm Hg. The client's level of consciousness is declining. The nurse should **first**:
☐ 1. call the PACU.
☐ 2. call the healthcare provider (HCP).
☐ 3. call the respiratory therapist.
☐ 4. call the rapid response team (RRT)/medical emergency team.

132. When completing the preoperative checklist on the nursing unit, the nurse discovers an allergy that the client has not reported. What should the nurse do **first**?
☐ 1. Administer the prescribed preanesthetic medication.
☐ 2. Note this new allergy prominently on the medical record.
☐ 3. Contact the scrub nurse in the operating room.
☐ 4. Inform the anesthesiologist.

133. Which activities should the nurse encourage the unlicensed assistive personnel (UAP) to assist with in the care of postoperative clients? Select all that apply.
☐ 1. Empty and measure indwelling urinary catheter collection bags.
☐ 2. Reposition clients for pain relief.
☐ 3. Teach clients the proper use of the incentive spirometer.
☐ 4. Tell the nurse if clients report they are having pain.
☐ 5. Assess IV insertion site for redness.

134. The client's identification armband was cut and removed to start an IV line as a part of the preoperative preparation. The transport team has arrived to transport the client to the operating room. The nurse notices that the client's identification band is not on either wrist. What should the nurse do?
☐ 1. Send the removed armband with the medical record and the client to the operating room.
☐ 2. Place a new identification armband on the client's wrist before transport.
☐ 3. Tape the cut armband back onto the client's wrist.
☐ 4. Send the client without an armband because the client is alert and can respond to questions about his or her identity.

135. On the 2nd day after surgery, the nurse assesses an elderly client and finds the following:
☐ 1. blood pressure, 148/92 mm Hg; heart rate, 98 bpm; respirations 32 breaths/min
☐ 2. O$_2$ saturation of 88% on 4 L/min of oxygen administered by nasal cannula
☐ 3. breath sounds are coarse and wet bilaterally with a loose, productive cough
☐ 4. client voided 100 mL very dark, concentrated urine during the last 4 hours
☐ 5. bilateral pitting pedal edema
Using the SBAR method to notify the healthcare provider (HCP) of current assessment findings, the nurse should recommend that the HCP write a prescription for a(n):
☐ 1. antihypertensive medication.
☐ 2. additional fluid intake.
☐ 3. diuretic medication.
☐ 4. increased oxygen liter flow rate.

136. Which prescription is entered correctly on the medical record?
☐ 1. fentanyl 50 mcg given IV every 2 hours as needed for pain greater than 6/10
☐ 2. give 4 U regular insulin IV now
☐ 3. .5 mg MS given IM for c/o pain
☐ 4. 60.0 mg ketorolac tromethamine given IM for c/o pain

137. The nurse has just received morning change-of-shift report on four clients. In what order from first to last should the nurse perform the actions? All options must be used.

1. Discuss the plan for the day with the unlicensed assistive personnel (UAP), delegating duties as appropriate.

2. Assess the client who has been vomiting according to the report from the night nurse.

3. Begin discharge paperwork for a client who is eager to go home.

4. Notify the healthcare provider (HCP) about a client who has a serum potassium level of 6.2.

138. While making rounds, the nurse observes that a client's primary bag of intravenous (IV) solution is light yellow. The label on the IV bag says the solution is D5W. What should the nurse do **first**?
- ☐ 1. Continue to monitor the bag of IV solution.
- ☐ 2. Ask another nurse to look at the solution.
- ☐ 3. Notify the healthcare provider (HCP).
- ☐ 4. Hang a new bag of D5W, and complete an incident report.

139. A client informs the nurse that the venipuncture site "hurts." The nurse should assess the site for what findings? Select all that apply.
- ☐ 1. redness
- ☐ 2. pain
- ☐ 3. coolness
- ☐ 4. blanching
- ☐ 5. firmness
- ☐ 6. edema

140. A client has accidentally received twice the normal dose of a medication that was administered on the previous shift. What should the nurse who discovers the error do **first**?
- ☐ 1. Call the person who made the error, and request that an incident report be completed.
- ☐ 2. Assess the client, and note any changes in condition.
- ☐ 3. Call the healthcare provider (HCP) to obtain a prescription for additional IV fluids to dilute the drug.
- ☐ 4. Administer a drug antidote per standing prescription.

141. A client is in the operating room having surgery to replace a hip. Prior to starting the surgery, there is confusion about the view of the hip on the x-ray. The surgical team requests a "time-out" and stops the surgery. When can surgery continue? Select all that apply.
- ☐ 1. The surgeon verifies the correct procedure.
- ☐ 2. The surgeon verifies correct surgical site.
- ☐ 3. The nurse reestablishes the sterile field.
- ☐ 4. The surgical team identifies the client using two sources of identification.
- ☐ 5. Another x-ray is obtained.

142. A client is being transferred from the recovery room to the medical-surgical nursing unit. The nurse from the recovery room should report which information to the nurse in the medical-surgical unit? Select all that apply.
- ☐ 1. type of surgery
- ☐ 2. name of insurance provider
- ☐ 3. current vital signs
- ☐ 4. names of all surgeons participating in the surgery
- ☐ 5. amount of blood loss
- ☐ 6. fluids infusing including rate and type of fluid

143. A client with a history of myocardial infarction 3 years ago was admitted at 0700 for a cholecystectomy scheduled at 0900. The client has been NPO since midnight. At 0830, the client reports having chest pains. At 0700, the client's vital signs were pulse, 80 bpm; respirations, 14 breaths/min; and blood pressure, 110/70 mm Hg. At 0830 the nurse takes the vital signs again: pulse is 110 bpm; respirations, 20 breaths/min; and blood pressure, 90/60 mm Hg. The nurse calls the surgeon and, using SBAR communication protocol, should discuss which information with the surgeon? Select all that apply.
- ☐ 1. that the client has remained NPO
- ☐ 2. history of myocardial infarction and current report of chest pains
- ☐ 3. the change in vital signs
- ☐ 4. the type of surgery scheduled
- ☐ 5. request for ECG
- ☐ 6. request to administer nitroglycerin tablet

144. When taking a client's vital signs on the first postoperative day, the unlicensed assistive personnel (UAP) reports to the nurse that the oral temperature is 100°F (37.8°C). After encouraging the client to use the incentive spirometer, the nurse should delegate which activity to the UAP?
- ☐ 1. Apply an ice cap to a client's forehead.
- ☐ 2. Bathe the client with cool water.
- ☐ 3. Place a hyperthermia blanket on the client's bed.
- ☐ 4. Continue to monitor the client's temperature.

145. A nurse is working with an unlicensed assistive personnel (UAP). Which clients should the nurse assign to the UAP? Select all that apply.
- ☐ 1. Adult client newly diagnosed with diabetes who is learning to administer insulin.
- ☐ 2. Older adult client who had hip replacement surgery and needs to walk in the hall with a walker.
- ☐ 3. Adult client who had abdominal surgery yesterday and requires a dressing change.
- ☐ 4. Young adult client who requires tube feedings.
- ☐ 5. Adult client who had a hysterectomy 3 days ago and requires vital sign checks every 4 hours.

146. A nurse is caring for a group of clients. After receiving shift report, the nurse should make rounds on the clients in which order? Place in order of the highest to lowest priority. All options must be used.

1. female client who is 34 years of age and just returning from the recovery room following an abdominal hysterectomy; IV running at 50 drops per minute with 100 mL remaining.

2. client who is 50 years of age and diagnosed with diabetes mellitus 3 days ago who is learning to administer insulin.

3. client who is 75 years of age with a fractured hip of 4 days who needs to be turned frequently.

4. client who is 79 years of age 2 days postsurgery for removal of cancer of the colon who has had a tracheotomy for 4 years.

| |
| |
| |
| |

147. A client scheduled for surgery is confused and shows signs of dementia. The nurse should ask which person to sign the consent for the client?
☐ **1.** minister
☐ **2.** nursing supervisor
☐ **3.** attorney
☐ **4.** spouse

Answers, Rationales, and Test-Taking Strategies

The answers and rationales for each question follow below, along with keys (🔑) to the client need (CN) and cognitive level (CL) for each question. In addition, you will also see a glossary icon (📖) highlighting specific terminology used on the licensing exam. As you check your answers, use the **Content Mastery and Test-Taking Skill Self-Analysis** *worksheet (tear-out worksheet in back of book) to identify the reason(s) for not answering the questions correctly. For additional information about test-taking skills and strategies for answering questions, refer to pages 12–23 and pages 35–36 in Part 1 of this book.*

The Client Who Is Preparing for Surgery

1. 4. The health history is conducted to ascertain a client's state of wellness or illness. A personal dialogue between a client and a nurse is conducted to obtain information. To achieve a relationship of mutual trust and respect, the nurse must have the ability to communicate a sincere interest in the client. The therapeutic communication must be adapted to the responses, problems, and needs of the client. Reassurance and the remaining options do not demonstrate that the nurse is genuinely interested in the client's needs.

🔑 CN: Psychosocial integrity; CL: Synthesize

2. 1,2,3. Treatment and diagnostic evaluation must be done in a latex-safe environment. Signs and symptoms of latex allergy may range from mild to anaphylaxis. Clients with latex allergy are advised to notify their **HCPs**📖 and to wear a medical ID; however, all metal and jewelry must be removed prior to surgery as they could conduct an electrical current. The surgery can be safely performed at a free-standing surgery center as long as latex precautions are observed.

🔑 CN: Safety and infection control; CL: Create

3. 3. It is the surgeon's responsibility to discuss the planned procedure and review the risks, benefits, and alternatives to the planned procedure. If the client verbalizes that he or she does not understand the procedure that is planned, it is the nurse's responsibility to notify the surgeon of this lack of understanding right away, prior to any other/additional nursing actions. In this case, when the client verbalizes a lack of understanding, the nurse should not teach about the procedure; the surgeon needs to do this. The nurse cannot assist the client to sign for **consent** 📖 and should not administer narcotics or sedatives until the client understands and agrees to the procedure.

🔑 CN: Management of care; CL: Synthesize

4. 3. Garlic has anticoagulant properties and may pose a problem with bleeding if enough has been taken too close to surgery. Therefore, the nurse must obtain more quantifiable details about the client's statement. The nurse should check the surgical procedure, anesthesia preference, and blood pressure status with the client. However, the part of the client's statement that needs further investigation concerns intake of a herb with anticoagulant properties before a surgical procedure.

🔑 CN: Pharmacological and parenteral therapies; CL: Synthesize

5. 1. The nurse should remove the face mask. The face mask contains nasal and oral droplets, which are easily transmitted to the hands as the mask dangles when left hanging around the neck. When a face mask is not worn over the mouth and nose, it should be completely removed.

⚷ CN: Safety and infection control;
CL: Synthesize

6. This is the correct surgical site.

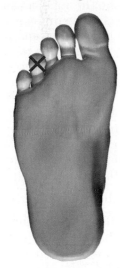

⚷ CN: Physiological adaptation; CL: Apply

7. 1. A pimple close to the incision site may be reason for the surgeon to cancel the surgical procedure because it increases the risk of infection. If the client had an abnormal ECG, the nurse would notify the anesthesiologist who will be administering the anesthesia. The anesthesiologist is the decision-maker regarding the implications of the anesthesia on the cardiac system. The surgical team should be notified of the client's hearing disability, but the surgeon, who has already met the client, does not need to be notified. The surgical team should be notified of the client's allergy to iodine, and it should be documented in all the appropriate places, but the surgeon would not need to be notified in advance of the surgical procedure.

⚷ CN: Safety and infection control;
CL: Synthesize

8. 4. The nurse serves as a client advocate when helping in addressing a client's concern. The nurse should call the operating room and inform the intraoperative nurse about the client's request. A special container with correct identification can be prepared so that when the client is anesthetized and her hearing aid is removed, it will not be lost or broken. It is usual policy not to send personal belongings to surgery because they are easily broken or lost in the transfer of an anesthetized client with higher priority needs, but special needs do exist. In some instances, the nurse does bring a

client's personal belongings to the postanesthesia care unit, but in this case, the item involves the client's ability to communicate. Because the trend is to use little premedication, clients are more alert and may want to talk with their surgical team before going to sleep. Decreasing the client's anxieties preoperatively affects the amount of medication used to induce the client and her overall psychological and physiologic status. Telling the client that she will not need to hear is insensitive.

⚷ CN: Basic care and comfort;
CL: Synthesize

9. 3. A least-restraint environment should always be provided as much as possible. Nursing staff are required to attempt lesser restrictive alternatives (e.g., use of family or sitter, reorientation, distraction, or a toileting schedule) prior to notifying the provider of the need for restraints. Nursing staff are also required to document clinical conditions requiring restraint, lesser restrictive alternatives attempted, and client/family education provided regarding restraint use. Provider prescriptions for restraints must be time limited and specific regarding the type of restraint. Additionally, if restraints are implemented, nursing staff must monitor clients for safety (including skin checks and range of motion) and provide frequent food/fluids/toileting.

⚷ CN: Safety and infection control;
CL: Synthesize

10. 4. The client has deficient knowledge if he smoked a cigarette after 0400 because, even though he did not have anything to eat or drink, smoking has increased the production of gastric hydrochloric acid, which can increase the risk of aspiration in an anesthetized client. The client consumed the gelatin dessert prior to the 0400 restriction for being NPO. Comfort measures, such as brushing the teeth without swallowing or holding a cold washcloth against the lips, are acceptable for a client who is to have nothing by mouth.

⚷ CN: Reduction of risk potential;
CL: Evaluate

11. 2. The antibiotic is most effective in preventing infection, according to research, if it is given 30 to 60 minutes before the operative incision is made. When the surgeon prescribes the antibiotic to be given at a specific time related to the scheduled time of the surgical procedure, it is imperative that the antibiotic is given on time. Legally, the nurse considers 30 minutes on either side of the scheduled time to be acceptable for administering medications; however, in this situation, giving the antibiotic 30 minutes too soon can make the prophylactic antibiotic ineffective. The postoperative dose of antibiotic is not timed according to the preoperative dose. Peak and titer levels are measured for some antibiotics, but in this case, the primary reason is to have the antibiotic infused before the time of the incision.

CN: Reduction of risk potential; CL: Apply

12. 3. Nurses should provide the preoperative client individual and sincere attention by meeting the client at eye level and introducing themselves by name and role. The nurse should ask the client to tell her full name rather than asking if she is Mrs. Smith because there might be another client by that name on the schedule. Nurses should not start the physical assessment or ask the client's name without first identifying themselves and their role out of courtesy and to relieve the client's anxiety in the new environment of the surgical experience.

CN: Psychosocial integrity; CL: Apply

13. 4. The nurse should notify the anesthesiologist because a serum potassium level of 5.8 mEq/L (5.8 mmol/L) places the client at risk for arrhythmias when under general anesthesia. It is not the role of the nurse to cancel surgery. The nurse should not automatically send a client with abnormal laboratory findings to surgery because the procedure may be canceled. Once the client is inside the operating room and sterile supplies have been opened up for the procedure, the client is usually charged. The nurse should call ahead of time to communicate the abnormal laboratory result instead of noting the finding on the client's record. The information on the record should not be reviewed until after the client has been transported to the operating room and the supplies have been opened.

CN: Reduction of risk potential;
CL: Synthesize

14. 4. Clients should be made aware that some questions are asked for verification and safety with each new phase of treatment. Indicating that the nurse is sorry, or needs to check several times, or telling the client that the question will be asked again does not tell the client why it is necessary to continue to verify information essential to the client's safety.

CN: Psychosocial integrity; CL: Synthesize

15. 3. The nurse should notify the **HCP** directly for specific prescriptions based on the client's glucose level. The nurse cannot ignore the elevated glucose level. The surgical experience is stressful, and the client needs specific insulin coverage during the perioperative period. The nurse should not administer the insulin without checking with the surgeon because there are specific prescriptions to withhold all medications. It is not necessary to notify the surgery department unless the HCP cancels the surgery.

CN: Pharmacological and parenteral therapies; CL: Synthesize

16. 3. Psychosocial integrity issues, including coping mechanisms, situational role changes, and body image changes, are more common in a client who undergoes elective cosmetic surgical procedures. Reduction of risk potential, physiologic adaptation, and health promotion and maintenance are greater needs for clients who are undergoing surgical correction of functional, anatomic, or physiologic defects in nonelective surgical procedures.

CN: Psychosocial integrity; CL: Analyze

17. 1. A client should not elect surgery to meet someone else's needs. The nurse should encourage the client to share his feelings and his perception of the deformity and to clarify his reasons for electing to have the surgery. It is normal to be somewhat afraid, and it is good if a client says he feels "OK" about the surgery. The fact that a client believes that his wife will help him after surgery and that he will also be relatively independent reflects appropriate adaptation. It is a common feeling among preoperative clients that they are ready to "get this over with," indicating that the waiting period is stressful.

CN: Psychosocial integrity; CL: Evaluate

18. 2. Brittle nails indicate poor nutrition. Poor posture indicates that the client does not stand up straight and use her muscles to support herself. A dull expression reflects the client's affect and emotional status. The client's weight of 128 lb (58.1 kg) is within normal range.

CN: Health promotion and maintenance;
CL: Analyze

19. 1,2,4. The nurse should explain and demonstrate the discharge instructions and then ask the client to give a return demonstration. The Joint Commission and Health Canada require that discharge instructions be written for the postoperative client. Clients need to be given discharge instructions orally and in written form because of stress, medications, and the volume of material to be learned. Explaining all the instructions to a family member and giving them a link to a video is important but does not replace the need for written instructions. Since the family does not live nearby, the nurse must be certain the client can manage the instructions by herself.

CN: Health promotion and maintenance;
CL: Synthesize

20. 1. The preadmission nurse, the first person in contact with the client, starts the discharge planning for the client undergoing surgery. All nurses involved with the client, from preadmission through postoperative recovery, should continue to reinforce the discharge plan.

CN: Health promotion and maintenance;
CL: Apply

21. 3. The nurse should have the client empty the bladder before the premedication is administered. This will be more comfortable and safe for the client.

The purpose of the premedication is to decrease anxiety and promote a relaxed state. The client must have an empty bladder before being transferred to the operating room, where the client will be immobilized and receive IV fluids. The family does not have to be present, but it is usually desired. Shaving the operative area is not generally recommended because it can cause small nicks that harbor bacteria. If the client must be shaved, it is usually done in the operating room holding area. The client should be comfortable at all times and offered a warm blanket before or after the premedication.

 ⚷ CN: Basic care and comfort;
 CL: Synthesize

22. 4. The nurse should immediately think of the congenital metabolic tendency for malignant hyperthermia, which occurs in the presence of certain kinds of anesthetics. Whenever a preoperative client states that a family member has had problems with anesthesia or surgery, the nurse should inquire about the nature of the problems and whether other family members have had similar problems. Reassuring the client that technology has changed will do little to affect her fears and misses the opportunity to evaluate the risk for malignant hyperthermia. Encouraging the client to further express her concerns and reassuring her that her feelings are normal are important, but missing a familial tendency of malignant hyperthermia could be fatal.

 ⚷ CN: Reduction of risk potential;
 CL: Synthesize

23. 3. The nurse should assess the vital signs of the client who exhibits urticaria, rhinitis, and conjunctivitis a few seconds after coming in contact with rubber gloves, a plastic catheter, plastic IV tubing, or a plastic IV solution bag. The nurse should recognize that these symptoms indicate that a type I allergic reaction is occurring. Although many healthcare agencies now use latex-free materials, it is possible that the products contain latex or other materials that might be precipitating the client's allergic response. The client does not need to be distracted or assessed for pain. It is not necessary to lower the head of the bed.

 ⚷ CN: Physiological adaptation;
 CL: Synthesize

24. 4. The nurse would ask the client whether he or she wears glasses to evaluate his or her preoperative cognitive-perceptual pattern. Asking about the client's swallowing pattern would evaluate his or her nutritional-metabolic pattern. Asking about the client's need for special equipment to walk would evaluate his or her activity-exercise pattern. Asking the client about his or her history of smoking would evaluate the client's health perception health management pattern.

 ⚷ CN: Physiological adaptation; CL: Analyze

25. 3. The client is at risk for a difficult intubation because the neck must be hyperextended to pass the endotracheal tube. Assessment of the pupils should not be limited. If the client is positioned appropriately during surgery, there is no risk of postoperative neck pain or limited neck movement.

 ⚷ CN: Reduction of risk potential;
 CL: Analyze

26. 3. The Universal Protocol is used to prevent wrong site, wrong procedure, and wrong person surgery. Actions included in the protocol are as follows: conduct a preprocedure verification process, mark the procedure site, and perform a **time-out**📖. Exceptions to the Universal Protocol are routine or "minor" procedures, such as venipuncture, peripheral IV line placement, insertion of oral/nasal drainage or feeding tubes, or Foley catheter insertion. Prior to closure, the surgeon or circulating nurse will initiate a time-out to verbally confirm a review of **informed consent**📖 and procedures completed; all specimens are identified, accounted for, and accurately labeled; and all foreign bodies have been removed. The chief of surgery and medical director are the ones who will verify the surgeons' levels of expertise.

 ⚷ CN: Safety and infection control;
 CL: Apply

27. 1,2,3,4. Splinting the incision is important to avoid stress on the surgical site and to promote comfort so that the client will adhere to the plan of care. Inhaling through the nostrils and exhaling through pursed lips are important to bring in adequate oxygen and clear out carbon dioxide; however, closing one nostril when inhaling would be inappropriate and ineffective. The most important step is asking the client to hold the inhaled breath for about 5 seconds, which keeps the alveoli expanded. This step should be stressed the most. Repeating the exercise 5 to 10 times hourly is the second most important point to emphasize in this teaching plan.

 ⚷ CN: Reduction of risk potential;
 CL: Create

28. 2. The nurse should call the surgeon for a serum creatinine level of 2.6 mg/dL (198 μmol/L), which is higher than the normal range of 0.1 to 0.4 mg/dL (8 to 31 μmol/L). An elevated serum creatinine value indicates that the kidneys are not filtering effectively and has important implications for the surgical client because many anesthesia and analgesia medications need to be filtered out through the renal system. The red blood cell count, hemoglobin level, and blood urea nitrogen level are within normal limits and do not need to be reported to the surgeon.

 ⚷ CN: Reduction of risk potential;
 CL: Analyze

weakness or numbness, especially in the legs. The nurse should also ask if the client has allergies before medication administration. It is not the nurse's responsibility to chart laboratory results; the results will be documented on the client's health record.

> **CN:** Safety and infection control;
> **CL:** Synthesize

50. 2,3,4,6. Complications may develop when a client is receiving medication via epidural, intrathecal, or continuous nerve block routes. The nurse should inform the **healthcare provider (HCP)**📖 if there is a dislodged catheter, disconnected tubing, or an occluded line. The nurse must also notify the HCP if the client has nausea or vomiting as the movement involved could dislodge the catheter. Numbness or weakness in the legs could also indicated a dislodged catheter, and the nurse must assess the client for these signs and report them if they occur. The client should call for assistance when getting out of bed or ambulating. The client should not take a shower or a bath while the catheter is in place. The client does not need to take shallow breaths, and the nurse should encourage the client to breathe normally and take deep breaths regularly.

> **CN:** Safety and infection control;
> **CL:** Synthesize

51. 4. Airway flow is always the first assessment. Once the nurse establishes that the client has a patent airway, the pulse oximeter is applied to measure the oxygen saturation, the respiratory rate is counted, and the breath sounds are auscultated bilaterally.

> **CN:** Physiological adaptation; **CL:** Analyze

52. 1. The last area to regain sensation is the perineal area, and the nurse should check the client for a distended bladder. The client has received a large volume of IV fluids since the epidural was inserted, and the client may not feel the urge to void or may be unable to void. In that case, the nurse should obtain a prescription to catheterize the client before the bladder becomes so distended as to cause bladder spasms. The nurse should assess for a spinal headache, postoperative pain, and the client's ability to move after determining whether the bladder is distended.

> **CN:** Reduction of risk potential;
> **CL:** Analyze

53. 3. Spinal anesthesia is an extensive conduction nerve block that is produced when a local anesthetic is introduced into the subarachnoid space at the lumbar level. A few minutes after induction of a spinal anesthetic, anesthesia and paralysis affect the toes and perineum and then, gradually, the legs and abdomen. When the autonomic nervous system is blocked, vasodilation occurs and hypotension occurs. The client will feel sensation to the toes before the perineal area. A spinal headache due to loss of fluid is a severe headache that occurs while in the upright position but is relieved in the lying position.

> **CN:** Physiological adaptation; **CL:** Analyze

54. 3. The nurse should check the client's baseline data to ascertain whether the client's pupil has always been enlarged or this is a new finding. The preoperative assessment is valuable as the baseline for comparison of all subsequent assessments made throughout the perioperative period. The nurse may determine that a more involved neurologic examination is indicated or may choose to assess other signs using the Glasgow Coma Scale, administer oxygen, or call the surgeon, but the nurse still needs to know the baseline data before proceeding.

> **CN:** Physiological adaptation;
> **CL:** Synthesize

55. 2. During the immediate postanesthesia period, the unconscious client should be positioned on the side to maintain an open airway and promote drainage of secretions; because of the type of surgery, the client should be positioned on the right side. Removing the oral airway and observing the surgical dressing are appropriate, but other actions should be implemented before these. Respiratory depression can occur in a client after a procedure requiring sedation. If the client cannot be aroused, the sedation drugs can be reversed by administering a sedation reversal agent, but this client's respiratory rate is 14, and the client is moaning, indicating expected recovery from anesthetics.

> **CN:** Physiological adaptation;
> **CL:** Synthesize

56. 1. The nurse should check the dressing for signs of bleeding to establish a baseline for future assessments of the dressing and to verify that there is no obvious sign of hemorrhage. The nurse does not need to empty peri-incisional drains at this time. All drains should have been emptied and reconstituted by the postanesthesia care nurse before the client was transferred to the surgical floor. Assessing the client's pain level and assessing the bladder are important; however, it is more important to assess the surgical site for bleeding because hemorrhage is a life-threatening complication of any surgical procedure.

> **CN:** Physiological adaptation;
> **CL:** Synthesize

57. 3. Sodium pentothal, a short-acting barbiturate, can cause hypotension, which may be especially problematic for the client with impaired cardiac functioning. Sodium pentothal does not cause bradycardia, complete muscle relaxation, hypertension, or tachypnea.

> **CN:** Pharmacological and parenteral therapies; **CL:** Apply

58. 1. Propofol, a nonbarbiturate anesthetic, causes less nausea and vomiting than do other induction agents because of a direct antiemetic action. It does not cause hypotension or skeletal muscle movement, and it does not act slowly.

CN: Pharmacological and parenteral therapies; CL: Analyze

59. 4. Desflurane and sevoflurane are volatile liquid anesthesia agents that are used for outpatient surgeries primarily because they are rapidly eliminated. They have the added benefits of being better tolerated and nonirritating to the respiratory tract, and they have predictable cardiovascular effects. However, rapid elimination is an important consideration for outpatient procedures.

CN: Pharmacological and parenteral therapies; CL: Apply

60. 3. A heart rate of 150 bpm or greater, hypotension, and muscle rigidity are early signs of malignant hyperthermia. The nurse should quickly assemble emergency supplies and personnel because malignant hyperthermia is potentially and rapidly fatal in more than 50% of cases. Rapid, extreme rise in temperature is a late sign. Another factor influencing the analysis is that the client has a large body frame, and having large, bulky muscles is a risk factor for malignant hyperthermia. The client's vital signs are well out of the range of normal; analysis of the data and swift intervention are indicated. Excessive blood loss is unlikely, and the data do not support this conclusion. Although clients do have changes in vital signs when in acute pain, the nurse would expect the client to be hypertensive, not hypotensive.

CN: Physiological adaptation; CL: Analyze

61. 2. One of the earliest signs of hypoxia is restlessness and agitation. Decreased level of consciousness and somnolence are later signs of hypoxia. Chills can be related to the anesthetic agent used but are not indicative of hypoxia. Urgency is not related to hypoxia.

CN: Physiological adaptation; CL: Analyze

62. 2,3,4,5. Flumazenil should be administered in small quantities such as 0.2 mg over 15 to 30 seconds but never as a bolus. Flumazenil may be given undiluted in incremental doses. Adverse effects of flumazenil may include shivering and hypotension. The nurse should monitor the client's level of consciousness while recovering from sedation. Flumazenil should be administered through a free-flowing IV line in a large vein because extravasation causes local irritation.

CN: Pharmacological and parenteral therapies; CL: Synthesize

63. 2. It is important for the nurse to cover this client with warm blankets because he is at high risk for hypothermia secondary to age, spinal anesthesia, placement in a lithotomy position in the cool operating room for 1.5 hours, instillation of 4,000 mL of room temperature bladder irrigation, and ongoing bladder irrigation. Spinal anesthesia causes vasodilation, which results in heat loss from the core to the periphery. The nurse will empty the catheter drainage bag and hang new bags of irrigation as needed, but the client's potential for hypothermia should be addressed first. The client will not be turned at this time.

CN: Reduction of risk potential; CL: Synthesize

64. 3. The client who is 5 feet 1 inch tall (155 cm) and weighs 200 lb (90.7 kg) would be expected to retain the anesthetic agents longer because adipose tissue absorbs the drug before the desired systemic effect is reached for anesthesia maintenance. Nursing interventions are aimed at encouraging the obese client to turn, cough, and deep breathe despite feeling sleepy and tired. The sooner this client ambulates, the sooner the retained anesthesia will be worked out of the adipose tissue.

CN: Reduction of risk potential; CL: Analyze

65. 1. The nurse should encourage the client to avoid holding the operated arm, the arm with the intravenous regional nerve block (Bier block), close to the face because the client does not have motor control over it. With the cast in place, the client could hit the eye, nose, or mouth and cause soft tissue damage. It is acceptable for the client to hold the operated arm with the unoperated arm or to use the unoperated arm. The nurse should administer the analgesic before the intravenous regional anesthetic completely wears off so that the pain does not peak before pain medication is administered.

CN: Reduction of risk potential; CL: Synthesize

66. 3. The nurse should monitor the client's respirations closely for 4 to 6 hours because naloxone has a shorter duration of action than do opioids. The client may need repeated doses of naloxone to prevent or treat a recurrence of the respiratory depression. Naloxone is usually effective in a few minutes; however, its effects last only 1 to 2 hours, and ongoing monitoring of the client's respiratory rate will be necessary. The client's dosage of morphine will be decreased or a new drug will be prescribed to prevent another instance of respiratory depression.

CN: Pharmacological and parenteral therapies; CL: Synthesize

67. 3. Abnormal coagulation test results have been associated with naloxone, and the nurse should monitor surgical clients closely for bleeding. Dizziness, biliary colic, and urine retention are not associated with naloxone.

    CN: Pharmacological and parenteral therapies; CL: Analyze

68. 3. The client who receives epidural anesthesia is at decreased risk for a headache because a noncutting needle is used instead of a side angle-cutting needle. The epidural needle is a 25- to 27-gauge needle, which is much smaller than a 17-gauge needle. Epidural anesthesia involves an extradural injection; a subarachnoid injection is used in spinal anesthesia. The onset of spinal anesthesia is faster because a larger dose of medication is usually administered.

    CN: Physiological adaptation; CL: Analyze

69. 3. Spinal anesthesia does not cause parasympathetic blockage. The spinal anesthetic agent usually is injected into the L2 subarachnoid space, where it produces sympathetic, sensory, and motor blockade.

    CN: Pharmacological and parenteral therapies; CL: Apply

70. 0.5 mL. To obtain the answer, treat the volume to be administered as X.

$$\frac{2.5 \text{ mg}}{X \text{ mL}} = \frac{5 \text{ mg}}{1 \text{ mL}}$$

$$5X = 2.5$$

$$X = \frac{2.5}{5} = 0.5$$

    CN: Pharmacological and parenteral therapies; CL: Apply

The Client Who Has Had Surgery

71. 4. Bowel sounds are not present until the 3rd or 4th postoperative day; the nurse should document the assessment findings. Since this is an expected finding it is not necessary to notify the HCP or have another nurse validate the findings. Too many ice chips may promote abdominal distention, especially if the client is not ambulating in the intermediate postoperative period.

    CN: Physiological adaptation; CL: Synthesize

72. 3,2,1,4. The nurse first auscultates the abdomen for bowel sounds to determine if peristalsis has resumed and is present. The nurse then administers hot liquids to stimulate peristalsis and promote expulsion of the gas that is causing the client to be uncomfortable. Positioning the client on the right side permits gas to rise along the transverse colon and facilitates its release. Abdominal distention may be minimized by early and frequent ambulation, which stimulates intestinal motility. The nurse also assists the client to ambulate.

    CN: Physiological adaptation; CL: Synthesize

73. 3. Restlessness in the immediate postoperative period may be a sign of cerebral hypoxia as a result of depression on the central nervous from anesthetic agents and sedatives. Administering sedatives would depress the central nervous system further. A client may aspirate ice chips when he or she is restless. Wrist restraints may increase agitation and cannot be used without justification.

    CN: Physiological adaptation; CL: Analyze

74. 2,3,1,4. The oncoming nurse should first assess the client for pain. Next, the nurse should check the documentation and then validate with the nurse who reported giving the medication that the medication had been given. Finally, the nurse should determine if there is a discrepancy between administration and documentation.

    CN: Management of care; CL: Synthesize

75. 3. Deep breathing and coughing help to increase lung expansion and prevent the accumulation of secretions in postoperative clients. An O_2 saturation of 89% is not an unexpected or emergent finding immediately following surgery. Frequent coughing and deep breathing will likely quickly remedy an O_2 saturation of 89% but will also effectively help to prevent atelectasis and pneumonia in the remainder of the postoperative period. It is not necessary to notify the **HCP** 📖 prior to intervening with coughing/deep breathing, and it is not appropriate to position this client with the head of the bed lower because this would make it more difficult for the client to expectorate secretions. Oxygen may be necessary, but the nurse should assist the client to cough and deep breathe first, in an attempt to improve his oxygenation and saturation.

    CN: Physiological integrity; CL: Synthesize

76. 4. Urinary retention is common following surgery with anesthesia, following childbirth, or as a result of specific medication use, for example, narcotics for pain. Clients should be assisted to an anatomically comfortable position to void prior to resorting to more invasive methods such as intermittent or indwelling catheterization to manage urinary retention. Difficulty voiding after childbirth is expected, and it is not necessary to notify the **HCP** 📖. While increasing fluid intake is important, it will not help the client void now.

    CN: Basic care and comfort; CL: Synthesize

77. 4. Following surgery, clients are at risk for respiratory complications and should take the necessary actions to prevent these. The nurse should first be sure that the client understands how to do the exercises and the potential complications if they are not done. It is not the wife's responsibility to make the client do the exercise, but she can help. Increasing fluid intake and frequent turning are appropriate, but not sufficient for aerating the lungs.

🔑 CN: Health promotion and maintenance; CL: Synthesize

78. 1. The nurse should first try to facilitate the client's ability to void by having the client stand at the bedside and use the urinal. Pouring running water over the perineum is a strategy that could be used if the client cannot void in a standing position. Ambulation will not help the client void. If such conservative methods fail, the nurse should obtain a prescription to catheterize the client, but an indwelling urinary catheter increases the risk of urinary tract infection because microbes ascend the catheter and travel to the bladder.

🔑 CN: Reduction of risk potential; CL: Synthesize

79. 4. The first cognitive response that returns after anesthesia is orientation to person. The nurse assesses this by asking the client his name. Orientation to place and time usually occurs after orientation by the nurse because of confusion from anesthesia and waking in an unfamiliar place. The nurse can then continue to assess and document the client's cognitive ability to remember information. The nurse does not need to notify the surgeon. The client's cognitive response is normal. It is not necessary to ask the wife to reorient the client; however, she can continue to talk to him and help him regain consciousness.

🔑 CN: Physiological adaptation; CL: Synthesize

80. 3. Potassium in an IV solution may be irritating to a vein. The nurse should assess the IV site before taking any of the other actions listed. The infusion may have to be slowed and/or stopped, and the HCP📖 contacted. An outdated parenteral fluid setup does not cause pain, but may be a source of infection.

🔑 CN: Pharmacological and parenteral therapies; CL: Synthesize

81. 2. The client's body temperature dropped 2.5°F (1.4°C) from the preoperative to postoperative phase. The client lost heat during the preoperative period. The client has not had time to regain the heat she has lost and should not be discharged postoperatively until her postoperative vital signs, which include body temperature, are closer to her preoperative vital signs. The client's pulse rate, respiratory rate, and blood pressure have compensated according to the client's hypothermic state and will reflect changes as the client warms up. There are no indications that the client needs more pain medication, oxygen, or IV fluids.

🔑 CN: Physiological adaptation; CL: Synthesize

82. 3. The client still has a respiratory rate of 8; the nurse should first assist the client to sit and stimulate the client to take deep breaths and cough. This action will also help the nurse to determine what the client's level of sedation is; if the client is too sedated to cooperate with coughing/deep breathing, it will be important to slow or stop the infusion of narcotics and to consider contacting the HCP📖 for a prescription for naloxone. The client is still breathing, so it is not necessary to call the rapid response team📖.

🔑 CN: Physiologic adaptation; CL: Synthesize

83. 3. The nurse is helping the client manage pain and comfort level. The nurse has completed the assessment of the client and should now dim the lights and create a quiet environment. Such non-pharmacologic measures as adjusting the light level in the room facilitate pain management. Decreasing stimulation from the environment, such as brightness to the optic nerve, promotes the client's ability to relax skeletal muscles and fall asleep. It is too soon to reassess vital signs. Checking that the family is comfortable is important but is not the next thing to do for this client. Increasing the oxygen flow rate is not indicated and, if needed, should have been done before repositioning the client.

🔑 CN: Management of care; CL: Synthesize

84. 4. When a postoperative client has a temperature elevation to >100°F (37.8°C) in the first 24 hours after surgery, the temperature elevation is usually related to atelectasis. Because this client had upper abdominal surgery with manipulation around the diaphragm, the client is more prone to guarding the operative site and shallow breathing. Encouraging the client to take deep breaths and use incentive spirometry is an appropriate measure to prevent atelectasis and pulmonary infection. The nurse must assist the client in filling the alveoli in the lower posterior lobes of the lungs. An incentive spirometer is a good visual biofeedback instrument that the client had practiced with preoperatively. Changing the client's position from lying to sitting for deep breathing will expand alveoli in the lower posterior lobes. There is no indication that a surgical wound infection is occurring. An antibiotic is not indicated at this time. Pain medication will decrease respirations, and the client is not indicating pain at the moment.

🔑 CN: Physiological adaptation; CL: Synthesize

85. 3. The client must be able to verbalize understanding about receiving no more pain medication than is prescribed no matter how many times the button is pushed. Only the client should press the button for the PCA. The client should administer the pain medication when the pain is first noticed, well before the pain is out of control. One of the advantages of the PCA is that the amount of pain medication is controlled; therefore, overdosing is not a client concern when using a PCA.

> **CN:** Pharmacological and parenteral therapies; **CL:** Evaluate

86. 3. The nurse should take the client's blood pressure. She is likely experiencing orthostatic hypotension. The PCA pump does not need to be discontinued because as soon as the blood pressure stabilizes the pain medication can be resumed. Administering oxygen is not necessary unless the oxygen saturation also drops. The client should sit in the chair until the blood pressure stabilizes.

> **CN:** Pharmacological and parenteral therapies; **CL:** Synthesize

87. 3. Urinary catheters should be limited in use and duration only as needed for client care. The guideline also specifies that if used, the catheter should be inserted using aseptic technique, secured to provide unobstructed flow and drainage, and maintained in a way that protects sterility of the catheter and the drainage system. It is not necessary to provide catheter care or cleanse the meatus as these can be a source of introducing an infection; it is not necessary to check for bladder distention if the catheter is draining correctly.

> **CN:** Safety and infection control; **CL:** Synthesize

88. 4,1,3,2. The client must first splint the incision to avoid increased intolerable pain, or he or she may not cooperate with the pulmonary ventilation. The next step is to inhale oxygen to expand the alveoli for a few seconds and then exhale carbon dioxide in successive steps 5 to 10 times. The client should try to cough on the end of the exhalation to remove retained secretions from the larger airways.

> **CN:** Reduction of risk potential; **CL:** Synthesize

89. 3. The client who has not had the gag reflex anesthetized is the client who had a repair of the carpal tunnel syndrome under local anesthesia because the area being anesthetized was the tissue in the wrist. The client who had a bronchoscopy received a local anesthetic on the vocal cords, and the nurse should check the gag reflex or ability to swallow before administering fluids. Clients who had general anesthesia or intravenous conscious sedation received medication for central nervous system sedation, and the nurse should assess the level of consciousness and ability to swallow before administering fluids.

> **CN:** Reduction of risk potential; **CL:** Analyze

90. 3. The client is experiencing activity intolerance, which is common following the first ambulation following surgery. The nurse should allow the client to rest and continue to monitor vital signs. Since the client is not dizzy or in pain, the nurse should wait to see if the client recovers from ambulating and reports having pain prior to administering pain medication. There is no need to request different activity prescriptions; it will still be important for the client to ambulate. The client is not having chest pain; it is not necessary to obtain a 12-lead ECG.

> **CN:** Basic care and comfort; **CL:** Synthesize

91. 3. When the urine output is <30 mL/h, the nurse should assess for potential causes such as hypovolemia or hemorrhage. The nurse should assess and evaluate the client's vital signs, intake and output, dressing, and available laboratory values and notify the **healthcare provider (HCP)** 📖. Bowel obstruction, although possible after surgery, is characterized most notably by abdominal distention and absent bowel sounds, not decreased urine output. The nurse would not expect the client to have hypertension, but rather hypotension.

> **CN:** Physiological adaptation; **CL:** Synthesize

92. 3. A client who had a left thoracoscopy is placed in the lateral position, in which the most common injury is an injury to the brachial plexus. Numbness and tingling in the arm suggests a brachial plexus injury. There is no undue pressure on the ankles or knees during thoracic surgery.

> **CN:** Physiological adaptation; **CL:** Analyze

93. 2,3,5,6. The client should be in an upright position when using the spirometer. The client should exhale fully prior to using the spirometer and then inhale to expand the lungs and continue inhaling for 3 more seconds. The client should relax and exhale before inhaling for the next use of the spirometer. The client should cough and clear retained secretions following the use of the spirometer. The client should use the spirometer every 2 hours during the immediate postoperative period.

> **CN:** Physiological adaptation; **CL:** Evaluate

94. 3. The nurse should inform the client that as the incision heals, uneven lumps might appear under the incision line because the collagen is growing new tissue at different rates. Eventually, the lumps will even out and the tissue will be smooth. The client can touch the incision with clean hands as needed to perform incisional care. The client should not clean the incision with hydrogen peroxide because it may dry out the natural skin oils. The surgeon will remove the staples for the client.

> **CN:** Reduction of risk potential; **CL:** Synthesize

95. 2. When a wound eviscerates (abdominal organs protruding through the opened incision), the nurse should cover the open area with a sterile dressing moistened with sterile normal saline and then cover it with a dry dressing. The surgeon should then be notified to take the client back to the operating room to close the incision under general anesthesia. The nurse should not press the emergency alarm because this is not a cardiac or respiratory arrest. The nurse should have the visitors and family leave the room to decrease the chance of airborne contamination, but the primary focus should be on covering the wound with a moist, sterile covering.

CN: Safety and infection control; CL: Synthesize

96. 4. The findings (WBC count above normal; inflammation and drainage at the incision site; and an elevated temperature) indicate that the client has an infection. The nurse should first notify the **HCP** 📖. Encouraging fluids will be helpful, but it is not the first action. The client may have incisional pain, and after the nurse has contacted the HCP, the nurse can determine if the client needs pain management. The nurse should not cleanse the site until the HCP writes a prescription to do so.

CN: Physiological adaptation; CL: Analyze

97. 3. The client is receiving oxygen using a partial rebreathing mask, which is positioned correctly. The correct flow rate for this type of oxygen mask is 6 to 10 L of oxygen per minute. To be effective, the mask must cover the client's face. The elastic band must be tight enough to secure the mask. When used correctly, the reservoir bag should inflate during the inspiratory phase.

CN: Physiological adaptation; CL: Synthesize

98. 4. A wet-to-dry dressing should be able to dry out between dressing changes. Thus, the dressing should be moist, not dry, when applied. As the moist dressing dries, the wound will be debrided of necrotic tissue and exudate. Normal saline is most commonly used to moisten the sponge; Burow's solution will irritate the wound. The sponge should not be packed into the wound tightly because the circulation to the site could be impaired. The moist sponge should be placed so that all surfaces of the wound are in contact with the dressing. Then the sponge is covered and protected by a dry sterile dressing to prevent contamination from the external environment.

CN: Safety and infection control; CL: Synthesize

99. 1. Common client misconceptions regarding pain and pain medication administration include a concern that taking pain medication regularly will lead to addiction. However, this misconception overstates the risk of addiction and greatly understates the risk of immobility due to poor pain control, including atelectasis, decubitus formation, and delayed healing. The nurse should assist the client to understand the importance of adequate pain medication to support and promote client mobilization following surgery and client/family satisfaction with care. There is a potential for dependence and addiction with all narcotic drugs, although not likely during the postoperative periods.

CN: Basic care and comfort; CL: Synthesize

100. 3. After emptying a Jackson-Pratt drainage bulb, the nurse should compress the bulb, plug it to establish suction, and then document the amount and type of drainage emptied. Irrigating a Jackson-Pratt drain is inappropriate because it could contaminate the wound. The Jackson-Pratt drain is not usually connected to wall suction. The purpose of the Jackson-Pratt drain is to remove bloody drainage from the deep tissues of the incision; clamping the drain would be counterproductive.

CN: Reduction of risk potential; CL: Synthesize

101. 1. Performing leg exercises, including ankle pumping, ankle rotation, and quadriceps setting exercises, will help prevent stasis of blood in the lower extremities, which can lead to blood clot formation. Encouraging the client to cough and deep breathe is an important postoperative intervention; however, it is directed at preventing pneumonia, not pulmonary emboli. The nurse should not massage the calves because a deep vein thrombus could dislodge and travel to the pulmonary vasculature. Antiembolism stockings should be worn continuously during the postoperative period.

CN: Physiological adaptation; CL: Synthesize

102. 2. Naloxone hydrochloride is the antidote for morphine sulfate. The signs of overdose on morphine sulfate are a respiration rate of 2 to 4 breaths/min, bradycardia, and hypotension. Flumazenil is the antidote for midazolam. Doxacurium is a nondepolarizing muscle relaxant. Remifentanil is an opioid used as an anesthetic adjunct.

CN: Pharmacological and parenteral therapies; CL: Synthesize

103. 4. The device is applied correctly, and the nurse should ensure the client's comfort. The client's legs should remain extended as shown while using the device; legs may be elevated, but it is not necessary to elevate the client's legs. The device should be placed directly on the client's legs; it is not necessary to apply antiembolic stockings under them. The client may move in bed as needed; active and isometric movement is encouraged to promote blood flow.

> 🔑 CN: Health promotion and maintenance; CL: Synthesize

104. 2. The client admitted for same-day surgery should not drive home after the surgical procedure because it is unsafe. Even without an anesthetic, the surgical event can be more stressful than anticipated. It is acceptable to have someone arrive after the surgery has started to take the client home. A taxi is permissible but not desirable.

> 🔑 CN: Reduction of risk potential; CL: Evaluate

105. 3. The urine output does not have to be checked every 15 minutes for a client who has had an arthroscopy because this client probably does not have a catheter in place. If the client voids, the output would be recorded. Assessments every 15 minutes during the first hour would include vital signs, pulse oximeter values, and pain to monitor the client's comfort level and check for compartment syndrome. Neurovascular checks distal to the operative site are especially vital because a tourniquet was used proximal to the operative site during the surgical procedure and because edema may develop during the postoperative period.

> 🔑 CN: Reduction of risk potential; CL: Analyze

106. 2. Hypotension and tachycardia are common adverse effects of droperidol and should be monitored closely by the nurse. Hypotension and tachycardia are not common adverse effects of ondansetron hydrochloride, prochlorperazine, or promethazine.

> 🔑 CN: Pharmacological and parenteral therapies; CL: Analyze

107. 1. The nurse should assess but not disturb the epidural dressing because the catheter can be easily dislodged and organisms can easily be transmitted into the central nervous system. The nurse should not have to change the dressing at all if a waterproof dressing is applied over the epidural site. Even with strict aseptic technique, a drain into a sterile cavity is a direct route for transmission of organisms and places a client at increased risk of infection, and the nurse should not handle the dressing or the catheter.

> 🔑 CN: Pharmacological and parenteral therapies; CL: Apply

108. 2. The client who has epidural pain management postoperatively can ambulate because a low concentration of local analgesia causes sensory blockage only. The catheter is placed so that constant pain management plus patient-controlled administration of an analgesic dose can block sensory innervation. Motor function should not be affected since the catheter is placed above the dura lining the spinal fluid. If the catheter would move through the dura sac, spinal analgesia would occur, affecting motor function as well as sympathetic nervous system function.

> 🔑 CN: Pharmacological and parenteral therapies; CL: Apply

109. 3. Portable wound suction units can be emptied and drained. The nurse should compress the unit after emptying to create suction before reinserting the plug. It is normal for the suction unit to be full 6 hours after surgery, and the nurse does not need to notify the surgeon. The drainage unit should be emptied when full or every 8 hours. The drain in the incision should remain in place until the surgeon removes it. While all drainage should be noted as output on the **medical record**⬚, recording the amount without emptying the drainage unit is not accurate, nor is it safe practice.

> 🔑 CN: Safety and infection control; CL: Synthesize

110. 1. The nurse should ask the client about having a bowel movement because acetaminophen with hydrocodone is an opioid, which can be constipating. By the 3rd day, many clients become constipated and are feeling distended, with sharp, cramping pain due to gas, which is treated with ambulation, not more opioids. The client's emptying the bladder should not affect the pain level. The nurse should look at the client's **medical record** 📖 to determine when the client's last dose of pain medication was administered, rather than asking the client. The client's statement regarding the pain level before the surgery is not relevant to whether the nurse should administer the acetaminophen and hydrocodone.

> 🔑 CN: Physiological adaptation; CL: Synthesize

111. 1. Blood and serous fluid is drained from the operative site to prevent hematoma formation or a collection of fluid that could become a site for infection. This also minimizes postoperative swelling, which can be painful. A simple explanation such as this is appropriate because the client is just waking up from surgery. Blood from the operative site can be collected through an autotransfusion system so that it can be transfused to the client during or immediately after surgery. However, strict guidelines about volume of blood lost, how quickly the device fills, and how long the blood has been out of the client's body govern whether the blood can be transfused. Therefore, although it is possible that the drainage system to which the client refers is an autotransfusion system, it is more likely that the client has a simple Hemovac drain. It is incorrect to tell a client not to worry about something even if he or she is in the drowsy state of awakening from anesthesia. It is inappropriate to ignore the client and give the client something to make him or her drowsy instead of addressing his or her concerns.

⚷ CN: Psychosocial integrity; CL: Synthesize

112. 1. The purpose of the Jackson-Pratt drainage tube is to drain off the purulent drainage from the sterile peritoneal cavity and prevent peritonitis. A Jackson-Pratt drain cannot prevent bleeding. The Jackson-Pratt drain has no effect on pressure on the bladder. There is no reason to be concerned about pressure on the gallbladder.

⚷ CN: Reduction of risk potential; CL: Apply

113. 2. Biliary drainage tubes (T tubes) are placed in the common bile duct and drain bile, which is dark yellow-orange. Serosanguineous drainage is thin and pinkish red. Bile is not clear and is not green unless it comes in contact with gastric fluid.

⚷ CN: Reduction of risk potential;
CL: Analyze

114. 1. Urinary elimination in the first 8 hours postoperatively is a requirement before the client who has had an inguinal hernia repair can be discharged from same-day surgery. Ingestion of fluids without nausea and vomiting is important, but eating solid foods is not a requirement for discharge from same-day surgery. Being completely pain free is an unrealistic expectation for the time frame and is not a requirement for leaving same-day surgery. However, the client should be comfortable, and his pain should be controlled. It is not a requirement for the client to ambulate in the hallway, but the client should be able to sit up and go to the bathroom without assistance.

⚷ CN: Reduction of risk potential;
CL: Analyze

115. 3. The ability to self-administer the drug is a requirement for the client to use PCA. Having a family member or advance directives is not a requirement for initiating PCA. The nurse teaches the client about how to use PCA and monitors effectiveness of the pain medication; however, it is not necessary for the nurse to assist with the administration of the drug.

⚷ CN: Pharmacological and parenteral therapies; CL: Evaluate

116. 2. The client's body temperature should be assessed every 4 hours during the first 24 hours because the client is still at risk for hypothermia or malignant hyperthermia. The client does not need to be checked every 2 hours unless indicated by an abnormal finding.

⚷ CN: Reduction of risk potential; CL: Apply

117. 1. The client's systolic blood pressure is dropping, and the pulse pressure is narrowing, indicating impending shock. The nurse should notify the surgeon. Elevating the head of the bed will not increase the blood pressure. Administering pain medication could cause the blood pressure to drop further. The intake and output record may indicate decreased urine output related to shock, but the nurse should first contact the **HCP**📖.

⚷ CN: Reduction of risk potential;
CL: Synthesize

118. 1. The client who has been positioned in the lithotomy position under general anesthesia may experience discomfort in the shoulders postoperatively because the client is placed in the Trendelenburg position to expose the perineal area. The client's weight is then shifted toward the shoulders, and the client experiences muscle soreness postoperatively. Although there may be pressure on the nerves in the thighs, legs, or feet from pressure from the stirrups, there should be no discomfort if the stirrups are well padded.

⚷ CN: Basic care and comfort; CL: Apply

119. 2. The client should drink a minimum of 2,500 mL of fluid per day (not 1,000 mL) to keep secretions liquefied and easier to cough up and eliminate from the upper respiratory tract. The client should use pain medication before coughing. The client should use the incentive spirometer every 2 to 4 hours. The nurse should monitor the client's breath sounds and temperature to detect early signs of infection. The nurse should assist with early ambulation.

⚷ CN: Reduction of risk potential;
CL: Synthesize

120. 3. The client should sit in an upright position when doing breathing exercises to allow for full chest expansion of both lungs and all fields and bases. Using an incentive spirometer every hour while awake is appropriate and allows the client visual feedback. Placing his hands lightly over the lower ribs and upper abdomen allows the client to see muscles of inspiration and expiration and is appropriate. Coughing deeply from the lungs after four deep breaths allows the client to effectively cough up secretions.

⚷ CN: Reduction of risk potential;
CL: Evaluate

121. 2. Muscle cramping is a sign of hypokalemia. Potassium is an electrolyte lost with nasogastric suctioning. Confusion is seen with hypercalcemia. Edema is seen with protein deficit or fluid volume overload. Tremors are seen with hypomagnesemia.

⚷ CN: Reduction of risk potential;
CL: Analyze

Legal and Ethical Issues Associated with Surgery

122. 3. The most critical piece of information is the client identification bracelet. Misidentification of clients can result in serious harm to the client. The nurse also needs the admitting records and any preprinted labels as part of verifying the client's identification. The location of the family is not included in verifying identification.

> CN: Reduction of risk potential; CL: Synthesize

123. 2. When the client cannot sign the operative **consent** 📖 and it is a true lifesaving emergency, consent may be obtained over the telephone from the client's next of kin or guardian. The surgeon must obtain the telephone consent, but if it is a true lifesaving emergency, the surgeon often is already in surgery, so the nurse makes the telephone call and another nurse witnesses the call. Some institutions have a special consent form for emergency surgery. Consent can be waived in situations in which no family is available; however, if the family can be reached by telephone before surgery, verbal consent is legally required.

> CN: Management of care; CL: Synthesize

124. 3. There are risks with both the surgical procedure and the general anesthesia required for a craniotomy. The risks involved in the procedure are a part of the **informed consent** 📖. Other information that is part of an informed consent includes potential complications, expected benefits, inability of the surgeon to predict results, irreversibility of the procedure (if applicable), and other available treatments. Talking about the effects of the diabetes on healing, explaining how the craniotomy is performed, and explaining the consequences of declining treatment (e.g., death if the tumor is not removed) represent appropriate actions to provide information to the client.

> CN: Management of care; CL: Evaluate

125. 3. The surgeon is responsible for explaining the surgical procedure to be performed and the risks of the procedure, as well as for obtaining the **informed consent** 📖 from the client. A nurse may be responsible for obtaining and witnessing a client's signature on the consent form. The nurse is the client's advocate, verifying that a client (or family member) understands the consent form and its implications and that consent for the surgery is truly voluntary.

> CN: Reduction of risk potential; CL: Apply

126. 2. When the client cannot read or write, the **consent** 📖 can be read to the client and the client can sign in the presence of two witnesses. The client (not the next of kin) should always sign for self unless he or she is a minor or not of sound mind. The court does not appoint a guardian for a person of sound mind just because he or she cannot read or write. Hospital personnel would not and could not sign a consent form for a client.

> CN: Management of care; CL: Apply

Managing Care, Quality, and Safety of Clients Having Surgery

127. 1,2,3. Clients who have diabetes mellitus controlled by diet, those with a high stress response to surgery, or those who have been on steroid treatment for the last 3 months should have their serum glucose level assessed. A client with a family history of diabetes receiving D_5LR IV fluids does not need to have the serum glucose level checked unless other clinical manifestations are present. The client who has a high-carbohydrate diet should be able to metabolize the glucose unless there are other health problems.

> CN: Reduction of risk potential; CL: Analyze

128. 1. Clients who have had long-term multiple exposures to latex products, such as would occur with six previous surgeries and recoveries, are at increased risk for latex allergies. The nurse should explore what types of surgeries these were, how involved the client's recoveries were, and whether signs of latex allergies have occurred in the past. Working as a sales clerk, having type 2 diabetes, and undergoing laser surgery do not expose a client to latex or increase the risk of latex allergy.

> CN: Health promotion and maintenance; CL: Analyze

129. 1,2,3,4. The root cause of wrong-site surgery involves a breakdown in communication between the client and family and the healthcare team. Information retrieved from the client in the preoperative assessment, such as the client's name, surgical site, and procedure, should be verbally assessed and verified with medical records and radiographic diagnostic reports. This information should be compiled in a checklist that the intraoperative team can recheck, thus avoiding unnecessary distraction and delay in the operating room. The nurse in the operating room is responsible for calling a **"time-out"** 📖 so that every surgical team member can double-check the correct site of surgery, verify the site using the operative **consent** 📖 form, and verify that the surgeon has marked the operative site on the client. Showing the client an anatomic model will assist the client in understanding the location of the surgery, but it will not prevent anyone from identifying the wrong site on the client.

    CN: Safety and infection control; CL: Apply

130. 4. The nurse should first contact the **HCP** 📖 because the prescription for the morphine is not complete. The Joint Commission of the United States and the Institute for Safe Medication Practices Canada recommend not to use MSO_4 because it can apply to morphine as well as to magnesium sulfate. There is no mention of an IV system being needed. The morphine should not be in the medication cabinet because the prescription is not complete. Although pharmacy may offer a suggestion as to what the medication prescribed is, the best means to confirm the intent of the prescription is to contact the HCP who wrote the prescription.

    CN: Safety and infection control; CL: Synthesize

131. 4. The nurse should first call the **rapid response team (RRT)** 📖 or medical emergency team that provides a team approach to evaluate and treat immediately clients with alterations in vital signs or neurological deterioration. The client's vital signs have changed since the client was in the PACU, and immediate action is required to manage the changes; the staff in PACU are not responsible for managing care once the client is transferred to the surgical unit. The respiratory therapist may be a part of the RRT but should not be called first.

    CN: Management of care; CL: Synthesize

132. 4. The anesthesiologist who administers the anesthetic agent and monitors the client's physical status throughout the surgery must have knowledge of all known allergies for client safety. The completed record (with the preoperative checklist) must be available to all members of the surgical team, and any unusual last-minute observations that may have a bearing on anesthesia or surgery are noted prominently at the front of the **medical record** 📖. The preanesthetic medication can cause light-headedness or drowsiness. The nurse in the scrub role provides sterile instruments and supplies to the surgeon during the procedure.

    CN: Safety and infection control; CL: Synthesize

133. 1,2,4. Nurses can delegate to the **UAP** 📖 to observe clients and promote their comfort following surgery and to empty and measure urinary catheter drainage bags. UAPs cannot teach clients; that is the responsibility of the **registered nurse (RN)** 📖 or respiratory therapist. UAPs cannot assess IV insertion sites, which is the responsibility of an RN.

    CN: Management of care; CL: Synthesize

134. 2. The client must have an identification bracelet properly secured on the wrist before being transported to the operating room to ensure correct identification. It is incorrect to send the client without a properly secured identification bracelet. The perioperative nurse must verify the client's identification by checking for the same name on the **medical record** 📖, armband, and schedule and by the client's statement. The preoperative nurse may be asked to physically identify the client and obtain a new armband.

    CN: Management of care; CL: Synthesize

135. 3. The client is experiencing a fluid overload and has vital signs that are outside of normal limits. The provider must be notified of the client's current status. It would be appropriate to recommend the provider administer a diuretic to correct the fluid overload. It is not appropriate to administer an antihypertensive medication or administer more fluids. It may be appropriate to administer additional oxygen, but because of the fluid volume excess the client exhibits, diuretic administration is most important.

    CN: Physiologic adaptation; CL: Analyze

136. 1. Prescriptions should be written clearly to avoid confusion or misinterpretation. Clearly written prescriptions do not use a "trailing" zero (a zero following a decimal point) and do use a "leading" zero (a zero preceding a decimal point). Additionally, the prescribed medication should be written in full and avoid abbreviations of the drug and the dosage, for example, "morphine sulfate" (avoiding use of "MS"), "mL" instead of "cc," and "micrograms" instead of "mcg."

    CN: Safety and infection control; CL: Apply

137. 4,2,1,3. The nurse should first notify the **HCP** 📖 of the high serum potassium level. Normal serum potassium level is 3.5 to 5.0; a level of 6.2 must be called to the HCP immediately because hyperkalemia may cause serious cardiac arrhythmias, potentially leading to death if left untreated. The nurse should next assess the client who has been vomiting and if necessary contact the HCP for a prescription for an antiemetic if none has been prescribed. After assessing all clients, the nurse should discuss the plan for the day, with the **UAP** 📖 delegating duties as appropriate. Though the client is eager to go home, the discharge paperwork must wait until all clients have been assessed and immediate needs met.

    CN: Reduction of risk potential; CL: Synthesize

138. 4. Maintenance of IV sites and systems includes regular assessment and rotation of the site and periodic changes of the dressing, solution, and tubing; these measures help prevent complications. The nurse should also observe the solution for discoloration, turbidity, and particulates. An IV solution is changed every 24 hours or as needed, and because the nurse noted an abnormal color, the nurse should change the bag of D5W and note this on an incident report. It is not necessary to verify this action with another nurse. Paging the **HCP** 📖 is not necessary; maintaining the IV and using the correct solutions is a nursing responsibility. Although the first action is to hang a new bag, hospital policy should be followed if there is a question as to whether there could have been an unknown substance in the bag that caused it to change color.

> 🔑 CN: Safety and infection control; CL: Synthesize

139. 1,2,3,4,5,6. The venipuncture site must be assessed for signs of infection (redness and pain at the puncture site), infiltration (coolness, blanching, and edema at the site), and thrombophlebitis (redness, firmness, pain along the path of the vein, and edema).

> 🔑 CN: Safety and infection control; CL: Analyze

140. 2. In any situation that involves a medication error, the nurse first assesses the client immediately to determine any changes in condition and the need for urgent interventions. Calling the **HCP** 📖 and/or administering an antidote is not done until the client is assessed and the necessary data are gathered. The nurse finding the error can complete an incident report after the client's safety is established and any emergency treatments are completed.

> 🔑 CN: Management of care; CL: Synthesize

141. 1,2,4. When a **"time-out"** 📖 is called prior to surgery, the surgical team must read back all prescriptions, verify the correct site, identify the client again, and double-check the echocardiogram. The sterile field has not been disrupted and does not need to be set up again. It is not necessary to obtain another x-ray as long as the confusion is clarified and the surgical team is satisfied that all are ready to begin the surgery.

> 🔑 CN: Management of care; CL: Apply

142. 1,3,5,6. Transfer reports must include information about the client's surgery; all current treatments and medications; vital signs, including pain level; fluid status, including blood loss; and current IV infusions. It is not necessary to identify the surgeons who were present during the surgery or report the name of the insurance provider.

> 🔑 CN: Management of care; CL: Apply

143. 2,3,5,6. Using SBAR (situation-background-assessment-recommendation), the nurse informs the surgeon of the current situation (chest pains), the background (history of myocardial infarction), and assessment (chest pains, vital signs changes, likelihood of having a myocardial infarction). The nurse should also discuss recommendations and suggestions for prescriptions such as the ECG and nitroglycerin tablet. The nurse is focusing on the chest pain and change in vital signs and communicating recommendations for managing the chest pain; it is not necessary to report at this time that the client has been NPO or the type of surgery the client will have.

> 🔑 CN: Management of care; CL: Synthesize

144. 4. Temperature variation in the postoperative period provides valuable information about a client's status. Fever may occur at any time during the postoperative period. A mild elevation (up to 100.4°F [38°C]) during the first 48 hours usually reflects the surgical stress response. After the first 48 hours, a moderate to marked elevation (higher than 99.9°F [37°C]) is usually caused by infection. It is not appropriate to do any of the other options to lower a client's temperature at this time.

> 🔑 CN: Management of care; CL: Synthesize

145. 2,5. The **UAP** 📖 can assist clients ambulate and take vital signs. It is within the RN scope of practice to teach the client to administer insulin, change dressings, and administer tube feedings.

> 🔑 CN: Management of care; CL: Synthesize

146. 1,4,3,2. The nurse establishes priorities based on airway, breathing, circulation, and disability as well as immediacy of client needs. The client who is just returning from surgery needs to be assessed; the nurse will also need to check the IV. The client with cancer of the colon also needs to have vital signs, pain, and dressings checked; the tracheotomy is established, and in the report there was no mention of distress. The client with the fractured hip is at risk for pressure ulcers and should be seen next. The nurse should then make rounds on the client with diabetes and schedule the time to continue teaching injection technique at that time.

> 🔑 CN: Management of care; CL: Synthesize

147. 4. Although practices for signing **informed consent** 📖 documents may vary across practice jurisdictions, generally, the spouse, or other responsible family member, may sign the consent form for a client with dementia. The minister, supervisor, and attorney cannot provide legal consent for surgery for this client.

> 🔑 CN: Management of care; CL: Synthesize

The Client with Health Problems of the Eyes, Ears, Nose, and Throat

- The Client with Cataracts
- The Client with a Retinal Detachment
- The Client with Glaucoma
- The Client with Adult Macular Degeneration
- The Client Undergoing Nasal Surgery
- The Client with a Hearing Disorder
- The Client with Ménière's Disease
- The Client with Cancer of the Larynx
- Managing Care, Quality, and Safety of Clients with Health Problems of the Eyes, Ears, Nose, and Throat
- Answers, Rationales, and Test-Taking Strategies

The Client with Cataracts

1. The nurse is observing a spouse administer eyedrops, as shown in the figure. What should the nurse instruct the spouse to do?
- ☐ 1. Move the dropper to the inner canthus.
- ☐ 2. Have the client raise the eyebrows.
- ☐ 3. Administer the drops in the center of the lower lid.
- ☐ 4. Have the client squeeze both eyes after administering the drops.

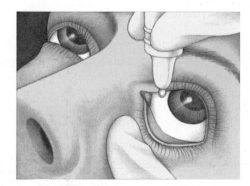

2. One day after cataract surgery, the client is having discomfort from bright light. The nurse should advise the client to:
- ☐ 1. dim lights in the house and stay inside for 1 week.
- ☐ 2. attach sun shields to existing eyeglasses when in direct sunlight.
- ☐ 3. use sunglasses that wrap around the side of the face when in bright light.
- ☐ 4. patch the affected eye when in bright light.

3. The nurse is discharging a client who just had cataract removal and intraocular lens implantation. The nurse is confident the client understands discharge instructions when the client states (select all that apply):
- ☐ 1. "I understand the schedule for my eyedrops and will use the medications."
- ☐ 2. "I feel good and am ready to drive home now."
- ☐ 3. "I will call in the morning if I cannot see clearly."
- ☐ 4. "I will wear the eye shield at night to protect my eye."
- ☐ 5. "I will avoid lifting or pulling anything over 15 lb (6.8 kg)."
- ☐ 6. "I will call if I still have eye pain after taking acetaminophen."

4. A client is having a cataract removed and will use eyeglasses after the surgery. What information should the nurse include in the teaching plan? Select all that apply.
- ☐ 1. Images will appear one-third larger.
- ☐ 2. Look through the center of the glasses.
- ☐ 3. The changes will be immediate.
- ☐ 4. Use handrails when climbing stairs.
- ☐ 5. Stay out of the sun for 2 weeks.

5. The client has had a cataract removed. The nurse's discharge instructions should include telling the client to:
- ☐ 1. keep the head aligned straight.
- ☐ 2. utilize bright lights in the home.
- ☐ 3. use an eye shield at night.
- ☐ 4. change the eye patch as needed.

6. The client with a cataract tells the nurse about being afraid of being awake during eye surgery. Which response by the nurse would be the **most** appropriate?
☐ **1.** "Have you ever had any reactions to local anesthetics in the past?"
☐ **2.** "What is it that disturbs you about the idea of being awake?"
☐ **3.** "By using a local anesthetic, you will not have nausea and vomiting after the surgery."
☐ **4.** "There is really nothing to fear about being awake. You will be given a medication that will help you relax."

7. A client tells the nurse about the vision being blurred and hazy throughout the entire day. The nurse should recommend that the client:
☐ **1.** purchase a pair of magnifying glasses.
☐ **2.** wear glasses with tinted lenses.
☐ **3.** schedule an appointment with an optician.
☐ **4.** schedule an appointment with an ophthalmologist.

8. The nurse is to instill drops of phenylephrine hydrochloride into the client's eye prior to cataract surgery. Which is the expected outcome?
☐ **1.** dilation of the pupil and blood vessels
☐ **2.** dilation of the pupil and constriction of blood vessels
☐ **3.** constriction of the pupil and constriction of blood vessels
☐ **4.** constriction of the pupil and dilation of blood vessels

9. A short time after cataract surgery, the client has nausea. The nurse should **first**:
☐ **1.** instruct the client to take a few deep breaths until the nausea subsides.
☐ **2.** explain that this is a common feeling that will pass quickly.
☐ **3.** tell the client to call the nurse promptly if vomiting occurs.
☐ **4.** medicate the client with an antiemetic, as prescribed.

10. Which complications can occur following cataract surgery? Select all that apply.
☐ **1.** acute bacterial endophthalmitis
☐ **2.** retrobulbar hemorrhage
☐ **3.** rupture of the posterior capsule
☐ **4.** suprachoroidal hemorrhage
☐ **5.** vision loss

11. The nurse is instructing the client about postoperative care following cataract removal. What position should the nurse teach the client to use?
☐ **1.** Remain in a semi-Fowler's position.
☐ **2.** Position the feet higher than the body.
☐ **3.** Lie on the operative side.
☐ **4.** Place the head in a dependent position.

12. After returning home, a client who has had cataract surgery will need to continue to instill eyedrops in the affected eye. The client is instructed to apply slight pressure against the nose at the inner canthus of the eye after instilling the eyedrops. The expected outcome of applying pressure is that the pressure:
☐ **1.** prevents the medication from entering the tear duct.
☐ **2.** prevents the drug from running down the client's face.
☐ **3.** allows the sensitive cornea to adjust to the medication.
☐ **4.** facilitates distribution of the medication over the eye surface.

13. To decrease intraocular pressure following cataract surgery, the nurse should instruct the client to avoid:
☐ **1.** lying supine.
☐ **2.** coughing.
☐ **3.** deep breathing.
☐ **4.** ambulation.

14. After cataract removal surgery, the client is instructed to report sharp pain in the operative eye because this could indicate which postoperative complication?
☐ **1.** detached retina
☐ **2.** prolapse of the iris
☐ **3.** extracapsular erosion
☐ **4.** intraocular hemorrhage

The Client with a Retinal Detachment

15. The client is diagnosed with a detached retina in the right eye. What should the nurse do **first**?
☐ **1.** Apply compresses to the eye.
☐ **2.** Instruct the client to lie prone.
☐ **3.** Remove all bed pillows.
☐ **4.** Promote measures that limit mobility.

16. A client with detachment of the retina is to patch both eyes. The expected outcome of patching is to:
☐ **1.** reduce rapid eye movements.
☐ **2.** decrease the irritation caused by light entering the damaged eye.
☐ **3.** protect the injured eye from infection.
☐ **4.** minimize eye strain on the uninvolved eye.

17. The client with retinal detachment in the right eye is extremely apprehensive and tells the nurse, "I am afraid of going blind. It would be so hard to live that way." What factor should the nurse consider before responding to this statement?
- [ ] 1. Repeat surgery is impossible, so if this procedure fails, vision loss is inevitable.
- [ ] 2. The surgery will only delay blindness in the right eye, but vision is preserved in the left eye.
- [ ] 3. More and more services are available to help newly blind people adapt to daily living.
- [ ] 4. Optimism is justified because surgical treatment has a 90% to 95% success rate.

18. Which statement would provide the **best** guide for activity during the rehabilitation period for a client who has been treated for retinal detachment?
- [ ] 1. Activity is resumed gradually; the client can resume usual activities in 5 to 6 weeks.
- [ ] 2. Activity level is determined by the client's tolerance; clients can be as active as they wish.
- [ ] 3. Activity level will be restricted for several months; the client should plan on being sedentary.
- [ ] 4. Activity level can return to normal; clients can resume regular aerobic exercises.

19. Which goal is a **priority** for a client who has undergone surgery for retinal detachment?
- [ ] 1. Control pain.
- [ ] 2. Prevent an increase in intraocular pressure.
- [ ] 3. Cleanse the eye with soap and water.
- [ ] 4. Maintain a darkened environment.

The Client with Glaucoma

20. A client with glaucoma is to receive 3 gtt of acetazolamide in the left eye. What should the nurse do?
- [ ] 1. Ask the client to close the right eye while administering the drug in the left eye.
- [ ] 2. Have the client look up while the nurse administers the eyedrops.
- [ ] 3. Have the client lift the eyebrows while the nurse positions the hand with the dropper on the client's forehead.
- [ ] 4. Wipe the eyes with a tissue following administration of the drops.

21. A client who has been treated for chronic open-angle glaucoma (COAG) for 5 years asks the nurse, "How does glaucoma damage my eyesight?" The nurse's reply should be based on the knowledge that COAG:
- [ ] 1. results from chronic eye inflammation.
- [ ] 2. causes increased intraocular pressure.
- [ ] 3. leads to detachment of the retina.
- [ ] 4. is caused by decreased blood flow to the retina.

22. The nurse should assess clients with chronic open-angle glaucoma (COAG) for:
- [ ] 1. eye pain.
- [ ] 2. excessive lacrimation.
- [ ] 3. colored light flashes.
- [ ] 4. decreasing peripheral vision.

23. What information should the nurse provide when preparing the client for tonometry?
- [ ] 1. Oral pain medication will be given before the procedure.
- [ ] 2. It is a painless procedure with no adverse effects.
- [ ] 3. Blurred or double vision may occur after the procedure.
- [ ] 4. Medication will be given to dilate the pupils before the procedure.

24. A client uses timolol maleate eyedrops. The expected outcome of this drug is to control glaucoma by:
- [ ] 1. constricting the pupils.
- [ ] 2. dilating the canals of Schlemm.
- [ ] 3. reducing aqueous humor formation.
- [ ] 4. improving the ability of the ciliary muscle to contract.

25. The nurse observes the client instill eyedrops. The client says, "I just try to hit the middle of my eyeball so the drops do not run out of my eye." The nurse explains to the client that this method may cause:
- [ ] 1. scleral staining.
- [ ] 2. corneal injury.
- [ ] 3. excessive lacrimation.
- [ ] 4. systemic drug absorption.

26. Which clinical manifestation should the nurse assess when a client has acute angle-closure glaucoma?
- [ ] 1. gradual loss of central vision
- [ ] 2. acute light sensitivity
- [ ] 3. loss of color vision
- [ ] 4. sudden eye pain

27. A client has been diagnosed with an acute episode of angle-closure glaucoma. The nurse plans the client's nursing care with the understanding that acute angle-closure glaucoma:
- [ ] 1. frequently resolves without treatment.
- [ ] 2. is typically treated with sustained bed rest.
- [ ] 3. is a medical emergency that can rapidly lead to blindness.
- [ ] 4. is most commonly treated with steroid therapy.

The Client with Adult Macular Degeneration

28. The nurse should assess an older adult with macular degeneration for:
- ☐ 1. loss of central vision.
- ☐ 2. loss of peripheral vision.
- ☐ 3. total blindness.
- ☐ 4. blurring of vision.

29. A client has a history of macular degeneration. While in the hospital, the **priority** nursing goal will be to:
- ☐ 1. provide education regarding community services for clients with adult macular degeneration (AMD).
- ☐ 2. provide health care related to monitoring the eye condition.
- ☐ 3. promote a safe, effective care environment.
- ☐ 4. improve vision.

30. Which measure should the nurse teach the client with adult macular degeneration (AMD) as a safety precaution?
- ☐ 1. Wear a patch over one eye.
- ☐ 2. Place personal items on the sighted side.
- ☐ 3. Lie in bed with the unaffected side toward the door.
- ☐ 4. Turn the head from side to side when walking.

31. The nurse is assessing a client with macular degeneration. Identify the illustration that **best** depicts what clients with this disorder typically see.

32. The nurse is assisting a client who has new-onset vision loss to transition to home from the hospital. The client can see shadow and light in the right eye only. When at home, the client is at **greatest** risk for:
- ☐ 1. loss of sensory perception.
- ☐ 2. injury from falls.
- ☐ 3. denial of changes in vision.
- ☐ 4. isolation from social activities.

The Client Undergoing Nasal Surgery

33. A young adult is admitted for elective nasal surgery for a deviated septum. Which sign would be an important indicator of bleeding even if the nasal drip pad remained dry and intact?
- ☐ 1. presence of nausea
- ☐ 2. repeated swallowing
- ☐ 3. rapid respiratory rate
- ☐ 4. feelings of anxiety

34. The client is ready for discharge after surgery for a deviated septum. Which instruction would be appropriate?
- ☐ 1. Avoid activities that elicit Valsalva's maneuver.
- ☐ 2. Take aspirin to control nasal discomfort.
- ☐ 3. Avoid brushing the teeth until the nasal packing is removed.
- ☐ 4. Apply heat to the nasal area to control swelling.

35. Which statement indicates that the client who has undergone repair of the nasal septum has understood the discharge instructions?
- ☐ 1. "I should not shower until my packing is removed."
- ☐ 2. "I will take stool softeners and modify my diet to prevent constipation."
- ☐ 3. "Coughing every 2 hours is important to prevent respiratory complications."
- ☐ 4. "It is important to blow my nose each day to remove the dried secretions."

The Client with a Hearing Disorder

36. To approach a deaf client, what should the nurse do **first**?
- ☐ 1. Knock on the room's door loudly.
- ☐ 2. Close and open the vertical blinds rapidly.
- ☐ 3. Talk while walking into the room.
- ☐ 4. Get the client's attention.

37. A 75-year-old client who has been taking furosemide regularly for 4 months tells the nurse about having trouble hearing. What should the nurse do?
- ☐ 1. Tell the client that at age 75 years, it is inevitable that there will be hearing loss.
- ☐ 2. Report the hearing loss to the healthcare provider (HCP).
- ☐ 3. Schedule the client for audiometric testing and a hearing aid.
- ☐ 4. Tell the client that the hearing loss is only temporary; when the body adjusts to the furosemide, hearing will improve.

38. The nurse is providing preoperative instructions to a client who is deaf. Which strategy is **most** effective in assuring that the client understands the information?
- ☐ 1. Stand in front of the client, and slowly explain the instructions.
- ☐ 2. Provide instructions to the spouse, and have the spouse explain them to the client.
- ☐ 3. Give the client written material to read, and follow up with time for questions.
- ☐ 4. Show the client a DVD with instructions.

39. A client who is prescribed by the healthcare provider (HCP) to take aspirin daily in order to prevent thrombus formation reports having ringing in the ears. The nurse advises the client to take which measure?
- ☐ 1. Increase fluid intake.
- ☐ 2. Stop taking the aspirin.
- ☐ 3. Use acetaminophen instead.
- ☐ 4. Contact the HCP.

40. The son of an older adult reports that his father just "stares off into space" more and more in the last several months but then eagerly smiles and nods once the son can get his attention. The nurse should assess the client further for:
- ☐ 1. dementia.
- ☐ 2. hearing loss.
- ☐ 3. anger.
- ☐ 4. depression.

41. The nurse has been assigned to a client who is hearing impaired and reads speech. Which strategies should the nurse incorporate when communicating with the client? Select all that apply.
- ☐ 1. Avoid being silhouetted against strong light.
- ☐ 2. Do not block out the person's view of the speaker's mouth.
- ☐ 3. Face the client when talking.
- ☐ 4. Have bright light behind so the individual can see.
- ☐ 5. Ensure the client is familiar with the subject material before discussing.
- ☐ 6. Talk to the client while doing other nursing procedures.

42. Eardrops have been prescribed to be instilled in the adult client's left ear to soften cerumen. To position the client, what should the nurse do?
- ☐ 1. Have the client lie on the left side.
- ☐ 2. Pull the auricle lobe up and back.
- ☐ 3. Pull the ear lobe down and back.
- ☐ 4. Chill the eardrops prior to administering.

43. Sensorineural hearing loss results from which condition?
- ☐ 1. presence of fluid and cerumen in the external canal
- ☐ 2. sclerosis of the bones of the middle ear
- ☐ 3. damage to the cochlear or vestibulocochlear nerve
- ☐ 4. emotional disturbance resulting in a functional hearing loss

44. What should the nurse instruct a client who has cerumen buildup in the ear to do? Select all that apply.
- ☐ 1. Wash the external ear with a washcloth.
- ☐ 2. Instill cerumenolytic drops in the ear canal.
- ☐ 3. Use cotton-tipped applicators to remove the wax from the ear canal.
- ☐ 4. Use small forceps to extract the wax.
- ☐ 5. Irrigate the ear with sterile water after softening the wax with a cerumenolytic solution.

45. A client is about to have a tympanoplasty and asks the nurse what the surgical procedure involves. The nurse begins the conversation by:
- ☐ 1. assessing the client's understanding of what the healthcare provider (HCP) has explained.
- ☐ 2. describing the surgical procedure.
- ☐ 3. educating the client that the procedure will close the perforation and prevent recurrent infection.
- ☐ 4. informing the client that the procedure will improve hearing.

46. An older adult takes two 81-mg aspirin tablets daily to prevent a heart attack. The client reports having a constant "ringing" in both ears. How should the nurse respond to the client's comment?
- ☐ 1. Tell the client that "ringing" in the ears is associated with the aging process.
- ☐ 2. Refer the client to have a Weber test.
- ☐ 3. Schedule the client for audiometric testing.
- ☐ 4. Explain to the client that the "ringing" may be related to the aspirin.

The Client with Ménière's Disease

47. An older adult has vertigo accompanied with tinnitus as the result of Ménière's disease. The nurse should instruct the client to restrict which dietary element?
- ☐ 1. protein
- ☐ 2. potassium
- ☐ 3. fluids
- ☐ 4. sodium

48. A client has vertigo. Which goal would be **most** appropriate to prevent injury related to altered immobility and gait disturbances? Select all that apply.
- ☐ 1. The client assumes a safe position when dizzy.
- ☐ 2. The client experiences no falls.
- ☐ 3. The client performs vestibular/balance exercises.
- ☐ 4. The client demonstrates family involvement.
- ☐ 5. The client keeps the head still when dizzy.

49. The client with Ménière's disease is instructed to modify the diet. The nurse should explain that the **most** frequently recommended diet modification for Ménière's disease is:
☐ 1. low sodium.
☐ 2. high protein.
☐ 3. low carbohydrate.
☐ 4. low fat.

50. Which statement indicates the client understands the expected course of Ménière's disease?
☐ 1. "The disease process will gradually extend to the eyes."
☐ 2. "Control of the episodes is usually possible, but a cure is not yet available."
☐ 3. "Continued medication therapy will cure the disease."
☐ 4. "Bilateral deafness is an inevitable outcome of the disease."

51. The risk for injury during an attack of Ménière's disease is high. The nurse should instruct the client to take which immediate action when experiencing vertigo?
☐ 1. "Place your head between your knees."
☐ 2. "Concentrate on rhythmic deep breathing."
☐ 3. "Close your eyes tightly."
☐ 4. "Assume a reclining or flat position."

The Client with Cancer of the Larynx

52. Following a laryngectomy, the nurse notices that the client has saliva collecting beneath the skin flaps. This finding is indicative of:
☐ 1. skin necrosis.
☐ 2. carotid artery rupture.
☐ 3. stomal stenosis.
☐ 4. development of a fistula.

53. The nurse is developing a care plan with a client who had a laryngectomy 3 days ago. To assure adequate nutrition, what should the nurse instruct the client to do? Select all that apply.
☐ 1. Weigh weekly and report weight loss.
☐ 2. When eating, sit and lean slightly forward.
☐ 3. Have serum albumin level checked regularly.
☐ 4. Administer enteral tube feedings as prescribed.
☐ 5. Manipulate the nasogastric tube daily.

54. The client with a laryngectomy is being discharged. The nurse should determine that the client understands to do which self-care measures? Select all that apply.
☐ 1. Provide humidification in the home.
☐ 2. Use a protective shield over the stoma for bathing.
☐ 3. Consume a liberal intake of fluids (2 to 3 L/day).
☐ 4. Limit spicy seasonings on food.
☐ 5. Follow a low-fiber diet.

55. After a total laryngectomy, the client has a feeding tube. The feeding tube is effective if the tube feedings:
☐ 1. meet the fluid and nutritional needs of the client.
☐ 2. prevent aspiration.
☐ 3. prevent fistula formation.
☐ 4. maintain an open airway.

56. Complications associated with having a tracheostomy tube include:
☐ 1. decreased cardiac output.
☐ 2. damage to the laryngeal nerve.
☐ 3. pneumothorax.
☐ 4. acute respiratory distress syndrome (ARDS).

57. A **priority** goal for the hospitalized client who 2 days earlier had a total laryngectomy with creation of a new tracheostomy is to:
☐ 1. decrease secretions.
☐ 2. learn to care for the tracheostomy.
☐ 3. relieve anxiety related to the tracheostomy.
☐ 4. maintain a patent airway.

Managing Care, Quality, and Safety of Clients with Health Problems of the Eyes, Ears, Nose, and Throat

58. The client with glaucoma is scheduled for a hip replacement. Which prescription would require clarification before the nurse carries it out?
☐ 1. Administer morphine sulfate.
☐ 2. Administer atropine sulfate.
☐ 3. Teach deep-breathing exercises.
☐ 4. Teach leg lifts and muscle-setting exercises.

59. To ensure safety for a hospitalized blind client, the nurse should:
☐ 1. require that the client has a sitter for each shift.
☐ 2. request that the client stays in bed until the nurse can assist.
☐ 3. orient the client to the room environment.
☐ 4. keep the side rails up when the client is alone.

60. The nurse is taking care of a client who had a laryngectomy yesterday. To assure client safety, the nurse should give "hand-off reports" at which times? Select all that apply.
☐ 1. change of shift
☐ 2. change of nurses
☐ 3. when the nurse goes to lunch
☐ 4. when the unit clerk goes to a staff meeting
☐ 5. when new medication prescriptions are written

61. The nurse is admitting a client with glaucoma. The client brings prescribed eyedrops from home and insists on using them in the hospital. The nurse should:
☐ 1. allow the client to keep the eyedrops at the bedside and use as prescribed on the bottle.
☐ 2. place the eyedrops in the hospital medication drawer and administer as labeled on the bottle.
☐ 3. explain to the client that the healthcare provider (HCP) will write a prescription for the eyedrops to be used at the hospital.
☐ 4. ask the client's wife to assist the client in administering the eyedrops while the client is in the hospital.

62. The nurse is assigned to care for a client with an ocular prosthesis who is having surgery under a local anesthetic. Prior to surgery, the nurse should:
☐ 1. maintain surgical asepsis when caring for the prosthesis.
☐ 2. leave the prosthesis in place.
☐ 3. cleanse the ocular prosthesis with full-strength hydrogen peroxide.
☐ 4. instruct the client to cleanse the prosthesis daily.

Answers, Rationales, and Test-Taking Strategies

The answers and rationales for each question follow below, along with keys (🔑) to the client need (CN) and cognitive level (CL) for each question. In addition, you will also see a glossary icon (📖) highlighting specific terminology used on the licensing exam. As you check your answers, use the **Content Mastery and Test-Taking Skill Self-Analysis** *worksheet (tear-out worksheet in back of book) to identify the reason(s) for not answering the questions correctly. For additional information about test-taking skills and strategies for answering questions, refer to pages 12–23 and pages 35–36 in Part 1 of this book.*

The Client with Cataracts

1. 3. The spouse has positioned the dropper and the client correctly to prevent injury to the client's eye. The spouse should administer the drops in the center of the lower lid. Following administration of the eyedrops, the client should blink the eyes to distribute the medication; squeezing or rubbing the eyes might cause the medication to drip out of the eye.

🔑 CN: Safety and infection control;
CL: Apply

2. 3. To prevent discomfort from bright light, the client should wear sunglasses that cover the front and side of the face, thus minimizing light that comes into the eye from any direction. It is not necessary to remain in dim light or inside. Attaching sun shields or sunglasses to existing glasses will not cover the eye sufficiently, and bright light will come in on the side of the face. It is not necessary to patch the affected eye.

🔑 CN: Basic care and comfort;
CL: Synthesize

3. 1,4,5,6. To promote success of lens implant without complication (infection, inflammation, hemorrhage), it is important for the client to instill eyedrops as prescribed, protect the eye, and avoid placing any stress on the eye by lifting, pulling, or pushing objects that weigh more than 15 lb. Pain should be minimal and relieved with acetaminophen; if not, the client should notify the **healthcare provider (HCP)** 📖. Clients should not expect to drive or see clearly immediately following lens implant; it may take several days for vision to clear, and limitations will be discussed at the follow-up appointment.

🔑 CN: Reduction of risk potential;
CL: Evaluate

4. 1,2,4. The use of glasses following cataract surgery does not totally restore binocular vision. Glasses will cause images to appear larger, and peripheral vision will be distorted; the client should look through the center of the glasses and turn his or her head to view objects in the periphery. The client should also use caution when walking or climbing stairs until he or she has adjusted to the change in vision. Changes in vision following cataract surgery are not immediate, and the nurse can instruct the client to be patient while adjusting to the changes. The client does not need to stay out of the sun but should wear dark glasses to prevent discomfort from photophobia.

🔑 CN: Physiological adaptation;
CL: Create

5. 3. Using an eye shield at night prevents rubbing the eye. The head should be turned to the side to scan the entire visual field to compensate for impaired peripheral vision. Eye medications may initially cause sensitivity to bright light. The surgeon changes the eye patch on the second postoperative day.

🔑 CN: Reduction of risk potential;
CL: Synthesize

6. 2. The nurse should give a client who seems fearful of surgery an opportunity to express his or her feelings. Only after identifying the client's concerns can the nurse intervene appropriately. Asking the client about previous reactions to local anesthetics may be warranted, but it does not address the client's concerns in this instance. Telling the client that he or she will not have nausea or vomiting ignores the client's feelings of fear and does not provide any data about the client's feelings. More data would help the nurse plan care. Telling the client that there is nothing to be afraid of minimizes the client's feelings and does not address his or her concerns. Premature explanations and clichés do not provide the needed assessment data and ignore the client's feelings.

☇ CN: Psychosocial integrity;
CL: Synthesize

7. 4. An ophthalmologist is a **healthcare provider (HCP)** 📖 who specializes in the treatment of disorders of the eye, and the nurse should advise the client to see an ophthalmologist. An optician makes glasses, and it is not known at this point what the best treatment for the client is. Magnifying glasses, or glasses with tinted lenses, do not correct hazy or blurred vision. If glasses are needed to correct refractive errors, they should be prescription glasses.

☇ CN: Health promotion and maintenance;
CL: Synthesize

8. 2. Instilled in the eye, phenylephrine hydrochloride acts as a mydriatic, causing the pupil to dilate. It also constricts small blood vessels in the eye.

☇ CN: Pharmacological and parenteral therapies; CL: Evaluate

9. 4. A prescribed antiemetic should be administered as soon as the client has nausea following a cataract extraction. Vomiting can increase intraocular pressure, which should be avoided after eye surgery because it can cause complications. Deep breathing is unlikely to relieve nausea. Postoperative nausea may be common; however, it does not necessarily pass quickly and can lead to vomiting. Telling the client to call only if vomiting occurs ignores the client's need for comfort and intervention to prevent complications.

☇ CN: Pharmacological and parenteral therapies; CL: Synthesize

10. 1,5. Acute bacterial endophthalmitis can occur in about 1 out of 1,000 cases. Organisms that are typically involved include Staphylococcus epidermidis, Staphylococcus aureus, and Pseudomonas and Proteus species. Vision loss is one result of acute bacterial infection. In addition, vision loss can be the result of malposition of the intraocular lens implant or opacification of the posterior capsule. Retrobulbar hemorrhage is a complication that may occur right before surgery and is a result of retrobulbar infiltration of anesthetic agents. Rupture of the posterior capsule and suprachoroidal hemorrhage are both complications that can result during surgery.

☇ CN: Physiological adaptation;
CL: Analyze

11. 1. The nurse should instruct the client to remain in a semi-Fowler's position or on the nonoperative side. Positioning the feet higher than the body does not affect the operative eye; placing the head in a dependent position could increase pressure within the eyes.

☇ CN: Reduction of risk potential;
CL: Synthesize

12. 1. Applying pressure against the nose at the inner canthus of the closed eye after administering eyedrops prevents the medication from entering the lacrimal (tear) duct. If the medication enters the tear duct, it can enter the nose and pharynx, where it may be absorbed and cause toxic symptoms. Eyedrops should be placed in the eye's lower conjunctival sac. Applying pressure will not prevent the drug from running down the face as long as the drops are instilled in the eye. Pressure does not affect the cornea or facilitate distribution of the medication over the eye surface.

☇ CN: Pharmacological and parenteral therapies; CL: Apply

13. 2. Coughing is contraindicated after cataract extraction because it increases intraocular pressure. Other activities that are contraindicated because they increase intraocular pressure include turning to the operative side, sneezing, crying, and straining. Lying supine, ambulating, and deep breathing do not affect intraocular pressure.

☇ CN: Physiological adaptation;
CL: Synthesize

14. 4. Sudden, sharp pain after eye surgery should suggest to the nurse that the client may be experiencing intraocular hemorrhage. The **healthcare provider (HCP)** 📖 should be notified promptly. Detached retina and prolapse of the iris are usually painless. Extracapsular erosion is not characterized by sharp pain.

☇ CN: Physiological adaptation;
CL: Analyze

The Client with a Retinal Detachment

15. 4. Promoting measures that limit mobility may prevent further injury. Following surgical repair of a detached retina, cool or warm compresses are applied to edematous eyelids, if prescribed. The client should avoid lying face down, stooping, or bending preoperatively. It is not necessary to remove all pillows.

⚷ CN: Physiological adaptation; CL: Synthesize

16. 1. Patching the eyes helps decrease random eye movements that could enlarge and worsen retinal detachment. Although clients with eye injuries frequently are light sensitive, and preventing infection is important, the specific goal is to reduce rapid eye movements. Using the uninvolved eye would not cause eye strain, but random movements of one eye will involve the other eye.

⚷ CN: Physiological adaptation; CL: Evaluate

17. 4. Untreated retinal detachment results in increasing detachment and eventual blindness, but 90% to 95% of clients can be successfully treated with surgery. If necessary, the surgical procedure can be repeated about 10 to 14 days after the first procedure. Many more services are available for newly blind people, but ideally this client will not need them. Surgery does not delay blindness.

⚷ CN: Physiological adaptation; CL: Synthesize

18. 1. The scarring of the retinal tear needs time to heal completely. Therefore, resumption of activity should be gradual; the client may resume usual activities in 5 to 6 weeks. Successful healing should allow the client to return to a previous level of functioning.

⚷ CN: Basic care and comfort; CL: Synthesize

19. 2. After surgery to correct a detached retina, prevention of increased intraocular pressure is the priority goal. Control of pain with analgesics is a secondary goal. The client should avoid getting soap and water in the eye when bathing. Maintaining a darkened environment is not necessary for this client.

⚷ CN: Physiological adaptation; CL: Synthesize

The Client with Glaucoma

20. 2. The client should look up while the nurse instills the eyedrops. The client will need to keep both eyes open while the nurse administers the drug. If the client raises the eyebrows while the nurse's hand is positioned on the eyebrows, the movement of the forehead may cause the dropper to move and injure the eye. The client should gently blink the eyes after the eyedrops have been instilled. Using a tissue to wipe the eyes could remove some of the medication; excess fluid can be removed with a cotton ball.

⚷ CN: Pharmacological and parenteral therapies; CL: Apply

21. 2. In COAG, there is an obstruction to the outflow of aqueous humor, leading to increased intraocular pressure. The increased intraocular pressure eventually causes destruction of the retina's nerve fibers. This nerve destruction causes painless vision loss. The exact cause of glaucoma is unknown. Glaucoma does not lead to retinal detachment.

⚷ CN: Physiological adaptation; CL: Analyze

22. 4. Although COAG is usually asymptomatic in the early stages, peripheral vision gradually decreases as the disorder progresses. Eye pain is not a feature of COAG but is common in clients with angle-closure glaucoma. Excessive lacrimation is not a symptom of COAG; it may indicate a blocked tear duct. Flashes of light are a common symptom of retinal detachment.

⚷ CN: Physiological adaptation; CL: Analyze

23. 2. Tonometry, which measures intraocular pressure, is a simple, noninvasive, and painless procedure that requires no particular preparation or postprocedure care and carries no adverse effects. It is not necessary to dilate the pupils for tonometry.

⚷ CN: Reduction of risk potential; CL: Synthesize

24. 3. Timolol maleate is commonly administered to control glaucoma. The drug's action is not completely understood, but it is believed to reduce aqueous humor formation, thereby reducing intraocular pressure. Timolol does not constrict the pupils; miotics are used for pupillary constriction and contraction of the ciliary muscle. Timolol does not dilate the canal of Schlemm.

⚷ CN: Pharmacological and parenteral therapies; CL: Evaluate

25. 2. The cornea is sensitive and can be injured by eyedrops falling onto it. Therefore, eyedrops should be instilled into the lower conjunctival sac of the eye to avoid the risk of corneal damage. The drops do not cause scleral staining or excessive lacrimation. Systemic absorption occurs when eyedrops enter the tear ducts.

CN: Pharmacological and parenteral therapies; CL: Evaluate

26. 4. Acute angle-closure glaucoma produces abrupt changes in the angle of the iris. Clinical manifestations include severe eye pain, colored halos around lights, and rapid vision loss. Gradual loss of central vision is associated with macular degeneration. The loss of color vision, or achromatopsia, is a rare symptom that occurs when a stroke damages the fusiform gyrus. It most often affects only half of the visual field.

CN: Physiological adaptation; CL: Analyze

27. 3. Acute angle-closure glaucoma is a medical emergency that rapidly leads to blindness if left untreated. Treatment typically involves miotic drugs and surgery, usually iridectomy or laser therapy. Both procedures create a hole in the periphery of the iris, which allows the aqueous humor to flow into the anterior chamber. Bed rest does not affect the progression of acute angle-closure glaucoma. Steroids are not a treatment for acute angle-closure glaucoma; in fact, they are associated with the development of glaucoma.

CN: Physiological adaptation; CL: Apply

The Client with Adult Macular Degeneration

28. 1. Macular degeneration generally involves loss of central vision. Gradual blurring of vision can occur as the disease progresses and may result in blindness; however, loss of central vision is the most common finding. Tiny yellowish spots, known as drusen, develop beneath the retina. Loss of peripheral vision is characteristic of glaucoma.

CN: Physiological adaptation; CL: Analyze

29. 3. AMD generally affects central vision. Confusion may result related to the changes in the environment and the inability to see the environment clearly. Therefore, providing safety is the priority goal in the care of this client. Educating him regarding community resources or monitoring his AMD may have been done at an earlier date or can be done after assessing his knowledge base and experience with the disease process. Improving his vision may not be possible.

CN: Safety and infection control;
CL: Synthesize

30. 4. To expand the visual field, the partially sighted client should be taught to turn the head from side to side when walking. Neglecting to do so may result in accidents. This technique helps maximize the use of remaining sight. A patch does not address the problem of hemianopsia. Appropriate client positioning and placement of personal items will increase the client's ability to cope with the problem but will not affect safety.

CN: Safety and infection control;
CL: Synthesize

31. In macular degeneration, the center vision is blackened out, and only the outer visual fields are clear.

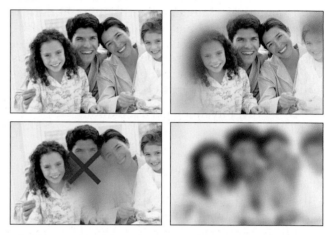

CN: Physiological adaptation; CL: Analyze

32. 2. Because of the client's recent vision loss, the client is at high risk for injury. Sensory alterations often affect other areas of functional ability, including leaving clients with sensory deficits at risk for injuries as a result. Disturbed sensory perception, denial and difficulty adjusting to the vision loss, and social isolation may also be of concern and may accompany changes in sensory function, but they are not of higher priority than risk for injury.

CN: Management of care; CL: Analyze

The Client Undergoing Nasal Surgery

33. 2. Because of the dense packing, it is relatively unusual for bleeding to be apparent through the nasal drip pad. Instead, the blood runs down the throat, causing the client to swallow frequently. The back of the throat can be assessed with a flashlight. An accumulation of blood in the stomach may cause nausea and vomiting but is not an initial sign of bleeding. Increased respiratory rate occurs in shock and is not an early sign of bleeding in the client after nasal surgery. Feelings of anxiety are not indicative of nasal bleeding.

CN: Physiological adaptation;
CL: Synthesize

34. 1. The client should be instructed to avoid any activities that cause Valsalva's maneuver (e.g., straining at stool, vigorous coughing, exercise) to reduce stress on suture lines and bleeding. The client should not take aspirin because of its antiplatelet properties, which may cause bleeding. Oral hygiene is important to rid the mouth of old dried blood and to enhance the client's appetite. Cool compresses, not heat, should be applied to decrease swelling and control discoloration of the area.

CN: Reduction of risk potential; CL: Synthesize

35. 2. Constipation can cause straining during defecation, which can induce bleeding. Showering is not contraindicated. The client should take measures to prevent coughing. The client should avoid blowing the nose for 48 hours after the packing is removed. Thereafter, the client should blow the nose gently using the open-mouth technique to minimize bleeding in the surgical area.

CN: Physiological adaptation; CL: Evaluate

The Client with a Hearing Disorder

36. 4. The nurse should avoid startling the client who is deaf and should obtain the attention of the client before speaking. The client who is deaf cannot hear knocking on the door or talking. Opening the blinds is not a helpful way to get the client's attention.

CN: Psychosocial integrity; CL: Synthesize

37. 2. Furosemide may cause ototoxicity. The nurse should tell the client to promptly report the hearing loss, dizziness, or tinnitus to help prevent permanent ear damage. Hearing loss is not inevitable, and it is inappropriate to make assumptions about the cause of symptoms without a thorough evaluation. The client's system will not "adjust," and hearing loss will not resolve.

CN: Pharmacological and parenteral therapies; CL: Synthesize

38. 3. A client who is deaf benefits most from reading information and then having an opportunity to ask questions and follow up. Verbal communication, while appropriate, may not be sufficient. The spouse can be included in the teaching, but the nurse is responsible for ensuring that the client understands the instructions. DVDs may be helpful, but unless they have closed captioning, key points may be missed in the audio portion.

CN: Physiological adaptation; CL: Synthesize

39. 4. Because aspirin is ototoxic, the ringing in the ears is likely caused by long-term aspirin use. The nurse advises the client to contact the **HCP** 📖; if the aspirin is to be discontinued, other drugs may be ordered. The client is not instructed to stop taking the drug without discussing the change with the HCP. Acetaminophen does not have the same antithrombotic properties as does aspirin. Increasing fluid intake will not stop the ringing in the ears.

CN: Physiological adaptation; CL: Synthesize

40. 2. Blank looks, decreased attention span, positioning of the head toward sound, and smiling/nodding in agreement once attention is gained are all behaviors that indicate hearing loss in adults. It is common to confuse sensory deficits for a change in cognitive status. The nurse should focus assessments of sensory function on considering any pathophysiology of existing or new-onset deficits and consider all client factors that might contribute to deficits. The blank looks do not indicate that this client is angry with his son.

CN: Basic care and comfort; CL: Analyze

41. 1,2,3,5. When working with a client who is hearing impaired and reads speech, the presenter must face the person directly and devote full attention to the communication process. In addition, it will be useful for the client that the speaker not be too silhouetted against strong light, that the speaker's mouth not be blocked from the client's view, and that there are no objects in the mouth of the speaker. Finally, it is recommended that the presenter provide the client with the needed information to study before reviewing. This will provide the client with the ability to use contextual clues in speech reading.

CN: Basic care and comfort; CL: Synthesize

42. 2. The nurse should have the client lie on the side opposite the affected ear. To straighten the client's ear canal, pull the auricle of the ear up and back for an adult. For an infant or a young child, gently pull the auricle down and back to the nasopharynx. The eardrops should be administered at body temperature.

CN: Pharmacological and parenteral therapies; CL: Apply

43. 3. A sensorineural hearing loss results from damage to the cochlear or vestibulocochlear nerve. Presence of fluid and cerumen in the external canal or sclerosis of the bones of the middle ear results in a conductive hearing loss. Hearing loss resulting from an emotional disturbance is called a psychogenic hearing loss.

CN: Physiological adaptation; CL: Apply

44. 1,2,5. The nurse can advise the client with cerumen that is impacted in the ear to use a washcloth to clean the exterior part of the ear. The client can also instill cerumenolytic drops to soften the earwax. The client can then irrigate the ear canal with sterile water using a small bulb syringe. The client should not use cotton-tipped applicators as they often push the cerumen further into the ear canal. The client should never put forceps in the ear.

🗝 CN: Pharmacological and parenteral therapies; CL: Synthesize

45. 1. The nurse should first assess the client's knowledge base. Working within the framework of the client's knowledge and educational level, the nurse then can describe the procedure and its benefits.

🗝 CN: Reduction of risk potential; CL: Synthesize

46. 4. Tinnitus (ringing in the ears) is an adverse effect of aspirin. Aspirin contains salicylate, which is an ototoxic drug that can induce reversible hearing loss and tinnitus. The nurse should explain this to the client and then encourage the client to inform the **healthcare provider (HCP)** 📖 of the symptom. Tinnitus is not a function of aging. The Weber test and audiometric testing are useful for determining hearing loss but are not necessarily helpful in the management or diagnosis of drug-induced tinnitus.

🗝 CN: Pharmacological and parenteral therapies; CL: Synthesize

The Client with Ménière's Disease

47. 4. Ménière's disease is commonly seen in older women; the disorder is caused by pressure within the labyrinth of the inner ear as a result of excess endolympha resulting in swelling in the cochlea. Therefore, the nurse should instruct the client about dietary restrictions of sodium to reduce fluid retention. Pharmacologic treatment includes antivertiginous drugs and diuretics. If the client is prescribed a diuretic, the fluid and electrolytes are monitored. The amount of protein does not have a direct influence in this disease process.

🗝 CN: Physiological adaptation; CL: Synthesize

48. 1,2,3,5. Assessment of vertigo, including history, onset, description of attacks, duration, frequency, and associated ear symptoms, is important. Vestibular/balance therapy or exercises should be taught and practiced. The client needs to be instructed to sit down when dizzy and decrease the amount of head movement. The client will benefit

from recognizing whether he or she experiences an "aura" before an attack so appropriate action can be taken. Finally, it is recommended that the client keep the eyes open and look straight ahead when lying down. These expected outcomes will prevent the problem of injury. Family involvement is essential when dealing with a client experiencing vertigo but is not essential for this client who must manage the vertigo with or without family involvement.

🗝 CN: Reduction of risk potential; CL: Synthesize

49. 1. A low-sodium diet is frequently an effective mechanism for reducing the frequency and severity of the disease episodes. About three-quarters of clients with Ménière's disease respond to treatment with a low-salt diet. A diuretic may also be prescribed. Other dietary changes, such as high protein, low carbohydrate, and low fat, do not have an effect on Ménière's disease.

🗝 CN: Basic care and comfort; CL: Apply

50. 2. There is no cure for Ménière's disease, but the wide range of medical and surgical treatments allows for adequate control in many clients. The disease often worsens, but it does not spread to the eyes. The hearing loss is usually unilateral.

🗝 CN: Physiological adaptation; CL: Evaluate

51. 4. The client needs to assume a safe and comfortable position during an attack, which may last several hours. The client's location when the attack occurs may dictate the most reasonable position. Ideally, the client should lie down immediately in a reclining or flat position to control the vertigo. The danger of a serious fall is real. Placing the head between the knees will not help prevent a fall and is not practical because the attack may last several hours. Concentrating on breathing may be a useful distraction, but it will not help prevent a fall. Closing the eyes does not help prevent a fall.

🗝 CN: Safety and infection control; CL: Synthesize

The Client with Cancer of the Larynx

52. 4. A salivary fistula is suspected when there is saliva collecting beneath skin flaps or leaking through the suture line or drain site. Salivary fistula or skin necrosis usually precedes carotid artery rupture. Stomal stenosis may be present when there are suprasternal and intercostal retractions and difficult breathing.

🗝 CN: Physiological adaptation; CL: Analyze

53. 1,2,3,4. The nurse should monitor nutritional status through frequent weighing and checking the serum albumin level. The nurse also should administer enteral tube feedings until there is sufficient healing of pharynx and the client can consume sufficient oral feedings to meet body needs. The nurse should avoid manipulation of the nasogastric tube during this time so it does not disrupt the suture line. The nurse should place the client in a sitting position, leaning slightly forward, which allows the larynx to move forward and the hypopharynx to partially open; the epiglottis normally prevents fluid and food from entering the larynx during swallowing.

🔑 CN: Physiological adaptation; CL: Create

54. 1,2,3. The nurse should advise the client to provide humidification at home. Instruct the client to use a protective shield for bathing, showering, or shampooing or cutting hair to prevent aspiration. The nurse can also encourage the client to obtain a fluid intake of 2 to 3 L daily to help liquefy secretions. To counteract any loss of smell and impairment of taste sensation, the client can add additional seasoning to food. The client should follow a high-fiber diet and use stool softeners because the client may not be able to hold the breath and bear down for bowel movements.

🔑 CN: Health promotion and maintenance; CL: Evaluate

55. 1. The goal of postoperative care is to maintain physiologic integrity. Therefore, inserting a feeding tube is a strategy to ensure the fluid and nutritional needs of the client as the surgical site is healing. The feeding tube does help prevent aspiration by preventing ingested fluid from leaking through the wound into the trachea before healing occurs; however, the primary rationale is to meet the client's nutritional and fluid needs. A tracheoesophageal fistula is a rare complication of total laryngectomy and may occur if radiation therapy has compromised wound healing. A feeding tube does not help maintain an open airway.

🔑 CN: Reduction of risk potential; CL: Evaluate

56. 2. Tracheostomy tubes carry several potential complications, including laryngeal nerve damage, bleeding, and infection. Tracheostomy tubes alone do not affect cardiac output or cause acute respiratory distress. The tube is inserted in the trachea, not the lung, so there is no risk of pneumothorax.

🔑 CN: Physiological adaptation; CL: Apply

57. 4. The main goal for a client with a new tracheostomy is to maintain a patent airway. A fresh tracheostomy frequently causes bleeding and excess secretions, and clients may require frequent suctioning to maintain patency. Decreasing secretions may be a component of a client's care after laryngectomy and tracheostomy, and relieving anxiety is always an important goal; however, the primary goal is to maintain a patent airway. Instruction in care of a tracheostomy is a priority later in the client's recovery.

🔑 CN: Physiological adaptation; CL: Synthesize

Managing Care, Quality, and Safety of Clients with Health Problems of the Eyes, Ears, Nose, and Throat

58. 2. Atropine sulfate causes pupil dilation. This action is contraindicated for the client with glaucoma because it increases intraocular pressure. The drug does not have this effect on intraocular pressure in people who do not have glaucoma. Morphine causes pupil constriction. Deep-breathing exercises will not affect glaucoma. The client should resume taking all medications for glaucoma immediately after surgery.

🔑 CN: Pharmacological and parenteral therapies; CL: Synthesize

59. 3. The priority goal of care for a client who is blind is safety and preventing injury. The initial action is to orient the client to a new environment. Taking time to identify the objects and where they are located in the room can achieve this goal. It is unrealistic to have someone stay with the client at all times or for the client to stay in bed until the nurse can assist. Using side rails creates unnecessary barriers and may be a safety hazard.

🔑 CN: Safety and infection control; CL: Synthesize

60. 1,2,3. Effective communication is essential when managing client safety and preventing errors. "Hand-off reports" should be made at shift change, when there is a change of nurses or when the nurse leaves the unit, and when the client is discharged or transfers to another unit. There does not need to be a hand-off report when the unit clerk leaves the unit or when new medication prescriptions are written.

🔑 CN: Safety and infection control; CL: Apply

61. 3. In order to prevent medication errors, clients may not use medications they bring from home; the **HCP** 📖 will prescribe the eyedrops as required. It is not safe to place the eyedrops in the client's medication box or to permit the client to use them at the bedside. The nurse should ask the wife to take the eyedrops home.

🔑 CN: Safety and infection control;
CL: Synthesize

62. 2. The nurse should maintain medical asepsis to care for an ocular prosthesis. Because the client will have a local anesthetic, the nurse should leave the prosthesis in place. Daily removal and cleansing is not necessary and may be irritating to the socket; removal for cleansing once or twice a month is sufficient. The nurse should never use anything stronger than liquid soap and water to cleanse an ocular prosthesis.

🔑 CN: Reduction of risk potential;
CL: Apply

TEST 16 The Client with Health Problems of the Integumentary System

- The Client with Burns
- The Older Adult with General Problems of the Integumentary System
- The Client with Shingles
- The Client with a Pressure Ulcer
- The Client with Skin Cancer
- Managing Care, Quality, and Safety of Clients with Health Problems of the Integumentary System
- Answers, Rationales, and Test-Taking Strategies

The Client with Burns

1. There has been a fire in an apartment building. All residents have been evacuated, but many are burned. Which clients should be transported to a burn center for treatment? Select all that apply.
☐ 1. an 8-year-old with third-degree burns over 10% of the body surface area (BSA)
☐ 2. a 20-year-old who inhaled the smoke of the fire
☐ 3. a 50-year-old diabetic with first- and second-degree burns on the left forearm (about 5% of the body surface area [BSA])
☐ 4. a 30-year-old with second-degree burns on the back of the left leg (about 9% of body surface area [BSA])
☐ 5. a 40-year-old with second-degree burns on the right arm (about 10% of BSA)

2. The nurse is assessing an 80-year-old client who has scald burns on the hands and both forearms (first- and second-degree burns on 10% of the body surface area). What should the nurse do **first**?
☐ 1. Clean the wounds with warm water.
☐ 2. Apply antibiotic cream.
☐ 3. Refer the client to a burn center.
☐ 4. Cover the burns with a sterile dressing.

3. During the emergent (resuscitative) phase of burn injury, which finding indicates that the client requires additional volume with fluid resuscitation?
☐ 1. serum creatinine level of 2.5 mg/dL (221 μmol/L)
☐ 2. little fluctuation in daily weight
☐ 3. hourly urine output of 60 mL
☐ 4. serum albumin level of 3.8 mg/dL (38 g/L)

4. A client is admitted to the hospital after sustaining burns to the chest, abdomen, right arm, and right leg. The shaded areas in the illustration indicate the burned areas on the client's body. Using the "rule of nines," estimate what percentage of the client's body surface has been burned.
☐ 1. 18%
☐ 2. 27%
☐ 3. 45%
☐ 4. 64%

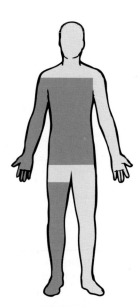

5. The nurse is caring for a client with severe burns who is receiving fluid resuscitation. Which finding indicates that the client is responding to the fluid resuscitation?
☐ 1. pulse rate of 112 bpm
☐ 2. blood pressure of 94/64 mm Hg
☐ 3. urine output of 30 mL/h
☐ 4. serum sodium level of 136 mEq/L (136 mmol/L)

6. At about one-half hour **before** the daily whirl-pool bath and dressing change, the nurse should:
☐ **1.** soak the dressing.
☐ **2.** remove the dressing.
☐ **3.** administer an analgesic.
☐ **4.** slit the dressing with blunt scissors.

7. The client with a major burn injury receives total parenteral nutrition (TPN). The expected outcome is to:
☐ **1.** correct water and electrolyte imbalances.
☐ **2.** allow the gastrointestinal tract to rest.
☐ **3.** provide supplemental vitamins and minerals.
☐ **4.** ensure adequate caloric and protein intake.

8. An advantage of using biologic burn grafts such as porcine (pigskin) grafts is that they:
☐ **1.** encourage the formation of tough skin.
☐ **2.** promote the growth of epithelial tissue.
☐ **3.** provide for permanent wound closure.
☐ **4.** facilitate the development of subcutaneous tissue.

9. Which factor would have the **least** influence on the survival and effectiveness of a burn victim's porcine grafts?
☐ **1.** absence of infection in the wounds
☐ **2.** adequate vascularization in the grafted area
☐ **3.** immobilization of the area being grafted
☐ **4.** use of analgesics as necessary for pain relief

10. The nurse should plan to begin rehabilitation efforts for the burn client:
☐ **1.** immediately after the burn has occurred.
☐ **2.** after the client's circulatory status has been stabilized.
☐ **3.** after grafting of the burn wounds has occurred.
☐ **4.** after the client's pain has been eliminated.

11. During the early phase of burn care, the nurse should assess the client for:
☐ **1.** hypernatremia.
☐ **2.** hyponatremia.
☐ **3.** metabolic alkalosis.
☐ **4.** hyperkalemia.

12. Which client with burns will **most** likely require an endotracheal or tracheostomy tube? A client who has:
☐ **1.** electrical burns of the hands and arms causing arrhythmias.
☐ **2.** thermal burns to the head, face, and airway resulting in hypoxia.
☐ **3.** chemical burns on the chest and abdomen.
☐ **4.** secondhand smoke inhalation.

13. A client is receiving fluid replacement with lactated Ringer's after 40% of the body was burned 10 hours ago. The assessment reveals temperature 97.1°F (36.2°C), heart rate 122 bpm, blood pressure 84/42 mm Hg, central venous pressure (CVP) 2 mm Hg, and urine output 25 mL for the last 2 hours. The IV rate is currently at 375 mL/h. Using the SBAR (Situation-Background-Assessment-Recommendation) technique for communication, the nurse calls the healthcare provider (HCP) with a recommendation for:
☐ **1.** furosemide.
☐ **2.** fresh frozen plasma.
☐ **3.** IV rate increase.
☐ **4.** dextrose 5%.

14. After the initial phase of the burn injury, the client's plan of care will focus **primarily** on:
☐ **1.** helping the client maintain a positive self-concept.
☐ **2.** promoting hygiene.
☐ **3.** preventing infection.
☐ **4.** educating the client regarding care of the skin grafts.

15. The rate at which IV fluids are infused is based on the burn client's:
☐ **1.** lean muscle mass and body surface area (BSA) burned.
☐ **2.** total body weight and BSA burned.
☐ **3.** total BSA and BSA burned.
☐ **4.** height and weight and BSA burned.

16. The nurse is conducting a focused assessment of the gastrointestinal system of a client with a burn injury. The nurse should assess the client for:
☐ **1.** paralytic ileus.
☐ **2.** gastric distention.
☐ **3.** hiatal hernia.
☐ **4.** Curling's ulcer.

17. In the acute phase of burn injury, which pain medication would **most** likely be given to the client to decrease the perception of the pain?
☐ **1.** oral analgesics such as ibuprofen or acetaminophen
☐ **2.** intravenous opioids
☐ **3.** intramuscular opioids
☐ **4.** oral antianxiety agents such as lorazepam

18. Using the Parkland formula, calculate the hourly rate of fluid replacement with lactated Ringer's solution during the first 8 hours for a client weighing 75 kg with total body surface area (TBSA) burn of 40%. Record your answer using a whole number.

_____ mL/h.

The Older Adult with General Problems of the Integumentary System

19. The nurse is assessing an older adult's skin. The assessment will involve inspecting the skin for color, pigmentation, and vascularity. The critical component in the nurse's assessment is noting the:
- ☐ 1. similarities from one side to the other.
- ☐ 2. changes from the normal expected findings.
- ☐ 3. appearance of age-related wrinkles.
- ☐ 4. skin turgor.

20. Which change in the integumentary system is associated with normal aging?
- ☐ 1. The outer layer of skin is replaced with new cells every 3 days.
- ☐ 2. Subcutaneous fat and extracellular water decrease.
- ☐ 3. The dermis becomes highly vascular and assists in the regulation of body temperature.
- ☐ 4. Collagen becomes elastic and strong.

21. Which findings should the nurse expect to assess as normal skin changes in an elderly client? Select all that apply.
- ☐ 1. diminished hair on scalp and pubic areas
- ☐ 2. dusky rubor of left lower extremity
- ☐ 3. solar lentigo
- ☐ 4. wrinkles
- ☐ 5. xerosis
- ☐ 6. yellow pigmentation

22. Which problem related to changes of the integumentary system can result for the older adult undergoing abdominal surgery?
- ☐ 1. increased scarring
- ☐ 2. decreased melanin and melanocytes
- ☐ 3. decreased healing
- ☐ 4. increased immunocompetence

23. Which activity reflects health maintenance for an otherwise healthy older adult?
- ☐ 1. drinks 1,500 mL of fluids per day
- ☐ 2. consumes a balanced diet of 1,200 cal/day
- ☐ 3. walks briskly for 10 minutes three times per week
- ☐ 4. sleeps at least 8 hours each night

24. Which factor puts an older adult at the **greatest** risk for impaired wound healing after abdominal surgery?
- ☐ 1. age 75 years
- ☐ 2. age 30 years, with poorly controlled diabetes
- ☐ 3. age 55 years, with myocardial infarction
- ☐ 4. age 60 years, with peripheral vascular disease

25. An older adult has several ecchymotic areas on the left arm. The nurse should further assess the client for (select all that apply):
- ☐ 1. elder abuse.
- ☐ 2. self-inflicted injury.
- ☐ 3. increased capillary fragility and permeability.
- ☐ 4. increased blood supply to the skin.
- ☐ 5. shingles

26. An older adult reports being cold in the room even though the thermostat is set at 75°F (24°C). The client may feel cold because older adults have:
- ☐ 1. increased cellular cohesion.
- ☐ 2. increased moisture content of the stratum corneum.
- ☐ 3. slower cellular renewal time.
- ☐ 4. decreased ability to thermoregulate.

27. What should the nurse instruct the client with tinea capitis to do? Select all that apply.
- ☐ 1. Place a dressing saturated with vinegar and water on the area.
- ☐ 2. Apply topical antibacterial ointment to the area.
- ☐ 3. Shampoo hair two or three times with selenium sulfide shampoo.
- ☐ 4. Use antibacterial soap for bathing.
- ☐ 5. Take antifungal medication as prescribed.

28. A **priority** for nursing care for an older adult who has pruritus, is continuously scratching the affected areas, and demonstrates agitation and anxiety regarding the itching is:
- ☐ 1. preventing infection.
- ☐ 2. instructing the client not to scratch.
- ☐ 3. increasing fluid intake.
- ☐ 4. avoiding social isolation.

29. The nurse is applying a hand mitt restraint for a client with pruritus (see figure). The nurse should **first**:
- ☐ 1. verify the prescription to use the restraint.
- ☐ 2. secure the mitt with ties around the wrist tied to the bed frame.
- ☐ 3. place a folded pillow under the wrist.
- ☐ 4. place the mitt on top of the hand.

30. An older adult client in stage 2 of Parkinson's disease is being discharged with cellulitis of the right lower extremity. The nurse should base the discharge plan on which information? Select all that apply.
- ☐ 1. The client has decreased tissue perfusion.
- ☐ 2. The client is at risk for skin breakdown.
- ☐ 3. The client is at risk for falls or injuries.
- ☐ 4. The client has difficulty communicating.
- ☐ 5. The client has limited activity.

31. An alert and oriented elderly client is admitted to the hospital for treatment of cellulitis of the left shoulder after an arthroscopy. Which fall prevention strategy is **most** appropriate for this client?
- ☐ 1. Keep all the lights on in the room at all times.
- ☐ 2. Use a night-light in the bathroom.
- ☐ 3. Keep all four side rails up at all times.
- ☐ 4. Place the client in a room with a camera monitor.

32. The nurse is discharging an older adult to home after hospitalization for cellulitis of the right foot. The client originally scraped the foot on a rock while walking barefoot outside; the scrape became infected and eventually required hospitalization for wound care and several days of IV antibiotics. After reviewing discharge instructions, what statement by the client indicates the need for further teaching by the nurse?
- ☐ 1. "I will eat lots of fruit and vegetables and take vitamin C to help this heal."
- ☐ 2. "I will be sure to wear shoes to protect my feet when I go out to get the mail."
- ☐ 3. "I will manage my pain by putting this foot up on a pillow when it hurts."
- ☐ 4. "I will take the antibiotics until the redness goes away and my foot feels better."

33. Prevention of skin breakdown and maintenance of skin integrity among older clients is important because they are at greater risk secondary to:
- ☐ 1. altered balance.
- ☐ 2. altered protective pressure sensation.
- ☐ 3. impaired hearing ability.
- ☐ 4. impaired visual acuity.

The Client with Shingles

34. The client has been diagnosed with herpes zoster (shingles). The nurse should include which information in a teaching plan? Select all that apply.
- ☐ 1. Instruct the client about taking antiviral agents as prescribed.
- ☐ 2. Demonstrate how to apply wet-to-dry dressings.
- ☐ 3. Explain how to follow proper hand hygiene techniques.
- ☐ 4. Assure the client that the pain from herpes zoster will be gone by 7 days.
- ☐ 5. Tell the client to remain in isolation in a bedroom until the lesions have healed.

35. Which client should receive a shingles vaccine? A client who:
- ☐ 1. has never had chickenpox.
- ☐ 2. is at risk for genital herpes.
- ☐ 3. is over 60 years of age.
- ☐ 4. has a compromised immune system.

36. A nurse is caring for an older adult with shingles. The client is experiencing considerable pain related to open blisters on the client's abdomen and back. The client is taking acyclovir and low-dose prednisone. The nurse has several prescriptions available. What additional medications or nursing care strategies to promote comfort may be helpful? Select all that apply.
- ☐ 1. diphenhydramine 25 mg by mouth every 6 hours prn
- ☐ 2. calamine lotion applied to the affected areas
- ☐ 3. cool, wet compresses to the affected areas
- ☐ 4. acetaminophen 325 mg by mouth every 6 hours prn
- ☐ 5. ondansetron 4 mg by mouth every 4 hours prn
- ☐ 6. diversionary activities to prevent client scratching

The Client with a Pressure Ulcer

37. The nurse is assessing a client with dark skin for the presence of a stage I pressure ulcer. The nurse should:
- ☐ 1. use a fluorescent light source to assess the skin.
- ☐ 2. inspect the skin only when the Braden score is above 12.
- ☐ 3. look for skin color that is darker than the surrounding tissue.
- ☐ 4. avoid touching the skin during inspection.

38. The nurse is assessing a client who is immobile and notes that an area of sacral skin is reddened, but not broken. The reddened area continues to blanch and refill with fingertip pressure. The **most** appropriate nursing action at this time is to:
- ☐ 1. apply a moist to moist dressing, being careful to pack just the wound bed.
- ☐ 2. consult with a wound-ostomy-continence nurse specialist.
- ☐ 3. reposition the client off of the reddened skin and reassess in a few hours.
- ☐ 4. complete and document a Braden skin breakdown risk score for the client.

39. The nurse is assessing a hospitalized older client for the presence of pressure ulcers. The nurse notes that the client has a 1" × 1" (3 cm × 3 cm) area on the sacrum in which there is skin breakdown as far as the dermis. What should the nurse note on the medical record?
- [ ] 1. stage I pressure ulcer
- [ ] 2. stage II pressure ulcer
- [ ] 3. stage III pressure ulcer
- [ ] 4. stage IV pressure ulcer

40. A stage II pressure ulcer is characterized by:
- [ ] 1. redness in the involved area.
- [ ] 2. muscle spasms in the involved area.
- [ ] 3. pain in the involved area.
- [ ] 4. tissue necrosis in the involved area.

41. The nurse is using home telehealth monitoring to manage care for an 80-year-old who is home bound. The client spends most of the day in bed. Two months ago, the nurse detected sacral redness from friction and shearing force of being in bed. Last month, the client had increased sacral redness, and the area was classified as a stage I pressure ulcer. On this visit, the nurse is assessing the sacral area using a video camera. The nurse compares the site from a visit made 1 month ago (see figure part **A**) to the assessment made at this visit (see figure part **B**). Upon comparing the change of the pressure ulcer from this visit to the previous visit, what should the nurse do **first**?
- [ ] 1. Instruct the home health aide to reposition the client every 2 hours while the client is awake.
- [ ] 2. Ask the client's daughter to observe the area and report changes to the nurse.
- [ ] 3. Contact the healthcare provider (HCP) to request a hydrocolloid dressing.
- [ ] 4. Make a home visit to verify the changes in the ulcer.

The Client with Skin Cancer

42. Which factor places a client at **greatest** risk for skin cancer?
- [ ] 1. fair skin and history of chronic sun exposure
- [ ] 2. Caucasian race and history of hypertension
- [ ] 3. dark skin and family history of skin cancer
- [ ] 4. dark skin and history of hypertension

43. A nurse is teaching a client about skin cancer. Which risk factors for skin cancer should the nurse explain? Select all that apply.
- [ ] 1. increasing age
- [ ] 2. exposure to chemical pollutants
- [ ] 3. long-term exposure to the sun
- [ ] 4. increased pigmentation
- [ ] 5. genetics
- [ ] 6. immunosuppression

44. The nurse is developing a program about skin cancer prevention for a community group. Which information should be included in the program? Select all that apply.
- [ ] 1. Purchase sunscreen containing benzophenones to block UVA and UVB rays.
- [ ] 2. Use sunscreen with a minimum of 30 sun protection factor (SPF).
- [ ] 3. Obtain genetic screening to identify risk of melanoma.
- [ ] 4. Apply sunscreen only on sunny days, especially between 1000 and 1400.
- [ ] 5. Have a pigmented lesion biopsied by shaving if it looks suspicious.
- [ ] 6. Rub baby oil to lubricate skin before going out in the sun.

45. A client with malignant melanoma asks the nurse about the prognosis. The nurse should base a response that informs the client that the prognosis depends on:
- [ ] 1. the amount of ulceration of the lesion.
- [ ] 2. the age of the client.
- [ ] 3. the location of the lesion on the body.
- [ ] 4. the thickness of the lesion.

Managing Care, Quality, and Safety of Clients with Health Problems of the Integumentary System

46. The nurse finds an unlicensed assistive personnel (UAP) massaging the reddened bony prominences of a client on bed rest. The nurse should:
- [ ] 1. Reinforce the UAP's use of this intervention over the bony prominences.
- [ ] 2. Explain that massage is effective because it improves blood flow to the area.
- [ ] 3. Inform the UAP that massage is even more effective when combined with lotion during the massage.
- [ ] 4. Instruct the UAP that massage is contraindicated because it decreases blood flow to the area.

47. The nurse manager on the orthopedic unit is reviewing a report that indicates that in the last month, five clients were diagnosed with pressure ulcers. The nurse manager should:

☐ **1.** use benchmarking procedures to compare the findings with other nursing units in the hospital.

☐ **2.** ask the staff education department to conduct an educational session about preventing pressure ulcers.

☐ **3.** institute a quality improvement plan that identifies contributing factors, proposes solutions, and sets improvement outcomes.

☐ **4.** conduct a chart audit to determine which nurses on which shifts were giving nursing care to the clients with pressure ulcers.

48. A client has been admitted to the hospital with draining foot lesions. What should the nurse do? Select all that apply.

☐ **1.** Place the client in a room with negative air pressure.

☐ **2.** Admit the client to a semiprivate room.

☐ **3.** Admit the client to a private room.

☐ **4.** Post a "contact isolation" sign on the door.

☐ **5.** Wear a protective gown when in the client's room.

☐ **6.** Wear gloves when providing direct care.

49. The nurse is to administer an antibiotic to a client with burns, but there is no medication in the client's medication box. What should the nurse do **first**?

☐ **1.** Inform the unit's shift coordinator.

☐ **2.** Contact the client's healthcare provider (HCP).

☐ **3.** Call the pharmacy department.

☐ **4.** Borrow the medication from another client.

50. A client has a wound on the ankle that is not healing. The nurse should assess the client for which risk factors for delayed wound healing? Select all that apply.

☐ **1.** atrial fibrillation

☐ **2.** advancing age

☐ **3.** type 2 diabetes mellitus

☐ **4.** hypertension

☐ **5.** smoking

51. The nurse is assessing the left lower extremity of a client with type 2 insulin-requiring diabetes and cellulitis. What should the nurse do?

☐ **1.** Instruct the client to elevate the left leg when sitting in the chair.

☐ **2.** Encourage the client to ambulate in the halls on the unit.

☐ **3.** Massage the left leg with alcohol to stimulate circulation.

☐ **4.** Cleanse the left lower leg with perfumed liquid soap.

52. A client is admitted with pneumonia and shingles with draining lesions over the right anterior and posterior chest wall. Of the nurses scheduled for the shift, which nurses may be assigned to care for this client? Select all that apply.

☐ **1.** 43-year-old female who had a preexposure varicella vaccination

☐ **2.** 48-year-old male who had shingles 1 year prior

☐ **3.** 32-year-old female who is in the first trimester of pregnancy

☐ **4.** 24-year-old female who has never had the pneumococcal vaccine

☐ **5.** 36-year-old male taking steroids for an autoimmune disease

Answers, Rationales, and Test-Taking Strategies

The answers and rationales for each question follow below, along with keys (🔑) to the client need (CN) and cognitive level (CL) for each question. In addition, you will also see a glossary icon (📖) highlighting specific terminology used on the licensing exam. As you check your answers, use the **Content Mastery and Test-Taking Skill Self-Analysis** *worksheet (tear-out worksheet in back of book) to identify the reason(s) for not answering the questions correctly. For additional information about test-taking skills and strategies for answering questions, refer to pages 12–23 and pages 35–36 in Part 1 of this book.*

The Client with Burns

1. 1,2,3. Clients who should be transferred to a burn center include children under age 10 or adults over age 50 with second- and third-degree burns on 10% or greater of their BSA, clients between ages 11 and 49 with second- and third-degree burns over 20% of their BSA, clients of any age with third-degree burns on more than 5% of their BSA, clients with smoke inhalation, and clients with chronic diseases, such as diabetes and heart or kidney disease.

🔑 CN: Management of care; CL: Analyze

2. 3. The nurse should have the client transported to a burn center. The client's age and the extent of the burns require care by a burn team, and the client meets triage criteria for referral to a burn center. Because of the age of the client and the extent of the burns, the nurse should not treat the burn. Scald burns are not at high risk for infection and do not need to be cleaned, covered, or treated with antibiotic cream at this time.

🔑 CN: Physiological adaptation; CL: Synthesize

3. 1. Fluid shifting into the interstitial space causes intravascular volume depletion and decreased perfusion to the kidneys. This would result in an increase in serum creatinine. Urine output should be frequently monitored and adequately maintained with intravenous fluid resuscitation that would be increased when a drop in urine output occurs. Urine output should be at least 30 mL/h. Fluid replacement is based on the Parkland or Brooke formula and also the client's response by monitoring urine output, vital signs, and CVP readings. Daily weight is important to monitor for fluid status. Little fluctuation in weight suggests that there is no fluid retention and the intake is equal to output. Exudative loss of albumin occurs in burns, causing a decrease in colloid osmotic pressure. The normal serum albumin is 3.5 to 5 g/dL (35 to 50 g/L).

🔑 CN: Physiological adaptation; CL: Analyze

4. 3. According to the rule of nines, this client has sustained burns on about 45% of the body surface. The right arm is calculated as being 9%, the right leg is 18%, and the anterior trunk is 18%, for a total of 45%.

🔑 CN: Physiological adaptation; CL: Apply

5. 3. Ensuring a urine output of 30 to 50 mL/h is the best measure of adequate fluid resuscitation. The heart rate is elevated, but is not an indicator of adequate fluid balance. The blood pressure is low, likely related to the hypervolemia, but urinary output is the more accurate indicator of fluid balance and kidney function. The sodium level is within normal limits.

🔑 CN: Physiologic adaptation; CL: Evaluate

6. 3. Removing dressings from severe burns exposes sensitive nerve endings to the air, which is painful. The client should be given a prescribed analgesic about one-half hour before the dressing change to promote comfort. The other activities are done as part of the whirlpool and dressing change process and not one-half hour beforehand.

🔑 CN: Reduction of risk potential; CL: Synthesize

7. 4. Nutritional support with sufficient calories and protein is extremely important for a client with severe burns because of the loss of plasma protein through injured capillaries and an increased metabolic rate. Gastric dilation and paralytic ileus commonly occur in clients with severe burns, making oral fluids and foods contraindicated. Water and electrolyte imbalances can be corrected by administration of IV fluids with electrolyte additives, although TPN typically includes all necessary electrolytes. Resting the gastrointestinal tract may help prevent paralytic ileus, and TPN provides vitamins and minerals; however, the primary reason for starting TPN is to provide the protein necessary for tissue healing.

🔑 CN: Pharmacological and parenteral therapies; CL: Evaluate

8. 2. Biologic dressings such as porcine grafts serve many purposes for a client with severe burns. They enhance the growth of epithelial tissues, minimize the overgrowth of granulation tissue, prevent loss of water and protein, decrease pain, increase mobility, and help prevent infection. They do not encourage growth of tougher skin, provide for permanent wound closure, or facilitate growth of subcutaneous tissue.

🔑 CN: Physiological adaptation; CL: Apply

9. 4. Analgesic administration to keep a burn victim comfortable is important but is unlikely to influence graft survival and effectiveness. Absence of infection, adequate vascularization, and immobilization of the grafted area promote an effective graft.

🔑 CN: Physiological adaptation; CL: Evaluate

10. 2. Rehabilitation efforts are implemented as soon as the client's condition is stabilized. Early emphasis on rehabilitation is important to decrease complications and to help ensure that the client will be able to make the adjustments necessary to return to an optimal state of health and independence. It is not possible to completely eliminate the client's pain; pain control is a major challenge in burn care.

🔑 CN: Basic care and comfort; CL: Synthesize

11. 4. Immediately after a burn, excessive potassium from cell destruction is released into the extracellular fluid. Hyponatremia is a common electrolyte imbalance in the burn client that occurs within the first week after being burned. Metabolic acidosis usually occurs as a result of the loss of sodium bicarbonate.

🔑 CN: Reduction of risk potential; CL: Analyze

12. 2. Airway management is the priority in caring for a burn client. Tracheostomy or endotracheal intubation is anticipated when significant thermal and smoke inhalation burns occur. Clients who have experienced burns to the face and neck usually will be compromised within 1 to 2 hours. Electrical burns of the hands and arms, even with cardiac arrhythmias, or a chemical burn of the chest and abdomen is not likely to result in the need for intubation. Secondhand smoke inhalation does influence an individual's respiratory status but does not require intubation unless the individual has an allergic reaction to the smoke.

🔑 CN: Physiological adaptation; CL: Analyze

13. 3. The decreased urine output, low blood pressure, low CVP, and high heart rate indicate hypovolemia and the need to increase fluid volume replacement. Furosemide is a diuretic that should not be given due to the existing fluid volume deficit. Fresh frozen plasma is not indicated. It is given for clients with deficient clotting factors who are bleeding. Fluid replacement used for burns is lactated Ringer's solution, normal saline, or albumin.

CN: Management of care; **CL:** Synthesize

14. 3. The inflammatory response begins when a burn is sustained. As a result of the burn, the immune system becomes impaired. There are a decrease in immunoglobulins, changes in white blood cells, alterations of lymphocytes, and decreased levels of interleukin. The human body's protective barrier, the skin, has been damaged. As a result, the burn client becomes vulnerable to infections. Education and interventions to maintain a positive self-concept would be appropriate during the rehabilitation phase. Promoting hygiene helps the client feel comfortable; however, the primary focus is on reducing the risk for infection.

CN: Safety and infection control; **CL:** Synthesize

15. 2. During the first 24 hours, fluid replacement for an adult burn client is based on total body weight and BSA burned. Lean muscle mass considers only muscle mass; replacement is based on total body weight. Total surface area is estimated by taking into account the individual's height and weight. Height is not a common variable used in formulas for fluid replacement.

CN: Physiological adaptation; **CL:** Apply

16. 4. Curling's ulcer, or gastrointestinal ulceration, occurs in about half of the clients with a burn injury. The incidence of ulceration appears proportional to the extent of the burns, and the ulceration is believed to be caused by hypersecretion of gastric acid and compromised gastrointestinal perfusion. Paralytic ileus and gastric distention do not result from hypersecretion of gastric acid and stress and thus are not expected findings at this time. Hiatal hernia is not necessarily a potential complication of a burn injury.

CN: Physiological adaptation; **CL:** Analyze

17. 2. The severe pain experienced by burn clients requires opioid analgesics. In addition, opioids such as morphine sedate and alleviate apprehension. Oral analgesics such as ibuprofen or acetaminophen are unlikely to be strong enough to effectively manage the intense pain experienced

by the client who is severely burned. Because of the altered tissue perfusion from the burn injury, intravenous medications are preferred. Antianxiety agents are not effective against pain.

CN: Pharmacological and parenteral therapies; **CL:** Synthesize

18. 750 mL/h. When calculating fluid replacement, only the burned portion of the TBSA is used to calculate fluid volume; thus, the nurse should administer the solution at 750 mL/h. Lactated Ringer's solution 4 mL × weight in kg × TBSA; half given over the first 8 hours and half given over the next 16 hours.

$$4 \text{ mL} \times 75 \text{ kg} \times 40 = 12{,}000 \text{ mL or}$$

$$\frac{4 \text{ mL} \times 75 \text{ kg} \times 40}{8 \text{ hours}} \times \frac{1}{2} = \frac{750 \text{ mL}}{\text{hour}}$$

$$12{,}000 \text{ mL} \times 21 = 6{,}000 \text{ mL}$$

$$\frac{6{,}000 \text{ mL}}{8 \text{ hours}} = 750 \text{ mL/h}$$

CN: Pharmacological and parenteral therapies; **CL:** Apply

The Older Adult with General Problems of the Integumentary System

19. 2. Noting changes from the normal expected findings is the most important component when assessing an older client's integumentary system. Comparing one extremity with the contralateral extremity (i.e., comparing one side with the other) is an important assessment step; however, the most important component is noting changes from an expected normal baseline. Noting wrinkles related to age is not of much consequence unless the client is admitted for cosmetic surgery to reduce the appearance of age-related wrinkling. Noting skin turgor is an assessment of fluid status, not an assessment of the integumentary system.

CN: Health promotion and maintenance; **CL:** Analyze

20. 2. With age, there is a decreased amount of subcutaneous fat, muscle laxity, degeneration of elastic fibers, and collagen stiffening. The outer layer of skin is almost completely replaced every 3 to 4 weeks. The vascular supply diminishes with age. Collagen thins and diminishes with age.

CN: Health promotion and maintenance; **CL:** Analyze

21. 1,3,4,5. Skin changes associated with aging include the following: diminished hair on scalp and pubic areas, solar lentigo (liver spots), wrinkles, and xerosis (dryness). Dusky rubor of the left lower extremity may indicate the individual has a venous stasis problem in the affected extremity and is generally associated with "unsuccessful aging." Yellow pigmentation of the skin that may be associated with liver inflammation is generally known as jaundice.

> CN: Health promotion and maintenance; CL: Analyze

22. 3. Normal aging consists of decreased proliferative capacity of the skin. Decreased collagen synthesis slows capillary growth, impairs phagocytosis among older clients, and results in slow healing. Increased scarring is not a result of age-related skin changes. Both melanin and melanocytes give color to the skin and hair but are increased with aging. There is a decrease in the immunocompetence of the aging client.

> CN: Health promotion and maintenance; CL: Analyze

23. 1. Drinking at least 1,500 mL of fluid per day helps the client stay well hydrated. Maintaining optimal fluid balance is important for all body systems. Caloric intake varies according to an individual's size and activity level. An intake of 1,200 cal/day may be insufficient for some older clients. Walking 10 minute/day is useful, but an otherwise healthy older client should try to walk 20 to 30 minute/day three or more times a week. It is important to get adequate rest; however, the amount of sleep needed varies with the individual.

> CN: Health promotion and maintenance; CL: Evaluate

24. 2. Poorly controlled diabetes is a serious risk factor for postoperative wound infection. Other factors that delay wound healing include advanced age, nutritional deficiencies (vitamin C, protein, zinc), inadequate blood supply, use of corticosteroid, infection, mechanical friction on the wound, obesity, anemia, and poor general health.

> CN: Reduction of risk potential; CL: Analyze

25. 1,2,3. The nurse should always assess an older adult who has signs of bruising (ecchymosis) for signs of abuse, self-inflicted injuries, or injuries that might have occurred from falls. Also, the aging process involves increased capillary fragility and permeability, and because older adults have a decreased amount of subcutaneous fat, it is also likely that there is an increased incidence of bruise-like lesions caused by collection of extravascular blood in the loosely structured dermis. In addition, older clients do not always realize that injury has occurred because of a diminished awareness of pain,

touch, and peripheral vibration. Blood supply to the skin decreases with aging and thus is not a cause of the ecchymotic areas. Shingles presents as a red rash and fluid-filled blisters.

> CN: Health promotion and maintenance; CL: Analyze

26. 4. Older clients have a decreased thermoregulation that is related to decreased blood supply and reabsorption of body fat. As a result, older adults are at risk for hypothermia. Cellular cohesion and moisture content diminish with age, and cellular renewal time is slowed; however, these do not result in impaired thermoregulation.

> CN: Health promotion and maintenance; CL: Analyze

27. 3,5. Tinea capitis is a contagious fungal infection of the hair shaft. The hair should be shampooed two or three times with selenium sulfide shampoo. An oral medication will typically be prescribed as well, since the shampoo alone will not cure tinea capitis. Vinegar and water may be used to treat tinea pedis. The most common fungal skin infection is tinea (also called ringworm because of its characteristic appearance of a ring or rounded tunnel under the skin). Tinea infections affect the head, body, groin, feet, and nails. Antibacterial ointment and soap are not effective for treating fungal infections.

> CN: Physiological adaptation; CL: Create

28. 1. The client is at risk for infection because of the pruritus, and the nurse should institute measures to help the client control the scratching such as cutting fingernails, using protective gloves or mitts, and, if necessary, using antianxiety medications. More information is required regarding the knowledge level of the client, but learning cannot take place when an individual's attention is distracted with pruritus. Increasing fluid intake is not a priority at this time. There are no data to indicate the client is experiencing social isolation.

> CN: Reduction of risk potential; CL: Synthesize

29. 1. Before using any restraints, the nurse must verify that a **healthcare provider (HCP)** has written a prescription for the restraint. The mitt does not need to be secured with ties. The client can move the hand as needed. It is not necessary to place a pillow under the wrist. The nurse should place the mitt on the palmar surface of the hand.

> CN: Safety and infection control; CL: Synthesize

30. 2,3. Usual aging is associated with dry skin; however, seborrhea (oily skin and dandruff) is one result of the biochemical changes associated with Parkinson's disease. The client with Parkinson's disease has a higher risk of skin breakdown due to the moist and oily skin. To maintain skin integrity, a client with Parkinson's disease needs frequent skin care and aeration of the skin. Gait instability in a client with Parkinson's disease is a result of muscle rigidity, change in the center of gravity, and gait shuffling. Because of these changes in gait and balance, the client is at higher risk for injuries in the environment, such as hitting furniture or obstacles in the client's path. As a result, the environment should be evaluated for potential injury or falls. Tissue perfusion and verbal communication are not problems typically associated with Parkinson's disease. The client should not experience activity intolerance from the cellulitis or Parkinson's disease.

CN: Pharmacological and parenteral therapies; CL: Analyze

31. 2. Many falls occur when older clients attempt to get to the bathroom at night. The risk is even greater in an unfamiliar environment. Use of a night-light in the bathroom enables the older adult client to see the way to the bathroom. Keeping the lights on in the room at all times may contribute to sensory overload and prevent adequate rest. Raised side rails paradoxically contribute to falls when the older client tries to climb over them to get to the bathroom. The upper side rails may be raised, but it is not recommended that all four side rails be elevated. Camera monitoring can be used but does nothing to prevent a fall.

CN: Safety and infection control; CL: Synthesize

32. 4. It is important for the client to understand the need to complete the entire course of oral antibiotics as prescribed in order to prevent recurrence/worsening of cellulitis. Further, if the pain and redness continue despite antibiotics, the client needs to understand the need to follow up with the healthcare provider. Extra vitamin C, protective footwear, and elevating the foot are strategies to promote healing.

CN: Management of care; CL: Synthesize

33. 2. Pressure ulcers usually occur over bony prominences. An alteration in the protective pressure sensation results from a decline in the number of Meissner's and pacinian corpuscles. Older adults do have altered balance that may result in falls but not skin breakdown. Impaired hearing and vision do not contribute to pressure ulcers.

CN: Reduction of risk potential; CL: Analyze

The Client with Shingles

34. 1,2,3. The nurse should instruct the client and family members about the importance of taking antiviral agents as prescribed. The client must be taught how to apply wet dressings or medication to the lesions and to follow proper hand hygiene techniques to avoid spreading the virus. The healing time varies from 7 to 26 days. The most common complication is postherpetic neuralgia, which may last longer than 6 months. It is not necessary for the client to remain in isolation.

CN: Health promotion and maintenance; CL: Create

35. 3. People older than 60 years should receive shingles vaccine to prevent the disease. The vaccine is not effective for genital herpes. The vaccine can be given to persons who have or have not had chickenpox. The vaccine is not advised for persons with a compromised immune system, for example, those receiving chemotherapy or radiation therapy.

CN: Health promotion and maintenance; CL: Apply

36. 1,2,3,4,6. Diphenhydramine is an antihistamine that reduces allergic reactions, calamine lotion is a topical antipruritic, and acetaminophen is an analgesic. These medications may help increase client comfort by reducing pain, inflammation, and itching, which, in turn, may reduce client scratching and potentially spreading the virus. Cool wet compresses also relieve itching and pain. Ondansetron is an antiemetic and would not be helpful for this client's discomfort.

CN: Physiological integrity; CL: Synthesize

The Client with a Pressure Ulcer

37. 3. When assessing a client with dark skin, the nurse should observe for skin that is darker, brownish, purplish, or bluish compared to surrounding skin. Fluorescent light casts a blue light, making skin assessment difficult; natural or halogen light sources help to accurately assess the skin. Risk assessment using the Braden Scale should be performed on all clients. A Braden score of 12 indicates a high risk for pressure ulcer, and the lower the Braden score, the higher the risk (no risk 19 to 23, at risk 15 to 18, moderate risk 13 to 14, high risk 10 to 12, and very high risk 9 or below). The nurse should touch the skin to assess consistency and temperature differences.

CN: Physiological adaptation; CL: Analyze

38. 3. A stage I ulcer presents as an area of intact, nonblanchable redness, usually over a bony prominence, caused by pressure. If a reddened area blanches and refills with fingertip pressure, it indicates that there is still some blood flow to the injured area, and the redness may be reversible. It may be appropriate to complete and document a Braden score or consult a wound nurse specialist, but it is imperative to reposition the client off the reddened skin area first. Since there is no break in the skin, it is not appropriate to apply a moist to moist dressing.

🔑 CN: Basic care and comfort; CL: Synthesize

39. 2. Stage I pressure ulcers appear as non-blanching macules that are red in color. Stage II ulcers have breakdown of the dermis. Stage III ulcers have full-thickness skin breakdown. In stage IV ulcers, the bone, muscle, and supporting tissue are involved. The nurse should immediately initiate plans to relieve the pressure, ensure good nutrition, and protect the area from abrasion.

🔑 CN: Reduction of risk potential; CL: Analyze

40. 3. A stage II skin breakdown involves epidermal sloughing and pain. Redness without blanching is noted in stage I. Stage III involves tissue necrosis with subcutaneous involvement. Stage IV involves muscle or bone destruction. Muscle spasm is not a criterion used in the staging process.

🔑 CN: Physiological adaptation; CL: Analyze

41. 3. The pressure ulcer has changed from stage I to stage II and requires the use of a protective dressing. Repositioning and use of foam mattresses are appropriate interventions for stage I pressure ulcers. While the daughter can assess the client and report changes, it is the nurse's responsibility to make decisions about needed care. Telehealth monitoring equipment is providing sufficient visualization of the skin changes; the nurse does not need to make a home visit at this time.

🔑 CN: Reduction of risk potential; CL: Synthesize

The Client with Skin Cancer

42. 1. Caucasians who have fair skin and a high exposure to ultraviolet light are at increased risk for malignant neoplasms of the skin. The other risk factors include exposure to tar and arsenicals and family history. History of hypertension is a coronary artery disease risk factor. Clients with dark skin have increased melanin and are not as prone to skin cancer.

🔑 CN: Health promotion and maintenance; CL: Analyze

43. 1,2,3,5,6. Risk factors associated with skin cancer include age, exposure to chemical pollutants, exposure to the sun, genetics, and immunosuppression. As individuals age, the risk of developing skin cancer increases. Longtime exposure to the sun and exposure to chemical pollutants (nitrates, coal, tar, etc.) increase the risk of skin cancer. Individuals who have less skin pigmentation (e.g., fair, blue-eyed people) have a higher risk of skin cancer because they tend to incur sunburns rather than tan. Family history plays a role in cancer. Regardless, immunosuppressed individuals are at a higher risk for the development of any type of cancer, as the body's defenses are not functioning properly.

🔑 CN: Health promotion and maintenance; CL: Apply

44. 1,2. Sunscreen should be applied 20 to 30 minutes before going outside, even in cloudy weather. Sunscreen with a minimum of 30 SPF should be used. Sunscreen containing benzophenones block both UVA and UVB rays. The rays of the sun are most dangerous between 1000 and 1400. Genetic screening is not indicated, although a mutated gene has been identified in some families with high incidence of melanoma. A prior diagnosis of melanoma and having a first-degree relative diagnosed with melanoma increase a person's risk. Lesions should not be shave biopsied; excisional biopsy technique is used. Baby oil will increase the adverse effects of sun exposure; sunscreen protection should be used.

🔑 CN: Health promotion and maintenance; CL: Create

45. 4. Tumor or lesion thickness is the predictive factor for survival. Cutaneous melanoma that is confined to the epidermis has a high cure rate. Asymmetry, border, color, and diameter are known as the "ABCDs" of melanoma. Thus, the amount of ulceration, age, and location are not clearly associated with the prognosis.

🔑 CN: Health promotion and maintenance; CL: Synthesis

Managing Care, Quality, and Safety of Clients with Health Problems of the Integumentary System

46. 4. Massaging areas that are reddened due to pressure is contraindicated because it further reduces blood flow to the area. The **UAP** 🔲 should not massage the bony prominences or use lotion on the area. Massage does improve circulation and blood flow to muscle areas; however, because the area is reddened, the client is at risk for further skin breakdown.

🔑 CN: Management of care; CL: Synthesize

47. 3. The problem of pressure ulcers in hospitalized clients is best addressed by using quality improvement techniques to identify the problem, determining strategies for improvement, and setting goals for outcomes. Benchmarking for comparison will indicate where this nursing unit compares with other units, but does not address the problem for this unit; having clients with pressure ulcers on any unit is not acceptable. Educational programs are more effective after there is an understanding of the problem. Chart audits and blaming do not solve the problem or address quality improvement measures.

⚷ CN: Management of care; CL: Synthesize

48. 3,4,5,6. Infection control policies must be followed to prevent the spread of infection. Until the pathogens are identified, the client must be isolated in a private room. Utilizing contact isolation and wearing a protective isolation gown and clean gloves, in addition to following isolation protocol to exit the room, may aid in the prevention of spread of infectious agents to others. A draining foot lesion does not require a negative air pressure room, which is primarily reserved for preventing spread of tuberculosis.

⚷ CN: Safety and infection control; CL: Synthesize

49. 3. By contacting the pharmacy to report the absence of the medication, the pharmacy can bring the medication to the client's medication box. From there on, the pharmacy can make sure the correct medications are present. Contacting the shift coordinator or the client's **HCP** 📖 will not correct the original cause of the variance. It is never appropriate to "borrow" a medication from another client.

⚷ CN: Management of care; CL: Synthesize

50. 2,3,5. Advancing age, type 2 diabetes mellitus, and smoking are risk factors for delayed healing. Advanced age slows collagen synthesis by fibroblasts, impairs circulation, and requires a longer time for epithelialization of the skin. Type 2 diabetes mellitus reduces supply of oxygen and nutrients secondary to vascular complications. Nicotine is a potent vasoconstrictor and impedes blood flow, which reduces the supply of oxygen and nutrients necessary for healing. Atrial fibrillation causes venous stasis in the atria, but does not have an effect on wound healing. Hypertension does not have an effect on healing.

⚷ CN: Reduction of risk potential; CL: Analyze

51. 1. The client has cellulitis and should elevate the affected area above heart level. Ambulation stimulates circulation and promotes deposition of pathogens in other areas of the body. Alcohol and perfumed soaps are drying to the skin. Massaging the lower extremities could dislodge a clot.

⚷ CN: Reduction of risk potential; CL: Synthesize

52. 1,2,4. While the 43-year-old female has not had chickenpox, she has been vaccinated against the disease. A person can have shingles twice, but there is nothing in the 48-year-old nurse's history that precludes him from caring for this client. Having or not having the pneumococcal vaccine does not preclude a healthcare worker for caring for someone with pneumonia or shingles. Anyone who is immunocompromised or pregnant is at an increased risk for contracting varicella and should not be assigned to care for a client with shingles. All healthcare workers should have evidence of immunity to varicella and, if not, should receive two doses of vaccine at the recommended intervals at the time of employment. However, in this scenario, the immunity status of the pregnant nurse is not given, and risk reduction is warranted.

⚷ CN: Management of care; CL: Synthesize

Responding to Emergencies, Mass Casualties, and Disasters

- Emergencies
- Mass Casualties
- Disasters
- Managing Care, Quality, and Safety of Clients
- Answers, Rationales, and Test-Taking Strategies

Emergencies

1. A client is admitted to the emergency department with a headache, weakness, and slight confusion. The healthcare provider (HCP) diagnoses carbon monoxide poisoning. What should the nurse do **first**?

- ☐ 1. Initiate gastric lavage.
- ☐ 2. Maintain body temperature.
- ☐ 3. Administer 100% oxygen by mask.
- ☐ 4. Obtain a psychiatric referral.

2. Three hours ago, a client was thrown from a car into a ditch and is now admitted to the emergency department in a stable condition with vital signs within normal limits, alert and oriented with good coloring, and an open fracture of the right tibia. For which sign should the nurse be especially alert?

- ☐ 1. hemorrhage
- ☐ 2. infection
- ☐ 3. deformity
- ☐ 4. shock

3. A client admitted to the emergency department with atrial fibrillation has a heart rate of 160 bpm. The nurse should implement which prescription **first**?

- ☐ 1. Administer a heparin bolus.
- ☐ 2. Administer a beta-blocker.
- ☐ 3. Administer oxygen via nasal cannula.
- ☐ 4. Prepare the client for an immediate cardioversion.

4. A client is admitted to the emergency department with atrial fibrillation and does not recall how long the rapid pulse and irregular heart rate has been occurring. The nurse should include which goals of care at this time? Select all that apply.

- ☐ 1. Convert the heart rate to sinus rhythm.
- ☐ 2. Decrease cardiac output and workload.
- ☐ 3. Increase exercise tolerance.
- ☐ 4. Maintain a ventricular response below 100 bpm.
- ☐ 5. Prevent an embolic stroke.

5. The nurse is discharging a client who had a fish hook embedded in the eye. The fish hook was removed surgically in the emergency department, but the client currently has no vision in that eye. The surgeon has informed the client that a corneal transplant may restore some vision but the surgery cannot be performed for 6 to 8 weeks and only if no infection occurs. A **priority** in the teaching plan includes:

- ☐ 1. resting to reduce strain to the eye and promote healing after surgery.
- ☐ 2. washing hands carefully to keep the area clean and decrease risk of infection.
- ☐ 3. verbalizing feelings regarding vision loss.
- ☐ 4. eating a healthy diet to promote healing and prevent constipation.

6. A client is admitted to the emergency department with sneezing and coughing. The client is in the triage area, waiting to be seen by a healthcare provider (HCP). To prevent spread of infection to others in the area and to the healthcare staff, the nurse should:

- ☐ 1. place the client in an isolation room.
- ☐ 2. ask the others in the area to move away from the client.
- ☐ 3. give the client a surgical mask to wear.
- ☐ 4. ask the client to wash the hands before being examined.

7. There has been a car accident involving four vehicles on a remote highway. The nearest emergency department is 15 minutes away. Which victim should be transported by helicopter rather than an ambulance to the nearest hospital?

- ☐ 1. a 10-year-old with a simple fracture of the femur, who is crying and cannot find his parents
- ☐ 2. a middle-aged female with cold, clammy skin, heart rate of 120 bpm, and is unconscious
- ☐ 3. middle-aged male with severe asthma, heart rate of 120 bpm, and is having difficulty breathing
- ☐ 4. an older adult with severe headache, but conscious

8. The nurse notices a fire in a wastebasket in a client's room. In which order of priority from first to last should the nurse perform the actions? All options must be used.

> **1.** Confine the fire by closing the door to the client's room.

> **2.** Extinguish the fire.

> **3.** Remove the client from the room.

> **4.** Pull the fire alarm at the alarm pull station.

>

>

>

>

9. A client is admitted to the emergency department with a full-thickness burn to the right arm. Upon assessment, the arm is edematous, fingers are mottled, and radial pulse is now absent. The client states that the pain is 8 on a scale of 1 to 10. The nurse should:
- ☐ **1.** administer morphine sulfate IV push for the severe pain.
- ☐ **2.** call the healthcare provider (HCP) to report the loss of the radial pulse.
- ☐ **3.** continue to assess the arm every hour for any additional changes.
- ☐ **4.** instruct the client to exercise the fingers and wrist.

10. A client is brought to the emergency department with abdominal trauma following an automobile accident. The vital signs are as follows: heart rate, 132 bpm; respirations, 28 breaths/min; blood pressure, 84/58 mm Hg; temperature, 97.0°F (36.1°C); and oxygen saturation 89% on room air. Which prescription should the nurse implement **first**?
- ☐ **1.** Administer 1 L 0.9% normal saline IV.
- ☐ **2.** Draw a complete blood count (CBC) with hematocrit and hemoglobin.
- ☐ **3.** Obtain an abdominal x-ray.
- ☐ **4.** Insert an indwelling urinary catheter.

11. A middle-aged man collapses in the emergency department waiting room. The triage nurse should **first**:
- ☐ **1.** Ask the client to state his name.
- ☐ **2.** Perform the head tilt/chin lift to open the victim's airway.
- ☐ **3.** Feel for any air movement from the victim's nose or mouth.
- ☐ **4.** Watch the client's chest for respirations.

12. A client is experiencing an allergic response. The nurse should perform the actions in which order from first to last? All options must be used.

> **1.** Assess for urticaria.

> **2.** Assess the airway and breathing pattern.

> **3.** Notify the healthcare provider (HCP).

> **4.** Activate the rapid response team.

>

>

>

>

13. Proper hand placement for chest compressions during cardiopulmonary resuscitation (CPR) is essential to reduce the risk of which complication?
- ☐ **1.** gastrointestinal bleeding
- ☐ **2.** myocardial infarction
- ☐ **3.** emesis
- ☐ **4.** rib fracture

14. Automated external defibrillators (AEDs) are used in cardiac arrest situations for:
- ☐ **1.** early defibrillation in cases of atrial fibrillation.
- ☐ **2.** cardioversion in cases of atrial fibrillation.
- ☐ **3.** pacemaker placement.
- ☐ **4.** early defibrillation in cases of ventricular fibrillation.

15. Indicate on the illustration where the nurse would place the other electrode of the automated external defibrillator (AED) on a victim who has collapsed and does not have a pulse.

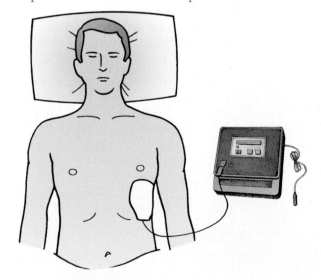

16. An adult has been admitted to the emergency department diagnosed with food poisoning following an outdoor picnic. What should the nurse do? Select all that apply.
☐ 1. Tell the family to discard contaminated food.
☐ 2. Collect specimens for laboratory examination.
☐ 3. Assess vital signs.
☐ 4. Initiate support for the respiratory system.
☐ 5. Monitor fluid and electrolyte status.
☐ 6. Provide antiemetics, as prescribed.

17. A client is admitted to the emergency department after being found in a daze walking away from her burning car after an accident. She was not injured in the accident, but the other driver died. She states, "I cannot handle it anymore. There is no point to it all." The crisis nurse recommends hospital admission based on the identification of which concern?
☐ 1. The client was walking around in a daze.
☐ 2. The client has a lack of knowledge of what to do next.
☐ 3. The client is having delusions and is not in touch with reality.
☐ 4. The client is expressing helplessness and hopelessness and is a risk for suicide.

18. A client is brought to the emergency department via ambulance accompanied by her sister. The sister states, "She was playing cards with us and had a seizure. Then she had another seizure just as the first one was stopping, so I called the ambulance." The client is currently not demonstrating any seizure activity, her eyes are closed, and she does not respond to commands. Which intervention should the nurse implement **first**?
☐ 1. Make sure suction equipment is set up bedside.
☐ 2. Draw blood for a phenytoin level.
☐ 3. Assess the client's vital signs.
☐ 4. Prepare the client for a head computed tomography (CT).

19. The nurse in the emergency department reports there is a possibility of having had direct contact with blood of a client who is suspected of having HIV/AIDS. The nurse requests that the client have a blood test. Consent for human immunodeficiency virus (HIV) testing can only be completed when which circumstances are present? Select all that apply.
☐ 1. An emergency medical provider has been exposed to the client's blood or body fluids.
☐ 2. Testing is prescribed by a healthcare provider (HCP) under emergency circumstances.
☐ 3. Testing is prescribed by a court, based on evidence that the client poses a threat to others.
☐ 4. Testing is done on blood collected anonymously in an epidemiologic survey.
☐ 5. A healthcare provider (HCP) who is taking care of a client suspected of having HIV/AIDS requests a blood test.

Mass Casualties

20. Thirty people are injured in a train derailment. Which client should be transported to the hospital **first**?
☐ 1. a 20-year-old who is unresponsive and has a high injury to his spinal cord
☐ 2. an 80-year-old who has a compound fracture of the arm
☐ 3. a 10-year-old with a laceration on his leg
☐ 4. a 25-year-old with a sucking chest wound

21. An explosion at a chemical plant produces flames and smoke. More than 20 persons have burn injuries. Which victims, all adults, should be transported to a burn center? Select all that apply.
☐ 1. the victim with chemical spills on both arms
☐ 2. the victim with third-degree burns of both legs
☐ 3. the victim with first-degree burns of both hands
☐ 4. the victim in respiratory distress
☐ 5. the victim who inhaled smoke

22. An apartment fire spreads to seven apartment units. Victims suffer burns, minor injuries, and broken bones from jumping from windows. Which client should be transported **first**?
☐ 1. a woman who is 5 months pregnant with no apparent injuries
☐ 2. a middle-aged man with no injuries who has rapid respirations and coughs
☐ 3. a 10-year-old with a simple fracture of the humerus who is in severe pain
☐ 4. a 20-year-old with first-degree burns on her hands and forearms

23. There is a shooting in a shopping mall. Three victims with gunshot wounds are brought to the emergency department. What should the nurse do to preserve forensic evidence? Select all that apply.
☐ 1. Cut around blood stains to remove clothing.
☐ 2. Place each item of clothing in a separate paper bag.
☐ 3. Hang wet clothing to dry.
☐ 4. Refrain from documenting client statements.
☐ 5. Place bullets in a sterile container.

24. An airplane crash results in mass casualties. The nurse is directing personnel to tag all victims. Which information should be placed on the tag? Select all that apply.
☐ 1. triage priority
☐ 2. identifying information when possible (such as name, age, and address)
☐ 3. medications and treatments administered
☐ 4. presence of jewelry
☐ 5. next of kin

25. Four people who have been injured in a car accident are admitted to the emergency department. Using the emergency severity index (ESI), in which order should the victims be seen by a healthcare provider (HCP)?

1. an adult with severe bleeding from a laceration in the leg

2. a child with lacerations on the arms and legs

3. an adult with a history of asthma and respirations of 30 breaths per minute.

4. an older adult with normal vital signs, but is confused

26. A small airplane crashes in a neighborhood of 10 houses. One of the victims appears to have a cervical spine injury. What should first aid for this victim include? Select all that apply.
☐ 1. Establish an airway with the jaw-thrust maneuver.
☐ 2. Immobilize the spine.
☐ 3. Logroll the victim to a side-lying position.
☐ 4. Elevate the feet 6 inches (15.2 cm).
☐ 5. Place a cervical collar around the neck.

27. Thirty-two children are brought to the emergency department after a school bus accident. Two children were killed along with the three people in the car that caused the crash. Before the victims arrive, in addition to ensuring that the hospital staff are prepared for the emergency, which step should the nurse anticipate carrying out?
☐ 1. calling the nearest crisis response team
☐ 2. alerting the news media
☐ 3. notifying the hospital volunteer office
☐ 4. calling the school to inform teachers of the accident

28. The nurse in the emergency department is triaging victims of an airplane crash. Prioritize the clients in the order in which they should be treated from first to last. All options must be used.

1. a 75-year-old with a 2-inch (5.1-cm) laceration to the left forearm

2. a 22-year-old with a 2-inch (5.1-cm) laceration to the left temple, slightly confused

3. a 14-year-old with a 2-inch (5.1-cm) laceration to the chin, history of asthma, respirations 26 breaths/min, audible wheezing

4. a 22-year-old female, 36 weeks pregnant with contractions every 10 to 15 minutes

Disasters

29. A suspected outbreak of anthrax has been transmitted by skin exposure. A client is admitted to the emergency department with lesions on the hands. The healthcare provider prescribes antibiotics and sends the client home. What should the nurse instruct the client to do? Select all that apply.
☐ 1. Take the prescribed antibiotics for 60 days.
☐ 2. Avoid contact with other members of the family during the treatment period.
☐ 3. Wear a mask for 60 days.
☐ 4. Expect the skin lesions to clear up within 1 to 2 weeks.
☐ 5. Wash hands frequently.

30. A severe acute respiratory syndrome (SARS) epidemic is suspected in a community of 10,000 people. As clients with SARS are admitted to the hospital, what type of precautions should the nurse institute?
☐ 1. enteric precautions
☐ 2. handwashing precautions
☐ 3. reverse isolation precautions
☐ 4. airborne precautions

31. Several clients who work in the same building are brought to the emergency department. They all have fever, headache, a rash over the entire body, and abdominal pain with vomiting and diarrhea. Upon initial assessment, the nurse finds that each client has low blood pressure and has developed petechiae in the area where the blood pressure cuff was inflated. Which isolation precautions should the nurse initiate?

- ☐ **1.** contact isolation with double gloving and shoe covers
- ☐ **2.** respiratory isolation with positive pressure rooms
- ☐ **3.** enteric precautions
- ☐ **4.** reverse isolation

32. Eight farm workers are admitted to the emergency department after they were splashed with "a couple of chemicals" at work 30 minutes ago. They have watery/itchy eyes, slight cough, diaphoresis, and constricted pupils and are conscious and oriented. Their clothes are wet. What action should the nurse do **first**?

- ☐ **1.** Apply oxygen at 3 L per nasal cannula.
- ☐ **2.** Remove their clothing.
- ☐ **3.** Begin decontamination shower.
- ☐ **4.** Isolate the clients.

33. The nurse is triaging victims of an earthquake who were removed from a building following its collapse. Which victims should be classified as red? Select all that apply.

- ☐ **1.** a 10-year-old male with crushing chest wound, tachypnea with labored breathing, unconscious, impaled object in the forehead
- ☐ **2.** a 49-year-old male with crushing chest pain radiating to the jaw, is diaphoretic, nauseated, and has an open fracture of the left wrist
- ☐ **3.** a 75-year-old female with obvious fracture of the femur, absent pedal pulses on the affected side; heart rate 110 bpm, respirations 34 breaths/min, skin diaphoretic; awake/alert, states pain is 10 on a scale of 1 to 10
- ☐ **4.** a 32-year-old female who is unconscious, 3-inch (7.6-cm) laceration to her forehead, ecchymosis behind the ears, respiratory rate 10 breaths/min and shallow; radial pulse is weak/thready/rapid; no breath sounds on the right side

34. The nurse is assessing the client (see photo) who has recently returned from a 2-month mission in Africa. What type of respiratory protection is appropriate for the staff?

- ☐ **1.** N95 particulate respirator
- ☐ **2.** double-layered surgical mask
- ☐ **3.** surgical mask with eye shield
- ☐ **4.** no respiratory protection needed

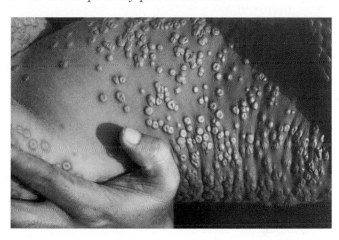

Managing Care, Quality, and Safety of Clients

35. A client who was a victim of a gunshot wound was treated in the emergency department and died. What should the nurse direct the unlicensed assistive personnel (UAP) to do during postmortem care? Select all that apply.

- ☐ **1.** Remove all tubes and IV lines.
- ☐ **2.** Cover the body with a sheet.
- ☐ **3.** Notify the family.
- ☐ **4.** Transport the body to the morgue.
- ☐ **5.** Notify the chaplain.

36. The nurse in the emergency department is administering a prescription for 20 mg intravenous furosemide, which is to be given immediately. The nurse scans the client's identification band and the medication barcode. The medication administration system does not verify that furosemide is prescribed for this client; however, the furosemide is prepared in the accurate unit dose for intravenous infusion. What should the nurse do **next**?

- ☐ **1.** Contact the pharmacist immediately to check the prescription and the barcode label for accuracy.
- ☐ **2.** Administer the medication now, knowing the medication is labeled and the client is identified.
- ☐ **3.** Report the problem to the information technology team to have the barcode system recalibrated.
- ☐ **4.** Ask another nurse to verify the medication and the client so the medication can be given now.

37. The nurse notices a pair of nervous-acting individuals entering the emergency department. When reporting suspicious activity, the nurse should include which information in the report? Select all that apply.
- ☐ 1. vehicle/vehicles description
- ☐ 2. current location of parties involved
- ☐ 3. names and phone numbers of parties involved
- ☐ 4. relationship to hospitalized client
- ☐ 5. tone of voice of each party involved

38. There has been an increase in medication errors and errors in prescribing laboratory studies in the emergency department. The nurse manager is conducting a staff education session on when to use "read-back" procedures. "Read-back" procedures should be performed in which situations? Select all that apply.
- ☐ 1. when a medication prescription or critical laboratory result is received verbally or over the telephone
- ☐ 2. when any verbal or phone prescription is received
- ☐ 3. whenever a written prescription or printed critical test result is received
- ☐ 4. when the unit secretary takes a phone prescription
- ☐ 5. when the agency uses computerized healthcare records

39. Which client admitted to the emergency department should the nurse see **first**? A client:
- ☐ 1. experiencing a "ripping" sensation in the chest.
- ☐ 2. with a blood pressure of 170/95 mm Hg.
- ☐ 3. with a urine output of 240 mL in 12 hours.
- ☐ 4. taking anticoagulants with bloody stool.

Answers, Rationales, and Test-Taking Strategies

*The answers and rationales for each question follow below, along with keys (🔑) to the client need (CN) and cognitive level (CL) for each question. In addition, you will also see a glossary icon (📖) highlighting specific terminology used on the licensing exam. As you check your answers, use the **Content Mastery and Test-Taking Skill Self-Analysis** worksheet (tear-out worksheet in back of book) to identify the reason(s) for not answering the questions correctly. For additional information about test-taking skills and strategies for answering questions, refer to pages 12–23 and pages 35–36 in Part 1 of this book.*

Emergencies

1. 3. Carbon monoxide poisoning develops when carbon monoxide combines with hemoglobin. Because carbon monoxide combines more readily with hemoglobin than oxygen does, tissue anoxia results. The nurse should administer 100% oxygen by mask to reduce the half-life of carboxyhemoglobin. Gastric lavage is used for ingested poisons. With tissue anoxia, metabolism is diminished, with a subsequent lowering of the body's temperature; thus, steps to increase body temperature would be required. Unless the carbon monoxide poisoning is intentional, a psychiatric referral would be inappropriate.

🔑 CN: Physiological adaptation; CL: Synthesize

2. 2. Because of the degree of contamination of the open fracture and the time that has passed since the accident, the risk of infection is very high. Therefore, the nurse should be especially alert for signs and symptoms of possible existing infection or early signs of infections, such as debris in the wound site, temperature abnormalities, results of laboratory studies (such as complete blood cell count and wound culture and sensitivities), or heat or redness around or in the wound. Because the client's vital signs and cardiovascular status are stable at this time, hemorrhage is not the primary concern. The client is talking coherently at this point, which does not suggest shock. However, the nurse should continue to assess the client for signs and symptoms of hemorrhage and shock. The fracture would be corrected by surgery as soon as possible, thereby minimizing the risk of deformity.

🔑 CN: Physiological adaptation; CL: Analyze

3. 3. The nurse should first administer oxygen; in atrial fibrillation, the workload of the heart is increased, and as a result, myocardial oxygen demands are also increased. A heparin bolus may be prescribed; it is not clear how long the client has been in atrial fibrillation, and it is critical to determine this before treatment is initiated. Beta-blockers and cardioversion are not primary interventions, and it is important first to determine if the client is hemodynamically stable and the length of time the client has had atrial fibrillation.

🔑 CN: Physiological integrity; CL: Analyze

4. 3,4,5. Clients who experience atrial fibrillation for more than 48 hours are at an increased risk of developing blood clots due to stasis of blood in the atria. Initially, it will be important to maintain a ventricular heart rate of <100 bpm and prevent complications related to clot formation including an embolic stroke. Decreasing heart rate will help to increase exercise tolerance. Atrial fibrillation causes a decrease in cardiac output, and a goal of therapy would be to increase cardiac output. It is imperative to determine the length of time a client has been in atrial fibrillation prior to performing a cardioversion. If a client has been in atrial fibrillation longer than 48 hours and a cardioversion is performed, a clot may be dislodged and find its way to the brain, lungs, or coronary arteries.

CN: Physiological integrity;
CL: Synthesize

5. 2. Infection prevention is the immediate priority for this client in order to promote healing and successful corneal transplant with potential restoration of vision. Rest and a diet rich in nutrients and fiber to prevent straining due to constipation are important considerations as well as allowing the client to discuss feelings regarding vision loss. However, these are currently lower priority than infection prevention.

CN: Reduction of risk potential;
CL: Analyze

6. 3. In order to prevent infections in hospitals, the nurse institutes measures to contain respiratory secretions in symptomatic clients. The nurse gives the client a mask to wear and tissues; the nurse instructs the client to dispose of used tissues in a no-touch receptacle. It is not necessary to place the client in isolation. It is not appropriate to ask others to move away from the client, but the nurse can ask the client to keep 3 feet away from others in the waiting room, if there is room. The nurse instructs the client to perform hand hygiene after blowing his nose or touching his nose or face, but doing so is not a prerequisite for being examined by the **HCP** . The nurse and HCP also use hand hygiene practices when caring for this client.

CN: Safety and infection control;
CL: Synthesize

7. 2. The middle-aged female is likely in shock; she is classified as a triage level I, requiring immediate care. The child with moderate trauma is classified as triage level III, urgent, and can be treated within 30 minutes. The man with asthma and the man with the severe headache are classified as emergent, triage level II, and can be transported by ambulance and reach the hospital within 15 minutes.

CN: Physiological adaptation;
CL: Synthesize

8. 3,4,1,2. The nurse uses the RACE procedure to manage a fire: Rescue, Alarm, Confine, Extinguish.

CN: Safety and infection control;
CL: Apply

9. 2. Circulation can be impaired by circumferential burns and edema, causing compartment syndrome. Early recognition and treatment of impaired blood supply is key. The **HCP** should be informed since an escharotomy (incision through full-thickness eschar) is frequently performed to restore circulation. Pain management is important for burn clients, but restoration of circulation is the priority. Assessments should be performed every 15 minutes while there is absence of the radial pulse. Exercise will not restore the obstructed circulation.

CN: Safety and infection control;
CL: Synthesize

10. 1. The client is demonstrating vital signs consistent with fluid volume deficit, likely due to bleeding and/or hypovolemic shock as a result of the automobile accident. The client will need intravenous fluid volume replacement using an isotonic fluid (e.g., 0.9% normal saline) to expand or replace blood volume and normalize vital signs. The other prescriptions can be implemented once the intravenous fluids have been initiated.

CN: Physiologic adaptation; CL: Analyze

11. 1. Calling the victim's name and gently shaking the victim is used to establish unresponsiveness. The head-tilt, chin-lift maneuver is used to open the victim's airway. Feeling for any air movement from the victim's nose or mouth indicates whether the victim is breathing on his own. The rescuer can watch the victim's chest for respirations to see if the victim is breathing.

CN: Physiological adaptation;
CL: Synthesize

12. 2,1,4,3. If a client is experiencing an allergic response, the nurse's initial action is to assess the client for signs/symptoms of anaphylaxis, first checking the airway, breathing pattern, and vital signs, with particular attention to signs of increasing edema and respiratory distress. The nurse should then assess for other indications of anaphylaxis, such as urticaria, feelings of impending doom or fright, weakness, sweating (because a severe systemic response to an allergen can result in massive vasodilation), increased capillary permeability, decreased perfusion, decreased venous return, and subsequent decreased cardiac output. The nurse should call the **rapid response team** and then notify the **HCP** .

CN: Reduction of risk potential;
CL: Synthesize

13. 4. Proper hand placement during chest compressions is essential to reduce the risk of rib fractures, which may lead to pneumothorax and other internal injuries. Gastrointestinal bleeding and myocardial infarction are generally not considered complications of CPR. Although the victim may vomit during CPR, this is not associated with poor hand placement, but rather with distention of the stomach.

CN: Physiological adaptation; CL: Apply

14. 4. AEDs are used for early defibrillation in cases of ventricular fibrillation. The AHA and Canadian Heart and Stroke Foundation place major emphasis on early defibrillation for ventricular fibrillation and use of the AED as a tool to increase sudden cardiac arrest survival rates.

CN: Reduction of risk potential; CL: Apply

15. One electrode is placed to the right of the upper sternum just below the right clavicle. The other is placed, as shown, over the fifth or sixth intercostal space at the left anterior axillary line.

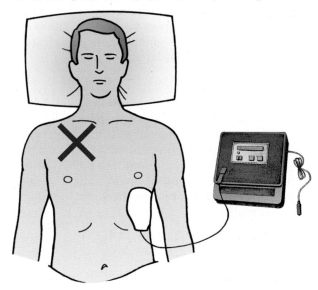

CN: Reduction of risk potential; CL: Apply

16. 2,3,4,5,6. Food poisoning is a sudden illness that occurs after ingestion of contaminated food or drink. The nurse should first assess vital signs and then ensure that the client is not in respiratory distress because death from respiratory paralysis can occur with botulism, fish poisoning, and other food poisonings. Measures to control nausea are important to prevent vomiting, which could exacerbate fluid and electrolyte imbalance. Because large volumes of electrolytes and water are lost by vomiting and diarrhea, fluid and electrolyte status needs to be continuously monitored. The key to treatment is determining the source and type of food poisoning. If possible, rather than discarding the food, the suspected food should be brought to the medical facility and a history obtained from the client or family.

CN: Physiological adaptation; CL: Synthesize

17. 4. The client is demonstrating helplessness and hopelessness during a crisis, as evidenced by her statement, "I cannot handle it. There is no point to it." Feelings of helplessness and hopelessness are common factors associated with suicidal ideation. Therefore, the client must be hospitalized to ensure safety to herself. There is not sufficient information to know if the client has a lack of knowledge of what to do next. The client is not having delusions, which would be evidenced by statements such as "The devil set my car on fire," not just the inability to think clearly.

CN: Psychosocial integrity; CL: Analyze

18. 1. Following a seizure (postictal stage), the client will most likely be tired and want to sleep. Maintaining the airway is the priority; the nurse should verify that suction equipment is available in case the client aspirates or chokes. Assessing vital signs and obtaining a phenytoin level are both appropriate actions by the nurse, but assuring safety is the first priority. There is no indication of a need to obtain a head CT at this time.

CN: Physiological integrity; CL: Synthesize

19. 1,2,3,4. Upon an **HCP's** 📖 written prescription requesting an HIV test for a client, **consent** 📖 for HIV testing must be obtained. Consent exceptions include the following: testing is prescribed by an HCP under emergency circumstances, and the test is medically necessary to diagnose or treat the client's condition; testing is prescribed by a court, based on clear and convincing evidence of a serious and present health threat to others posed by an individual; testing is done on blood collected or tested anonymously as part of an epidemiologic survey; or an emergency medical provider has been exposed to the client's blood or body fluids.

CN: Safety and infection control; CL: Apply

Mass Casualties

20. 4. During a disaster, the nurse must make difficult decisions about which persons to treat first. The guidelines for triage offer general priorities for immediate, delayed, minimal, and expectant care. The client with a sucking chest wound needs immediate attention and will likely survive. The 80-year-old is classified as delayed; emergency response personnel can immobilize the fracture and cover the wound. The 10-year-old has minimal injuries and can wait to be treated. The client with a spinal cord injury is not likely to survive and should not be among the first to be transported to the healthcare facility.

CN: Management of care; CL: Analyze

21. 1,2,4,5. Victims with chemical burns, second- and third-degree burns over more than 20% of their body surface area, and those with inhalation injuries should be transported to a burn center. The victim with first-degree burns of the hands can be treated with first aid on the scene and referred to a healthcare facility.

CN: Management of care; CL: Analyze

22. 2. The man with respiratory distress and coughing should be transported first because he is probably experiencing smoke inhalation. The pregnant woman is not in imminent danger or likely to have a precipitous birth. The 10-year-old is not at risk for infection and could be treated in an outpatient facility. First-degree burns are considered less urgent.

CN: Management of care; CL: Analyze

23. 2,3. Preserving forensic evidence is essential for investigative purposes following injuries that may be caused by criminal intent. The nurse should put each item of clothing in a separate paper bag and label it; wet clothing should be hung to dry. The nurse should not cut or otherwise unnecessarily handle clothing, particularly clothing with such evidence as blood or body fluids. The nurse should document carefully the client's description of the incident and use quotes around the client's exact words where possible. The documentation will become a part of the client's record and can be subpoenaed for subsequent investigation. The nurse should not handle bullets from the client because they are an important piece of forensic evidence.

CN: Management of care; CL: Apply

24. 1,2,3. Tracking victims of disasters is important for casualty planning and management. All victims should receive a tag, securely attached, that indicates the triage priority, any available identifying information, and what care, if any, has been given along with time and date. Tag information should be recorded in a disaster log and used to track victims and inform families. It is not necessary to document the presence of jewelry or next of kin.

CN: Management of care; CL: Apply

25. 1,3,2,4. Using the emergency severity index, the nurse should triage the clients to be seen by an **HCP** as follows: the adult with severe bleeding is categorized as level 1, life threatening and should be seen first; the adult with asthma and rapid bleeding is in the emergent category and should be seen next; the child with lacerations is categorized as less urgent and can be seen next; and the older adult has vital signs within normal range and is assessed as being nonurgent and can be seen last.

CN: Management of care; CL: Analyze

26. 1,2. The victim of a neck injury should be immobilized and moved as little as possible. It is also important to ensure an open airway; this can be accomplished with the jaw-thrust maneuver, which does not require tilting the head. The victim should not be rolled to a side-lying position nor have his feet elevated. Both actions can cause additional injury to the spinal cord. Placing a cervical collar causes movement of the spinal column and should not be done as a first aid measure.

CN: Management of care; CL: Synthesize

27. 1. The children and their families are at risk for experiencing a crisis. Disaster teams are available for crisis intervention in such emergencies. Usually, the news media monitors emergency radio frequencies and most likely are aware of the accident already. Although volunteers may help in some ways, they are not responsible for crisis intervention. Calling the school might be done, but the emergency issues take precedence.

CN: Psychosocial integrity; CL: Synthesize

28. 3,2,4,1. The 14-year-old with asthma needs immediate, lifesaving interventions for the wheezing and should be seen first. The 22-year-old who is confused should be seen next to assess for head injury; the location of the laceration could indicate a significant blunt force traumatic injury. The pregnant female requires assessment but is not urgent unless other symptoms appear. The 75-year-old is nonurgent and can wait safely for several hours.

CN: Management of care; CL: Evaluate

Disasters

29. 1,4. Anthrax is treated with antibiotics, and the client must continue the prescription for 60 days, even if symptoms do not persist. The client may have skin lesions at the point of contact, with macula or papule formation; the eschar will fall off in 1 to 2 weeks. Clients with anthrax are not contagious; the client does not need to follow isolation procedures at home. Anthrax from skin exposure is not transmitted by respiratory contact, and the client does not need to wear a mask.

CN: Safety and infection control; CL: Synthesize

30. 4. Transmission of SARS can be contained by airborne precautions that include an isolation room with negative pressure, use of N95 respirator, and use of personal protective equipment. The disease is spread by the respiratory, not enteric, route. Handwashing alone is not sufficient to prevent transmission. Reverse isolation (protection of the client) is not sufficient to prevent transmission.

∽ CN: Safety and infection control;
CL: Synthesize

31. 1. The nurse should institute treatment for hemorrhagic fever viruses, including contact isolation with double gloving and shoe covers, strict hand hygiene, and protective eyewear. The nurse should start respiratory isolation with negative pressure rooms, not positive pressure rooms. Enteric precautions are not needed because the virus is spread by droplet and contact. Reverse isolation protects the client; in this situation, the healthcare team also needs protection.

∽ CN: Reduction of risk potential;
CL: Synthesize

32. 4. Safety of the staff and others is the first priority. Isolating reduces the chance of contaminating others (secondary contamination). Vital signs can be obtained when it is safe—after protecting staff, clients, and visitors from secondary contamination. Oxygen is not indicated for any of the listed symptoms. Removing clothing is important to prevent further exposure to the client, but must be done in a safe manner to prevent secondary contamination to others. The clients can remove their own clothes and place them in plastic bags. After the safety of the staff and others is addressed, and the facility is prepared and properly trained staff is ready, the clients can be given a decontamination shower. If the staff is not trained, 911 may be the most appropriate response. Finding out which chemicals were involved is important but does not take priority over preventing secondary contamination.

∽ CN: Management of care; CL: Synthesize

33. 2,3. The client with crushing chest pain has an acute cardiac condition and can have a successful outcome if immediate interventions are initiated. The client with the open fracture could be stabilized and is not a significant factor in triage in a mass casualty incident. The client with a displaced femur fracture can also be classified as immediate because the fracture can impair circulation. There are also signs of shock and severe pain. All conditions can improve with interventions. In a mass casualty incident, the goal is to do the greatest good for the greatest number—which sometimes means that limited resources are not allocated to the very critically injured who have a very low probability of survival. The other two clients are categorized as "black"/expectant because of their critical injuries and the unavailability of advance trauma care.

∽ CN: Management of care; CL: Analyze

34. 1. Any type of blistering lesion, such as smallpox, requires extreme care to prevent exposure. Transmission-based precautions for smallpox

includes airborne, droplet, and contact precautions. The N95 mask filters at least 95% of airborne particles. To prevent exposure through the respiratory tract, the N95 mask must be fitted and worn properly.

∽ CN: Safety and infection control;
CL: Synthesize

Managing Care, Quality, and Safety of Clients

35. 2,4. The UAP 🔲 can cover the body and transport it to the morgue. Deaths by gunshot wound are considered reportable deaths. All evidence in a reportable death, including tubes and IV lines, should remain intact until the coroner has been contacted. The **healthcare provider (HCP)** 🔲 should be the one to notify the family. The nurse should be the one to notify the chaplain.

∽ CN: Management of care; CL: Synthesize

36. 1. The nurse should contact the pharmacist first to be sure the medication is labeled for administration to this client. The nurse should not administer the drug until all safety precautions have been observed; the nurse should also not ask another nurse to verify the medication or client. Later, if the problem cannot be resolved with relabeling the medication, the nurse or pharmacist can contact the information technology team to check the barcode system.

∽ CN: Safety and infection control;
CL: Synthesize

37. 1,2. All suspicious individuals or activities should be reported as soon as possible to the security department. When reporting an incident, nurses/employees should provide the following: (a) type of incident, (b) persons involved/physical description, (c) vehicles involved and description, (d) date and time the incident occurred, (e) location where the incident occurred, (f) weapons involved, and (g) current location of parties involved. All reports of threats, actual episodes of violence, or suspicious individuals or activities must be investigated.

∽ CN: Safety and infection control;
CL: Synthesize

38. 1,2. A goal of client safety is to improve the effectiveness of communication among caregivers. For verbal or telephone prescriptions, or for telephone reporting of critical test results, one must verify the complete prescription or test result by having the individual receiving the information record "read-back" the complete prescription or test result. The unit secretary is not a licensed health-care professional who has a scope of practice or the authority to receive prescriptions or results. The type of charting system used by the health-care agency is not a factor in using "read-back" prescriptions.

  CN: Safety and infection control; CL: Synthesize

39. 1. A client experiencing a "ripping" sensation in the chest is indicative of a ruptured thoracic aneurysm and warrants an immediate intervention. While a blood pressure of 170/95 mm Hg is high, there is not enough information that suggests that this client is a higher priority than the others. A urine output of 240 mL in 12 hours is <30 mL/h; however, this is this client's only problem now, and the nurse can investigate the cause next. A client experiencing bloody stools will need to be seen; however, no other information is present that would warrant this client being seen first.

  CN: Management of care; CL: Analyze

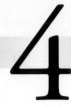

The Nursing Care of Clients with Psychiatric Disorders and Mental Health Problems

TEST 1

Mood Disorders

- **The Client with Major Depression**
- **The Client with Bipolar Disorder, Manic Phase**
- **The Client with Suicidal Ideation and Suicide Attempt**
- **The Client with Psychosexual Disorders**
- **Managing Care, Quality, and Safety of Clients with Psychiatric Disorders and Mental Health Problems**
- **Answers, Rationales, and Test-Taking Strategies**

The Client with Major Depression

1. The nurse is planning care with a Latino client who is diagnosed with a depressive disorder. The client believes in "mal de ojo" (the evil eye) and uses treatment by a root healer. Which intervention is **most** indicated?
- ☐ **1.** Avoid talking to the client about the root healer.
- ☐ **2.** Explain to the client that Western medicine has a scientific, not mystical, basis.
- ☐ **3.** Explain that such beliefs are superstitious and should be forgotten.
- ☐ **4.** Involve the root healer in a consultation with the client, healthcare provider (HCP), and nurse.

2. After a period of unsuccessful treatment with amitriptyline, a client diagnosed with depression is switched to tranylcypromine. Which statement by the client indicates the client understands the side effects of tranylcypromine?
- ☐ **1.** "I need to increase my intake of sodium."
- ☐ **2.** "I must refrain from strenuous exercise."
- ☐ **3.** "I must refrain from eating aged cheese or yeast products."
- ☐ **4.** "I should decrease my intake of foods containing sugar."

3. A client is scheduled for the first electroconvulsive therapy (ECT) treatment in the morning and has been unable to sleep. In what order should the nurse perform the interventions from first to last? All options must be used.

1. Sit quietly with the client.

2. Encourage the use of prescribed PRN temazepam.

3. Offer use of an audio recording with relaxing music.

4. Discuss specific concerns.

4. A client visits the mental health clinic and tells the nurse that she is lethargic, experiences pain in her back, cannot concentrate, and is depressed. The nurse observes patches of hair loss on the client's scalp. Which referral should the nurse make **first**?
- ☐ **1.** occupational therapist
- ☐ **2.** physical therapist
- ☐ **3.** psychologist
- ☐ **4.** a healthcare provider (HCP)

5. A client has been taking 30 mg of duloxetine twice daily for 2 months because of depression and vague aches and pains. While interacting with the nurse, the client discloses a pattern of drinking a six-pack of beer daily for the past 10 years to help with sleep. What should the nurse do **first**?
- ☐ **1.** Refer the client to the concurrent disorders program at the clinic.
- ☐ **2.** Share the information at the next interdisciplinary treatment conference.
- ☐ **3.** Report the client's beer consumption to the healthcare provider (HCP).
- ☐ **4.** Teach the client relaxation exercises to perform before bedtime.

6. A client was admitted to the inpatient unit 3 days ago with a flat affect, psychomotor retardation, anorexia, hopelessness, and suicidal ideation. The healthcare provider (HCP) prescribed 75 mg of venlafaxine extended release to be given every morning. The client interacted minimally with the staff and spent most of the day in his room. As the nurse enters the unit at the beginning of the evening shift, the client is smiling and cheerful and appears to be relaxed. What should the nurse interpret as the **most** likely cause of the client's behavior?
- ☐ **1.** The venlafaxine is helping the client's symptoms of depression significantly.
- ☐ **2.** The client's sudden improvement calls for close observation by the staff.
- ☐ **3.** The staff can decrease their observation of the client.
- ☐ **4.** The client is nearing discharge due to the improvement of his symptoms.

7. The client is taking 50 mg of lamotrigine daily for bipolar disorder. The client shows the nurse a rash on his arm. What should the nurse do?
- ☐ **1.** Report the rash to the healthcare provider (HCP).
- ☐ **2.** Explain that the rash is a temporary adverse effect.
- ☐ **3.** Give the client an ice pack for his arm.
- ☐ **4.** Question the client about recent sun exposure.

8. The nurse is reviewing the laboratory report with the client's lithium level prior to administering the 1700 hours dose. The lithium level is 1.8 mEq/L (1.8 mmol/L). The nurse should:
- ☐ **1.** administer the 1700 hours dose of lithium.
- ☐ **2.** hold the 1700 hours dose of lithium.
- ☐ **3.** give the client 240 mL of water with the lithium.
- ☐ **4.** give the lithium after the client's supper.

9. A nurse is conducting a psychoeducational group for family members of clients hospitalized with depression. Which family member's statement indicates a need for additional teaching?
- ☐ **1.** "My husband will slowly feel better as his medicine takes effect over the next 2 to 4 weeks."
- ☐ **2.** "My wife will need to take her antidepressant medicine and go to group to stay well."
- ☐ **3.** "My son will only need to attend outpatient appointments when he starts to feel depressed again."
- ☐ **4.** "My mother might need help with grocery shopping, cooking, and cleaning for a while."

10. A 16-year-old client is prescribed 10 mg of paroxetine at bedtime for major depression. The nurse should instruct the client and parents to monitor the client closely for which adverse effect?
- ☐ **1.** headache
- ☐ **2.** nausea
- ☐ **3.** fatigue
- ☐ **4.** agitation

11. A client diagnosed with major depression spends most of the day lying in bed with the sheet pulled over his head. Which approach by the nurse is **most** therapeutic?
- ☐ **1.** Wait for the client to begin the conversation.
- ☐ **2.** Initiate contact with the client frequently.
- ☐ **3.** Sit outside the client's room.
- ☐ **4.** Question the client until the client responds.

12. The client exhibits a flat affect, psychomotor retardation, and depressed mood. The nurse attempts to engage the client in an interaction, but the client does not respond to the nurse. Which response by the nurse is **most** appropriate?
- ☐ **1.** "I will sit here with you for 15 minutes."
- ☐ **2.** "I will come back a little bit later to talk."
- ☐ **3.** "I will find someone else for you to talk with."
- ☐ **4.** "I will get you something to read."

13. After a few minutes of conversation, a female client who is depressed wearily asks the nurse, "Why pick me to talk to? Go talk to someone else." Which reply by the nurse is **best**?
- ☐ **1.** "I am assigned to care for you today, if you will let me."
- ☐ **2.** "You have a lot of potential, and I would like to help you."
- ☐ **3.** "I will talk to someone else later."
- ☐ **4.** "I am interested in you and want to help you."

14. A client is receiving paroxetine 20 mg every morning. After taking the first three doses, the client tells the nurse that the medication upsets the stomach. What instructions should the nurse give to the client?
- ☐ **1.** "Take the medication an hour before breakfast."
- ☐ **2.** "Take the medication with some food."
- ☐ **3.** "Take the medication at bedtime."
- ☐ **4.** "Take the medication with 4 oz (120 mL) of orange juice."

15. The healthcare provider (HCP) prescribes fluoxetine orally every morning for a 72-year-old client with depression. Which transient adverse effect of this drug requires **immediate** action by the nurse?
- ☐ **1.** nausea
- ☐ **2.** dizziness
- ☐ **3.** sedation
- ☐ **4.** dry mouth

16. Which statement by a client taking trazodone as prescribed by the healthcare provider (HCP) indicates to the nurse that further teaching about the medication is needed?
- ☐ **1.** "I will continue to take my medication after a light snack."
- ☐ **2.** "Taking trazodone at night will help me to sleep."
- ☐ **3.** "My depression will be gone in about 5 to 7 days."
- ☐ **4.** "I will not drink alcohol while taking trazodone."

17. A 62-year-old female client with severe depression and psychotic symptoms is scheduled for electroconvulsive therapy (ECT) tomorrow morning. The client's daughter asks the nurse, "How painful will the treatment be for Mom?" The nurse should respond with which statement?
- ☐ **1.** "Your mother will be given something for pain before the treatment."
- ☐ **2.** "The healthcare provider (HCP) will make sure your mother does not suffer needlessly."
- ☐ **3.** "Your mother will be asleep during the treatment and will not be in pain."
- ☐ **4.** "Your mother will be able to talk to us and tell us if she is in pain."

18. During a group session, a client who is depressed tells the group that he lost his job. Which response by the nurse is **best**?
- ☐ **1.** "It must have been very upsetting for you."
- ☐ **2.** "Would you tell us about your job?"
- ☐ **3.** "You will find another job when you are better."
- ☐ **4.** "You were probably too depressed to work."

19. A client who is very depressed exhibits psychomotor retardation, a flat affect, and apathy. The nurse observes the client to be in need of grooming and hygiene. Which nursing action is **most** appropriate?
- ☐ **1.** explaining the importance of hygiene to the client
- ☐ **2.** asking the client if he is ready to shower
- ☐ **3.** waiting until the client's family can participate in the client's care
- ☐ **4.** stating to the client that it is time for him to take a shower

20. Which interventions should the nurse include in the plan of care to prepare a client for ECT? Select all that apply.
- ☐ **1.** Maintain NPO status.
- ☐ **2.** Verify if consent is signed.
- ☐ **3.** Orient the client to place and time.
- ☐ **4.** Remove dentures.
- ☐ **5.** Request the client to void.
- ☐ **6.** Assess client vital signs every 30 minutes.

21. Which comment indicates that a client understands the nurse's teaching about sertraline?
- ☐ **1.** "Sertraline will probably cause me to gain weight."
- ☐ **2.** "This medicine can cause delayed ejaculations."
- ☐ **3.** "Dry mouth is a permanent side effect of sertraline."
- ☐ **4.** "I can take my medicine with St. John's wort."

22. The client with recurring depression will be discharged from the psychiatric unit. What instructions for the family are **most** important to include in the plan of care?
- ☐ **1.** Discourage visitors while the client is at home.
- ☐ **2.** Provide for a schedule of activities outside the home.
- ☐ **3.** Involve the client in usual at-home activities.
- ☐ **4.** Encourage the client to sleep as much as possible.

23. A client with major depression and psychotic features is admitted involuntarily to the hospital. He will not eat because his "bowels have turned to jelly," which the client states is punishment for his wickedness. The client requests to leave the hospital. The nurse denies the request because commitment papers have been initiated by the healthcare provider (HCP). The nurse understands this client legally committable based on which criterion?
☐ 1. evidence of psychosis
☐ 2. being gravely disabled
☐ 3. risk of harm to self or others
☐ 4. diagnosis of mental illness

24. The client who has been taking venlafaxine 25 mg PO three times a day for the past 2 days states, "This medicine is not doing me any good. I am still so depressed." Which response by the nurse is **most** appropriate?
☐ 1. "Perhaps we will need to increase your dose."
☐ 2. "Let us wait a few days and see how you feel."
☐ 3. "It takes about 2 to 4 weeks to receive the full effects."
☐ 4. "It is too soon to tell if your medication will help you."

25. The client states to the nurse, "I take citalopram 40 mg every day as my healthcare provider (HCP) prescribed. I have also been taking St. John's wort 750 mg daily for the past 2 weeks." Which findings would indicate that the client is developing serotonin syndrome? Select all that apply.
☐ 1. confusion
☐ 2. restlessness
☐ 3. constipation
☐ 4. diaphoresis
☐ 5. ataxia

26. Which food should the nurse tell the client to avoid while taking phenelzine?
☐ 1. roasted chicken
☐ 2. salami
☐ 3. fresh fish
☐ 4. hamburger

27. A client is taking phenelzine 15 mg PO three times a day. The nurse is about to administer the next dose when the client tells the nurse about having a throbbing headache. Which action should the nurse do **first**?
☐ 1. Give the client an analgesic prescribed PRN.
☐ 2. Call the healthcare provider (HCP) to report the symptom.
☐ 3. Administer the client's next dose of phenelzine.
☐ 4. Obtain the client's vital signs.

28. A client with severe depression and weight loss has not eaten since admission to the hospital 2 days ago. Which approach should the nurse include when developing the plan of care to ensure that the client eats?
☐ 1. serving the client her meal trays in her room
☐ 2. sitting with the client and spoon-feeding if required
☐ 3. calling the family to bring the client food from home
☐ 4. explaining the importance of nutrition in recovery

29. After administering a prescribed medication to a client who becomes restless at night and has difficulty falling asleep, which nursing action is **most** appropriate?
☐ 1. sitting quietly with the client at the bedside until the medication takes effect
☐ 2. engaging the client in interaction until the client falls asleep
☐ 3. reading to the client with the lights turned down low
☐ 4. encouraging the client to watch television until the client feels sleepy

30. Which behavior if exhibited by a client with a depressive disorder should lead the nurse to determine that the client is ready for discharge?
☐ 1. interactions with staff and peers
☐ 2. sleeping for 4 hours at a time
☐ 3. verbalization of feeling in control of self and situations
☐ 4. statements of dissatisfaction over not being able to perform at work

31. The client with major depression and suicidal ideation has been taking bupropion 100 mg PO 3 times daily for 5 days. Assessment reveals the client to be somewhat less withdrawn, able to perform activities of daily living with minimal assistance, and eating 50% of each meal. At this time, the nurse should monitor the client specifically for which behavior?
☐ 1. seizure activity
☐ 2. suicide attempt
☐ 3. visual disturbances
☐ 4. increased libido

32. Which outcome should the nurse include in the initial plan of care for a client who is exhibiting psychomotor retardation, withdrawal, minimal eye contact, and unresponsiveness to the nurse's questions?
☐ 1. The client will initiate interactions with peers.
☐ 2. The client will participate in milieu activities.
☐ 3. The client will discuss adaptive coping techniques.
☐ 4. The client will interact with the nurse.

33. When preparing a teaching plan for a client about imipramine, which substance should the nurse tell the client to avoid while taking the medication?
- ☐ 1. caffeinated coffee
- ☐ 2. sunscreen
- ☐ 3. alcohol
- ☐ 4. artificial tears

34. The client with depression who is taking imipramine states to the nurse, "My psychiatrist wants me to have an electrocardiogram (ECG) in 2 weeks, but my heart is fine." Which response by the nurse is **most** appropriate?
- ☐ 1. "It is routine practice to have an ECG periodically because there is a slight chance that the drug may affect the heart."
- ☐ 2. "It is probably a precautionary measure because I am not aware that you have a cardiac condition."
- ☐ 3. "Try not to worry too much about this. Your healthcare provider is just being very thorough in monitoring your condition."
- ☐ 4. "You had an ECG before you were prescribed imipramine, and the procedure will be the same."

35. When assessing a client who is receiving tricyclic antidepressant therapy, which finding should alert the nurse to the possibility that the client is experiencing anticholinergic effects?
- ☐ 1. tremors and cardiac arrhythmias
- ☐ 2. sedation and delirium
- ☐ 3. respiratory depression and convulsions
- ☐ 4. urine retention and blurred vision

36. The healthcare provider (HCP) prescribes mirtazapine 30 mg PO at bedtime for a client diagnosed with depression. The nurse should:
- ☐ 1. give the medication as prescribed.
- ☐ 2. question the HCP's prescription.
- ☐ 3. request to give the medication in the morning.
- ☐ 4. give the medication in three divided doses.

37. A client taking mirtazapine is disheartened about a 20-lb (9 kg) weight gain over the past 3 months. The client tells the nurse, "I stopped taking my mirtazapine 15 days ago. I do not want to get depressed again, but I feel awful about my weight." Which response by the nurse is **most** appropriate?
- ☐ 1. "Focusing on diet and exercise alone should control your weight."
- ☐ 2. "Your depression is much better now, so your medication is helping you."
- ☐ 3. "Look at all the positive things that have happened to you since you started mirtazapine."
- ☐ 4. "I hear how difficult this is for you and will help you approach your healthcare provider about it."

38. When developing a teaching plan for a client about the medications prescribed for depression, which component is **most** important for the nurse to include?
- ☐ 1. pharmacokinetics of the medication
- ☐ 2. current research related to the medication
- ☐ 3. management of common adverse effects
- ☐ 4. dosage regulation and adjustment

39. The client diagnosed with severe major depression has been taking escitalopram 10 mg daily for the past 2 weeks. Which parameter should the nurse monitor **most** closely at this time?
- ☐ 1. suicidal ideation
- ☐ 2. sleep
- ☐ 3. appetite
- ☐ 4. energy level

40. A client taking paroxetine 40 mg PO every morning tells the nurse that her mouth "feels like cotton." Which statement by the client necessitates further assessment by the nurse?
- ☐ 1. "I am sucking on ice chips."
- ☐ 2. "I am using sugarless gum."
- ☐ 3. "I am sucking on sugarless candy."
- ☐ 4. "I am drinking 12 glasses of water every day."

41. The client with a depressive disorder has been consistent with taking 12.5 mg of paroxetine extended release daily. The nurse judges the client to be benefiting from this drug therapy when the client demonstrates which behaviors? Select all that apply.
- ☐ 1. takes 2-hour evening naps daily
- ☐ 2. completes homework assignments
- ☐ 3. decreases pacing
- ☐ 4. increases somatization
- ☐ 5. verbalizes feelings

42. A client diagnosed with major depression has sleep and appetite disturbances and a flat affect and is withdrawn. The client has been taking fluvoxamine 50 mg twice daily for 5 days. Which client behavior is **most** important to report to the next shift?
- ☐ 1. client's flat affect
- ☐ 2. client's interacting with a visitor
- ☐ 3. client sleeping from 2300 hours to 0600 hours
- ☐ 4. client spending the entire evening in her room

43. When educating a client who has been diagnosed with dysthymia about possible treatment for the disorder, which information should the nurse include?
- ☐ 1. "Antidepressants offer you the best treatment for your dysthymia."
- ☐ 2. "You are a good candidate for electroconvulsive therapy (ECT)."
- ☐ 3. "Dysthymia often responds to the combination of psychotherapy and antidepressants."
- ☐ 4. "Your condition will most likely need long-term psychoanalysis."

44. A client with a major depressive disorder comes to the mental health clinic for a follow-up visit. The client has been taking escitalopram for 3 months and tells the nurse that he is feeling "like my old self again." Now the client wants to stop taking medication. "I do not want to be dependent on meds like my father." What is the nurse's **best** initial response to him?
- [ ] 1. "After another 3 months of stability, it might be safe for you to go off the escitalopram."
- [ ] 2. "After two significant episodes, you will need to take an antidepressant indefinitely."
- [ ] 3. "Research indicates that individuals who have had two major depressive episodes have a 70% chance of having a third episode."
- [ ] 4. "It is likely that you can learn to manage your depression with a regular exercise regime and a healthy diet."

45. Which statement made by an adolescent who has just begun taking an antidepressant would indicate the need for further teaching?
- [ ] 1. "Now that I have been taking my antidepressant for a week, I am going to feel better about myself."
- [ ] 2. "A week ago when I started my antidepressant, I did not care about eating, but now I want to eat a bit more."
- [ ] 3. "After a week of taking my antidepressant, I can sleep a little better—6 hours or so each night."
- [ ] 4. "Now that I have had a week of my antidepressant, it is a little easier to get up in the morning."

The Client with Bipolar Disorder, Manic Phase

46. A client comes to the mental health clinic saying that he feels so down and lacking in energy with "loss of interest in everything." He tells the nurse that he received some samples of a new medication from his healthcare provider (HCP) last week to relieve his depression. The nurse recalls that this client has a history of bipolar disorder with hospitalization for a significant manic episode. With this knowledge, the nurse would have special concern if he is taking which category of medication?
- [ ] 1. atypical antipsychotics
- [ ] 2. mood stabilizers/antimanics
- [ ] 3. antianxiety agents/benzodiazepines
- [ ] 4. selective serotonin reuptake inhibitor antidepressants

47. In a predischarge program to educate clients with bipolar disorder and their family members, the nurse emphasizes which symptom is the **most** significant indicator for the onset of relapse?
- [ ] 1. a sense of pleasure and motivation for new endeavors
- [ ] 2. decreased need for sleep and racing thoughts
- [ ] 3. self-concern about increase in energy
- [ ] 4. leaving a good job to start a new business

48. Which statement by a client taking lithium **most** indicates a need for more teaching?
- [ ] 1. "My healthcare provider tells me that my lithium level is 1.0, so I do not have to worry about my levels."
- [ ] 2. "I have been getting a lot of good exercise playing on a local soccer team."
- [ ] 3. "I am trying hard to watch my diet and eat healthy."
- [ ] 4. "I have learned to take my lithium even when I am not feeling well, like when I had the stomach flu."

49. A young woman comes to the mental health clinic for her routine medication follow-up. She has been married for 2 years and reports that she and her husband are ready to start a family. She has a diagnosis of bipolar disorder and has been well managed on divalproex for at least 3 years. What is the **most** essential counsel for the nurse to give her?
- [ ] 1. "Schedule an appointment for a complete gynecological exam if you have not had one in the past year."
- [ ] 2. "Pay careful attention to eating healthy from this point on in order to maximize the health of both mother and baby."
- [ ] 3. "Check with your prescriber today as divalproex carries an increased risk for birth defects."
- [ ] 4. "Learning to reduce stress now is important to reduce your chances of developing postpartum depression."

50. A healthcare provider (HCP) has prescribed valproic acid for a client with bipolar disorder who has achieved limited success with lithium carbonate. Which information should the nurse teach the client about taking valproic acid?
- [ ] 1. Follow-up blood tests are necessary while on this medication.
- [ ] 2. The extended-release tablet can be crushed if necessary for ease of swallowing.
- [ ] 3. Tachycardia and upset stomach are common side effects.
- [ ] 4. Consumption of a moderate amount of alcohol is safe if the medication is taken in the morning.

51. A young adult client diagnosed with bipolar disorder has been managing the disorder effectively with medication and treatment for several years. The client suddenly becomes manic. The nurse reviews the client's medication record. Which new medication may have contributed to the development of his manic state?

> **Medication Record**
>
> Amitriptyline 50 mg PO daily at bedtime
> Prednisone 20 mg PO daily
> Buspirone HCl 5 mg PO three times a day
> Gabapentin 300 mg PO three times a day

- ☐ **1.** amitriptyline
- ☐ **2.** prednisone
- ☐ **3.** buspirone
- ☐ **4.** gabapentin

52. The client with acute mania has been admitted to the inpatient unit voluntarily. The nurse approaches the client with medication to be taken orally as prescribed by the healthcare provider (HCP). The client states, "I do not need that stuff." Which response by the nurse is **best**?
- ☐ **1.** "You cannot refuse to take this medication."
- ☐ **2.** "If you do not take it orally, I will give you a shot."
- ☐ **3.** "The medication will help you feel calmer."
- ☐ **4.** "I will get you some written information about the medication."

53. A nurse observes a male client who is hyperactive and intrusive sitting very close to a female client with his arm around her shoulders. The nurse hears the male client tell a sexually explicit joke. The nurse approaches the client and asks him to walk down the hallway. Which statement by the nurse should benefit the client?
- ☐ **1.** "She will not want to be around you with that kind of talk."
- ☐ **2.** "Telling sexual jokes and touching others is not permitted here."
- ☐ **3.** "You need to be careful about what you say to other people."
- ☐ **4.** "I think a time-out in your room would be appropriate now."

54. A client with acute mania fails to respond to a nurse's interventions to decrease his agitation. The nurse has attempted to defuse the client's anger, but the client refuses to participate in interventions that would lower anxiety. Which action should the nurse take **next**?
- ☐ **1.** Seclude the client.
- ☐ **2.** Restrain the client.
- ☐ **3.** Medicate the client.
- ☐ **4.** Control the client.

55. The client with mania is irritable and insulting to an unlicensed assistive personnel (UAP). The UAP states, "I cannot believe Mark is so rude. Should he not be overly happy?" Which response by the nurse should help the UAP understand the client's behavior?
- ☐ **1.** "It is our responsibility to listen to him even though we might not like what he is saying."
- ☐ **2.** "We must reprimand Mark for doing that, because there is no reason for him to behave like that."
- ☐ **3.** "I will go and speak to him about his behavior and make sure he understands that he needs to control what he is saying."
- ☐ **4.** "I know it is difficult, but Mark is a client whose irritable mood is a symptom of his mania."

56. Which milieu activity should the nurse recommend to a client with acute mania? Select all that apply.
- ☐ **1.** scheduled rest periods
- ☐ **2.** relaxation exercises
- ☐ **3.** listening to soft music
- ☐ **4.** watching television
- ☐ **5.** aerobic exercise

57. A nurse is assessing a client experiencing hypomania who wants to stop her mood-stabilizing medication because she is "feeling good," has a high energy level, and thinks she is productive at work. Which response by the nurse is **most** appropriate?
- ☐ **1.** "Are you thinking about hurting yourself?"
- ☐ **2.** "If you stop your medication, your behavior will quickly spiral out of control."
- ☐ **3.** "I believe you were hospitalized the last time you stopped your medication."
- ☐ **4.** "Why do you not cut your medication dosage in half for a while and see how you respond?"

58. The client with acute mania is prescribed 600 mg of lithium PO three times per day. The healthcare provider (HCP) also prescribes 5 mg of haloperidol PO at bedtime. Which action should the nurse take?
- ☐ **1.** Administer the medication as prescribed.
- ☐ **2.** Question the HCP about the prescription.
- ☐ **3.** Administer the haloperidol but not the lithium.
- ☐ **4.** Consult with the nursing supervisor before administering the medications.

59. The client with a diagnosis of bipolar disorder, manic phase, states to the nurse, "I am the Queen of England. Bow before me." The nurse interprets this statement as important to document as which area of the mental status examination?
- ☐ **1.** psychomotor behavior
- ☐ **2.** mood and affect
- ☐ **3.** attitude toward the nurse
- ☐ **4.** thought content

60. The client is laughing and telling jokes to a group of clients. Suddenly, the client is crying and talking about a death in the family. A moment later, the client is laughing and joking again. The nurse should:
☐ 1. call the healthcare provider (HCP) for a prescription for lorazepam as needed.
☐ 2. place the client in seclusion and call the HCP for a prescription for the seclusion.
☐ 3. ignore the client's behavior in order not to give the client too much attention.
☐ 4. ask the client to come to a quiet area to talk to the nurse individually.

61. A client with acute mania exhibits euphoria, pressured speech, and flight of ideas. The client has been talking to the nurse nonstop for 5 minutes, and lunch has arrived on the unit. What should the nurse do **next**?
☐ 1. Excuse oneself while telling the client to come to the dining room for lunch.
☐ 2. Tell the client he needs to stop talking because it is time to eat lunch.
☐ 3. Do not interrupt the client, but wait for him to finish talking.
☐ 4. Walk away, and approach the client in a few minutes before the food gets cold.

62. A female client with acute mania brings six suitcases and three shopping bags of personal belongings on admission to the unit. When informed that some of the suitcases and bags need to be returned home with her husband because of a lack of storage space, the client begins to use profanity against the nurse. Which response by the nurse is **most** therapeutic?
☐ 1. "You are acting inappropriately."
☐ 2. "I will not tolerate your talking to me like that."
☐ 3. "Swearing and profanity are unacceptable here."
☐ 4. "We do not want to put you in seclusion yet."

63. The husband of a client who is experiencing acute mania and is swearing and using profanity apologizes to the nurse for his wife's behavior. Which of the reply by the nurse is **most** therapeutic?
☐ 1. "This must be difficult for you."
☐ 2. "It is okay. We have heard worse."
☐ 3. "How long has she been like this?"
☐ 4. "She needs some medication."

64. The nurse is caring for a client with acute mania who is euphoric and flirtatious. The nurse overhears the client describing a sexual exploit with a group of clients seated at a table. What should the nurse do **next**?
☐ 1. Continue walking down the hall, ignoring the conversation.
☐ 2. Speak to the client later in private while saying nothing at this time.
☐ 3. Tell the client others may not want to hear about sex, and invite him to play a game of ping-pong.
☐ 4. Inform the client that if he continues to talk about sex, no one will want to be around him.

65. The client with acute mania states to the nurse, "I am the prince of peace and can save the world. Those against me will find me and take me to another world. They will come. I know it." The client is beginning to scan the room and starts to repeat his delusion. Which response by the nurse is **most** therapeutic?
☐ 1. "Describe the people who will come."
☐ 2. "The staff and I will protect you."
☐ 3. "You are not the prince of peace. Your name is Joe."
☐ 4. "Let us walk around the unit for a while."

66. A client with bipolar disorder, manic phase, is scheduled for a chest x-ray. Before taking the client to the radiology department, the nurse should:
☐ 1. give a thorough explanation of the procedure.
☐ 2. explain the procedure in simple terms.
☐ 3. call security to be on standby for possible problems.
☐ 4. cancel the appointment until the client can go unescorted.

67. The client with bipolar disorder, manic phase, appears at the nurse's station wearing a transparent shirt, miniskirt, high heels, 10 bracelets, and 8 necklaces. Her makeup is overdone, and she is not wearing underwear. What should the nurse do?
☐ 1. Tell the client to dress appropriately while out of her room.
☐ 2. Ask the client to put on hospital pajamas until she can dress appropriately.
☐ 3. Instruct the client to go to her room and change clothes.
☐ 4. Escort the client to her room, and assist with choosing appropriate attire.

68. A client diagnosed with bipolar disorder and experiencing acute mania states to the nurse, "Where is my son? I love Lucy. Rain, rain go away. Dogs eat dirt." Another client approaches the nurse and says, "Man, is he ever nuts! He is driving me crazy with all his weird talk." Which response by the nurse to the second client is **most** appropriate?
- ☐ **1.** "I agree. He is a little hard to take sometimes."
- ☐ **2.** "Just walk away and leave him alone. There is nothing else you can do."
- ☐ **3.** "I realize his behavior bothers you, but he cannot control it right now."
- ☐ **4.** "I will give him some medication so he will not bother you."

69. The client with mania is skipping up and down the hallway, nearly running into other clients. The nurse should include which activity in the client's plan of care?
- ☐ **1.** leading a group activity
- ☐ **2.** watching television
- ☐ **3.** reading the newspaper
- ☐ **4.** cleaning the dayroom tables

70. A client admitted to the nursing unit with bipolar disorder, manic phase, is accompanied by his wife. The wife states that her husband has been overly energetic and happy, talking constantly, purchasing many unneeded items, and sleeping about 4 hours a night for the past 5 days. When completing the client's daily assessment, the nurse should be especially alert for which finding?
- ☐ **1.** exhaustion
- ☐ **2.** vertigo
- ☐ **3.** gastritis
- ☐ **4.** bradycardia

71. The wife of a client with bipolar disorder, manic phase, states to the nurse, "He is acting so crazy. What did he do to get this way?" The nurse bases the response on which understanding of this disorder?
- ☐ **1.** It is caused by underlying psychological difficulties.
- ☐ **2.** It is caused by disturbed family dynamics in the client's early life.
- ☐ **3.** It is the result of an imbalance of chemicals in the brain.
- ☐ **4.** It is the result of a genetic inheritance from someone in the family.

72. A client diagnosed with bipolar disorder asks the nurse why it is necessary to have a serum lithium level drawn every 3 to 4 months. The nurse's response should be based on which factor?
- ☐ **1.** to monitor compliance with the medication
- ☐ **2.** to prevent toxicity related to the drug's therapeutic range
- ☐ **3.** to monitor the client's white blood cell count
- ☐ **4.** to comply with governmental safety requirements

73. The healthcare provider (HCP) prescribes a serum lithium level tomorrow for a client with bipolar disorder, manic phase, who has been receiving lithium 300 mg PO three times daily for the past 5 days. At what time should the nurse plan to have the blood specimen obtained?
- ☐ **1.** before bedtime
- ☐ **2.** after lunch
- ☐ **3.** before breakfast
- ☐ **4.** during the afternoon

74. A client will be discharged on lithium carbonate 600 mg three times daily. When teaching the client and his family about lithium therapy, the nurse determines that teaching has been effective if the client and family state that they will notify the prescribing healthcare provider (HCP) immediately with which symptoms? Select all that apply.
- ☐ **1.** nausea
- ☐ **2.** muscle weakness
- ☐ **3.** vertigo
- ☐ **4.** fine hand tremor
- ☐ **5.** vomiting
- ☐ **6.** anorexia

75. After the nurse teaches a client with bipolar disorder about lithium therapy, which client statement indicates the need for additional teaching?
- ☐ **1.** "It is important to keep using a regular amount of salt in my diet."
- ☐ **2.** "It is okay to double my next dose of lithium if I forget a dose."
- ☐ **3.** "I should drink about 8 to 10 eight-ounce (240 to 300 mL) glasses of water each day."
- ☐ **4.** "I need to take my medicine at the same time each day."

76. A client with acute mania is to receive lithium carbonate 600 mg PO three times daily and 2 mg of haloperidol PO at bedtime. The nurse should:
- ☐ **1.** refuse to give the medications as prescribed.
- ☐ **2.** give the lithium only.
- ☐ **3.** request a decreased dosage of lithium.
- ☐ **4.** give the medications as prescribed.

77. After the nurse teaches a client about bipolar disorder, which statement indicates that the client has developed insight about the diagnosis?
- ☐ **1.** "I enjoy feeling high. I do not need much sleep then and get really creative."
- ☐ **2.** "My medicine really helped me. I know I will not need it in about another week."
- ☐ **3.** "I am cured now. I was really wild for a while even though I got into trouble."
- ☐ **4.** "I know I am getting sick when I do not need much sleep and start buying things."

78. During morning community meeting, a client with bipolar disorder, manic phase, interrupts others to the point where no one can finish their statements. The nurse should tell the client:
☐ 1. "Please stop interrupting others. You can speak when it is your turn."
☐ 2. "Stop talking. It is time for you to leave the meeting."
☐ 3. "If you cannot control yourself, we will have to take action."
☐ 4. "Please behave like an adult. Your behavior is childish."

79. The client with bipolar disorder, manic phase, has a valproic acid level of 15 mg/mL (104 mmol/L). Which client behaviors should the nurse judge to be due to this level of valproic acid? Select all that apply.
☐ 1. irritability
☐ 2. grandiosity
☐ 3. anhedonia
☐ 4. hypersomnia
☐ 5. flight of ideas

80. The client with rapid-cycling bipolar disorder who is about to receive his 1700 hours dose of carbamazepine tells the nurse he has a sore throat and chills. What should the nurse do **next**?
☐ 1. Administer the prescribed dose of carbamazepine.
☐ 2. Give the client acetaminophen as prescribed PRN.
☐ 3. Report the symptoms to the healthcare provider (HCP) in the morning.
☐ 4. Call the HCP to report changes.

81. A client's wife states, "I do not know what to do sometimes. It is so hard having a husband with a mental illness like bipolar disorder." After talking with the client's wife about her feelings and difficulties, which action is **most** appropriate?
☐ 1. Suggest that the wife see her healthcare provider (HCP).
☐ 2. Give the wife information about a support group.
☐ 3. Recommend that the wife talk with her close friend.
☐ 4. Have the wife share her feelings with her husband.

82. The client with bipolar disorder is approaching discharge after being hospitalized with her first episode of acute mania. The client's husband asks the nurse what he can do to help her. What recommendation for the husband should the nurse anticipate including in the teaching plan?
☐ 1. Help the client to be free from worry and anxiety.
☐ 2. Communicate openly and offer support.
☐ 3. Relieve the client of all responsibilities.
☐ 4. Remind the client to control her symptoms.

83. A client experiencing a manic episode has been talking loudly, pacing the unit and trying to draw other clients into debates about the value of self-determination. Arrange in order the steps a nurse should take to help calm this client. All options must be used.

1. Use oral medication to decrease anxiety and increase appropriate social interaction.
2. Talk with the client about the anxiety and stress the client is feeling.
3. Take client to a quiet area, such as his or her room, to decrease stimuli.
4. Teach the client coping strategies to deal with stressors.

84. The client with bipolar disorder, manic phase, states, "You are looking good. I am taking you out to dinner." What reply by the nurse is **most** therapeutic?
☐ 1. "I do not want to go out to dinner."
☐ 2. "I cannot go out to dinner with you."
☐ 3. "It does not matter how I look; the answer is no."
☐ 4. "I am Chris Smith, a nurse working on this unit."

85. After the nurse administers haloperidol 5 mg PO to a client with acute mania, the client refuses to lie down on her bed, runs out on the unit, pushes clients in her vicinity out of the way, and screams threatening remarks to the staff. What should the nurse do **next**?
☐ 1. Follow the client and ask her to calm down.
☐ 2. Tell the client to lie down on the sofa in the community room.
☐ 3. Seclude the client and use restraints if necessary.
☐ 4. Tell the staff to ignore the client's remarks.

86. As the nurse is turning off the television, a client with bipolar disorder, manic phase, says, "I want the television on so I can watch the late show. I am not tired, and you cannot tell me what to do. I want it on!" The nurse should tell the client:

☐ 1. "I will let you watch television just this once, but you have to turn the sound off."

☐ 2. "I will turn the television off when you get sleepy. Do not ask me to do this again."

☐ 3. "Television hours are from 1900 hours to 2200 hours. It is 2200, and the television goes off so everyone can sleep."

☐ 4. "The television goes off at 2200 hours. I have been telling you this for the past three evenings."

The Client with Suicidal Ideation and Suicide Attempt

87. Which strategies would be helpful in preventing suicide for clients about to be discharged from a psychiatric inpatient unit? Select all that apply.

☐ 1. At discharge, give all depressed clients a card containing the crisis phone line number for their area.

☐ 2. Have all clients who have expressed suicidal ideation just prior to or during hospitalization make a written personal suicide prevention plan.

☐ 3. Require that all clients who have had previous suicidal ideation, plans, or attempts refill their medication every 2 weeks rather than monthly.

☐ 4. Educate family and friends of previously suicidal clients in ways to help clients remain safe after discharge.

☐ 5. Suggest that family and friends of previously suicidal clients know the client's whereabouts at all times.

88. The nurse manager in the emergency department (ED) is conducting an in-service for the nursing staff about screening clients for suicide. One of the nurses states, "Questioning adolescents about suicide will only increase their thinking about self-harm, and they would not admit it to me anyhow." How should the nurse manager respond?

☐ 1. "You could be correct. Let us assess only adults because they will be more honest."

☐ 2. "We will limit the assessment to adolescents with psychiatric diagnoses."

☐ 3. "It is a myth that talking about suicide leads to suicide attempts. Adolescents will disclose suicidal thoughts when asked directly."

☐ 4. "If you think the adolescent is not telling you the truth, you can question the parents."

89. When assessing a client for suicidal risk, which method of suicide should the nurse identify as **most** lethal?

☐ 1. aspirin overdose

☐ 2. use of a gun

☐ 3. head banging

☐ 4. wrist cutting

90. The nurse manager overhears two staff members talking in the snack room. One of the staff members states, "Her superficial cuts are just a means of getting our attention. She never should have been admitted. I hope she is out of here soon." Which response by the nurse manager is **most** appropriate?

☐ 1. "It is our job to help her no matter how we feel about her or what she did. She will be discharged soon."

☐ 2. "I will not tolerate that kind of discussion from my staff. Now, it is time for you to go back to work."

☐ 3. "I know it is hard to understand, but we need to do the best we can even though she will be back."

☐ 4. "No matter what the intent, all suicidal behavior is serious and deserves our serious consideration."

91. The history of a female client who has just been admitted to the unit and is very depressed reveals a weight loss of 10 lb (4.5 kg) in 2 weeks, sleeping 3 hours a night, and poor hygiene. The client states, "I am no good to anyone. Everyone would be better off without me." Which question should the nurse ask **first**?

☐ 1. "What do you mean?"

☐ 2. "Are you thinking about hurting yourself?"

☐ 3. "Does your family not care about you?"

☐ 4. "What happened to make you think that?"

92. When developing the plan of care for a client with suicidal ideation, developing goals to address which issue is a **priority**?

☐ 1. self-esteem

☐ 2. sleep

☐ 3. stress

☐ 4. safety

93. Which question should the nurse ask to **best** determine the seriousness of a client's suicidal ideation?

☐ 1. "How are you planning on harming yourself?"

☐ 2. "Have you made out a will?"

☐ 3. "Does your family know you are here?"

☐ 4. "How long have you been thinking about harming yourself?"

94. The unlicensed assistive personnel (UAP) states to the nurse, "My client talks about how awful and useless she is. Sometimes, she sounds angry for no reason. I am tired of listening to her." Which response by the nurse is **most** appropriate?
- ☐ 1. "I will switch your assignment to someone who is less depressed and less tiring."
- ☐ 2. "It is important for you to listen to her because she needs to verbalize how she is feeling."
- ☐ 3. "Do not worry about it. I know you have not done anything to make her angry."
- ☐ 4. "Clients with depression are hard to deal with, but do not take what they say seriously."

95. A client who was recently discharged from the psychiatric unit telephones the unit to speak to the nurse. The client states that she took her children to the neighbors' house and has turned on the gas to kill herself. She is home alone and gives the nurse her address. Which action should the nurse take **next**?
- ☐ 1. Refer the caller to a 24-hour suicide hotline.
- ☐ 2. Tell the caller that another nurse will telephone the police.
- ☐ 3. Ask the caller whether she telephoned her healthcare provider (HCP).
- ☐ 4. Instruct the caller to telephone her family for help.

96. A client walks into the clinic and tells the nurse she wants to die because her boyfriend broke up with her. The client states, "I will show him. He will be sorry." The nurse notes which underlying theme and method to deal with the client?
- ☐ 1. Sadness—ask the client to reveal how long she has felt this way.
- ☐ 2. Escape—ask the client to indicate what she wants to escape.
- ☐ 3. Loneliness—ask the client to state who she believes to be her friends.
- ☐ 4. Retaliation—ask the client about her specific plans to harm herself and/or her boyfriend.

97. The client has been hospitalized for major depression and suicidal ideation. Which statement indicates to the nurse that the client is improving?
- ☐ 1. "I could not kill myself because I do not want to go to hell."
- ☐ 2. "I do not think about killing myself as much as I used to."
- ☐ 3. "I am of no use to anyone anymore."
- ☐ 4. "I know my kids do not need me anymore since they are grown."

98. The client states to the nurse at the outpatient clinic, "I do not feel ready to go back to work. It has only been a week since I left the hospital." Assessment reveals a flat affect, disheveled appearance, poor posture, and minimal eye contact during interaction. The nurse asks the client whether he is thinking about harming himself. The client tells the nurse he has a loaded revolver at home and will probably use it. What should the nurse do **next**?
- ☐ 1. Tell the client to go and remove the gun from his home.
- ☐ 2. Ask the client to call the nurse every hour when he gets home.
- ☐ 3. Ask the client to promise not to harm himself.
- ☐ 4. Initiate plans for hospitalization immediately.

99. The widow of a client who successfully completed suicide tearfully says, "I feel guilty because I am so angry at him for killing himself. It must have been what he wanted." After assisting the widow with dealing with her feelings, which intervention is **most** helpful?
- ☐ 1. Referring her to a group for survivors of suicide.
- ☐ 2. Encouraging her to receive counseling from a chaplain.
- ☐ 3. Providing her with the local suicide hotline number.
- ☐ 4. Suggesting she receive individual therapy by the nurse.

100. The husband of a client to be discharged from the hospital after an episode of major depression and a suicide attempt asks, "What can I do if she tries to kill herself again?" Which response is **most** appropriate?
- ☐ 1. "Do not worry. She will be okay as long as she takes her medication."
- ☐ 2. "She told me she wants to live, so I do not think she will try again."
- ☐ 3. "Let us talk about some behavioral clues and resources that can help."
- ☐ 4. "Tell her about your concern, and just take care of her."

101. A client with depression is exhibiting a brighter affect and an ability to attend to hygiene and grooming tasks and is beginning to participate in group activities. The nurse asks the client to identify three of her strengths. After much hesitation and thinking, the client can state she is usually a nice person, a good cook, and a hard worker. What should the nurse do **next**?
- ☐ 1. Ask the client to identify additional three strengths.
- ☐ 2. Volunteer the client to lead the cooking group later in the day.
- ☐ 3. Educate the client about the importance of medication.
- ☐ 4. Reinforce the client for identifying and sharing her strengths.

102. The friend of a client with depression and suicidal ideation asks the nurse, "How should I act around her?" Which response by the nurse is **best**?
☐ **1.** "Try to cheer her up."
☐ **2.** "Be caring and genuine."
☐ **3.** "Control your expressions."
☐ **4.** "Avoid asking how she is feeling."

103. A client with depression and suicidal ideation voices feelings of self-doubt and powerlessness and is very dependent on the nurse for most aspects of her care. According to Erikson's stages of growth and development, the nurse determines the client to be manifesting problems in which stage?
☐ **1.** trust versus mistrust
☐ **2.** autonomy versus shame/doubt
☐ **3.** initiative versus guilt
☐ **4.** industry versus inferiority

104. A client who overdosed on barbiturates is being transferred to the inpatient psychiatric unit from the intensive care unit. Assessing the client for which need should be a **priority** for the nurse receiving the client?
☐ **1.** nutrition
☐ **2.** sleep
☐ **3.** safety
☐ **4.** hygiene

105. A client is brought to the psychiatric unit from the emergency department (ED) escorted by ED staff and a security officer. The client's shoulder is bandaged and his arm is in a sling because of a self-inflicted gunshot wound to his shoulder. Later, the client's wife follows with a bag of her husband's belongings. Which nursing action is **most** appropriate at this time?
☐ **1.** Tell the wife to take her husband's things home because he is suicidal.
☐ **2.** Instruct the wife to unpack the bag and put her husband's things in the dresser.
☐ **3.** Ask the wife whether the bag contains anything dangerous.
☐ **4.** Inspect the bag and its contents in the presence of the client and his wife.

106. A suicidal client is placed in the seclusion room and given lorazepam because she tried to harm herself by banging her head against the wall. After 10 minutes, the client starts to bang her head against the wall in the seclusion room. Which action should the nurse take **next**?
☐ **1.** Call hospital security for assistance.
☐ **2.** Place the client in restraints.
☐ **3.** Call the healthcare provider (HCP) for additional medication prescriptions.
☐ **4.** Instruct a staff member to sit in the room with the client.

107. A client lives in a group home and visits the community mental health center regularly. During one visit with the nurse, the client states, "The voices are telling me to hurt myself again." Which question by the nurse is **most** important to ask?
☐ **1.** "When do you hear the voices?"
☐ **2.** "Are you going to hurt yourself?"
☐ **3.** "How long have you heard the voices?"
☐ **4.** "Why are the voices starting again?"

108. A 20-year-old client diagnosed with paranoid schizophrenia is recovering from his first psychotic break. Before discharge from the hospital, the client becomes depressed and states, "I do not want this illness. I am about to begin my junior year in college." Which issue would be **most** important for the nurse to address at this time?
☐ **1.** disturbed thought process
☐ **2.** disturbed sensory perceptions
☐ **3.** communication problems
☐ **4.** potential for medication noncompliance

109. The nurse is teaching two unlicensed assistive personnel (UAP) who are new to the inpatient unit about caring for a client who is suicidal. The nurse determines that additional teaching is needed when which statement is made?
☐ **1.** "I need to check the client precisely at 15-minute intervals."
☐ **2.** "Documenting suicide checks is absolutely necessary."
☐ **3.** "Clients on one-to-one suicide precautions can never be left alone."
☐ **4.** "All clients using razors must be supervised by staff."

110. Which activity should the nurse recommend to the client on an inpatient unit when thoughts of suicide occur?
☐ **1.** keeping track of feelings in a journal
☐ **2.** engaging in physical activity
☐ **3.** talking with the nurse
☐ **4.** playing a card game with other clients

111. For the client receiving outpatient treatment for depression and suicidal ideation, what is the correct amount of imipramine to have at one time?
☐ **1.** a 30-day supply
☐ **2.** a 21-day supply
☐ **3.** a 14-day supply
☐ **4.** a 7-day supply

112. The client with recurrent depression and suicidal ideation tells the nurse, "I cannot afford this medicine anymore. I know I will be okay without it." The nurse should:
☐ **1.** inform the healthcare provider (HCP) of the client's statement.
☐ **2.** ask the social worker to find financial assistance for the client.
☐ **3.** schedule a follow-up appointment in 2 weeks.
☐ **4.** ask the client whether a family member could help.

113. Which statement by the nurse reflects the **best** understanding about suicide in an individual with depression?
- [ ] 1. "The more severe the depression, the greater the probability for suicidal behavior."
- [ ] 2. "The person who talks about suicide is less likely to try it."
- [ ] 3. "Every client with depression is potentially suicidal."
- [ ] 4. "Suicide is less likely when the individual is receiving antidepressant therapy."

The Client with Psychosexual Disorders

114. A couple informs the nurse that they have been having some "problems in the bedroom." What is **most** appropriate response by the nurse?
- [ ] 1. "I can refer you to a therapist."
- [ ] 2. "I need to obtain your admission history first."
- [ ] 3. "I would like to hear your concerns."
- [ ] 4. "Let me refer you to a marriage counselor."

115. A client who is admitted to the adult unit of a mental healthcare facility with depression tells the nurse that he has pedophilia. The nurse should:
- [ ] 1. be aware of personal opinions and views.
- [ ] 2. recognize that because the client is depressed, the client will not be able to discuss the pedophilia.
- [ ] 3. ensure that the client is never alone with other clients on the unit.
- [ ] 4. refer the client to group therapy.

116. A client and her partner come to the clinic stating they have been unable to have sexual intercourse. The female client states she has pain and her "vagina is too tight." The client was raped at age 15 years of age. Which nursing problem is **most** appropriate for this client?
- [ ] 1. Dysfunctional Grieving related to loss of self-esteem because of lack of sexual intimacy
- [ ] 2. Risk for Trauma related to fear of vaginal penetration
- [ ] 3. Vaginismus related to vaginal constriction
- [ ] 4. Sexual Dysfunction related to sexual trauma

117. A client with erectile disorder is taking sildenafil. What instructions should the nurse give the client?
- [ ] 1. Take the medication 8 hours before having intercourse.
- [ ] 2. Use nitroglycerin if chest pains occur during intercourse.
- [ ] 3. Take up to three tablets within 24 hours.
- [ ] 4. Expect an erection that may last up to 4 hours.

Managing Care, Quality, and Safety of Clients with Psychiatric Disorders and Mental Health Problems

118. The nurse is caring for a client with bipolar disorder who was recently admitted to an inpatient unit and is experiencing a manic episode. What is a **priority** nursing intervention for this client?
- [ ] 1. Order and administer all medications in a liquid form.
- [ ] 2. Base permission for family visits on the client's attendance at therapy groups.
- [ ] 3. Closely monitor the client's eating and sleeping habits.
- [ ] 4. Encourage the client to keep a journal about feelings and emotions.

119. Which reaction to learning about a diagnosis of being HIV positive would put the client at the greatest need of intervention by the nurse?
- [ ] 1. A person who is angry, hostile, and alienated from the family.
- [ ] 2. A person who is obsessed with cleanliness and showers many times a day.
- [ ] 3. A person who is unable to make decisions and is helpless and tearful.
- [ ] 4. A person who says, "I have found a solution for this mess."

120. Which represents a breach of the nursing Code of Ethics regarding the rights of clients in psychiatric care situations?
- [ ] 1. The nurse discusses client's care with out-of-town family members who the client has formally indicated are allowed to know about the client's hospital care.
- [ ] 2. The nurse discusses the client's history and hospital course of treatment with a consulting healthcare provider (HCP).
- [ ] 3. The nurse discusses with peers in the hospital cafeteria the progress of a well-known client being cared for at the hospital.
- [ ] 4. The nurse discusses the client's care with the admission coordinator of a retirement home that the client plans to enter after discharge from the hospital.

121. A client diagnosed with schizophrenia for the last 2 years tells the nurse who has brought the morning medications, "That is not my pill! My pill is blue, not green." What should the nurse tell the client?
- [ ] 1. "Go ahead and take it. You can trust me. I am watching out for your safety and well-being."
- [ ] 2. "I know I took the correct medication out of the dispenser. Do you not trust me?"
- [ ] 3. "Do not worry; your medication is generic, and sometimes the manufacturers change the color of the pills without letting us know."
- [ ] 4. "I will go back and check the drawer as well as telephone the pharmacy to check about any possible changes in the medication color."

122. A colleague tells the nurse that she is feeling stressed and believes that she may be depressed. Healthy workplaces protect and promote the health and well-being of workers. What workplace strategies would **most** likely support the health and well-being of workers? Select all that apply.
- ☐ **1.** workshops for workers nearing retirement
- ☐ **2.** counseling for workers exposed to traumatic events
- ☐ **3.** interventions for workers with substance-related problems
- ☐ **4.** standard work hours that include scheduled rest periods
- ☐ **5.** education for workers regarding customary workplace practices

123. When developing appropriate assignments for the staff, which client should the nurse manager judge to be at **highest** risk for suicide completion?
- ☐ **1.** an 85-year-old Caucasian man who lives alone after his wife's death
- ☐ **2.** a 34-year-old single Latino woman who has recently been diagnosed with cancer
- ☐ **3.** a 15-year-old girl of African descent whose boyfriend broke up with her
- ☐ **4.** a 52-year-old Asian man who was terminated from his job because of downsizing

124. A high school student tells a nurse in an outpatient clinic the reason he is depressed and suicidal is that he is being bullied at school. While discussing the circumstances of the bullying, the student indicates he is gay, which he thinks contributes to his being bullied. He tells the nurse his sexual orientation in confidence, stating that his parents do not know and that he does not want that information revealed to them. Which actions should the nurse take? Select all that apply.
- ☐ **1.** Give him the crisis phone line number and contact information for a support group for gay teens.
- ☐ **2.** Notify the student's parents despite his objections because of the risk to him.
- ☐ **3.** Question him about the bullying and his current status regarding suicidal thoughts/plans.
- ☐ **4.** Help him develop a safety plan regarding suicidal thoughts/plans.
- ☐ **5.** Notify the school about the bullying without identifying the specific student.

125. A wife brings her husband to the emergency department with a bleeding gunshot wound to the leg. The wife tells the nurse that her husband was trying to commit suicide. In what order should the nurse perform the actions from first to last? All options must be used.

1. Assess current suicide risk.

2. Ensure constant observation.

3. Remove potentially harmful objects from the area.

4. Assess the gunshot wound.

Answers, Rationales, and Test-Taking Strategies

The answers and rationales for each question follow below, along with keys (🔑) to the client need (CN) and cognitive level (CL) for each question. In addition, you will also see a glossary icon (📖) highlighting specific terminology used on the licensing exam. As you check your answers, use the **Content Mastery and Test-Taking Skill Self-Analysis** *worksheet (tear-out worksheet in back of the book) to identify the reason(s) for not answering the questions correctly. For additional information about test-taking skills and strategies for answering questions, refer to pages 12–23 and pages 35–36 in Part 1 of this book.*

The Client with Major Depression

1. 4. Including the root healer gives credibility and respect to the client's cultural beliefs. Avoiding talking about the healer demonstrates either ignorance or disregard for the client's cultural values. Negative comparison of root healing with Western medicine not only denigrates the client's beliefs but also is likely to alienate and cause the client to end treatment.

🔑 CN: Psychosocial integrity; CL: Create

2. 3. Cheese and yeast products contain tyramine, which the client should avoid to prevent a negative interaction with tranylcypromine, a monoamine oxidase (MAO) inhibitor. Sodium will not interact with tranylcypromine, and neither exercise nor sugar needs to be limited.

CN: Pharmacological and parenteral therapies; CL: Evaluate

3. 1,4,3,2. The client is likely anxious about the procedure. The nurse should first spend time with the client and then discuss the client's concerns about the procedure. Next, the nurse could suggest the client listen to relaxing music. The use of the sleeping medication would only be considered as a last resort since it might interfere with the effectiveness of the seizure required for the treatment.

CN: Psychosocial integrity; CL: Synthesize

4. 4. The client is exhibiting signs of hypothyroidism, which includes hair loss, pain, fatigue, and increased sensitivity to cold. Hypothyroidism may be impacting the client's mood, ability to concentrate, physical sensations, and energy levels. Resolving potential biological causes of her symptoms takes priority over rehabilitation strategies or psychological approaches.

CN: Management of care; CL: Synthesize

5. 3. The nurse should report the client's beer consumption to the **HCP** ▢. Duloxetine should not be administered to a client with renal or hepatic insufficiency because the medication can elevate liver enzymes and, together with substantial alcohol use, can cause liver injury. Referring the client to the concurrent diagnosis program, sharing information at the next interdisciplinary treatment conference, and teaching the client relaxation exercises are helpful interventions for the nurse to implement. However, reporting the findings to the HCP is most important.

CN: Pharmacological and parenteral therapies; CL: Synthesize

6. 2. The client's sudden improvement and decrease in anxiety most likely indicate that the client is relieved because he has made the decision to kill himself and may now have the energy to complete the suicide. Symptoms of severe depression do not suddenly abate because most antidepressants work slowly and take 2 to 4 weeks to provide a maximum benefit. The client will improve slowly due to the medication. The sudden improvement in symptoms does not mean the client is nearing discharge, and decreasing observation of the client compromises the client's safety.

CN: Psychosocial adaptation; CL: Analyze

7. 1. The nurse should immediately report the rash to the **HCP** ▢ because lamotrigine can cause Stevens-Johnson syndrome, a toxic epidermal necrolysis. The rash is not a temporary adverse effect. Giving the client an ice pack and questioning the client about recent sun exposure are irresponsible nursing actions because of the possible seriousness of the rash.

CN: Pharmacological and parenteral therapies; CL: Synthesize

8. 2. The nurse should hold the 1700 hours dose of lithium because a level of 1.8 mEq/L (1.8 mmol/L) can cause adverse reactions, including diarrhea, vomiting, drowsiness, muscle weakness, and lack of coordination, which are early signs of lithium toxicity. The nurse should report the lithium level to the **healthcare provider (HCP)** ▢, including any symptoms of toxicity. Administering the 1700 hours dose of lithium, giving the client the lithium with 240 mL of water, or giving it after supper would result in an increase of the lithium level, thus increasing the risk of lithium toxicity.

CN: Pharmacological and parenteral therapies; CL: Synthesize

9. 3. Additional teaching is needed for the family member who states her son will only need to attend outpatient appointments when he starts to feel depressed again. Compliance with medication and outpatient follow-up are key in preventing relapse and rehospitalization. The statements expressing expectations of feeling better as medication takes effect, needing medicine and group therapy to stay well, and needing help with grocery shopping, cooking, and cleaning for a while indicate the families' understanding of depression, medication, and follow-up care.

CN: Psychosocial integrity; CL: Evaluate

10. 4. The nurse closely monitors the client taking paroxetine for the development of agitation, which could lead to self-harm in the form of a suicide attempt. Headache, nausea, and fatigue are transient adverse effects of paroxetine.

CN: Pharmacological and parenteral therapies; CL: Synthesize

11. 2. The nurse should initiate brief, frequent contacts throughout the day to let the client know that he is important to the nurse. This will positively affect the client's self-esteem. The nurse's action conveys acceptance of the client as a worthwhile person and provides some structure to the seemingly monotonous day. Waiting for the client to begin the conversation with the nurse is not helpful because the depressed client resists interaction and involvement with others. Sitting outside of the client's room is not productive and not necessary in this situation. If the client were actively suicidal, then a one-on-one client-to-staff assignment would be necessary. Questioning the client until he responds would overwhelm him because he could not meet the nurse's expectations to interact.

CN: Psychosocial integrity; CL: Synthesize

12. 1. The most appropriate action is for the nurse to remain with the client even if the client does not engage in conversation with the nurse. A client with severe depression may be unable to engage in an interaction with the nurse because the client feels worthless and lacks the necessary energy to do so. However, the nurse's presence conveys acceptance and caring, thus helping to increase the client's self-worth. Telling the client that the nurse will come back later, stating that the nurse will find someone else for the client to talk with, or telling the client that the nurse will get her something to read conveys to the client that she is not important, reinforcing the client's negative view of herself. Additionally, such statements interfere with the client's development of a sense of security and trust in the nurse.

CN: Psychosocial integrity; CL: Synthesize

13. 4. The nurse tells the client that the nurse is interested in her to increase the client's sense of importance, worth, and self-esteem. Also, stating that the nurse wants to help conveys to the client that she is worthwhile and important. Telling the client that the nurse is assigned to care for her is impersonal and implies that the client is being uncooperative. Telling the client that the nurse is there because the client has potential for improvement will not help the client with low self-esteem because most people develop a sense of self-worth through accomplishment. Simply saying that the client has a lot of potential will not convince her that she is worthwhile. Telling the client that the nurse will talk to someone else later is not client focused and does not address the client's question or concern.

CN: Psychosocial integrity; CL: Synthesize

14. 2. Nausea and gastrointestinal upset are common, but usually temporary, side effects of paroxetine. Therefore, the nurse would instruct the client to take the medication with food to minimize nausea and stomach upset. Other more common side effects are dry mouth, constipation, headache, dizziness, sweating, loss of appetite, ejaculatory problems in men, and decreased orgasms in women. Taking the medication an hour before breakfast would most likely lead to further gastrointestinal upset. Taking the medication at bedtime is not recommended because paroxetine can cause nervousness and

interfere with sleep. Because orange juice is acidic, taking the medication with it, especially on an empty stomach, may lead to nausea or increase the client's gastrointestinal upset.

CN: Pharmacological and parenteral therapies; CL: Synthesize

15. 2. The presence of dizziness could indicate orthostatic hypotension, which may cause injury to the client from falling. Nausea, sedation, and dry mouth do not require immediate intervention by the nurse.

CN: Pharmacological and parenteral therapies; CL: Analyze

16. 3. Symptom relief can occur during the first week of therapy, with optimal effects possible within 2 weeks. For some clients, 2 to 4 weeks is needed for optimal effects. The client's statement that the depression will be gone in 5 to 7 days indicates to the nurse that clarification and further teaching is needed. Trazodone should be taken after a meal or light snack to enhance its absorption. Trazodone can cause drowsiness, and therefore, the major portion of the drug should be taken at bedtime. The depressant effects of central nervous system depressants and alcohol may be potentiated by this drug.

CN: Pharmacological and parenteral therapies; CL: Evaluate

17. 3. The nurse should explain that ECT is a safe treatment and that the client is given an ultra-short-acting anesthetic to induce sleep before ECT and a muscle relaxant to prevent musculoskeletal complications during the convulsion, which typically lasts 30 to 60 seconds to be therapeutic. Atropine is given before ECT to inhibit salivation and respiratory tract secretions and thereby minimize the risk of aspiration. Medication for pain is not necessary and is not given before or during the treatment. Some clients experience a headache after the treatment and may request and be given an analgesic such as acetaminophen. Telling the daughter that the **HCP** 🖳 will ensure that the client does not suffer needlessly would not provide accurate information about ECT. This statement also implies that the client will have pain during the treatment, which is untrue.

CN: Reduction of risk potential; CL: Synthesize

18. 1. By stating "It must have been very upsetting for you," the nurse conveys empathy to the client by recognizing the underlying meaning of a painful occurrence. The nurse's statement invites the client to verbalize feelings and thoughts and lets the client know that the nurse is listening to and respects the client. Telling the client to talk about the job disregards the client's feelings and is nontherapeutic for the depressed client because of underlying feelings of worthlessness and guilt that are commonly present. Telling the client that he will find another job when he is better or that he was probably too depressed to work is inappropriate because it disregards the client's feelings and may promote additional feelings of failure and inadequacy in the client.

🔑 CN: Psychosocial integrity;
CL: Synthesize

19. 4. The client with depression is preoccupied, has decreased energy, and cannot make decisions, even simple ones. Therefore, the nurse presents the situation, "It is time for a shower," and assists the client with personal hygiene to preserve his dignity and self-esteem. Explaining the importance of good hygiene to the client is inappropriate because the client may know the benefits of hygiene but is too fatigued and preoccupied to pay attention to self-care. Asking the client if he is ready for a shower is not helpful because the client with depression commonly cannot make even simple decisions. This action also reinforces the client's feeling about not caring about showering. Waiting for the family to visit to help with the client's hygiene is inappropriate and irresponsible on the part of the nurse. The nurse is responsible for making basic decisions for the client until the client can make decisions for himself.

🔑 CN: Psychosocial integrity;
CL: Synthesize

20. 1,2,4,5. NPO status, a signed **consent** 📖, removal of dentures, and preprocedure voiding are all preparations prior to a procedure involving anesthesia, such as ECT. Orientation and frequent assessment of vital signs occur after the procedure.

🔑 CN: Reduction of risk potential;
CL: Synthesize

21. 2. Sertraline, like other selective serotonin reuptake inhibitors (SSRIs), can cause decreased libido and sexual dysfunction such as delayed ejaculation in men and an inability to achieve orgasm in women. SSRIs do not typically cause weight gain but may cause loss of appetite and weight loss. Dry mouth is a possible side effect, but it is temporary. The client should be told to take sips of water, suck on ice chips, or use sugarless gum or candy. St. John's wort should not be taken with SSRIs because a severe reaction could occur.

🔑 CN: Pharmacological and parenteral therapies; CL: Evaluate

22. 3. It is best to involve the client in usual at-home activities as much as the client can tolerate them. Discouraging visitors may not be in the client's best interest because visits with supportive significant others will help reinforce supportive relationships, which are important to the client's self-worth and self-esteem. Providing for a schedule of activities outside the home may be overwhelming for the client initially. Involving the client in planning for outside activities would be appropriate. Encouraging the client to sleep as much as possible is nontherapeutic and promotes withdrawal from others.

🔑 CN: Management of care; CL: Synthesize

23. 2. Criteria for commitment include being gravely disabled and posing a harm to self or others. This client is not threatening to harm himself in the form of suicide or to harm others. The client is gravely disabled because of his inability to care for himself—namely, not eating because of his delusion. Evidence of psychosis or psychotic symptoms or diagnosis of a mental illness alone does not make the client legally eligible for commitment.

🔑 CN: Management of care; CL: Apply

24. 3. The client needs to be informed of the time lag involved with antidepressant therapy. Although improvement in the client's symptoms will occur gradually over the course of 1 to 2 weeks, typically it takes 2 to 4 weeks to get the full effects of the medication. This information will help the client be compliant with medication and will also help in decreasing any anxiety the client has about not feeling better. The client's dose may not need to be increased; it is too early to determine the full effectiveness of the drug. Additionally, such a statement may increase the client's anxiety and diminish self-worth. Telling the client to wait a few days discounts the client's feelings and is inappropriate. Although it is too soon to tell whether the medication will be effective, telling this to the client may cause the client undue distress. This statement is somewhat negative because it is possible that the medication will not be effective, possibly further compounding the client's anxiety about not feeling better.

🔑 CN: Pharmacological and parenteral therapies; CL: Synthesize

25. 1,2,4,5. Serotonin syndrome can occur if a selective serotonin reuptake inhibitor is combined with a monoamine oxidase inhibitor, a tryptophan-serotonin precursor, or St. John's wort. Signs and symptoms of serotonin syndrome include mental status changes (such as confusion, restlessness, or agitation), headache, diaphoresis, ataxia, myoclonus, shivering, tremor, diarrhea, nausea, abdominal cramps, and hyperreflexia. Constipation is not associated with serotonin syndrome.

🔑 CN: Pharmacological and parenteral therapies; CL: Analyze

26. 2. Phenelzine is a monoamine oxidase inhibitor (MAOI). MAOIs block the enzyme monoamine oxidase, which is involved in the decomposition and inactivation of norepinephrine, serotonin, dopamine, and tyramine (a precursor to the previously stated neurotransmitters). Foods high in tyramine—those that are fermented, pickled, aged, or smoked—must be avoided because, when they are ingested in combination with MAOIs, a hypertensive crisis occurs. Some examples include salami, bologna, dried fish, sour cream, yogurt, aged cheese, bananas, pickled herring, caffeinated beverages, chocolate, licorice, beer, red wine, and alcohol-free beer.

⚿⬌ CN: Pharmacological and parenteral therapies; CL: Apply

27. 4. The nurse should first take the client's vital signs because the client could be experiencing a hypertensive crisis, which requires prompt intervention. Signs and symptoms of a hypertensive crisis include occipital headache, a stiff or sore neck, nausea, vomiting, sweating, dilated pupils and photophobia, nosebleed, tachycardia, bradycardia, and constricting chest pain. Giving this client an analgesic without taking his vital signs first is inappropriate. After the client's vital signs have been obtained, the nurse would call the **HCP** 📖 to report the client's problems and vital signs. Administering the client's next dose of phenelzine before taking his vital signs could result in a dangerous situation if the client is experiencing a hypertensive crisis.

⚿⬌ CN: Pharmacological and parenteral therapies; CL: Synthesize

28. 2. A depressed client commonly is not interested in eating because of the psychopathology of the disorder. Therefore, the nurse must take responsibility to ensure that the client eats, including spoon-feeding the client (placing the food on the spoon, putting the food near the client's mouth, and asking her to eat) if necessary. Serving the client her tray in her room does not ensure that she will eat. Calling the family to bring the client food from home usually is allowed, but it is still the nurse's responsibility to ensure that the client eats. Explaining the importance of nutrition in recovery is not helpful. The client may intellectually know that eating is important but may not be interested in eating or want to eat.

⚿⬌ CN: Psychosocial integrity; CL: Synthesize

29. 1. To promote adequate rest (6 to 8 hours per night) and to eliminate hyposomnia, the nurse should sit with the client at the bedside until the medication takes effect. The presence of a caring nurse provides the client with comfort and security and helps to decrease the client's anxiety. Engaging the client in interaction until the client falls asleep, reading to the client, or encouraging the client to watch television may be too stimulating for the client, consequently increasing rather than decreasing the client's restlessness.

⚿⬌ CN: Psychosocial integrity; CL: Synthesize

30. 3. The client who verbalizes feeling in control of self and situations no longer feels powerless to affect an outcome but realizes that one's actions can have an impact on self and situations. It is common for the client with depression to feel powerless to affect an outcome and to feel a lack of control over a situation. Although interacting with staff and peers is a positive action, the client could be conversing in a negative or nontherapeutic manner. Sleeping only 4 hours at a time is evidence of symptomatology and does not indicate improvement or recovery. Verbalizing dissatisfaction over not being able to perform at work indicates that the client is most likely focusing on shortcomings and powerlessness.

⚿⬌ CN: Psychosocial integrity; CL: Analyze

31. 2. The nurse must monitor the client for a suicide attempt at this time when the client is starting to feel better because the depressed client may now have enough energy to carry out an attempt. Bupropion inhibits dopamine reuptake; it is an activating antidepressant and could cause agitation. Although bupropion lowers the seizure threshold, especially at doses greater than 450 mg/day, and visual disturbances and increased libido are possible adverse effects, the nurse must closely monitor the client for a suicide attempt. As the client with major depression begins to feel better, the client may have enough energy to carry out an attempt.

⚿⬌ CN: Psychosocial integrity; CL: Analyze

32. 4. In the initial plan of care, the most appropriate outcome would be that the client will interact with the nurse. First, the client would begin interacting with one individual, the nurse. The nurse would gradually assist the client to engage in interactions with other clients in one-on-one contacts, progressing toward informal group gatherings and eventually taking part in structured group activities. The client needs to experience success according to the client's level of tolerance. Initiating interactions with peers occurs when the client can gain a measure of confidence and self-esteem instead of feeling intimidated or unduly anxious. Discussing adaptive coping techniques is an outcome the client may be able to reach when symptoms are not as severe and the client can concentrate on improving coping skills.

⚿⬌ CN: Psychosocial integrity; CL: Synthesize

33. 3. Imipramine, a tricyclic antidepressant, in combination with alcohol will produce additive central nervous system depression. Although caffeinated coffee is safe to use when the client is taking imipramine, it is not recommended for a client with depression who may be experiencing sleep disturbances. Imipramine may cause photosensitivity, so the client would be instructed to use sunscreen and protective clothing when exposed to the sun. Reduced lacrimation may occur as a side effect of imipramine. Therefore, the use of artificial tears may be recommended.

☘ CN: Pharmacological and parenteral therapies; CL: Create

34. 1. Telling the client that ECGs are done routinely for all clients taking imipramine, a tricyclic antidepressant, is an honest and direct response. Additionally, it provides some reassurance for the client. Commonly, a client with depression will ruminate, leading to needless increased anxiety. Tricyclic antidepressants may cause tachycardia, ECG changes, and cardiotoxicity. Telling the client that it is probably a precautionary measure because the nurse is not aware of a cardiac condition instills doubt and may cause undue anxiety for the client. Telling the client not to worry because the **HCP** 📖 is very thorough dismisses the client's concern and does not give the client adequate information. Explaining that the client had an ECG before initiating therapy with imipramine and that the procedure will be the same does not answer the client's question.

☘ CN: Pharmacological and parenteral therapies; CL: Synthesize

35. 4. Anticholinergic effects, which result from blockage of the parasympathetic nervous system, include urine retention, blurred vision, dry mouth, and constipation. Tremors, cardiac arrhythmias, and sexual dysfunction are possible side effects, but they are caused by increased norepinephrine availability. Sedation and delirium are not anticholinergic effects. Sedation may be a therapeutic effect because many clients with depression experience agitation and insomnia. Delirium, typically not a side effect, would indicate toxicity, especially in elderly clients. Respiratory depression, convulsions, ataxia, agitation, stupor, and coma indicate tricyclic antidepressant toxicity.

☘ CN: Pharmacological and parenteral therapies; CL: Analyze

36. 1. The nurse should give the medication as prescribed. Mirtazapine is given once daily, preferably at bedtime to minimize the risk of injury resulting from postural hypotension and sedative effects. The usual dosage ranges from 15 to 45 mg. There is no reason to question the **HCP's** 📖 prescriptions.

The nurse should administer the medication as prescribed. Requesting to give the medication in three divided doses is inappropriate and demonstrates the nurse's lack of knowledge about the drug.

☘ CN: Pharmacological and parenteral therapies; CL: Synthesize

37. 4. The nurse should express concern for the client and offer to help the client speak with the **HCP** 📖, which will lend support to the client's concerns. The client who has stopped the medication must be taken seriously because medication noncompliance could result in a recurrence of symptoms of depression. Telling the client to focus on diet and exercise ignores the client's feelings and subtly implies the weight gain is the client's fault. Pointing out that the medication has helped and that positive things have happened since the depression lifted may be true, but it does not address the client's current feelings or needs.

☘ CN: Pharmacological and parenteral therapies; CL: Synthesize

38. 3. Compliance with medication therapy is crucial for the client with depression. Medication noncompliance is the primary cause of relapse among psychiatric clients. Therefore, the nurse needs to teach the client about managing common adverse effects to promote compliance with medication. Teaching the client about the medication's pharmacokinetics may help the client to understand the reason for the drug. However, teaching about how to manage common adverse effects to promote compliance is crucial. Current research about the medication is more important to the nurse than to the client. Teaching about dosage regulation and adjustment of medication may be helpful, but typically, the **HCP** 📖, not the client, is the person in charge of this aspect.

☘ CN: Pharmacological and parenteral therapies; CL: Create

39. 1. After about 2 weeks of medication therapy, the nurse should expect improvements in sleep, appetite, and energy though mood may not have improved significantly yet. The increased energy related to better sleep and food intake gives the client the ability to act on thoughts to harm self (suicide) since the depressed mood has not completely lifted.

☘ CN: Pharmacological and parenteral therapies; CL: Analyze

40. 4. Dry mouth is a common, temporary side effect of paroxetine. The nurse needs to further assess the client's water intake when the client states she is drinking lots of water. Excessive intake of water could be harmful to the client and could lead to electrolyte imbalance. Dry mouth is caused by the medication, and drinking a lot of water will not eliminate it. Sucking on ice chips or using sugarless gum or candy is appropriate to ease the discomfort of dry mouth associated with paroxetine.

> CN: Pharmacological and parenteral therapies; CL: Evaluate

41. 2,3,5. Symptoms of depression include depressed mood, anhedonia, appetite disturbance, sleep disturbance, psychomotor disturbance, fatigue, feelings of worthlessness, excessive or inappropriate guilt, decreased concentration, and recurrent thoughts of death or suicide. Paroxetine is a selective serotonin reuptake inhibitor antidepressant that also can be used to treat anxiety. Improved concentration, verbalization of feelings, and decreased agitation or pacing are signs of improvement. Taking 2-hour evening naps daily is still a sign of fatigue or lack of energy, and the increased use of somatization (bodily problems) could be signs of continued symptoms of depression.

> CN: Pharmacological and parenteral therapies; CL: Evaluate

42. 3. The most important behavior to report to the next shift is that the client was able to sleep from 2300 to 0600. This indicates that improvement in the symptoms of depression is occurring as a result of pharmacologic therapy. The nurse would expect to observe improvement in sleep, appetite, and psychomotor behavior first before improvement in cognitive symptoms. The client's flat affect is still a symptom of depression. The fact that the client had a visitor is not as important as changes in the client's behavior. Spending the evening in her room is a continuation of the client's withdrawn behavior and is important to report but not as important as the improvement in sleep.

> CN: Psychosocial integrity; CL: Analyze

43. 3. Dysthymia is a milder, persistent type of depression in which sufferers are able to minimally carry on their work. The combination of psychotherapy with antidepressants is more effective in treating this order than using either treatment alone. ECT is a treatment used for occurrences of major depression as a last resort when several medications fail. Psychoanalysis is a very involved, long-term treatment rarely used now due to its cost and the long period of treatment required for results.

> CN: Psychosocial integrity; CL: Synthesize

44. 3. After two episodes of a major depressive disorder, the likelihood of a third episode increases to 70%. This information would be useful to convey prior to discussing the importance of continuing his medication. This client also has a family history of depression. A healthy diet and exercise are very significant adjuncts to the therapeutic plan but may not be sufficient as stand-alone therapy.

> CN: Physiological integrity; CL: Analyze

45. 1. In the first week or so of taking an antidepressant, the vegetative symptoms of depression (poor sleep, appetite, and energy level) improve. However, it takes 3 to 4 weeks for improvement in self-concept/self-esteem to take place.

> CN: Pharmacological and parenteral therapies; CL: Evaluate

The Client with Bipolar Disorder, Manic Phase

46. 4. The most urgent consideration for intervention and for teaching is the fact that for individuals with a history of bipolar disorder, antidepressants when taken alone can push the person into mania. Antipsychotics are sometimes prescribed for clients with bipolar disorder and would not pose a special concern. Individuals with bipolar disorder are typically treated with mood stabilizers, and benzodiazepines are sometimes used in the short term to give a client relief before the mood stabilizers can take effect.

> CN: Pharmacological and parenteral therapies; CL: Analyze

47. 2. Decreased need for sleep and racing thoughts are the most prominent hallmarks of mania. Feelings of pleasure, motivation, and increased energy, within reason, are desired experiences. Also, leaving a job to start a new business is not, in itself, a sign of impending illness.

> CN: Psychosocial integrity; CL: Apply

48. 4. The therapeutic serum level for lithium is 0.6 to 1.2 mEq/L (0.6 to 1.2 mmol/L). Levels do fluctuate with fluid intake and output, however. Therefore, the most urgent matter for teaching is the client's comment about taking his lithium during excessive loss of fluids during an episode of "stomach flu" with diarrhea. Exercising is only concerning if the client becomes dehydrated. A healthy diet is indicated while taking lithium.

> CN: Pharmacological and parenteral therapies; CL: Analyze

49. 3. All of these options need to be addressed. However, it is vital that this young woman receive counseling about the serious birth defects that have an increased incidence with the taking of divalproex during the first trimester of pregnancy. These problems include craniofacial abnormalities (cleft palate), organ malformations (holes in the heart and urinary tract problems), limb deficiencies, and developmental delays. The chances of preeclampsia and premature labor are also increased.

> CN: Reduction of risk potential; CL: Analyze

50. 1. Valproic acid can cause hepatotoxicity, so regular liver function tests are needed. Other side effects include nausea and drowsiness. Extended-release tablets should not be split or crushed; doing so changes their absorption. Alcohol should never be mixed with this medication. There will be medication in the client's body at all times. Nausea and tachycardia are not common side effects of valproic acid.

CN: Pharmacological and parenteral therapies; CL: Synthesize

51. 2. The use of prednisone or other steroids can initiate a manic state in a bipolar client even if he is well controlled on medication. The other medications would decrease the client's depression, mood swings, and anxiety, making him calmer rather than more agitated.

CN: Pharmacological and parenteral therapies; CL: Analyze

52. 3. The nurse should first attempt a collaborative approach to increasing adherence to the prescribed medication regimen. Giving written medication information to a client with acute mania is poor nursing judgment because a client with acute mania cannot benefit from written information as a result of impaired ability to focus and concentrate. The client was a voluntary admission and has the right to refuse any medication. Giving the medication as an injection against the client's **consent** 📖 constitutes battery.

CN: Management of care; CL: Synthesize

53. 2. The nurse clearly informs the client about behavior that is unacceptable on the unit, such as voicing jokes with sexual content and touching others. Setting limits on behavior provides safety and security to the client and conveys to the client that he is worthy of help. Saying "She will not want to be around you with that kind of talk" and "You need to be careful about what you say to others" does not clearly inform the client about behaviors that are unacceptable and implies that the client can control behaviors if he chooses. A time-out in the client's room does not inform the client about the inappropriateness of his behaviors and could be interpreted by the client as punitive as well as diminishing his self-esteem.

CN: Psychosocial integrity; CL: Synthesize

54. 3. The nurse should medicate the client who does not respond to verbal interventions and whose anxiety is escalating. This will reduce the client's anxiety and agitation and prevent harm or injury to the client and others. Seclusion, restraint, and controlling the client are a last resort and require a **healthcare provider's (HCP's)** 📖 prescription and close assessment for when the prescriptions can be discontinued.

CN: Psychosocial integrity; CL: Synthesize

55. 4. The nurse should help the **unlicensed assistive personnel (UAP)** 📖 understand the client's behavior by stating that his irritable mood is a symptom of mania. Not all clients with mania are euphoric or have an expansive mood. Saying "It is our responsibility to listen to him even though we might not like what he is saying" does not help the UAP understand the client with mania. Reprimanding the client for his behavior and asking him to control his behavior are inappropriate actions and show poor nursing judgment and a lack of understanding of the manic client.

CN: Psychosocial integrity; CL: Synthesize

56. 1,2,3,5. Scheduled rest periods, relaxation exercises, and listening to soft music are activities that reduce environmental stimuli for the client who is hyperactive, talkative, easily distracted, irritable, and angry. Aerobic exercise is also beneficial to discharge some of the client's need to be active. Watching television is not therapeutic because it would stimulate the client with acute mania.

CN: Psychosocial integrity; CL: Apply

57. 3. Reminding the client of past consequences of stopping the medication may help her realize the risks of stopping the medication again. While increases in energy may precipitate suicide attempts, the priority here is to reinforce the need for maintenance medications. Encouraging the client to reduce her medication dose reinforces the client's misperception that she only needs medication when she feels depressed or manic rather than recognizing that her mood stabilizer can prevent her from experiencing those extreme highs and lows. Saying she will "spiral out of control" if she stops her medication is not as specific as identifying the need for hospitalization.

CN: Pharmacological and parenteral therapies; CL: Synthesize

58. 1. The nurse should administer the medication as prescribed. Lithium has a clinical response lag time of 1 to 2 weeks. Haloperidol is prescribed temporarily to produce a neuroleptic effect until the lithium starts to produce a clinical response. Haloperidol is usually discontinued when the lithium starts to take effect. There is no need to contact the HCP or supervisor as the prescription is appropriate.

CN: Pharmacological and parenteral therapies; CL: Synthesize

59. 4. The client's statement "I am the Queen of England. Bow before me" is an example of a grandiose delusion and refers to thought content of the mental status examination. Examples of psychomotor behavior to be documented would include excited, typically exaggerated, and repetitive physical movements, and excessive talking and gesturing. Mood is a subjective state, and affect is an observable expression of emotion. Mood is what a client tells you she is feeling, and affect is what you see the client feeling. For example, the client may state that she feels sad or happy in reference to mood. Affect refers to the display of physical emotion, commonly described as "appropriate" or "flat." Attitude toward the nurse refers to the client's behavior in the presence of the nurse during the mental status examination (pleasant and cooperative, irritable, and guarded).

    CN: Psychosocial integrity; CL: Analyze

60. 4. Decreasing external stimuli is the intervention most likely to decrease the emotional lability and minimize its effect on other clients. While the client is displaying emotional lability, this behavior has not reached the level where involuntary isolation (seclusion) or physical restraint is needed. The client is not totally out of control or threatening others. However, ignoring the behavior will not result in a decrease in the lability. Lorazepam can be used, but benzodiazepines can lead to dependence and should not be used before other measures have been tried.

    CN: Psychosocial integrity;
CL: Synthesize

61. 1. The nurse would request to be excused, showing respect and regard for the client, while telling the client to come to the dining room for lunch. Acutely manic clients need clear, concise comments and directions. Telling the client that he needs to stop talking because it is lunchtime is disrespectful and does not give the client directions for what he needs to do. Using the familiar skill of waiting without interrupting until the person pauses would not be effective with the very talkative, manic client. Walking away and approaching the client after a few minutes before the food gets cold is not helpful because the client would probably continue talking.

    CN: Psychosocial integrity;
CL: Synthesize

62. 3. By stating to the client "Swearing and profanity is unacceptable here," the nurse is setting limits in a nonpunitive manner for behavior that is inappropriate or threatening to other clients and staff. Setting limits helps the client regain self-control, prevents alienation from others, and preserves self-esteem. It is common for the irritable manic client to misperceive the nurse's and other's statements and intentions, feel threatened, and respond in a manner that is out of character for the client when not in a manic phase. Stating that the client is acting very inappropriately or that the nurse will not tolerate the client's swearing and profanity or threatening to put the client in seclusion is threatening and punitive and thus nontherapeutic.

    CN: Psychosocial integrity;
CL: Synthesize

63. 1. Stating that this must be difficult for the husband conveys empathy and understanding and offers him the opportunity to voice his feelings to the nurse. Telling the husband that it is okay and that the nurse has heard worse is inappropriate and minimizes the impact of the wife's illness on the husband. Asking about the length of the client's illness or telling the husband that his wife needs some medication ignores the husband's feelings, thereby minimizing his self-respect.

    CN: Psychosocial integrity;
CL: Synthesize

64. 3. Telling the client that others may not want to hear about sex and inviting him to play a game of ping-pong with the nurse informs the client that even though his behavior is unacceptable, the nurse considers him worthy of help. The client's thoughts and actions are out of control, and directing him to an activity with the nurse is an appropriate way of regaining control. The nurse is responsible for providing safety and security to this client and others on the unit. Continuing to walk down the hall while ignoring the conversation does nothing to meet the needs of this or other clients. Doing so also diminishes trust in the nurse. Speaking to the client later in private while saying nothing at the time allows the client to continue his provocative behavior instead of focusing his energy toward productive activity. Informing the client that if he continues to talk about sex, no one will want to be around him is not helpful because his behavior is a symptom of his illness and the statement diminishes his self-worth.

    CN: Psychosocial integrity;
CL: Synthesize

65. 4. The nurse suggests an activity such as walking around the unit to distract the client from the paranoid grandiose delusion that could result in loss of control. This action interrupts the client's anxious state and helps to redirect energy and focus on an activity based in reality. The focus must be on the underlying need or feeling of the delusion and not on the content. Asking the client to describe the people who will come challenges the client and forces the client to cling to the delusion. Stating that the nurse and staff will protect the client conveys agreement with the client's belief system, reinforcing the client's delusion. Telling the client that he is not the prince of peace and repeating his name challenges the client and his present belief system. Doing so may lead to decreased trust in the nurse and an aggressive response, or it may force the client to defend his beliefs.

🔑 CN: Psychosocial integrity;
CL: Synthesize

66. 2. The nurse needs to explain the procedure in simple terms because the client in a manic phase has difficulty concentrating, is easily distracted, and can misinterpret what the nurse states. Giving a thorough explanation of the procedure is not helpful and can confuse the client. Calling security to be on standby is inappropriate. If the nurse judges that the client might elope or become agitated, the nurse should schedule the appointment for another time. Canceling the appointment until the client can go unescorted is impractical and may not follow unit or hospital policy and the client's treatment plan.

🔑 CN: Psychosocial integrity;
CL: Synthesize

67. 4. The nurse escorts the client to her room and assists with choosing appropriate attire to preserve the client's dignity and self-esteem and prevent ridicule from others on the unit. It is common for a client with bipolar disorder, manic phase, to exhibit poor judgment, provocative behavior, and hyperactivity. The client in the manic phase commonly dresses inappropriately and changes clothes many times throughout the day. The nurse needs to assist the client with hygiene, grooming, and proper attire until her judgment improves. Telling the client to dress appropriately while out of her room may be perceived by the client as an attack. Additionally, the client may be incapable of making that decision. Asking the client to put on hospital pajamas until she can dress appropriately is punitive and demeaning. Because of the client's cognitive difficulties, the client may not understand the instructions to go to her room to change clothes. Additionally, the client may become distracted by stimuli on the unit and may not reach her room.

🔑 CN: Psychosocial integrity;
CL: Synthesize

68. 3. While the client who is psychotic can upset other clients, the nurse must respond to the second client with both empathy for his feelings and a general explanation that the behavior is out of the psychotic client's control. Agreeing with the second client or giving medication to the psychotic client does not help the complaining client gain empathy for his peer and only temporarily deals with the problem.

🔑 CN: Psychosocial integrity;
CL: Synthesize

69. 4. The client with mania is very active and needs to have this energy channeled in a constructive task such as cleaning or tidying the dayroom. Because the client is distracted easily and can concentrate only for short periods, the successful completion of a helpful task would give the nurse the opportunity to thank the client for the help, thereby enhancing the client's self-esteem. Leading a group activity is too stimulating for the client. Participating in this type of activity also may cause the client to be disruptive. Watching television or reading the newspaper would be inappropriate for the client who cannot sit for a period of time.

🔑 CN: Psychosocial integrity;
CL: Synthesize

70. 1. The client in the manic phase experiences insomnia, as evidenced by his sleeping only for about 4 hours a night for the past 5 days. The client experiencing an acute manic episode is not capable of judging the need for sleep. Therefore, the nurse should assess the amount of rest the client is receiving daily to prevent exhaustion. The development of vertigo, gastritis, or bradycardia typically does not result from acute mania.

🔑 CN: Psychosocial integrity; CL: Analyze

71. 3. Bipolar disorder is a biochemical disorder caused by an imbalance of neurotransmitters in the brain. Manic episodes seem to be related to excessive levels of norepinephrine, serotonin, and dopamine. Psychopharmacologic therapy aims to restore the balance of neurotransmitters. In the past, it was thought that bipolar disorder may have been caused by early psychodynamics or disturbed families, but the current view emphasizes the role of biology. Bipolar disorder could be genetic or inherited from someone in the family, but it is best for the client and family to understand the disease concept related to neurotransmitter imbalance. This understanding also helps them to refrain from placing blame on anyone. Siblings and close relatives have a higher incidence of bipolar disorder and mood disorders in general when compared with the general population.

🔑 CN: Psychosocial integrity; CL: Apply

72. 2. The serum lithium level has nothing to do with the client's white blood cell count, and there are no governmental safety regulations for blood testing. While a periodic serum lithium level could monitor whether or not a client was taking the prescribed medication, the most important reason for the blood test is to periodically assess the client's lithium level and prevent even mild toxicity on an ongoing basis.

🔑 CN: Pharmacological and parenteral therapies; CL: Apply

73. 3. Because lithium reaches peak blood levels in 1 to 3 hours, blood specimens for serum lithium concentration determinations are usually drawn before the first dose of lithium in the morning (which is usually 8 to 12 hours after the previous dose) or before breakfast. Stat lithium levels can be drawn at any time, usually when toxicity is suspected.

🔑 CN: Pharmacological and parenteral therapies; CL: Apply

74. 2,3,5. Serious side effects that may indicate lithium toxicity include muscle weakness, vertigo, vomiting, extreme hand tremor, and sedation. The prescribing **HCP** 📖 should be notified immediately when these symptoms occur. When lithium is initiated, mild or transient side effects can occur, such as nausea, fine hand tremor, anorexia, increased thirst and urination, and diarrhea or constipation.

🔑 CN: Pharmacological and parenteral therapies; CL: Evaluate

75. 2. The therapeutic and toxic range of lithium is very narrow. If the client forgets to take a scheduled dose of lithium, the client needs to wait until the next scheduled time to take it because taking twice the amount of lithium can cause lithium toxicity. The client needs to maintain a regular diet and regular salt intake. Lithium and sodium are eliminated from the body through the kidneys. An increase in salt intake leads to decreased plasma lithium levels because lithium is excreted more rapidly. A decrease in salt intake leads to increased plasma lithium levels. The client needs to drink 8 to 10 eight-ounce (240 to 300 mL) glasses of water daily to maintain fluid balance and decrease thirst. Decreased water intake can lead to an increase in the lithium level and consequently a risk of toxicity. Lithium must be taken on a regular basis at the same time each day to ensure maximum therapeutic effect.

🔑 CN: Pharmacological and parenteral therapies; CL: Evaluate

76. 4. Lithium commonly is combined with an antipsychotic agent, such as haloperidol, or a benzodiazepine such as lorazepam. Antipsychotic agents, such as haloperidol, are prescribed to produce a neuroleptic effect until the lithium produces a clinical response. After a clinical response is achieved, the antipsychotic agent usually is discontinued. Additionally, the dosages of each drug listed are appropriate. Therefore, the nurse would administer the drugs as prescribed.

🔑 CN: Pharmacological and parenteral therapies; CL: Synthesize

77. 4. The client's statement "I know I am getting sick when I do not need much sleep and start buying things" indicates insight into her illness because the client recognizes symptoms that can lead to relapse. The statement "I enjoy feeling high; I do not need much sleep then and get really creative" gives no indication that the client recognizes the detrimental effects of bipolar disorder. The statements about not needing medicine in another week and being cured indicate the client's lack of understanding about the chronic nature of the disorder. The client is not cured from bipolar disorder, but symptoms of the disorder are usually managed when she is stabilized on medication. Medication may be needed by the client for many years or throughout her life.

🔑 CN: Psychosocial integrity; CL: Evaluate

78. 1. For this client, the nurse needs to set limits on the client's intrusive, interruptive behavior by saying "Please stop interrupting others; you can speak when it is your turn." This statement also clearly points out to the client the specific unacceptable behavior. The nurse helps the client to attain control and helps the other clients become more tolerant of the situation. Saying "Stop talking; it is time for you to leave the meeting" is not helpful because it leaves the client unaware of what has happened or the behavior that is unacceptable. Also, such a statement may seem punitive. The statement, "If you cannot control yourself, we will have to take action," is threatening to the client and diminishes the client's self-worth. Using the statement "Please behave like an adult. Your behavior is childish" is demeaning and scolding to the client, thereby diminishing the client's self-esteem.

🔑 CN: Psychosocial integrity; CL: Synthesize

79. 1,2,5. The therapeutic level of valproic acid is 50 to 100 mg/mL (347 to 693 mmol/L). A level of 15 mg/mL (104 mmol/L) is not considered therapeutic. Therefore, the client would be manifesting symptoms of mania. Irritability, euphoria, grandiosity, pressured speech, flight of ideas, distractibility, and a decreased need for sleep are some characteristics of a manic episode. Anhedonia and hypersomnia are related to a depressive illness and not mania.

🔑 CN: Pharmacological and parenteral therapies; CL: Analyze

80. 4. The nurse should call the **HCP** 📖 to report symptoms of a sore throat, fever, and chills because these symptoms may be signs of serious adverse effects of the medication, including potentially fatal hematologic, cardiovascular, and hepatic complications. Giving the dose of carbamazepine is contraindicated in this situation. Giving the acetaminophen would be inappropriate and potentially detrimental to the client's health. Waiting until morning to report the client's symptoms is a serious error in judgment.

🔑 CN: Pharmacological and parenteral therapies; CL: Synthesize

81. 2. The nurse's most appropriate action is to give the wife information about a support group in her area. Family members need and want education and support. Suggesting that the wife see an **HCP** 📖 is not necessary in this situation. She needs support and education. Recommending that she talk with her close friend may be helpful if she so chooses. However, this is not as helpful as attending a support group. Here, the wife can learn, share, obtain support from, and provide support to others with similar situations. Having the wife share her feelings with her husband may or may not be appropriate or helpful to her or her husband. The husband may be unable to help his wife with adaptive coping, and therefore, the client's self-esteem could be diminished.

🔑 CN: Psychosocial integrity;
CL: Synthesize

82. 2. The nurse should encourage the husband to support and communicate openly with his wife to maintain effective family-client interactions. During any illness, open communication and support helps the relationship between husband and wife. It is unrealistic for any individual to be free from anxiety or worry and impossible for the husband to be able to control what his wife may think or feel. Relieving the client of all responsibilities is unrealistic and not helpful. The client needs to resume activities as soon as she can manage them. Reminding his wife to control her symptoms is not appropriate and indicates that the husband needs further teaching about this condition.

🔑 CN: Psychosocial integrity; CL: Create

83. 3,1,2,4. None of the other interventions will be successful unless the stimuli that fuel the client's mania are removed or decreased. Once the client is in a quieter setting, oral medication will help calm the client so he or she can be calmer. Once the medication has taken effect, the nurse can help the client explore the client's feelings and problem. Finally, teaching coping techniques can be effective to address client problems after he or she has become calmer.

🔑 CN: Psychosocial integrity;
CL: Synthesize

84. 4. The nurse should state her name and purpose on the unit to clarify her identity and to counteract other beliefs the client may have. Stating that the nurse does not want to or cannot go out to dinner is not therapeutic because it fails to clarify the client's misperceptions or erroneous beliefs, as is the statement "It does not matter how I look; the answer is no."

🔑 CN: Psychosocial integrity;
CL: Synthesize

85. 3. The client is visibly out of control, and other measures have not helped. Therefore, the nurse needs to seclude the client and use restraints if necessary to protect the client and others from harm. Following the client and asking her to calm down or telling the client to lie down on the sofa is not helpful because the client's level of anxiety is too high for her to attempt to calm down on her own and she cannot control her behavior. Telling the staff to ignore the client's remarks is not helpful because the client needs external means of control to protect the client, other clients on the unit, and the staff. Safety is the priority.

🔑 CN: Safety and infection control;
CL: Synthesize

86. 3. When the client in a manic state attempts to manipulate the nurse or demands privileges, the nurse must restate the unit rules in a calm and matter-of-fact manner. "The television hours are from 1900 hours to 2200 hours. It is 2200, and the television goes off so everyone can sleep" is the most therapeutic response because it restates the rules and is nonthreatening. During a manic phase, the client is impulsive and has difficulty concentrating. The client needs consistency and structure from the staff. The statement "I will let you watch television just this once" allows the client to manipulate the nurse, as does "I will turn the television off when you get sleepy. Do not ask me to do this again." In addition, the last portion of the statement is a threat. The statement, "The television goes off at 2200 hours; I've been telling you this for the past three evenings," is inappropriate because it is authoritative and demeaning to the client.

🔑 CN: Psychosocial integrity;
CL: Synthesize

The Client with Suicidal Ideation and Suicide Attempt

87. 1,2,4. Having resources such as a crisis phone line number and a specific prevention plan helps clients know what to do if they begin to feel they want to harm themselves. Likewise, having support people educated about how to help the client stay safe also improves the client's safety. Not all medications are lethal enough that access to a month's supply of medication should be limited. Further, such a limitation is likely to increase costs for the clients, which may increase the client's stress. It is unrealistic and potentially distressing to the client and family/friends to have the client under constant surveillance.

🔑 CN: Safety and infection control;
CL: Apply

88. 3. It is important to assess clients in the ED for suicide risk so that those with the potential can receive help prior to discharge. Many visitors to the ED have no other source for health care. It is a myth that talking about suicide will cause young people to think about suicide, and evidence exists that they will talk about suicide if asked directly. Assessing adults only because they will be more honest is an incorrect assumption. Limiting the assessment of suicide risk only to adolescents with psychiatric diagnoses falsely assumes that other young people are not at risk for suicide. Questioning the parents about their adolescent's suicide risk may be an unreliable method because the parents may not be aware that suicide risk is present.

⚲— CN: Psychosocial integrity;
CL: Synthesize

89. 2. A crucial factor in determining the lethality of a method is the amount of time that occurs between initiating the method and the delivery of the lethal impact of the method. Lethal methods of suicide include using a gun, jumping from a high place, hanging, drowning, carbon monoxide poisoning, and overdose with certain drugs, such as central nervous system depressants, alcohol, and barbiturates. The more detailed the suicide plan, the more lethal and accessible the method, and the more effort exerted to block rescue, the greater the chance is for the suicide to be completed. Impulsive attempts at suicide even with rescuers in sight may be lethal depending on the method. Less lethal methods may include overdosing on aspirin and wrist cutting. Head banging is a self-injurious behavior that requires intervention and is not to be taken lightly; however, it is not considered a lethal method of suicide.

⚲— CN: Psychosocial integrity; CL: Apply

90. 4. The statement "No matter what the intent, all suicidal behavior is serious and deserves our serious consideration" is most appropriate because it provides accurate information for the staff. Superficial cuts may be termed *suicide gestures*. Nevertheless, they still are a cry for help and may indicate ambivalence about dying. Clients have accidentally and unintentionally killed themselves because previous attempts were not taken seriously, they acted on impulse, or rescue attempts were foiled. Stating "It is our job to help her no matter how we feel about her or what she did; she will be discharged soon" is inappropriate because it does not provide the staff members with accurate information. Stating "I will not tolerate that kind of discussion from my staff; now it is time for you to go back to work" is authoritarian and punitive. Additionally, it does not help the staff members gain insight. Stating "I know it is hard to understand, but we need to do the best

we can even though she will be back" voices agreement with the staff's bias and lack of knowledge. As such, this statement is inappropriate.

⚲— CN: Management of care; CL: Synthesize

91. 2. On hearing the client's statement, the nurse must ask the client directly if she plans to kill herself. It is erroneous to think that talking to the client about suicide will drive her to it. Asking directly about suicidal intent is absolutely necessary. Commonly, doing so provides the client with a sense of relief. In addition, the nurse conveys concern for and a sense of worth to the client, thus enabling appropriate planning for care. Asking "What do you mean?" is an indirect method of inquiry that provides the client with the opportunity to evade the nurse's intent. Asking "Does your family not care about you?" shows poor judgment on the nurse's part and is demeaning to the client. Asking "What happened to make you think that?" conveys a lack of knowledge of psychopathology.

⚲— CN: Psychosocial integrity; CL: Analyze

92. 4. For the client with suicidal ideation, client safety is the priority. The nurse protects the client from self-harm or self-destruction. Although self-esteem, sleep, and stress are common areas that require intervention for a client with suicidal ideation, ensuring the client's safety is the most immediate and serious concern.

⚲— CN: Safety and infection control;
CL: Synthesize

93. 1. To determine the seriousness of the suicidal ideation, the nurse must ask directly about the intent and the plan. The nurse needs to determine whether the client has a concrete plan and will act on his or her thoughts. Then, the nurse assesses the lethality of the method, immediacy, means to complete suicide, and possibility of rescue. Asking the client "Have you made out a will?" is not as important and does not necessarily imply that he or she is planning self-harm. Many individuals have made out wills without planning self-harm. Asking the client "Does your family know you are here?" provides no information about the client's intent and plan. Asking the client "How long have you been thinking about harming yourself?" does provide information that the client is thinking about self-harm. However, it does not provide information about the client's immediate intent and plan.

⚲— CN: Psychosocial integrity; CL: Analyze

94. 2. The nurse's best response is to teach the UAP □ about the appropriate intervention and why it is important for the client. Staff members need to be client focused and to understand why a specific intervention is important and appropriate. Telling the UAP that the assignment will be switched or not to worry about it is not appropriate because it does not teach the UAP about the client's illness and appropriate client care. The statement "Clients who are depressed are hard to deal with, but do not take what they say seriously" does not help the staff member understand why listening is important and may jeopardize the client's safety.

🔑 CN: Management of care; CL: Synthesize

95. 2. The immediate priority is to save the caller's life. Therefore, the nurse should tell the caller that another nurse will telephone the police. The immediate goal is to rescue the caller because the suicide attempt has begun. Referring the caller to a 24-hour suicide hotline or instructing the caller to telephone her family for help may be appropriate as part of discharge planning. Asking the caller whether she has telephoned her **IICP** 📖 is not appropriate. The nurse is responsible for notifying the HCP.

🔑 CN: Psychosocial integrity; CL: Synthesize

96. 4. The statement refers to the suicidal client's wish to use her own death to retaliate or get even with her boyfriend. If a client wishes to retaliate, discovering the specific plans would be important to maintaining her safety as well as possibly her boyfriend's. Though sadness, escape, and loneliness can all be themes expressed by a suicidal client, they do not apply to the comment made by this client.

🔑 CN: Psychosocial integrity; CL: Analyze

97. 2. The statement "I do not think about killing myself as much as I used to" indicates a lessening of suicidal ideation and improvement in the client's condition. The statement "I could not kill myself because I do not want to go to hell" indicates that the client will not attempt suicide but could still be thinking about death. The statements "I am of no use to anyone anymore" and "I know my kids do not need me anymore since they are on their own" indicate that the client feels worthless and may be experiencing suicidal ideation.

🔑 CN: Psychosocial integrity; CL: Evaluate

98. 4. Based on the client's statement, the nurse must initiate plans for hospitalization immediately because the client has suicidal ideation with a definite plan, lethal method, and immediate access to the method. Telling the client to remove the gun, call the nurse, or promise not to hurt himself does not sufficiently reduce the risk of suicide.

🔑 CN: Psychosocial integrity; CL: Synthesize

99. 1. The survivor of suicide, in this situation, would be referred to a group for survivors of suicide to help her with her feelings and to work through the grief reaction. This group provides support and understanding of what the individual is experiencing by members who are experiencing similar reactions, including anger and guilt. Depression and unresolved grief can occur when the survivor does not receive appropriate help. Counseling by a chaplain or individual therapy by the nurse may be appropriate in addition to referral to the group. Giving the survivor the suicide hotline number would be appropriate if the survivor herself were thinking about suicide.

🔑 CN: Psychosocial integrity; CL: Synthesize

100. 3. The most appropriate response is to discuss the behavioral clues and resources because it provides the husband with important information that he needs to cope with his wife's condition. Family members are commonly afraid of future suicidal activity and need helpful information and resources to turn to in a crisis. Telling the husband not to worry minimizes the husband's concern and is not necessarily true. Additionally, past suicide attempts need to be considered when evaluating the client's future risk of suicide. The statement "She told me she wants to live, so I do not think she will try again" ignores the husband's request and concerns. Additionally, there is no way for the nurse to know whether the client will attempt suicide again. The statement "Tell her about your concern, and just take care of her" is not helpful because the husband needs information and resources to turn to should a crisis develop.

🔑 CN: Psychosocial integrity; CL: Synthesize

101. 4. After the client identifies and shares her strengths, the nurse reinforces the client for her ability to evaluate herself in a positive manner. Doing so promotes self-esteem and offers hope for improvement. Asking the client to identify three additional strengths or volunteering the client to lead the cooking group could be too overwhelming for the client at this time and may increase her anxiety and feelings of worthlessness. Although educating the client about the importance of medication is important, doing so at another time would be more appropriate.

🔑 CN: Psychosocial integrity; CL: Synthesize

102. 2. The best response would be for the nurse to advise the visitor to be caring and genuine to the client as a friend normally would. Family and friends are commonly afraid or at a loss about how to act or what to say to someone with a mental illness or to someone who may voice thoughts of self-harm. The statement "Try to cheer her up" is inappropriate because the client may feel overwhelmed and thus become more despondent when she cannot meet or match the cheerful demeanor. The statement "Control your expressions" is inappropriate because the client is not helped when

6. The police bring a client to the emergency department after she threatens to kill her ex-husband. The client states emphatically, "The police should bring him in, not me. He is paranoid about my dating and has been stalking me for weeks. He is probably off his medicines. His case manager and the police will not do anything." In what order should the following nursing actions be done from first to last? All options must be used.

1. Ask about the marital problems leading to the divorce.

2. Assess the client's risk for harm to self and others.

3. Obtain the name of her ex-husband's case manager.

4. Interview the client about her current needs and situation.

7. A client who has been stabilized on medications for several months is at the clinic for a medication check. During a conversation with the nurse, the client suddenly jumps up, begins pacing, and wrings her hands. In what order should the nurse do the following interventions from first to last? All options must be used.

1. Walk with the client to help decrease her anxiety.

2. Discuss productive ways to solve her problems causing anxiety.

3. Share observations about her anxiety-related behaviors.

4. Ask the client about the sources of her anxiety.

8. A client on haloperidol has stiff muscles, restlessness, and internal jumpiness. The client has all of the following medications prescribed as needed. Which one would be **most** appropriate for the nurse to administer to decrease the client's symptoms?
- ☐ **1.** lorazepam
- ☐ **2.** benztropine
- ☐ **3.** trazodone
- ☐ **4.** olanzapine

9. The parents of a 20-year-old female client diagnosed with paranoid schizophrenia admitted 4 days ago are attending a family psychoeducation group in the hospital. Which statement by the mother indicates that she understands her daughter's illness and management?
- ☐ **1.** "I know that I will have to do everything for my daughter when she comes home."
- ☐ **2.** "Tasks as simple as getting out of bed and showering in the morning may be difficult for her."
- ☐ **3.** "I know that visits from her friends at home should be discouraged for a while."
- ☐ **4.** "She will not experience a relapse as long as she takes her prescribed medication."

10. During a home visit for a client diagnosed with paranoid schizophrenia discharged 1 week ago, the client's mother tearfully states, "I can hardly sleep because I am so worried about my daughter. I am afraid to leave her alone in the house. What if something should happen while I am gone?" Which caregiver problem would be the **most** inclusive one for the nurse to incorporate into the client's plan of care?
- ☐ **1.** caregiver role strain
- ☐ **2.** anxiety
- ☐ **3.** fear
- ☐ **4.** disturbed sleep pattern

11. When conducting a mental status examination with a newly admitted client who has a diagnosis of paranoid schizophrenia, the client states, "I am being followed; it is not safe. They are monitoring my every move." In which area of the mental status examination should the nurse document this information?
- ☐ **1.** thought content
- ☐ **2.** quality of speech
- ☐ **3.** insight
- ☐ **4.** judgment

12. The wife of a client admitted for treatment of newly diagnosed paranoid schizophrenia visits 2 days after her husband's admission and states to the nurse, "Why is he not eating? He is still talking about his food being poisoned." Which appraisal by the nurse is **most** accurate?
- ☐ **1.** The wife's inquiry is reasonable.
- ☐ **2.** Education about her husband's medications is needed.
- ☐ **3.** Her expectations of her husband are realistic.
- ☐ **4.** An increase in the client's medication is indicated.

13. A client states that she hears God's voice telling her that she has sinned and needs to punish herself. Which response by the nurse is **most** important?
- ☐ **1.** "How do you think you will be punished?"
- ☐ **2.** "Do you think you need to punish yourself now?"
- ☐ **3.** "What exactly do you think you have done to be punished?"
- ☐ **4.** "Let us talk about your strengths."

14. When developing the plan of care for a client who is staying in his room because he perceives that staff want to harm him, which outcome of care planning is **most** realistic?
- ☐ **1.** Within 2 days, the client will complete activities of daily living.
- ☐ **2.** Within 3 days, the client will participate in recreation with other clients.
- ☐ **3.** Within 4 days, the client will demonstrate an absence of verbal aggression.
- ☐ **4.** Within 5 days, the client will seek out staff to talk about feelings.

15. A client diagnosed with paranoid schizophrenia is still withdrawn, unkempt, and unmotivated to get out of bed. An unlicensed assistive personnel (UAP) asks the nurse why the client is behaving this way after being on fluphenazine 10 mg for 7 days. The nurse should tell the UAP:
- ☐ **1.** "Fluphenazine is most effective with the positive symptoms of schizophrenia."
- ☐ **2.** "The client will be less withdrawn and unmotivated when the fluphenazine takes effect."
- ☐ **3.** "The client's fluphenazine dose probably needs to be increased again."
- ☐ **4.** "Lack of motivation is a common side effect of fluphenazine."

16. A pregnant client in her third trimester is started on chlorpromazine 25 mg 4 times daily. Which instructions are **most** important for the nurse to include in the client's teaching plan?
- ☐ **1.** "Do not drive because there is a possibility of seizures occurring."
- ☐ **2.** "Avoid going out in the sun without a sunscreen with a sun protection factor of at least 30."
- ☐ **3.** "Stop the medication immediately if constipation occurs."
- ☐ **4.** "Tell your healthcare provider (HCP) if you experience an increase in blood pressure."

17. A client reports that men in blue clothes keep looking in her window and talking about her. Which response by the nurse is **most** appropriate?
- ☐ **1.** "Those men are groundskeepers. They are talking about their work, not you."
- ☐ **2.** "Do not take things so personally. Not everyone who is talking is talking about you."
- ☐ **3.** "Let us not pay attention to the men. Let us play cards instead."
- ☐ **4.** "I will close the drapes so you cannot see the men."

18. When preparing the teaching plan for a client who is to start clozapine, which information is crucial to include?
- ☐ **1.** description of akathisia and drug-induced parkinsonism
- ☐ **2.** measures to relieve episodes of diarrhea
- ☐ **3.** the importance of reporting insomnia
- ☐ **4.** an emphasis on the need for weekly blood tests

19. A client is sitting in the corner of the dayroom cocking his head to one side as if he hears something, but no one is nearby. The nurse suspects he is having auditory hallucinations. Which question should the nurse ask **first**?
- ☐ **1.** "Are you seeing someone other than me?"
- ☐ **2.** "What are you hearing right now?"
- ☐ **3.** "What is going on with you right now?"
- ☐ **4.** "Do you want to go to the recreation room?"

20. A client who is newly diagnosed with paranoid schizophrenia tells the nurse, "The aliens are telling me that I am defective and need to be eliminated." Which response by the nurse is **most** appropriate initially?
- ☐ **1.** "I know those voices are real to you, but I do not hear them."
- ☐ **2.** "You are having hallucinations as a result of your illness."
- ☐ **3.** "I want you to agree to tell staff when you hear these voices."
- ☐ **4.** "Your medications will help control these voices you are hearing."

21. An outpatient client who has a history of paranoid schizophrenia and chronic alcohol dependency has been taking risperidone for several months. She reports that she stopped drinking 4 days ago. The client is very frightened by the tactile hallucinations of bugs crawling under her skin. Which factor should the nurse incorporate into the plan of care when explaining the tactile hallucinations?
- ☐ **1.** alcohol intoxication
- ☐ **2.** ineffectiveness of risperidone
- ☐ **3.** alcohol withdrawal
- ☐ **4.** interaction of alcohol and risperidone

22. A client with a long history of paranoid schizophrenia is readmitted voluntarily after missing his last two injections of haloperidol. He reports, "I am not sleeping much, and my friend says I smell from not showering. God is telling me to protect myself from others. My parents are sick and tired of me and my illness. They wish I were dead." Which admission notes by the nurse contains assumptions and potentially false accusations? Select all that apply.
- [ ] 1. Client has been noncompliant with his medications, causing decreased sleep and activities of daily living, increased auditory hallucinations, and paranoid delusions about his parents harming him.
- [ ] 2. Client has missed two injections of haloperidol and was admitted voluntarily. He reports he has decreased sleep and showering and that he hears God's voice telling him to protect himself from others. He stated, "My parents are sick and tired of me and my illness. They wish I were dead."
- [ ] 3. Client has missed two doses of haloperidol. He is not sleeping and showering. Has a strained relationship with his parents and delusions that they want him dead. Voluntary admission to restart haloperidol.
- [ ] 4. Client admitted for noncompliance with haloperidol injections, sleep disturbance, poor hygiene, auditory hallucinations, and suspiciousness of his parents. Needs to be monitored for suicidal and homicidal ideation.
- [ ] 5. Client admitted because of hallucinations and delusions. His parents may be abusing him. He states he has not taken his medications for 2 days.

23. A newly admitted client diagnosed with paranoid schizophrenia is pacing rapidly and wringing his hands. He states that another client is out to get him. Then he says, "Protect me, select me, reject me." The nurse should **next**:
- [ ] 1. administer his oral PRN lorazepam and haloperidol.
- [ ] 2. place the client in temporary seclusion before he has a chance to hurt others.
- [ ] 3. call the healthcare provider (HCP) for a prescription for restraints.
- [ ] 4. ask the other clients to leave the immediate area.

24. A new nurse is coleading a family education group for those who have relatives with paranoid schizophrenia. Which statement by the new nurse indicates the need for further teaching about symptom management?
- [ ] 1. "When the clients get overwhelmed, it is best if they spend some time in their room."
- [ ] 2. "The more we push the clients to spend time with friends, the more their voices decrease."
- [ ] 3. "Until we get the clients up and going, they seem to have no motivation to do anything."
- [ ] 4. "We still have to remind the clients that we do not hear the voices they do."

25. A client is being successfully treated with clozapine. Which statement by the client reflects a need for further teaching about managing the drug's adverse effects?
- [ ] 1. "If I eat too many fruits, I will get constipated."
- [ ] 2. "I need to take the medicine with food to avoid nausea."
- [ ] 3. "I have to get up slowly so I do not get dizzy."
- [ ] 4. "Sometimes I have to push myself because I am sleepy."

26. Which statement indicates increased insight by the client about her newly diagnosed paranoid schizophrenia being stabilized on medications?
- [ ] 1. "Now that the voices are gone, I can decrease my medicines."
- [ ] 2. "I would feel better if I knew there was not poison in my food."
- [ ] 3. "Since I feel better, I know I can restart school next week."
- [ ] 4. "The voices go away when I tell them to, except if I am really nervous."

27. A client who is suspicious of others, including the staff, is brought to the hospital wearing a wrinkled dress with stains on the front. Assessment also reveals a flat affect, confusion, and slow movements. Which goal should the nurse identify as the **initial priority** when planning this client's care?
- [ ] 1. helping the client feel safe and accepted
- [ ] 2. introducing the client to other clients
- [ ] 3. giving the client information about the program
- [ ] 4. providing the client with clean, comfortable clothes

28. The parent of a young adult client diagnosed with paranoid schizophrenia is asking questions about his son's antipsychotic medication, ziprasidone. Which statement by the parent reflects a need for further teaching?
- [ ] 1. "If he experiences restlessness or muscle stiffness, he should tell his healthcare provider (HCP)."
- [ ] 2. "I should give him benztropine to help prevent constipation from the ziprasidone."
- [ ] 3. "If he becomes dizzy, I will make sure he does not drive."
- [ ] 4. "The ziprasidone should help him be more motivated and less withdrawn."

29. While the nurse is performing an admission assessment, the client stops talking in the middle of a sentence, tips his head to the side, and listens carefully. The nurse recognizes that the client is most likely experiencing which problem?
- [ ] 1. somatic delusions
- [ ] 2. pseudoparkinsonism
- [ ] 3. delusions of reference
- [ ] 4. auditory hallucinations

30. A client diagnosed with schizophrenia gained 50 lb (22.7 kg) in 6 months while taking olanzapine. After a prescription change from olanzapine to ziprasidone, the client tells the nurse, "I do not want to take this ziprasidone either. I cannot gain any more weight." Which response by the nurse is **most** appropriate for this client?
- ☐ **1.** "Ziprasidone causes less weight gain than do the other atypical antipsychotics."
- ☐ **2.** "We can give it to you as an injection rather than in capsule form."
- ☐ **3.** "Abnormal movements are not as common with ziprasidone."
- ☐ **4.** "You can take it just before bedtime, so you will not need a snack."

31. As hospital-based care has become more oriented to crisis intervention, criteria for admission to the hospital have also changed. Which clients have **priority** for admission to an acute care facility? Select all that apply.
- ☐ **1.** clients who live alone
- ☐ **2.** clients who are acutely psychotic
- ☐ **3.** clients who are acutely depressed
- ☐ **4.** clients who are dangerous to self or others
- ☐ **5.** clients who are not sleeping and have a lack of appetite
- ☐ **6.** clients who are not complying with medication regimens

32. A 79-year-old woman is brought to the outpatient clinic by her daughter for a routine medication evaluation. The daughter reports that her mother is quite stable and has no adverse effects from the risperidone she is taking. Then, the daughter says, "I just think my mother could be even better if she was on a larger dosage. My son takes 1 mg of risperidone every day and my mother is only on 0.5 mg." What is the **most** helpful response by the nurse?
- ☐ **1.** "Maybe your son is sicker than your mother is."
- ☐ **2.** "We could increase your mother's dosage if you want."
- ☐ **3.** "Older clients generally need lesser doses than do younger people."
- ☐ **4.** "I am not seeing any symptoms of illness in your mother. Let us wait until the next visit."

33. At an outpatient visit 3 months after discharge from the hospital, a client says he has stopped his olanzapine even though it controls his symptoms of schizophrenia better than other medications. "I have gained 20 lb (9.1 kg) already. I cannot stand anymore." Which response by the nurse is **most** appropriate?
- ☐ **1.** "I do not think you look fat; why do you think so?"
- ☐ **2.** "I can help you with a diet and exercise plan to keep your weight down."
- ☐ **3.** "You can be switched to another medicine."
- ☐ **4.** "Your weight gain will level off if you stay on the medication 3 more months."

34. A client diagnosed with schizophrenia is being switched to risperidone long-acting injection. The client is told that he will remain on his oral dose of risperidone daily for approximately 1 month. The client says, "I did not have to take pills when I was on fluphenazine shots in the past." The nurse should tell the client:
- ☐ **1.** "Taking fluphenazine orally and by injection would not be as effective as the injection alone."
- ☐ **2.** "Risperidone is less potent than fluphenazine."
- ☐ **3.** "Your healthcare provider did not believe you would take both the pills and fluphenazine injections."
- ☐ **4.** "Risperidone initially takes a little longer to reach the ideal blood level."

35. The nurse is developing a care plan with a client who is receiving ziprasidone and has stopped taking the drug. Which side effects that may occur and be a reason the client is noncompliant with taking this medication should the nurse discuss? Select all that apply.
- ☐ **1.** somnolence
- ☐ **2.** weight gain
- ☐ **3.** urticaria
- ☐ **4.** constipation
- ☐ **5.** headache

36. A client has been perceiving her roommate's stuffed animal as her own dog at home. The nurse determines that this misperception of reality (illusion) is improving when the client makes which statement?
- ☐ **1.** "Jan's stuffed dog looks somewhat like my dog, Trixie."
- ☐ **2.** "Jan's dog and my dog could be twins."
- ☐ **3.** "I wish Jan had not had my dog stuffed."
- ☐ **4.** "I guess Jan needs a dog as much as I do."

37. When asked about her stresses before admission, an anxious client stares blankly at the nurse and mutters unintelligibly. Which description of the client's behaviors should the nurse document in the client's medical record?
- ☐ **1.** "Client cannot answer any questions asked at this time."
- ☐ **2.** "Client is uncooperative during the admission procedure, refusing to answer any questions."
- ☐ **3.** "Client responded to questions with a blank look and incomprehensible mumble."
- ☐ **4.** "Client stared at the wall when asked questions and was disoriented and incoherent."

38. When planning care for a client with schizophrenia who lacks motivation to shower and dress, which outcome should the nurse expect the client to achieve by the end of 4 days?
- ☐ 1. Verbalize the need to shower and dress herself.
- ☐ 2. Recognize the need to shower and dress herself.
- ☐ 3. Explain reasons for showering and dressing herself.
- ☐ 4. Perform showering and dressing for herself.

39. A client diagnosed with schizophrenia is brought to the hospital from a group home where he became agitated, threw a chair at another client, and has been refusing medication for 8 weeks. The client exhibits a flat affect, is not caring for his hygiene, and has become increasingly withdrawn and asocial. The healthcare provider (HCP) prescribes treatment with risperidone to improve the client's negative and positive symptoms of schizophrenia. When evaluating the drug's effectiveness on the client's negative symptoms, the nurse should expect improvement in which symptom?
- ☐ 1. apathy, affect, social isolation
- ☐ 2. agitation, delusions, hallucinations
- ☐ 3. hostility, ideas of reference, tangential speech
- ☐ 4. aggression, bizarre behavior, illusions

40. A 77-year-old client is brought to the emergency department by her son. The client has a severe headache and lack of sleep because "I am so worried about everything." Her son says that she has heart failure and chronic schizophrenia. "In addition to all of her heart medicines, she is on aripiprazole, which was increased to 30 mg by her healthcare provider (HCP) 3 days ago." In addition to documenting all of the client's medications and exact dosages, the nurse should particularly investigate which factors? Select all that apply.
- ☐ 1. the qualifications of the client's HCP
- ☐ 2. the client's symptoms of schizophrenia
- ☐ 3. the dose of aripiprazole
- ☐ 4. the client's symptoms of heart failure
- ☐ 5. the client's relationship with her son

41. A client with schizophrenia comes to the outpatient mental health clinic 5 days after being discharged from the hospital. The client was given a 1-week supply of clozapine. The client tells the nurse that she has too much saliva and frequently needs to spit. The nurse interprets the client's statement as being consistent with which factor?
- ☐ 1. delusion, requiring further assessment
- ☐ 2. unusual reaction to clozapine
- ☐ 3. expected adverse effect of clozapine
- ☐ 4. unresolved symptom of schizophrenia

42. The client with a diagnosis of schizophrenia is acutely psychotic and exhibits religious delusions and hallucinations, loose associations, and concrete thinking. When the nurse offers the client her medication, the client states, "I do not need that. God will heal me." The nurse should respond to the client by saying:
- ☐ 1. "God helps those who help themselves."
- ☐ 2. "God wants you to take your medicine."
- ☐ 3. "God is important in your life, but the medicine will help you too."
- ☐ 4. "This medicine will help clear your thoughts and decrease anxiety."

43. The nurse hands the medication cup to a client who is psychotic and exhibiting concrete thinking and tells the client to take his medicine. The client takes the cup, holds it in hand, and stares at it. What should the nurse do **next**?
- ☐ 1. Tell the client to put the medicine in the mouth and swallow it with some water.
- ☐ 2. Instruct the client to sit in the dayroom and wait for the nurse to assist him.
- ☐ 3. Ask another staff member to stay with the client until the client takes the medication.
- ☐ 4. Say nothing and wait for the client to put the medication in the mouth and swallow it.

44. Which action by the nurse is likely to increase the anxiety and suspiciousness of a client who is delusional?
- ☐ 1. informing the client of schedule changes
- ☐ 2. whispering with others where the client can observe
- ☐ 3. telling the client gently that the nurse does not share the client's view
- ☐ 4. inviting the client to join in leisure activities

45. A client with schizophrenia tells the nurse that he does not go out much because he does not have anywhere to go and he does not know anyone in the apartment where he is staying. Which action is **most** beneficial for the client at this time?
- ☐ 1. encouraging him to call his family to visit more often
- ☐ 2. making an appointment for the client to see the nurse daily for 2 weeks
- ☐ 3. thinking about the need for rehospitalization for the client
- ☐ 4. arranging for the client to attend day treatment at the clinic

46. The plan of care for an outpatient client with schizophrenia includes risperidone therapy. The nurse prepares to administer this drug based on the understanding of which factor?
- ☐ 1. The positive symptoms of schizophrenia are usually more prominent than the negative symptoms.
- ☐ 2. Agranulocytosis is less of a risk with risperidone therapy than with clozapine.
- ☐ 3. Typical antipsychotics help with negative symptoms, but not as well as risperidone does.
- ☐ 4. Risperidone is less expensive than traditional antipsychotics.

47. A client diagnosed with schizophrenia is being discharged on aripiprazole 5 mg every night. When developing the teaching plan about the most common adverse effects, which information should the nurse include? Select all that apply.
- ☐ 1. headaches
- ☐ 2. transient mild anxiety
- ☐ 3. insomnia
- ☐ 4. torticollis
- ☐ 5. pill rolling movements

48. A newly admitted client with an acute exacerbation of psychotic symptoms of schizophrenia is having trouble deciding whether to live in a group home or a supervised apartment. Based on the client's current cognitive functioning, which activity is **most** appropriate for the nurse to ask the client to do initially?
- ☐ 1. List the pros and cons of each housing option.
- ☐ 2. Choose between apple and orange juice for breakfast.
- ☐ 3. Identify why the client cannot live in an unsupervised apartment.
- ☐ 4. Decide which staff member the client would like to have today.

49. An outpatient client who has been receiving haloperidol for 2 days develops muscular rigidity, altered consciousness, a temperature of 103°F (39.4°C), and trouble breathing on day 3. The nurse interprets these findings as indicating which complication?
- ☐ 1. neuroleptic malignant syndrome
- ☐ 2. tardive dyskinesia
- ☐ 3. extrapyramidal adverse effects
- ☐ 4. drug-induced parkinsonism

50. A client with schizophrenia reports doing very little all day except sleeping and eating. The nurse should:
- ☐ 1. have three meals per day brought in to increase the amount of time the client spends out of bed.
- ☐ 2. ask a relative to call the client at least 10 times a day to decrease the sleeping.
- ☐ 3. help the client set up a daily activity schedule to include setting a wake-up alarm.
- ☐ 4. arrange for the client to move to a group home with structured activities.

51. The nurse notes that a client sitting in a chair has not gotten up in 1 hour. The client does not respond to verbal directions, and her arm has been extended over the armrest for 30 minutes. What should the nurse do **next**?
- ☐ 1. Assist the client out of the chair to lead her back to bed.
- ☐ 2. Give PRN-prescribed doses of haloperidol and lorazepam.
- ☐ 3. Ask the client to describe what she is experiencing right now.
- ☐ 4. Sit quietly with the client until she begins to respond.

52. What is the most appropriate long-term goal for an outpatient client with schizophrenia who has been withdrawn from friends and family for 3 weeks?
- ☐ 1. calling the client's mother once a day
- ☐ 2. attending day therapy three times a week
- ☐ 3. allowing two friends to visit every day
- ☐ 4. remaining out of bed for 10 hours a day

53. For the client with catatonic behaviors, which outcome would indicate a medication has been most effective in improving long-term behavior?
- ☐ 1. The client can move all extremities occasionally.
- ☐ 2. The client walks with the nurse to the client's room.
- ☐ 3. The client responds to verbal directions to eat.
- ☐ 4. The client initiates simple activities without directions.

54. The mother of a client with schizophrenia calls the visiting nurse in the outpatient clinic to report that her daughter has not answered the phone in 10 days. "She was doing so well for months. I do not know what is wrong. I am worried." Which response by the nurse is **most** appropriate?
- ☐ 1. "Maybe she is just mad at you. Did you have an argument?"
- ☐ 2. "She may have stopped taking her medications. I will check on her."
- ☐ 3. "Do not worry about this. It happens sometimes."
- ☐ 4. "Go over to her apartment and see what is going on."

55. During a home visit, the nurse discovers that the client is less verbal, less active, less responsive to directions, severely anxious, and more stuporous. The nurse interprets these findings to indicate that the client needs which intervention?
- ☐ 1. a sleep aid
- ☐ 2. a clinic appointment
- ☐ 3. an increase in medication
- ☐ 4. immediate medical evaluation

56. A client admitted with a diagnosis of schizoaffective disorder, manic phase, who is currently taking fluoxetine, valproic acid, and olanzapine as prescribed, has had an increase in manic symptoms in the past week. The healthcare provider (HCP) prescribes a valproic acid blood level to be drawn at once. What does the nurse understand is the rationale for this prescription?
- [ ] 1. All clients taking valproic acid need periodic valproic acid levels drawn.
- [ ] 2. Fluoxetine can decrease the effectiveness of the valproic acid.
- [ ] 3. A decrease in the level of valproic acid could explain the increase in manic symptoms.
- [ ] 4. The valproic acid level is needed before a short course of lorazepam for agitation can be prescribed.

57. A 22-year-old client is being admitted with a diagnosis of brief psychotic disorder. Which finding would the nurse expect to find during the admission interview that is consistent with the client's diagnosis?
- [ ] 1. current treatment for pneumonia
- [ ] 2. regular use of alcohol or marijuana
- [ ] 3. evidence of delusions or hallucinations
- [ ] 4. a history of chronic depression

58. A successful real estate agent brought to the clinic after being arrested for harassing and stalking his ex-wife denies any other symptoms or problems except anger about being arrested. The ex-wife reports to the police, "He is fine except for this irrational belief that we will remarry." When collaborating with the healthcare provider (HCP) about a plan of care, which intervention would be most effective for the client at this time?
- [ ] 1. a prescription for olanzapine 10 mg daily
- [ ] 2. a joint session with the client and his ex-wife
- [ ] 3. a prescription for fluoxetine 20 mg every morning
- [ ] 4. referral to an outpatient counselor

Clients and Families Affected by Chronic Mental Illnesses

59. A nurse working at an outpatient mental health center primarily with chronically mentally ill clients receives a telephone call from the mother of a client who lives at home. The mother reports that the client has not been taking her medication and now is refusing to go to the work center where she has worked for the past year. What should the nurse do **first**?
- [ ] 1. Call the director of the work center for information about the client.
- [ ] 2. Reserve an inpatient bed in preparation for the client's admission.
- [ ] 3. Ask to speak to the client directly on the phone.
- [ ] 4. Make an appointment for the client to see the healthcare provider (HCP).

60. A nurse is teaching the families of clients with chronic mental illnesses about causes of relapse and rehospitalization. What should the nurse include as the **primary** cause?
- [ ] 1. loss of family support
- [ ] 2. noncompliance with medications
- [ ] 3. sudden changes in medications
- [ ] 4. nonattendance at treatment programs

61. The director of an outpatient rehab program tells the nurse that the client with schizophrenia had done well for 6 months until last week, when a new person started the program. This new person worked faster than the client did and took his place as leader of the group. Based on this information, which intervention is **most** appropriate?
- [ ] 1. Make a home visit, and tell the client that if he does not return to the program, he will lose his place there.
- [ ] 2. Ask the director to assign the client to another group when he returns to the program.
- [ ] 3. Make an appointment to meet the client at the mental health center, and ask him about the situation.
- [ ] 4. Arrange for the placement of the client in a skill training program.

62. A 25-year-old client diagnosed with chronic schizophrenia states, "I stopped my medications a week ago. I was just tired of not being able to drink with my friends. Besides, I feel fine without them." Which response by the nurse is **most** appropriate?
- [ ] 1. "It is important for you to go back on your medicines."
- [ ] 2. "I hear how difficult it must be to live with the changes caused by your illness."
- [ ] 3. "You will have to talk to your health-care provider (HCP) about stopping your medications."
- [ ] 4. "Your buddies will understand that you cannot drink anymore."

63. A 23-year-old client diagnosed with schizophrenia cheerfully announces, "My mom and I are so excited that I am pregnant. She is willing to help us take care of the baby too." Which reason should cause the nurse to be concerned about this situation?
- [ ] 1. The client did not say that the father of the baby was excited about this.
- [ ] 2. The mother is not likely to provide enough help for what the client needs.
- [ ] 3. Symptom management will be difficult in early pregnancy without medications.
- [ ] 4. The client will have difficulty financially supporting the baby.

64. The nurse is reviewing laboratory values of a client receiving clozapine. Which of the following laboratory values does the nurse **immediately** report to the healthcare provider (HCP)?
- ☐ 1. WBC of 3,500
- ☐ 2. hemoglobin of 11.9 g/dL (119 g/L)
- ☐ 3. sodium level of 136 mEq/L (136 mmol/L)
- ☐ 4. hyaline casts in the urinalysis

65. A client is being discharged before complete stabilization of symptoms. When developing a discharge plan for this client, the nurse should ensure that the client will have:
- ☐ 1. more medical consultations after discharge.
- ☐ 2. monthly outpatient visits.
- ☐ 3. many coordinated services.
- ☐ 4. a caring and supportive family.

66. Which facility would the nurse rank as the lowest **priority** to expand when developing a community-based service program for clients with chronic mental illnesses?
- ☐ 1. partial hospitalization programs
- ☐ 2. psychiatric home care
- ☐ 3. residential services
- ☐ 4. long-term hospitals

67. Crisis intervention plays a major role in the management of care for clients with chronic mental illnesses. Although the safety of the client and others is always a priority, these clients typically need crisis intervention in which situations? Select all that apply.
- ☐ 1. inability to keep outpatient appointments
- ☐ 2. signs of relapse and decompensation
- ☐ 3. threat of eviction from housing
- ☐ 4. unpaid bills and lack of food
- ☐ 5. occasionally missing a dose of medication

68. The most common reason given by mentally ill clients for noncompliance with medications is their uncomfortable adverse effects. When teaching the families, what need should the nurse identify as the **greatest**?
- ☐ 1. alternative ways to manage the adverse effects
- ☐ 2. home visits to set up a week's supply of medications
- ☐ 3. family monitoring of the administration of medication
- ☐ 4. outpatient monitoring of medication compliance

69. The stigma related to having a mental illness, especially a chronic illness, persists despite improvements in the management of illnesses and an increase in public education. Which view **most** perpetuates the stigma?
- ☐ 1. Mental illness is hereditary.
- ☐ 2. Mental illnesses have biochemical bases.
- ☐ 3. Clients cannot prevent mental illness if they want to do so.
- ☐ 4. Clients can recover from mental illness if they have willpower.

The Client with Cognitive Disorders

70. An elderly woman experiences short-term memory problems and occasional disorientation a few weeks after her husband's death. She also is not sleeping, has urinary frequency and burning, and sees rats in the kitchen. The home care nurse calls the woman's healthcare provider (HCP) to discuss the client's situation and background, assess, and give recommendations. The nurse concludes that the woman:
- ☐ 1. is experiencing the onset of Alzheimer's disease.
- ☐ 2. is having trouble adjusting to living alone without her husband.
- ☐ 3. is having delayed grieving related to her Alzheimer's disease.
- ☐ 4. is experiencing delirium and a urinary tract infection (UTI).

71. An elderly client was prescribed lorazepam 1 mg three times a day to help calm her anxiety after her husband's death. The next day, the client calls her daughter asking when she is picking her up to go to the graveside. The client says she has been walking up and down the driveway for the past hour waiting for her daughter. Noting the client's agitation, hyperactivity, and insistence, the daughter calls the nurse to report her mother's behavior. Which finding would the nurse suspect as the cause of the mother's behavior, and what action would she suggest?
- ☐ 1. The client is manic and may need a sleeping pill.
- ☐ 2. The client is experiencing a medication interaction and should go to the emergency department.
- ☐ 3. The client is experiencing a paradoxical reaction to the lorazepam and should stop the new medication immediately.
- ☐ 4. The client is overcome by grief and probably needs an antidepressant.

72. The son of an elderly client who has cognitive impairments approaches the nurse and says, "I'm so upset. The healthcare provider (HCP) says I have 4 days to decide on where my dad is going to live." The nurse responds to the son's concerns, gives him a list of types of living arrangements, and discusses the needs, abilities, and limitations of the client. The nurse should intervene further if the son makes which comment?
- ☐ 1. "Boy, I have a lot to think about before I see the social worker tomorrow."
- ☐ 2. "I think I can handle most of Dad's needs with the help of some home health care."
- ☐ 3. "I am so afraid of making the wrong decision, but I can move him later if I need to."
- ☐ 4. "I want the social worker to make this decision so Dad will not blame me."

73. A client has been transferred to the hospital's psychiatric unit from a nursing home for increasing confusion. The client's behavior is found to be the result of cerebral arteriosclerosis. Which nursing staff actions should positively influence the client's behavior? Select all that apply.
- ☐ 1. limiting the client's choices
- ☐ 2. accepting the client as he is
- ☐ 3. allowing the client to do as he wishes
- ☐ 4. acting nonchalantly
- ☐ 5. explaining to the client what he needs to do step-by-step

74. The nurse observes a client in a group who is reminiscing about his past. Which effect should the nurse expect reminiscing to have on the client's functioning in the hospital?
- ☐ 1. Increase the client's confusion and disorientation.
- ☐ 2. Cause the client to become sad.
- ☐ 3. Decrease the client's feelings of isolation and loneliness.
- ☐ 4. Keep the client from participating in therapeutic activities.

The Client with Delirium

75. A 69-year-old client is admitted and diagnosed with delirium. Later in the day, he tries to get out of the locked unit. He yells, "Unlock this door. I have got to go see my doctor. I just cannot miss my monthly Friday appointment." Which of the following responses by the nurse is **most** appropriate?
- ☐ 1. "Please come away from the door. I will show you your room."
- ☐ 2. "It is 5 o'clock Tuesday, and you are in the hospital. I am Anne, a nurse."
- ☐ 3. "The door is locked to keep you from getting lost."
- ☐ 4. "I want you to come eat your lunch before you go for your appointment."

76. An 83-year-old woman is admitted to the unit after being examined in the emergency department (ED) and diagnosed with delirium. After the admission interviews with the client and her grandson, the nurse explains that there will be more laboratory tests and x-rays done that day. The grandson says, "She has already been stuck several times and had a brain scan or something. Just give her some medicine and let her rest." What should the nurse tell the grandson? Select all that apply.
- ☐ 1. "I agree she needs to rest, but there is no one specific medicine for your grandmother's condition."
- ☐ 2. "The healthcare provider will look at the results of those tests in the ED and decide what other tests are needed."
- ☐ 3. "Delirium commonly results from underlying medical causes that we need to identify and correct."
- ☐ 4. "Tell me about your grandmother's behaviors, and maybe I could figure out what medicine she needs."
- ☐ 5. "I will ask the healthcare provider to postpone more tests until tomorrow."

77. The nurse is attempting to draw blood from a client with a diagnosis of delirium who was admitted last evening. The client yells out, "Stop; leave me alone. What are you trying to do to me? What is happening to me?" Which response by the nurse is **most** appropriate?
- ☐ 1. "The tests of your blood will help us figure out what is happening to you."
- ☐ 2. "Please hold still so I do not have to stick you a second time."
- ☐ 3. "After I get your blood, I will get some medicine to help you calm down."
- ☐ 4. "I will tell you everything after I get your blood tests to the laboratory."

78. A 90-year-old client diagnosed with major depression is suddenly experiencing sleep disturbances, inability to focus, poor recent memory, altered perceptions, and disorientation to time and place. Lab results indicate the client has a urinary tract infection (UTI) and dehydration. After explaining the situation and giving the background and assessment data, the nurse should make which recommendation to the client's healthcare provider (HCP)?
- ☐ 1. a prescription to place the client in restraints
- ☐ 2. a reevaluation of the client's mental status
- ☐ 3. the transfer of the client to a medical unit
- ☐ 4. a transfer of the client to a nursing home

79. When caring for the client diagnosed with delirium, which condition is the **most** important for the nurse to investigate?
☐ 1. cancer of any kind
☐ 2. impaired hearing
☐ 3. prescription drug intoxication
☐ 4. heart failure

80. Which characteristic would make the nurse suspect that a client with changes in cognition has delirium?
☐ 1. disturbances in cognition and consciousness that fluctuate during the day
☐ 2. the failure to identify objects despite intact sensory functions
☐ 3. significant impairment in social or occupational functioning over time
☐ 4. memory impairment to the degree of being called amnesia

81. What intervention is essential when caring for a client who is experiencing delirium?
☐ 1. controlling behavioral symptoms with low-dose psychotropics
☐ 2. identifying the underlying causative condition or illness
☐ 3. manipulating the environment to increase orientation
☐ 4. decreasing or discontinuing all previously prescribed medications

82. What is a realistic short-term goal to be accomplished in 2 to 3 days for a client with delirium?
☐ 1. Explain the experience of having delirium.
☐ 2. Resume a normal sleep-wake cycle.
☐ 3. Regain orientation to time and place.
☐ 4. Establish normal bowel and bladder function.

83. What should the nurse expect to include as a **priority** in the plan of care for a client with delirium based on the nurse's understanding of the disturbances in orientation associated with this disorder?
☐ 1. identifying self and making sure that the nurse has the client's attention
☐ 2. eliminating the client's napping in the daytime as much as possible
☐ 3. engaging the client in reminiscing with relatives or visitors
☐ 4. avoiding arguing with a suspicious client about his perceptions of reality

84. A client has been in the critical care unit for 3 days following a severe myocardial infarction. Although he is medically stable, he has begun to have fluctuating episodes of consciousness, illogical thinking, and anxiety. He is picking at the air to "catch these baby angels flying around my head." While waiting for medical and psychiatric consults, which needs have the highest **priority**? Select all that apply.
☐ 1. decreasing as much "foreign" stimuli as possible
☐ 2. avoiding challenging the client's perceptions about "baby angels"
☐ 3. orienting the client about his medical condition
☐ 4. gently presenting reality as needed
☐ 5. calling the client's family to report his onset of dementia

The Client with Dementia

85. The nurse is assessing an older adult for signs of dementia using the Mini Mental Status Exam. The nurse gives the client three words to remember: "cat," "crackers," and "toys." After having the client perform a short task, the nurse asks the client to repeat the words. The client says "toys," "boys," and "joys." The nurse should **next**:
☐ 1. ask the client to repeat the original words one more time.
☐ 2. note on the medical record that the client has echolalia.
☐ 3. refer the client to a healthcare provider (HCP) for further follow-up.
☐ 4. repeat the test when a family member is present.

86. The nurse is caring for a hospitalized client who has a disorder of the amygdala. Which of symptoms can the nurse anticipate that the client will have?
☐ 1. impulsive acts of aggression
☐ 2. sleep disturbance
☐ 3. unable to recognize objects by touch
☐ 4. difficulties with speech

87. A client has been admitted to the emergency department. The client's family tells the nurse that the client has suddenly become lethargic and is "not making sense." The client has not had anything to eat or drink for the last 8 hours. The nurse further assesses the client using the Confusion Assessment Method (CAM). The client's responses to questions are rambling, and the client is not able to focus clearly to answer the nurse's questions. Based on these findings, the nurse should report that the client has:
☐ 1. dementia.
☐ 2. depression.
☐ 3. delirium.
☐ 4. dehydration.

88. A nurse on the geropsychiatric unit receives a call from the son of a recently discharged client. He reports that his father just got a prescription for memantine to take "on top of his donepezil." The son then asks, "Why does he have to take extra medicines?" The nurse should tell the son:

☐ 1. "Maybe the donepezil alone is not improving his dementia fast enough or well enough."

☐ 2. "Memantine and donepezil are commonly used together to slow the progression of dementia."

☐ 3. "Memantine is more effective than donepezil. Your father will be tapered off the donepezil."

☐ 4. "Donepezil has a short half-life, and memantine has a long half-life. They work well together."

89. An elderly client diagnosed with dementia wanders the halls of the locked nursing unit during the day. To ensure the client's safety while walking in the halls, what should the nurse do?

☐ 1. Administer PRN haloperidol to decrease the need to walk.

☐ 2. Assess the client's gait for steadiness.

☐ 3. Restrain the client in a geriatric chair.

☐ 4. Administer PRN lorazepam to provide sedation.

90. A client with dementia who prefers to stay in his room has been brought to the dayroom. After 10 minutes, the client becomes agitated and retreats to his room again. The nurse decides to assess the conditions in the dayroom. Which is the **most** likely occurrence that is disturbing to this client?

☐ 1. There is only one other client in the dayroom; the rest are in a group session in another room.

☐ 2. There are three staff members and one healthcare provider (HCP) in the nurse's station working on charting.

☐ 3. A relaxation tape is playing in one corner of the room, and a television airing a special on crime is playing in the opposite corner.

☐ 4. A housekeeping staff member is washing off the countertops in the kitchen, which is on the far side of the dayroom.

91. Nursing staff are trying to provide for the safety of an elderly client with moderate dementia. The client is wandering at night and has trouble keeping her balance. She has fallen twice but has had no resulting injuries. The nurse should:

☐ 1. move the client to a room near the nurse's station and install a bed alarm.

☐ 2. have the client sleep in a reclining chair across from the nurse's station.

☐ 3. help the client to bed and raise all four bedrails.

☐ 4. ask a family member to stay with the client at night.

92. During a home visit to an elderly client with mild dementia, the client's daughter reports that she has one major problem with her mother. She says, "She sleeps most of the day and is up most of the night. I cannot get a decent night's sleep anymore." Which suggestions should the nurse make to the daughter? Select all that apply.

☐ 1. Ask the client's healthcare provider (HCP) for a strong sleep medicine.

☐ 2. Establish a set routine for rising, hygiene, meals, short rest periods, and bedtime.

☐ 3. Engage the client in simple, brief exercises or a short walk when she gets drowsy during the day.

☐ 4. Promote relaxation before bedtime with a warm bath or relaxing music.

☐ 5. Have the daughter encourage the use of caffeinated beverages during the day to keep her mother awake.

93. A client with agnosia as a result of vascular dementia is staring at dinner and utensils without trying to eat. Which intervention should the nurse attempt **first?**

☐ 1. Pick up the fork and feed the client slowly.

☐ 2. Say, "It is time for you to start eating your dinner."

☐ 3. Hand the fork to the client and say, "Use this fork to eat your green beans."

☐ 4. Save the client's dinner until her family comes in to feed her.

94. A client with early dementia exhibits disturbances in mental awareness and orientation to reality. The nurse should expect to assess a loss of ability in what other areas?

☐ 1. speech

☐ 2. judgment

☐ 3. endurance

☐ 4. balance

95. The client with dementia states to the nurse, "I know you. You are Margaret, the girl who lives down the street from me." Which response by the nurse is **most** therapeutic?

☐ 1. "Mrs. Jones, I am Rachel, a nurse here at the hospital."

☐ 2. "Now Mrs. Jones, you know who I am."

☐ 3. "Mrs. Jones, I told you already, I am Rachel, and I do not live down the street."

☐ 4. "I think you forgot that I am Rachel, Mrs. Jones."

96. While assessing a client diagnosed with dementia, the nurse notes that her husband is concerned about what he should do when she uses vulgar language with him. The nurse should:

☐ 1. tell her that she is very rude.

☐ 2. ignore the vulgarity and distract her.

☐ 3. tell her to stop swearing immediately.

☐ 4. say nothing and leave the room.

97. The nurse understands that the client with severe dementia and motor apraxia may be able to perform which action?
- ☐ 1. Balance a checkbook accurately.
- ☐ 2. Brush the teeth when handed a toothbrush.
- ☐ 3. Use confabulation when telling a story.
- ☐ 4. Find misplaced car keys.

98. When communicating with the client who is experiencing dementia and exhibiting decreased attention and increased confusion, which intervention should the nurse employ as the **first** step?
- ☐ 1. using gentle touch to convey empathy
- ☐ 2. rephrasing questions the client does not understand
- ☐ 3. eliminating distracting stimuli such as turning off the television
- ☐ 4. asking the client to go for a walk while talking

99. During family teaching, the daughter of a client with dementia mentions to the nurse that her mother distorts things. The nurse understands that the daughter needs further teaching about dementia when she makes which statement?
- ☐ 1. "I tell her reality, such as 'That noise is the wind in the trees.'"
- ☐ 2. "I understand the misperceptions are part of the disease."
- ☐ 3. "I turn off the radio when we are in another room."
- ☐ 4. "I tell her she is wrong, and then I tell her what is right."

The Client with Alzheimer's Disease

100. The client in the early stage of Alzheimer's disease and his adult son attend an appointment at the community mental health center. While conversing with the nurse, the son states, "I am tired of hearing about how things were 30 years ago. Why does Dad always talk about the past?" The nurse should tell the son:
- ☐ 1. "Your dad lost his short-term memory, but he still has his long-term memory."
- ☐ 2. "You need to be more accepting of your dad's behavior."
- ☐ 3. "I want you to understand your dad's level of anxiety."
- ☐ 4. "Reminding your dad that you have heard that story will help him stop."

101. The nurse discusses the possibility of a client's attending day treatment for clients with early Alzheimer's disease. What is the **best** rationale for encouraging day treatment?
- ☐ 1. The client would have more structure to his day.
- ☐ 2. The staff are excellent in the treatment they offer clients.
- ☐ 3. The client would benefit from increased social interaction.
- ☐ 4. The family would have more time to engage in their daily activities.

102. The nurse is planning care for a client admitted for vascular dementia. Which action is **most** appropriate in assisting the client with activities of daily living?
- ☐ 1. Perform activities for the client during hospitalization.
- ☐ 2. Document all activities the nurse expects the client to complete during the shift.
- ☐ 3. Inform the client that if morning care is not completed by 0830 hours, the UAP will complete it.
- ☐ 4. Encourage the client to complete as many activities as possible, and provide ample time to complete them.

103. The family of a client diagnosed with Alzheimer's disease wants to keep the client at home. They say that they have the most difficulty in managing his wandering. What should the nurse instruct the family to do? Select all that apply.
- ☐ 1. Ask the healthcare provider (HCP) for a sleeping medication.
- ☐ 2. Install motion and sound detectors.
- ☐ 3. Have a relative sit with the client all night.
- ☐ 4. Have the client wear a Medical Alert bracelet.
- ☐ 5. Install door alarms and high door locks.

104. What is a **priority** to include in the plan of care for a client with Alzheimer's disease who is experiencing difficulty processing and completing complex tasks?
- ☐ 1. repeating the directions until the client follows them
- ☐ 2. asking the client to do one step of the task at a time
- ☐ 3. demonstrating for the client how to do the task
- ☐ 4. maintaining routine and structure for the client

increased delusions and hallucinations. Also, the client did not say that his parents wanted to harm him directly. Stating that the client's relationship with his parents is strained is an assumption, even if he did indeed state that they wanted him dead. The client does not state a wish to be dead or harm others, although further assessment would be necessary. Documenting that his parents may be abusing him makes an assumption, although the nurse should further assess for this possibility.

🔑 CN: Management of care; CL: Evaluate

23. 1. The client's anxiety as reflected in rapid pacing and clang associations is rising as a result of his paranoid delusions. Administering the lorazepam and haloperidol will help the anxiety and delusions. The client is not threatening others at this point, so seclusion, restraints, and asking clients to leave the area are not necessary.

🔑 CN: Pharmacological and parenteral therapies; CL: Synthesize

24. 2. Pushing a suspicious client into social situations is likely to increase anxiety, which increases, not decreases, the hallucinations. The statement about spending some time alone if the client is overwhelmed indicates awareness and understanding of how to intervene when the client is exposed to stress. The statement about lack of motivation indicates awareness and understanding of avolition. The statement about reminding the client that the family does not hear the voices indicates awareness and understanding of the client's hallucinations.

🔑 CN: Psychosocial integrity; CL: Evaluate

25. 1. Clozapine is the one atypical antipsychotic associated with severe anticholinergic adverse effects such as constipation. Consuming fruits would not be the cause of the client's constipation. The client should take clozapine with food to avoid nausea. Getting up slowly indicates that the client understands that postural hypotension may occur with clozapine. The statement about sleepiness indicates that the client understands that sedation may occur with this drug.

🔑 CN: Pharmacological and parenteral therapies; CL: Evaluate

26. 4. The statement about the voices occurring if the client is nervous reflects awareness that stress and anxiety can increase the positive symptoms of schizophrenia. Decreasing the medications because the voices are gone reveals a lack of awareness about the need for the medications to control the client's symptoms. Stating that there is still poison in her food demonstrates a lack of insight into the client's delusions. Restarting school in a week reflects an unrealistic expectation for a client who is newly diagnosed and being stabilized on medications.

🔑 CN: Psychosocial integrity; CL: Evaluate

27. 1. The initial priority for this client is to help her overcome suspiciousness of others, including staff, and thereby feel safe and accepted. Introducing the client to others, giving the client information about the program, and providing clean clothes are important, but these are of lower priority than helping the client feel safe and accepted.

🔑 CN: Psychosocial integrity; CL: Create

28. 2. Constipation caused by medication is best managed by diet, fluids, and exercise. Benztropine can increase constipation. However, it may be prescribed for restlessness and stiffness. Restlessness and stiffness should be reported to the **HCP** 📖. Drowsiness and dizziness are adverse effects of ziprasidone. Clients should not drive if they are experiencing dizziness. Ziprasidone does help improve the negative symptoms of schizophrenia such as avolition.

🔑 CN: Pharmacological and parenteral therapies; CL: Evaluate

The Client with Other Types of Schizophrenia and Psychotic Disorders

29. 4. When the client is listening to the voices, it is most likely an auditory hallucination. Somatic delusions are false beliefs about the functioning of the client's own body. Pseudoparkinsonism is another name for the extrapyramidal symptoms of the medications. Delusions of reference involve events within the environment.

🔑 CN: Psychosocial Integrity; CL: Analyze

30. 1. Most clients experience less weight gain when taking ziprasidone. Although ziprasidone can be administered intramuscularly, it can be used only on an as-needed basis by this route. Ziprasidone has fewer extrapyramidal side effects, but that is not this client's major concern. Ziprasidone is better absorbed when taken with food, so a bedtime snack is needed.

🔑 CN: Pharmacological and parenteral therapies; CL: Synthesize

31. 2,4. Safety issues, including protection of the client and others, are the priorities for admission. Acute psychosis commonly involves issues of safety. Living alone is not a sufficient reason to be admitted to a healthcare facility. Depression, insomnia, lack of appetite, and noncompliance are important issues but not sufficient for admission unless combined with one of the other criteria.

🔑 CN: Management of care; CL: Analyze

32. 3. Elderly clients are typically on lower dosages of antipsychotic medications due to the metabolic changes of aging. Comparing dosages is not relevant. Each client is unique in metabolizing medications. Changing medication dosages is based on an assessment of illness symptoms and the adverse effect profile, not on family preferences. Urging the daughter to wait discounts her concerns and gives no rationale for waiting.

CN: Pharmacological and parenteral therapies; CL: Synthesize

33. 2. Helping the client control his weight is the most appropriate approach. The nurse's contradiction of the client's statement is inappropriate. Most atypical antipsychotics cause weight gain and are not a solution to the weight gain. There is little evidence that weight gain from taking olanzapine decreases with time.

CN: Pharmacological and parenteral therapies; CL: Synthesize

34. 4. Achieving a therapeutic blood level is a slower process with risperidone long-acting injection. Oral fluphenazine does not decrease the effectiveness of the intramuscular version and might increase the incidence of adverse effects. There is no evidence that the potency of the two medications is significantly different. Blaming the client for noncompliance with these two medications is inappropriate.

CN: Pharmacological and parenteral therapies; CL: Synthesize

35. 1,2,4,5. Ziprasidone can cause somnolence, drowsiness, weight gain (can be excessive), constipation, and headache; these side effects may preclude noncompliance with this medication. Urticaria is not a common side effect of ziprasidone.

CN: Pharmacological and parenteral therapies; CL: Synthesize

36. 1. Recognition by the client that there is a difference between the stuffed animal and her live dog indicates that the client perceives the reality of the situation. Stating that the stuffed animal and the client's dog could be twins reflects the client's continued misperception of reality, thinking that the stuffed animal and her dog are one and the same. Stating that she wishes her dog had not been stuffed reflects her continued misperception of reality. Stating that the roommate needs a dog as much as she does is unrelated to the client's perception or misperception of reality.

CN: Psychosocial integrity; CL: Evaluate

37. 3. The nurse must be objective in documenting the client's behavior, recording exactly what the client did or did not say or do in a particular situation. Recording that the client could not answer any questions, was uncooperative and refused to answer questions, or was disoriented and incoherent is not described and is a subjective interpretation on the nurse's part.

CN: Management of care; CL: Create

38. 4. By the end of 4 days, the client should be able to perform showering and dressing for herself. The client with schizophrenia commonly appears to be apathetic and lack initiative. Therefore, demonstrating the ability to complete the tasks indicates improvement. Although the client may be able to recognize, verbalize, or explain the need to shower and dress herself, she may be unable to do so because of the ambivalence associated with schizophrenia that impedes the client's ability to initiate and complete self-care. Therefore, evidence of improvement would be lacking.

CN: Management of care; CL: Create

39. 1. When determining the effectiveness of risperidone, the nurse would expect improvement in the client's negative symptoms of apathy, flat affect, and social withdrawal. Delusions, hallucinations, illusions, and ideas of reference are positive symptoms of schizophrenia. Agitation, hostility, and aggression are also the result of the positive symptoms.

CN: Pharmacological and parenteral therapies; CL: Evaluate

40. 2,3,4. The client's symptoms are likely to be adverse effects of aripiprazole, especially at the reported dose. The normal adult dose is 5 to 10 mg. The elderly client commonly needs a lower dose compared with other adults. The anxiety and sleep disturbance could be symptoms of schizophrenia or medication adverse effects. A holistic approach would include assessing the client's heart failure. Questioning the qualifications of the family **HCP** ▭ is unproductive. There are no indications of problems in the client's relationship with her son.

CN: Pharmacological and parenteral therapies; CL: Analyze

41. 3. Excessive salivation, or sialorrhea, is commonly associated with clozapine therapy. The client can use a washcloth to wipe the saliva instead of spitting. It is an expected adverse effect of the drug, not a delusion, an unusual reaction, or an unresolved symptom of schizophrenia.

CN: Pharmacological and parenteral therapies; CL: Analyze

42. 3. Stating that God is important in the client's life recognizes the client's cognitive and perceptual disturbances and level of anxiety and acknowledges the client's message in a respectful and neutral manner, while adding that the medicine also will help clearly and directly states the need for medication. Stating "God helps those who help themselves" challenges the client. Stating "God wants you to take your medicine" is deceitful. Stating "Medicine will help clear your thinking and decrease anxiety" would be helpful to the client later when she is less acutely psychotic and anxious.

🔑 CN: Psychosocial integrity; CL: Apply

43. 1. The nurse instructs the client clearly and directly to put the medication in the mouth and then to swallow it with some water. Clear, step-by-step directions assist the client to process what the nurse is saying. Telling the client to sit in the dayroom and wait, asking another staff member to stay with the client, or saying nothing is not helpful.

🔑 CN: Pharmacological and parenteral therapies; CL: Synthesize

44. 2. Whispering and laughing with another person where the client can see or observe the nurse but not hear the conversation increases the client's anxiety and suspiciousness. Therefore, this action should be avoided. Informing the client of schedule changes, telling the client gently that the nurse does not share the client's interpretation of an event, and inviting the client to participate in leisure activities help the client to decrease anxiety and suspiciousness and to focus on actual or realistic events.

🔑 CN: Psychosocial integrity; CL: Synthesize

45. 4. Because the client can live in an apartment setting, further development of independent functioning and the skills to gain as much independence as he is capable of need to be fostered, including getting out and developing new friendships. Arranging for participation in day treatment is most beneficial at this time. Family visits and daily nursing visits do not encourage the client to do this. Making an appointment for 2 weeks later puts the client's needs off. Lack of social relationships is not a sufficient reason for rehospitalization.

🔑 CN: Psychosocial integrity; CL: Synthesize

46. 2. One advantage of using risperidone is that it is not associated with agranulocytosis like clozapine and does not require the same lab monitoring. In schizophrenia negative symptoms are more prominent than positive. Negative symptoms do not respond to typical antipsychotics such as haloperidol. Agranulocytosis is commonly associated with clozapine. Because it is a newer drug, risperidone usually is more expensive than typical antipsychotics.

🔑 CN: Pharmacological and parenteral therapies; CL: Apply

47. 1,2,3. Headaches, transient anxiety, and insomnia are the most common adverse effects of aripiprazole. Torticollis and pill rolling are more common with the older antipsychotics.

🔑 CN: Pharmacological and parenteral therapies; CL: Create

48. 2. The client is in an acute psychotic state and cannot process complex decisions or explain complex situations. Therefore, the nurse would focus on decision making involving simple choices. Listing the pros and cons of each housing option and identifying why the client cannot live in an unsupervised apartment involve complex decision-making skills. Deciding which staff member to have today is a difficult and threatening decision for a client who is psychotic.

🔑 CN: Management of care; CL: Synthesize

49. 1. The client is exhibiting hallmark signs and symptoms of life-threatening neuroleptic malignant syndrome induced by the haloperidol. Tardive dyskinesia usually occurs later in treatment, typically months to years later. Extrapyramidal adverse effects (dystonia, akathisia) and drug-induced parkinsonism, although common, are not life threatening.

🔑 CN: Reduction of risk potential; CL: Analyze

50. 3. The client with schizophrenia needs more structure every day to improve functioning. Therefore, helping the client to set up a daily activity schedule is most appropriate. However, a group home is not necessary. The client is already eating. Having meals brought in would increase the client's dependence, not his activity level. Asking a relative to call the client 10 times per day is unrealistic given the typical daily responsibilities of a healthy relative.

🔑 CN: Psychosocial integrity; CL: Synthesize

51. 2. The client is exhibiting catatonic behavior, an acutely serious result of severe anxiety and psychosis. In this situation, the nurse needs to administer the PRN-prescribed doses of haloperidol and lorazepam; they can be given together safely. Assisting the client out of the chair to go back to bed or sitting quietly until the client responds ignores the seriousness of the client's condition. It is unlikely that the client can describe what is being experienced.

🔑 CN: Psychosocial integrity; CL: Synthesize

52. 2. Attending day therapy three times per week is a long-term goal that will show the most progress in overcoming withdrawal. The client's calling his or her mother is a first step in getting out of a severe withdrawal. Allowing two friends to visit every day would be appropriate if the client is successful with calling his or her mother once a day. Insufficient information is presented in the scenario to indicate that excessive sleep is a problem.

> CN: Psychosocial integrity; CL: Synthesize

53. 4. Although all the actions indicate improvement, the ability to initiate simple activities without directions indicates the most improvement in the catatonic behaviors. Moving all extremities occasionally, walking with the nurse to the client's room, and responding to verbal directions to eat represent single steps toward the client initiating his or her own actions.

> CN: Pharmacological and parenteral therapies; CL: Evaluate

54. 2. Noncompliance with medications is common in the client with schizophrenia. The nurse has the responsibility to assess this situation. Asking the mother if they've argued or if the client is mad at the mother or telling the mother to go over to the apartment and see what's going on places the blame and responsibility on the mother and therefore is inappropriate. Telling the mother not to worry ignores the seriousness of the client's symptoms.

> CN: Management of care; CL: Synthesize

55. 4. The client is exhibiting symptoms of becoming catatonic and unable to care for himself and needs immediate evaluation and possible hospitalization. A sleep aid is not sufficient to treat this client. The client's worsening condition dictates action without waiting for a clinic appointment. An increase in medication may be indicated, but hospitalization is required first for safety.

> CN: Management of care; CL: Analyze

56. 3. Valproic acid is commonly used to treat manic symptoms. Therefore, a decrease in the valproic acid level could explain the increase in manic symptoms. Periodic determinations of the valproic acid level are necessary to determine the effectiveness of the drug. However, the stat nature of the specimen to be drawn indicates an immediate problem. Fluoxetine is not known to decrease the effectiveness of valproic acid. The valproic acid level is not needed before beginning a short course of therapy with lorazepam.

> CN: Pharmacological and parenteral therapies; CL: Apply

57. 3. A diagnosis of brief psychotic disorder is made when the client exhibits delusions, hallucinations, and disorganized speech or behaviors in the absence of a mood disorder, substance-induced disorder, or general medical condition.

> CN: Reduction of risk potential; CL: Analyze

58. 4. Follow-up counseling is appropriate because of the client's anger and inappropriate behaviors. The goal is to help the client deal with the end of his marriage. A joint session might have been useful before the divorce and arrest, but not after. The client is exhibiting no signs or symptoms of schizophrenia or psychosis, so olanzapine is not indicated. The client is not exhibiting signs of depression, so fluoxetine is not indicated.

> CN: Management of care; CL: Synthesize

Clients and Families Affected by Chronic Mental Illnesses

59. 3. The first thing that the nurse should do is to speak with the client on the phone and question her about perceptions or reasons that are interfering with her going to the sheltered workshop. This conveys that the nurse is interested and willing to help the client. The nurse should call the director of the work center for information only if the nurse receives the client's permission. Making preparations for the client's admission is inappropriate and would not be done until the client's needs have been assessed and it is determined that the client requires hospitalization. Making an appointment with the **healthcare provider (HCP)** is inappropriate until the nurse has assessed the client's needs.

> CN: Management of care; CL: Synthesize

60. 2. Noncompliance with medications is documented as the primary cause of relapse. Although loss of family support, sudden changes in medications, and nonattendance at treatment programs may contribute to relapse, these factors are not as significant as medication noncompliance as causes of relapse.

> CN: Psychosocial integrity; CL: Analyze

61. 3. The most therapeutic action at this time is for the nurse to make an appointment with the client at the mental health center to explore his feelings and behavior. Doing so acknowledges the client's importance and makes him a partner in resolving the problem. The nurse needs to determine what is going on in the situation first, and then plan accordingly. Threatening the client with loss of the position, asking for a new assignment for the client, or arranging for the placement of the client in a skill training program is inappropriate and premature.

> CN: Management of care; CL: Synthesize

62. 2. By acknowledging the difficulties of living with the illness, the nurse conveys empathy for the client's feelings and opens up the lines of communication. Although it is important for the client to maintain compliance with medication therapy, telling the client that it is important to start taking them again or to talk with the **HCP** 📖 about stopping the medications ignores the underlying feelings of the client's initial statements. Stating that the client's buddies will understand may or may not be true. Additionally, this statement ignores the underlying feelings.

🔑 CN: Psychosocial integrity;
CL: Synthesize

63. 3. Because antipsychotic agents cross the placental barrier and can be teratogenic, they are to be avoided during pregnancy, especially during the first trimester. Later in the pregnancy, low doses of medications may be given if necessary. Although the degree of excitement by the father, the mother's ability to provide help, and the client's financial situation may or may not be of concern, the priority in this situation is the safety of the fetus and risks associated with the need for antipsychotic therapy.

🔑 CN: Reduction of risk potential;
CL: Analyze

64. 1. A side effect of clozapine is leukopenia. A WBC count is drawn every week, and if it starts to drop, the **HCP** 📖 is notified. Slightly low hemoglobin levels or a normal sodium level is not significant. Hyaline casts occur because of protein in the urine, and a small amount is normally found in the urine, especially after exercise.

🔑 CN: Reduction of risk potential;
CL: Analyze

65. 3. Many coordinated services are needed, including medication management, more frequent outpatient visits, day treatment, or some combination of these, to decrease the risk of relapse, which is common among chronically ill clients. Medical consultations (if needed) would be included in the coordinated services provided. Chronically mentally ill clients, who are discharged early before becoming truly stable, typically require more than monthly outpatient visits because of the high risk of relapse. A caring and supportive family is ideal for all clients but not always available.

🔑 CN: Management of care; CL: Create

66. 4. For a community-based program, the need for long-term hospitalization is least needed if the other services, such as partial hospitalization programs, psychiatric home care, and residential services, are available and accessible.

🔑 CN: Management of care; CL: Apply

67. 2,3,4. Although all of the situations require immediate attention, the inability to keep outpatient appointments is less critical than signs of relapse and decompensation, threat of eviction, and unpaid bills and lack of food. Occasionally missing a dose of medication usually will not precipitate a crisis for a client.

🔑 CN: Psychosocial integrity; CL: Analyze

68. 1. Providing ways to decrease or manage adverse effects without additional medications is crucial. Although home visits, family monitoring, and outpatient monitoring may help, if the adverse effects are not controlled, the client is less likely to take the drug, which would interfere with its effectiveness.

🔑 CN: Pharmacological and parenteral therapies; CL: Analyze

69. 4. Many still believe that recovery from mental illness is a matter of willpower—for example, "pull yourself up by your bootstraps" or "just get over it." This belief persists despite awareness that mental illness can be hereditary and has a biochemical basis. Mental illness can be prevented only if there is early intervention. Clients cannot prevent it just by the desire to do so.

🔑 CN: Psychosocial integrity;
CL: Evaluate

The Client with Cognitive Disorders

70. 4. Delirium is commonly due to a medical condition such as a UTI in the elderly. Delirium often involves memory problems, disorientation, and hallucinations. It develops rather quickly. There are not enough data to suggest Alzheimer's disease especially given the quick onset of symptoms. Delayed grieving and adjusting to being alone are unlikely to cause hallucinations.

🔑 CN: Reduction of risk potential;
CL: Analyze

71. 3. Paradoxical responses to benzodiazepines are more common in children and the elderly than other age groups and generally occur at the beginning of treatment. Grief and depression in the elderly is more likely to result in fatigue and withdrawal than hyperactivity and agitation. Treatment with a sleeping medication chemically related to the benzodiazepines is likely to result in an increase rather than decrease in agitation symptoms in elderly clients. A medication interaction is possible, but less likely since most pharmacies screen for drug interactions when filling prescriptions.

🔑 CN: Pharmacological and parenteral therapies; CL: Analyze

72. 4. Expecting the social worker to make the decision indicates that the son is avoiding participating in decisions about his father. The other responses convey that the son understands the importance of a careful decision, the availability of resources, and the ability to make new plans if needed.

🔑 CN: Management of care; CL: Synthesize

73. 1,2,5. Confused clients need fewer choices, acceptance as a person, and step-by-step directions. Allowing the client to do as he wishes can lead to substandard care and the risk of harm. Acting nonchalantly conveys a lack of caring.

🔑 CN: Psychosocial integrity; CL: Synthesize

74. 3. Reminiscing can help reduce depression in an elderly client and lessens feelings of isolation and loneliness. Reminiscing encourages a focus on positive memories and accomplishments as well as shared memories with other clients. An increase in confusion and disorientation is most likely the result of other cognitive and situational factors, such as loss of short-term memory, not reminiscing. The client will not likely become sad because reminiscing helps the client connect with positive memories. Keeping the client from participating in therapeutic activities is less likely with reminiscing.

🔑 CN: Psychosocial integrity; CL: Evaluate

The Client with Delirium

75. 2. Loss of orientation, especially for time and place, is common in delirium. The nurse should orient the client by telling him the time, date, place, and who the client is with. Taking the client to his room and telling him why the door is locked do not address his disorientation. Telling the client to eat before going to his medical appointment reinforces his disorientation.

🔑 CN: Psychosocial integrity; CL: Synthesize

76. 1,2,3. The client does need rest and it is true that there is no specific medicine for delirium, but it is crucial to identify and treat the underlying causes of delirium. Other tests will be based on the results of already completed tests. Although some medications may be prescribed to help the client with her behaviors, this is not the primary basis for medication prescriptions. Because the underlying medical causes of delirium could be fatal, treatment must be initiated as soon as possible. It is not the nurse's role to determine medications for this client. Postponing tests until the next day is inappropriate.

🔑 CN: Psychosocial integrity; CL: Apply

77. 1. Explaining why blood is being taken responds to the client's concerns or fears about what is happening. Threatening more pain or promising to explain later ignores or postpones meeting the client's need for information. The client's statements do not reflect loss of self-control requiring medication intervention.

🔑 CN: Psychosocial integrity; CL: Synthesize

78. 3. The client is showing symptoms of delirium, a common outcome of UTI in older adults. The nurse can request a transfer to a medical unit for acute medical intervention. The client's symptoms are not just due to a worsening of the depression. There are not indications that the client needs restraints or a transfer to a nursing home at this point.

🔑 CN: Management of care; CL: Synthesize

79. 3. Polypharmacy is much more common in the elderly. Drug interactions increase the incidence of intoxication from prescribed medications, especially with combinations of analgesics, digoxin, diuretics, and anticholinergics. With drug intoxication, the onset of the delirium typically is quick. Although cancer, impaired hearing, and heart failure could lead to delirium in the elderly, the onset would be more gradual.

🔑 CN: Reduction of risk potential; CL: Analyze

80. 1. In addition to developing over a period of hours or days, fluctuating symptoms are characteristic of delirium. The failure to identify objects despite intact sensory functions, significant impairment in social or occupational functioning over time, and memory impairment to the degree of being called amnesia all indicate dementia.

🔑 CN: Physiological adaptation; CL: Analyze

81. 2. The most critical aspect of caring for the client with delirium is to institute measures to correct the underlying causative condition or illness. Controlling behavioral symptoms with low-dose psychotropics, manipulating the environment, and decreasing or discontinuing all medications may be dangerous to the client's health.

🔑 CN: Reduction of risk potential; CL: Apply

82. 3. In approximately 2 to 3 days, the client should be able to regain orientation and thus become oriented to time and place. Being able to explain the experience of having delirium is something that the client is expected to achieve later in the course of the illness, but ultimately before discharge. Resuming a normal sleep-wake cycle and establishing normal bowel and bladder function probably will take longer, depending on how long it takes to resolve the underlying condition.

🔑 CN: Psychosocial integrity; CL: Synthesize

83. 1. Identifying oneself and making sure that the nurse has the client's attention address the difficulties with focusing, orientation, and maintaining attention. Eliminating daytime napping is unrealistic until the cause of the delirium is determined and the client's ability to focus and maintain attention improves. Engaging the client in reminiscing and avoiding arguing are also unrealistic at this time.

∞ CN: Psychosocial integrity; CL: Apply

84. 1,2,4. The abnormal stimuli of the critical care unit can aggravate the symptoms of delirium. Arguing with hallucinations is inappropriate. When a client has illogical thinking, gently presenting reality is appropriate, but orienting the client to his condition is unlikely to be helpful. Dementia is not the likely cause of the client's symptoms. The client is experiencing delirium, not dementia.

∞ CN: Psychosocial integrity; CL: Synthesize

The Client with Dementia

85. 3. That the client is not able to recall the three words is a likely indicator of dementia; the nurse should make a referral for further testing. It is recommended not to repeat the test a second time if the client is not able to recall the words. Although the client repeated rhyming words, echolalia refers to repletion of the same word. It is not necessary to have a family member present when conducting the test, but the nurse should communicate the findings to the family and encourage them to seek follow-up assessment.

∞ CN: Reduction of risk potential; CL: Analyze

86. 1. Impulsive acts of aggression and violence have been linked to dysregulation of the amygdala. The hypothalamus regulates basic human activities such as sleep-rest patterns. The parietal lobe contains the primary somatosensory area. The temporal lobes contain the primary auditory areas.

∞ CN: Management of care; CL: Analyze

87. 3. Based on CAM's assessment tool, the client has an acute onset of behaviors, is inattentive, has disorganized thinking, and is lethargic (decreased level of consciousness). This cluster of behaviors constitutes delirium. Dementia has a slow onset, the client's level of consciousness is usually normal, and the client can focus attention. Clients who are depressed are alert and oriented and able to focus attention, although they may be easily distracted. Further assessment is needed to determine if the client also is dehydrated.

∞ CN: Reduction of risk potential; CL: Analyze

88. 2. Memantine and donepezil are commonly given together. Neither medicine will improve dementia, but they may slow the progression. Neither medicine is more effective than the other; they act differently in the brain. Both medicines have a half-life of 60 or more hours.

∞ CN: Pharmacological and parenteral therapies; CL: Apply

89. 2. Elderly clients with dementia have increased risk for falls due to balance problems, medication use, and decreased eyesight. Haloperidol may cause extrapyramidal side effects, which increase the risk for falls. The client is not agitated, so restraints are not indicated. Lorazepam may increase fall risk and cause paradoxical excitement.

∞ CN: Reduction of risk potential; CL: Synthesize

90. 3. The tape and television are competing, even conflicting, stimuli. Crime events portrayed on television could be misperceived as a real threat to the client. A low number of clients and the presence of a few staff members quietly working are less intense stimuli for the client and not likely to be disturbing.

∞ CN: Management of care; CL: Analyze

91. 1. Using a bed alarm enables the staff to respond immediately if the client tries to get out of bed. Sleeping in a chair at the nurse's station interferes with the client's restful sleep and privacy. Using all four bedrails is considered a restraint and unsafe practice. It is not appropriate to expect a family member to stay all night with the client.

∞ CN: Safety and infection control; CL: Synthesize

92. 2,3,4. A set routine and brief exercises help decrease daytime sleeping. Decreasing caffeine and fluids and promoting relaxation at bedtime promote nighttime sleeping. A strong sleep medicine for an elderly client is contraindicated due to changes in metabolism, increased adverse effects, and the risk of falls. Using caffeinated beverages may stimulate metabolism but can also have long-lasting adverse effects and may prevent sleep at bedtime.

∞ CN: Management of care; CL: Synthesize

93. 3. Agnosia is the lack of recognition of objects and their purpose. The nurse should inform the client about the fork and what to do with it. Feeding the client does not address the agnosia or give the client specific directions. It should only be attempted if identifying the fork and explaining what to do with it is ineffective. Waiting for the family to care for the client is not appropriate unless identifying the fork and explaining or feeding the client is not successful.

∞ CN: Management of care; CL: Synthesize

94. 2. Clients with chronic cognitive disorders experience defects in memory orientation and intellectual functions, such as judgment and discrimination. Loss of other abilities, such as speech, endurance, and balance, is less typical.

⚷ CN: Psychosocial integrity; CL: Analyze

95. 1. Because of the client's short-term memory impairment, the nurse gently corrects the client by stating her name and who she is. This approach decreases anxiety, embarrassment, and shame and maintains the client's self-esteem. Telling the client that she knows who the nurse is or that she forgot can elicit feelings of embarrassment and shame. Saying "I told you already" sounds condescending, as if blaming the client for not remembering.

⚷ CN: Psychosocial integrity; CL: Synthesize

96. 2. Vulgar language is common in clients with dementia when they are having trouble communicating about a topic. Ignoring the vulgarity and distracting her is appropriate. Telling the client she is rude or to stop swearing will have no lasting effect and may cause agitation. Just leaving the room is abandonment that the client will not understand.

⚷ CN: Psychosocial integrity; CL: Synthesize

97. 2. Highly conditioned motor skills, such as brushing tooth, may be retained by the client who has dementia and motor apraxia. Balancing a checkbook involves calculations, a complex skill that is lost with severe dementia. Confabulation is fabrication of details to fill a memory gap. This is more common when the client is aware of a memory problem, not when dementia is severe. Finding keys is a memory factor, not a motor function.

⚷ CN: Psychosocial integrity; CL: Analyze

98. 3. Competing and excessive stimuli lead to sensory overload and confusion. Therefore, the nurse should first eliminate any distracting stimuli. After this is accomplished, then using touch and rephrasing questions are appropriate. Going for a walk while talking has little benefit on attention and confusion.

⚷ CN: Psychosocial integrity; CL: Synthesize

99. 4. Telling the client that she is wrong and then telling her what is right is argumentative and challenging. Arguing with or challenging distortions is least effective because it increases defensiveness. Telling the client about reality indicates awareness of the issues and is appropriate. Acknowledging that misperceptions are part of the disease indicates an understanding of the disease and an awareness of the issues. Turning off the radio helps to limit environmental stimuli and indicates an awareness of the issues.

⚷ CN: Psychosocial integrity; CL: Evaluate

The Client with Alzheimer's Disease

100. 1. The son's statements regarding his father's recalling past events is typical for family members of clients in the early stage of Alzheimer's disease, when recent memory is impaired. Telling the son to be more accepting is being critical and not an attempt to educate. Understanding the client's level of anxiety is unrelated to the memory loss of Alzheimer's disease. The client cannot stop reminiscing at will.

⚷ CN: Psychosocial integrity; CL: Apply

101. 3. The best rationale for day treatment for the client with Alzheimer's disease is the enhancement of social interactions. More daily structure, excellent staff, and allowing caregivers more time for themselves are all positive aspects, but they are less focused on the client's needs.

⚷ CN: Psychosocial integrity; CL: Apply

102. 4. By fostering independence and providing as much time as possible, the nurse is helping the client to continue to complete as many tasks as possible. Performing activities for the client is counterproductive. A list may cause the client to become frustrated if the list is not completed or if it becomes lost. Informing the client that the **UAP** 🖵 will complete activities may be perceived as a threat.

⚷ CN: Basic care and comfort; CL: Apply

103. 2,4,5. Motion and sound detectors, a Medical Alert bracelet, and door alarms and locks are all appropriate interventions for wandering. Sleep medications do not prevent wandering before and after the client is asleep and may have negative effects. Having a relative sit with the client is usually an unrealistic burden.

⚷ CN: Psychosocial integrity; CL: Synthesize

104. 2. Because the client is experiencing difficulty processing and completing complex tasks, the priority is to provide the client with only one step at a time, thereby breaking the task up into simple steps, ones that the client can process. Repeating the directions until the client follows them or demonstrating how to do the task is still too overwhelming to the client because of the multiple steps involved. Although maintaining structure and routine is important, it is unrelated to task completion.

⚷ CN: Psychosocial integrity; CL: Synthesize

105. 3. The therapeutic communication technique of asking the client to describe the forgetfulness seeks clarification and provides the client an opportunity to tell more about the problem. A client who is 75 years of age may take a prolonged time to remember as a result of normal cognitive changes of aging, but telling the client it is normal to forget is diminishing the importance of the comment. Referring to the nurse's self is also diminishing the importance of the client's concern. It is not the nurse's role to indicate that the client does or does not have Alzheimer's disease; the nurse uses communication techniques that obtain sufficient information to determine if a referral is needed.

⚷ CN: Psychosocial integrity; CL: Apply

106. 1. The vulgar or sexual behaviors are commonly expressions of anger or more sensual needs that can be addressed directly. Therefore, the families should be encouraged to ignore the behaviors but attempt to identify their purpose. Then the purpose can be addressed, possibly leading to a decrease in the behaviors. Because of impaired cognitive function, the client is not likely to be able to process the inappropriateness of the behaviors if given feedback. Likewise, anger management strategies would be ineffective because the client would probably be unable to process the inappropriateness of the behaviors. Risperidone may decrease agitation, but it does not improve social behaviors.

⚷ CN: Psychosocial integrity; CL: Apply

107. 4. The statement about expecting that the old Dad would be back conveys a lack of acceptance of the irreversible nature of the disease. The statement about not realizing that the deterioration would be so incapacitating is based in reality. The statement about the Alzheimer's group is based in reality and demonstrates the son's involvement with managing the disease. Stating that reminiscing is important reflects a realistic interpretation on the son's part.

⚷ CN: Psychosocial integrity; CL: Evaluate

108. 1. When compared with other similar medications, donepezil has fewer adverse effects. Donepezil is effective primarily in the early stages of the disease. The drug helps to slow the progression of the disease if started in the early stages. After the client has been diagnosed for 6 years, improvement to the level seen 6 years ago is highly unlikely. Data are not available to support the drug's effectiveness for clients in the terminal phase of the disease.

⚷ CN: Pharmacological and parenteral therapies; CL: Apply

109. 3. Antipsychotics are most effective with agitation and assaultiveness. Antipsychotics have little effect on sleep disturbances, concomitant depression, or confusion and withdrawal.

⚷ CN: Pharmacological and parenteral therapies; CL: Apply

110. 1. Although all of the side effects listed are possible with lorazepam, paradoxical excitement is cause for immediate discontinuation of the medication. (Paradoxical excitement is the opposite reaction to lorazepam than is expected.) The other side effects tend to be minor and usually are transient.

⚷ CN: Pharmacology and parental therapies; CL: Apply

111. 4. Change increases stress. Therefore, the most important and relevant suggestion is to maintain consistency in the client's environment, routine, and caregivers. Although rest periods are important, going to bed interferes with the sleep-wake cycle. Rest in a recliner chair is more useful. Testing cognitive functioning and reality orientation are not likely to be successful and may increase stress if memory loss is severe.

⚷ CN: Psychosocial integrity; CL: Apply

Managing Care, Quality, and Safety of Clients with Schizophrenia, Other Psychoses, and Cognitive Disorders

112. 4. The neighbor could be harmed as well as the daughter if she should try to stop her father from using the gun, so both should be notified. Any use of firearms against another person requires the involvement of the police. The nurse has a legal/ethical responsibility to warn potential victims and other involved parties as well as law enforcement authorities when one person makes a threat against another person. This duty supersedes confidentiality statutes. Failure to do so and to document it can result in civil penalties. The client's early dementia would likely not prevent him from carrying through his threat.

⚷ CN: Management of care; CL: Analyze

113. 4. Benztropine has a common side effect of blurred vision. After evaluating the relative doses of haloperidol and benztropine, the *assessment* would be that the higher dose of benztropine compared to the dose of haloperidol is responsible for the blurred vision. (High doses of haloperidol can cause blurred vision at times.) Reporting that Mr. Roberts has blurred vision is the *situation*. Listing the medications and doses is describing the *background*. The *recommendation* would be a lower dose of benztropine.

⚷ CN: Management of care; CL: Synthesize

114. 2. Nurses are required to document that clients have been given information about their status and rights. Seclusion is not related to people becoming involuntary or certified clients. Including details contained within the certificates, such as a **healthcare provider (HCP)** 📖 signing the certificates, is not required.

🔑 CN: Management of care; CL: Apply

115. 4. The client exhibits aggression against his perceived adversary when he names another client as his adversary. The staff will need to watch him carefully for signs of impending violent behavior that may injure others. Crying about a divorce would be appropriate, not pathologic, behavior demonstrating grief over a loss. A petition to delay bedtime would be a positive, direct action aimed at a bothersome situation. Although declining to attend group therapy needs follow-up, there may be any number of unknown reasons for this action.

🔑 CN: Safety and infection control; CL: Synthesize

116. 2. When caring for a client with cognitive impairment, the priority is to ensure that all objects in the client's path are removed to prevent the client from falling. Additional measures, such as having two people accompany the client when he ambulates, placing his favorite things in safekeeping, and giving medications in a liquid form to be sure he swallows them, are less crucial.

🔑 CN: Safety and infection control; CL: Synthesize

117. 1. The most common reason for the nurse's discomfort with elderly clients is that she has not examined her own fears and conflicts about aging. Until nurses resolve their fears, it is unlikely that they will feel comfortable with elderly clients. A dislike of physical contact with older people, a desire to be surrounded by beauty and youth, and recent experiences with a parent's elderly friends are possible explanations, but not common or likely.

🔑 CN: Management of care; CL: Analyze

Personality Disorders, Substance-Related Disorders, Anxiety Disorders, and Anxiety-Related Disorders

- The Client with a Personality Disorder
- The Client with an Alcohol-Related Disorder
- The Client with Disorders Related to Other Addictive Substances
- The Client with Anxiety Disorders and Anxiety-Related Disorders
- The Client with a Somatoform Disorder
- Managing Care, Quality, and Safety of Clients with Personality Disorders, Substance-Related Disorders, Anxiety Disorders, and Anxiety-Related Disorders
- Answers, Rationales, and Test-Taking Strategies

The Client with a Personality Disorder

1. A client has been diagnosed with avoidant personality disorder. He reports loneliness, but has fears about making friends. He also reports anxiety about being rejected by others. In a long-term treatment plan, in what order, from first to last, should the nurse list her goals for the client? All options must be used.

1. Teach the client anxiety management and social skills.

2. Ask the client to join one of his chosen activities with the nurse and two other clients.

3. Talk with the client about his self-esteem and his fears.

4. Help the client make a list of small group activities at the center he would find interesting.

2. A client diagnosed with borderline personality disorder has self-inflicted cuts on her arms. The nurse is assessing the client for the risk of suicide. What should the nurse ask the client **first**?
- ☐ 1. about medications she has taken recently
- ☐ 2. if she is taking antidepressants
- ☐ 3. if she has a suicide plan
- ☐ 4. why she cut herself

3. When developing the plan of care for a client diagnosed with a personality disorder, the nurse plans to assist the client **primarily** with what factor?
- ☐ 1. specific dysfunctional behaviors
- ☐ 2. psychopharmacologic compliance
- ☐ 3. examination of developmental conflicts
- ☐ 4. manipulation of the environment

4. A client diagnosed with paranoid personality disorder is hospitalized for physically threatening his wife because he suspects her of having an affair with a coworker. What approach should the nurse employ with this client?
- ☐ 1. authoritarian
- ☐ 2. parental
- ☐ 3. matter of fact
- ☐ 4. controlling

5. When planning care for a client diagnosed with schizotypal personality disorder, which intervention helps the client become involved with others?
- ☐ 1. participating solely in group activities
- ☐ 2. being involved with primarily one-to-one activities
- ☐ 3. leading a sing-along in the afternoon
- ☐ 4. attending an activity with the nurse

6. A client is complaining to other clients about not being allowed by staff to keep food in her room. The nurse should:
☐ **1.** ignore the client's behavior.
☐ **2.** set limits on the behavior.
☐ **3.** reprimand the client.
☐ **4.** allow the snack to be kept in her room.

7. A client with a diagnosis of antisocial personality disorder has a potential for violence and aggressive behavior. Which short-term client outcome is **most** appropriate for the nurse to include in the plan of care?
☐ **1.** Use humor when expressing anger.
☐ **2.** Discuss feelings of anger with staff.
☐ **3.** Ask the nurse for medication when upset.
☐ **4.** Use indirect behaviors to express anger.

8. A new client on the psychiatric unit has been diagnosed with depression and obsessive-compulsive personality disorder (OCPD). During visiting hours, her husband states to the nurse that he does not understand this OCPD and what can be done about it. What information should the nurse share with the client and her husband? Select all that apply.
☐ **1.** Perfectionism and overemphasis on tasks usually interfere with friendships and leisure time.
☐ **2.** It will help to interrupt her tasks and tell her you are going out for the evening.
☐ **3.** There are medicines, such as clomipramine or fluoxetine, that may help.
☐ **4.** Remind your wife that it is "OK" to be human and make mistakes.
☐ **5.** Reinforce with her that she is not allowed to expect the whole family to be perfect too.
☐ **6.** This disorder typically involves inflexibility and a need to be in control.

9. A client diagnosed with paranoid personality disorder is being admitted on an involuntary 24-hour hold after a physical altercation with a police officer who was investigating the client's threatening phone calls to his neighbors. He states that his neighbors are spying on him for the government, saying, "I want them to stop and leave me alone. Now they have you nurses and doctors involved in their conspiracy." Which nursing approaches are **most** appropriate? Select all that apply.
☐ **1.** Approach the client in a professional, matter-of-fact manner.
☐ **2.** Avoid intrusive interactions with the client.
☐ **3.** Gently present reality to counteract the client's current paranoid beliefs.
☐ **4.** Develop trust consistently with the client.
☐ **5.** Do not pressure the client to attend any groups.

10. A 28-year-old client with a diagnosis of major depression and dependent personality disorder has been living at home with very supportive parents. The client is thinking about independent living on the recommendation of the treatment team. The client states to the nurse, "I do not know if I can make it in an apartment without my parents." The nurse should respond by saying to the client:
☐ **1.** "You are a 28-year-old adult now, not a child who needs to be cared for."
☐ **2.** "Your parents will not be around forever. After all, they are getting older."
☐ **3.** "Your parents need a break, and you need a break from them."
☐ **4.** "Your parents have been supportive and will continue to be even if you live apart."

11. A client moves in with her family after her boyfriend of 4 weeks told her to leave. She is admitted to the subacute unit after reporting feeling empty and lonely, being unable to sleep, and eating very little for the last week. Her arms are scarred from frequent self-mutilation. What should the nurse do in order of priority from first to last? All options must be used.

1. Monitor for suicide and self-mutilation.

2. Discuss the issues of loneliness and emptiness.

3. Monitor sleeping and eating behaviors.

4. Discuss her housing options for after discharge.

12. The client approaches various staff with numerous requests and needs to the point of disrupting the staff's work with other clients. The nurse meets with the staff to decide on a consistent, therapeutic approach for this client. Which approach will be **most** effective?
☐ **1.** telling the client to stay in his room until staff approach him
☐ **2.** limiting the client to the dayroom and dining area
☐ **3.** giving the client a list of permissible requests
☐ **4.** having the client discuss needs with the staff person assigned

13. The client with diagnosed borderline personality disorder tells the nurse, "You are the best nurse here. I can talk to you and you listen. You are the only one here that can help me." Which response by the nurse is **most** therapeutic?
- [ ] 1. "Thank you; you are a good person."
- [ ] 2. "All of the nurses here provide good care."
- [ ] 3. "Other clients have told me that too."
- [ ] 4. "Mary and Sam are good nurses too."

14. The nurse assesses a client to be at risk for self-mutilation and implements a safety contract with the client. Which client behavior indicates that the contract is working?
- [ ] 1. The client withdraws to his room when feeling overwhelmed.
- [ ] 2. The client notifies staff when anxiety is increasing.
- [ ] 3. The client suppresses his feelings when angry.
- [ ] 4. The client displaces his feelings onto the healthcare provider (HCP).

15. The client diagnosed with borderline personality disorder who is to be discharged soon threatens to "do something" to herself if discharged. The nurse should **first**:
- [ ] 1. request that the client's discharge be canceled.
- [ ] 2. ignore the client's statement because it is a sign of manipulation.
- [ ] 3. ask a family member to stay with the client at home temporarily.
- [ ] 4. discuss the meaning of the client's statement with her.

16. A 19-year-old client is admitted to a psychiatric unit with a diagnosis of alcohol abuse and personality disorder. The client's mother states, "He is always in trouble, just like when he was a boy. Now he is just a bigger prankster and out of control." In view of the client's history, which intervention is **most** important initially?
- [ ] 1. letting the client know the staff has the authority to subdue him if he gets unruly
- [ ] 2. keeping the client isolated from other clients until he is better known by the staff
- [ ] 3. emphasizing to the client that he will have to pay for any damage he causes
- [ ] 4. closely observing the client's behavior to establish a baseline pattern of functioning

17. The client tells the nurse at the outpatient clinic that she does not need to attend groups because she is "not a regular like these other people here." The nurse should respond to the client by saying:
- [ ] 1. "Because you are not a regular client, sit in the hall when the others are in group."
- [ ] 2. "Your family wants you to attend, and they will be very disappointed if you do not."
- [ ] 3. "I will have to mark you absent from the clinic today and speak to the healthcare provider (HCP) about it."
- [ ] 4. "You say you are not a regular here, but you are experiencing what others are experiencing."

18. The client who has a history of angry outbursts when frustrated begins to curse at the nurse during an appointment after being informed that she will have to wait to have her medication refilled. Which response by the nurse is **most** appropriate?
- [ ] 1. "You are being very childish."
- [ ] 2. "I am sorry if you cannot wait."
- [ ] 3. "I will not continue to talk with you if you curse."
- [ ] 4. "Come back tomorrow and your medication will be ready."

19. Which behavior indicates to the nurse that the client diagnosed with avoidant personality disorder is improving?
- [ ] 1. interacting with two other clients
- [ ] 2. listening to music with headphones
- [ ] 3. sitting at a table and painting
- [ ] 4. talking on the telephone

20. One evening, the client takes the nurse aside and whispers, "Do not tell anybody, but I am going to call in a bomb threat to this hospital tonight." Which action is the **priority**?
- [ ] 1. warning the client that his telephone privileges will be taken away if he abuses them
- [ ] 2. offering to disregard the client's plan if he does not go through with it
- [ ] 3. notifying the proper authorities after saying nothing until the client has actually completed the call
- [ ] 4. explaining to the client that this information will have to be shared immediately with the staff and the healthcare provider (HCP)

21. When teaching an unlicensed assistive personnel (UAP) new to the unit about the principles for the care of a client diagnosed with a personality disorder, the nurse should explain that:
- [ ] 1. the clients are accepted, although their behavior may not be.
- [ ] 2. the clients need limits on their behavior.
- [ ] 3. the staff members are the primary ones left to care about these clients.
- [ ] 4. the staff should use minimal humor when working with these clients.

22. The nurse is talking with a client who has been diagnosed with antisocial personality disorder about how to socialize during activities without being seductive. The nurse should focus the discussion on which area?
- ☐ 1. explaining the negative reactions of others toward his behavior
- ☐ 2. suggesting he apologize to others for his behavior
- ☐ 3. asking him to explain the reasons for his seductive behavior
- ☐ 4. discussing his relationship with his mother

23. Which approach is **most** appropriate to use with a client diagnosed with a narcissistic personality disorder when discrepancies exist between what the client states and what actually exists?
- ☐ 1. limit setting
- ☐ 2. supportive confrontation
- ☐ 3. consistency
- ☐ 4. rationalization

24. The client with histrionic personality disorder is melodramatic and responds to others and situations in an exaggerated manner. The nurse should recommend which activity for this client?
- ☐ 1. party planning
- ☐ 2. music group
- ☐ 3. cooking class
- ☐ 4. role-playing

The Client with an Alcohol-Related Disorder

25. A client has been diagnosed with dementia related to chronic and heavy alcohol consumption. In a family meeting with the client, discharge plans are being discussed. Which points should the nurse share with the family and client? Select all that apply.
- ☐ 1. Even after all alcohol has been removed from the home, clients frequently find ways to get more.
- ☐ 2. Without continued alcohol intake, the client will gradually get better.
- ☐ 3. With the memory loss, answer the client's question once, and then ignore that question when asked again.
- ☐ 4. Safety alarms on the doors will help to keep the client from wandering off.
- ☐ 5. As the need for supervision increases, it may be necessary for the client to be placed in an extended care facility.

26. In an outpatient addiction group, a recovering client said that before her treatment, her husband drank on social occasions. "Now he drinks at home, from the time he comes home from work and drinks until he goes to bed. He says that he does not like me anymore and that I expect him to do more work on the house and yard. I use to ignore that stuff. I do not know what to do." In which order of priority from first to last would the nurse make the comments? All options must be used.

1. "What do you think you could do to have your husband come in for an evaluation?"

2. "I hear how confused and frustrated you are."

3. "It can happen that as one person sobers up, the spouse deteriorates."

4. "What have you tried to do about your husband's behaviors?"

27. For the client who has difficulty falling asleep at night because of withdrawal symptoms from alcohol, which are abating, which nursing intervention is likely to be **most** effective?
- ☐ 1. inviting the client to play a board game with the nurse
- ☐ 2. allowing the client to sit in the community room until the client feels sleepy
- ☐ 3. advising the client to take multiple short naps during the day until symptoms improve
- ☐ 4. teaching the client relaxation exercises to use before bedtime

28. Which symptoms are expected indications that a client has alcohol withdrawal delirium? Select all that apply.
- ☐ 1. tachycardia
- ☐ 2. tachypnea
- ☐ 3. dry, flushed skin
- ☐ 4. thirst
- ☐ 5. hypertension
- ☐ 6. abdominal cramping

29. A client known to have alcohol dependence is admitted to the emergency department with a temperature of 99°F (37.2°C), a pulse of 110 beats/min, respirations of 26 breaths/min, and blood pressure of 150/98 mm Hg. The blood alcohol level is 0.25%. Now, the client is becoming belligerent and uncooperative. In which order, from first to last, should the nursing and medical prescriptions be implemented? All options must be used.

1. Administer lorazepam 2 mg IM.

2. Draw blood for a magnesium level.

3. Take vital signs every 15 minutes.

4. Place the client in a quiet room with dimmed lights.

30. A client has been admitted to the emergency department with alcohol withdrawal delirium. The nurse is assessing the client for signs of withdrawal. At 0900 hours on 10/25, the nurse notes that the client is confused. Vital signs are T = 99°F (37.2°C), P = 50, R = 10, and BP = 100/60. The nurse compares these findings to the nurses' progress notes from admission 24 hours ago (see exhibit). What should the nurse do **first**?
☐ 1. Contact the healthcare provider (HCP).
☐ 2. Increase the rate of the IV infusion.
☐ 3. Attempt to arouse the client.
☐ 4. Administer magnesium sulfate.

Progress Notes

Date	Time	Progress Notes
10/24	2100	T = 99° F (37.2°C); P = 110; R = 18; BP = 140/90; Client has IV D₅W keep open rate started; diazepam administered as prescribed. Client oriented × 3.
10/25	0100	T = 99.2° F (37.3°C); P = 90; R = 14; BP = 130/80; Client resting.
10/25	0500	T = 99° F (37.2°C); P = 70; R = 14; BP = 126/80; Client oriented × 3.

31. An intoxicated client is admitted to the hospital for alcohol withdrawal. What should the nurse do to help the client become sober?
☐ 1. Give the client black coffee to drink.
☐ 2. Walk the client around the unit.
☐ 3. Have the client take a cold shower.
☐ 4. Provide the client with a quiet room to sleep in.

32. The client is admitted to the hospital for alcohol detoxification. Which interventions should the nurse use? Select all that apply.
☐ 1. taking vital signs
☐ 2. monitoring intake and output
☐ 3. placing the client in restraints as a safety measure
☐ 4. reinforcing reality if the client is disoriented or hallucinating
☐ 5. explaining to the client that the symptoms of withdrawal are temporary

33. The nurse is assessing a client who has fallen twice in the last 2 days. The client has been diagnosed with delirium tremens (DTs) following withdrawal from alcohol use. The nurse should further evaluate the client for which complications? Select all that apply.
☐ 1. disorientation
☐ 2. paralysis
☐ 3. elevated temperature
☐ 4. diaphoresis
☐ 5. visual or auditory hallucinations

34. A client was discharged from an alcohol rehabilitation program on clonazepam 0.5 mg three times a day. Several months later, he reports having insomnia, shakiness, sweating, and one seizure. The nurse should **first** ask the client if he:
☐ 1. has been drinking alcohol with the clonazepam.
☐ 2. has developed tolerance to the clonazepam and needs to increase the dose.
☐ 3. has stopped taking the clonazepam suddenly.
☐ 4. has increased his clonazepam without consulting his healthcare provider (HCP).

35. A client is entering the chemical dependency unit for treatment of alcohol dependency. Which of the client's possessions should the nurse place in a locked area?
☐ 1. toothpaste
☐ 2. dental floss
☐ 3. shaving cream
☐ 4. antiseptic mouthwash

36. A client is entering rehabilitation for alcohol dependency as an alternative to going to jail for multiple DUIs (driving under the influence). While obtaining the client's history, the nurse asks about the amount of alcohol he consumes daily. He responds, "I just have a few drinks with the guys after work." Which response by the nurse is **most** therapeutic?

- ☐ **1.** "That is what all the clients here say at first."
- ☐ **2.** "Then you should have had a designated driver for yourself."
- ☐ **3.** "I guess you just cannot handle a few drinks."
- ☐ **4.** "You say you have a few drinks, but you have multiple arrests."

37. While admitting a client to the alcohol treatment program, the nurse asks the client how long she has been drinking, how much she has been drinking, and when she had her last drink. The client replies that she has been drinking about a liter of vodka a day for the past week and her last drink was about an hour ago. This information helps the nurse to determine which factor?

- ☐ **1.** the severity of the disease
- ☐ **2.** the severity of withdrawal symptoms
- ☐ **3.** the possibility of alcoholic hallucinosis
- ☐ **4.** the occurrence of delirium tremens

38. A client who is experiencing alcohol withdrawal exhibits tremors, diaphoresis, and hyperactivity. Blood pressure is 190/87 mm Hg and pulse is 92 bpm. Which medication should the nurse expect to administer?

- ☐ **1.** haloperidol
- ☐ **2.** lorazepam
- ☐ **3.** benztropine
- ☐ **4.** naloxone

39. Which assessment provides the **best** information about the client's physiologic response and the effectiveness of the medication prescribed specifically for alcohol withdrawal?

- ☐ **1.** nutritional status
- ☐ **2.** evidence of tremors
- ☐ **3.** vital signs
- ☐ **4.** sleep pattern

40. A client who had been drinking heavily over the weekend could not remember specific events of where he had been or what he had done. The nurse interprets this information as indicating that the client experienced which condition?

- ☐ **1.** blackout
- ☐ **2.** hangover
- ☐ **3.** tolerance
- ☐ **4.** delirium tremens

41. A client is entering the alcohol treatment program for the fourth time in 5 years. Which statement by the nurse will be **most** helpful to the client?

- ☐ **1.** "I hope you are serious about maintaining your sobriety this time."
- ☐ **2.** "I am Maria, a nurse here. I do not know you from past attempts, but you will get it right this time."
- ☐ **3.** "I know someone who was successful after the fifth program."
- ☐ **4.** "I am Maria, a nurse in the program. The staff and I will help you through the program."

42. The wife of a client with alcohol dependency tells the nurse, "I am tired of making excuses for him to his boss and coworkers when he cannot make it into work. I believe him every time he says he is going to quit." The nurse recognizes the wife's statement as indicating which behavior?

- ☐ **1.** helpfulness
- ☐ **2.** self-defeat
- ☐ **3.** enabling
- ☐ **4.** masochism

43. Which statement by the nurse participating in a group confrontation of a coworker is **most** helpful in reducing the coworker's denial about alcohol being a problem?

- ☐ **1.** "Your behavior is unprofessional."
- ☐ **2.** "As a nurse, you should have sought help earlier."
- ☐ **3.** "Nurses are the worst when it comes to asking for help."
- ☐ **4.** "You have alcohol on your breath."

44. A nurse working in an alcohol rehabilitation program is teaching staff how to give clients constructive feedback. Which statement given as an example illustrates that the staff member understands the nurse's teaching regarding the use of constructive feedback?

- ☐ **1.** "I think you are a real con artist."
- ☐ **2.** "You are dominating the conversation."
- ☐ **3.** "You interrupted Terry twice in 4 minutes."
- ☐ **4.** "You do not give anyone a chance to finish talking."

45. A client ashamedly tells the nurse that he hit his wife while intoxicated and asks the nurse if his wife will ever forgive him. The nurse should reply to the client by saying:

- ☐ **1.** "Perhaps you could ask her and find out."
- ☐ **2.** "That is something you can explore in family therapy."
- ☐ **3.** "It would depend on how much she really cares for you."
- ☐ **4.** "You seem to have some feelings about hitting your wife."

46. While meeting with the nurse, a client's wife states, "I do not know what else to do to make him stop drinking." The nurse should refer the wife to which organization?
☐ **1.** Alateen
☐ **2.** Al-Anon
☐ **3.** employee assistance program
☐ **4.** Alcoholics Anonymous

47. Which nursing action is contraindicated for the client who is experiencing severe symptoms of alcohol withdrawal?
☐ **1.** helping the client walk
☐ **2.** monitoring intake and output
☐ **3.** assessing vital signs
☐ **4.** using short, concrete statements

48. Which client statement indicates to the nurse that the client needs further teaching about disulfiram?
☐ **1.** "I can drink one or two beers and not get sick while on disulfiram."
☐ **2.** "I can take disulfiram at bedtime if it makes me sleepy."
☐ **3.** "A metallic or garlic taste in my mouth is normal when starting on disulfiram."
☐ **4.** "I will read the labels on cough syrup and mouthwash for possible alcohol content."

49. While receiving disulfiram therapy, the client becomes nauseated and vomits severely. Which question should the nurse ask **first**?
☐ **1.** "How long have you been taking disulfiram?"
☐ **2.** "Do you feel like you have the flu?"
☐ **3.** "How much alcohol did you drink today?"
☐ **4.** "Have you eaten any foods cooked in wine?"

50. The expected outcome for using thiamine for a client being treated for an alcohol addiction is to:
☐ **1.** prevent the development of Wernicke's encephalopathy.
☐ **2.** decrease client's withdrawal symptoms.
☐ **3.** aid the client in regaining strength sooner.
☐ **4.** promote elimination of alcohol from the body faster.

51. Which client statement indicates an understanding of the risk of alcohol relapse?
☐ **1.** "I know I can stay dry if my wife keeps alcohol out of the house."
☐ **2.** "Stopping Alcoholics Anonymous (AA) and not expressing feelings can lead to relapse."
☐ **3.** "I will have my sponsor at AA keep the list of symptoms for me."
☐ **4.** "If someone tells me I am about to relapse, I will be sure to do something about it."

52. The client sees no connection between her liver disorder and her alcohol intake. She believes that she drinks very little and that her family is making something out of nothing. The nurse interprets these behaviors as indicative of the client's use of which defense mechanisms?
☐ **1.** denial
☐ **2.** displacement
☐ **3.** rationalization
☐ **4.** reaction formation

53. Which food should the nurse eliminate from the diet of a client in alcohol withdrawal?
☐ **1.** milk
☐ **2.** regular coffee
☐ **3.** orange juice
☐ **4.** eggs

54. A client with alcohol dependency has peripheral neuropathy. The nurse should develop a teaching plan that emphasizes:
☐ **1.** washing and drying the feet daily.
☐ **2.** massaging the feet with lotion.
☐ **3.** trimming the toenails carefully.
☐ **4.** avoiding use of an electric blanket.

55. A client is experiencing alcohol withdrawal. He wakes up and screams "There is something crawling under my skin. Help me." What should the nurse do in order of priority from first to last? All options must be used.

1. Remind the client that he is having withdrawal symptoms and that these will be treated.

2. Administer a dose of lorazepam depending on the severity of the withdrawal symptoms.

3. Assess the client for other withdrawal symptoms.

4. Take the client's vital signs.

5. Chart the details of the episode in the medical record.

56. Which measure should the nurse include in the plan of care for a client with alcohol withdrawal delirium?
☐ 1. using restraints continuously
☐ 2. touching the client before saying anything
☐ 3. remaining with the client when she is confused or disoriented
☐ 4. informing the client about alcohol treatment programs

57. What is an accurate response when a client asks the nurse about requirements to become a member of Alcoholics Anonymous (AA)?
☐ 1. "You must be sober for at least a month before joining."
☐ 2. "AA is open to anyone who wants sobriety."
☐ 3. "The members will interview you and decide if you can join the group."
☐ 4. "AA requires daily attendance at meetings."

58. A client is to be discharged from an alcohol rehabilitation program. What should the nurse emphasize in the discharge plan as a **priority**?
☐ 1. supportive friends
☐ 2. a list of goals
☐ 3. returning to work
☐ 4. follow-up care

59. The client is to be discharged from the hospital after a safe, medically supervised withdrawal from alcohol. Which outcomes indicate client readiness for an outpatient alcohol treatment program? Select all that apply.
☐ 1. The client states the need to cut down on his alcohol intake.
☐ 2. The client verbalizes the damaging effects of alcohol on his body.
☐ 3. The client plans to attend Alcoholics Anonymous meetings.
☐ 4. The client takes naltrexone daily.
☐ 5. The client says he is indestructible.

60. A client diagnosed with major depression and substance dependence is being admitted to the concurrent disorder treatment unit. In explaining the focus of this program, the nurse should tell what information to the client?
☐ 1. The addiction will be treated first, then the depression.
☐ 2. The depression will be treated first, then the addiction.
☐ 3. There will be simultaneous treatment of the addiction and depression.
☐ 4. As the addiction is treated, the depression will clear up on its own.

61. While caring for a client who has a bipolar disorder and alcohol dependency, which area is the **priority** for daily assessment?
☐ 1. sleep pattern
☐ 2. mental status
☐ 3. eating habits
☐ 4. self-care ability

62. The nurse is caring for a client admitted to the emergency department after being found lying on the bathroom floor with several empty pill bottles around her. While waiting for a psychiatric consult, the nurse discovers that the client's boyfriend has recently broken up with her. Which response is **most** likely to build and maintain a therapeutic relationship within the emergency department?
☐ 1. "You will have other boyfriends."
☐ 2. "I know that this hurts."
☐ 3. "Why did you try to kill yourself?"
☐ 4. "What can I do to help while you are here?"

The Client with Disorders Related to Other Addictive Substances

63. A client is being admitted to the hospital following an inadvertent overdose with oxycodone. He reveals that he has chronic back pain that resulted from an injury on a construction site. He states, "I know I took too much oxycodone at once, but I cannot live with this pain without them. You cannot take them away from me." Which response by the nurse is **most** appropriate?
☐ 1. "Once you are tapered off the oxycodone, you will find that nonaddictive pain medicines will be enough to control your pain."
☐ 2. "You are going to be switched from the oxycodone to methadone for long-term pain management."
☐ 3. "The oxycodone will be stopped tomorrow, but you will have lorazepam to help you with the withdrawal symptoms."
☐ 4. "Your pain will be controlled by tapering doses of oxycodone, with other pain management strategies and medicines."

64. A school nurse is planning a program for parents on "Drugs Commonly Abused by Teenagers." Which information should be included about inhalants? Select all that apply.
☐ 1. Monitor for paper bags and rags that may have been used for breathing inhalants.
☐ 2. Brain damage is unlikely with the use of inhalants.
☐ 3. Use of inhalants by teens is on the decline.
☐ 4. Deaths from inhalants occur from asphyxiation, suffocation, and aspiration of vomit.
☐ 5. Inhalants usually cause depression of the central nervous system.
☐ 6. The basic groups of inhalants are hydrocarbon solvents such as glue, aerosol propellants from spray cans, and anesthetics/gases.

65. The friend of a client brought to the emergency department states, "I guess she had some bad junk (heroin) today." The client is drowsy and verbally nonresponsive. Which finding is of **immediate** concern to the nurse?
- ☐ **1.** respiratory rate of 9 breaths/min
- ☐ **2.** urinary retention
- ☐ **3.** hypotension
- ☐ **4.** reduced pupil size

66. A client is brought to the emergency department by a friend who states, "He was using a lot of heroin until he ran out of money about 2 days ago." The nurse judges the client to be in opioid withdrawal if he exhibits which sign or symptom? Select all that apply.
- ☐ **1.** rhinorrhea
- ☐ **2.** diaphoresis
- ☐ **3.** piloerection
- ☐ **4.** synesthesia
- ☐ **5.** formication

67. An unconscious client in the emergency department is given IV naloxone due to an overdose of heroin. Which findings would indicate a therapeutic response to the naloxone? Select all that apply.
- ☐ **1.** decreased pulse rate
- ☐ **2.** warm moist skin
- ☐ **3.** dilated pupils
- ☐ **4.** increased respirations
- ☐ **5.** consciousness

68. Which findings should the nurse expect to assess for a client who is exhibiting late signs of heroin withdrawal?
- ☐ **1.** vomiting and diarrhea
- ☐ **2.** yawning and diaphoresis
- ☐ **3.** lacrimation and rhinorrhea
- ☐ **4.** restlessness and irritability

69. After administering naloxone, an opioid antagonist, the nurse should monitor the client carefully for which problem?
- ☐ **1.** cerebral edema
- ☐ **2.** kidney failure
- ☐ **3.** seizure activity
- ☐ **4.** respiratory depression

70. When teaching a client who is to receive methadone therapy for opioid addiction, the nurse should instruct the client that methadone is useful primarily for what reason?
- ☐ **1.** It is not an addictive substance.
- ☐ **2.** A maintenance dose is taken twice a day.
- ☐ **3.** The client will no longer be addicted to opioids.
- ☐ **4.** The client may work and live normally.

71. A client states to the nurse, "I am not going anymore to Narcotics Anonymous meetings. I felt out of place there." Which response by the nurse is **best**?
- ☐ **1.** "Try attending a meeting at a different location; you may feel more comfortable there."
- ☐ **2.** "Maybe it just was not a good day for you. Everybody has bad days now and then."
- ☐ **3.** "Perhaps you were not paying close enough attention to what they were saying."
- ☐ **4.** "Sometimes the meetings can seem like a waste of time, but you need to attend to stay clean."

72. Which outcome should the nurse use as the **best** measure to determine a client's progress in rehabilitation?
- ☐ **1.** The kinds of friends he makes.
- ☐ **2.** The number of drug-free days he has.
- ☐ **3.** The way he gets along with his parents.
- ☐ **4.** The amount of responsibility his job entails.

73. Which finding would lead the nurse to suspect that a client is addicted to heroin?
- ☐ **1.** hilarity
- ☐ **2.** aggression
- ☐ **3.** labile mood
- ☐ **4.** hypoactivity

74. A client brought by ambulance to the emergency department after taking an overdose of barbiturates is comatose. The nurse should assess the client for:
- ☐ **1.** kidney failure.
- ☐ **2.** cerebrovascular accident.
- ☐ **3.** status epilepticus.
- ☐ **4.** respiratory failure.

75. The client's spouse reports that the client has been taking about eight "reds" or 800 mg of secobarbital daily, besides drinking more alcohol than usual. The spouse asks anxiously, "Do you think she will live?" Which response by the nurse is **most** appropriate?
- ☐ **1.** "We can only wait and see. It is too soon to tell."
- ☐ **2.** "This must be quite a shock. How long have you been married?"
- ☐ **3.** "She is very ill and may not live. Some do not pull through."
- ☐ **4.** "Her condition is serious. You sound very worried about her."

76. Before his hospitalization, a client needed increasingly larger doses of barbiturates to achieve the same euphoric effect he initially realized from their use. From this information, the nurse develops a plan of care that takes into account that the client is likely suffering from what problem?
- ☐ **1.** tolerance
- ☐ **2.** addiction
- ☐ **3.** abuse
- ☐ **4.** dependence

77. Which statement by the nurse is **most** appropriate when addressing a client with a barbiturate overdose who awakens in a confused state and exhibits stable vital signs?
☐ 1. "I am here to help you beat your drug habit. But it is you who will need to work hard."
☐ 2. "It is time to get straight and stay clean and put an end to your torture."
☐ 3. "I am glad you pulled through; it was touch and go with you for a while."
☐ 4. "You are in the hospital because of a drug problem; I am one of the nurses who will help you."

78. A client states that her "life has gone down the tubes" since her divorce 6 months ago. Then, after she lost her job and apartment, she took an overdose of barbiturates so she "could go to sleep and never wake up." Which statement by the nurse should be made **first**?
☐ 1. "It seems as if your self-esteem has been affected by all your losses."
☐ 2. "I know you took an overdose of barbiturates. Are you thinking of suicide now?"
☐ 3. "Helplessness is common after losing a job. Are you having trouble making decisions?"
☐ 4. "You sound hopeless about the future since your divorce."

79. A client who has experienced the loss of her husband through divorce, the loss of her job and apartment, and the development of drug dependency is suffering situational low self-esteem. Which outcome is **most** appropriate initially?
☐ 1. The client will discuss her feelings related to her losses.
☐ 2. The client will identify two positive qualities.
☐ 3. The client will explore her strengths.
☐ 4. The client will prioritize problems.

80. The nurse notices that a client recovering from a barbiturate overdose spends most of his time with other young adults who have substance-related problems. This group of clients is a dominant force on the unit, keeping the nondrug users entertained with stories of their "highs." Which method is **best** to use when dealing with this problem?
☐ 1. providing additional recreation
☐ 2. breaking up drug-oriented discussions
☐ 3. speaking with the clients individually about their behavior
☐ 4. discussing the behavior at the daily community meeting

81. A client recovering from a drug overdose is interacting with the nurse and recounting her exploits at numerous parties she has attended. Which action is **most** therapeutic?
☐ 1. allowing the client to continue with her stories
☐ 2. telling the client you've heard the stories before
☐ 3. questioning the client further about her exploits
☐ 4. directing the conversation to realistic concerns

82. The nurse is speaking to a sixth grade class about drugs. A student states, "I know someone who smokes marijuana, and he says it is safe." The nurse should tell the student:
☐ 1. "Marijuana is not safe, and it is illegal in many places."
☐ 2. "Do you really believe him?"
☐ 3. "That drug impairs short-term memory and judgment and distorts perception."
☐ 4. "Marijuana usage can lead to using other chemicals."

83. When developing a teaching plan for a group of middle school children about the drug 3,4-methylenedioxymethamphetamine (Ecstasy), what information should the nurse expect to include? Select all that apply.
☐ 1. Using Ecstasy is similar to using speed.
☐ 2. Ecstasy is used at all-night parties.
☐ 3. Teeth grinding is seen with cocaine, not Ecstasy use.
☐ 4. It can cause death.
☐ 5. It reduces self-consciousness.

84. A young client is being admitted to the psychiatric unit after her obstetrician's staff suspected she was experiencing a postpartum psychosis. Her husband said she was doing fine for 2 weeks after the birth of the baby, except for pain from the C-section and trouble sleeping. These symptoms subsided over the next 4 weeks. Three days ago, however, the client started having anxiety, irritability, vomiting, diarrhea, and delirium, resulting in her inability to care for the baby. The husband says, "I saw that my bottles of alprazolam and oxycodone were empty even though I have not been taking them." What should the nurse do in order of priority from first to last? All options must be used.

| 1. Call the healthcare provider (HCP) for prescriptions for appropriate treatment for opiate and benzodiazepine withdrawal. |

| 2. Immediately place the client on withdrawal precautions. |

| 3. Confirm with the client that she has in fact been using her husband's medications. |

| 4. Assess the client for prior and current use of any other substances. |

| |

| |

| |

| |

85. A 68-year-old client is admitted to the addiction unit after treatment in the emergency department for an overdose of oxycodone. Her son calls the unit and expresses intense anger that his mother is being treated as a "common street addict." He says she has severe back pain and was given that prescription by her healthcare provider (HCP). "She just accidentally took a few too many pills last night." Which reply by the nurse is **most** therapeutic?

☐ 1. "I understand that your mother may not have intentionally taken too many pills. This medication can cause one to forget how many have been taken."

☐ 2. "It may be appropriate for your mother to be referred to a pain management program."

☐ 3. "Unfortunately, it is fairly common for clients with pain to increase their use of pain pills over time."

☐ 4. "I can hear how upset you are. You sound very concerned about your mother."

86. A client is being admitted to the addiction unit for a confirmed and long-term addiction to alprazolam. She continues to strongly deny her addiction, stating she was prescribed the alprazolam to control her "panic attacks." Which procedures would be the **most** important during the admission process? Select all that apply.

☐ 1. Assess the client for suicide, escape, and aggression risks.

☐ 2. With the client present, search the client's clothes and belongings for contraband and restricted items.

☐ 3. Initiate withdrawal precautions.

☐ 4. Explain the unit routine and types of groups.

☐ 5. Obtain a urine specimen for a urine drug screen.

87. A client is returning to the healthcare provider's (HCP's) office for follow-up on his diagnosis of coronary artery disease. After all the appropriate exams and assessments are completed, the nurse asks the client about how well he is sleeping. The client states, "Oh, that is not a problem anymore. I take a couple of my wife's diazepam and sleep like a baby." Which information should the nurse obtain? Select all that apply.

☐ 1. the reason the client's wife is taking diazepam

☐ 2. the dose of the diazepam he is taking and how long he has been taking it

☐ 3. exactly how much diazepam he takes at night and during the day

☐ 4. whether he intends to stop the diazepam use

☐ 5. what was interfering with his sleep prior to starting the diazepam

88. A client is admitted to the emergency department having just used cocaine. The nurse should assess this client for which factors? Select all that apply.

☐ 1. mood swings

☐ 2. feeling of euphoria

☐ 3. constricted pupils

☐ 4. increased blood pressure

☐ 5. tachycardia

89. A client who chronically snorts cocaine is brought to the emergency department due to a cocaine overdose. The client is experiencing delusions, hallucinations, mild respiratory distress, and mild tachycardia initially. What should the nurse do? Select all that apply.

☐ 1. induce vomiting

☐ 2. place seizure pads on the bed

☐ 3. administer PRN haloperidol as prescribed

☐ 4. monitor for respiratory acidosis

☐ 5. encourage deep breathing

☐ 6. monitor for metabolic acidosis

90. A client walks into the clinic and tells the nurse she has run out of money for crack, has crashed, and wants something to help her feel better. Which factor is **most** important for the nurse to assess?

☐ 1. suspiciousness

☐ 2. loss of appetite

☐ 3. drug craving

☐ 4. suicidal ideation

91. A client in the emergency department is diagnosed as having amphetamine psychosis. What should the nurse do in order of priority from first to last? All options must be used.

1. Transfer the client to the psychiatric unit.

2. Monitor cardiac and respiratory status.

3. Place seizure pads on the bed.

4. Administer IM haloperidol as prescribed.

92. A client has been taking increased amounts of alprazolam for about 6 months for anxiety. She asks the nurse how she can "get off the alprazolam." What is the nurse's **best** response?
- ☐ 1. "There will be an immediate discontinuation of the alprazolam, and haloperidol will be available if needed."
- ☐ 2. "Instead of alprazolam, you will take lorazepam in decreasing doses and frequency over a period of 3 to 4 days."
- ☐ 3. "The alprazolam will be tapered down over a period of 48 hours."
- ☐ 4. "Alprazolam will be available on an as-needed basis for 4 to 5 days."

93. The client is fidgeting and has trouble sitting still. He has difficulty concentrating and is tangential. Which intervention should help decrease this client's level of anxiety? Select all that apply.
- ☐ 1. refocusing attention
- ☐ 2. allowing ventilation
- ☐ 3. suggesting a time-out
- ☐ 4. giving intramuscular medication
- ☐ 5. assisting with problem solving

94. When caring for a client who has overdosed on phencyclidine (PCP), the nurse should be especially cautious about which client behavior?
- ☐ 1. visual hallucinations
- ☐ 2. violent behavior
- ☐ 3. bizarre behavior
- ☐ 4. loud screaming

95. Which liquid should the nurse administer to a client who is intoxicated on phencyclidine (PCP) to hasten excretion of the chemical?
- ☐ 1. water
- ☐ 2. milk
- ☐ 3. cranberry juice
- ☐ 4. grape juice

96. When assessing a client with possible alcohol poisoning, the nurse should investigate the client's use of which substance while drinking alcohol?
- ☐ 1. marijuana
- ☐ 2. lysergic acid diethylamide
- ☐ 3. peyote
- ☐ 4. psilocybin

97. A client with a cocaine dependency is irritable, anxious, highly sensitive to stimuli, and over reactive to clients and staff on the unit. Which action is **most** therapeutic for this client?
- ☐ 1. secluding and restraining the client as needed
- ☐ 2. telling the client to stay in his room until he can control himself
- ☐ 3. providing the client with frequent "time-outs"
- ☐ 4. confronting the client about his behaviors

98. A client with symptoms of amphetamine psychosis that are improving is anxious and still experiencing some delusions. When developing the client's plan of care, which measure should the nurse include?
- ☐ 1. Assign the client to a group meeting about the physiologic effects of drugs.
- ☐ 2. Advise the client to watch television.
- ☐ 3. Wait for the client to approach the nurse.
- ☐ 4. Invite the client to play a game of ping-pong with the nurse.

99. In consultation with his outpatient psychiatrist, a client is admitted for detoxification from methadone. He states, "I got addicted to morphine for my chronic knee pain. Methadone worked for a long time. Since I had my knee replacement surgery 3 months ago and physical therapy, I do not think I need methadone anymore." It is important to discuss which information with this client? Select all that apply.
- ☐ 1. "Detoxification will likely occur with slowly decreasing doses of methadone."
- ☐ 2. "Oxycodone will be available if needed for breakthrough pain."
- ☐ 3. "You will be monitored closely for withdrawal symptoms and treated as needed."
- ☐ 4. "Physical therapy and nonchemical pain management techniques can be prescribed if needed."
- ☐ 5. "If you have knee stiffness or pain, it is likely to be managed by nonnarcotic pain medicines."

100. A client approaches the medication nurse and states, "I cannot believe you are NOT helping me with my cravings for my fentanyl patches! When I got off alcohol 2 years ago, they gave me naltrexone for my cravings, and it really helped. I cannot stand the cravings and back pain anymore, and I am getting angry." Which responses by the nurse would be helpful for this client? Select all that apply.
- ☐ 1. "Naltrexone does help decrease the cravings for alcohol."
- ☐ 2. "Naltrexone can interfere with opiate cravings in some clients."
- ☐ 3. "Cravings are hard to deal with, especially when you are in pain too."
- ☐ 4. "I hear your frustration about how your detoxification is going."
- ☐ 5. "I am positive naltrexone can help with your cravings for fentanyl."
- ☐ 6. "I can ask your healthcare provider (HCP) if he thinks naltrexone might help you."

The Client with Anxiety Disorders and Anxiety-Related Disorders

101. A 17-year-old female client who has been treated for an anxiety disorder since middle school with behavioral treatment and as-needed (PRN) anxiety medication is preparing to go to college. The parents are concerned that she will experience an exacerbation of symptoms if she attends college out of town and want their daughter to attend the local community college and live at home. The girl believes she can handle the challenge of leaving home for college. How should the nurse in the outpatient clinic respond to the family's concerns?
☐ 1. "Your parents have a point; transitions have been hard for you in the past."
☐ 2. "There are many pros and cons here that we all need to discuss together."
☐ 3. "Every high school graduate deserves the chance to take on new challenges."
☐ 4. "It may be premature for you to think of college at this point in time."

102. A 16-year-old boy who is academically gifted is about to graduate from high school early since he has completed all courses needed to earn a diploma. Within the last 3 months, he has begun to experience panic attacks that have forced him to leave classes early and occasionally miss a day of school. He is concerned that these attacks may hinder his ability to pursue a college degree. What would be the **best** response by the school nurse who has been helping him deal with his panic attacks?
☐ 1. "It is natural to be worried about going into a new environment. I am sure with your abilities you will do well once you get settled."
☐ 2. "You are putting too much pressure on yourself. You just need to relax more, and things will be alright."
☐ 3. "It might be best for you to postpone going to college. You need to get these panic attacks controlled first."
☐ 4. "It sounds like you have real concern about transitioning to college. I can refer you to a healthcare provider (HCP) for assessment and treatment."

103. A client has been diagnosed with posttraumatic stress disorder (PTSD) because he experienced childhood sexual abuse (CSA) by his babysitter and her boyfriend from ages 4 to 10. He is admitted for the second time after physically assaulting a woman he said was a prostitute. "She is no better than my babysitter and deserves to be dead. I would like to kill the sitter too." With the knowledge of PTSD and CSA, which nursing interventions should be implemented at admission? Select all that apply.
☐ 1. Institute precautions for suicide, assault, and escape.
☐ 2. Ask him to sign a no-harm contract.
☐ 3. Provide safe outlets for his anger and rage.
☐ 4. Encourage him to express his attitude toward prostitutes during unit group sessions.
☐ 5. In one-to-one staff talks, encourage him to safely verbalize his anger toward his babysitter and her boyfriend.

104. A client is taking diazepam while establishing a therapeutic dose of antidepressants for generalized anxiety disorder. Which instruction should the nurse give to this client? Select all that apply.
☐ 1. to consult with his healthcare provider (HCP) before he stops taking the drug
☐ 2. to avoid eating cheese and other tyramine-rich foods
☐ 3. to take the medication on an empty stomach
☐ 4. not to use alcohol while taking the drug
☐ 5. to stop taking the drug if he experiences swelling of the lips and face and difficulty breathing

105. An adult client diagnosed with anxiety disorder becomes anxious when she touches fruits and vegetables. What should the nurse do?
☐ 1. Instruct the woman to avoid touching these foods.
☐ 2. Ask the woman why she becomes anxious in these situations.
☐ 3. Assist the woman to make a plan for her family to do the food shopping and preparation.
☐ 4. Teach the woman to use cognitive-behavioral approaches to manage her anxiety.

106. A client who is pacing and wringing his hands states, "I just need to walk" when questioned by the nurse about what he is feeling. Which response by the nurse is **most** therapeutic?
☐ 1. "You need to sit down and relax."
☐ 2. "Are you feeling anxious?"
☐ 3. "Is something bothering you?"
☐ 4. "You must be experiencing a problem now."

107. A client brought to the emergency department is perspiring profusely, breathing rapidly, and having dizziness and palpitations. Problems of a cardiovascular nature are ruled out, and the client's diagnosis is tentatively listed as a panic attack. After the symptoms pass, the client states, "I thought I was going to die." Which is the nurse's **best** response?
☐ 1. "It was very frightening for you."
☐ 2. "We would not have let you die."
☐ 3. "I would have felt the same way."
☐ 4. "But you are okay now."

108. A client commonly jumps when spoken to and reports feeling uneasy. The client says, "It is as though something bad is going to happen." In which order, from first to last, should the nursing actions be done? All options must be used.

1. Teach problem-solving strategies.

2. Ask the client to deep breathe for 2 minutes.

3. Discuss the client's feelings in more depth.

4. Reduce environmental stimuli.

109. A client with panic disorder is taking alprazolam 1 mg PO three times daily. The nurse understands that this medication is effective in blocking the symptoms of panic because of its specific action on which neurotransmitters?
☐ 1. gamma-aminobutyrate
☐ 2. serotonin
☐ 3. dopamine
☐ 4. norepinephrine

110. A client is diagnosed with generalized anxiety disorder (GAD) and given a prescription for venlafaxine. Which information should the nurse include in a teaching plan for this client? Select all that apply.
☐ 1. various strategies for reducing anxiety
☐ 2. the benefits and mechanisms of actions of venlafaxine in treating GAD
☐ 3. how venlafaxine will eliminate his anxiety at home and work
☐ 4. the management of the common side effects of venlafaxine
☐ 5. substituting adaptive coping strategies for maladaptive ones
☐ 6. the positive effects of venlafaxine being evident in 4 to 5 days

111. While a client is taking alprazolam, which food should the nurse instruct the client to avoid?
☐ 1. chocolate
☐ 2. cheese
☐ 3. alcohol
☐ 4. shellfish

112. Which statement by a client who has been taking buspirone as prescribed for 2 days indicates the need for further teaching?
☐ 1. "This medication will help my tight, aching muscles."
☐ 2. "I may not feel better for 7 to 10 days."
☐ 3. "The drug does not cause physical dependence."
☐ 4. "I can take the medication with food."

113. A week ago, a tornado destroyed the client's home and seriously injured her husband. The client has been walking around the hospital in a daze without any outward display of emotions. She tells the nurse that she feels like she is going crazy. Which intervention should the nurse use **first**?
☐ 1. Explain the effects of stress on the mind and body.
☐ 2. Reassure the client that her feelings are typical reactions to serious trauma.
☐ 3. Reassure the client that her symptoms are temporary.
☐ 4. Acknowledge the unfairness of the client's situation.

114. After being discharged from the hospital with acute stress disorder, a client is referred to the outpatient clinic for follow-up. What is **most** important for the client to use for continued alleviation of anxiety?

☐ 1. recognizing when she is feeling anxious
☐ 2. understanding reasons for her anxiety
☐ 3. using adaptive and palliative methods to reduce anxiety
☐ 4. describing the situations preceding her feelings of anxiety

115. A client with acute stress disorder states to the nurse, "I keep having horrible nightmares about the car accident that killed my daughter. I should not have taken her with me to the store." Which response by the nurse is **most** therapeutic?

☐ 1. "Do not keep torturing yourself with such horrible thoughts."
☐ 2. "Stop blaming yourself. It is only hurting you."
☐ 3. "Let us talk about something that is a bit more pleasant."
☐ 4. "The accident just happened and could not have been predicted."

116. The client, who is a veteran and has posttraumatic stress disorder, tells the nurse about the horror and mass destruction of war. He states, "I killed all of those people for nothing." Which response by the nurse is appropriate?

☐ 1. "You did what you had to do at that time."
☐ 2. "Maybe you did not kill as many people as you think."
☐ 3. "How many people did you kill?"
☐ 4. "War is a terrible thing."

117. A client with acute stress disorder has avoided feelings of anger toward her rapist and cannot verbally express them. The nurse suggests which activity to assist the client with expressing her feelings?

☐ 1. working on a puzzle
☐ 2. writing in a journal
☐ 3. meditating
☐ 4. listening to music

118. When developing the plan of care for a client with acute stress disorder who lost her sister in a boating accident, which intervention should the nurse initiate?

☐ 1. helping the client to evaluate her sister's behavior
☐ 2. telling the client to avoid details of the accident
☐ 3. facilitating progressive review of the accident and its consequences
☐ 4. postponing discussion of the accident until the client brings it up

119. A soldier on his second tour of duty was notified of the date that he will be redeployed. As this date approaches, he is showing signs of excess anxiety and irritability and inability to sleep at night because of nightmares of IED (improvised explosive devices) tragedies, all leading to poor work performance. His commanding officer refers him to the base hospital for an evaluation. What should the nurse do in order of priority from first to last? All options must be used.

1. Remind him that any feelings and problems he is having are typical in his current situation.

2. Ask him to talk about his upsetting experiences.

3. Remove any weapons and dangerous items he has in his possession.

4. Acknowledge any injustices/unfairness related to his experiences, and offer empathy and support.

120. A newly admitted 20-year-old client, diagnosed with posttraumatic stress disorder (PTSD), reluctantly reveals that she escaped from a cult 2 years ago. The client says, "Nobody will ever believe the horrible things the men did to me, and no one never stopped them." Which response is appropriate for the nurse to make?

☐ 1. "I will believe anything you tell me. You can trust me."
☐ 2. "I cannot understand why members did not protect you. It is not right."
☐ 3. "Tell me about the cult. I did not know there were any near here."
☐ 4. "It must be difficult to talk about what happened. I am willing to listen."

121. A 15-year-old client diagnosed with post-traumatic stress disorder (PTSD) is admitted to the unit after slicing both arms with a razor blade. He says, "Maybe my mother will listen to me now. She tells me I am just crazy when I say I am screwed up because my stepdad had sex with me for years." What should the nurse do in order of priority from first to last? All options must be used.

1. Ask the client about the stepdad possibly abusing younger children in the family.

2. Ask the client to be specific about what he means by "screwed up."

3. Ask the client to sign a no-harm contract related to suicide and self-mutilation.

4. Ask the client to talk about appropriate ways to express anger toward his mother.

122. A client diagnosed with posttraumatic stress disorder is readmitted for suicidal thoughts and continued trouble sleeping. She states that when she closes her eyes, she has vivid memories about being awakened at night. "My dad would be on top of me trying to have sex with me. I could not breathe." Which suggestions would be appropriate for the nurse to make for the insomnia? Select all that apply.
- ☐ 1. trying relaxation techniques to help decrease her anxiety before bedtime
- ☐ 2. taking the quetiapine 25 mg as needed as prescribed by the healthcare provider (HCP)
- ☐ 3. staying in the dayroom and trying to sleep in the recliner chair near staff
- ☐ 4. listening to calming music as she tries to fall asleep
- ☐ 5. processing the content of her flashbacks no less than an hour before bedtime
- ☐ 6. leaving her door slightly open to decrease noise during the nightly checks

123. A client with posttraumatic stress disorder needs to find new housing and wants to wait for a month before setting another appointment to see the nurse. How should the nurse interpret this action?
- ☐ 1. a method of avoidance
- ☐ 2. a detriment to progress
- ☐ 3. the end of treatment
- ☐ 4. a necessary break in treatment

124. The nurse should warn a client who is taking a benzodiazepine about using which medication in combination with his current medication?
- ☐ 1. antacids
- ☐ 2. acetaminophen
- ☐ 3. vitamins
- ☐ 4. aspirin

125. Which client statement indicates the need for additional teaching about benzodiazepines?
- ☐ 1. "I cannot drink alcohol while taking diazepam."
- ☐ 2. "I can stop taking the drug anytime I want."
- ☐ 3. "Diazepam can make me drowsy, so I should not drive for a while."
- ☐ 4. "Diazepam will help my tight muscles feel better."

126. A client is diagnosed with agoraphobia without panic disorder. Which type of therapy would **most** the nurse expect to see included in the plan of care?
- ☐ 1. insight therapy
- ☐ 2. group therapy
- ☐ 3. behavior therapy
- ☐ 4. psychoanalysis

127. The client diagnosed with a fear of eating in public places or in front of other people has finished eating lunch in the dining area in the nurse's presence. Which statement by the nurse should reinforce the client's positive action?
- ☐ 1. "It was not so hard, now was it?"
- ☐ 2. "At supper, I hope to see you eat with a group of people."
- ☐ 3. "You must have been hungry today."
- ☐ 4. "It is progress for you to eat in the dining room with me."

128. The client diagnosed with agoraphobia refuses to walk down the hall to the group room. Which response by the nurse is **most** appropriate?
- ☐ 1. "I know you can do it."
- ☐ 2. "Try holding onto the wall as you walk."
- ☐ 3. "You can miss group this one time."
- ☐ 4. "I will walk with you."

129. A client diagnosed with obsessive-compulsive disorder has been taking sertraline but would like to have more energy every day. At his monthly checkup, he reports that his massage therapist recommended he take St. John's wort to help his depression. The nurse should tell the client:
- ☐ 1. "St. John's wort is a harmless herb that might be helpful in this instance."
- ☐ 2. "Combining St. John's wort with the sertraline can cause a serious reaction called serotonin syndrome."
- ☐ 3. "If you take St. John's wort, we will have to decrease the dose of your sertraline."
- ☐ 4. "St. John's wort is not very effective for depression, but we can increase your sertraline dose."

130. A client diagnosed with obsessive-compulsive disorder arrives late for an appointment with the nurse at the outpatient clinic. During the interview, he fidgets restlessly, has trouble remembering what topic is being discussed, and says he thinks he is going crazy. Which statement by the nurse **best** deals with the client's feelings of "going crazy?"
- ☐ 1. "What do you mean when you say you think you are going crazy?"
- ☐ 2. "Most people feel that way occasionally."
- ☐ 3. "I do not know you well enough to judge your mental state."
- ☐ 4. "I have not heard you make a crazy statement."

131. A client with obsessive-compulsive disorder reveals that he was late for his appointment "because of my dumb habit. I have to take off my socks and put them back on 41 times! I cannot stop until I do it just right." The nurse interprets the client's behavior as **most** likely representing an effort to obtain:
- ☐ 1. relief from anxiety.
- ☐ 2. control of his thoughts.
- ☐ 3. attention from others.
- ☐ 4. safe expression of hostility.

132. A client with obsessive-compulsive disorder, who was admitted early yesterday morning, must make his bed 22 times before he can have breakfast. Because of his behavior, the client missed having breakfast yesterday with the other clients. Which action should the nurse institute to help the client be on time for breakfast?
- ☐ 1. Tell the client to make his bed one time only.
- ☐ 2. Wake the client an hour earlier to perform his ritual.
- ☐ 3. Insist that the client stop his activity when it is time for breakfast.
- ☐ 4. Advise the client to have breakfast first before making his bed.

133. The nurse notices that a client diagnosed with major depression and social phobia must get up and move to another area when someone sits next to her. Which action by the nurse is appropriate?
- ☐ 1. Ignore the client's behavior.
- ☐ 2. Question the client about her avoidance of others.
- ☐ 3. Convey awareness of the client's anxiety about being around others.
- ☐ 4. Have nursing staff follow the client as moves away.

134. The nurse is developing a long-term care plan for an outpatient client diagnosed with dissociative identity disorder. Which interventions should be included in this plan? Select all that apply.
- ☐ 1. learning how to manage feelings, especially anger and rage
- ☐ 2. joining several outpatient support groups that are process oriented
- ☐ 3. identifying resources to call when there is a risk of suicide or self-mutilation
- ☐ 4. selecting a method for alter personalities to communicate with each other, such as journaling
- ☐ 5. trying different medicines to find one that eliminates the dissociative process
- ☐ 6. helping each alter accept the goal of sharing and integrating all their memories

135. A client with a long history of experiencing dissociative identity disorder is admitted to the unit after the cuts on her legs were sutured in the emergency department. During the admission interview, the client tearfully states that she does not know what happened to her legs. Then, a stronger, alter personality states that the client is useless, weak, and needs to be eliminated completely. The nurse should do which action **first**?
- ☐ 1. Explore the alter personalities' attitudes toward the client more thoroughly.
- ☐ 2. Place the client in restraints when the alter personality emerges.
- ☐ 3. Contract with the alter personality to tell the nurse when he has the urge to harm the client and the body they both share.
- ☐ 4. Keep the client in a stress-free environment so that the stronger alter personality does not get a chance to emerge.

The Client with a Somatoform Disorder

136. At 1000 hours, a client with a diagnosis of pain disorder demands that the nurse call the healthcare provider (HCP) for more pain medication because she is still in pain after the 0900 analgesic. What should the nurse do **next**?
☐ **1.** Call the HCP as the client requests.
☐ **2.** Suggest the client lie down while she is waiting for her next dose.
☐ **3.** Tell the client that the HCP will be in later to talk to her about it.
☐ **4.** Inform the client that the nurse cannot give her additional medication at this time.

137. The unlicensed assistive personnel (UAP) tells the nurse that the client with a somatoform disorder is sick and is not coming to the dining room for lunch. The nurse should direct the UAP to do which intervention?
☐ **1.** Take the client a lunch tray, and let him eat in his room.
☐ **2.** Tell the client he will need to wait until supper to eat if he misses lunch.
☐ **3.** Invite the client to lunch and accompany him to the dining room.
☐ **4.** Inform the client that he has 10 minutes to get to the dining room for lunch.

138. The client diagnosed with conversion disorder has a paralyzed arm. A staff member states, "I would just tell the client her arm is paralyzed because she had an affair and neglected her baby's care to the point where the baby had to be hospitalized for dehydration." Which response by the nurse is **best**?
☐ **1.** "Ignore the client's behaviors and treat her with respect."
☐ **2.** "Pushing insight will increase the client's anxiety and the need for physical symptoms."
☐ **3.** "Pushing awareness will be helpful and further the client's recovery."
☐ **4.** "We will meet with the client and confront her with her behavior."

139. The healthcare provider (HCP) refers a client diagnosed with somatization disorder to the outpatient clinic because of problems with nausea. The client's past symptoms involved back pain, chest pain, and problems with urination. The client tells the nurse that the nausea began when his wife asked him for a divorce. Which intervention is **most** appropriate?
☐ **1.** asking the client to describe his problem with nausea
☐ **2.** directing the client to describe his feelings about his impending divorce
☐ **3.** allowing the client to talk about the HCPs he has seen and the medications he has taken
☐ **4.** informing the client about a different medication for his nausea

140. A client diagnosed with pain disorder is talking with the nurse about fishing when he suddenly reverts to talking about the pain in his arm. What should the nurse do next?
☐ **1.** Allow the client to talk about his pain.
☐ **2.** Ask the client if he needs more pain medication.
☐ **3.** Get up and leave the client.
☐ **4.** Redirect the interaction back to fishing.

141. Which statement indicates to the nurse that the client is progressing toward recovery from a somatoform disorder?
☐ **1.** "I understand my pain will feel worse when I am worried about my divorce."
☐ **2.** "My stomach pain will go away once I get properly diagnosed."
☐ **3.** "My headache feels better when I time my medication dose."
☐ **4.** "I need to find a healthcare provider (HCP) who understands what my pain is like."

Managing Care, Quality, and Safety of Clients with Personality Disorders, Substance-Related Disorders, Anxiety Disorders, and Anxiety-Related Disorders

142. A client is brought to the emergency department (ED) by a friend who states that the client recently ran out of his lorazepam and has been having a grand mal seizure for the last 10 minutes. The nurse observes that the client is still seizing. What should the nurse do in order of priority from first to last? All options must be used.

1. Monitor the client's safety, and place seizure pads on the cart rails.

2. Record the time, duration, and nature of the seizures.

3. Page the ED healthcare provider (HCP), and prepare to give diazepam intravenously.

4. Ask the friend about the client's medical history and current medications.

143. The client is in the emergency department with her boyfriend. She is just recovering from a "bad trip" from lysergic acid diethylamide (LSD). She is still frightened and a little suspicious. Which nursing action is **most** appropriate?
- ☐ 1. having an unlicensed assistive personnel (UAP) stay with the client to decrease her fear
- ☐ 2. placing the client next to the nursing desk
- ☐ 3. leaving the client alone until the "trip" is over
- ☐ 4. having the boyfriend check on the client frequently

144. A client on a stretcher in the emergency department begins to thrash around, slap the sheets, and yell, "Get these bugs off of me." She is disoriented and has a blood pressure of 189/75 mm Hg and a pulse of 96 bpm. The friend who is with her says, "She was drinking *a lot* 3 days ago and asked me for money to get more vodka, but I did not have any." What should the nurse do in order of priority from first to last? All options must be used.

1. Obtain a prescription to place the client in restraints, if needed.

2. Implement constant observation.

3. Monitor vital signs every 15 minutes.

4. Administer haloperidol and lorazepam IM as prescribed.

5. Remind the client that she is in the hospital and the nurse is with her.

6. Chart the client's response to the interventions.

145. The nurse is teaching unlicensed staff about caring for the client with alcohol dependency. Which statement by the staff indicates the need for additional teaching?
- ☐ 1. "Alcohol dependency affects the entire family."
- ☐ 2. "The client is a weak individual and could stop if he desires."
- ☐ 3. "Alcohol is a problem when it interferes with the client's daily life."
- ☐ 4. "The client who cannot stop drinking, even though he wants to, is alcohol dependent."

146. The nurse is serving on the hospital ethics committee that is considering the ethics of a proposal for the nursing staff to search the room of a client diagnosed with substance abuse while he is off the unit and without his knowledge. What should be considered concerning the relationship of ethical and legal standards of behavior?
- ☐ 1. Ethical standards are generally higher than those required by law.
- ☐ 2. Ethical standards are equal to those required by law.
- ☐ 3. Ethical standards bear no relationship to legal standards for behavior.
- ☐ 4. Ethical standards are irrelevant when the health of a client is at risk.

147. A client with a history of cocaine abuse is receiving intravenous therapy and exits the hospital "to visit a friend." The client returns to the nursing unit 1 hour later, agitated, aggressive, combative, and reporting "chest pain." Place the nurse's actions in priority order from first to last. All options must be used.

1. Contact the security department.

2. Obtain an ECG.

3. Initiate a referral to obtain drug rehabilitation counseling.

4. Obtain a urine sample.

148. During a unit meeting attended by clients and staff, several clients are criticizing their primary nurses. These clients have also been intimidating two other clients who have recently been admitted to the unit, and now, the new clients have stopped sharing their opinions during the meeting. What is the **first** action for the nurse to take?
- ☐ 1. Help the new clients express the reasons they have stopped sharing their ideas.
- ☐ 2. Ask the clients criticizing their nurses to suggest some possible solutions for the practices they are criticizing.
- ☐ 3. Give the clients who are publically criticizing the nurses a verbal warning that this behavior is not acceptable.
- ☐ 4. Use the next unit meeting to discuss respect and the importance of collaboration with the treatment team.

149. Two nurses disagree on what is the **most** important information for the client with addictions to have during a discharge teaching session. How should the nurse assigned to provide the discharge teaching proceed?
- ☐ 1. Share all the information that both nurses thought was important.
- ☐ 2. Review the policies related to required discharge teaching.
- ☐ 3. Be aware of different interpretations and personal biases held by nurses.
- ☐ 4. Ask the client what is most important for her as she prepares for discharge.

Answers, Rationales, and Test-Taking Strategies

*The answers and rationales for each question follow below, along with keys (🔑) to the client need (CN) and cognitive level (CL) for each question. In addition, you will also see a glossary icon (📖) highlighting specific terminology used on the licensing exam. As you check your answers, use the **Content Mastery and Test-Taking Skill Self-Analysis** worksheet (tear-out worksheet in back of book) to identify the reason(s) for not answering the questions correctly. For additional information about test-taking skills and strategies for answering questions, refer to pages 12–23 and pages 35–36 in Part 1 of this book.*

The Client with a Personality Disorder

1. 3,1,4,2. The client needs a stepwise plan for developing a social life. He needs to first work on his self-esteem and reduce his fears of rejection before talking about how to decrease his anxiety and learning new social skills. Helping him chose interesting activities is important before suggesting an activity for him. Then, he will be ready to try a structured activity with the nurse present for support and role modeling.

🔑 CN: Psychosocial integrity; CL: Synthesize

2. 3. The client is at risk for suicide, and the nurse should determine how serious the client is, including if she has a plan and the means to implement the plan. While medication history may be important, the nurse should first attempt to determine suicide risk. Asking the client why she cut herself will likely cause the client to respond with insufficient information to determine suicide risk.

🔑 CN: Reduction of risk potential; CL: Synthesize

3. 1. The nurse should plan to assist the client who has a personality disorder primarily with specific dysfunctional behaviors that are distressing to the client or others. The client with a personality disorder has lifelong, inflexible, and dysfunctional patterns of relating and behaving. The client commonly does not view his behavior as distressful to himself. The client becomes distressed because of others' reactions and behaviors toward him, which cause the client emotional pain and discomfort. Psychopharmacologic compliance is not a primary need because medication does not cure a personality disorder. Medication is prescribed if the client has a severe symptom that interferes with functioning, such as severe anxiety or depression. Examination of developmental conflicts usually is not helpful because of the ingrained dysfunctional ways of thinking and behaving. It is more useful to help the client with changing dysfunctional behaviors. Although milieu management is a component of care, the client usually is proficient enough in the manipulation of the environment to meet his needs.

🔑 CN: Psychosocial integrity; CL: Synthesize

4. 3. For this client, the nurse needs to use a calm, matter-of-fact approach to create a nonthreatening and secure environment because the client is experiencing problems with suspiciousness and trust. Use of "I" statements and responses would be therapeutic to reduce the client's suspiciousness and increase his trust in the staff and the environment. An authoritarian approach is nontherapeutic and inappropriate because the client may perceive this approach as an attack, subsequently responding with anger and threatening behavior. A parental or controlling approach may be perceived as authoritarian, and the client may become defensive and angry.

🔑 CN: Safety and infection control; CL: Synthesize

5. 4. Attending an activity with the nurse assists the client to become involved with others slowly. The client with a schizotypal personality disorder needs support, kindness, and gentle suggestion to improve social skills and interpersonal relationships. The client commonly has problems in thinking, perceiving, and communicating and appears similar to clients with schizophrenia except that psychotic episodes are infrequent and less severe. Participation solely in group activities or leading a sing-along would be too overwhelming for the client, subsequently increasing the client's anxiety and withdrawal. Engaging primarily in one-to-one activities would not be helpful because of the client's difficulty with social skills and interpersonal relationships. However, activities with the nurse could be used to establish trust. Then, the client could proceed to activities with others.

🔑 CN: Psychosocial integrity;
CL: Synthesize

6. 2. The nurse needs to set limits on the client's manipulative behavior to help the client control dysfunctional behavior. The manipulative client bends rules to have her needs met without regard for rules or the needs or rights of others. A consistent approach by the staff is necessary to decrease manipulation. Ignoring the client's behavior reinforces or promotes the continuation of the client's manipulative behavior. Reprimanding the client may be perceived as a threat, resulting in aggressive behavior. Allowing the client to keep a snack in her room reinforces the dysfunctional behavior.

🔑 CN: Psychosocial integrity;
CL: Synthesize

7. 2. The nurse assists the client with identifying and putting feelings into words during one-to-one interactions. This helps the client express her feelings in a nonthreatening setting and avoid directing anger toward other clients. A client with an antisocial personality disorder needs to understand how others feel and react to her behaviors and why they react the way they do. The client also needs to understand the consequences of her behaviors. Using humor or indirect behaviors to express anger is a passive-aggressive method that will not help the client learn how to express her anger appropriately. Asking the nurse for medication when upset is a way to avoid dealing with feelings and is not helpful. However, medication may be necessary if talking, and engaging in a physical activity has not been effective in lowering anxiety or if the client is about to lose control of her behavior.

🔑 CN: Psychosocial integrity;
CL: Synthesize

8. 1,3,4,6. Inflexibility, need to be in control, perfectionism, overemphasis on work or tasks, and a fear of making mistakes are common symptoms of OCPD. Clomipramine and fluoxetine may help with the obsessive symptoms. Interrupting the client's tasks is likely to increase her anxiety even more. Telling her that she cannot expect the family to be perfect is likely to create a power struggle.

🔑 CN: Psychosocial integrity; CL: Apply

9. 1,2,4,5. A professional, matter-of-fact approach and developing trust are the most effective with this client. A friendly approach, intrusiveness, and attempting to counteract the client's beliefs will increase the client's paranoia; he will present more false beliefs to prove he is right about the conspiracy. Placing the client in group settings may be counterproductive because questions and emotionality from peers, as well as confrontations with reality, will increase the client's anxiety.

🔑 CN: Management of care; CL: Analyze

10. 4. Some characteristics of a client with a dependent personality are an inability to make daily decisions without advice and reassurance and the preoccupation with fear of being alone to care for oneself. The client needs others to be responsible for important areas of his life. The nurse should respond "Your parents have been supportive of you and will continue to be supportive even if you live apart" to gently challenge the client's fears and suggest that they may be unwarranted. Stating "You are a 28-year-old adult now, not a child who needs to be cared for" or "Your parents need a break, and you need a break from them" is reprimanding and would diminish the client's self-worth. Stating "Your parents will not be around forever; after all, they are getting older" may be true, but it is an insensitive response that may increase the client's anxiety.

🔑 CN: Psychosocial integrity; CL: Apply

11. 1,3,2,4. Safety is the priority concern, and then, eating and sleeping patterns need to be reestablished. After intervening to meet basic needs, delving into the loneliness and emptiness are important for determining underlying issues that need to be followed up in outpatient counseling. Although the client is living with her family currently, other options might be appropriate for her to consider.

🔑 CN: Safety and infection control;
CL: Synthesize

12. 4. For the client with attention-seeking behaviors, the nurse would institute a behavioral contract with the client to help decrease dysfunctional behaviors and promote self-sufficiency. Having the client approach only his assigned staff person sets limits on his attention-seeking behavior. Telling the client to stay in his room until staff approach him, limiting the client to a certain area, or giving the client a list of permissible requests is punitive and does nothing to help the client gain control over the dysfunctional behavior.

    CN: Management of care; CL: Synthesize

13. 2. The most therapeutic response is "All of the nurses here provide good care." This statement corrects the client's unrealistic and exaggerated perception. "Splitting," defined as the inability to integrate good and bad aspects of an individual and the self, is a hallmark behavior of a client with borderline personality disorder. The client sees himself and others as all good or all bad. Components of "splitting" include behaviors that idealize and devalue others. It is a defense that allows the client to avoid pain and feelings associated with past abuse or a current situation involving the threat of rejection or abandonment. The other statements promote the client's idealistic view and do nothing to help correct the client's distortion.

    CN: Psychosocial integrity; CL: Apply

14. 2. For the client who is at risk for self-mutilation, the nurse develops a contract to assist the client with assuming responsibility for his behavior and to help the client develop adaptive methods of coping with feelings. Self-mutilation is usually an expression of intense anxiety, anger, helplessness, or guilt or a means to block psychological pain by inducing physical pain. A typical contract helpful to the client would have the client notify staff when anxiety is increasing. Withdrawing to his room when feeling overwhelmed, suppressing feelings when angry, or displacing feelings onto the **HCP** is not an adaptive method to help the client deal with his feelings and could still result in self-mutilation.

    CN: Safety and infection control; CL: Evaluate

15. 4. Any suicidal statement must be assessed by the nurse. The nurse should discuss the client's statement with her to determine its meaning in terms of suicide, overwhelming feelings of anxiety, abandonment, or other need that the client cannot express appropriately. It is not uncommon for a client with borderline personality disorder to make threatening comments before discharge. Extending the hospital stay is inappropriate because it would encourage dependency and manipulation. Ignoring the client's statement on the assumption that it is a sign of manipulation is an error in judgment. Asking a family member to stay with the client temporarily at home is not appropriate and places the responsibility for the client on the family instead of the client.

    CN: Psychosocial integrity; CL: Synthesize

16. 4. The best initial course of action when admitting a client is to observe him to establish baseline information. This assessment provides valuable information about the client's behavior and forms the basis for the plan of care. Telling the client that the staff has authority to subdue him if he gets unruly or that he will have to pay for any damage he causes is threatening and may incite or provoke trouble. Isolating a client is not recommended unless there is a very good reason for it, such as a very active, combative client who is dangerous to himself and others.

    CN: Psychosocial integrity; CL: Synthesize

17. 4. The best response is "You say you are not a regular here, but you are experiencing what others are experiencing." This statement helps the client to identify factors that precipitate denial by helping her to confront that which inhibits compliance. Denial is used to help a client feel better and more secure when a situation provokes a high level of anxiety and is threatening to the client. The statement "Because you are not a regular client, sit in the hall when the others are in group" agrees with and promotes denial in the client and interferes with treatment. The statement "Your family wants you to attend and they will be disappointed if you do not" causes the client to feel guilty and decreases her self-esteem. The statement "I will have to mark you absent from the clinic today and speak to the **healthcare provider** about it" is punitive and threatening to the client, subsequently decreasing her self-esteem.

    CN: Psychosocial integrity; CL: Synthesize

18. 3. Stating "I will not continue to talk with you if you curse" sets limits on the client's behavior and points out the negative effects of her behavior. Therefore, this response is most appropriate and therapeutic. The statement "You are being very childish" reprimands the client, possibly causing the anger to escalate. The statement "I am sorry if you cannot wait" fails to provide feedback to the client about her behavior. The statement "Come back tomorrow and your medication will be ready" ignores the client's behavior, failing to provide feedback to the client about the behavior. It also shows poor nursing judgment because the client may need her medication before tomorrow or may not return to the clinic the following day.

    CN: Psychosocial integrity; CL: Synthesize

19. 1. The client with avoidant personality disorder is showing signs of improvement when interacting with two other clients. A client with avoidant personality disorder is timid, socially uncomfortable, withdrawn, and hypersensitive to criticism.

Social contact with others decreases isolation and withdrawal. Listening to music with headphones, sitting at a table and painting, and talking on the telephone are solitary activities and therefore do not indicate improvement, which is evidenced by social contact.

🔑 CN: Psychosocial integrity; CL: Analyze

20. 4. The priority is to explain to the client that this information has to be shared immediately with the staff and the **HCP** 📖 because of its serious nature. Safety of all is crucial regardless of whether the client follows through on his plan. It is possible that the client is asking to be stopped and that he is indirectly pleading for help in a dysfunctional manner. Bargaining with the client, such as warning him that his telephone privileges will be taken away if he abuses them, or offering to disregard his plan if he does not go through with it, is inappropriate. Saying nothing to anyone until the client has actually completed the call and then notifying the proper authorities represent serious negligence on the part of the nurse.

🔑 CN: Safety and infection control; CL: Synthesize

21. 1. The most basic and important idea to convey to a client is that, as a person, he or she is accepted, although his or her behavior may not be. Empathy is conveyed for emotional pain regardless of the client's behavior. Although some clients need limits placed on their behavior, not all clients require limit setting. That the staff members are the primary ones left to care about these clients is not necessarily true, nor is it true that the staff should use very little humor with these clients. Clients who are rigid and perfectionists and who have a restricted affect may need help with displaying humor.

🔑 CN: Management of care; CL: Apply

22. 1. The nurse should explain the negative reactions of others toward the client's behaviors to make him aware of the impact of his seductive behaviors on others. Suggesting that the client apologize to others for his behavior is futile because the client cannot feel remorse for wrongdoing. Asking him to explain reasons for his seductive behavior is not helpful because this client is skillful at using projection and rationalization. Discussing his relationship with his mother is not helpful because the focus should be oriented to the present situation and managing his behavior at the present time.

🔑 CN: Psychosocial integrity; CL: Synthesize

23. 2. The nurse would specifically use supportive confrontation with the client to point out discrepancies between what the client states and what actually exists to increase responsibility for self.

Limit setting and consistency also may be used. However, limit setting helps the client control unacceptable behavior, and consistency helps reduce the frequency of negative behaviors; they do not point out discrepancies. Rationalization is typically used by the client, not the nurse, to blame others, make excuses, and provide alibis for self-centered behaviors.

🔑 CN: Psychosocial integrity; CL: Synthesize

24. 4. The nurse should use role-playing to teach the client appropriate responses to others in various situations. This client dramatizes events, draws attention to self, and is unaware of and does not deal with feelings. The nurse works to help the client clarify true feelings and learn to express them appropriately. Party planning, music group, and cooking class are therapeutic activities but will not help the client specifically learn how to respond appropriately to others.

🔑 CN: Psychosocial integrity; CL: Synthesize

The Client with an Alcohol-Related Disorder

25. 1,4,5. As with any dementia, there is a need to protect the client from wandering off and risking harm to self. Dementia is progressive and eventually requires 24-hour supervision. The client will find a way to get more alcohol if quitting is not a personal goal. Not answering the client's question will generally increase the client's anger. Once the dementia is evident, lack of alcohol intake will not reverse the condition.

🔑 CN: Psychosocial integrity; CL: Synthesize

26. 2,3,4,1. The client's feelings and concerns need to be validated so she will open up more. She also should know that the changes in her husband are not unusual. It helps to know the client has tried with her husband to determine if they are appropriate or not. Then, there can be a discussion about getting help for her husband so that her efforts to stay sober are not compromised.

🔑 CN: Reduction of risk potential; CL: Synthesize

27. 4. The best action by the nurse to help a client who has difficulty falling asleep would be to teach the client relaxation exercises to use before bedtime to reduce anxiety and promote relaxation. This activity will also be useful for the client when out of the hospital. Inviting the client to play a board game is inappropriate because this activity can be competitive and thus stimulate the client. Allowing the client to sit in the community room until she feels sleepy is inappropriate because it does nothing to help the client relax. Taking frequent naps can worsen the ability to fall asleep at night.

⚷ CN: Basic care and comfort;
CL: Synthesize

28. 1,2,5. When a client is developing impending alcohol withdrawal delirium, the initial symptoms are a fast pulse and respiratory rate, and an elevated blood pressure. Red, flushed, dry skin and complaints of thirst occur with diabetic ketoacidosis. Abdominal cramping and severe diarrhea are symptoms of opiate withdrawal.

⚷ CN: Reduction of risk potential;
CL: Analyze

29. 4,1,2,3. The nurse should first place the client in a quieter, darkened room with dimmer lights to decrease the stimuli from the busy emergency department (ED) and create a more calming environment. Next, the nurse should administer the lorazepam to help decrease agitation and reduce the risk of seizures. Drawing the blood will be easier as the client becomes less agitated. Depending on the magnesium blood level, the client may need an intramuscular (IM) dose of magnesium sulfate to prevent seizures. The nurse can then obtain the vital sign every 15 minutes to determine if the client is becoming stabilized and if the client needs further doses of lorazepam.

⚷ CN: Management of care; CL: Synthesize

30. 1. The nurse should first contact the HCP 📖. The client's vital signs and level of consciousness are deteriorating, indicating complications of withdrawal, which can be life threatening. Increasing the rate of the infusion may cause fluid overload and has not been prescribed by the HCP. Arousing the client will not address the underlying problems. Magnesium sulfate is used to treat seizures precipitated by alcohol withdrawal, but the client is not demonstrating signs of actual or impending seizures.

⚷ CN: Safety and infection control;
CL: Synthesize

31. 4. The nurse should provide the client with a quiet room to sleep in. Alcohol is destroyed and oxidized in the body at a slow, steady rate. The rate of alcohol metabolism is not influenced by drinking black coffee, walking around the unit, or taking a cold shower. Therefore, it is best to have the client sleep off the effects of the alcohol.

⚷ CN: Reduction of risk potential;
CL: Synthesize

32. 1,2,4,5. For the client experiencing symptoms of alcohol withdrawal, the nurse monitors vital signs and intake and output; reinforces reality for the client who is confused, disoriented, or hallucinating; explains that the symptoms of withdrawal are temporary; reduces stimulation; and stays with the client if he is confused or agitated. The nurse administers medications to prevent the progression of symptoms, such as seizures and delirium tremens, and to ensure the client's safety. Restraints are not used as a precautionary measure. Restraints are used only as a least restrictive measure to protect the client and others when the client is a danger to himself or others.

⚷ CN: Psychosocial integrity;
CL: Synthesize

33. 1,3,4,5. Two or three days after cessation of alcohol, clients may experience delirium tremens (DTs), as evidenced by disorientation, nightmares, abdominal pain, nausea, and diaphoresis, as well as elevated temperature, pulse, and blood pressure, and visual and auditory hallucinations. If the client had a traumatic brain injury after falling, the client might have paralysis, but there is no association of paralysis from DTs.

⚷ CN: Physiologic adaptation;
CL: Synthesize

34. 3. The nurse should first confirm that the client has stopped taking the clonazepam because the client is reporting symptoms of benzodiazepine withdrawal from stopping the clonazepam abruptly. The client would report symptoms of being sedated if he took alcohol with the clonazepam. Tolerance symptoms would be increased anxiety, not these physical symptoms. The client symptoms are consistent with clonazepam withdrawal not excess; thus, asking about increased use is not relevant.

⚷ CN: Pharmacological and parenteral therapies; CL: Analyze

35. 4. Antiseptic mouthwash commonly contains alcohol and should be kept in a locked area unless labeling clearly indicates that the product does not contain alcohol. A client with an intense craving for alcohol may drink mouthwash that contains alcohol. Personal care items, such as toothpaste, dental floss, and shaving cream, do not contain alcohol, and the client would be allowed to keep them in the room.

⚷ CN: Safety and infection control;
CL: Synthesize

36. 4. The best way to intervene with a client's minimization or denial of alcohol problems is to point out the consequences of the drinking—the multiple arrests. The other responses are superficial and discount the seriousness of the client's problem.

⚷ CN: Psychosocial integrity; CL: Synthesize

71. 1. Suggesting that the client try attending a meeting at a different location is a supportive, positive response and encourages the client to continue participating in treatment. Saying "Maybe it just was not a good day for you" or "Perhaps you were not paying close enough attention" places blame on the client and is not helpful. The statement "Sometimes the meetings can seem like a waste of time, but you need to attend to stay clean" diminishes the importance of the self-help group and offers little support to the client.

⚷ CN: Management of care; CL: Synthesize

72. 2. The best measure to determine a client's progress in rehabilitation is the number of drug-free days he has. The longer the client abstains, the better the prognosis is. Although the kinds of friends the client makes, the way he gets along with his parents, and the degree of responsibility his job requires could influence his decision to stay clean, the number of drug-free days is the best indicator of progress.

⚷ CN: Management of care; CL: Evaluate

73. 4. The client who is addicted to heroin is most likely to exhibit hypoactivity. Initially, the client feels euphoric. This is followed by drowsiness, hypoactivity, anorexia, and a decreased sex drive. Hilarity, aggression, and a labile mood usually are not associated with heroin addiction.

⚷ CN: Psychosocial integrity; CL: Analyze

74. 4. Because barbiturates are central nervous system depressants, the nurse should be especially alert for the possibility of respiratory failure. Respiratory failure is the most likely cause of death from barbiturate overdose. Kidney failure, cerebrovascular accident, and status epilepticus are not associated with barbiturate overdose.

⚷ CN: Reduction of risk potential; CL: Analyze

75. 4. When a spouse asks whether a seriously ill client will live, it is best for the nurse to respond by explaining the seriousness of the client's condition and acknowledging the spouse's concern. This type of comment does not offer false hope. Telling the spouse to wait and see and that it is too soon to tell is a stereotypical statement that offers no support. Asking the spouse to describe the length of his or her relationship with the client ignores the spouse's concern and does not focus on the problem. Simply saying that the client is very ill and may not live and that some do not pull through is harsh and not supportive.

⚷ CN: Psychosocial integrity; CL: Synthesize

76. 1. Tolerance for a drug occurs when a client requires increasingly larger doses to obtain the desired effect. Therefore, the plan of care would address the client's state of tolerance. The term addiction refers to psychological and physiologic symptoms indicating that an individual cannot control his or her use of psychoactive substances. This term has been replaced with the term dependence. Abuse refers to the excessive use of a substance that differs from societal norms. Drug dependence occurs when the client must take a usual or increasing amount of the drug to prevent the onset of abstinence symptoms, cannot keep drug intake under control, and continues to use even though physical, social, and emotional processes are compromised.

⚷ CN: Physiological adaptation; CL: Analyze

77. 4. For a client who is confused when awakening after taking a large dose of barbiturates, the nurse should speak in concrete terms using simple statements in a calm, nonjudgmental, gentle manner to assist the client with cognitive-perceptual impairment, enhance understanding, and decrease anxiety. The other statements contain abstract information and some slang terms that may further confuse the client and thus increase the client's anxiety.

⚷ CN: Psychosocial integrity; CL: Synthesize

78. 2. The highest priority is assessing for suicide risk. When the client is safe, then the self-esteem, helplessness, and hopelessness issues can be addressed.

⚷ CN: Psychosocial integrity; CL: Synthesize

79. 1. The most appropriate initial outcome for the client is to discuss thoughts and feelings related to her losses. The nurse should help the client identify and verbalize her feelings so that she can externalize her thoughts and emotions and begin to deal with them. This prevents the client from internalizing feelings, which leads to depression and self-harm. The ability to identify two positive qualities, explore strengths, and prioritize problems would be appropriate after the client has explored her thoughts and feelings, gained awareness of the issues, and then can participate in the treatment plan.

⚷ CN: Psychosocial integrity; CL: Evaluate

80. 4. The best method to deal with the problem is to discuss observations with clients at the daily community meeting because the problem involves all of the clients, and this provides them with the opportunity to offer their views. Peer pressure is valuable in confronting self-defeating and destructive behaviors. Providing additional recreation avoids or ignores the problem and is damaging to all clients because it decreases trust in the nurse. Breaking up drug-oriented discussions would not be sufficient to stop the behavior. Speaking with the clients individually about their behavior is not as effective as dealing with the problem openly and directly with everyone.

🔑 CN: Psychosocial integrity;
CL: Synthesize

81. 4. The nurse directs the conversation to realistic concerns or issues to decrease denial and focus on rebuilding a substance-free life. Allowing the client to continue with the stories or questioning the client further about her exploits reinforces the denial. Telling the client you have heard the stories before is nondirective. Additionally, these actions do nothing to help the client focus on rebuilding a substance-free life.

🔑 CN: Psychosocial integrity;
CL: Synthesize

82. 3. The statement that marijuana impairs short-term memory and judgment and distorts perceptions is a direct, correct, educational response to the student's statement that does not decrease the student's or the friend's self-worth. Telling the student that marijuana is unsafe and illegal, or that using marijuana leads to using other chemicals, does not provide the student with factual information to answer the student's question. Asking whether the student really believes the friend challenges the student and may lead to defensive behavior.

🔑 CN: Psychosocial integrity; CL: Apply

83. 1,2,4,5. Ecstasy is chemically related to methamphetamine (speed) and is used at all-night parties (also known as "raves") to enhance dancing, closeness to others, affection, and the ability to communicate. Euphoria, heightened sexuality, disinhibition, and diminished self-consciousness can occur. Adverse effects include tachycardia, elevated blood pressure, anorexia, dry mouth, and teeth grinding. Pacifiers, including candy-shaped pacifiers and lollipops, are used to ease the discomfort associated with teeth grinding and jaw clenching. Hyperthermia, dehydration, renal failure, and death can occur.

🔑 CN: Reduction of risk potential;
CL: Create

84. 3,4,2,1. It is crucial to confirm that the client was taking her husband's opiates and benzodiazepines and that her symptoms are due to the sudden withdrawal from these medications. It is also important to know if she has been using other substances (such as alcohol) that may cause other withdrawal symptoms. Even before calling for prescriptions, the nurse can initiate withdrawal precautions for client safety.

🔑 CN: Safety and infection control;
CL: Apply

85. 4. Acknowledging the client's son's feelings is the most therapeutic intervention because he is not likely to hear the nurse's information until his anger and other feelings are addressed and subside. Then, it is important to acknowledge that oxycodone, especially in older clients, can interfere with remembering how many pills were taken. It is common for clients with chronic pain to inadvertently overuse or become addicted to pain medications. Pain management programs help clients to withdraw from the offending medication and start on a multifaceted system for controlling the pain.

🔑 CN: Psychosocial integrity;
CL: Synthesize

86. 1,2,3,5. Clients who deny an addiction and the need for treatment can be at risk for a suicide attempt, efforts to escape the unit, and aggression directed at staff. A contraband search is a safety measure to look for concealed drugs and dangerous items. Depending on the last use of the substance, withdrawal symptoms can begin quickly. A urine drug screen is crucial to determine what other substances the client may be using that may cause other withdrawal symptoms. Explaining the unit routines and groups can wait until the client is calmer and more receptive.

🔑 CN: Safety and infection control;
CL: Analyze

87. 2,3,5. The dose, length of use, and the number of diazepam taken per day are important for assessing the severity of the substance abuse and potential withdrawal. Determining sleep interferences is necessary for treating the underlying causes of the insomnia. The reason his wife takes diazepam is confidential information and is not critical to his situation. Getting off the diazepam is essential for the client and is not an option, especially with his cardiac issues. This needs to be done safely if he has been taking diazepam for more than a week or two.

🔑 CN: Psychosocial integrity; CL: Analyze

88. 1,2,4,5. The client who has used cocaine experiences mood swings, a feeling of euphoria, and an elevation in heart rate and blood pressure. The client with cocaine use will have dilated pupils.

🔑 CN: Reduction of risk potential;
CL: Synthesize

89. 2,3,4,5,6. The cocaine was not swallowed, so inducing vomiting is not indicated. A cocaine overdose can produce seizures, paranoia, and respiratory and/or metabolic acidosis. Deep breathing will help decrease the respiratory distress and pulse rate.

🔑 CN: Pharmacological and parenteral therapies; CL: Synthesize

90. 4. The nurse assesses the client for feelings of depression and suicidal ideation. After experiencing an instantaneous high from crack, a crash immediately follows, and the client has an intense craving for more crack. A crash commonly leads to a cocaine-induced depression when additional crack is unavailable. At times, the depression is so severe that users attempt suicide. Although suspiciousness, loss of appetite, and drug craving are also associated with cocaine use, they are less of a priority than suicidal ideation.

⚷ CN: Psychosocial integrity; CL: Analyze

91. 3,2,4,1. The risk of seizures is an immediate safety issue, and the nurse should first place seizure pads on the bed. Amphetamine overdose can produce cardiac arrhythmias and respiratory collapse; the nurse should next monitor the client. After monitoring is initiated, the haloperidol is indicated to antagonize the amphetamine affects. When the client is medically stable, the nurse can transfer the client to a psychiatric unit. Haloperidol would be stopped as the psychotic symptoms subside.

⚷ CN: Reduction of risk potential; CL: Synthesize

92. 2. Lorazepam, as opposed to alprazolam, is available in dosage ranges that allow more gradual tapering down of doses over 3 to 4 days. Haloperidol is not effective for benzodiazepine withdrawal. Tapering alprazolam in 48 hours is too rapid. Offering alprazolam as a PRN does not deal with the need to gradually reduce the dose and frequency over time.

⚷ CN: Pharmacological and parenteral therapies; CL: Synthesize

93. 1,2,5. The client is exhibiting symptoms of moderate anxiety. At this level of anxiety, the nurse should help the client to decrease anxiety by allowing ventilation, crying, exercise, and relaxation techniques. The nurse would further assist the client by refocusing his attention, relating behaviors and feelings to anxiety, and then assisting with problem solving. Oral medication may be needed if the client's anxiety is prolonged or does not decrease with the nurse's interventions. Suggesting a time-out and giving intramuscular medication are possible interventions for a client whose anxiety level is severe.

⚷ CN: Psychosocial integrity; CL: Synthesize

94. 2. The nurse must be especially cautious when providing care to a client who has taken phencyclidine (PCP) because of unpredictable, violent behavior. The client can appear to be in a calm state or even in a coma, then become violent, and then return to a calm or comatose state. Visual hallucinations, bizarre behavior, and loud screaming are associated with PCP-intoxicated clients. However, the unpredictable, violent behavior presents a major issue of safety for clients and staff.

⚷ CN: Safety and infection control; CL: Analyze

95. 3. An acid environment aids in the excretion of PCP. Therefore, the nurse should give the client with PCP intoxication cranberry juice to acidify the urine to a pH of 5.5 and accelerate excretion. Water, milk, or grape juice will not acidify the urine.

⚷ CN: Reduction of risk potential; CL: Synthesize

96. 1. Smoking marijuana while using alcohol can lead to alcohol poisoning because marijuana masks the nausea and vomiting associated with excessive alcohol consumption. Marijuana contains tetrahydrocannabinol (THC), which is responsible for suppressing nausea. With dangerous levels of alcohol in the body, respiratory depression, coma, and death can occur. Lysergic acid diethylamide, peyote, and psilocybin do not contain THC.

⚷ CN: Reduction of risk potential; CL: Analyze

97. 3. Providing frequent "time-outs" when the client is highly anxious, sensitive, irritable, and over reactive is needed to calm the client and reduce the possibility of escalating behaviors and violence. Secluding and restraining the client is not appropriate and would only be used if the client was threatening others and other alternative actions had been unsuccessful. Telling the client to stay in his room until he can control himself is unrealistic and futile because the client cannot eliminate behaviors induced by chemicals. Confronting the client about his behaviors would most likely lead to aggression and possibly violent behavior.

⚷ CN: Safety and infection control; CL: Synthesize

98. 4. The nurse should invite the client who is anxious to participate in an activity that involves gross motor movements. Doing so helps to direct energy toward a therapeutic activity. Appropriate activities include walking, riding a stationary bicycle, or playing volleyball. Assigning the client to an educational group is not helpful because the anxious client would be unable to sit in a group setting and concentrate on what was occurring in the group. Watching television may be too stimulating for the client, possibly increasing anxiety. Additionally, the client may be too anxious to sit and focus. Waiting for the client to approach the nurse is not helpful or appropriate. The nurse is responsible for initiating contact with the client.

⚷ CN: Psychosocial integrity; CL: Synthesize

99. 1,3,4,5. Since methadone is an addictive medication, the client will be gradually tapered off of it, while being monitored for withdrawal symptoms. Any residual pain is likely to be controlled with other pain management techniques and non-narcotic pain medication. It is very unlikely that oxycodone would be prescribed PRN since it is a very addictive medication.

🔑 CN: Reduction of risk potential; CL: Apply

100. 1,2,3,4,6. Acknowledgment of the client's frustration, pain, and cravings is important to decrease the client's anger. Naltrexone can help with detoxification from alcohol and opiates. Asking the **healthcare provider (HCP)** 📖 about the possibility of adding naltrexone is appropriate. The nurse can never promise that a medication will help this client, since naltrexone is effective with only 20% to 30% of clients with opiate cravings.

🔑 CN: Pharmacological and parental therapies; CL: Analyze

The Client with Anxiety Disorders and Anxiety-Related Disorders

101. 2. The nurse cannot appear to take the side of either the student or her parent, so discussing the situation together where all points of view can be presented and evaluated is the best option. To avoid college altogether is likely to only escalate both parties' anxiety.

🔑 CN: Psychosocial integrity; CL: Apply

102. 4. The client's concerns are real and serious enough to warrant assessment by an **HCP** 📖 rather than being dismissed as trivial. Though he is very intelligent, his intelligence cannot overcome his anxiety, and in fact, his anxiety is likely to interfere with his ability to perform in college if no assessment and treatment is received. Just postponing college is likely to increase the client's anxiety rather than lower it since it does not address the panic he is experiencing.

🔑 CN: Psychosocial integrity; CL: Analyze

103. 1,2,3,5. Anger and rage could be directed at self and others. He implies that he did nothing wrong in assaulting the woman (denial) and may try to leave without treatment. A no-harm contract is essential for everyone's safety. He needs safe outlets, including staff talks, for his anger. Talking about his views of prostitutes in unit groups may be upsetting to female clients who have sexual abuse issues as well, so this needs to occur in private.

🔑 CN: Safety and infection control; CL: Create

104. 1,4,5. The nurse should instruct the client who is taking diazepam to take the medication as prescribed; stopping the medication suddenly can cause withdrawal symptoms. This medication is used for a short term only. The drug dose can be potentiated by alcohol, and the client should not drink alcoholic beverages while taking this drug. Swelling of the lips and face and difficulty breathing are signs and symptoms of an allergic reaction. The client should stop taking the drug and seek medical assistance immediately. The client does not need to avoid eating foods containing tyramine because it interacts with monoamine oxidase inhibitors, not benzodiazepines. The client can take the medication with food.

🔑 CN: Health promotion and maintenance; CL: Synthesize

105. 4. Cognitive-behavioral therapy is effective in treating anxiety disorders. The nurse can assist the client in identifying the onset of the fears that cause the anxiety and develop strategies to modify the behavior associated with the fears. Avoiding touching foods, asking about reasons for the anxiety, and providing ways to work around touching the foods do not deal with the anxiety and are not interventions that will help this client.

🔑 CN: Psychosocial integrity; CL: Synthesize

106. 2. Asking "Are you feeling anxious?" helps the client to specifically label the feeling as anxiety so that he can begin to understand and manage it. Some clients need assistance with identifying what they are feeling so they can recognize what is happening to them. Stating "You need to sit down and relax" is not appropriate because the client needs to continue his pacing to feel better. Asking if something is bothering the client or saying that he must be experiencing a problem is vague and does not help the client identify his feelings as anxiety.

🔑 CN: Psychosocial integrity; CL: Synthesize

107. 1. The nurse responds with the statement "It was very frightening for you" to express empathy, thus acknowledging the client's discomfort and accepting his feelings. The nurse conveys respect and validates the client's self-worth. The other statements do not focus on the client's underlying feelings, convey active listening, or promote trust.

🔑 CN: Psychosocial integrity; CL: Synthesize

108. 4,2,3,1. Immediate anxiety-reducing strategies are decrease stimuli and perform deep breathing. Once the anxiety is lessened, the client's feelings can be explored for triggers and underlying issues.

Then, problem-solving strategies can be discussed to handle the triggers and issues appropriately.

🔑 CN: Psychosocial integrity; CL: Synthesize

109. 1. Alprazolam, a benzodiazepine used on a short-term or temporary basis to treat symptoms of anxiety, increases gamma-aminobutyrate (GABA), a major inhibitory neurotransmitter. Because GABA is increased and the reticular activating system is depressed, incoming stimuli are muted, and the effects of anxiety are blocked. Alprazolam does not directly target serotonin, dopamine, or norepinephrine.

🔑 CN: Pharmacological and parenteral therapies; CL: Apply

110. 1,2,4,5. It is appropriate to provide education on medication mechanisms, benefits, and managing side effects. No medication will eliminate all anxiety, so teaching about anxiety reduction and adaptive coping is needed. Venlafaxine is a serotonin-norepinephrine reuptake inhibitor antidepressant, and it will take 2 to 4 weeks to feel the effects.

🔑 CN: Pharmacological and parenteral therapies; CL: Create

111. 3. Using alcohol or any central nervous system depressant while taking a benzodiazepine, such as alprazolam, is contraindicated because of additive depressant effects. Ingestion of chocolate, cheese, or shellfish is not problematic.

🔑 CN: Pharmacological and parenteral therapies; CL: Apply

112. 1. Buspirone, a nonbenzodiazepine anxiolytic, is particularly effective in treating the cognitive symptoms of anxiety, such as worry, apprehension, difficulty with concentration, and irritability. Buspirone is not effective for the somatic symptoms of anxiety (muscle tension). Therapeutic effects may be experienced in 7 to 10 days, with full effects occurring in 3 to 4 weeks. This drug is not known to cause physical or psychological dependence. It can be taken with food or small meals to reduce gastrointestinal upset.

🔑 CN: Pharmacological and parenteral therapies; CL: Evaluate

113. 2. The nurse initially reassures the client that her feelings and behaviors are typical reactions to serious trauma to help decrease anxiety and maintain self-esteem. Explaining the effects of stress on the body may be helpful later. Telling the client that her symptoms are temporary is less helpful. Acknowledging the unfairness of the client's situation does not address the client's needs at this time.

🔑 CN: Psychosocial integrity; CL: Synthesize

114. 3. The client with anxiety may be able to learn to recognize when she is feeling anxious, understand the reasons for her anxiety, and be able to describe situations that preceded her feelings of anxiety. However, she is likely to continue to experience symptoms unless she has also learned to use adaptive and palliative methods to reduce anxiety.

🔑 CN: Psychosocial integrity; CL: Synthesize

115. 4. Saying "The accident just happened and could not have been predicted" provides the client with an objective perception of the event instead of the client's perceived role. This type of statement reflects active listening and helps to reduce feelings of blame and guilt. Saying "Do not keep torturing yourself" or "Stop blaming yourself" is inappropriate because it tells the client what to do, subsequently delaying the therapeutic process. The statement "Let us talk about something that is a bit more pleasant" ignores the client's feelings and changes the subject. The client needs to verbalize feelings and decrease feelings of isolation.

🔑 CN: Psychosocial integrity; CL: Synthesize

116. 1. The nurse states "You did what you had to do at that time" to help the client evaluate past behavior in the context of the trauma. Clients commonly feel guilty about past behaviors when viewing them in the context of current values. The other statements are inappropriate because they do not help the client to evaluate past behavior in the context of the trauma.

🔑 CN: Psychosocial integrity; CL: Synthesize

117. 2. Writing in a journal can help the client safely express feelings, particularly anger, when the client cannot verbalize them. Listening to music, meditating, and working on a puzzle may be relaxing, but will not help the client express their feelings. Safely externalizing anger by writing in a journal helps the client to maintain control over her feelings.

🔑 CN: Psychosocial integrity; CL: Synthesize

118. 3. The nurse should facilitate progressive review of the accident and its consequences to help the client integrate feelings and memories and to begin the grieving process. Helping the client to evaluate her sister's behavior, telling the client to avoid details of the accident, or postponing the discussion of the accident until the client brings it up is not therapeutic and does not facilitate the development of trust in the nurse. Such actions do not facilitate review of the accident, which is necessary to help the client integrate feelings and memories and begin the grieving process.

🔑 CN: Management of care; CL: Create

119. **3,1,4,2.** Safety is the first priority in clients experiencing acute stress disorder (ASD). ASD symptoms are typical reactions to an abnormal situation that are not being handled effectively. When the client believes he is "normal," being accepted, understood, and supported, then he will be able to discuss his thoughts and feelings related to the traumas of the war.

> CN: Safety and infection control;
> CL: Synthesize

120. **4.** Survivors of trauma/torture have a lot of difficulty with trust and do not readily talk about the horrible events. Therefore, empathy and a willingness to listen without pressuring the client are crucial. Believing everything may or may not be possible and does not convey the empathy. It is sometimes difficult to believe what satanic cults can do to children. Saying that it was not right that members did not help diverts attention from the client to the member. Asking to hear about the cult shows more interest in the cult than the client.

> CN: Psychosocial integrity;
> CL: Synthesize

121. **3,1,2,4.** The nurse should first assure the client's safety after the client's self-mutilation. Another safety issue is whether the stepdad possibly may be abusing younger children; if so, a police report may need to be filed. Then, it is important to know what the client means exactly by "screwed up" to identify other emotions and behaviors that need attention. It is very common for survivors of childhood sexual abuse to have intense anger at those who did not stop or prevent the abuse, and once the other steps have been taken, the nurse can begin to help the client manage his anger.

> CN: Reduction of risk potential;
> CL: Synthesize

122. **1,2,4,6.** Relaxation techniques and listening to calming music decrease anxiety and promote sleep. Quetiapine is often effective in decreasing nightmare and flashbacks and has a beneficial side effect of drowsiness. Leaving her door slightly open will decrease the noise of making 15-minute checks at night. Staying in the dayroom in a recliner with all the noise and lights is not likely to help. Processing memories an hour or two before bedtime does not allow enough time to calm down before sleep.

> CN: Psychosocial integrity;
> CL: Synthesize

123. **4.** The nurse judges the client's request for an interruption in treatment as a necessary break in treatment. A "time-out" is common and necessary to enable the client to focus on pressing problems and solutions. It is not necessarily a method of avoidance, a detriment to progress, or the end of treatment.

A problem like housing can be very stressful and require all of the client's energy and attention, with none left for the emotional stress of treatment.

> CN: Management of care; CL: Analyze

124. **1.** Combining a benzodiazepine with an antacid impairs the absorption rate of the benzodiazepine. Acetaminophen, vitamins, and aspirin are safe to take with a benzodiazepine because no major drug interactions occur.

> CN: Pharmacological and parenteral
> therapies; CL: Synthesize

125. **2.** Diazepam, like any benzodiazepine, cannot be stopped abruptly. The client must be slowly tapered off of the medication to decrease withdrawal symptoms, which would be similar to withdrawal from alcohol. Alcohol in combination with a benzodiazepine produces an increased central nervous system depressant effect and therefore should be avoided. Diazepam can cause drowsiness, and the client should be warned about driving until tolerance develops. Diazepam has muscle relaxant properties and will help tight, tense muscles feel better.

> CN: Pharmacological and parenteral
> therapies; CL: Evaluate

126. **3.** The nurse should suggest behavior therapy, which is most successful for clients with phobias. Systematic desensitization, flooding, exposure, and self-exposure treatments are most therapeutic for clients with phobias. Self-exposure treatment is being increasingly used to avoid frequent therapy sessions. Insight therapy, exploration of the dynamics of the client's personality, is not helpful because the process of anxiety underlies the disorder. Group therapy or psychoanalysis, which deals with repressed, intrapsychic conflicts, is not helpful for the client with phobias because it does not help to manage the underlying anxiety or disorder.

> CN: Psychosocial integrity; CL: Apply

127. **4.** Saying "It is a sign of progress to eat in the dining area with me" conveys positive reinforcement and gives the client hope and confidence, thus reinforcing the adaptive behavior. Stating "It was not so hard, now was it" decreases the client's self-worth and minimizes his accomplishment. Stating "At supper, I hope to see you eat with a group of people" will overwhelm the client and increase anxiety. Stating "You must have been hungry today" ignores the client's positive behavior and shows the nurse's lack of understanding of the dynamics of the disorder.

> CN: Psychosocial integrity;
> CL: Synthesize

128. **4.** The nurse should walk with the client to activate adaptive coping for the client experiencing high anxiety and decreased motivation and energy.

Stating "I know you can do it," "Try holding on to the wall," or "You can miss group this one time" maintains the client's avoidance, thus reinforcing the client's behavior, and does not help the client begin to cope with the problem.

⚷— CN: Psychosocial integrity; CL: Synthesize

129. 2. The effectiveness of St. John's wort with depression is unconfirmed. The critical issue is that the combination of St. John's wort and sertraline (an SSRI antidepressant) can produce serotonin syndrome, which can be fatal. The client should not take the St. John's wort while taking sertraline.

⚷— CN: Pharmacological and parenteral therapies; CL: Apply

130. 1. When the client says he thinks he is "going crazy," it is best for the nurse to ask him what "crazy" means to him. The nurse must have a clear idea of what the client means by his words and actions. Using an open-ended question facilitates client description to help the nurse assess his meaning. The other statements minimize and dismiss the client's concern and do not give him the opportunity to openly discuss his feelings, possibly leading to increased anxiety.

⚷— CN: Psychosocial integrity; CL: Synthesize

131. 1. A client who is exhibiting compulsive behavior is attempting to control his anxiety. The compulsive behavior is performed to relieve discomfort and to bind or neutralize anxiety. The client must perform the ritual to avoid an extreme increase in tension or anxiety even though the client is aware that the actions are absurd. The repetitive behavior is not an attempt to control thoughts; the obsession or thinking component cannot be controlled. It is not an attention-seeking mechanism or an attempt to express hostility.

⚷— CN: Psychosocial integrity; CL: Analyze

132. 2. The nurse should wake the client an hour earlier to perform his ritual so that he can be on time for breakfast with the other clients. The nurse provides the client with time needed to perform rituals because the client needs to keep his anxiety in check. The nurse should never take away a ritual, because panic will ensue. The nurse should work with the client later to slowly set limits on the frequency of the action.

⚷— CN: Pharmacological and parenteral therapies; CL: Synthesize

133. 3. The nurse conveys empathy and awareness of the client's need to reduce anxiety by showing acceptance and understanding to the client, thereby promoting trust. Ignoring the behavior, questioning

the client about her avoidance of others, or telling other clients to follow her when she moves is not therapeutic or appropriate.

⚷— CN: Psychosocial integrity; CL: Synthesize

134. 1,3,4,6. Managing suicidal thought, urges to self-mutilate, and the intense anger are critical safety issues. Then, the focus can switch to communication methods for each alter and the integration issues. Process groups can be overwhelming when too much is revealed or when child alters are unable to understand the group content. There are no known medicines to stop the process of dissociating.

⚷— CN: Management of care; CL: Create

135. 3. The no-harm contract with any destructive alters is essential along with the reminder that the alters share the same body. Later, the alter's attitudes about the client can be explored in more depth. When alter personalities emerge, their behaviors are not predictable. Restraints could not be placed on the client soon enough. There are no behaviors to justify restraints at this point. Creating a stress-free environment is not possible.

⚷— CN: Safety and infection control; CL: Synthesize

The Client with a Somatoform Disorder

136. 4. The nurse sets limits by informing the client in a matter-of-fact manner that the nurse cannot give her additional pain medication at this time. The nurse can then invite the client to participate in another activity, such as a card game, to decrease rumination about pain by directing the client's attention to an activity. By telling the client the nurse will call the **HCP** 📖 as requested, the nurse is manipulated to do what the client demands. Suggesting that the client lie down because she has to wait for the next dosage or telling the client that the HCP will be in later ignores the client and her needs and is not helpful in decreasing rumination about her pain.

⚷— CN: Psychosocial integrity; CL: Synthesize

137. 3. The nurse instructs the **UAP** 📖 to invite the client to lunch and accompany him to the dining room to decrease manipulation, secondary gain, dependency, and reinforcement of negative behavior while maintaining the client's self-worth. Taking the client a lunch tray and allowing him to eat in his room reinforces negative behaviors and secondary gain. Telling the client he will need to wait until supper to eat if he misses lunch or informing the client that he has 10 minutes to get to the dining room challenges the client and may increase feelings of anger and the need for physical complaints.

>🔑 CN: Management of care; CL: Synthesize

138. 2. Pushing insight or awareness into conflicts or problems increases anxiety and the need for physical symptoms to handle or take care of the anxiety. Awareness or insight must be developed slowly as the client's need for symptoms diminishes. Saying "Ignore the client's behavior and treat her with respect" is not helpful to the staff member or the client. This statement fails to educate the staff member about the client's disorder and simply dismisses the needs of both. It is not true that pushing awareness will be helpful and further the client's recovery; this is the opposite of what is needed. Meeting with the client to confront her behavior is not therapeutic and will greatly increase the client's anxiety and the need for the conversion symptoms.

>🔑 CN: Management of care; CL: Synthesize

139. 2. The nurse helps the client to focus on his feelings about his impending divorce to decrease the client's anxiety and decrease his focus on physical ailments. The client with a somatoform disorder typically has problems with identifying, describing, and dealing with feelings. Internalizing feelings leads to increased anxiety and the need for protective mechanisms. Asking the client to describe his problem with nausea, allowing the client to talk about the many HCP 📖 he has seen and the medications he has taken, and informing the client about a different medication for nausea are counterproductive toward recovery because they reinforce the focus on the symptoms.

>🔑 CN: Psychosocial integrity; CL: Synthesize

140. 4. The nurse should redirect the interaction back to fishing or another focus whenever the client begins to ruminate about physical symptoms or impairment. Doing so helps the client talk about topics that are more therapeutic and beneficial to recovery. Allowing the client to talk about his pain or asking if he needs additional pain medication is not therapeutic because it reinforces the client's need for the symptom. Getting up and leaving the client is not appropriate unless the nurse has set limits previously by saying "I will get up and leave if you continue to talk about your pain."

>🔑 CN: Psychosocial integrity; CL: Synthesize

141. 1. The client who states "I understand my pain will feel worse when I am worried about my divorce" recognizes the connection between his pain and the divorce and indicates developing insight into his problem. The nurse should then be able to assist the client with developing adaptive

coping strategies. The other statements indicate a lack of insight into his disorder and lack of progress toward recovery. The client is still searching for the "right" diagnosis, medication, and HCP 📖.

>🔑 CN: Psychosocial integrity; CL: Evaluate

Managing Care, Quality, and Safety of Clients with Personality Disorders, Substance-Related Disorders, Anxiety Disorders, and Anxiety-Related Disorders

142. 3,1,2,4. The nurse should first obtain a prescription for and administer diazepam to stop the status epilepticus. The nurse should next prevent injury by using seizure pads. Recording the time, duration, and nature of the seizures will be important for ongoing treatment. Finally, the nurse can attempt to obtain information about medication use and abuse history from the friend until the client is able to do so for himself.

>🔑 CN: Safety and infection control; CL: Synthesize

143. 1. Having a UAP 📖 stay with the client provides for reassurance and safety. Being next to the nursing desk will increase stimuli and confusion. Being alone will increase the client's fears and anxiety. It is inappropriate to ask the boyfriend to provide client supervision for the nurse.

>🔑 CN: Safety and infection control; CL: Synthesize

144. 5,2,4,3,1,6. After orienting the client to time and place, the nurse should assure constant observation of the client to prevent the client from getting hurt. The administration of the haloperidol and lorazepam is needed to quickly decrease the symptoms of delirium tremens (DTs) and lower the vital signs. Monitoring vital signs assesses the client's stability and need for additional medications. The nurse can ask another staff to contact the **healthcare provider (HCP)** 📖 to request a prescription for restraints in case the client becomes violent toward self or others. After the DT symptoms subside, the haloperidol would be stopped due to the decrease in the seizure threshold. Other detoxification protocols would then begin. Last, chart the client's response.

>🔑 CN: Safety and infection control; CL: Synthesize

145. 2. The statement "The client is a weak individual and could stop if he desires" is false and indicates a lack of understanding regarding alcohol dependency. Criteria for substance dependency include the inability to stop using even when wanting to do so. The client cannot stop or control the amount used when dependent on a substance. Alcohol dependency affects individuals from every culture and socioeconomic background and has nothing to do with being a "weak" individual. The devastating effects of alcohol dependency are felt by every member of the family and not just the individual with the alcohol problem. Family members need education about the physical, physiologic, and psychological effects of alcohol and referrals to self-help groups for support. They have felt and lived with the devastating effects of the disease. A simple and commonly held view of alcoholism is that alcohol is a problem when it interferes with life or disrupts family, work, or social relationships.

CN: Management of care; CL: Evaluate

146. 1. Some behavior that is legally allowed might not be considered ethically appropriate. Legal and ethical standards are often linked, such as in the commandment "Thou shalt not kill." Ethical standards are never irrelevant, though a client's safety or the safety of others may pose an ethical dilemma for healthcare personnel. Searching a client's room when he or she is not there is a violation of privacy. Room searches can be done with an **HCP's** 📖 prescription and generally are done with the client present.

CN: Management of care; CL: Apply

147. 1,2,4,3. The nurse should first provide for safety of the client and the staff by requesting assistance from the security department. Next, the nurse should obtain an ECG because the client reports having chest pain. The nurse should then obtain a urine sample to identify if the client has been using illegal drugs. When the client is stabilized, the nurse

can develop a care plan that includes treatment goals to support the respiratory and cardiovascular functions and enhance clearance of the agent and initiate a referral for treatment where access to the drug is eliminated and drug rehabilitation is provided as part of therapeutic management of clients with substance abuse and/or a drug overdose.

CN: Reduction of risk potential; CL: Analyze

148. 2. Recognizing that the clients are part of the solution to the issues they are presenting demonstrates a client-centered approach to care. Having the new clients challenge the behaviors of other clients does not facilitate the development of a therapeutic milieu. Warning clients that behaviors are unacceptable reinforces a sense of client powerlessness and does not build a therapeutic relationship. Discussing respect and collaboration would happen after the criticisms have been acknowledged and the clients have been asked for their opinions.

CN: Management of care; CL: Synthesize

149. 4. The discharge teaching session will be most effective if the nurse uses a client-centered approach to better assess what the client needs and, therefore, what information to share. Sharing all the information does not respect the knowledge that the client already has. Reviewing the policies is one area to help identify important areas for teaching, but in order to ensure that client needs are met, further assessment is required. Awareness of personal biases should not be used to determine what is important for the client.

CN: Management of care; CL: Synthesize

TEST 4

Stress, Crisis, Anger, and Violence

- The Client Managing Stress
- The Client Coping with Physical Illness
- The Client in Crisis
- The Client with Problems Expressing Anger
- The Client with Interpersonal Violence
- Managing Care, Quality, and Safety of Clients with Stress, Crisis, Anger, and Violence
- Answers, Rationales, and Test-Taking Strategies

The Client Managing Stress

1. The nurse cares for a middle-aged client with a below-the-knee amputation. Which statement indicates the need for further assessment of the client's body image?
- ☐ **1.** "When I get my prosthesis, I want to learn to walk so I can participate in walkathons."
- ☐ **2.** "I hope to get skilled enough at using my prosthesis to help others like me adjust."
- ☐ **3.** "Whenever I start to feel sorry for myself, I remember that my buddy died in that accident."
- ☐ **4.** "I hope I can handle having a prosthesis, but I am really wondering what my wife will think."

2. A 75-year-old client is newly diagnosed with diabetes. The nurse is instructing him about blood glucose testing. After the session, the client states, "I cannot be expected to remember all this stuff." The nurse should recognize this response as **most** likely related to which factor?
- ☐ **1.** moderate to severe anxiety
- ☐ **2.** disinterest in the illness
- ☐ **3.** early-onset dementia
- ☐ **4.** normal reaction to learning a new skill

3. A client in a general hospital is to undergo surgery in 2 days. He is experiencing moderate anxiety about the procedure and its outcome. To help the client reduce his anxiety, the nurse should:
- ☐ **1.** tell the client to distract himself with games and television.
- ☐ **2.** reassure the client that he will come through surgery without incident.
- ☐ **3.** explain the surgical procedure to the client and what happens before and after surgery.
- ☐ **4.** ask the surgeon to refer the client to a psychiatrist who can work with the client to diminish his anxiety.

4. Anxiety occurs in degrees, from a level that stimulates productive problem solving to a level that is severely debilitating. At a mild, productive level of anxiety, the nurse should expect to see what cognitive characteristic of mild anxiety?
- ☐ **1.** slight muscle tension
- ☐ **2.** occasional irritability
- ☐ **3.** accurate perceptions
- ☐ **4.** loss of contact with reality

5. As a client's level of anxiety increases to a debilitating degree, the nurse should expect which psychomotor behavior as indicating a panic level of anxiety?
- ☐ **1.** suicide attempts and violence
- ☐ **2.** desperation and rage
- ☐ **3.** disorganized reasoning
- ☐ **4.** loss of contact with reality

6. Nursing interventions with an anxious client change as the anxiety level increases. At a low level of anxiety, what is the primary focus of intervention?
- ☐ **1.** taking control of the situation for the client
- ☐ **2.** learning and problem solving
- ☐ **3.** reducing stimuli and pressure
- ☐ **4.** using tension reduction activities

7. When coping becomes dysfunctional enough to require the client to be admitted to the hospital, the nurse expects that the client would be exhibiting what behaviors?
- ☐ **1.** objective and rational problem solving
- ☐ **2.** tension reduction activities and then problem solving
- ☐ **3.** anger management strategies with no problem solving
- ☐ **4.** minimal functioning with new problems developing

8. In addition to teaching assertiveness and problem-solving skills when helping the client cope effectively with stress and anxiety, the nurse should also address the client's ability to:
- ☐ 1. suppress anger.
- ☐ 2. balance a checkbook.
- ☐ 3. follow step-by-step directions.
- ☐ 4. use conflict resolution skills.

9. Which client statement indicates that the client has coped effectively with a relationship problem?
- ☐ 1. "My wife will be happy to know that I can spend less time at work now."
- ☐ 2. "My wife and I are talking about our likes and dislikes in activities."
- ☐ 3. "I can understand how my wife and I see things differently."
- ☐ 4. "We are really listening to each other about our different views on issues."

10. In an ongoing assessment, the nurse should identify the client's thoughts and feelings about a situation in addition to what other factors?
- ☐ 1. whether the client's behavior is appropriate in the context of the current situation
- ☐ 2. whether the client is motivated to decrease dysfunctional behaviors
- ☐ 3. which of the client's problems have the highest priority
- ☐ 4. which of the client's behaviors necessitates a no-harm contract

11. What short-term goal for a client hospitalized with a stress-related disorder is **most** realistic?
- ☐ 1. The client will demonstrate a positive self-image.
- ☐ 2. The client will describe plans for how to get back into school.
- ☐ 3. The client will write a list of strengths and needs.
- ☐ 4. The client will practice assertiveness skills in confronting his mother.

12. A nurse is counseling a client with cancer who is experiencing anxiety. Which goal will provide the **best** long-term client outcome?
- ☐ 1. Keep follow-up appointments with mental health providers.
- ☐ 2. Understand medication effects and adverse effects.
- ☐ 3. Take medication as prescribed.
- ☐ 4. Solve problems independently.

13. When integrating the concepts underlying the cognitive-behavioral model into a client's plan of care, the nurse should focus on what area?
- ☐ 1. substitution of rational beliefs for self-defeating thinking and behaving
- ☐ 2. insight into unconscious conflicts and processes
- ☐ 3. analysis of fears and barriers to growth
- ☐ 4. reduction of bodily tensions and stress management

14. Which client statement indicates that the client has gained insight into his use of the defense mechanism of displacement?
- ☐ 1. "I cannot think about the weekend right now. I have got to study for the exam."
- ☐ 2. "I know I am not good in sports, but I feel good about my grades."
- ☐ 3. "Now when I am mad at my wife, I talk to her instead of taking it out on the kids."
- ☐ 4. "For years I could not remember being molested; now I know I have to face it."

15. In which situation can a client's confidentiality be breached legally?
- ☐ 1. to answer a request from a client's spouse about the client's medication
- ☐ 2. in a student nurse's clinical paper about a client
- ☐ 3. when a client near discharge is threatening to harm an ex-partner
- ☐ 4. when a client's employer requests the client's diagnosis to initiate medical claims

16. A client is admitted after the police found he had been sleeping in his car for three nights. The client says, "My wife kicked me out and is divorcing me. It was not my fault I was fired from work. My wife and boss are plotting against me because I am smarter than they are." He then pounds the table and says, "I am not staying here, and you cannot stop me." What should be included in the client's **immediate** plan of care? Select all that apply.
- ☐ 1. collateral information from his wife and boss
- ☐ 2. anxiety and anger management
- ☐ 3. appropriate housing
- ☐ 4. divorce counseling
- ☐ 5. assault and escape precautions
- ☐ 6. suspiciousness and grandiosity issues

17. What is a crucial goal of therapeutic communication when helping the client deal with personal issues and painful feelings?
- ☐ 1. communicating empathy through gentle touch
- ☐ 2. conveying client respect and acceptance even if not all of the client's behaviors are tolerated
- ☐ 3. mutual sharing of information, spontaneity, emotions, and intimacy
- ☐ 4. guaranteeing total confidentiality and anonymity for the client

18. An 18-year-old pregnant college student presented at the prenatal clinic for an initial visit at 14 weeks' gestation. The client's history revealed that when she was 12, she and her mother survived a plane crash that killed her father and sister. Since that time, she has taken fluoxetine 20 mg orally daily for posttraumatic stress disorder (PTSD) and depression. Her medication was recently increased to 40 mg daily because of reports of increased stress and suicide ideation. Which side effect of fluoxetine would the nurse judge to be the greatest risk for the client and her developing fetus at this stage in her pregnancy?
- ☐ **1.** insomnia
- ☐ **2.** nausea/anorexia
- ☐ **3.** headache
- ☐ **4.** decreased libido

19. Which probe should the nurse use to encourage client evaluation of his or her own behavior?
- ☐ **1.** "I can hear that it is still hard for you to talk about this."
- ☐ **2.** "So what does this all mean to you now?"
- ☐ **3.** "What did you do differently with your coworker this time?"
- ☐ **4.** "What will it take to carry out your new plans?"

20. Even when the client understands problems and is motivated to change, the client may have fears about failing. Which intervention is **most** likely to facilitate change?
- ☐ **1.** reality testing about the need for change
- ☐ **2.** asking the client about fears that need to be overcome
- ☐ **3.** teaching new communication skills
- ☐ **4.** having client practicing new behaviors

The Client Coping with Physical Illness

21. A mastectomy is recommended for a 68-year-old client diagnosed with breast cancer a week ago. When approached about giving consent for the mastectomy, the client says, "What is the use in trying to get rid of the cancer? It will just come back! I cannot handle another thing—having diabetes is enough. Besides, I am getting old. It would be different if I were younger and had more energy." What should the nurse do?
- ☐ **1.** Accept the client's decision since it is her right to choose to obtain treatment or not.
- ☐ **2.** Give the client information about the 5- and 10-year survival rates for breast cancer clients who underwent mastectomies.
- ☐ **3.** Call the chaplain to speak with the client about her hopeless attitude about the future.
- ☐ **4.** Explore with the client her feelings about her health problems and proposed surgery.

22. An 18-year-old client is recently diagnosed with leukemia. What is the **most** appropriate short-term goal for the nurse and client to establish?
- ☐ **1.** accepting the client's death as imminent
- ☐ **2.** expressing the client's angry feelings to the nurse
- ☐ **3.** decreasing interaction with peers to conserve energy
- ☐ **4.** gaining an intellectual understanding of the illness

23. The nurse has been asked to develop a medication education program for clients with chronic mental illness in the rehabilitation program. When developing the course outline, which topic is **most** important to include?
- ☐ **1.** a categorization of many psychotropic drugs
- ☐ **2.** interventions for common side effects of psychotropic drugs
- ☐ **3.** the role of medication in the treatment of acute illness
- ☐ **4.** effects of combining common street drugs with psychotropic medication

24. The healthcare provider (HCP) recommends that a client have a partial bowel resection and an ileostomy. Later, the client says to the nurse, "That doctor of mine surely likes to play big. I will bet the more he can cut, the better he likes it." Which reply by the nurse is **most** therapeutic?
- ☐ **1.** "I can tell you more about the surgery if you like."
- ☐ **2.** "What do you mean by that statement?"
- ☐ **3.** "Why do you not think about getting a second opinion?"
- ☐ **4.** "Does that remark have something to do with the operation he wants you to have?"

25. A client becomes increasingly irritable after being told that she has cancer. She is rude to visitors and pushes nurses away when they attempt to give her medications and treatments. What should the nurse do when the client has a hostile outburst?
- ☐ **1.** Offer the client positive reinforcement each time she cooperates.
- ☐ **2.** Encourage the client to discuss her immediate concerns and feelings.
- ☐ **3.** Continue with the assigned tasks and duties as though nothing has happened.
- ☐ **4.** Limit visitation until the client is less irritable.

26. Arrangements are made for a member of the colostomy support group to meet with a client before bowel surgery. What is accomplished by having a representative from the group meet the client preoperatively?
- ☐ **1.** letting the client know that he has resources in the community to help him
- ☐ **2.** providing support for the healthcare provider's (HCP's) plan of therapy for the client
- ☐ **3.** providing the client with support and realistic information on the colostomy
- ☐ **4.** convincing the client that he will not be disfigured and can lead a full life

27. The client hospitalized for diagnosis and treatment of atrial fibrillation states to the nurse, "Please hand me the telephone. I need to check on my stocks and bonds." Which response by the nurse is **most** therapeutic?

☐ 1. "You will get more upset if you make that call."

☐ 2. "You have atrial fibrillations. Let us talk about what that means."

☐ 3. "You really do not care about the fact that you are sick, do you?"

☐ 4. "Do you realize you have a life-threatening condition?"

28. Which statement would lead the nurse to determine that a client lacks understanding of her acute cardiac illness and the ability to make changes in her lifestyle?

☐ 1. "I already have my airline ticket, so I will not miss my meeting tomorrow."

☐ 2. "These relaxation tapes sound okay; I will see if they help me."

☐ 3. "No more working 10 hours a day for me unless it is an emergency."

☐ 4. "I talked with my husband yesterday about working on a new budget together."

29. A client has been rehospitalized with a severe exacerbation of lupus. Her husband approaches the nurse and says, "My wife is scaring me. She says she does not want to live with this illness anymore. Our kids are grown, and she feels useless as a mother and a wife." Which statements are the **most** appropriate responses to the husband? Select all that apply.

☐ 1. "I will have a talk with your wife to see if she is suicidal."

☐ 2. "You need to be strong and optimistic when you are with her."

☐ 3. "I am glad you shared this with me. I can imagine that this is scary for you."

☐ 4. "I am sure she will feel differently when we get this episode under control."

☐ 5. "We can talk about what you can say to her that may help."

30. The client with kidney stones refuses to eat lunch and rudely tells the nurse to get out of his room. Which response by the nurse is **most** appropriate?

☐ 1. "I will leave, but you need to eat."

☐ 2. "I will get you something for your pain."

☐ 3. "Your anger does not bother me. I will be back later."

☐ 4. "You sound angry. What is upsetting you?"

31. A client diagnosed with ulcerative colitis also experiences obsessive-compulsive anxiety disorder (OCD). In helping the client understand her illness, the nurse should respond with which statement?

☐ 1. "Your ulcerative colitis has made you perfectionistic, and it has caused your OCD."

☐ 2. "There is no relationship at all between your colitis and your OCD. They are separate disorders."

☐ 3. "The perfectionism and anxiety related to your obsessions and compulsions have led to your colitis."

☐ 4. "It is possible that your desire to have everything be perfect has caused stress that may have worsened your colitis, but there is no proof that either disorder caused the other."

32. A client receiving dialysis directs profanities at the nurse and then abruptly hangs his head and pleads, "Please forgive me. Something just came over me. Why do I say those things?" The nurse interprets this as which finding?

☐ 1. neologism

☐ 2. confabulation

☐ 3. flight of ideas

☐ 4. emotional lability

33. On an oncology unit, the nurse hears noises coming from a client's room. The client is found throwing objects at the walls and has just picked up the phone and is screaming, "How can God do this to me? It is the third type of cancer I have had. I have gone through all the treatment for nothing." In what order of priority from first to last should the nurse make the interventions? All options must be used.

1. "Tell me what you are feeling right now."

2. "Please put the telephone down so we can talk."

3. "I can hear how upset you are about the cancer."

4. "I wonder if you would like to talk to a clergyman."

34. A client who has had AIDS for years is being treated for a serious episode of pneumonia. A psychiatric nurse consult was arranged after the client stated that he was tired of being in and out of the hospital. "I am not coming in here anymore. I have other options." The nurse would evaluate the psychiatric nurse consult as helpful if the client makes which statements?

- ☐ 1. "Nobody wants me to commit suicide."
- ☐ 2. "If I talk about suicide, I will be transferred to the psychiatric unit."
- ☐ 3. "I realize that I really do have more time to enjoy my family and friends."
- ☐ 4. "I would probably screw up suicide anyway."

The Client in Crisis

35. The nurse's overall goal in planning to assist the client responding to a loss is to:

- ☐ 1. make sure the client progresses through all of the stages of the grief process.
- ☐ 2. encourage the client to work to resolve lingering family conflicts.
- ☐ 3. assist the client to engage in the work associated with the normal grieving process.
- ☐ 4. allow the client to express anger.

36. The nurse working at the site of a severe flood sees a woman, standing in knee-deep water, staring at an empty lot. The woman states, "I keep thinking that this is a nightmare and that I will wake up and see that my house is still there." Which crisis intervention strategies are **most** needed at this time? Select all that apply.

- ☐ 1. Ask the client about any physical injuries she may have.
- ☐ 2. Determine if any of her family are injured or missing.
- ☐ 3. Allow the client to talk about her fears, anger, and other feelings.
- ☐ 4. Tell her that groups are being formed at the shelter for flood survivors.
- ☐ 5. Refer her to the shelter for dry clothes and food.
- ☐ 6. Assess her for risk of suicide and other signs of decompensation.

37. The nurse is assessing a client who has just experienced a crisis. The nurse should **first** assess this client for which behavior?

- ☐ 1. effective problem solving
- ☐ 2. level of anxiety
- ☐ 3. attention span
- ☐ 4. help seeking

38. The nurse is working with a family in crisis. What should the nurse do in order of priority from first to last? All options must be used.

1. Make a plan for managing the crisis.

2. Develop strategies to reduce symptoms.

3. Assess the family's resources.

4. Identify the family member in crisis.

39. An anxious young adult is brought to the interviewing room of a crisis shelter, sobbing and saying that she thinks she is pregnant but does not know what to do. Which nursing intervention is **most** appropriate at this time?

- ☐ 1. Ask the client about the type of things that she had thought of doing.
- ☐ 2. Give the client some ideas about what to expect to happen next.
- ☐ 3. Recommend a pregnancy test after acknowledging the client's distress.
- ☐ 4. Question the client about her feelings and possible parental reactions.

40. A potentially pregnant 16-year-old client says that she has been "hooking up" with a boy she considers to be her boyfriend. Which response should the nurse make **first**?

- ☐ 1. "You mean you have had sexual intercourse?"
- ☐ 2. "Describe what you mean by hooking up."
- ☐ 3. "I think we need to talk about what is involved in sexual intercourse."
- ☐ 4. "All you have been doing with your boyfriend is hooking up?"

41. A 40-year-old client who is quite anxious says that she would "rather die than be pregnant." Which response by the nurse is **most** helpful?
- ☐ 1. "Try not to worry until after the pregnancy test."
- ☐ 2. "You know, pregnancy is a normal event."
- ☐ 3. "You are only 40 years old and not too old to have a baby."
- ☐ 4. "I see you are upset. Take some deep breaths to relax a little."

42. On a crisis shelter hotline, the nurse talks to two 11-year-old boys who think a friend sniffs glue. They say his breath sometimes smells like glue and he acts drunk. They say they are afraid to tell their parents about the friend. When formulating a reply, what is **most** important factor for the nurse to consider?
- ☐ 1. The boys probably fear punishment.
- ☐ 2. Sniffing glue is illegal.
- ☐ 3. The boys' observations could be wrong.
- ☐ 4. Glue sniffing is a minor form of substance abuse.

43. While the nurse is teaching a group of volunteers for a crisis hotline, a volunteer asks, "What if I am not sure why someone is calling?" Which statement by the nurse is **most** helpful?
- ☐ 1. "Ask the caller to tell you why he or she is calling you today."
- ☐ 2. "Tell the caller to make an appointment at the walk-in crisis clinic."
- ☐ 3. "Instruct the caller to go to the nearest emergency department."
- ☐ 4. "Tell the caller to let you speak to anyone else in the house."

44. After teaching a group of students who are volunteering for a local crisis hotline, the nurse judges that further education about crisis and intervention is needed when a student makes which statement?
- ☐ 1. "Callers to a crisis line use this service when they are overwhelmed and exhausted."
- ☐ 2. "People use crisis hotlines when they are in the most pain and nothing is working for them."
- ☐ 3. "Most people in crisis will be calling the line once every day for at least a year."
- ☐ 4. "One benefit is that a person will know how to handle stressful situations better in the future."

45. An adolescent woman, whose family is living in a cult, ran away from the group's compound to her aunt's house. The aunt brought the girl to the emergency department after finding multiple knife cuts in various stages of healing on the girl's body. She is admitted to the unit because of many trauma-related symptoms. What actions should the nurse take? Select all that apply.
- ☐ 1. Ask her to describe her experiences in a discussion group with other teens.
- ☐ 2. Teach her emotion management skills to help her deal with her "normal reactions to an abnormal situation."
- ☐ 3. Assess her for other possible injuries, pregnancy, and sexually transmitted infections.
- ☐ 4. Teach her ways to control self-destructive behaviors such as suicide attempts, self-mutilation, and rage outbursts.
- ☐ 5. Obtain a sample for a urine drug screen and routine urinalysis.
- ☐ 6. Help her process her emotions and memories as she is willing to share these.

46. A true crisis state, involving a period of severe disorganization, is difficult to endure emotionally and physically. The nurse recognizes that a client will only be able to tolerate being in crisis for how long?
- ☐ 1. 1 to 2 weeks
- ☐ 2. 4 to 6 weeks
- ☐ 3. 12 to 14 weeks
- ☐ 4. 24 to 26 weeks

47. The nurse incorporates the underlying premise of crisis intervention, about providing "the right kind of help at the right time," to achieve which initial goal?
- ☐ 1. regaining emotional security and equilibrium
- ☐ 2. resolution of underlying emotional problems
- ☐ 3. development of insight and personal growth
- ☐ 4. formulation of more effective support systems

48. The nurse understands that with the right help at the right time, a client can successfully resolve a crisis and function better than before the crisis, based primarily on which factor?
- ☐ 1. relinquishment of dysfunctional coping
- ☐ 2. reestablishment of lost support systems
- ☐ 3. acquisition of new coping skills
- ☐ 4. gain of crisis prevention knowledge

49. A client is being discharged after 3 days of hospitalization for a suicide attempt that followed the receipt of a divorce notice. Which client finding indicates to the nurse that the client is ready for discharge?
- ☐ 1. Expresses a readiness for discharge.
- ☐ 2. Has the names and phone numbers of two divorce lawyers.
- ☐ 3. Has a list of support persons and community resources.
- ☐ 4. Displays emotional stability.

50. A distraught father is waiting for his son to come out of surgery. He accidentally backed the car into his son, causing multiple fractures and a serious head injury. Which statement by the father would **most** alert the nurse to the need for a psychiatric consultation?
- [ ] 1. "My son will be fine, but I may be charged with reckless driving."
- [ ] 2. "This accident will probably cost me my marriage."
- [ ] 3. "I just did not see him run behind the car."
- [ ] 4. "If he dies, there will be nothing for me to do but join him."

51. A grandson calls the crisis center expressing concern about his grandmother, who lost her husband a month ago. He states, "She has been in bed for a week and is not eating or showering. She told me that she did not want to kill herself, but it is not like her to do nothing for herself. She will not even talk to me when I visit her." The nurse encourages the grandson to bring his grandmother to the center for evaluation based on which reason?
- [ ] 1. The behaviors may reflect passive suicidal thoughts.
- [ ] 2. The behaviors reflect altered role performance.
- [ ] 3. Seeing the grandson and grandmother together will be helpful.
- [ ] 4. Refusing to talk to the grandson alone indicates a major problem.

52. A 16-year-old client who is being seen by the crisis nurse after making several superficial cuts on her wrist states that all her friends are siding with her ex-boyfriend and will not talk to her anymore. She says she knows that the relationship is over, but "If I cannot have him, no one else will." Which client problem takes the **highest priority**?
- [ ] 1. situational low self-esteem
- [ ] 2. risk for other-directed violence
- [ ] 3. risk for suicide
- [ ] 4. risk-prone health behavior

53. A client who comes to the crisis center in a very distressed state tells the nurse, "I just cannot get over being fired last week. I have asked for help. I have talked to friends. I have tried everything to get through this, but nothing is working. Help me!" Which initial crisis intervention strategy should the nurse use?
- [ ] 1. referral for counseling
- [ ] 2. support system assessment
- [ ] 3. emotion management
- [ ] 4. unemployment assistance

54. A major role in crisis intervention is getting a client's family and friends involved in helping with the immediate crisis as soon as possible. The nurse should determine that the support persons are prepared to help when they verbalize what information?
- [ ] 1. the name and phone number of the client's healthcare provider (HCP)
- [ ] 2. emergency resources and when to use them
- [ ] 3. the coping strategies they are using
- [ ] 4. long-term solutions they plan to tell the client to use

55. During the interview at a crisis center, a newly widowed client reveals the wish "to join my husband in Heaven." After the nurse asks the client to sign a no-harm contract, which question is appropriate to use **next**?
- [ ] 1. "What feelings you have been experiencing?"
- [ ] 2. "Have you considered taking antidepressants?"
- [ ] 3. "What was the cause of your husband's death?"
- [ ] 4. "Do you have children who are willing to help you?"

56. A nurse manager of the crisis access center of a psychiatric facility in a major city notices a sudden increase in the number of incoming calls one afternoon. After quickly surveying the call sheets, the nurse finds that most callers are very anxious after military aircraft flew very low over the city. Which strategies would be **most** appropriate in this situation? Select all that apply.
- [ ] 1. Instruct the crisis workers to additionally screen callers about where they were on 9/11/01 and their memories of that event.
- [ ] 2. Give the crisis workers a list of symptoms of posttraumatic stress disorder (PTSD) and techniques for dealing with these symptoms.
- [ ] 3. Ask for an emergency meeting with the managers of the inpatient and outpatient services to formulate a contingency plan for increased services if needed.
- [ ] 4. Ask the major media outlets in the city to make a scripted public service announcement about the possible recurrence of symptoms experienced after the events of 9/11/01.
- [ ] 5. Prepare for a scripted interview with the local media about PTSD symptoms and techniques for dealing with these symptoms.
- [ ] 6. Ask the director of psychiatric services to call the military to issue an apology for the flyover.

The Client with Problems Expressing Anger

57. A 35-year-old man was experiencing marital discord with his wife of 4 years. When his wife walked out, he became angry, throwing things, and breaking dishes. A friend talked him into seeking help at the local mental health center. Which of these questions should the nurse ask **initially** to begin to assess this man's immediate problem?
- ☐ 1. "Do you feel in control of yourself at this time?"
- ☐ 2. "What did you do to cause your wife to leave?"
- ☐ 3. "In hindsight, how might you have managed this situation differently?"
- ☐ 4. "What led you to come in for help today?"

58. A client is being admitted to a psychiatric outpatient program for counseling for his ongoing emotional symptoms. He is asked to rate the severity of his depression, anxiety, and anger. He states, "I do not have any anger any more. I lost my temper once and nearly hurt my wife. I never got angry again." In which order of priority from first to last should the principles related to anger be shared with this client? All options must be used.

1. "You can learn effective ways to discuss anger with others and still maintain control."

2. "Anger is a natural emotion occurring in all human relationships."

3. "Holding your anger inside contributes to your depression."

4. "Unexpressed anger has a negative effect on the human body and mind."

59. The father of a soldier who was killed 2 days ago is admitted after a serious suicide attempt. He is medically stable and has signed a no-harm contract. During a talk with the nurse, he says, "Terrorism and war are holding me and the whole world hostage. It is so unfair. I would rather be dead than live alone in constant fear." Which nursing interventions are important in the next few days? Select all that apply.
- ☐ 1. discussing effective ways to express justifiable anger
- ☐ 2. teaching stress management and relaxation techniques
- ☐ 3. identifying community groups for relatives of military personnel
- ☐ 4. recommending an antiwar advocacy group
- ☐ 5. strategizing about ways to increase a personal sense of security

60. In developing a plan of care for a client who has had previous episodes of angry verbal outbursts, the nurse plans to take an educational approach to the problem. Arrange the steps the nurse should take from first to last. All options must be used.

1. Assist the client to recognize the early cues that he is angry.

2. Help the client identify triggers for his anger.

3. Practice with the client appropriate ways to express his anger.

4. Identify alternate ways to express his anger.

61. The treatment team recommends that a client take an assertiveness training class offered in the hospital. Which behavior indicates that the client is becoming more assertive?
- ☐ 1. The client arrives late for unit activities, and when asked why he is late, he says, "Because I feel like it!"
- ☐ 2. The client asks the nurse to call his employer about his insurance.
- ☐ 3. The client asks his roommate to put away his dirty clothes because the untidiness bothers him.
- ☐ 4. The client follows the nurse's advice of asking his healthcare provider (HCP) about being passive aggressive.

62. Which physiologic response should the nurse expect as **unlikely** to occur when a client is angry?
- ☐ 1. increased respiratory rate
- ☐ 2. decreased blood pressure
- ☐ 3. increased muscle tension
- ☐ 4. decreased peristalsis

63. When planning the care of a client experiencing aggression, the nurse incorporates the principle of "least restrictive alternative," meaning that less restrictive interventions must be tried before more restrictive measures are employed. What measures should the nurse consider to be the **most** restrictive?
- ☐ 1. tension reduction strategies
- ☐ 2. haloperidol given orally
- ☐ 3. voluntary seclusion or time-out
- ☐ 4. haloperidol given intramuscularly

64. As an angry client becomes more agitated while talking about his problems, the nurse decides to ask for staff assistance in taking control of the situation when the client demonstrates which behavior?
- ☐ 1. swearing about his wife's behaviors when discussing marital problems
- ☐ 2. picking up a pool cue stick and telling the nurse to get out of his way
- ☐ 3. making a fist and pounding loudly on the table
- ☐ 4. coming out of his room instead of staying in time-out

65. The nurse is advising a client with schizophrenia about what to do when she begins to get agitated. The client has been compliant with taking her medications and has worked with clinic staff on dealing with her illness and recognizing when she is becoming agitated. Indicate the order from first to last in which the nurse should suggest the actions be taken. All options must be used.

1. "Take your oral lorazepam."

2. "Take your oral haloperidol."

3. "Go to a quiet place."

4. "Tell trusted people that you are becoming upset."

66. When a client is about to lose control, the extra staff who come to help commonly stay at a distance from the client unless asked to move closer by the nurse who is talking to the client. What **best** explains the primary rationale for staying at a distance initially?
- ☐ 1. The client is more likely to act out if there is an audience, even additional staff.
- ☐ 2. The nurse talking to the client makes the decisions about other staff actions.
- ☐ 3. The client is likely to perceive others as being closer than they are and feel threatened.
- ☐ 4. When the extra staff is visible, the client is less likely to regain self-control.

67. When preparing to use seclusion as an alternative to restraint for a client who has not yet lost control, the nurse expects to use a room with limited furniture and no access to dangerous articles. What should the nurse also consider as critical for the safety of the client?
- ☐ 1. a security window in the door or a room camera
- ☐ 2. lights that can be dimmed from outside the room
- ☐ 3. a staff member to stay in the room with the client
- ☐ 4. a prescription for the seclusion before it is initiated

68. The nurse is required initially to restrain all four of a client's extremities. For what reason would the nurse anticipate the need to add a full-length restraint blanket?
- ☐ 1. The client states that restraints are tight and uncomfortable.
- ☐ 2. The staff want extra protection for themselves.
- ☐ 3. The client is at risk for injury from fighting the restraints.
- ☐ 4. Staff assessment reveals that the client will feel more secure under the blanket.

69. Which nursing intervention is the **highest priority** when a client is placed in restraints?
- ☐ 1. monitoring the client every 15 minutes
- ☐ 2. assisting with nutrition and elimination
- ☐ 3. performing range-of-motion exercise for each limb, one at a time
- ☐ 4. changing the client's position every 2 hours

70. According to hospital protocol, after a client is restrained, the staff meet and discuss the restraint situation. In addition to sharing feelings and offering support, what should the nurse identify as the long-term goal for the debriefing?
- ☐ 1. providing feedback to each other on how procedures were handled
- ☐ 2. comparing the perceptions of the various staff members
- ☐ 3. deciding when to release the client from restraints
- ☐ 4. improving the staff's use of restraint procedures

The Client with Interpersonal Violence

71. A client was brought to the unit and admitted involuntarily. During visiting the next day, the client's brother demands that the client be released immediately. The brother says he might have to hurt staff if the unit door is not opened. In which order of priority from first to last should the nursing actions be implemented? All options must be used.

1. Call security officers to the unit for the protection of all on the unit.

2. Calmly restate to the client and his brother that the client cannot be released without a healthcare provider's (HCP's) prescription.

3. Quietly ask the other clients and visitors to move to another area of the unit with a staff member.

4. Ask the client's brother to leave the unit quietly when he repeats his demands.

72. Based on a client's history of violence toward others and inability to cope with anger, what should the nurse use as the **most** important indicator of goal achievement before discharge?
- ☐ 1. acknowledgment of the client's angry feelings
- ☐ 2. ability to describe situations that provoke angry feelings
- ☐ 3. development of a list of how anger has been handled in the past
- ☐ 4. verbalization of her feelings in an appropriate manner

73. A client is admitted to the psychiatric hospital for evaluation after numerous incidents of threatening others, angry outbursts, and two episodes of hitting a coworker at the grocery store where he works. The client is very anxious and tells the nurse who admits him, "I did not mean to hit him. He made me so mad that I just could not help it. I hope I do not hit anyone here." To ensure a safe environment, the nurse should **first:**
- ☐ 1. let other clients know that he has a history of hitting others so that they will not provoke him.
- ☐ 2. put him in a private room, and limit his time out of the room to when staff can be with him.
- ☐ 3. tell him that hitting others is unacceptable behavior, and ask him to tell a staff member when he begins feeling angry.
- ☐ 4. obtain a prescription for a medication to be administered to decrease his anxiety and threatening behavior.

74. A client loses control and throws two chairs toward another client. What should the nurse do **next**?
- ☐ 1. Ask the client to go to the quiet area and talk about the behavior.
- ☐ 2. Administer an oral PRN tranquilizer, and prepare for a show of determination.
- ☐ 3. Process the incident with the client and discuss alternative behaviors.
- ☐ 4. Call for assistance to restrain the client and administer a PRN intramuscular tranquilizer.

75. A woman who was raped in her home was brought to the emergency department by her husband. After being interviewed by the police, the husband talks to the nurse. "I do not know why she did not keep the doors locked like I told her. I cannot believe she has had sex with another man now." The nurse should respond by saying:
- ☐ 1. "Let us talk about how you feel. Maybe it would help to talk to other men who have been through this."
- ☐ 2. "Maybe the doors were locked, but the man broke in anyway."
- ☐ 3. "Your wife needs your support right now, not your criticism."
- ☐ 4. "It was not consensual sex. Let us see if your wife was physically injured."

76. A young man makes an appointment to see the psychiatric nurse at the employee assistance program of a large corporation because his boss is sending him provocative emails and making seductive remarks on his voice mail at home. The nurse informs him about corporate workplace violence guidelines, and he agrees to work with corporate security on the issue. What should the nurse do **next**?
☐ 1. Refer the client to his boss's supervisor to file a report.
☐ 2. Suggest the client to contact human resources to request a job transfer.
☐ 3. Ask the client about his reactions to this situation.
☐ 4. Report the incident to the client's coworkers who are at risk for similar harassment.

77. A 75 year old woman was brought to the crisis center by her husband. The husband reports that his wife has been in shock and anxious since her purse was stolen outside of their home. The woman blames herself for being robbed, is worried about her stolen wallet and credit cards, and is afraid to go home. What nursing actions are indicated? Select all that apply.
☐ 1. Request a prescription for lorazepam to decrease her anxiety.
☐ 2. Encourage her to talk about the robbery and her feelings.
☐ 3. Discuss what changes at home would help her feel safe.
☐ 4. Investigate if she has physical injuries from the robbery.
☐ 5. Ask her what she thinks she could have done to prevent the robbery.

78. A 35-year-old has been killed as a result of a terrorist attack. What should the nurse advise the friends and relatives of the victim to do during the early stages of the recovery process? Select all that apply.
☐ 1. Keep in contact with other family and friends.
☐ 2. Attend memorial or religious services.
☐ 3. Use relaxation techniques and physical activities.
☐ 4. Speak out publicly about the impact of the loss.
☐ 5. Attend community meetings with others who have lost loved ones.

Managing Care, Quality, and Safety of Clients with Stress, Crisis, Anger, and Violence

79. When the client is involuntarily committed to a hospital because he is assessed as being dangerous to himself or others, which client rights are lost?
☐ 1. the right to access health care
☐ 2. the right to send and receive uncensored mail
☐ 3. freedom from seclusion and restraints
☐ 4. the right to leave the hospital against medical advice

80. The nurse manager on a psychiatric unit is reviewing the outcomes of staff participation in an aggression management program. What indicator would the nurse used to evaluate the effectiveness of such a program?
☐ 1. fewer client injuries during restraint procedures
☐ 2. a reduction of complaints by clients' relatives
☐ 3. fewer staff injuries during restraint procedures
☐ 4. a reduction in the total number of restraint procedures

81. A young woman has been stalked and then beaten by an ex-boyfriend. Treatment of her injuries is complete, and she is ready for discharge. What should the nurse do to ensure the woman's safety and security prior to discharge? Select all that apply.
☐ 1. Determine if the client knows the location of the ex-boyfriend.
☐ 2. Ask if she plans to see the ex-boyfriend again.
☐ 3. Provide information on resources and a safety plan.
☐ 4. Ensure that she has a safe place to stay after discharge.
☐ 5. Obtain consent to send her emergency department records to her family healthcare provider (HCP).

82. Detention center staff asked for a mental health evaluation of a 21-year-old woman after she stabbed herself with a fork and woke from nightmares in fits of rage. The evaluation revealed that she was kidnapped and held from ages 8 to 16 by a convicted child pornographer. She said she never contacted her family after her release from captivity. In what order of priority from first to last should the nurse implement the steps? All options must be used.

1. Initiate suicide precautions and a no-harm contract.

2. Ask the client if she wishes to contact her family while hospitalized.

3. Offer empathy and support, and be nonjudgmental and honest with her.

4. Encourage safe verbalizations of her emotions, especially anger.

83. The nurse is planning care for a group of clients. Which client should the nurse identify as needing the **most** assistance in accepting being ill?

☐ 1. an 8-year-old boy who alternately cries for his mother and is angry with the nurse about being hospitalized after a bike accident

☐ 2. a 32-year-old woman diagnosed with depression related to lupus erythematosus who discusses her medication's adverse effects with the nurse

☐ 3. a 45-year-old man who just suffered a severe myocardial infarction and talks to the nurse about concerns regarding resuming sexual relations with his wife

☐ 4. a 60-year-old woman diagnosed with chronic obstructive pulmonary disease who refuses to wear an oxygen mask even though poor oxygenation makes her confused

84. The nurse is managing the care for a client in a disaster shelter who broke a femur and has lost her family home in a hurricane. What measures should the nurse take? Select all that apply.

☐ 1. Supervise the care provided to the client during the crisis.

☐ 2. Obtain an order for antipsychotic medications for the client.

☐ 3. Act as a client advocate for the client in crisis.

☐ 4. Discuss with the interdisciplinary team available community resources for the client.

☐ 5. Obtain accurate identification including name, age, address, contact information, and names of relatives.

85 Which client outcome **best** indicates effective mental healthcare coordination when the nurse uses a client-centered approach?

☐ 1. The level of client engagement is based on agency mandate and policy.

☐ 2. There are no further admissions to an acute care hospital.

☐ 3. The client is compliant with the treatment plan.

☐ 4. Preferred client outcomes vary from client to client.

86. How does participation in self-help groups benefit the client? Select all that apply.

☐ 1. It increases knowledge about mental illness.

☐ 2. It develops stronger social networks and support.

☐ 3. It is more cost-effective than in-client treatment.

☐ 4. It increases the client's sense of well-being.

☐ 5. It facilitates the development of advocacy skills.

87. During a unit meeting attended by clients and staff, several clients are criticizing their primary nurses. These clients have also been intimidating two other clients who have recently been admitted to the unit, and now, the new clients have stopped sharing their opinions during the meeting. What is the **first** action for the nurse to take?

☐ 1. Help the new clients express the reasons they have stopped sharing their ideas.

☐ 2. Ask the clients criticizing their nurses to suggest some possible solutions for the practices they are criticizing.

☐ 3. Give the clients who are publically criticizing the nurses a verbal warning that this behavior is not acceptable.

☐ 4. Use the next unit meeting to discuss respect and the importance of collaboration with the treatment team.

88. Two nurses disagree on what is the most important information for the client with a stress-related illness to have during a discharge teaching session. How should the nurse assigned to provide the discharge teaching proceed?

☐ 1. Share all the information that both nurses thought was important.

☐ 2. Review the policies related to required discharge teaching.

☐ 3. Be aware of different interpretations and personal biases held by nurses.

☐ 4. Ask the client what is most important for them as they prepare for discharge.

89. Despite education and role-play practice of restraint procedures, a staff member is injured when actually restraining a client. When helping the uninjured staff deal with the incident, the nurse should address which factor?

☐ 1. The emotional responses may be similar to those of other crime victims.

☐ 2. The member is likely to resign after experiencing such an injury.

☐ 3. Legal action against the client will take time and energy.

☐ 4. The member must debrief with the assaultive client before returning.

90. A nurse calls the unit manager to report that her purse has been stolen from the locked break room. The nurse says she thinks she knows which of the staff stole the purse. Which actions by the nurse manager would be appropriate? Select all that apply.

☐ 1. Confront the person the nurse suspects stole the purse.

☐ 2. Call hospital security to initiate an investigation.

☐ 3. Ask the nurse to document all the facts related to the stolen purse.

☐ 4. Alert nursing administration that a staff's purse has been stolen.

☐ 5. Ask other staff to report any suspicious activity they may have observed.

91. A nurse's ex-boyfriend enters the unit and states, "If I cannot have her, then no one will." Hospital security escorts him out of the building and warned him not to return. The unit manager holds a staff meeting to confirm that which workplace violence policies and procedures will be implemented? Select all that apply.

☐ 1. Give a quick overview of the hospital's workplace violence policies and procedures.

☐ 2. Offer counseling for the nurse and any other staff threatened by her ex-boyfriend.

☐ 3. Work with security and the nurse to initiate workplace precautions related to the ex-boyfriend.

☐ 4. Ask security to help the nurse understand how to initiate a protective order against her ex-boyfriend.

☐ 5. Ask the nurse to take a leave of absence until her ex-boyfriend is notified of the protective order.

Answers, Rationales, and Test-Taking Strategies

The answers and rationales for each question follow below, along with keys (🔑) to the client need (CN) and cognitive level (CL) for each question. In addition, you will also see a glossary icon (📖) highlighting specific terminology used on the licensing exam. As you check your answers, use the **Content Mastery and Test-Taking Skill Self-Analysis** *worksheet (tear-out worksheet in back of book) to identify the reason(s) for not answering the questions correctly. For additional information about test-taking skills and strategies for answering questions, refer to pages 12–23 and pages 35–36 in Part 1 of this book.*

The Client Managing Stress

1. 4. The client expressing doubts about his wife's response to his amputation as well as possible doubt on his part is still struggling with body image issues. Looking forward to participating in walkathons and helping others indicate plans for the future that imply an acceptance of his amputee status. Remembering that his friend died in the accident that caused his amputation indicates that the client is aware that there was a worse end result to the accident than his amputation.

🔑 CN: Psychosocial integrity; CL: Evaluate

2. 1. Anxiety, especially at higher levels, interferes with learning and memory retention. After the client's anxiety lessens, it will be easier for him to learn the steps of the blood glucose monitoring. Because the client's illness is a chronic, lifelong illness that severely changes his lifestyle, it is unlikely that he is uninterested in the illness or how to treat it. It is also unlikely that dementia would be the cause of the client's frustration and lack of memory. The client's response indicates anxiety. Client responses that would indicate lessening anxiety would be questions to the nurse or requests to repeat part of the instruction.

🔑 CN: Psychosocial integrity; CL: Analyze

3. 3. An explanation of what to expect decreases anxiety about upcoming events that could be seen as traumatic by the client. Distraction, such as with games or television, only decreases anxiety temporarily and does not fulfill the client's need for information about the procedure. Reassurance about an uncomplicated outcome is not appropriate; the nurse cannot guarantee that the client will come through surgery without problems. Referring the client to a psychiatrist is not indicated for moderate, expected preoperative anxiety.

🔑 CN: Psychosocial integrity; CL: Synthesize

4. 3. With mild anxiety, perceptions are accurate. Slight muscle tension reflects a motor response. Occasional irritability is an emotional response. Loss of contact with reality is a cognitive characteristic of severe anxiety.

🔑 CN: Psychosocial integrity; CL: Analyze

5. 1. Suicide attempts and violence are psychomotor responses to a panic level of anxiety. Desperation and rage are emotional responses. Disorganized reasoning and loss of contact with reality are cognitive responses.

🔑 CN: Psychosocial integrity; CL: Analyze

6. 2. Mild anxiety motivates the client to focus on issues and resolve them. Therefore, learning and problem solving can occur at a mild level of anxiety. Taking control for the client is reserved for a near-panic level of anxiety. Severe anxiety interferes with reasoning and functioning. Therefore, reducing stimuli and pressure is crucial at a severe level. Tension reduction is appropriate at a moderate level to help the client think more clearly and engage in problem solving.

🔑 CN: Psychosocial integrity; CL: Analyze

7. 4. Minimal functioning, which can cause new problems to develop, is a reflection of dysfunctional coping. The ability to objectively and rationally solve problems demonstrates adaptive coping. Tension reduction activities demonstrate palliative coping. However, such activities alone do not solve problems; they must be followed by problem solving.

Anger management alone may prevent new problems, such as violence toward oneself or others, but it does not solve problems directly. It is considered maladaptive coping.

CN: Psychosocial integrity; CL: Analyze

8. 4. Because relationships inherently lead to stress and anxiety, conflict resolution skills are essential for solving relationship problems. Dealing with anger is more effective than suppressing it. Suppression is a mechanism that avoids the issue rather than solving it. Balancing a checkbook involves calculations, not coping skills. Following directions is a passive activity that reflects a lack of problem solving by the client.

CN: Psychosocial integrity; CL: Analyze

9. 4. The client's statement that he and his wife listen to each other reflects improved efforts at communicating about issues. The other statements provide some insight into the need for better communication. However, they are but steps along the way to coping effectively with the problem.

CN: Psychosocial integrity; CL: Evaluate

10. 1. Assessment examines the client's thoughts, feelings, and behaviors within a context. Whether the client's behavior is appropriate for the situation is important assessment data. Setting priorities is part of making nursing diagnoses and planning; motivation to change and identifying the need for a no-harm contract are part of the planning stage.

CN: Psychosocial integrity; CL: Analyze

11. 3. Writing a list of strengths and needs is short term, achievable, and measurable. Achieving positive self-esteem would occur over the long term. Going to school involves complex future steps to a long-term goal. Using skills is likely to be stressful and is best attempted after the client has done a self-assessment.

CN: Psychosocial integrity;
CL: Synthesize

12. 4. The ultimate outcome is to have the client solve problems by himself, collaborating in his own care. Client follow-up with the mental health providers, while desirable, does not ensure that the client will fully comply with treatment or medication. Knowledge of the medication's effects and adverse effects and compliance can help the client but alone will not ensure success unless the client knows how to address and solve problems independently.

CN: Health promotion and maintenance;
CL: Synthesize

13. 1. Substituting rational beliefs is a major goal when using cognitive-behavioral models, which focus more on thinking and behaviors than feelings.

Unconscious processes are the focus of psychoanalytic models. Analysis of fears and barriers to growth is the focus of developmental models. Tension and stress are targets of the stress models.

CN: Psychosocial integrity; CL: Apply

14. 3. Displacement refers to a defense mechanism that involves taking feelings out on a less-threatening object or person instead of tackling the issue or problem directly. Talking to his wife directly reflects insight into the client's use of the defense mechanism and his ability to overcome it. Not thinking about the weekend is suppression. Here, the client is focusing on the issue with the highest priority. Focusing on academic rather than athletic achievement is compensation, highlighting one's strengths instead of weaknesses. Not remembering the molestation is repression.

CN: Psychosocial integrity; CL: Evaluate

15. 3. Legally, there is a duty to warn a potential victim of a client's intent to harm. Staff can be held accountable if the client injures the ex-partner and the staff failed to warn that person. The client's permission is needed to share information with a spouse. Student papers should not contain identifying information. Release of information is made directly to the client's insurance company, not to the employer.

CN: Management of care; CL: Apply

16. 2,5. The client is showing increased anxiety and anger as well as refusing to stay in the hospital, which are immediate and crucial concerns at admission. The client is not likely to give permission to talk to his wife and boss at this point. Housing issues and divorce counseling may be relevant before discharge, but not initially. Suspiciousness and grandiosity may be relevant after the client's anxiety and anger are under control.

CN: Management of care; CL: Synthesize

17. 2. The nurse is required to set limits on inappropriate behavior while conveying respect and acceptance of that person. Doing so conveys to the client that he is worthy without posing any harm or embarrassment to the client. Touch is a complex issue that must be used cautiously. Touch may be misinterpreted or misperceived by a client who has been abused or who has perceptual or thought disturbances. Mutual sharing reflects a social friendship, not a therapeutic one. Total confidentiality is not desirable. For example, treatment team members and insurance companies need selected information to ensure quality services.

CN: Psychosocial integrity; CL: Apply

18. 2. Growth of the fetus is important, so nausea and anorexia that would interfere with the young woman's nutrition would cause the most harm to the developing fetus. It could also lead to electrolyte imbalance if she did not take in enough fluid. While insomnia could cause problems long term, this side effect could be mitigated through adjustment of the dosing time (earlier in the day), by decreasing the dosage to her former 20 mg daily, or by changing to every other day dosing of 40 mg, since fluoxetine has a long half-life. Headaches are uncomfortable but can be treated with mild analgesics or other treatments, such as cold cloths, that would not harm the fetus. Decreased libido, while not enjoyable for the client or her sexual partner, does not pose any risks for the fetus.

🗝 CN: Pharmacological and parenteral therapy; CL: Analyze

19. 3. Asking for descriptions of changes in behavior (what the client did differently) encourages evaluation. Conveying empathy, such as stating that it is still hard for the client to talk about it, encourages data collection. Asking for meaning helps with the nursing diagnosis. Asking the client about what it will take to follow out a plan is part of planning.

🗝 CN: Psychosocial integrity; CL: Apply

20. 4. Practicing new behaviors builds confidence and reinforces appropriate behaviors. Reality testing, asking about fears, and teaching new communication skills are some of the many steps when trying out new behaviors.

🗝 CN: Psychosocial integrity; CL: Apply

The Client Coping with Physical Illness

21. 4. While the client does have a right to accept or reject treatment, she has not explored her feelings, her possible mastectomy, or the future. The nurse should assist the client in exploring her feelings and moving toward a fuller understanding of her options. Giving the client survival rates indicates that the nurse feels she should have the surgery and negates her fears and concerns. While the chaplain might be helpful, this step should be done after the client has explored her feelings.

🗝 CN: Management of care; CL: Synthesize

22. 2. Diagnosis of a serious illness would be a shock to anyone but particularly a young person. Feelings of anger are normal and should be expressed. Gaining an intellectual understanding of his illness would also be necessary, but such learning will not take place if the client's feelings have not been addressed. There is no indication that the client needs to conserve energy because of his condition, nor is it clear that death is imminent. Neither situation is likely at the point of first diagnosis

unless the disease is well advanced, which is not indicated here.

🗝 CN: Management of care; CL: Apply

23. 2. The psychotropic drugs used to treat chronic mental illnesses have side effects that can lead to noncompliance. Therefore, teaching the clients measures to deal with the common side effects would be most important. Teaching should be focused on the need for compliance and the specific interests of the target audience. Teaching should concentrate on the medications commonly used to treat chronic mental illness, not on many psychotropic drugs or those used in acute illness. Such topics as the role of medication in the treatment of chronic mental illness and the effects of using common street drugs with psychotropic medication should be discussed after the issue of compliance is addressed.

🗝 CN: Health promotion and maintenance; CL: Create

24. 2. When the client seems to be questioning the **HCP's** 📖 goals, it is best for the nurse to present an open statement and ask the client what he means. This technique helps the client express his feelings. Telling the client about the surgery is less therapeutic when he is upset. While it is the client's right to get a second opinion, this suggestion does not address the client's feelings. Making assumptions can also interfere with communication, especially if the assumption is incorrect.

🗝 CN: Psychosocial integrity; CL: Synthesize

25. 2. When the client has hostile outbursts, it is best for the nurse to help her express her feelings. This serves as a release valve for the client. Offering positive reinforcement for cooperation does not help the client express herself appropriately. Continuing with assigned tasks ignores the client's feelings and may lead to further escalation. Limiting visitation reduces the client's support systems and does not address the underlying problem.

🗝 CN: Psychosocial integrity; CL: Synthesize

26. 3. Preoperative visits and talks with others who have made successful adjustments to colostomies are helpful and tend to make the client less fearful of the operation and its consequences. Knowing about resources in the community will be helpful as the client approaches discharge. Supporting the **HCP** 📖 is less important than supporting the client and giving him information. The client will have a change in body image, with disfigurement due to the creation of a colostomy. However, the client should be able to lead a full life.

🗝 CN: Management of care; CL: Apply

27. 2. The nurse must present reality to the client about his condition to help decrease his denial about his physical status. By stating the name of the condition and talking about what it means, the nurse provides the client with information and conveys concerns about him and a willingness to help him understand his illness. It may not be true that the client would be made more upset by the call; the news might be good. However, this statement does not provide the client with the reality of his condition. Telling the client that he really does not care or asking the client if he realizes that he has a life-threatening condition is belittling and may make the client defensive.

CN: Psychosocial integrity; CL: Synthesize

28. 1. Leaving the hospital and immediately flying to a meeting indicate poor judgment by the client and little understanding of what she needs to change regarding her lifestyle. The other statements show that the client understands some of the changes she needs to make to decrease her stress and lead a healthier lifestyle.

CN: Psychosocial integrity; CL: Evaluate

29. 1,3,5. Suicide is a risk with chronic illnesses. The husband needs validation of his feelings and support as well as suggestions for helping his wife with her concerns. Telling him to be strong and optimistic ignores the client's needs. It is false to assume that the client will no longer be suicidal when the lupus is under control.

CN: Safety and infection control; CL: Synthesize

30. 4. The nurse's best response is one that directly expresses the nurse's observations to the client and offers the client the opportunity to talk about his feelings or concerns to decrease somatization (the need to express feelings through physical symptoms). Leaving, offering to provide pain medication, and stating that anger does not bother the nurse ignore the client's needs.

CN: Psychosocial integrity; CL: Synthesize

31. 4. Though ulcerative colitis and OCD have some features in common, and stress can make both illnesses worse; there is no definitive cause-effect relationship between ulcerative colitis and OCD. Therefore, the only appropriate nursing response would be to acknowledge the effect of stress on both illnesses and indicate there is no proof that either illness causes the other.

CN: Physiological adaptation; CL: Synthesize

32. 4. This type of behavior illustrates *emotional lability*, which is a readily changeable or unstable emotional affect. *Neologism* is using a word when it can have two or more meanings, or a play on words. *Confabulation* involves replacing memory loss by fantasy to hide confusion; it is unconscious behavior. *Flight of ideas* refers to a rapid succession of verbal expressions that jump from one topic to another and are only superficially related.

CN: Psychosocial integrity; CL: Analyze

33. 2,3,1,4. The first priority is a safe environment so the client and nurse are not hurt by the phone. Then, it is important to acknowledge the client's anger to help diffuse it. As the client calms down, the nurse can explore the client's feeling in more depth. Since the client implies anger at God, a clergy consult may be appropriate.

CN: Safety and infection control; CL: Analyze

34. 3. Focusing on enjoying time with family and friends conveys a renewal of hope for the future and a decreased risk of suicide. Simply saying that no one wants him to commit suicide does not say he does not want to do it. Avoiding a transfer to a psychiatric unit does not mean he is no longer suicidal. Fear of not being successful with suicide usually is not a deterrent.

CN: Reduction of risk potential; CL: Evaluate

The Client in Crisis

35. 3. Individuals progress through the stages of loss at their own pace. Not everyone experiences each phase, and no one can be forced to advance to the next stage until ready. The overall goal for helping the client to work through the pain of loss is to assist the client in processing and engaging in the pain of loss. This process may involve working on family conflicts and/or anger issues but is not the primary goal.

CN: Health promotion and maintenance; CL: Synthesize

36. 1,2,3,6. The immediate needs for this client are for safety and security, so it is important to assess for injuries, safety of her family, suicide risk, and signs of emotional decompensation. Needs for food, clothing, and support are important later, after safety and security are addressed.

CN: Reduction of risk potential; CL: Analyze

37. 2. During the first phase of crisis, the client exhibits elevated anxiety. A client who can use problem-solving capabilities is not in crisis. A short-ened attention span is characteristic of the fourth phase of crisis. Reaching out to others for help is indicative of the third phase of crisis.

🔑 CN: Management of care; CL: Synthesize

38. 4,2,3,1. The nurse must first identify which member is exhibiting crisis symptoms. Next, the nurse identifies strategies to reduce the most severe symptoms. The nurse then assesses the family's resources. The family member in crisis may have such overwhelming feelings that he or she is unable to identify or describe the feelings.

🔑 CN: Psychosocial integrity; CL: Synthesize

39. 3. Before any interventions can occur, know-ing whether the client is pregnant is crucial in formulating a plan of care. Asking the client about what things she had thought about doing, giving the client some ideas about what to expect next, and questioning the client about her feelings and possi-ble parental reactions would be appropriate after it is determined that the client is pregnant.

🔑 CN: Psychosocial integrity; CL: Synthesize

40. 2. Because of the client's potential pregnancy, the nurse needs to determine exactly what the client means by the term "hooking up" by asking the client to describe what she has been doing in sexual encounters with her boyfriend. Asking the client if she means sexual intercourse or telling the client that they need to talk about sexual intercourse makes an assumption that may or may not be appro-priate. The nurse needs to determine exactly what the client means by the terms used. Repeating the client's statement does not elicit the necessary infor-mation to interpret the client's statement. Addition-ally, this type of response assumes an understanding of what the client has said.

🔑 CN: Psychosocial integrity; CL: Synthesize

41. 4. Because people in an emotional crisis find it difficult to focus their thinking, the goal is to return the client to noncrisis functioning. Pointing out and decreasing the client's level of anxiety is the first step in attaining this goal. Telling an obviously distressed person not to worry is ineffective because it ignores the client's distress and concerns. Although preg-nancy is a normal event, and 40 years of age may not be too old for a pregnancy, these responses also ignore the client's distress and feelings.

🔑 CN: Psychosocial integrity; CL: Synthesize

42. 1. Telephoning the crisis shelter indicates that the boys are alarmed but are reluctant to talk with their parents. The boys may fear that their parents will assume that they have been sniffing glue and punish them. The nurse should focus on helping the boys talk with their parents. The legality of sniffing glue varies, but crisis hotlines are geared at providing supportive services. To prove that the observations are incorrect requires an intervention beginning with the boys' parents. Sniffing glue is classified as inhalant abuse, a very dangerous, not minor, form of substance abuse.

🔑 CN: Management of care; CL: Synthesize

43. 1. The crisis worker needs to use active focusing techniques to determine the crisis-precipitating event or the immediate problem. Asking the caller, "Why are you calling today?" or "What is the immediate problem?" will assist the caller to focus on the specific need or event. Telling the client to make an appointment is inappropriate because the problem might be life threatening. Tell-ing the caller to go to the nearest emergency depart-ment is precipitous and may be unnecessary. Asking to speak to someone else in the home may be futile because the caller might be alone. This action also ignores the caller and his or her feelings.

🔑 CN: Management of care; CL: Synthesize

44. 3. The concern that someone may call the cri-sis hotline every day for a year indicates that further understanding about crisis and crisis intervention is needed. A crisis situation is time limited, typically resolving in 4 to 6 weeks if handled effectively. If a person calls the line daily for a year, that person has not been properly dealt with or is probably in a highly disorganized state requiring an alternative intervention. The nurse needs to further review and clarify the material presented. Callers are typically in pain, overwhelmed, and exhausted when they call. A crisis can help an individual cope better in the future if he learns to handle the situation.

🔑 CN: Management of care; CL: Evaluate

45. 2,3,4,5,6. Controlling self-destructive behav-iors is a priority, but developing emotion manage-ment skills and processing emotions and memories are also important. Assessing for injuries, preg-nancy, sexually transmitted infections, and drugs in her system is important due to the fact that most cults foster sex and pregnancy in young teens and often use drugs to achieve compliance from the girls. It is not appropriate to ask the client to share her experiences in a group of teens. It could be more damaging to the client unless the other teens are also trauma/torture survivors.

🔑 CN: Psychosocial integrity; CL: Synthesize

46. 2. Generally, 4 to 6 weeks is viewed as the length of time a client can tolerate the severe level of disturbance of a true crisis. In the first week or two, the client usually is still trying to use normal coping skills and support systems. After 6 weeks of continuous crisis, a client is probably becoming so physically and emotionally drained that he has sought or has been brought by others for medical or psychiatric care.

⚷ CN: Management of care; CL: Apply

47. 1. The initial goal in crisis intervention is helping the client regain emotional security and equilibrium. Resolution of the underlying emotional problems, development of insight and personal growth, and formulation of more effective support systems are goals to address as the crisis subsides.

⚷ CN: Psychosocial integrity; CL: Apply

48. 3. Learning new coping skills is the major factor necessary for higher functioning. Better coping is likely to lead to regaining support systems, giving up dysfunctional coping, and awareness of how to prevent future crises.

⚷ CN: Psychosocial integrity; CL: Apply

49. 3. The risk of suicide can persist for 2 to 3 months even after a crisis has abated. Therefore, it is important for the client to be able to verbalize information about appropriate support persons and community resources and to have this information readily available. Although the client may state that she is ready to be discharged, this is not the most reliable indicator. A divorce lawyer may not be appropriate at this point. At 3 days after a suicide attempt, emotional stability is not likely.

⚷ CN: Management of care; CL: Evaluate

50. 4. The statement about joining the son if he dies indicates potential for self-harm and subsequent suicide, always a risk during crisis. Although the father may be charged with reckless driving, this is not an indication for a psychiatric consultation. Verbalizing that the accident may lead to divorce may or may not be a real risk; however, this situation is not urgent. The statement about not seeing the son run behind the car illustrates the father's attempts at trying to process the situation.

⚷ CN: Psychosocial integrity; CL: Evaluate

51. 1. Passive suicidal thoughts, such as a wish to die or giving up on self-care, can be as much of a risk as active suicidal ideation (the idea of killing one's self directly), especially for older clients because they commonly lack the means, energy, and motivation for an active suicide attempt. Seeing the grandson and grandmother together may help later. Not talking to the grandson and experiencing altered role performance may be real issues, but these are not as critical as the risk of indirect (passive) suicide.

⚷ CN: Psychosocial integrity; CL: Analyze

52. 2. The threat toward the ex-boyfriend is the most immediate concern now, as the client turns her anger toward him instead of herself. Although situational low self-esteem, risk for suicide, and risk-prone health behavior are evident, these problems are less of a concern at this time.

⚷ CN: Safety and infection control; CL: Analyze

53. 3. Letting the client express his feelings (emotion management) is essential before trying to solve the problem or deciding what kind of referral is appropriate. A referral for counseling, assessment of the client's support system, and unemployment assistance may be appropriate after the client's anxiety is reduced.

⚷ CN: Psychosocial integrity; CL: Apply

54. 2. During a crisis, support persons demonstrate preparedness to help the client by verbalizing the emergency resources available and knowing when to use them. Follow-up medical care may be helpful as the crisis subsides. The coping strategies used by the support persons may or may not be relevant to the client's needs and situation. Long-term solutions and advice may or may not be appropriate. The focus needs to be on the client's immediate needs and situation.

⚷ CN: Psychosocial integrity; CL: Analyze

55. 1. The nurse needs to focus on the client and address her feelings. Talking about her feelings helps to decrease the risk of self-harm. Doing so takes precedence over questions about the cause of death and her children's support. Antidepressant medications may be indicated, but more information is needed about the client's emotional state.

⚷ CN: Psychosocial integrity; CL: Synthesize

56. 1,2,3,4,5. All of the options are correct and in an appropriate sequence of actions except for option 6. The flyover is likely to trigger vivid memories and emotions in those living near the city related to the tragedy of the Twin Towers on 9/11/01. The severity of the flashbacks will vary in degree, just as they did after the original event. Asking the military for an apology will not address the caller's symptoms.

⚷ CN: Management of care; CL: Synthesize

The Client with Problems Expressing Anger

57. 4. Beginning with an open-ended question that brings out the client's view of his situation and reasons for seeking treatment is the most neutral beginning and helps to gain the client's perception of events. Blaming the client for his problems is accusatory and nonproductive. A time for reviewing what could be done differently will come later.

🔑 CN: Psychosocial integrity; CL: Apply

58. 2,4,3,1. The clients need to understand that anger is a normal emotion, but if not expressed can have negative effects on the body and mind. Then, the nurse begins to focus on the client's personal situation and help the client understand that holding anger can aggravate his depressive symptoms as well. One focus of outpatient counseling will be learning safe, effective ways to express anger.

🔑 CN: Reduction of risk potential; CL: Analyze

59. 1,2,3,5. Dealing with anger, stress, and anxiety; identifying resources and support groups; and increasing a sense of safety and security are appropriate interventions at this time. However, recommending an antiwar advocacy group may or may not be appropriate, even much later in the client's recovery.

🔑 CN: Psychosocial integrity; CL: Synthesize

60. 2,1,4,3. Angry clients may not realize what makes them angry and the cues that their behavior is becoming out of control. The nurse should first help the client identify what triggered the anger. Once the cause of the anger and cues to the loss of control are discovered, the nurse should assist the client in identifying safe and appropriate alternative expressions of anger and then practice those techniques prior to facing a real anger-producing situation.

🔑 CN: Psychosocial integrity; CL: Synthesize

61. 3. By requesting that the roommate respect his rights (asking the roommate to put the dirty clothes on the floor away after telling him that this bothers him), the client is asserting himself. Arriving late is commonly passive resistance and thus not an indicator that the client is becoming assertive. Asking the nurse to call is dependent behavior. Although asking the **HCP** 🖵 is more assertive, the client is relying on the nurse's direction to do so.

🔑 CN: Psychosocial integrity; CL: Analyze

62. 2. Blood pressure, as well as respiratory rate and muscle tension, increases during anger because of the autonomic nervous system response to epinephrine secretion. Peristalsis decreases.

🔑 CN: Physiological adaptation; CL: Apply

63. 4. When given intramuscularly, haloperidol is considered most restrictive because it is intrusive and a client usually does not receive the drug voluntarily. Oral haloperidol is considered less restrictive because the client usually accepts the pill voluntarily. Tension reduction strategies and voluntary seclusion are considered less restrictive because they are not intrusive and the client usually **consents** 🖵 to their use.

🔑 CN: Safety and infection control; CL: Apply

64. 2. Asking the staff for assistance is appropriate when the client demonstrates behaviors that involve the direct threat of violence. Holding a stick and telling the nurse to move is the most direct threat of violence. Swearing and pounding on a table may be disturbing, but these actions are less of a threat. Coming out of his room may indicate noncompliance with directions. However, further assessment is needed to determine whether this behavior was a direct threat of violence.

🔑 CN: Management of care; CL: Analyze

65. 3,4,1,2. Since external stimuli can greatly contribute to agitation, the nurse should teach the client that the first step is to go to a quiet area, then enlist the help of others, and finally take medication. Taking the lorazepam first would help decrease anxiety quickly, thus diminishing agitation. If the lorazepam is not successful, the client could take the oral haloperidol to help clear the client's thoughts and decrease agitation.

🔑 CN: Management of care; CL: Synthesize

66. 3. The client who is about to lose control is experiencing a high degree of anxiety or agitation, which alters the client's ability to perceive reality. Initially, the client may feel threatened by the presence of others. A client who is out of control is not thinking about having an audience. Although the nurse with the client who is about to lose control is generally the one giving directions, this is not a rationale for staying at a distance. When seeing extra staff, the client may or may not be able to gain self-control.

🔑 CN: Safety and infection control; CL: Apply

67. 1. When using seclusion, the safety of the client is paramount. Therefore, staff must be able to see the client in seclusion at all times, such as through a security window in the door or with a room camera. Although outside access for dimming the lights to decrease stimuli may be appropriate, it is not critical for the client's safety. Having one staff member stay in a room alone with a potentially violent client is unsafe. A prescription for seclusion can be obtained before or after it is initiated.

CN: Safety and infection control;
CL: Synthesize

68. 3. A full-length restraint blanket is added when the client is at risk for injury from fighting the restraints. The increased degree of restriction is justified only when the risk of client injury increases. Feeling more secure is not a sufficient cause for using a more restrictive measure. Client statements that restraints are tight and uncomfortable require the nurse to assess the situation and adjust the restraints if necessary to ensure adequate circulation. Four-way restraints already provide adequate protection for the staff.

CN: Safety and infection control;
CL: Apply

69. 1. Safety of the client and staff is the utmost priority. Therefore, the client must be monitored closely and frequently, such as every 15 minutes, to ensure that the client is safe and free from injury. Assisting with nutrition and elimination, performing range-of-motion exercises on each limb, and changing the client's position every 2 hours are important after the safety of the client and staff is ensured by close, frequent monitoring.

CN: Safety and infection control;
CL: Synthesize

70. 4. The long-term goal of the debriefing after restraining a client is to improve aggression management procedures so that prevention of aggression improves and the frequency of restraint use decreases. Providing feedback and comparing perceptions are single aspects that would eventually lead to the ultimate goal of improving aggression management procedures. When a client can be released from restraints is not immediately predictable.

CN: Management of care; CL: Synthesize

The Client with Interpersonal Violence

71. 2,4,3,1. The first step is to calmly present the reality that the client cannot be released at this time. Next, the brother should be asked to leave the unit quietly. When he does not, protecting the other clients and visitors is essential for their safety. (The staff member can help them process what is happening on the unit.) Calling security to the unit is a last resort when less restrictive measures have not worked. Calling them before setting limits with the brother and giving him a choice of actions will

likely escalate the situation. Security can legally escort the brother off the unit and hospital grounds.

CN: Safety and infection control;
CL: Synthesize

72. 4. Verbalizing feelings, especially feelings of anger, in an appropriate manner is an adaptive method of coping that reduces the chance that the client will act out these feelings toward others. The client's ability to verbalize feelings indicates a change in behavior, a crucial indicator of goal achievement. Although acknowledging feelings of anger and describing situations that precipitate angry feelings are important in helping the client reach her goal, they are not appropriate indicators that behavior has changed. Asking the client to list how anger has been handled in the past is helpful if the nurse discusses coping methods with the client. However, based on this client's history, this would not be helpful because the nurse and client are already aware of the client's aggression toward others.

CN: Safety and infection control;
CL: Evaluate

73. 3. The nurse must clearly address behavioral expectations, such as telling the client that hitting is unacceptable, and also provide alternatives for the client, such as letting staff members know when he begins to feel angry. Making others responsible for the client's behavior or isolating the client in his room is inappropriate because it does not include the client in managing his behavior. Although medication may be helpful, this action does not give the client responsibility for his behavior and is not warranted at this time.

CN: Safety and infection control;
CL: Synthesize

74. 4. The client is in the crisis phase of the assault cycle. Therefore, the nurse must act immediately, using restraints and an intramuscular tranquilizer to prevent injury to others or further property damage. It is too late to ask the client to go to a quiet area to talk because the client's behavior is past the triggering phase. Giving the client an oral tranquilizer and preparing for a show of determination are nursing interventions used in the escalation phase. Processing the incident with the client and discussing alternative behaviors are interventions used in the postcrisis phase.

CN: Safety and infection control;
CL: Synthesize

75. 1. The nurse should respond to the husband's needs and concerns and should offer support. Protecting or defending the wife against his criticism ignores the husband's needs.

CN: Psychosocial integrity;
CL: Synthesize

76. 3. It is important to know the client's reactions in order to plan appropriate interventions. Until the client's reactions are known, it is premature to suggest a job transfer, file a report to his boss's supervisor, or alert his coworkers.

⚿ CN: Management of care; CL: Synthesize

77. 2,3,4. After the impact of a crime, the client's most important needs are for physical safety and emotional security. There is no indication that the client has a severe level of anxiety; therefore, lorazepam is not indicated. Asking her how she could have prevented the robbery implies that she could be at fault.

⚿ CN: Psychosocial integrity; CL: Synthesize

78. 1,2,3,5. Receiving support from family, friends, other survivors, and community services is generally helpful after such events. Relaxation and participation in activities help manage stress reactions. Speaking out publicly may or may not be helpful later in the recovery process but may actually hinder recovery in the early stages.

⚿ CN: Psychosocial integrity; CL: Synthesize

Managing Care, Quality, and Safety of Clients with Stress, Crisis, Anger, and Violence

79. 4. When a client is committed involuntarily, the right to leave against medical advice is forfeited. All the other rights are preserved unless there is further court action or a case of imminent danger to self or others (hitting staff, cutting self).

⚿ CN: Management of care; CL: Apply

80. 4. The primary goal of an aggression management program is to prevent violence. This goal is evidenced by a reduction in the total number of restraint procedures used or needed. Although fewer client and staff injuries are important, these goals are secondary to prevention. Reduction in the number of complaints by clients' relatives is affected by more variables than just restraint procedures.

⚿ CN: Management of care; CL: Evaluate

81. 1,2,3,4. The crucial interventions involve safety and support. Asking for **consent** 📖 is a health privacy issue, not a safety issue, and is not essential to the discharge process.

⚿ CN: Safety and infection control; CL: Synthesize

82. 1,3,4,2. Safety is a priority after the client stabbed herself. A survivor of trauma/torture needs empathy, support, honesty, and a nonjudgmental stance from the nurse. Then, the client is more willing to learn safe ways to express feeling, especially anger. It will be the client's decision if she wants to contact her family and, if so, under what conditions. She would need extensive preparation before any contact with her family.

⚿ CN: Safety and infection control; CL: Synthesize

83. 4. The 60-year-old woman is acting in a way that worsens her physical and mental condition because she does not want to be sick. The 8-year-old child is acting normally for someone his age who is unexpectedly hospitalized. The cooperation demonstrated by the client with lupus and the client who had a myocardial infarction indicates a level of acceptance of their illnesses and of their role as being ill.

⚿ CN: Management of care; CL: Analyze

84. 1,3,4,5. The nurse who is managing the care of the client in a disaster shelter provides for the management of care by supervising the care for the client in crisis. In a disaster, the nurse also must be sure that the client is identified and contact information about the client is documented. The nurse also acts as a client advocate for the client in crisis and discusses available community resources for the client with the interdisciplinary team assigned to this client. There are no data to indicate that antipsychotic medications are needed for this client at this time.

⚿ CN: Management of Care; CL: Apply

85. 4. In order to be effective in the role of case manager or care coordinator, the nurse must practice with the philosophy that recovery is defined by the client, not the service provider. Using a predefined outcome measure to determine effectiveness or recovery does not demonstrate the belief that well-being is possible for all people living with a mental illness.

⚿ CN: Management of care; CL: Evaluate

86. 1,2,4. Participation in self-help groups has been shown to increase knowledge, coping skills, self-esteem, confidence, sense of well-being, and a sense of being in control. Improving social and support networks is also a common outcome of client engagement in self-help groups. If symptoms are severe and/or life threatening, in-client treatment may be the most appropriate and as a result potentially more cost-effective. Development of personal advocacy skills is not a primary outcome of client participation in self-help groups.

⚿ CN: Management of care; CL: Analyze

87. 2. Recognizing that the clients are part of the solution to the issues they are presenting demonstrates a client-centered approach to care. Having the new clients challenge the behaviors of other clients does not facilitate the development of a therapeutic milieu. Warning clients that behaviors are unacceptable reinforces a sense of client powerlessness and does not build a therapeutic relationship. Discussing respect and collaboration would happen after the criticisms have been acknowledged and the clients have been asked for their opinions.

CN: Management of care; CL: Synthesize

88. 4. The discharge teaching session will be most effective if the nurse uses a client-centered approach to better assess what the client needs and, therefore, what information to share. Sharing all the information does not respect the knowledge that the client already has. Reviewing the policies is one area to help identify important areas for teaching, but in order to ensure that client needs are met, further assessment is required. Awareness of personal biases should not be used to determine what is important for the client.

CN: Management of care; CL: Synthesize

89. 1. Being injured by a client can result in emotional responses similar to those of other crime victims. A resignation after being injured is relatively rare. Legal action against the client is sometimes discussed but rarely initiated. Debriefing with the client may be inappropriate or unnecessary to resolve the situation.

CN: Management of care; CL: Synthesize

90. 2,3,4,5. It is appropriate for the nurse manager to initiate a security investigation and ask the nurse to document all the facts about the missing purse. Alerting nursing administration is required. Seeking information from other staff will help with the investigation. It is inappropriate to confront any possible suspects while the investigation is ongoing.

CN: Management of care; CL: Analyze

91. 1,2,3,4. National guidelines exist for managing workplace violence. Unit staff, hospital administration, and hospital security personnel develop and enforce the resulting policies. These include training all staff about workplace violence, processes for reporting of such violence, and counseling for the staff victim. Protecting staff and clients may include posting the ex-boyfriend's picture at employee entrances and a protective order initiated by the nurse. With these policies and procedures in place, it is counterproductive to ask the nurse to take a leave of absence.

CN: Management of care; CL: Analyze

Abuse and Mental Health Problems of Children, Adolescents, and Families

- ■ The Client Experiencing Abuse
- ■ The Adolescent with Eating Disorders
- ■ Children and Adolescents with Behavioral Problems
- ■ The Child and Adolescent with Adjustment Disorders
- ■ Managing Care-Clients with Abuse and Mental Health Problems
- ■ Answers, Rationales, and Test-Taking Strategies

The Client Experiencing Abuse

1. A married female client has been referred to the mental health center because she is depressed. The nurse notices bruises on her upper arms and asks about them. After denying any problems, the client starts to cry and says, "He did not really mean to hurt me, but I hate for the kids to see this. I am so worried about them." What is the **most** crucial information for the nurse to determine?
- ☐ 1. the type and extent of abuse occurring in the family
- ☐ 2. the potential of immediate danger to the client and her children
- ☐ 3. the resources available to the client
- ☐ 4. whether the client wants to be separated from her husband

2. A client with suspected abuse describes her husband as a good man who works hard and provides well for his family. She does not work outside the home and states that she is proud to be a wife and mother just like her own mother. The nurse interprets the family pattern described by the client as **best** illustrating which characteristic of abusive families?
- ☐ 1. tight, impermeable boundaries
- ☐ 2. unbalanced power ratio
- ☐ 3. role stereotyping
- ☐ 4. dysfunctional feeling tone

3. When planning the care for a client who is being abused, which measure is **most** important to include?
- ☐ 1. being compassionate and empathetic
- ☐ 2. teaching the client about abuse and the cycle of violence
- ☐ 3. explaining to the client about the client's personal and legal rights
- ☐ 4. helping the client develop a safety plan

4. A nurse is assessing a client who is being abused. The nurse should assess the client for which characteristic(s)? Select all that apply.
- ☐ 1. assertiveness
- ☐ 2. self-blame
- ☐ 3. alcohol abuse
- ☐ 4. suicidal thoughts
- ☐ 5. guilt

5. After months of counseling, a client abused by her husband tells the nurse that she has decided to stop treatment. There has been no abuse during this time, and she feels better able to cope with the needs of her husband and children. In discussing this decision with the client, the nurse should:
- ☐ 1. tell the client that this is a bad decision that she will regret in the future.
- ☐ 2. find out more about the client's rationale for her decision to stop treatment.
- ☐ 3. warn the client that abuse commonly stops when one partner is in treatment, only to begin again later.
- ☐ 4. remind the client of her duty to protect her children by continuing treatment.

6. A third-grade child is referred to the mental health clinic by the school nurse because he is fearful, anxious, and socially isolated. After meeting with the client, the nurse talks with his mother, who says, "It is that school nurse again. She has done nothing but try to make trouble for our family since my son started school. And now you are in on it." The nurse should respond by saying:
- ☐ 1. "The school nurse is concerned about your son and is only doing her job."
- ☐ 2. "You do not need to feel singled out. We see a number of children who go to your son's school."
- ☐ 3. "You sound pretty angry with the school nurse. Tell me what has happened."
- ☐ 4. "Let me tell you why your son was referred, and then you can tell me about your concerns."

7. The parent of a school-aged child tells the nurse that, "For most of the past year, my husband was unemployed and I worked a second job. Twice during the year I spanked my son repeatedly when he refused to obey. It has not happened again. Our family is back to normal." After assessing the family, the nurse decides that the child is still at risk for abuse. Which observation **best** supports this conclusion?
☐ 1. The parents say they are taking away privileges when their son refuses to obey.
☐ 2. The child has talked about family activities with the nurse.
☐ 3. The parents are less negative toward the nurse.
☐ 4. The child wears long-sleeved shirts and long pants, even in warm weather.

8. When caring for a client who was a victim of a crime, the nurse is aware that recovery from any crime can be a long and difficult process depending on the meaning it has for the client. What should the nurse establish as a victim's ultimate goal in reconstructing his or her life?
☐ 1. getting through the shock and confusion
☐ 2. carrying out home and work routines
☐ 3. resolving grief over any losses
☐ 4. regaining a sense of security and safety

9. A client tells the nurse that she has been raped but has not reported it to the police. After determining whether the client was injured, whether it is still possible to collect evidence, and whether the client wants to file a report, the nurse's **next priority** is to offer which intervention to the client?
☐ 1. legal assistance
☐ 2. crisis intervention
☐ 3. a rape support group
☐ 4. medication for disturbed sleep

10. In working with a rape victim, which intervention is **most** important?
☐ 1. continuing to encourage the client to report the rape to the legal authorities
☐ 2. recommending that the client resume sexual relations with her partner as soon as possible
☐ 3. periodically reminding the client that she did not deserve and did not cause the rape
☐ 4. telling the client that the rapist will eventually be caught, put on trial, and jailed

11. In the process of dealing with intense feelings about being raped, victims commonly verbalize that they were afraid they would be killed during the rape and wish that they had been. The nurse should decide that further counseling is needed if the client makes which statement?
☐ 1. "I did not fight him, but I guess I did the right thing because I am alive."
☐ 2. "Suicide would be an easy escape from all this pain, but I could not do it to myself."
☐ 3. "I wish they gave the death penalty to all rapists and other sexual predators."
☐ 4. "I get so angry at times that I have to have a couple of drinks before I sleep."

12. One of the myths about sexual abuse of young children is that it usually involves physically violent acts. Which behavior is more likely to be used by the abusers?
☐ 1. tying the child down
☐ 2. bribery with money
☐ 3. coercion as a result of the trusting relationship
☐ 4. asking for the child's consent for sex

13. A preadolescent child is suspected of being sexually abused because he demonstrates the self-destructive behaviors of self-mutilation and attempted suicide. Which common behavior should the nurse also expect to assess?
☐ 1. inability to play
☐ 2. truancy and running away
☐ 3. head banging
☐ 4. overcontrol of anger

14. Adolescents and adults who were sexually abused as children commonly mutilate themselves. The nurse interprets this behavior as:
☐ 1. the need to make themselves less sexually attractive.
☐ 2. an alternative to binging and purging.
☐ 3. use of physical pain to avoid dealing with emotional pain.
☐ 4. an alternative to getting high on drugs.

15. A young child who has been sexually abused has difficulty putting feelings into words. Which approach should the nurse employ with the child?
☐ 1. engaging in play therapy
☐ 2. role-playing
☐ 3. giving the child's drawings to the abuser
☐ 4. reporting the abuse to a prosecutor

16. When working with a group of adult survivors of childhood sexual abuse, dealing with anger and rage is a major focus. Which strategies should the nurse expect to be successful? Select all that apply.
☐ 1. directly confronting the abuser
☐ 2. using a foam bat while symbolically confronting the abuser
☐ 3. keeping a journal of memories and feelings
☐ 4. writing letters to the abusers but not sending them
☐ 5. writing letters to the adults who did not protect them but not sending them

17. After a client reveals a history of childhood sexual abuse, what question should the nurse ask **first**?
☐ 1. "What other forms of abuse did you experience?"
☐ 2. "How long did the abuse go on?"
☐ 3. "Was there a time when you did not remember the abuse?"
☐ 4. "Does your abuser still have contact with young children?"

18. Which parental characteristic is **least** likely to be a risk factor for child abuse?
- ☐ **1.** low self-esteem
- ☐ **2.** history of substance abuse
- ☐ **3.** inadequate knowledge of normal growth and development patterns
- ☐ **4.** being a member of a large family

19. When obtaining a nursing history from parents who are suspected of abusing their child, which characteristic about the parents should the nurse particularly assess?
- ☐ **1.** attentiveness to the child's needs
- ☐ **2.** self-blame for the injury to the child
- ☐ **3.** ability to relate the child's developmental achievements
- ☐ **4.** difficulty with controlling aggression

20. A 3-year-old child with a history of being abused has blood drawn. The child lies very still and makes no sound during the procedure. Which comment by the nurse would be **most** appropriate?
- ☐ **1.** "It is okay to cry when something hurts."
- ☐ **2.** "That really did not hurt, did it?"
- ☐ **3.** "We must seem mean to hurt you that way."
- ☐ **4.** "You were very good not to cry with the needle."

21. While interviewing a 3-year-old girl who has been sexually abused about the event, which approach would be **most** effective?
- ☐ **1.** Describe what happened during the abusive act.
- ☐ **2.** Draw a picture and explain what it means.
- ☐ **3.** "Play out" the event using anatomically correct dolls.
- ☐ **4.** Name the perpetrator.

22. Which observation by the nurse should suggest that a 15-month-old toddler has been abused?
- ☐ **1.** The child appears happy when personnel work with him.
- ☐ **2.** The child plays alongside others contentedly.
- ☐ **3.** The child is underdeveloped for his age.
- ☐ **4.** The child sucks his thumb.

23. When planning interventions for parents who are abusive, the nurse should incorporate knowledge of which factor as a common parental indicator?
- ☐ **1.** lower socioeconomic group
- ☐ **2.** unemployment
- ☐ **3.** low self-esteem
- ☐ **4.** loss of emotional family attachments

24. A 15-year-old boy has been shy and quiet throughout his schooling. In the past, he has been teased about being "big" and "fat," leading him to get angry and fight those who called him names. This school year, he joined the wrestling team and showed some promise, though he had to lose weight to compete in a lower weight class. This spring, his mother called the nurse and said she had noticed that her son was wearing long-sleeved shirts all the time and spending a lot of time in the bathroom at home. She has seen scars on his wrists that the boy attributes to wrestling although the season has been over for several weeks. She and the boy's father are going through a contentious divorce that she thinks may be upsetting her son. In what order of priority from first to last should the nurse initiate the actions? All options must be used.

1. Interview the teen about how he is handling the divorce, any bullying he may be experiencing, and his current grades.

2. Interview the mother further about the child's early childhood and any potential antecedents to his current behavior.

3. Interview the father about his awareness of his son's behavior and perspective concerning it as well as the relationship between him and his son.

4. Ask the boy about self-injury, depression, and suicidality in connection with the scars on his wrists.

25. A shy middle school student set up a social network site. A popular student sent a message that included a suggestive picture of himself and suggested the student send a similar picture. When the student sent back a picture of himself dressed only in his boxers, the popular student sent it to all his friends and encouraged them to pass it along. Soon, the whole school had seen the picture identified as "Joe's Crotch." The student was so humiliated that he tried to hang himself but was found by his parent before he succeeded. Which outcomes would be **most** realistic and appropriate with regard to this situation? Select all that apply.
- ☐ 1. The social network privileges of all those who forwarded the message are revoked for a year.
- ☐ 2. All students in the school are educated about the risks of cyberbullying and how to respond to it.
- ☐ 3. The popular student who sent the message to his friends is disciplined by the school authorities.
- ☐ 4. The student can use the Internet safely after being educated about cyberbullying and completing a safety plan.
- ☐ 5. Through therapy, the student learns social skills to improve his confidence level and help him relate to peers more easily.

The Adolescent with Eating Disorders

26. The nurse is planning an eating disorder protocol for hospitalized clients experiencing bulimia and anorexia. Which elements should be included in the protocol? Select all that apply.
- ☐ 1. Clients must eat within view of a staff member.
- ☐ 2. Clients are not told their weight and cannot see their weight while being weighed.
- ☐ 3. Clients are not allowed to discuss food or eating in groups or informal conversation with peers.
- ☐ 4. Clients must rest within view of a staff member for one-half hour to an hour after eating.
- ☐ 5. Clients may not go to the bathroom for one-half hour to an hour after eating.
- ☐ 6. Clients cannot participate in any groups after admission until they gain 1 lb (0.5 kg).

27. A hospitalized adolescent diagnosed with anorexia nervosa refuses to comply with her daily before-breakfast weigh-in. She states that she just drank a glass of water, which she feels will unfairly increase her weight. What is the nurse's **best** response to the client?
- ☐ 1. "You are here to gain weight so that will work in your favor."
- ☐ 2. "Do not drink or eat for 2 hours, and then I will weigh you."
- ☐ 3. "You must weigh in every day at this time. Please step on the scale."
- ☐ 4. "If you do not get on the scale, I will be forced to call your healthcare provider."

28. The nurse discovers that an adolescent client with anorexia nervosa is taking diet pills rather than complying with the diet. What should the nurse do **first**?
- ☐ 1. Explain to the client how diet pills can jeopardize health.
- ☐ 2. Listen to the client discuss fears of losing control of eating while being treated.
- ☐ 3. Talk with the client about how weight loss and emaciation worry the healthcare providers (HCPs).
- ☐ 4. Inquire about worries of the client's family concerning the client's physical and emotional health.

29. When teaching a group of adolescents about anorexia nervosa, the nurse should describe this disorder as being characterized by which factors?
- ☐ 1. excessive fear of becoming obese, near-normal weight, and a self-critical body image
- ☐ 2. obsession with the weight of others, chronic dieting, and an altered body image
- ☐ 3. extreme concern about dieting, calorie counting, and an unrealistic body image
- ☐ 4. intense fear of becoming obese, emaciation, and a disturbed body image

30. The nurse reviews laboratory work for a client who is admitted to the acute psychiatric unit for an eating disorder.

History	Physical	Labs	Prescriptions

Test	Result Traditional Units	Result SI Units
Albumin level	2.8 g/dl	28 g/L
Sodium level	145 mEq/L	145 mmol/L
Hemoglobin level	10.8 g/dL	108 g/L
Potassium level	2.7 mEq/L	2.7 mmol/L
Hematocrit level	37%	0.37

Which finding does the nurse report to the healthcare provider (HCP)? Select all that apply.
- ☐ 1. albumin level
- ☐ 2. sodium level
- ☐ 3. hemoglobin level
- ☐ 4. potassium level
- ☐ 5. hematocrit level

31. The parents of a 15-year-old newly diagnosed with anorexia nervosa are meeting with the nurse during the admission process. Which remarks should the nurse interpret as typical for parents of a client with anorexia nervosa?
- ☐ 1. "We have given her everything, and look how she repays us!"
- ☐ 2. "She has had behavior problems for the past year both at home and at school."
- ☐ 3. "She has been a model child. We have never had any problems with her."
- ☐ 4. "We have five children, all normal kids with some problems at times."

32. A young adult female client is brought to the emergency department by her roommate to seek treatment for gastrointestinal problems. The client reveals that she attends college and works at a coffee shop each evening. A diet history indicates that the client has unhealthy eating habits, commonly eating large amounts of carbohydrates and junk food with few fruits and vegetables. "Her stomach is upset a lot," the roommate says. She further reports that the client is "in the bathroom all the time." The nurse should refer the client to:
- ☐ 1. a mental health clinic.
- ☐ 2. a weight loss program.
- ☐ 3. an overeating support group.
- ☐ 4. the client's family healthcare provider (HCP).

33. A nurse is working with a client with bulimia. Which goals should be included in the care plan? Select all that apply.
- ☐ 1. The client will maintain normal weight.
- ☐ 2. The client will comply with medication therapy.
- ☐ 3. The client will achieve a positive self-concept.
- ☐ 4. The client will acknowledge the disorder.
- ☐ 5. The client will never have the desire to purge again.

34. A nurse works with a client diagnosed with bulimia. What is the **most** appropriate long-term client goal for this client?
- ☐ 1. Eat meals at home without binging or purging.
- ☐ 2. Be able to eat out without binging or purging.
- ☐ 3. Manage stresses in life without binging or purging.
- ☐ 4. Be able to attend college without binging or purging.

35. A client newly diagnosed with bulimia is attending the nurse-led group at the mental health center. She tells the group that she came only because her husband said he would divorce her if she did not get help. Which response by the nurse is appropriate?
- ☐ 1. "You sound angry with your husband. Is that correct?"
- ☐ 2. "You will find that you like coming to group. These people are a lot of fun."
- ☐ 3. "Tell me more about why you are here and how you feel about that."
- ☐ 4. "Tell me something about what has caused you to be bulimic."

36. A client diagnosed with bulimia tells the nurse she only eats excessively when upset with her best friend, and then she vomits to avoid gaining a lot of weight. The nurse should **next**:
- ☐ 1. schedule daily family therapy sessions.
- ☐ 2. enroll client in a coping skills group.
- ☐ 3. work with the client to limit her purging.
- ☐ 4. have client take lorazepam 1 mg as needed whenever she feels the urge to binge.

37. A community health nurse working with a group of fifth-grade girls is planning a primary prevention to help the girls avoid developing eating disorders during their teen years. The nurse should focus on which factor?
- ☐ 1. working with the school nurse to closely monitor the girls' weight during middle school
- ☐ 2. limiting the girls' access to media images of very thin models and celebrities
- ☐ 3. telling the girls' parents to monitor their daughter's weight and media access
- ☐ 4. helping the girls accept and appreciate their bodies and feel good about themselves

Children and Adolescents with Behavioral Problems

38. A 17-year-old client who has been taking an antidepressant for 6 weeks has returned to the clinic for a medication check. When the nurse talks with the client and her parent, the mother reports that she has to remind the client to take her antidepressant every day. The client says, "Yeah, I am pretty bad about remembering to take my meds, but I never miss a dose because Mom always bugs me about taking it." Which response would be effective for the nurse to make to the client?
- ☐ 1. "It is a good thing your mom takes care of you by reminding you to take your meds."
- ☐ 2. "It seems there are some difficulties with being responsible for your medications that we need to address."
- ☐ 3. "You will never be able to handle your medication administration at college next year if you are so dependent on her."
- ☐ 4. "I am surprised your mother allows you to be so irresponsible."

39. The nurse assesses a 10-year-old girl who excessively cleans and categorizes. Her parents report that she has always been orderly, but since her brother died of cancer 6 months ago, her cleaning and categorizing have escalated. In school, she reads instead of playing with other children. These behaviors are now interfering with homework and leisure activities. To bolster her self-esteem, the nurse should encourage the child to:
☐ 1. be a library helper.
☐ 2. organize a party for the class.
☐ 3. be in charge of a group project with four peers.
☐ 4. be captain of the kickball team.

40. A 15-year-old is a heavy user of marijuana and alcohol. When the nurse confronts the client about his drug and alcohol use, he admits previous heavy use in order to feel more comfortable around peers and achieve social acceptance. He says he has been trying to stay clean since his parents found out and had him seek treatment. When the nurse develops a plan of care with the client, what should be the **highest priority** to help him maintain sobriety?
☐ 1. peer recognition that does not involve substance use
☐ 2. support and guidance from his parents
☐ 3. a strict no drug policy at his high school
☐ 4. the threat of legal charges if caught drinking or smoking marijuana

41. A 17-year-old is admitted to a psychiatric day treatment program due to severe lower back pain since her mother's death 3 years ago. Medical examinations have not discovered a physical cause for her pain. She cares for her four younger siblings after school and on weekends because of her father's long work hours. Which predischarge statement indicates that treatment for her condition has been successful?
☐ 1. "I understand now why my father spends so much time away from home."
☐ 2. "My back pain is worse on weekends with more responsibility and homework."
☐ 3. "I do not want to talk about my family. It is my back that is hurting."
☐ 4. "I just need more rest and relaxation and then my back will feel fine."

42. When collaborating with the healthcare provider (HCP) to develop the plan of care for a child diagnosed with attention deficit hyperactivity disorder (ADHD), the treatment plan will likely include which treatments?
☐ 1. antianxiety medications, such as buspirone, and homeschooling
☐ 2. antidepressant medications, such as imipramine, and family therapy
☐ 3. anticonvulsant medications, such as carbamazepine, and monthly blood levels
☐ 4. psychostimulant medications, such as methylphenidate, and behavior modification

43. The nurse meets with the mother of a child diagnosed with attention deficit hyperactivity disorder. The mother states, "I feel so guilty that he has this disease, like I did something wrong. I feel like I need to be with him constantly in order for him to get better. But still sometimes I feel like I am going to lose control and hurt him." The nurse should suggest which intervention to the mother?
☐ 1. arranging for respite care to watch her child and give herself a regular break
☐ 2. taking a job to allow herself to feel some success because her child will not ever improve
☐ 3. arranging to have coffee with friends daily as a way to begin a support group
☐ 4. considering foster care if she feels that she cannot handle her child's problems

44. The nurse is with the parents of a 16-year-old boy who recently attempted suicide. The nurse cautions the parents to be especially alert for which changes in their son?
☐ 1. expression of a desire to date
☐ 2. decision to try out for an extracurricular activity
☐ 3. giving away valued personal items
☐ 4. desire to spend more time with friends

45. A 19-year-old has struggled academically throughout high school and realizes during her last semester in school that she is not going to graduate with her class, which will delay her admission to college. In the past, she has intermittently used drugs and alcohol to deal with her anxiety, but now, her involvement with substances escalates to daily use. In what order of priority from first to last should the nurse, who has become aware of the problem, take the actions? All options must be used.

1. Refer her to the school authorities to address her academic issues so she can graduate next semester.

2. Refer her to a program at the local community college to improve the client's readiness for college and decrease her anxiety.

3. Refer her to an outpatient program that treats clients with chemical dependency issues.

4. Refer her to a psychiatric clinic so she can get an appropriate diagnosis and medication for her anxiety.

46. A mother states to the nurse in her healthcare provider's (HCP's) office that she is frustrated regarding her 7-year-old son's nightly enuresis for the past 3 years. She says she has limited his evening fluids, eliminated all caffeine and soft drinks from his diet, and has had him wash his own sheets, but he still wets the bed almost every night. Her husband has told her he was a bed wetter as a child. He thinks the son will "get over it." The mother is worried that it could negatively affect the son's peer relationships as he grows older. Which action should the nurse take?
- ☐ 1. Tell the mother her husband is correct and she should be patient since her husband's enuresis stopped without intervention.
- ☐ 2. Suggest asking the HCP about medication treatment to deal with the enuresis.
- ☐ 3. Discuss a behavioral treatment plan for the child focusing on the improvement of his social skills.
- ☐ 4. Suggest the mother ask the HCP about hospitalization for a complete renal workup since the enuresis has gone on a long time.

47. A parent of a 7-year-old diagnosed with attention deficit hyperactivity disorder (ADHD) since he was 5 years old is talking to the nurse about her concerns about the son's physical condition. The parent states that his medication, methylphenidate, extended release, controls his symptoms well but is causing him to lose weight. It is difficult to get him up and ready for school in the morning unless he is given the medication as soon as he awakens. He does not eat breakfast or very much of his lunch at school; he eats dinner, but only an average amount of food. He has lost 3 lb (1.4 kg) in the last 2 weeks. Which action should the nurse suggest the parent do **first**?
- ☐ 1. Have the child eat a breakfast bar, banana, and a glass of milk at his bedside at the same time he takes his medication every morning.
- ☐ 2. Monitor the child's weight closely for a month since he is likely to stop losing weight when the school year ends in 2 weeks.
- ☐ 3. Suggest a change of medication to a nonstimulant drug that will treat his ADHD without causing the appetite decrease.
- ☐ 4. Suggest that the parent supplement the child's dinner with a high-protein drink or other food that will increase his caloric intake.

48. An adolescent is brought to the emergency department (ED) after accidentally taking an overdose of heroin. The adolescent is semiconscious, unable to respond appropriately to questions, slurs his words, and has constricted pupils; his vital signs are blood pressure 60/50 mm Hg, pulse 50 beats/min, and respirations 8 breaths/min. Naloxone is administered to temporarily reverse the effects of the heroin. Which finding would **first** indicate that the naloxone administration has been effective?
- ☐ 1. The client's blood opiate level drops to a nontoxic level.
- ☐ 2. The client becomes talkative and physically active.
- ☐ 3. The client's memory and attention become normal.
- ☐ 4. The client's respirations improve to 12/min.

49. Assessment of suicidal risk in children and adolescents requires the nurse to know what information?
- ☐ 1. Children rarely commit suicide unless one of their parents has already committed suicide, especially in the past year.
- ☐ 2. The risk of suicide increases during adolescence, with those who have recently suffered a loss, abuse, or family discord being most at risk.
- ☐ 3. Children do have a suicidal risk that coincides with some significant event such as a recent gun purchase in the family.
- ☐ 4. Adolescents typically do not choose suicide unless they live in certain geographical regions of the United States and Canada.

50. A child is being seen at the clinic for an attention deficit hyperactivity disorder (ADHD) assessment. What symptoms the nurse would expect to find? Select all that apply.
- ☐ 1. excessive climbing and running
- ☐ 2. excessive fidgeting
- ☐ 3. pouting behaviors
- ☐ 4. cannot wait to take turns
- ☐ 5. easily distracted

51. The mother of a 14-year-old girl who is diagnosed with oppositional defiant disorder tells the nurse that she has read extensively on this disorder and does not believe the diagnosis is correct for her daughter. Which response by the nurse is appropriate?
- ☐ 1. "It sounds like you are very interested in your daughter. Let us focus on what is best for her."
- ☐ 2. "Tell me what you have found in your reading that is leading you to that conclusion."
- ☐ 3. "Your healthcare provider (HCP) has had many years of education and experience, so you can believe he is right."
- ☐ 4. "That does not matter now because we just need to help her get better."

52. The parents of a preschool child diagnosed with autism must take their child on a plane flight and are concerned about how they can make the experience less stressful for her and their fellow travelers. The nurse suggests a dry run to the airport in which they simulate going through security and boarding a plane. In addition, the nurse suggests taking items to help the child be calm during the flight. In what order of priority from first to last should the parents employ the items listed below? All options must be used.

| 1. a DVD player with headphones and favorite games, cartoons, and child films |

| 2. a favorite stuffed toy animal or other soft toy |

| 3. a favorite nonelectronic game |

| 4. medication that can be given as needed to calm the child |

| |

| |

| |

| |

53. A young school-age girl whose mother and aunt have been diagnosed as having bipolar disorder and whose father is diagnosed with depression is brought to the clinic because of problems with behavior and attention in school and inability to sleep at night. The child says, "My brain does not turn off at night." The child is diagnosed as experiencing attention deficit hyperactivity disorder (ADHD) with a possibility of bipolar disorder as well. What should the nurse say to the father to explain what the provider said? Select all that apply.
- ☐ 1. "Your child was diagnosed as having ADHD because of her attention and behavior problems at school."
- ☐ 2. "ADHD involves difficulty with attention, impulse control, and hyperactivity at school, home, or in both settings."
- ☐ 3. "Your provider does not know how to diagnose your child's illness since she has symptoms of both bipolar disorder and ADHD."
- ☐ 4. "The child's description of her inability to sleep is irrelevant to diagnosing her condition since she stays up late."
- ☐ 5. "Your provider is considering a bipolar diagnosis because of your child's family history of bipolar disorder and her sleep issues."

54. At the admission interview, the father of a 4-year-old boy with attention deficit hyperactivity disorder (ADHD) says to the nurse, "I know that my wife or I must have caused this disease." What is the nurse's **best** response?
- ☐ 1. "ADHD is more common within families, but there is no evidence that problems with parenting cause this disorder."
- ☐ 2. "What do you think you might have done that could have led to causing this disorder to develop in your son?"
- ☐ 3. "Many parents feel this way, but I doubt there is anything that you did that caused ADHD to develop in your child."
- ☐ 4. "Let us not focus on the cause but rather on what needs to be done to help your son get better. I know that you and your wife are very interested in helping him to improve his behavior."

55. A member of a nurse-led group for depressed adolescents tells the group that she is not coming back because she is taking medication and no longer needs to talk about her problems. Which response by the nurse is **most** appropriate?
- ☐ 1. "I am glad that you are taking your medication, but how can we know that you will continue to take it? After all, you have not been on it for very long, and you might decide to stop taking it."
- ☐ 2. "I think that it is important to let everyone respond to what you said, so let us go around the group and let everyone give their thoughts about what you have decided."
- ☐ 3. "The purpose of the group is to provide each of you with a place to discuss the problems of being a teenager with depression with others who also are experiencing a similar situation."
- ☐ 4. "You do not have to stay in the group if you do not want to, but if you choose to leave, then you will not be able to change your mind later and return to the group."

56. Which question is **most** appropriate to use when assessing a 17-year-old client with depression for suicide risk?
- ☐ 1. "What movies about death have you watched lately?"
- ☐ 2. "Can you tell me what you think about suicide?"
- ☐ 3. "Has anyone in your family ever committed suicide?"
- ☐ 4. "Are you thinking about killing yourself?"

57. A teacher is talking to the nurse about a child in her classroom who has a tic disorder. The teacher mentions that the boy frequently trips other children although no one has ever been hurt. The teacher then further states that she ignores him when that happens because it is part of his disorder. The nurse should tell the teacher:
- ☐ 1. "Tripping other children is not a tic, so you can respond to that as you would in any other child."
- ☐ 2. "I cannot believe that you actually allow him to get away with that!"
- ☐ 3. "I think that is the best choice unless some parents of the other children start to protest about it."
- ☐ 4. "If no one else is getting hurt, then it seems harmless and might prevent the development of a worse behavior."

58. A 15-year-old boy being successfully treated for Tourette's syndrome tells the nurse, "I am not going to take this medication anymore. Anyone who is really my friend will accept me as I am, tics and all!" What is the nurse's **best** response?
- ☐ 1. "You and your family came to the clinic for treatment, so you can terminate it whenever you wish."
- ☐ 2. "Will your lack of medication cause more tics and make you less attractive to girls?"
- ☐ 3. "Let us talk about what brought you into treatment and why you now want to stop taking medication."
- ☐ 4. "I think that is a very unwise decision, but you are entitled to do whatever you wish."

59. The nurse is leading a group session for parents of children diagnosed with oppositional defiant disorder. The nurse should give which recommendation for discipline?
- ☐ 1. Avoid limiting the child's use of the television and computer for punishment.
- ☐ 2. Be consistent with discipline while assisting with ways for the child to more positively express anger and frustration.
- ☐ 3. Use primarily positive reinforcement for good behavior while ignoring any demonstrated bad behavior.
- ☐ 4. Use time-out as the primary means of punishment for the child regardless of what the child has done.

60. A 15-year-old girl is sent to the school nurse with dizziness and nausea. While assessing the girl, who denies any health problems, the nurse smells alcohol on her breath. Which response by the nurse is **most** appropriate?
- ☐ 1. "Do not tell me that you have been drinking alcohol before you came to school this morning!"
- ☐ 2. "What is the real reason that you are feeling sick this morning?"
- ☐ 3. "Tell me everything that you have had to eat and drink yesterday and today."
- ☐ 4. "I know that high school is stressful, but drinking alcohol is not the best way to handle it."

61. What should the nurse include in the teaching plan for the parents of a child who is receiving methylphenidate?
- ☐ 1. Give the medication at the same time every evening.
- ☐ 2. Have the child take two doses at the same time if the last dose was missed.
- ☐ 3. Give the single-dose form of the medication early in the day.
- ☐ 4. Allow concurrent use of any over-the-counter medications with this drug.

62. An 8-year-old child was recently hospitalized at a child psychiatric unit for inattention and acting out behavior at school and home. His provider prescribed the methylphenidate patch to control his attention deficit hyperactivity disorder symptoms, and inpatient unit staff worked with him on behavioral control measures. During his first office visit after his discharge from the hospital, the office nurse discovers that the boy has been taking off his patch during the day, which is causing problems at school and at home. In which order of priority from first to last should the nurse take the actions? All options must be used.

1. Explain to the family, in terms the child can understand, the benefits of his medication in dealing with school and home problems he is experiencing.

2. Explore the parents' attitudes about medication administration in general and their child's medication in particular.

3. Explore the child's reasons for removing the patch during the day rather than at the end of the day.

4. Have the provider discuss with the child and parents a trial of a different medication.

74. A new client has just been admitted to an adolescent psychiatric inpatient unit. The charge nurse and an unlicensed assistive personnel (UAP) are discussing the client's needs. The UAP says, "She is just showing off to try and get our sympathy. There is no need for her to cut herself. Why would adolescents want to do such a thing to themselves?" What response by the charge nurse would **most** help the UAP understand the client and her illness?

☐ 1. "She is not doing the cutting for attention since she always wears clothing that covers up her injuries and further, she is not willing to talk about it."

☐ 2. "It is hard to see a young person harm herself as she does, but she has serious family issues and does not know better ways to handle them, so we have to help her with that."

☐ 3. "You do not understand her problems and do not take them seriously, so you should not be allowed to work with her during her hospitalization."

☐ 4. "Perhaps you should transfer to another unit where you are able to have empathy for the clients."

75. A teenage client is admitted to the psychiatric unit with both bulimia nervosa and anorexia nervosa. Which initial interventions are appropriate for this client? Select all that apply.

☐ 1. Assign a staff member to accompany the client when using the bathroom.

☐ 2. Have the client keep a self-monitoring journal as a coping strategy.

☐ 3. Weigh the client in same amount of clothing and facing away from scale readout at daily scheduled intervals (e.g., 0645 on Tuesdays and Fridays).

☐ 4. Inform the client that parenteral nutrition will be necessary if the client does not gain weight.

☐ 5. Assign a staff member to sit with client during meals and for 1½ hour after meals.

☐ 6. Provide liquid protein supplements when client is unable to eat meals.

76. A young adult female who was admitted to the psychiatric hospital 2 months ago with an eating disorder is being discharged. Which action indicates the client understands discharge instructions?

☐ 1. Client returns to the same living situation as she had prior to hospitalization.

☐ 2. Client attends a social club at her local church.

☐ 3. Client returns to the lab for routine lab tests.

☐ 4. Client enrolls in a health club.

Answers, Rationales, and Test-Taking Strategies

*The answers and rationales for each question follow below, along with keys (🔑) to the client need (CN) and cognitive level (CL) for each question. In addition, you will also see a glossary icon (📖) highlighting specific terminology used on the licensing exam. As you check your answers, use the **Content Mastery and Test-Taking Skill Self-Analysis** worksheet (tear-out worksheet in back of book) to identify the reason(s) for not answering the questions correctly. For additional information about test-taking skills and strategies for answering questions, refer to pages 12–23 and pages 35–36 in Part 1 of this book.*

The Client Experiencing Abuse

1. 2. The safety of the client and her children is the most immediate concern. If there is immediate danger, action must be taken to protect them. The other options can be discussed after the client's safety is assured.

🔑 CN: Psychosocial integrity; CL: Analyze

2. 3. The traditional and rigid gender roles described by the client are examples of role stereotyping. Impermeable boundaries, unbalanced power ratio, and dysfunctional feeling tone are also common in abusive families.

🔑 CN: Safety and infection control; CL: Analyze

3. 4. The client's safety, including the need to stay alive, is crucial. Therefore, helping the client develop a safety plan is most important to include in the plan of care. Being empathetic, teaching about abuse, and explaining the person's rights are also important after safety is ensured.

🔑 CN: Psychosocial integrity; CL: Synthesize

4. 2,3,4,5. The victim of abuse is usually compliant with the spouse and feels guilt, shame, and some responsibility for the battering. Self-blame, substance abuse, and suicidal thoughts and attempts are possible dysfunctional coping methods used by abuse victims. The victim of abuse is not likely to demonstrate assertiveness.

🔑 CN: Psychosocial integrity; CL: Analyze

5. 2. The nurse needs more information about the client's decision before deciding what intervention is most appropriate. Judgmental responses could make it difficult for the client to return for treatment should she want to do so. Telling the client that this is a bad decision that she will regret is inappropriate because the nurse is making an assumption. Warning the client that abuse commonly stops when one partner is involved in treatment may be true for some clients. However, until the nurse determines the basis for the client's decision, this type of response is an assumption and therefore inappropriate. Reminding the client about her duty to protect the children would be appropriate if the client had talked about episodes of current abuse by her partner and the fear that her children might be hurt by him, but the scenario offers no evidence that the husband has threatened the children.

🔑 CN: Psychosocial integrity;
CL: Synthesize

6. 3. The mother's feelings are the priority here. Addressing the mother's feelings and asking for her view of the situation is most important in building a relationship with the family. Ignoring the mother's feelings will hinder the relationship. Defending the school nurse and the school puts the client's mother on the defensive and stifles communication.

🔑 CN: Psychosocial integrity;
CL: Synthesize

7. 4. Parental use of nonviolent discipline, the child's talk about what the family is doing, and the easing of the parent's negativity toward the school nurse are all signs of progress. Avoidance and wearing clothes inappropriate for the weather implies that the child has something to hide, likely signs of physical abuse.

🔑 CN: Psychosocial integrity; CL: Analyze

8. 4. Ultimately, a victim of a crime needs to move from being a victim to being a survivor. A reasonable sense of safety and security is key to this transition. Getting through the shock and confusion, carrying out home and work routines, and resolving grief over any losses represent steps along the way to becoming a survivor.

🔑 CN: Psychosocial integrity;
CL: Synthesize

9. 2. The experience of rape is a crisis. Crisis intervention services, especially with a rape crisis nurse, are essential to help the client begin dealing with the aftermath of a rape. Legal assistance may be recommended if the client decides to report the rape and only after crisis intervention services have been provided. A rape support group can be helpful later in the recovery process. Medications for sleep disturbance, especially benzodiazepines, should

be avoided if possible. Benzodiazepines are potentially addictive and can be used in suicide attempts, especially when consumed with alcohol.

🔑 CN: Psychosocial integrity;
CL: Synthesize

10. 3. Guilt and self-blame are common feelings that need to be addressed directly and frequently. The client needs to be reminded periodically that she did not deserve and did not cause the rape. Continually encouraging the client to report the rape pressures the client and is not helpful. In most cases, resuming sexual relations is a difficult process that is not likely to occur quickly. It is not necessarily true that the rapist will be caught, tried, and jailed. Most rapists are not caught or convicted.

🔑 CN: Psychosocial integrity; CL: Apply

11. 4. Use of alcohol reflects unhealthy coping mechanisms. The client's report of needing alcohol to calm down needs to be addressed. Survival is the most important goal during a rape. The client's acknowledging this indicates that she is aware that she made the right choice. Although suicidal thoughts are common, the statement that suicide is an easy escape but the client would be unable to do it indicates low risk. Fantasies of revenge, such as giving the death penalty to all rapists, are natural reactions and are a problem only if the client intends to carry them out directly.

🔑 CN: Psychosocial integrity; CL: Evaluate

12. 3. Coercion is the most common strategy used because the child commonly trusts the abuser. Tying the child down usually is not necessary. Typically, the abusive person can control the child by his or her size and weight alone. Bribery usually is not necessary because the child wants love and affection from the abusive person, not money. Young children are not capable of giving consent for sex before they develop an adult concept of what sex is.

🔑 CN: Psychosocial integrity; CL: Apply

13. 2. Truancy and running away are common symptoms for young children and adolescents. The stress of the abuse interferes with school success, leading to the avoidance of school. Running away is an effort to escape the abuse and/or lack of support at home. Rather than an inability to play or a lack of play, play is likely to be aggressive with sexual overtones. Children tend to act out anger rather than control it. Head banging is a behavior typically seen with very young children who are abused.

🔑 CN: Psychosocial integrity; CL: Analyze

14. 3. Dealing with the physical pain associated with mutilation is viewed as easier than dealing with the intense anger and emotional pain. The client fears an aggressive outburst when anger and emotional pain increase. Self-mutilation seems easier and safer. Additionally, self-mutilation may occur if the client feels unreal or numb or is dissociating. Here, the mutilation proves to the client that he or she is alive and capable of feeling. The client may want to be less sexually attractive, but this aspect usually is not related to self-mutilation. Binging and purging is commonly done in addition to, not instead of, self-mutilation. Although a few clients report an occasional high with self-mutilation, usually the experience is just relief from anger and rage.

CN: Psychosocial integrity; CL: Analyze

15. 1. The dolls and toys in a play therapy room are useful props to help the child remember situations and reexperience the feelings, acting out the experience with the toys rather than putting the feelings into words. Role-playing without props commonly is more difficult for a child. Although drawing itself can be therapeutic, having the abuser see the pictures is usually threatening for the child. Reporting abuse to authorities is mandatory but does not help the child express feelings.

CN: Psychosocial integrity; CL: Synthesize

16. 2,3,4,5. Using a foam bat while symbolically confronting the abuser, keeping a journal of memories and feelings, and writing letters about the abuse but not sending them are appropriate strategies because they allow anger to be expressed safely. Directly confronting the abuser is likely to result in further harm because the abusers commonly deny the abuse, rationalize about it, or blame the victim.

CN: Psychosocial integrity; CL: Synthesize

17. 4. The safety of other children is a primary concern. It is critical to know whether other children are at risk for being sexually abused by the same perpetrator. Asking about other forms of abuse, how long the abuse went on, and if the victim did not remember the abuse are important questions after the safety of other children is determined.

CN: Psychosocial integrity; CL: Synthesize

18. 4. From documented cases of child abuse, a profile has emerged of a high-risk parent as a person who is isolated, impulsive, impatient, and single with low self-esteem, a history of substance abuse, a lack of knowledge about a child's normal growth and development, and multiple life stressors. Just because a parent comes from a large family, there is no increase in the incidence of the parent abusing their own children unless they possess the other risk factors.

CN: Psychosocial integrity; CL: Apply

19. 4. Parents of an abused child have difficulty controlling their aggressive behaviors. They may blame the child or others for the injury, may not ask questions about treatment, and may not know developmental information.

CN: Psychosocial integrity; CL: Analyze

20. 1. It is not normal for a preschooler to be totally passive during a painful procedure. Typically, a preschooler reacts to a painful procedure by crying or pulling away because of the fear of pain. However, an abused child may become "immune" to pain and may find that crying can bring on more pain. The child needs to learn that appropriate emotional expression is acceptable. Telling the child that it really did not hurt is inappropriate because it is untrue. Telling the child that nurses are mean does not build a trusting relationship. Praising the child will reinforce the child's response not to cry, even though it is acceptable to do so.

CN: Psychosocial integrity; CL: Synthesize

21. 3. A 3-year-old child has limited verbal skills and should not be asked to describe an event, explain a picture, or respond verbally or nonverbally to questions. More appropriately, the child can act out an event using dolls. The child is likely to be too fearful to name the perpetrator or will not be able to do so.

CN: Psychosocial integrity; CL: Synthesize

22. 3. An almost universal finding in descriptions of abused children is underdevelopment for age. This may be reflected in small physical size or in poor psychosocial development. The child should be evaluated further until a plausible diagnosis can be established. A child who appears happy when personnel work with him is exhibiting normal behavior. Children who are abused often are suspicious of others, especially adults. A child who plays alongside others is exhibiting normal behavior, that of parallel play. A child who sucks his thumb contentedly is also exhibiting normal behavior.

CN: Psychosocial integrity; CL: Analyze

23. 3. Parents who are abusive often suffer from low self-esteem, commonly because of the way they were parented, including not being able to develop trust in caretakers and not being encouraged or offered emotional support by parents. Therefore, the nurse works to bolster the parents' self-esteem. This can be achieved by praising the parents for appropriate parenting. Employment and socioeconomic status are not indicators of abusive parents. Abusive parents usually are attached to their children and do not want to give them up to foster care. Parents who are abusive usually love their children and feel close to them emotionally.

🔑 CN: Psychosocial integrity; CL: Analyze

24. 1,4,2,3. The nurse should talk to the boy directly about how he is dealing with the stresses in his life, but he may not be forthcoming if the nurse approaches the self-injury first. Once the nurse has established rapport and learned about the client's view of his situation, it will be more likely that the client will be honest about his self-injury and any depression or suicidal thoughts or plans he may have. Since the mother called the nurse with her concerns about her son, a further interview with the mother would be the next step to take. Because there is conflict in the home, it would be necessary to also interview the father for his perspective of the situation. If he is not aware of his son's self-injury, he needs to be informed of it.

🔑 CN: Safety and infection control; CL: Synthesize

25. 2,3,4,5. Education of all students in the school about cyberbullying is appropriate and possible as programs exist to educate students in many communities. That education and his therapy should enable the student to eventually return to using the Internet safely and to feel more confidence interacting with classmates. Disciplining of the student who posted the picture by school authorities is appropriate and can be helpful in reducing further incidents of cyberbullying. It is unrealistic to think that all those who forwarded the message could be identified, much less taken off a social network.

🔑 CN: Psychosocial integrity; CL: Evaluate

The Adolescent with Eating Disorders

26. 1,2,4,5. In hospital settings, clients are not allowed to know their weight at the time they are being weighed to decrease obsessing about weight gain. They must also eat and rest in staff view and cannot use the bathroom for a period to prevent discarding food or vomiting ingested food (purging). The rest prevents the client from exercising off the calories they just consumed. Barring clients from ever talking about food or attending groups until they have gained weight diminishes the therapeutic value of the inpatient hospital stay.

🔑 CN: Psychosocial integrity; CL: Create

27. 3. In responding to the client, the nurse must be nonjudgmental and matter of fact. Telling her that weight gain is in her favor ignores the client's extreme fear of gaining weight. Putting off the weigh-in for 2 hours allows the client to manipulate the nurse and interferes with the need to weigh the client at the same time each day. Threatening to call the care provider is not likely to build rapport or a working relationship with the client.

🔑 CN: Psychosocial integrity; CL: Synthesize

28. 2. A client with anorexia nervosa commonly has an extreme fear of not being able to control weight. The nurse should address this fear. Explaining the dangers of diet pills or discussing **HCP** 📖 or family concerns focuses on the effect of the client's weight loss on other people rather than the client. Unless the client is motivated to stop, the client will likely not be successful.

🔑 CN: Psychosocial integrity; CL: Synthesize

29. 4. An intense fear of becoming obese, emaciation, and a disturbed body image all are considered to be characteristics of anorexia nervosa. Near-normal weight is not associated with anorexia. The weight of others is not a primary factor. "Concern about dieting" is not strong enough language to describe the control of food intake in the individual with anorexia nervosa.

🔑 CN: Psychosocial integrity; CL: Apply

30. 1,3,4. The normal albumin level is 3.5 to 5 g/dL (35 to 50 g/L), the normal hemoglobin level is 12 to 16 g/dL (120 to 160 g/L), and the normal potassium is 3.5 to 5 mEq/L (3.5 to 5 mmol/L). These levels are all low. The client is likely not eating a sufficient amount of protein; therefore, the albumin and hemoglobin are low. The potassium level would be low if the client was purging. The sodium level is normally 136 to 145 mEq/L (136 to 145 mmol/L), so this is in the normal range; however, it can be high in a client with an eating disorder. The normal hematocrit level is 37% to 47% (0.37 to 0.47) in an adult.

🔑 CN: Reduction of risk potential; CL: Analyze

31. 3. Parents commonly describe their child as a model child who is a high achiever and compliant. These adolescents are typically well liked by teachers and peers. It is not typical for behavior problems to be reported. The description about having given the child everything and being repaid is more likely to describe an adolescent who is exhibiting behavior problems.

🔑 CN: Psychosocial integrity; CL: Analyze

32. 1. The large carbohydrate intake and significant time in the bathroom are characteristics of bulimia. To address the problem, the client must obtain an evaluation of her physical and psychological status. Suggesting going to a weight loss program or overeating support group frames the problem as strictly a weight issue and ignores the psychological etiology of the problem. Seeing the family's **HCP** 📖 does not address the psychological aspect of the client's illness, and the client must make the appointment herself.

🔑 CN: Psychosocial integrity; CL: Apply

33. **1,2,3,4.** Because of the large number of calories ingested in a binge and the fact that a purge does not eliminate all calories consumed, the client with bulimia is of more normal weight but still must have a goal of maintaining that weight. Research has shown that selective serotonin reuptake inhibitors are effective in treating bulimia, and the client is usually amenable to taking the medication. The client with an eating disorder (bulimia and anorexia) has negative self-concepts that fuel her disordered eating, and attaining a positive self-concept is an appropriate goal. The nurse should work with the client with bulimia to help her recognize her eating as disordered. That recognition can make the client more amenable to treatment. It is not realistic to establish a goal that the client with bulimia will never have the desire to purge again.

🔑 CN: Psychosocial integrity; CL: Create

34. **3.** A successful outcome for a bulimic client is to avoid using the eating disorder as a coping measure when dealing with stress. Being able to attend college, eat at home, and eat out without binging and purging are important goals, but they do not address the primary problem of stress management and its connection to eating.

🔑 CN: Psychosocial integrity; CL: Create

35. **3.** Encouraging the client to talk about why she is here and her feelings may reveal more information about what led her to come to the group and what led to her diagnosis. It also provides the nurse with valuable information needed to develop an appropriate plan of care. The comment that the client sounds angry presumes what the client is feeling and focuses the talk on her husband. The focus should be on the client, not the husband. Telling the client that she will like coming to group imposes the nurse's view onto the client. The statement also focuses on having fun in the group instead of stressing the therapeutic value. Having the client tell the nurse something about the cause of her bulimia ignores the client's original statement. In addition, it requires the client to have insight into the cause of her disease, which may not be possible at this point. Also, it may be too early in the relationship to discuss this disorder.

🔑 CN: Psychosocial integrity; CL: Synthesize

36. **2.** Because the client eats excessively when upset, the best treatment would be a group to help her learn alternative coping skills. Trying to limit purging without controlling binging would result in weight gain and likely increase the client's purging. Daily family therapy sessions are not realistic. Taking lorazepam whenever she feels she needs to binge may temporarily calm the client but does not address the cause of the binging and purging and will lead to drug dependence with long-term use.

🔑 CN: Psychosocial integrity; CL: Synthesize

37. **4.** The goal of a primary prevention program for eating disorders is for the girls to have positive feelings about themselves and their bodies. Monitoring of weight by parents and/or nurses might note eating disorders early, particularly anorexia, but will not address the cause of the disorder. Limiting the girls' access to media would be impossible and does not prevent distress with one's body image.

🔑 CN: Psychosocial integrity; CL: Synthesize

Children and Adolescents with Behavioral Problems

38. **2.** The client and mother need to address the issue of responsibility for medication administration. Reinforcing the mother's overinvolvement in medication taking or making negative comments about the client and mother is unlikely to engage them in problem solving about the matter.

🔑 CN: Psychosocial integrity; CL: Synthesize

39. **1.** This child is demonstrating signs of anxiety and withdrawal. Being a library helper enables the client to use an interest (reading) when interacting with others and gaining pride in helping others. Most interaction will be one-to-one and with adults, which is likely to be more comfortable for her in her state of anxiety. Organizing a class party, a group project with her peers, and a kickball team involve multiple peer interactions, which are likely to be difficult for her at this time. Also, there is no mention of the child liking sports, so kickball would not be an appropriate activity.

🔑 CN: Psychosocial integrity; CL: Synthesize

40. **1.** Peer acceptance and recognition is a very powerful force in the lives of adolescents, leading to positive or negative behavior depending on the child's peers. While the influence of parents remains strong, peer acceptance combined with the adolescent's desire for independence can lead to disobeying the parents. The sanctions provided at school and in the community by law enforcement will support those teens that have other support in their lives but are generally not sufficient to prevent substance use in adolescents lacking support at home and with peers.

🔑 CN: Psychosocial integrity; CL: Create

41. 2. This statement indicates insight into possible emotional causes for her pain. After insight is achieved, the client can make behavior changes to effectively cope with her anxiety-related disorder. Saying that she understands why her father is away so often demonstrates insight into her father's actions rather than her own. Wanting to discuss her pain and not her family indicates denial of any connection between her pain and her stress, which perpetuates her current situation. While rest may help her back, the client's statement does not address psychological issues related to the back pain.

🔑 CN: Psychosocial integrity;
CL: Evaluate

42. 4. ADHD is typically managed by psychostimulant medications, such as methylphenidate and pemoline, along with behavior modification. Antianxiety medications, such as buspirone, are not appropriate for treating ADHD. Homeschooling commonly is not a possibility because both parents work outside the home. Antidepressants, such as imipramine, are indicated for major depressive disorders and must be used with extreme caution in children because they carry the risk of suicidal thinking. Family therapy may be a part of the treatment. Anticonvulsant medications, such as carbamazepine, are not appropriate for ADHD. Also, carbamazepine levels are obtained weekly early during therapy to avoid toxicity and ascertain therapeutic levels.

🔑 CN: Pharmacological and parenteral therapies; CL: Apply

43. 1. Suggesting that the mother arrange for respite care so that she can have a regular break would help to alleviate some of the stress that she feels when she is with her child constantly. The mother also could use family and friends to provide some care, thereby helping with giving her a break. The child may improve, so suggesting that the mother take a job to provide a feeling of success would be inappropriate. Having coffee daily with friends may provide some opportunities for socialization. However, friends may not be able to provide the verbal support that the mother needs. Rather, attending a support group of other parents with children with attention deficit hyperactivity disorder might be helpful. Placing the child in foster care is an extreme measure that may damage the therapeutic relationship with the nurse and dramatically

and negatively affect the relationship between the mother and child.

🔑 CN: Psychosocial integrity;
CL: Synthesize

44. 3. Giving away personal items has consistently been shown to be an indicator of suicide plans in a depressed and suicidal individual. Expression of a desire to date, trying out for an extracurricular activity, or the desire to spend more time with friends indicates a return of interest in normal adolescent activities.

🔑 CN: Psychosocial integrity; CL: Analyze

45. 4,3,1,2. The client's anxiety seems to fuel her substance abuse, so treatment for her anxiety is paramount, followed by treatment for substance abuse. Those two interventions should increase her readiness to profit from academic aid offered by the school. Referral to a community college program would help her get ready for college, which will likely decrease her anxiety.

🔑 CN: Psychosocial integrity; CL: Create

46. 2. The mother's distress and length of time the problem has existed combined with the efforts she has made to address the problem demonstrate that medication treatment should be considered. The absence of any other symptoms makes a renal workup unnecessary at this time. It is unlikely that social skills training alone will change his nocturnal enuresis. Just waiting for the behavior to stop is likely to further tax the mother and son.

🔑 CN: Psychosocial integrity; CL: Create

47. 1. Because weight loss is a common side effect of methylphenidate and because the child's symptoms are controlled with the stimulant, the first action should be to increase the child's oral intake before the medication's side effects begin. Weight should be monitored, but since the child has already lost weight, a remedy is needed as well as monitoring. The weight loss is directly due to the medication's side effects, so the child will continue to lose weight unless an intervention is made whether or not he is enrolled in school or on summer vacation. A high-protein drink could work, but then, the child is taking in all his calories in the evening, which is not best nutritionally. A change of medication should be the last resort since methylphenidate is the most effective medication for ADHD and has been successful with this child.

🔑 CN: Pharmacological and parenteral therapies; CL: Analyze

48. 4. Decreased respirations and coma are the two most dangerous effects of heroin overdose, so an increase in respirations after administration of the naloxone demonstrates initial effectiveness of the medication. Changes in cognition and psychomotor activity will take more time to become apparent. The client's blood opioid level may not drop to a nontoxic level for a few days.

🔑 CN: Pharmacological and parenteral therapies; CL: Evaluate

49. 2. Adolescents are more likely than children to attempt or commit suicide. Loss, abuse, and family discord remain significant risk factors. There is no evidence to support that children rarely commit suicide. Additionally, evidence fails to support the belief that children who have lost a parent to suicide will attempt it themselves. Significant events, such as a recent firearm purchase, have not been linked to suicide attempts in children. No geographical region in the United States or Canada is free from adolescent suicide.

🔑 CN: Psychosocial integrity; CL: Apply

50. 1,2,4,5. A child with ADHD will manifest excessive climbing and running, excessive fidgeting, inability to take turns, and distractibility. This child does not exhibit pouting or moody behaviors.

🔑 CN: Psychosocial integrity; CL: Analyze

51. 2. The nurse needs to find out what exactly the mother knows and has read. Reviewing what the mother has found in her reading that is leading her to doubt the diagnosis will help direct the nurse's teaching and clarify any misperceptions or misinformation that the mother may have. The **HCP** 📖 may indeed have many years of education and experience, and the focus should be on the daughter, but the nurse needs to address the mother's concerns at this time.

🔑 CN: Psychosocial integrity; CL: Synthesize

52. 1,3,2,4. Electronic games and stories are favorites of most children but are particularly enjoyed by children on the autism spectrum. The headphones block out some of the noises that might be upsetting to a child on the autism spectrum. If the child cannot be engaged electronically, a favorite nonelectronic toy would be the next choice. Stuffed animals or other soft toys can soothe a child who is starting to become upset. Medication should be a last resort as it can have a paradoxical effect if it is an antianxiety medication or may cause too much sedation during the flight.

🔑 CN: Psychosocial integrity; CL: Synthesize

53. 1,2,5. The client's school problems, the presence of first-degree relatives diagnosed with bipolar disorder and depression, and her inability to sleep at night mirror aspects of both ADHD and bipolar disorder, which are difficult to distinguish from each other in children. **Healthcare providers (HCPs)** 📖 are reluctant to diagnose young children as bipolar at this age. She may have only one disorder or the other or both. Further monitoring and her response to medication will differentiate whether she is suffering from one of the disorders or both. Any comments indicating that the provider does not know what he or she is doing or that the child's perceptions of her illness are not valid will undermine any trust the father and child might be developing in their caregiver and so should be avoided.

🔑 CN: Psychosocial integrity; CL: Apply

54. 1. Stating that attention deficit hyperactivity disorder occurs more commonly in families takes the opportunity for teaching while also helping the father realize that he and his wife are not to blame. Parents who are commonly blamed by society for their child's behavior need help with education. Questioning the father on what he thinks he may have done implies that the parents played some role in this disorder, possibly contributing to the father's guilt. Telling the father that many parents feel this way and that the nurse does not think the parents are at fault is premature at this point. Telling the father that he should focus on what needs to be done, rather than what caused the disorder, minimizes the father's concerns and feelings.

🔑 CN: Psychosocial integrity; CL: Synthesize

55. 3. Focusing on the purpose of the group is the best response. Adolescents are greatly influenced by their peers. Medication alone is not typically the most successful treatment strategy. Questioning whether the client will continue the medication is negative and is not the reason for her to stay in the group. Asking the rest of the group to respond may or may not give the nurse support for the teenager remaining in the group. Groups commonly have rules regarding movement of members in and out of the group, but this does not address the reasons for the client to remain in the group.

🔑 CN: Psychosocial integrity; CL: Synthesize

56. 4. Asking whether the client is thinking about killing himself is the most direct and therefore the best way to assess suicidal risk. Knowing whether the client has watched movies on suicide and death, what the client thinks about suicide, and whether other family members have committed suicide will not tell the nurse whether the client is thinking about committing suicide right now.

🔑 CN: Psychosocial integrity; CL: Analyze

57. 1. The teacher needs to be informed that this behavior is inappropriate. Therefore, educating the teacher and encouraging her to respond to misbehavior consistently are correct. Telling the teacher that the nurse can't believe the teacher lets the child get away with the behavior is demeaning and condescending. Allowing the child to continue the misbehavior is counterproductive to discipline and could create other problems.

CN: Psychosocial integrity; CL: Synthesize

58. 3. When an adolescent wants to stop treatment with medication, it represents a desire for more control over his/her life as well as a wish to be free of the disorder with which they have been diagnosed. If the caregiver merely acknowledges the client's right to stop treatment or warns of consequences if the client stops medication, he or she abdicates the adult role of healthcare advisor. Before any action is taken, the nurse should explore the client's reasoning to see if anything in the medication regimen could be changed to make it more palatable for the client. The client also needs to know that if his current objections cannot be overcome, he can return later to restart his medication.

CN: Psychosocial integrity; CL: Synthesize

59. 2. Consistent discipline and alternative methods of anger management are two important tools for parents who have a child with oppositional defiant disorder. Consistent discipline sets limits for the child. Helping the child learn more appropriate ways to manage anger assists the child in living within societal expectations. Avoiding restriction of television and computer time for punishment or using time-out as the primary means of punishment has not been suggested as an appropriate management method. Typically, using many strategies is more effective. Ignoring bad behavior could be dangerous and does not reinforce to the child that limits on behavior exist in society.

CN: Psychosocial integrity; CL: Synthesize

60. 3. Asking the client to report everything that she has had to eat and drink yesterday and today is the least judgmental approach and also provides helpful information. Confronting the client about drinking alcohol or asking her to admit the real reason for feeling sick can put the client on the defensive and block further communication. The nurse should avoid putting the client on the defensive to facilitate communication that may eventually enable the nurse to get the truth and identify interventions.

CN: Psychosocial integrity; CL: Synthesize

61. 3. The single-dose form of methylphenidate should be taken 10 to 14 hours before bedtime to prevent problems with insomnia, which can occur when the daily or last dose of the medication is taken within 6 hours (for multiple dosing) or 10 to 14 hours (for single dosing) before bedtime. It is recommended that a missed dose be taken as soon as possible; the dose is skipped if it is not remembered until the next dose is due. Any other medication, including over-the-counter medications, should be discussed with the **healthcare provider (HCP)** before use to eliminate the risk of a possible drug interaction.

CN: Pharmacological and parenteral therapies; CL: Create

62. 3,2,1,4. First, the child's reasons for removing the patch need to be explored to determine what needs to be done to solve the problem of inadequate medication administration. Since the child is probably heavily influenced by his parents' attitudes about taking medications, their attitudes need to be addressed next to determine if they openly or subtly oppose the medication or its method of administration. Once the knowledge of the child's and parent's feelings about medication are known, education can be offered to be sure the child understands how the medication can help him cope better in school and home. If the child continues to take off his patch or demonstrates an allergic response to the patch, or if it is determined that his parents are not supportive of the patch, discussion of a trial of another medication to treat the child's symptoms should occur.

CN: Pharmacological and parenteral therapies; CL: Create

63. 1,2,3,4. The crucial elements of a behavioral contract include compliance with the medication regimen if medication is prescribed, appropriate anger management, consequences for unacceptable behaviors, and rules for interactions with others. Personal possessions may be limited by unit rules but are not part of an individualized behavioral contract.

CN: Psychosocial integrity; CL: Create

64. 1. While all the occurrences could upset the client in the early stage of treatment, the one involving the most risk to safety is the suicide completion of a peer. Adolescents are susceptible to "copycat" suicides. The fact that she knows the method of suicide of the acquaintance and is at a critical period in treatment, when her antidepressant may have given her increased energy while still experiencing low self-esteem, can put her at significant risk for suicide.

CN: Safety and infection control; CL: Analyze

The Child and Adolescent with Adjustment Disorders

65. 3. A client who has endured serious chronic illness (both psychiatric and medical) would be well aware of his shortened life span, particularly if he is unable to get a lung transplant. It would not be unusual for him to want to plan ahead so his wishes would be honored in the event of his death. In the absence of other physical signs, an exacerbation of CF or delirium is not demonstrated. Likewise, his successful bipolar treatment in the absence of any other signs rules depression out as a reason for his behavior. Though it may be difficult to think about a young person in terms of dying, the client's consideration of the future is a rational decision.

   CN: Psychosocial integrity; CL: Analyze

66. 1,2,4,5. Young children cannot be sad all the time after a loss, but that does not mean they grieve less. Their moods change more quickly, and they often work out their issues through play rather than talking. Because young children do not have a full understanding of death's finality, they may talk to a deceased loved one as if they are present. They also may not understand the circumstances of the death and so may think the loved one left voluntarily and be angry at the deceased for leaving them. Play involving a dangerous object such as a rope, coupled with a stated desire to join the deceased parent, would be cause for alarm as the child could harm himself either purposely or accidentally.

   CN: Psychosocial integrity; CL: Apply

67. 1. Five-year-old children view death as reversible, so talking about seeing her mother again is a normal statement for a child of this age. A child of this age would not usually state that she was glad Jesus took her mom but instead might be afraid that God would also take her or her dad. The idea of replacing her mother with a new one, as hinted in the statement that they got another dog after the dog died, has not been supported by studies of grieving children. Stating that mommy went to heaven and that the child will see her someday when the child dies is reflective of more advanced abstract thinking than a 5-year-old would demonstrate.

   CN: Health promotion and maintenance; CL: Analyze

68. 2,3,4. The development of friendships and good grades with moderate amounts of study are positive signs since friends and grades in the new school were sources of stress and anxiety for the girl. The ability to wear clothes appropriate to the weather rather than hiding her arms is a sign she is no longer injuring her arms. Joining three clubs and being an officer in one of them is unlikely and

would probably be an additional source of stress for the girl as would be pushing herself to extraordinary academic achievement to secure a place in college when she has just entered junior high.

   CN: Psychosocial integrity; CL: Evaluate

Managing Care-Clients with Abuse and Mental Health Problems

69. 4. Children who experience serious losses, especially multiple losses, such as old friends or a parent, are more at risk for depression. Girls also are at greater risk than boys during the adolescent years. While doing poorly in school is a risk factor for depression, it is not as great as having two sudden losses. Being upset over not being selected over being a cheerleader indicates represents a loss, but not multiple or serious losses. Not doing well in school is a risk, but developing new friends shows a positive perspective.

   CN: Health promotion and maintenance; CL: Analyze

70. 3. The nurse manager needs to focus on the frustration that the nurse is expressing. Additionally, the nurse manager needs to correct any misinformation or misinterpretation that the staff nurse has. Saying that the nurse sounds burned out and asking about a vacation do not focus on the nurse's frustration or address the inaccuracy of the nurse's statement. There is no evidence to suggest that children with conduct disorder have more than the average adult's risk of depression or anxiety. Therefore, this response is inaccurate and inappropriate. Anecdotal information from personal experience does not supply the nurse with accurate, reliable information.

   CN: Management of care; CL: Synthesize

71. 4. Indifference to other people and mutism may be indicators of autism and would require further investigation. A 2-year-old who talks to himself and refuses to cooperate with toilet training is displaying behaviors typical for this age. Occasional thumb sucking and not having spent the night with a friend would be normal at age 6. Threatening to run away when angry is considered within the range of normal behaviors for a 10-year-old child.

   CN: Health promotion and maintenance; CL: Analyze

72. 1. The severe emotional trauma the girl has experienced will likely make it difficult for her to be successful in an adoptive placement at the present time, whether that placement is with someone she knows (the nurse) or another adoptive family. Additionally, adoption by the nurse is inappropriate because it blurs the lines between her professional and personal life and is likely to confuse the client. It is clear that the client has many issues and that love alone is not likely to solve all her problems. Treatment at the residential facility will allow her to work through emotional issues in a more therapeutic environment. Though not currently ready for adoption, she may be ready for adoption in the future after sufficient treatment.

🔑 CN: Management of care; CL: Evaluate

73. 3. Restricting intake to lose weight is a first step toward an eating disorder for males as well as females, so this behavior should be investigated further, especially since males of this age are usually unconcerned about their weight. Quick mood changes are common in young adolescents, particularly girls. Such mood changes should not be considered problematic if the adolescent is not experiencing trouble in major areas of his/her life. Experimenting with alcohol or other substances is fairly common in the teen years, but one or two uses do not generally lead to addiction. The negative effect of the coughing may be a deterrent to further use. Religious questioning and exploration of "dark" subjects is common among teens and is part of the development of mature thinking. In the absence of other signs of depression, it does not warrant further evaluation.

🔑 CN: Management of care; CL: Evaluate

74. 2. The UAP 📖 is concerned about the behavior of the client and confused about why it is occurring, so the nurse needs to explain a bit about the issues involved as well as demonstrate empathy for the aide. It is appropriate to explain that the client

is not cutting for attention, but the nurse's response does not address the reason for the teen's behavior and is therefore inadequate. It could also appear that the nurse is denigrating the UAP, which will not encourage the aide to listen to what she has to say. The comments that the UAP cannot work with the client or that she should transfer are punitive and do nothing to help the UAP understand self-mutilation.

🔑 CN: Management of care; CL: Analyze

75. 1,2,3,5,6. Interventions for the client with both bulimia nervosa and anorexia nervosa involve assigning a staff member to accompany the client to the bathroom; promoting a self-monitoring journal as a nonfood coping strategy; providing daily weight measurement in the same clothing at the same times of the week, while facing the client away from the scale readout; assigning a staff member to sit with the client during meals and stay with the client for 1½ hour after meals; and providing liquid protein supplements when the client is unable to eat meals. Telling the client that parenteral nutrition will be necessary may be perceived as a threat and is not an appropriate initial intervention.

🔑 CN Management of care; CL Apply

76. 3. The client with an eating disorder is instructed to receive regular lab tests to monitor nutritional compliance. Frequently, the living situation from before hospitalization was dysfunctional, and returning to the situation can result in recurrent health problems. Attending a social club is not a priority for the client, and enrolling in a health club could result in the client exercising excessively.

🔑 CN: Management of care; CL: Evaluate

Postreview Tests

This test has 75 questions. Time yourself as you take the test so you can determine the approximate amount of time it takes to complete this many questions. This test reflects the minimum number of questions you might receive on the actual licensing exam.

1. A client with human immunodeficiency virus (HIV) and acquired immunodeficiency syndrome confides that he is homosexual and his employer does not know his HIV status. Which response by the nurse is **best**?

☐ **1.** "Would you like me to help you tell them?"

☐ **2.** "The information you confide in me is confidential."

☐ **3.** "I must share this information with your family."

☐ **4.** "I must share this information with your employer."

2. An elderly client is being admitted to same-day surgery for cataract extraction. The client has several diamond rings. The nurse should explain to the client that:

☐ **1.** the rings will be taped before the surgery.

☐ **2.** the rings will be placed in an envelope, the client will sign the envelope, and the envelope will be placed in a safe.

☐ **3.** the rings will be locked in the narcotic box.

☐ **4.** the nursing supervisor will hold onto the rings during the surgery.

3. Under which circumstance may a nurse communicate medical information without the client's consent?

☐ **1.** when certifying the client's absence from work

☐ **2.** when requested by the client's family

☐ **3.** when treating the client with a sexually transmitted infection

☐ **4.** when prescribed by another healthcare provider (HCP)

4. A 22-year-old client is brought to the emergency department with his fiancée after being involved in a serious motor vehicle accident. His Glasgow Coma Scale score is 7, and he demonstrates evidence of decorticate posturing. Which action is appropriate for obtaining permission to place a catheter for intracranial pressure (ICP) monitoring?

☐ **1.** The nurse will obtain a signed consent from the client's fiancée because he is of legal age and they are engaged to be married.

☐ **2.** The healthcare provider (HCP) will get a consultation from another healthcare provider and proceed with placement of the ICP catheter until the family arrives to sign the consent.

☐ **3.** Two nurses will receive a verbal consent by telephone from the client's next of kin before inserting the catheter.

☐ **4.** The healthcare provider will document the emergency nature of the client's condition and that an ICP catheter for monitoring was placed without consent.

5. The nurse notices that a cart being used to transport a client has a nonfunctioning clasp on the safety belt. The nurse should:

☐ **1.** call the safety/security department to report the problem.

☐ **2.** use a draw sheet to secure the client during transport.

☐ **3.** contact the clinical engineering department to repair the clasp.

☐ **4.** request that the transporter bring a different cart with a functional clasp.

6. When coaching clients to improve their health, which strategy is the **most** effective for the nurse to use to help clients take an active role in their health care?

☐ **1.** Ask clients to complete a questionnaire.

☐ **2.** Provide clients with written instructions.

☐ **3.** Ask clients for their views of their health and health care.

☐ **4.** Ask clients if they have any questions about their health.

7. The nurse is planning care for a client who chews the fingers constantly. Before applying mitten restraints, the nurse could try which interventions? Select all that apply.
- ☐ **1.** Ask the client to rub lotion over the hands every day after bathing.
- ☐ **2.** Encourage physical activity, such as ambulation.
- ☐ **3.** Provide frequent contacts for communication and socialization.
- ☐ **4.** Provide family education.
- ☐ **5.** Encourage involvement of family and friends.

8. A client with major depression states, "Life is not worth living anymore. Nothing matters." Which response by the nurse is **best**?
- ☐ **1.** "Are you thinking about killing yourself?"
- ☐ **2.** "Things will get better, you know."
- ☐ **3.** "Why do you think that way?"
- ☐ **4.** "You should not feel that way."

9. A client with bipolar 1 disorder has been prescribed olanzapine 5 mg two times a day and lamotrigine 25 mg two times a day. Which adverse effects should the nurse report to the healthcare provider (HCP) immediately? Select all that apply.
- ☐ **1.** rash
- ☐ **2.** nausea
- ☐ **3.** sedation
- ☐ **4.** hyperthermia
- ☐ **5.** muscle rigidity

10. The nurse is planning care for an older adult with a pressure ulcer (see figure). What should the nurse do? Select all that apply.

- ☐ **1.** Elevate the head of the bed to 50 degrees.
- ☐ **2.** Obtain daily cultures.
- ☐ **3.** Cover with protective dressing.
- ☐ **4.** Reposition the client every 2 hours.
- ☐ **5.** Request an alternating pressure mattress.

11. A client takes hydrochlorothiazide (HCTZ) for treatment of hypertension. The nurse should instruct the client to report which effects? Select all that apply.
- ☐ **1.** muscle twitching
- ☐ **2.** abdominal cramping
- ☐ **3.** diarrhea
- ☐ **4.** confusion
- ☐ **5.** lethargy
- ☐ **6.** muscle weakness

12. A client has been taking imipramine for depression for 2 days. His sister asks the nurse, "Why is he still so depressed?" Which response by the nurse is **most** appropriate?
- ☐ **1.** "Your brother is experiencing a very serious depression."
- ☐ **2.** "I will be sure to convey your concern to his healthcare provider"
- ☐ **3.** "It takes 2 to 4 weeks for the drug to reach its full effect."
- ☐ **4.** "Perhaps we need to change his medication."

13. Which finding requires immediate intervention when planning care for an adolescent with cystic fibrosis (CF)?
- ☐ **1.** delayed puberty
- ☐ **2.** chest pain with dyspnea
- ☐ **3.** poor weight gain
- ☐ **4.** large, foul-smelling, bulky stools

14. Assessment of a client starting on lithium reveals dry mouth, nausea, thirst, and mild hand tremor. Based on an analysis of these findings, what should the nurse do **next**?
- ☐ **1.** Withhold the lithium, and obtain a lithium level to determine therapeutic effectiveness.
- ☐ **2.** Continue the lithium, and immediately notify the healthcare provider (HCP) about the assessment findings.
- ☐ **3.** Continue the lithium, and reassure the client that these temporary side effects will subside.
- ☐ **4.** Withhold the lithium, and monitor the client for signs and symptoms of increasing toxicity.

15. A client asks the nurse how long it will be necessary to take the medicine for hypothyroidism. The nurse's response is based on the knowledge that:
- ☐ **1.** lifelong daily medicine is necessary.
- ☐ **2.** the medication is expensive, and the dose can be reduced in a few months.
- ☐ **3.** the medication can be gradually withdrawn in 1 to 2 years.
- ☐ **4.** the medication can be discontinued after the client's thyroid-stimulating hormone (TSH) level is normal.

16. The nurse should advise which client who is taking lithium to consult with the healthcare provider (HCP) regarding a potential adjustment in lithium dosage?
- ☐ **1.** a client who continues work as a computer programmer
- ☐ **2.** a client who attends college classes
- ☐ **3.** a client who can now care for her children
- ☐ **4.** a client who is beginning training for a tennis team

17. A client admitted with a gastric ulcer has been vomiting bright red blood. The hemoglobin level is 5.11 g/dL (51.1 g/L), and blood pressure is 100/50 mm Hg. The client and family state that their religious beliefs do not support the use of blood products and refuse blood transfusions as a treatment for the bleeding. The nurse should collaborate with the healthcare provider (HCP) and family to **next**:
- ☐ **1.** discontinue all measures.
- ☐ **2.** notify the hospital attorney.
- ☐ **3.** attempt to stabilize the client through the use of fluid replacement.
- ☐ **4.** give enough blood to keep the client from dying.

18. Nonsteroidal anti-inflammatory drugs (NSAIDs) are commonly used in the treatment of musculoskeletal conditions. It is important for the nurse to remind the client to:
- ☐ **1.** take NSAIDs at least three times per day.
- ☐ **2.** exercise the joints at least 1 hour after taking the medication.
- ☐ **3.** take antacids 1 hour after taking NSAIDs.
- ☐ **4.** take NSAIDs with food.

19. When using a Z-track injection technique, the nurse holds the gauze pledget against an IM injection site while removing the needle from the muscle. This technique helps to:
- ☐ **1.** seal off the track left by the needle in the tissue.
- ☐ **2.** speed the spread of the medication in the tissue.
- ☐ **3.** avoid the discomfort of the needle pulling on the skin.
- ☐ **4.** prevent organisms from entering the body through the skin puncture.

20. When a client with alcohol dependency begins to talk about not having a problem with alcohol, what is the **best** approach for the nurse to use?
- ☐ **1.** Question the client about how much alcohol the client consumes each day.
- ☐ **2.** Confront the client about being intoxicated 2 days ago.
- ☐ **3.** Point out how alcohol has gotten the client into trouble.
- ☐ **4.** Ask the client about his or her reasons for not staying sober.

21. The nurse is caring for a toddler in contact isolation for respiratory syncytial virus (RSV). In what order from first to last should the nurse remove personal protective equipment (PPE)? All options must be used.

1. gloves

2. goggles

3. gown

4. mask

22. The nurse is preparing a teaching plan for a 45-year-old client recently diagnosed with type 2 diabetes mellitus. What is the **first** step in this process?
- ☐ **1.** Establish goals.
- ☐ **2.** Choose video materials and brochures.
- ☐ **3.** Assess the client's learning needs.
- ☐ **4.** Set priorities of learning needs.

23. A client with newly diagnosed type 1 diabetes mellitus has a finger stick blood sugar (FSBS) of 483 dL/mL (483 mmol/L). The nurse should **first**:
- ☐ **1.** start an intravenous infusion.
- ☐ **2.** repeat the finger stick in 30 minutes.
- ☐ **3.** notify the healthcare provider (HCP) of the results.
- ☐ **4.** obtain a serum glucose level as prescribed.

24. A female client who has diagnosis of borderline personality disorder is manipulative and very disruptive on the hospital unit. She is not dangerous to herself or others but is clearly not making any therapeutic progress. She consistently refuses any medications. The nurse realizes that legally, this client has which option?
- ☐ **1.** Refuse treatment.
- ☐ **2.** Receive forced treatment if the nursing team concurs.
- ☐ **3.** Be medicated if her family signs permission for treatment.
- ☐ **4.** Be guided to accept treatment recommendations by threatening loss of privileges.

25. A client admitted in an acute psychotic state hears terrible voices in the head and thinks a neighbor is upset with the client. What is the nurse's **best** response?
- ☐ **1.** "What has your neighbor been doing that bothers you?"
- ☐ **2.** "How long have you been hearing these terrible voices?"
- ☐ **3.** "We will not let your neighbor visit, so you will be safe."
- ☐ **4.** "What exactly are these terrible voices saying to you?"

26. A client who has a prescription to receive nothing by mouth (NPO) is constantly asking for a drink of water. Which nursing intervention is the **most** appropriate?
- ☐ **1.** Reexplain why it is not possible to have a drink of water.
- ☐ **2.** Offer ice chips every hour to decrease thirst.
- ☐ **3.** Offer the client frequent oral hygiene care.
- ☐ **4.** Divert the client's attention by turning on the television.

27. An older adult who is to be on bed rest has become incontinent of urine. To prevent pressure ulcers, the nurse should do which tasks? Select all that apply.
- ☐ **1.** Use a sanitary napkin to absorb urine.
- ☐ **2.** Institute a turning schedule.
- ☐ **3.** Inspect the groin for wetness.
- ☐ **4.** Have client wear incontinence briefs.
- ☐ **5.** Anchor a Foley catheter.

28. A mother tells the nurse that her 10-year-old daughter has an increase in hair growth and breast enlargement. The nurse explains to the mother and daughter that after the symptoms of puberty are noticed, menstruation typically occurs within which time frame?
- ☐ **1.** 6 months
- ☐ **2.** 12 months
- ☐ **3.** 30 months
- ☐ **4.** 36 months

29. A nurse is teaching a new mother how to prevent burns in the home. Which statement by the mother indicates more teaching is required?
- ☐ **1.** "I will set my hot water heater to 49°C (120°F)."
- ☐ **2.** "I will not hold my infant while drinking coffee."
- ☐ **3.** "I will heat my infant's formula in the microwave."
- ☐ **4.** "I will keep loose appliance cords tied up on the counter."

30. After teaching a primigravid client at 10 weeks' gestation about the recommendations for exercise during pregnancy, which client statement indicates successful teaching?
- ☐ **1.** "While pregnant, I should avoid contact sports."
- ☐ **2.** "Even though I am pregnant, I can learn to ski next month."
- ☐ **3.** "While we are on vacation next month, I can continue to scuba dive."
- ☐ **4.** "Sitting in a hot tub after exercise will help me to relax."

31. The healthcare provider (HCP) has prescribed a chemotherapy drug to be administered to a client every day for the next week. The client is on an adult medical-surgical floor, but the nurse assigned to the client has not been trained to handle chemotherapy agents. What is the nurse's **most** appropriate response?
- ☐ **1.** Send the client to the oncology floor for administration of the medication.
- ☐ **2.** Ask a nurse from the oncology floor to come to the client and administer the medication.
- ☐ **3.** Ask another nurse to help mix the chemotherapy agent.
- ☐ **4.** Ask the pharmacy to mix the chemotherapy agent and administer it.

32. Which is an appropriate outcome for a client with rheumatoid arthritis?
- ☐ **1.** The client will manage joint pain and fatigue to perform activities of daily living.
- ☐ **2.** The client will maintain full range of motion in joints.
- ☐ **3.** The client will prevent the development of further pain and joint deformity.
- ☐ **4.** The client will take anti-inflammatory medications as indicated by the presence of disease symptoms.

33. A healthcare provider (HCP) has been exposed to hepatitis B through a needlestick. Which drug should the nurse anticipate administering as postexposure prophylaxis?
- ☐ **1.** hepatitis B immune globulin
- ☐ **2.** interferon
- ☐ **3.** hepatitis B surface antigen
- ☐ **4.** amphotericin B

34. When instilling ear drops on a 2-year-old child, the nurse should pull the pinna in which directions?
- ☐ **1.** down and back
- ☐ **2.** down and slightly forward
- ☐ **3.** up and back
- ☐ **4.** up and forward

35. A client is in the compensatory stage of shock. Which finding indicates the client is entering the progressive stage of shock?
- ☐ **1.** urinary output of 20 mL/h
- ☐ **2.** blood pressure of 110/70 mm Hg
- ☐ **3.** heart rate of 110 bpm
- ☐ **4.** temperature of 99°F

36. A client has been prescribed hydrochlorothiazide to treat heart failure. The nurse should tell the client to report:
- ☐ **1.** urinary retention.
- ☐ **2.** muscle weakness.
- ☐ **3.** confusion.
- ☐ **4.** diaphoresis.

37. The son of a client with Alzheimer's disease excitedly tells the nurse, "Mom was singing one of her favorite old songs. I think she is getting her memory back!" What response by the nurse is **most** appropriate?
- ☐ **1.** "She still has long-term memory, but her short-term memory will not return."
- ☐ **2.** "I am so happy to hear that. Maybe she is getting better."
- ☐ **3.** "Do not get your hopes up. This is only a temporary improvement."
- ☐ **4.** "I am glad she can sing even if she cannot talk to you."

38. A client has the leg immobilized in a long leg cast. Which finding indicates the beginning of circulatory impairment?
- ☐ **1.** inability to move toes
- ☐ **2.** cyanosis of toes
- ☐ **3.** sensation of cast tightness
- ☐ **4.** tingling of toes

39. A multigravid client at 34 weeks' gestation who is leaking amniotic fluid has just been hospitalized with a diagnosis of preterm premature rupture of membranes and preterm labor. The client's contractions are 20 minutes apart, lasting 20 to 30 seconds. Her cervix is dilated to 2 cm. The nurse reviews prescriptions (see chart). Which prescription should the nurse initiate **first**?

Prescription

Continuous external fetal and contraction monitoring
IV of D5LR @ 125 mL/h
I&O catheterization for urinalysis and culture and
sensitivity
Betamethasone 12 mg IM daily × 2 days

- ☐ **1.** Initiate fetal and contraction monitoring.
- ☐ **2.** Start the intravenous infusion.
- ☐ **3.** Obtain the urine specimen.
- ☐ **4.** Administer betamethasone.

40. The nurse caring for a client with diabetes realizes that the client has a higher risk of developing cataracts and should also assess the client for indications of:
- ☐ **1.** background retinopathy.
- ☐ **2.** proliferative retinopathy.
- ☐ **3.** neuropathy.
- ☐ **4.** diabetic retinopathy.

41. The nurse is developing an education plan for clients with hypertension. The nurse should emphasize which long-term goal?
- ☐ **1.** Develop a plan to limit stress.
- ☐ **2.** Participate in a weight reduction program.
- ☐ **3.** Commit to lifelong therapy.
- ☐ **4.** Monitor blood pressure regularly.

42. When developing a plan of care to manage a client's pain from cancer, what should the nurse plan to do?
- ☐ **1.** Individualize the pain medication regimen for the client.
- ☐ **2.** Select medications that are least likely to lead to addiction.
- ☐ **3.** Administer pain medication as soon as the client requests it.
- ☐ **4.** Change pain medications periodically to avoid drug tolerance.

43. After explaining to a multigravid client at 36 weeks' gestation who is diagnosed with severe hydramnios about the possible complications of this condition, which client statement indicates the need for further instruction?
- ☐ **1.** "Because I have hydramnios, I may gain weight."
- ☐ **2.** "Hydramnios has been associated with gastrointestinal disorders in the fetus."
- ☐ **3.** "I should continue to eat high-fiber foods and avoid constipation."
- ☐ **4.** "I can continue to work at my job at the automobile factory until labor starts."

44. The nurse is instructing a client on how to care for skin that has become dry after radiation therapy. Which statement by the client indicates that the client understands the teaching?
- ☐ **1.** "I should take antihistamines to decrease the itching I am experiencing."
- ☐ **2.** "It is safe to apply a nonperfumed lotion to my skin."
- ☐ **3.** "A heating pad, set on the lowest setting, will help decrease my discomfort."
- ☐ **4.** "I can apply an over-the-counter cortisone ointment to relieve the dryness."

45. The antidote for heparin is:
- ☐ **1.** vitamin K.
- ☐ **2.** warfarin.
- ☐ **3.** thrombin.
- ☐ **4.** protamine sulfate.

46. Which measure should be implemented promptly after a client's nasogastric (NG) tube has been removed?
- [ ] 1. Provide the client with oral hygiene.
- [ ] 2. Offer the client liquids to drink.
- [ ] 3. Encourage the client to cough and deep breathe.
- [ ] 4. Auscultate the client's bowel sounds.

47. The nurse is assessing an older adult who is living with his son's family. The client has scald burns on the hands and both forearms (10% first- and second-degree burns). The nurse should **first**:
- [ ] 1. cleanse the wounds with warm water.
- [ ] 2. apply antibiotic cream.
- [ ] 3. call for transport to a hospital.
- [ ] 4. cover the burns with sterile dressing.

48. An infant is to receive the diphtheria, tetanus, and acellular pertussis (DTaP) and inactivated polio vaccine (IPV) immunizations. The child is recovering from a cold and is afebrile. The child's sibling has cancer and is receiving chemotherapy. Which action is **most** appropriate?
- [ ] 1. Give the DTaP and withhold the IPV.
- [ ] 2. Administer the DTaP and IPV immunizations.
- [ ] 3. Postpone both immunizations until the sibling is in remission.
- [ ] 4. Withhold both immunizations until the infant is well.

49. When creating a program to decrease the primary cause of disability and death in children, the nurse should:
- [ ] 1. encourage legislators to draft legislation to promote prenatal care.
- [ ] 2. require all children to be immunized.
- [ ] 3. teach accident prevention and safety practices to children and their parents.
- [ ] 4. hire a nurse practitioner for each of the schools in the community.

50. A tour bus has overturned on an exit ramp. Many passengers are injured, but there are no fatalities. While the emergency department nurse prepares for treating the injured, the nurse also anticipates that:
- [ ] 1. the accident victims will be experiencing grief and mourning.
- [ ] 2. many of the passengers may be experiencing feelings of victimization.
- [ ] 3. there is a need for someone to coordinate calls from relatives about the passengers.
- [ ] 4. some of the passengers will need psychiatric hospitalization.

51. The nurse teaches the parents of an infant who has had surgery to correct imperforate anus how to position the infant to prevent tension on the perineum. The nurse determines more teaching is needed when the parents put the infant in which position?
- [ ] 1. abdomen, with legs pulled up under the body
- [ ] 2. back, with legs suspended at a 90-degree angle
- [ ] 3. left side, with hips elevated
- [ ] 4. right side, with hips elevated

52. When developing the plan of care for a 14-year-old boy who is bored due to being immobilized in a cast, which activity is **most** appropriate?
- [ ] 1. playing a card game with a boy the same age
- [ ] 2. putting together a puzzle with his mother
- [ ] 3. playing video games with a 9-year-old
- [ ] 4. watching a movie with his younger brother

53. After surgery to create a urinary diversion, the client is at risk for a urinary tract infection. The nurse should:
- [ ] 1. clamp the urinary appliance at night.
- [ ] 2. empty the urinary appliance before it is one-third full.
- [ ] 3. limit the client's walking with the appliance.
- [ ] 4. change the urinary appliance daily.

54. When suctioning a client's tracheostomy tube, what should the nurse do?
- [ ] 1. Oxygenate the client before suctioning.
- [ ] 2. Insert the suction catheter about 2 inches (5 cm) into the cannula.
- [ ] 3. Use a bolus of sterile water to stimulate cough.
- [ ] 4. Use clean gloves during the procedure.

55. A 14-month-old child has a severe diaper rash. Which recommendation should the nurse provide to the parents?
- [ ] 1. Continue to use the baby wipes.
- [ ] 2. Change the diaper every 4 to 6 hours.
- [ ] 3. Wash the buttocks using mild soap.
- [ ] 4. Apply powder to the diaper area.

56. An adolescent thinks she has infectious mononucleosis. For which symptoms should the nurse assess the client? Select all that apply.
- [ ] 1. sore throat
- [ ] 2. malaise
- [ ] 3. weight loss
- [ ] 4. rash
- [ ] 5. swollen lymph glands

57. While assessing the fundus of a multiparous client on the first postpartum day, the nurse performs handwashing and puts on clean gloves. What should the nurse do **next**?
- ☐ 1. Place the nondominant hand above the symphysis pubis and the dominant hand at the umbilicus.
- ☐ 2. Ask the client to assume a side-lying position with the knees flexed.
- ☐ 3. Perform massage vigorously at the level of the umbilicus if the fundus feels boggy.
- ☐ 4. Place the client on a bedpan in case the uterine palpation stimulates the client to void.

58. What should be the nurse's **priority** assessment after an epidural anesthetic has been given to a nulligravid client in active labor?
- ☐ 1. level of consciousness
- ☐ 2. blood pressure
- ☐ 3. cognitive function
- ☐ 4. contraction pattern

59. The nurse monitors the serum electrolyte levels of a client who is taking digoxin. Which electrolyte imbalance is a common cause of digoxin toxicity?
- ☐ 1. hyponatremia
- ☐ 2. hypomagnesemia
- ☐ 3. hypocalcemia
- ☐ 4. hypokalemia

60. After abdominal surgery, a client has a prescription for meperidine IM 100 mg every 3 to 4 hours and acetaminophen with codeine 30 mg. The client has been taking meperidine every 4 hours for the past 48 hours but tells the nurse that the meperidine is no longer lasting 4 hours and that the client needs to have it every 3 hours. Which nursing measure is **most** appropriate?
- ☐ 1. Realizing that the client is developing tolerance to the meperidine, the nurse administers the meperidine every 3 hours.
- ☐ 2. The nurse urges the client to take the acetaminophen with codeine to prevent addiction to the meperidine.
- ☐ 3. The nurse requests a prescription from the healthcare provider (HCP) to change the dose to an equianalgesic dose of morphine.
- ☐ 4. The nurse encourages the client to do relaxation exercises to provide distraction from the pain.

61. The nurse assesses a 7-month-old infant's growth and development. Which behavior should the nurse consider unusual?
- ☐ 1. drinking from a cup and spilling little of the liquid
- ☐ 2. raising the chest and upper abdomen off the bed with the hands
- ☐ 3. imitating sounds that the nurse makes
- ☐ 4. crying loudly in protest when the mother leaves the room

62. A 13-year-old client is dying of cancer. When providing care for this client, the nurse should incorporate the developmental tasks for this age. According to Erikson's developmental model, the child normally is expected to be working on which psychosocial issue?
- ☐ 1. lifetime vocation
- ☐ 2. social conscience
- ☐ 3. personal values
- ☐ 4. sense of competence

63. The nurse is performing Leopold's maneuvers on a woman who is in her 8th month of pregnancy. The nurse is palpating the uterus as shown below. Which maneuver is the nurse performing?
- ☐ 1. First maneuver
- ☐ 2. Second maneuver
- ☐ 3. Third maneuver
- ☐ 4. Fourth maneuver

64. The nurse is instructing an unlicensed assistive personnel (UAP) on the prevention of postoperative pulmonary complications. Which statement indicates that the UAP has understood the nurse's instructions?
- ☐ 1. "I will turn the client every 2 hours."
- ☐ 2. "I will keep the client's head elevated."
- ☐ 3. "I should suction the client every 2 hours."
- ☐ 4. "I will have the client take 5 to 10 deep breaths every hour."

65. During an appointment with the nurse, a client says, "I could hate God for that flood." The nurse responds, "Oh, do not feel that way. We are making progress in these sessions." The nurse's statement demonstrates a failure to do what?
- ☐ 1. Look for meaning in what the client says.
- ☐ 2. Explain to the client why he may think as he does.
- ☐ 3. Add to the strength of the client's support system.
- ☐ 4. Give the client credit for solving his own problems.

66. The nurse observes that the client with multiple sclerosis looks untidy and sad. The client suddenly says, "I cannot even find the strength to comb my hair," and bursts into tears. Which response by the nurse is **best**?

- ☐ 1. "It must be frustrating not to be able to care for yourself."
- ☐ 2. "How many days have you been unable to comb your hair?"
- ☐ 3. "Why has your husband not been helping you?"
- ☐ 4. "Tell me more about how you are feeling."

67. The nurse is planning care for an obese female client. The client experiences dribbling urine when she coughs, sneezes, and changes positions. The nurse should instruct the client to promote urinary health by encouraging which actions? Select all that apply.

- ☐ 1. Increase consumption of fluids such as coffee and tea.
- ☐ 2. Use a Foley catheter.
- ☐ 3. Participate in a weight loss program.
- ☐ 4. Perform muscle-strengthening exercises (Kegel exercises).
- ☐ 5. Use adult diapers as needed.

68. A term primigravida was involved in a car accident 3 hours ago. She is having labor contractions every 4 minutes, and her cervical exam is dilated 3 cm, 100% effaced, and station −1. She is crying uncontrollably and states her pain is constant and severe, rating it at 10/10. The **priority** action by the nurse is to:

- ☐ 1. reassure the woman and assist with nonpharmacologic pain interventions.
- ☐ 2. assess intensity of contractions and determine if she would like an epidural.
- ☐ 3. notify the provider of the pain and request an assessment for potential abruption.
- ☐ 4. perform a vaginal exam and coach the woman with breathing exercise for pain control.

69. A nurse interviews the parent of a middle school student who is exhibiting behavioral problems, including substance abuse, following a sibling's suicide. The parent says, "I am a single parent who has to work hard to support my family, and now I have lost my only son, and my daughter is acting out and making me crazy! I just cannot take all this stress!" Which issue is the **priority**?

- ☐ 1. parent's ability to emotionally support the adolescent in this crisis
- ☐ 2. potential suicidal thoughts/plans of both family members
- ☐ 3. the adolescent's anger
- ☐ 4. the parent's frustration

70. Following surgery, the nurse is to apply sequential compression device to the client's legs. Prior to applying the device, the nurse should **first**:

- ☐ 1. confirm the client's identity using two client identifiers.
- ☐ 2. position the client in the bed.
- ☐ 3. explain the sequential compression therapy to the client.
- ☐ 4. determine the size of sleeve that is needed.

71. The nurse is caring for a previously healthy, independent 28-year-old client who is alert and oriented and is being admitted to the hospital for unexplained vomiting and abdominal pain. The client has intravenous fluids infusing through a saline lock and has been ambulating in the hallway with a steady gait. Using the Morse Fall Risk Scale (see chart), what is this client's total score and risk level?

Morse Fall Risk/Scale		
Item	**Scale**	**Scoring**
1. History of falling, immediate or within 3 months	No 0 Yes 25	
2. Secondary diagnosis	No 0 Yes 15	

3. Ambulatory aid
    Bed rest/nurse assist
    Crutches/cane/walker
    Furniture
	
	0
	15
	30	

4. IV/heparin lock	No 0 Yes 20	

5. Gait/transferring
    Normal/bed rest/
      immobile
    Weak
    Impaired
	
	0
	
	10
	20	

6. Mental status
    Oriented to own ability
    Forgets limitations
	
	0
	15	

Score _____ Risk _____.

72. Which statements made by a pregnant woman in the first trimester are consistent with this stage of pregnancy? Select all that apply.

- ☐ 1. "My husband told his friends we will have to give up the convertible for a minivan."
- ☐ 2. "Oh my, how did this happen? I do not need this now."
- ☐ 3. "I cannot wait to see my baby. Do you think it will have my blond hair and blue eyes?"
- ☐ 4. "I used a princess theme for decorating the room."
- ☐ 5. "I wonder how it will feel to buy maternity clothes and be fat."
- ☐ 6. "We went to the mall yesterday to buy a crib and dressing table."

73. A client is diagnosed with syndrome of inappropriate antidiuretic hormone (SIADH). The nurse should assess the client for which alteration in fluid and electrolyte balance?
☐ **1.** increased osmolality of the plasma
☐ **2.** decreased serum sodium level
☐ **3.** increased urine output
☐ **4.** decreased blood pressure

74. A client is admitted to the emergency department with crushing chest injuries sustained in a car accident. Which sign indicates a possible pneumothorax?
☐ **1.** Cheyne-Stokes respirations
☐ **2.** increased fremitus
☐ **3.** diminished or absent breath sounds on the affected side
☐ **4.** decreased sensation on the affected side

75. A primigravid client at 35 weeks' gestation is scheduled for a biophysical profile. After instructing the client about the test, which client statement about what the test measures indicates effective teaching?
☐ **1.** amniotic fluid volume
☐ **2.** placement of the placenta
☐ **3.** amniotic fluid color
☐ **4.** fetal gestational age

Answers, Rationales, and Test-Taking Strategies

The answers and rationales for each question follow below, along with keys (🔑) to the client need (CN) and cognitive level (CL) for each question. In addition, you will also see a glossary icon (📖) highlighting specific terminology used on the licensing exam. As you check your answers, use the **Content Mastery and Test-Taking Skill Self-Analysis** *worksheet (tear-out worksheet in back of book) to identify the reason(s) for not answering the questions correctly. For additional information about test-taking skills and strategies for answering questions, refer to pages 12–23 and pages 35–36 in Part 1 of this book.*

1. 2. The nurse is responsible for maintaining confidentiality of this disclosure by the client. The nurse cannot discuss the client's health problems with the family or employer. It is the client's reprehensibility to inform others if he or she chooses to do so.

🔑 CN: Psychosocial integrity; CL: Synthesize

2. 2. Under the policy for valuables, the nurse documents the description on an envelope with the client, the client and nurse sign the envelope, and the valuables envelope is locked in the safe. The other options increase the risk of loss or damage to the client's valuables.

🔑 CN: Management of care; CL: Synthesize

3. 3. Sexually transmitted infections are communicable diseases that must be reported. The nurse is responsible for reporting these diseases to the appropriate public health agency and to otherwise maintain the client's confidentiality. The client's family cannot request release of medical information without the client's **consent** 📖. An **HCP's** 📖 prescription is not a substitute for a client's consent to release medical information in the absence of a communicable disease.

🔑 CN: Management of care; CL: Synthesize

4. 4. In a life-threatening emergency where time is of the essence in saving life or limb, **consent** 📖 is not required. This client has a Glasgow Coma Scale score of 7, which indicates a comatose state. The client cannot be aroused, withdraws in a purposeless manner from painful stimuli, exhibits decorticate posturing, and may or may not have brain stem reflexes intact. The placement of the ICP monitor is crucial to determine cerebral blood flow and prevent herniation. The client's fiancée cannot sign the consent because, until she is his wife or has designated power of attorney, she is not considered his next of kin. The **HCP** 📖 should insert the catheter in this emergency. He does not need to get a consultation from another HCP. When consent is needed for a situation that is not a true emergency, two nurses can receive a verbal consent by telephone from the client's next of kin.

🔑 CN: Management of care; CL: Apply

5. 4. The nurse ensures client safety during transport and therefore requests another cart for transport. The other options do not ensure client safety. Method of transportation and person transporting the client are documented by the nurse responsible for the transfer. The clasp needs to be repaired. Contacting the security department is not appropriate.

🔑 CN: Safety and infection control; CL: Synthesize

6. 3. One of the best strategies to help empower clients to manage their health is to ask them their view of situations and to respond to what they say. This technique acknowledges that clients' opinions have value and relevance to the interview. It also promotes an active role for clients in the process. Use of a questionnaire or written instructions is a means of obtaining information but promotes a passive client role. Asking whether clients have questions encourages participation, but alone, it does not acknowledge their views.

🔑 CN: Management of care; CL: Synthesize

7. 2, 3, 4, 5. Socialization and communication, in addition to increased activity, are all means to aid in prevention of self-injury. Education of family members may foster development of strategies to prevent self-injury; hence, mitten restraints could be avoided. Applying lotion after bathing may not be appropriate when the skin is broken and not intact.

🔑 CN: Management of care; CL: Synthesize

8. 1. When the client verbalizes that life is not worth living anymore, the nurse needs to ask the client directly about suicide by saying, "Are you thinking about killing yourself?" Asking directly does not provoke suicide but conveys concern, understanding, and the worth of the client. Commonly, the client experiences a sense of relief that someone finally hears him. It also helps the nurse plan responsible care by identifying the client who is at risk for suicide. The nurse should then evaluate the seriousness of the suicidal ideation by inquiring about the intent and plan. Stating "Things will get better" offers hope too soon without first evaluating the intent of the suicidal ideation. Asking "Why do you think that way?" implies a lack of understanding and knowledge on the part of the nurse. Major depression usually is endogenous and biochemically based. Therefore, the client may not know why he does not want to live. Saying "You should not feel that way" admonishes the client, decreases self-worth, and conveys a lack of understanding.

🔑 CN: Psychosocial integrity;
CL: Synthesize

9. 1, 4, 5. Lamotrigine, an antiepileptic, is used as a mood stabilizer for clients with bipolar disorder and has been found to be effective for the depressive phase of bipolar disorder. Common adverse effects are dizziness, headache, sedation, tremors, nausea, vomiting, and ataxia. The development of a rash needs to be reported and evaluated by the healthcare provider because it could indicate the start of a severe systemic rash known as Stevens-Johnson syndrome, a toxic epidermal necrolysis, which would necessitate the discontinuation of lamotrigine. Hyperthermia in conjunction with muscle rigidity suggests the development of neuroleptic malignant syndrome, a life-threatening complication associated with olanzapine.

🔑 CN: Pharmacological and parenteral therapies; CL: Analyze

10. 3, 4, 5. The client has a stage II pressure ulcer. The nurse should take measures to relieve the pressure, treat the local infection, and protect the wound. The nurse should keep the ulcer covered with a protective dressing. The client should turn every 2 hours and use an alternating pressure mattress to relieve pressure on the buttocks. The head of the bed should be elevated no more than 30 degrees. All wounds have bacteria, and obtaining frequent cultures (unless prescribed otherwise) is not necessary.

🔑 CN: Safety and infection control;
CL: Synthesize

11. 2, 5, 6. HCTZ is a thiazide diuretic used in the management of mild to moderate hypertension and in the treatment of edema associated with heart failure, renal dysfunction, cirrhosis, corticosteroid therapy, and estrogen therapy. It increases the excretion of sodium and water by inhibiting sodium reabsorption in the distal tubule of the kidneys. It promotes the excretion of chloride, potassium, magnesium, and bicarbonate. Side effects include drowsiness, lethargy, and muscle weakness but not muscle twitching. Although there may be abdominal cramping, there is no diarrhea. The client does not become confused as a result of taking this drug.

🔑 CN: Health promotion and maintenance;
CL: Analyze

12. 3. The nurse needs to inform the sister that it takes 2 to 4 weeks before a full clinical effect occurs with the drug. The nurse should let her know that her brother will gradually get better and symptoms of depression will improve. Telling the sister that her brother is experiencing a very serious depression does not give the sister important information about the medication. Additionally, this statement may cause alarm and anxiety. Conveying the sister's concern to the **healthcare provider (HCP)** 📖 does not provide her with the necessary information about the client's medication. Telling the sister that the client's medication may need to be changed is inappropriate because a full clinical effect occurs after 2 to 4 weeks.

🔑 CN: Pharmacological and parenteral therapies; CL: Synthesize

13. 2. Chest pain and dyspnea are signs of a pneumothorax and should be treated immediately. Delayed puberty is common in adolescents with CF and is caused by poor nutrition. Poor weight gain is common in children with CF because so little is absorbed in the small intestine. Large, foul-smelling stools indicate noncompliance with taking enzymes and should be addressed, but respiratory complications are the greatest concern.

🔑 CN: Physiological adaptation;
CL: Analyze

14. 3. The client is exhibiting temporary side effects associated with beginning lithium therapy. Therefore, the nurse should continue the lithium and explain to the client that the temporary side effects of lithium will subside. Common side effects of lithium are nausea, dry mouth, diarrhea, thirst, mild hand tremor, weight gain, bloating, insomnia, and light-headedness. Immediately notifying the **HCP** 📖 about these common side effects is not necessary.

🔑 CN: Pharmacological and parenteral therapies; CL: Synthesize

15. 1. Thyroid replacement is a lifelong maintenance therapy. The medication is usually given as one dose in the morning. It cannot be tapered or discontinued because the client needs thyroid supplementation to maintain health. The medication cannot be discontinued after the TSH level is normal; the dose will be maintained at the level that normalizes the TSH concentration.

CN: Pharmacological and parenteral therapies; CL: Apply

16. 4. A client who is beginning training for a tennis team would most likely require an adjustment in lithium dosage because excessive sweating can increase the serum lithium level, possibly leading to toxicity. Adjustments in lithium dosage would also be necessary when other medications have been added, when an illness with high fever occurs, and when a new diet begins.

CN: Pharmacological and parenteral therapies; CL: Analyze

17. 3. The most appropriate response is to continue all treatments and attempt to stabilize the client using fluid replacement without administering blood or blood products. It is imperative that the healthcare team respects the client's religious beliefs and wishes, even if they are not those of the healthcare team. Discontinuing all measures is not an option. The healthcare team should continue to provide the best care possible and does not need to notify the attorney.

CN: Management of care; CL: Synthesize

18. 4. NSAIDs irritate the gastric mucosa and should be taken with food. NSAIDs are usually taken once or twice daily. Joint exercise is not related to the drug administration. Antacids may interfere with the absorption of NSAIDs.

CN: Pharmacological and parenteral therapies; CL: Synthesize

19. 1. When administering an injection using the Z-track method, holding the gauze pledget against the site while removing the needle from the muscle helps to seal off the track left by the needle in the tissue. The Z-track technique does not speed the spread of the medication or lessen the discomfort of an injection. Wiping the skin with alcohol prior to administering the injection prevents the likelihood of microorganisms from entering the body.

CN: Pharmacological and parenteral therapies; CL: Apply

20. 3. When a client talks about not having a problem with alcohol, the nurse needs to point out how alcohol has gotten the client into trouble. Concrete facts are helpful in decreasing the client's denial that alcohol is a problem. The other approaches allow the client to use defense mechanisms, such as rationalization, projection, and minimization, to explain his or her actions. Therefore, these approaches are not helpful.

CN: Psychosocial integrity; CL: Synthesize

21. 1, 3, 2, 4. There are two acceptable ways of removing PPE. The nurse should remove the dirtiest items first. Typically, these items are the gloves followed by the gown. In the alternative method, the gloves and gown may be removed at the same time. It is then recommended that the nurse perform hand hygiene and remove the goggles, which may fit over the mask. Finally, the mask is removed from behind. The nurse should then again perform hand hygiene when all PPE has been removed.

CN: Safety and infection control; CL: Apply

22. 3. Before development and implementation of the teaching plan, it is vital to determine what the client currently knows regarding diabetes and what the client needs to know.

CN: Management of care; CL: Create

23. 4. The nurse should first obtain a serum glucose level for a more accurate information about the client's blood sugar level. The nurse should not wait for 30 minutes to obtain another fingerstick blood sugar when more accurate information will be obtained with a blood glucose level. The nurse should have more information about the glucose level before contacting the **HCP** 📖. It is not necessary to start an intravenous infusion at this point.

CN: Management of care; CL: Synthesize

24. 1. A client who has not been deemed a danger to self or others or who has not been declared incompetent retains the right to refuse treatment. Legal protocols need to be followed to initiate treatment against an adult client's wishes, even if the family wishes treatment to occur. Punitive threats of retaliation or loss of privileges are ethically unacceptable in administering treatment.

CN: Management of care; CL: Analyze

25. 4. The nurse needs to collect additional information about the client's report about hearing voices. Assessing the content of hallucinations is essential to determine whether they are command hallucinations that the client might act on. Asking about what the neighbor has been doing or telling the client that the neighbor will not visit indirectly reinforces the delusion about the neighbor. Although determining the onset and duration of the voices is important, the nurse needs to assess the content of the hallucinations first.

🔑 CN: Psychosocial integrity;
CL: Synthesize

26. 3. The most appropriate intervention is to offer the client frequent mouth care to moisten the dry oral mucosa. Reexplaining why the client cannot drink may be helpful but will not relieve the thirst. Ice chips cannot be given to a client who is on NPO status. Diverting the client's attention does not help manage the thirst.

🔑 CN: Basic care and comfort;
CL: Synthesize

27. 2, 3, 4. This client is at risk for pressure ulcers because of age, being on bed rest, and being incontinent. The nurse assesses all pressure points and the groin area, assures that the client changes positions every 2 hours, and has the client wear incontinence pads containing absorbent material (specially designed to absorb many times its weight in water) or disposable incontinence briefs. Sanitary napkins are not designed to contain/absorb urine. Anchoring a Foley catheter increases the risk for infection.

🔑 CN: Physiological adaptation;
CL: Synthesize

28. 3. After the symptoms of puberty, such as increased hair growth and enlargement of the breasts, are noticed, menstruation typically begins within 30 months.

🔑 CN: Health promotion and maintenance;
CL: Apply

29. 3. Infant formula should never be heated in the microwave; the formula may heat at different temperatures and can burn the infant's mouth. Plastic bottle liners may also burst with the heat. Setting your hot water heater a couple of degrees cooler will help keep hot water in the house cooler (recommended since 1974 by the Consumer Product Safety Commission). Small children are at risk for scald injury from hot tap water due to their decreased reaction time, their curiosity, and the thermal sensitivity of their skin. Avoiding holding infants while drinking coffee can prevent possible spills onto children. Keeping cords tied up on the counter prevents children from pulling on dangling cords and spilling hot liquids over themselves.

🔑 CN: Safety and infection control;
CL: Evaluate

30. 1. The client understands the instructions when she says she should avoid contact sports because they may result in injury to the client and the fetus. Learning to ski while pregnant is not rec-

ommended because injury may occur. Scuba diving should be avoided because depth pressures could cause fetal damage. Hot tubs should be avoided during the first trimester because sitting in them can result in fetal hyperthermia and fetal hypoxia. Mild exercises, such as walking, can help strengthen the muscles and prevent some discomforts such as backache.

🔑 CN: Health promotion and maintenance;
CL: Evaluate

31. 1. The nurse should call the oncology unit to institute a transfer. The nurse handling chemotherapy agents should be specially trained. It is an unwise use of nursing resources to send a nurse from one unit to administer medications to a client on another unit. It is better to centralize and send the client who needs chemotherapy to one unit. Even if the pharmacy mixes the agent, the drug must be administered by a specially trained nurse.

🔑 CN: Management of care; CL: Synthesize

32. 1. An appropriate outcome for the client with rheumatoid arthritis is that the client will adopt self-care behaviors to manage joint pain, stiffness, and fatigue and be able to perform activities of daily living. Range-of-motion (ROM) exercises can help maintain mobility, but it may not be realistic to expect the client to maintain full ROM. Depending on the disease progression, there may be further development of pain and joint deformity, even with appropriate therapy. It is important for the client to understand the importance of taking the prescribed drug therapy even if symptoms have abated.

🔑 CN: Reduction of risk potential;
CL: Synthesize

33. 1. Hepatitis B immune globulin is given as prophylactic therapy to individuals who have been exposed to hepatitis B. Interferon has been approved to treat hepatitis B. Hepatitis B surface antigen is a diagnostic test used to detect current infection. Amphotericin B is an antifungal.

🔑 CN: Pharmacological and parenteral therapies; CL: Apply

34. 1. When instilling ear drops on a child younger than age 3 years, the nurse should pull the pinna down and back. This helps open the ear canal to ensure drops reach the tympanic membrane. For an older child, the nurse should pull the pinna up and back.

🔑 CN: Reduction of risk potential;
CL: Apply

35. 1. In the compensatory stage of shock, the client exhibits moderate tachycardia, but as the shock continues to the progressive stage, the client will have a decreased urinary output, hypotension, and mental confusion as a result of failure to perfuse and ineffective compensatory mechanisms. The body temperature initially may remain normal. These findings are indications that the body's compensatory mechanisms are failing.

CN: Reduction of risk potential;
CL: Analyze

36. 2. Hydrochlorothiazide is a thiazide diuretic. Muscle weakness can be an indication of hypokalemia. Polyuria is associated with this diuretic, not urinary retention. Confusion and diaphoresis are not side effects of hydrochlorothiazide.

CN: Pharmacological and parenteral therapies; CL: Analyze

37. 1. The ability to remember an old song is related to long-term memory, which persists after short-term memory is lost. Therefore, the nurse should respond by providing the son with this information. Stating that the nurse is happy to hear about the change and that the client is getting better is inappropriate and inaccurate. This statement ignores the issue of long-term versus short-term memory. Telling the client not to get his hopes up because the improvement is only temporary is inappropriate. The information provided does not indicate that the client has expressive aphasia, which would be suggested by the statement that the client cannot talk to the son.

CN: Psychosocial integrity; CL: Analyze

38. 4. Tingling and numbness of the toes would be the earliest indication of circulatory impairment. Inability to move the toes and cyanosis are later indicators. Cast tightness should be investigated because cast tightness can lead to circulatory impairment; it is not, however, an indicator of impairment.

CN: Reduction of risk potential;
CL: Analyze

39. 1. The nurse should initiate fetal and contraction monitoring for this client upon arrival to the unit. This gives the nurse data regarding changes in fetal and maternal contraction status before completing the other prescriptions. Next, the betamethasone would be given to begin the maturation process for the fetal lungs. The nurse should then start an intravenous infusion to provide a line for immediate intravenous access, if needed, and provide hydration for the client. The nurse should obtain the urine specimen prior to administering any antibiotic therapy, if prescribed.

CN: Management of care; CL: Synthesize

40. 4. Diabetic retinopathy involves background and proliferative retinopathy. Both forms are associated with vascular changes in the basement membrane of the arterioles and capillaries of the choroid and retina. Neuropathy is usually associated with the lower extremities.

CN: Reduction of risk potential;
CL: Analyze

41. 3. The most appropriate long-term goal for the client with hypertension is to commit to life-long therapy. A significant problem in the long-term management of hypertension is compliance with the treatment plan. It is essential that the client understand the reasons for modifying lifestyle, taking prescribed medications, and obtaining regular health care. Limiting stress, losing weight, and monitoring blood pressure are important aspects of care for the client with hypertension; however, the treatment plan must be individualized to include aspects of care that are appropriate for each client.

CN: Health promotion and maintenance;
CL: Synthesize

42. 1. The nurse should work with the client to individualize the plan of care for managing pain. Cancer pain is best managed with a combination of medications, and each client needs to be worked with individually to find the treatment regimen that works best. Cancer pain is commonly undertreated because of fear of addiction. The client who is in pain needs the appropriate level of analgesic and needs to be reassured that addiction is unlikely. Cancer pain is best treated with regularly scheduled doses of medication. Administering the medication only when the client asks for it will not lead to adequate pain control. As drug tolerance develops, the dosage of the medication can be increased.

CN: Basic care and comfort;
CL: Synthesize

43. 4. The client needs further instructions when she says, "I can continue to work at my job at the automobile factory until labor starts." The goal is to avoid preterm labor. Because the client is experiencing severe hydramnios, she will most likely be maintained on bed rest to increase uteroplacental circulation and reduce pressure on the cervix. Hydramnios has been associated with increased weight gain caused by increased amniotic fluid volume. Hydramnios has been associated with gastrointestinal disorders in the fetus, such as tracheoesophageal fistula with stenosis or intestinal obstruction. The client should continue to eat high-fiber foods and should avoid straining, which could lead to ruptured membranes. Stool softeners may also be prescribed. The client should report any symptoms of fluid rupture or labor.

CN: Reduction of risk potential;
CL: Evaluate

44. 2. Irradiated skin can become dry and irritated, resulting in itching and discomfort. The client should be instructed to clean the skin gently and apply nonperfumed, nonirritating lotions to help relieve dryness. Taking an antihistamine does not relieve the skin dryness that is causing the itching. Heat should not be applied to the area because it can cause further irritation. Medicated ointments should not be applied to the skin without the prescription of the radiation therapist.

🔑 CN: Reduction of risk potential;
CL: Evaluate

45. 4. The antidote for heparin is 1% protamine sulfate. Vitamin K is the antidote for warfarin, an oral anticoagulant. Thrombin is a topical anticoagulant.

🔑 CN: Pharmacological and parenteral therapies; CL: Apply

46. 1. The nurse's first action after the removal of an NG tube is to provide the client with oral hygiene. Then it is appropriate to give the client liquids to drink if the client is no longer on nothing-by-mouth status. There is no association between removal of an NG tube and having the client cough and deep breathe. Auscultating the client's bowel sounds should be done before removal of the NG tube.

🔑 CN: Basic care and comfort;
CL: Synthesize

47. 3. The nurse has the client transported to a hospital. The client's age and the extent of the burns require care by a healthcare team. Additionally, the nurse considers that the client may be a victim of elder abuse and investigates further as needed. The nurse should refrain from cleansing the wound, applying cream, or covering the area.

🔑 CN: Physiological adaptation;
CL: Synthesize

48. 2. At this time, the infant can be given the vaccines. The fact that the child's sibling is immunosuppressed because of chemotherapy is not a reason to withhold the vaccines. The fact that the child has a cold is not grounds for delaying the immunizations. However, if the child had a high fever, the immunizations would be delayed.

🔑 CN: Health promotion and maintenance;
CL: Synthesize

49. 3. The primary cause of disability and death in children is injury from accidents. Teaching safety measures to children and their parents is the best way to decrease injury and accidents. Legislation for prenatal care is not a primary prevention for accidents. Communicable diseases are not the primary cause of disability and death in children; therefore requiring immunizations is not an appropriate strategy for this health problem. Having nurse practitioners in schools is not a primary prevention measure for accidents.

🔑 CN: Management of care; CL: Synthesize

50. 2. Major accidents can induce feelings similar to those of victims of other kinds of disasters and crime. Therefore, the nurse should also be prepared to assist the passengers with their feelings of victimization. Passengers may mourn the loss of a vacation, but with no fatalities, major grief reactions are not expected. Other personnel can take calls from relatives while the nurse helps the passengers. Psychiatric hospitalization is a premature assumption.

🔑 CN: Psychosocial integrity; CL: Analyze

51. 1. When placed on the abdomen, a neonate pulls the legs up under the body, which puts tension on the perineum. Therefore, after surgery, the neonate should be positioned either supine with the legs suspended at a 90-degree angle or on either side with the hips elevated.

🔑 CN: Reduction of risk potential;
CL: Evaluate

52. 1. Teenagers usually enjoy activities with peers in preference to socializing with their parents or siblings. Peer relationships help the adolescent develop self-identity.

🔑 CN: Health promotion and maintenance;
CL: Synthesize

53. 2. The urinary appliance should be emptied before the pouch is one-third full to prevent urinary reflux. The appliance should be attached to a leg bag at night to allow for adequate drainage. The urinary appliance is not changed daily. If no leakage occurs and the client's skin remains free from irritation, the appliance can be left in place for 1 week or more. The client can ambulate as tolerated.

🔑 CN: Basic care and comfort;
CL: Synthesize

54. 1. Preoxygenating the client before suctioning helps prevent the development of hypoxia during the procedure. The suction catheter is inserted about 5 to 6 inches (12.7 to 15. cm) into the cannula. A bolus of 3 to 5 mL of sterile normal saline solution may be inserted into the cannula before suctioning to stimulate coughing and loosen secretions. The nurse uses sterile technique when suctioning a client.

🔑 CN: Reduction of risk potential;
CL: Apply

55. 3. Because the toddler has a severe diaper rash, it may be best to change all that the parents are doing. The buttocks need to be washed thoroughly with mild soap and dried well. In fact, it is helpful to leave the diaper off and expose the buttocks to the air. Baby wipes commonly contain additives and perfumes that may be irritating to the baby's sensitive skin. The diaper needs to be changed more often than every 4 to 6 hours. Otherwise, the moist diaper environment will continue to irritate the skin, causing the rash to worsen. Powder has limited absorbing ability and will most likely irritate the area more. In addition, some powders contain perfumes or are scented and can irritate the skin.

⚷ CN: Basic care and comfort;
CL: Synthesize

56. 1, 2, 5. The common presenting symptoms of infectious mononucleosis vary greatly but commonly include fever, malaise, sore throat, and lymphadenopathy. Skin rash, cold symptoms, abdominal pain, and weight loss are rarely presenting symptoms.

⚷ CN: Reduction of risk potential;
CL: Analyze

57. 1. The nurse should place the nondominant hand above the symphysis pubis and the dominant hand at the umbilicus to palpate the fundus. This prevents uterine inversion and trauma, which can be very painful to the client. The nurse should ask the client to assume a supine, not side-lying, position with the knees flexed. The fundus can be palpated in this position, and the perineal pads can be evaluated for lochia amounts. The fundus should be massaged gently if the fundus feels boggy. Vigorous massaging may fatigue the uterus and cause it to become firm and then boggy again. The nurse should ask the client to void before fundal evaluation. A full bladder can cause discomfort to the client, the uterus to be deviated to one side, and postpartum hemorrhage.

⚷ CN: Health promotion and maintenance;
CL: Apply

58. 2. Administration of an epidural anesthetic can result in a hypotensive effect on maternal blood pressure. Therefore, the priority assessment is the mother's blood pressure. Ephedrine or wedging the client to a position to keep pressure off the vena cava, such as on the left side, can be used to elevate maternal blood pressure should it drop too low. Epidural anesthesia has no effect on the level of consciousness or the client's cognitive function. Although the client's contraction pattern may decrease in frequency after administration of the anesthesia, the priority assessment is the client's blood pressure. After blood pressure is maintained, contractions can be assessed.

⚷ CN: Pharmacological and parenteral therapies; CL: Analyze

59. 4. Hypokalemia is one of the most common causes of digoxin toxicity. It is essential that the nurse carefully monitor the potassium levels of clients taking digoxin to avoid toxicity. Low serum potassium levels can cause cardiac dysrhythmias. Sodium, magnesium and calcium levels are not significantly affected by the use of digoxin.

⚷ CN: Pharmacological and parenteral therapies; CL: Apply

60. 3. Current pain guidelines recommend the removal of meperidine from formularies and the substitution of morphine commonly administered by patient-controlled analgesia. Meperidine can be prescribed for severe pain, but its use is limited by the high incidence of neurotoxicity (seizures) associated with the accumulation of its metabolite, normeperidine. It is contraindicated in clients with acute pain lasting more than 2 days and in those for whom large daily doses (more than 600 mg) are needed. It would be inappropriate to urge the client to take the acetaminophen and codeine to prevent addiction. Addiction is a psychological condition in which a client is driven to take drugs for reasons that are not therapeutic. The client is in pain, and her need for the morphine is therapeutic. Although the client may obtain some relief from relaxation exercises, this alone is not sufficient to provide pain relief.

⚷ CN: Pharmacological and parenteral therapies; CL: Synthesize

61. 1. Infants at age 7 months are not capable of drinking from a cup without spilling. At age 6 months, infants can partially lift their weight on the hands, enjoy imitating sounds, and are developing separation anxiety.

⚷ CN: Health promotion and maintenance;
CL: Analyze

62. 3. According to Erikson, a child of 13 years is normally seeking to meet the need to develop personal identity. Personal values are a component of this identity. Developing a conscience is a component of achieving initiative during the preschool years. Developing a sense of competence is a component of achieving industry in the school-age years. Developing a lifetime vocation is a component of achieving generativity in adulthood.

⚷ CN: Psychosocial integrity; CL: Analyze

63. 3. The third maneuver is used to identify the presenting part. This maneuver is used to identify the part of the fetus that lies over the inlet to the pelvis. While facing the client, the nurse places the tips of the first three fingers on the side of the woman's abdomen above the symphysis pubis and palpates deeply around the presenting part to identify its contour and size. The first maneuver involves using the tips of the fingers of both hands to palpate the uterine fundus. The second maneuver identifies the back of the fetus, and the fourth maneuver identifies the cephalic prominence.

CN: Reduction of risk potential; CL: Apply

64. 4. Having the client deep breathe hourly is the most appropriate action for the **UAP** 📖 to take to help prevent pulmonary complications. The client should be turned at least every 2 hours or as needed for this particular client. Keeping the client's head elevated will not prevent pulmonary complications. Suctioning the client is not a UAP's responsibility, nor does it prevent pulmonary complications.

CN: Management of care; CL: Evaluate

65. 1. The nurse's response fails to identify the meaning in what the client has said. The nurse needs to explore the client's statement about hating God for that flood because the meaning of the client's statement is unclear. Also, clichés such as "Do not feel that way" are not helpful because they ignore the client's feelings and his interpretation of the situation in which he finds himself. Explaining to the client why he may think as he does (offering a rationale) is inappropriate. The nurse's response fails to identify the meaning in what the client has said and is not supportive. There is no evidence that the client is solving his problems.

CN: Psychosocial integrity; CL: Analyze

66. 4. By asking the client to tell more about how she is feeling, the nurse is not making any assumptions about what is troubling the client. The nurse should acknowledge the client's feelings and encourage her to discuss them. Saying that this situation must be frustrating involves assumptions by the nurse about why the client is crying and is not a therapeutic response. Asking how long the client has been unable to comb her hair takes the focus off her feelings and inhibits therapeutic communication. Inquiring why the client's husband has not helped insinuates that the husband is not helping enough, which is inappropriate, takes the focus off the client's feelings, and inhibits therapeutic communication.

CN: Psychosocial integrity; CL: Synthesize

67. 3. The goal is to promote health in this client who has stress incontinence. Participating in a weight loss program or support group may decrease the intra-abdominal pressure contributing to the incontinence. Participating in swimming, bicycling, or low-impact exercise is beneficial to weight loss. Kegel exercises are helpful in developing muscle control. Wearing adult diapers will absorb leaked urine and prevent excoriation. Clients with urinary stress incontinence are encouraged to avoid drinks with caffeine and alcohol. Perineal care is essential to prevent skin breakdown, but the client does not require a Foley or straight catheter at this time.

CN: Physiological adaptation; CL: Synthesize

68. 3. The woman is at risk for placental abruption due to her recent car accident. Symptoms of a placental abruption include unrelenting pain and a rigid board-like abdomen. She may or may not have vaginal bleeding. In contrast, labor contractions are intermittent. The priority action by the nurse should be to ensure that this client is further evaluated by her **HCP** 📖. Subsequent actions could include assisting with pain control measures, assessing contractions, and checking cervical dilation.

CN: Management of care; CL: Analyze

69. 2. The parent's expressions of stress and grief and the adolescent's behavior and drug use could be preludes to suicide, especially since another member of the family succeeded in suicide. Suicide attempts are more likely in families in which there has been a previous suicide attempt or suicide death, especially for young people. Though the family's emotional states are important, one is not more important than the other. Obviously, the parent's ability to emotionally support the adolescent in this crisis has been compromised, but the safety of both supersedes this concern.

CN: Safety and infection control; CL: Analyze

70. 1. The nurse must use at least two ways to identify clients. This is done to make sure that each client gets the correct medication/s and/or treatment/s. Although all of the remaining actions need to be done, none of the others would be the first action.

CN: Physiological adaptation; CL: Apply

71. 20, Low Risk. This client's only risk factor is IV access, making this client low risk for a fall. The nurse must remember to reevaluate a client's risk for fall after any change in condition, upon transfer to another unit within the hospital, or after a fall. In most acute care facilities, a fall risk is completed at least every 24 hours, if not every shift.

CN: Safety and infection control; CL: Evaluate

72. 1, 2, 5. The first trimester is when the couple works through the psychological task of accepting the pregnancy. These statements describe the client and her partner coping with the pregnancy, how it feels, and how it will impact their lives. The feelings include pleasure, excitement, and ambivalence. Wondering what the baby will look like and planning for the baby's room occur later in the pregnancy.

⚷ CN: Health promotion and maintenance;
CL: Analyze

73. 2. SIADH is characterized by excess antidiuretic hormone (ADH, vasopressin) secretion, despite low plasma osmolality. Excess ADH causes water to be retained. As blood volume expands, plasma becomes diluted resulting in dilutional hyponatremia. Aldosterone is suppressed, resulting in increased renal sodium excretion. Water moves from the hypotonic plasma and the interstitial spaces into the cells.

⚷ CN: Physiological adaptation;
CL: Analyze

74. 3. Accumulation of air in the pleural cavity after a crushing chest injury may be assessed by unilateral diminished or absent breath sounds. Cheyne-Stokes respirations with periods of apnea commonly precede death. They indicate heart failure or brain death. Fremitus is increased with lung consolidation and decreased with pleural effusion or pneumothorax. Pain occurs at the injury site and increases with inspiration.

⚷ CN: Physiological adaptation;
CL: Analyze

75. 1. The biophysical profile typically measures five parameters to assess the fetus: fetal breathing, movement, and tone; amniotic fluid volume; and fetal heart reactivity. The test uses a scale of 0 to 2 for each parameter with a maximum score of 10.

⚷ CN: Physiological adaptation;
CL: Evaluate

This test has 110 questions. Time yourself as you take the test so you can determine the approximate amount of time it takes to complete this many questions. This test is close to the average number of questions you might receive on the actual licensing exam.

1. The unit secretary who transcribes the healthcare provider's (HCP's) prescriptions asks the nurse to interpret an illegible prescription. The nurse should clarify the prescription with the:
- ☐ **1.** client.
- ☐ **2.** pharmacist.
- ☐ **3.** HCP.
- ☐ **4.** client's family.

2. A client with cholecystitis is taking propantheline bromide. The expected outcome of this drug is:
- ☐ **1.** increased bile production.
- ☐ **2.** decreased biliary spasm.
- ☐ **3.** absence of infection.
- ☐ **4.** relief from nausea.

3. The nurse refers the parents of a child with cystic fibrosis to an organization that helps families with children who have this disease. Such organizations are especially beneficial for parents by helping them:
- ☐ **1.** find tutors to educate their children at home.
- ☐ **2.** obtain genetic counseling.
- ☐ **3.** meet with other parents of children with cystic fibrosis for mutual support.
- ☐ **4.** obtain financial assistance to purchase medications for their children.

4. A client tells the nurse that "the hospital food is horrible." What should the nurse tell the client?
- ☐ **1.** "The staff is doing the best it can to cook in such large quantities."
- ☐ **2.** "I will report this to the healthcare provider (HCP)."
- ☐ **3.** "Would you like to speak with the dietitian about the food and meal selection?"
- ☐ **4.** "I do not like the hospital cafeteria food either."

5. An elderly client had a thrombotic cerebrovascular accident and now has flaccid hemiplegia of the right side. When planning care for this client, the nurse understands that rehabilitation begins:
- ☐ **1.** as soon as anticoagulant therapy is started.
- ☐ **2.** when the client is admitted to the hospital.
- ☐ **3.** when the client can first work cooperatively with healthcare personnel.
- ☐ **4.** as directed by the physical therapist.

6. A client has been involuntarily committed to a hospital because he has been assessed as being dangerous to self or others. The client has lost which right?
- ☐ **1.** the right to refuse medications and treatments
- ☐ **2.** the right to send and receive uncensored mail
- ☐ **3.** freedom from seclusion and restraints
- ☐ **4.** the right to leave the hospital against medical advice

7. Which statement by a client taking valproic acid for bipolar disorder indicates that further teaching about this medication is necessary?
- ☐ **1.** "I need to take the pills at the same time each day."
- ☐ **2.** "I can chew the pills if necessary."
- ☐ **3.** "I can take the pills with food."
- ☐ **4.** "I need to call my healthcare provider (HCP) if I start bruising easily."

8. The nurse is making rounds and observes a client who is unconscious (see figure). The unlicensed assistive personnel (UAP) has just turned the client from lying on her back. Before raising the side rail, the nurse should:

- ☐ **1.** elevate the head of the bed to 30 degrees.
- ☐ **2.** ask the nursing assistant to add a pillow under the right arm.
- ☐ **3.** inspect the skin at pressure points from the back-lying position.
- ☐ **4.** help the nursing assistant move the client closer to the head of the bed.

9. A client is having elective surgery under general anesthesia. Who is responsible for obtaining the informed consent?
☐ **1.** the nurse
☐ **2.** the surgeon
☐ **3.** the anesthesiologist
☐ **4.** the social worker

10. The family of an elderly client with terminal cancer inquires about hospice services. The nurse explains that hospice care:
☐ **1.** focuses only on the needs of the client.
☐ **2.** can only be provided in the inpatient setting.
☐ **3.** is staffed exclusively by professional health-care workers.
☐ **4.** focuses on supportive care for the client and family.

11. When caring for a child who has been receiving long-term steroid therapy, the nurse should assess the child for:
☐ **1.** usual behavior and temperament.
☐ **2.** loss of weight from baseline.
☐ **3.** development of truncal obesity.
☐ **4.** demonstration of a growth spurt.

12. The nurse manager has assigned a nurse as the circulating nurse for a surgical abortion. The nurse has a religious objection and wishes to refuse to participate in an abortion. The nurse manager of the operating room should:
☐ **1.** require the nurse to do this assignment.
☐ **2.** change the assignment and record the behavior on the nurse's evaluation.
☐ **3.** change the assignment without comment.
☐ **4.** change the assignment to circulate but have the nurse prepare the equipment.

13. A client is taking phenytoin as an antiepileptic medication. The nurse should instruct the client to obtain:
☐ **1.** increased iron.
☐ **2.** increased calcium.
☐ **3.** frequent dental examinations.
☐ **4.** frequent eye examinations.

14. A hospitalized 5-year-old is pulseless, and after verifying the child is not breathing, the nurse begins chest compressions. The nurse should apply pressure:
☐ **1.** on the lower sternum with the heel of one hand.
☐ **2.** midway on the sternum with the tips of two fingers.
☐ **3.** over the apex of the heart with the heel of one hand.
☐ **4.** on the upper sternum with the heels of both hands.

15. The nurse instructs a client with coronary artery disease in the proper use of nitroglycerin. The client has had two previous episodes of coronary artery disease. At the onset of chest pain, what should the client do?
☐ **1.** Call 911 when three nitroglycerin tablets taken every 5 minutes are not effective.
☐ **2.** Call 911 when five nitroglycerin tablets taken every 5 minutes are not effective.
☐ **3.** Take one tablet and then immediately call 911.
☐ **4.** Go to the emergency department if two nitroglycerin tablets taken 5 minutes apart are not effective.

16. The nurse is coaching an older adult who has been diagnosed with high serum lipids and leads a sedentary lifestyle. The goal is to increase the amount of exercise this client currently performs. After assessing the client's interests and setting an acceptable goal with the client, which exercise will offer the client the **most** health benefits while being practical to implement?
☐ **1.** jogging three to five times per week for 30 to 60 minutes
☐ **2.** playing golf three times per week for 60 minutes
☐ **3.** walking three to five times per week for 30 to 60 minutes
☐ **4.** swimming once a week for 30 minutes

17. During the health history, a client bluntly states, "I think I am better off dead." What is the **best** response by the nurse?
☐ **1.** "Has a family member ever committed suicide?"
☐ **2.** "When did these feelings begin?"
☐ **3.** "Do you have someone at home to help you?"
☐ **4.** "Are you thinking about suicide?"

18. A client is taking methotrexate for severe rheumatoid arthritis. The nurse instructs the client that it will be necessary to monitor:
☐ **1.** serum glucose.
☐ **2.** serum electrolytes.
☐ **3.** complete blood count (CBC) with differential and platelet count.
☐ **4.** sedimentation rate.

19. An elderly client is constipated and tells the nurse that this has not happened before. What should the nurse tell the client?
☐ **1.** "Constipation is an expected problem at your age. Wait to see if this continues."
☐ **2.** "You need to eat more fiber. I will tell the dietician."
☐ **3.** "You need to drink more water. I will start a record so you can keep track"
☐ **4.** "This may be a sign of a more serious problem; I will report this to your healthcare provider (HCP)."

20. A nurse is interviewing a client who will begin rehabilitation for alcohol dependency. Which approach by the nurse is **most** helpful to the client before starting the program?

☐ **1.** "You need to be very serious about this program."

☐ **2.** "You need to want to be alcohol-free before we can help you."

☐ **3.** "This program requires you to do a lot of hard work."

☐ **4.** "We will help you be successful so that you can stay alcohol-free."

21. A client who has been newly diagnosed with type 1 diabetes asks the nurse, "Why do I have to take two shots of insulin? One shot is not enough?" The nurse should tell the client:

☐ **1.** "A single shot of long-acting insulin would be preferable."

☐ **2.** "You might be able to change to oral medications soon."

☐ **3.** "Two shots will give you better control and decrease complications."

☐ **4.** "I will ask the healthcare provider (HCP) to change your insulin schedule."

22. The nurse reviews the peak and trough serum levels from a client who is receiving gentamicin sulfate in order to:

☐ **1.** adjust the dosage to the therapeutic range.

☐ **2.** avoid allergic reactions.

☐ **3.** prevent side effects.

☐ **4.** reach therapeutic levels more quickly.

23. The nurse who is caring for a client with type 1 diabetes mellitus should use which report to determine how well the insulin, diet, and exercise are balanced?

☐ **1.** fasting serum glucose level

☐ **2.** 1-week dietary recall

☐ **3.** home log of blood glucose levels

☐ **4.** glycosylated hemoglobin level

24. The nurses have instituted a falls prevention program. Which strategy will have the **highest** likelihood of preventing falls?

☐ **1.** putting a falls risk sign on the clients' doors

☐ **2.** having the client wear a color-coded armband

☐ **3.** making rounds of the unit and clients' rooms

☐ **4.** keeping all beds in low position

25. A client is receiving a unit of packed red blood cells. Before the transfusion started, the client's blood pressure was 90/50 mm Hg, pulse rate 100 bpm, respirations 20 breaths/min, and temperature 98°F (36.7°C). Fifteen minutes after the transfusion starts, the client's blood pressure is 92/54 mm Hg, pulse 100 bpm, respirations 18 breaths/min, and temperature is 101.4°F (38.6°C). The nurse should **first**:

☐ **1.** stop the transfusion.

☐ **2.** raise the head of the bed.

☐ **3.** obtain a prescription for antibiotics.

☐ **4.** offer the client a cool washcloth.

26. A client is receiving opioid epidural analgesia. The nurse should notify the healthcare provider (HCP) if the client has which findings? Select all that apply.

☐ **1.** blood pressure of 80/40 mm Hg and baseline blood pressure of 110/60 mm Hg

☐ **2.** respiratory rate of 14 breaths/min and baseline respiratory rate of 18 breaths/min

☐ **3.** report of crushing headache

☐ **4.** 1.5 mL of blood aspirated from the catheter before the bolus injection

☐ **5.** pain rating of 3 on a scale of 1 to 10

27. Which dietary strategy **best** meets the nutritional needs of a client with acquired immunodeficiency syndrome (AIDS)?

☐ **1.** Tell the client to eat large meals frequently.

☐ **2.** Encourage mega doses of nutritional supplements.

☐ **3.** Instruct the client to cook foods thoroughly and adhere to safe food-handling practices.

☐ **4.** Tell the client to prepare food in advance and leave it out to eat small amounts throughout the day.

28. The nurse is examining a 6-week-old dark-skinned infant. There are large spots of deep blue pigmentation across the infant's buttocks. The nurse should identify this sign as characteristic of:

☐ **1.** vascular disease.

☐ **2.** telangiectatic nevi.

☐ **3.** infant milia.

☐ **4.** Mongolian spots.

29. A nulliparous client has been given a prescription for oral contraceptives. The nurse should instruct the client to report which sign to the healthcare provider (HCP) immediately?

☐ **1.** blurred vision

☐ **2.** nausea

☐ **3.** weight gain

☐ **4.** mild headache

30. An 80-year-old client is admitted with nausea and vomiting. The client has a history of heart failure and is being treated with digoxin. The client has been nauseated for a week and began vomiting 2 days ago. Laboratory values indicate hypokalemia. Because of these clinical findings, the nurse should assess the client carefully for:

☐ **1.** chronic renal failure.

☐ **2.** exacerbation of heart failure.

☐ **3.** digoxin toxicity.

☐ **4.** metabolic acidosis.

31. The nurse instructs the client with osteoporosis that food products high in calcium include:

☐ **1.** rice.

☐ **2.** broccoli.

☐ **3.** apples.

☐ **4.** meat.

32. A woman is using progestin injections for contraception. The nurse instructs the client to return for an appointment in:
- ☐ **1.** 1 month.
- ☐ **2.** 3 months.
- ☐ **3.** 4 months.
- ☐ **4.** 6 months.

33. While the nurse is caring for a multigravid client at 39 weeks' gestation in active labor whose cervix is dilated to 7 cm and completely effaced at +1 station, the client says, "I need to push!" What should the nurse do **next**?
- ☐ **1.** Turn the client to her left side.
- ☐ **2.** Tell her to push when she has the urge.
- ☐ **3.** Have her pant quickly during the contraction.
- ☐ **4.** Tell her to focus on an object in the room to relax.

34. When teaching a client with chronic renal failure who is taking antibiotics about signs and symptoms of potential nephrotoxicity to report, the nurse should encourage the client to promptly report which changes in the color of the urine? Select all that apply.
- ☐ **1.** straw colored
- ☐ **2.** cloudy
- ☐ **3.** smoky
- ☐ **4.** pink

35. The nurse is coaching a client with heart failure about reducing fluid retention. Which strategy will be **most** effective in reducing a client's fluid retention?
- ☐ **1.** low-sodium diet
- ☐ **2.** walking for 20 minutes 3 times a week
- ☐ **3.** restricting fluid intake
- ☐ **4.** elevating the feet

36. During a physical examination, the nurse observes a copper bracelet on a client's wrist. The client states that she is wearing it to treat her arthritis. The nurse should:
- ☐ **1.** recognize that the client is wearing a protective object she believes wards off illness.
- ☐ **2.** inform the client that this is a not a helpful practice and ask her to remove the bracelet.
- ☐ **3.** tell the client that wearing the bracelet is a form of quackery and not to use the bracelet as a treatment.
- ☐ **4.** continue to wear the copper bracelet because this is a medically supported treatment for arthritis.

37. The heart rate of a newly born term neonate is regular at 142 bpm. What should the nurse do **next**?
- ☐ **1.** Notify the neonate's healthcare provider (HCP).
- ☐ **2.** Check for the presence of cyanosis.
- ☐ **3.** Assess the heart rate again in 3 hours.
- ☐ **4.** Document this as a normal neonatal finding.

38. The nurse is teaching a client with diabetes insipidus about using desmopressin nasal spray. The therapeutic effects of desmopressin nasal spray are obtained when the client no longer has:
- ☐ **1.** polydipsia.
- ☐ **2.** nasal congestion.
- ☐ **3.** headache.
- ☐ **4.** blurred vision.

39. A client is recovering from an infected abdominal wound. Which foods should the nurse encourage the client to eat to support wound healing and recovery from the infection?
- ☐ **1.** chicken and orange slices
- ☐ **2.** cheeseburger and French fries
- ☐ **3.** cheese omelet and bacon
- ☐ **4.** gelatin salad and tea

40. The nurse teaches the client with iron deficiency anemia that food sources with high iron content include:
- ☐ **1.** cheese.
- ☐ **2.** squash.
- ☐ **3.** apples
- ☐ **4.** beef.

41. A toddler admitted in respiratory distress keeps pulling at the oxygen mask, trying to remove it. Which interventions are indicated? Select all that apply.
- ☐ **1.** Restrain the child.
- ☐ **2.** Have the parent read to the child.
- ☐ **3.** Administer a sedative.
- ☐ **4.** Encourage the parent to hold the child.
- ☐ **5.** Tell the child the mask will help him breathe better.
- ☐ **6.** Ask the parent to leave the child's bedside.

42. The nurse is developing a plan of care for a client who has joint stiffness due to rheumatoid arthritis. Which measure will be the **most** effective in relieving stiffness?
- ☐ **1.** a warm shower before performing activities of daily living
- ☐ **2.** aspirin after activity to decrease inflammation
- ☐ **3.** a 10-lb (4.5-kg) weight loss to limit stress on joints
- ☐ **4.** cold compresses to joints for 30 minutes to relieve stiffness

43. A client is taking large doses of aspirin daily to treat rheumatoid arthritis. The nurse should instruct the client to tell the healthcare provider (HCP) when having:
- ☐ **1.** abdominal cramps.
- ☐ **2.** tinnitus.
- ☐ **3.** rash.
- ☐ **4.** low blood pressure.

44. A client is transferred from the coronary care unit to the step-down unit. Which information should be included in the transfer report? Select all that apply.
☐ **1.** The client needs oxygen at 2 L/min.
☐ **2.** The client has a "do-not-resuscitate" prescription.
☐ **3.** The client uses the bedpan.
☐ **4.** The client has four grandchildren.
☐ **5.** The client has been in normal sinus rhythm for 6 hours.

45. A multigravid client at 26 weeks' gestation with a history of pregnancy-induced hypertension (PIH) asks the nurse about traveling from North America to a village in India by airplane to visit her father, who wishes to see her before she gives birth. Which response by the nurse is **most** appropriate?
☐ **1.** "Air travel at this point in your pregnancy can lead to preterm labor."
☐ **2.** "You can travel by airplane as long as you take frequent walks during the trip."
☐ **3.** "You need to avoid traveling because of your history of PIH."
☐ **4.** "You would be placing yourself and your fetus at risk for communicable diseases common in India."

46. A pregnant woman does not have funds to purchase adequate, nutritious food. She works part time at a low-wage job and has two other children. The nurse can refer the client to which type of assistance?
☐ **1.** home-delivered meals
☐ **2.** neighbors who can provide food
☐ **3.** the pregnant woman's employer
☐ **4.** food bank

47. The client has various sensory impairments associated with type 1 diabetes. The nurse determines that the client needs further instruction when the client says:
☐ **1.** "I will carefully test the temperature of my bathwater."
☐ **2.** "I will avoid kitchen activities."
☐ **3.** "I will avoid hot water bottles or heating pads."
☐ **4.** "I will inspect my skin daily for pressure points and injury."

48. The nurse is providing discharge instructions to the client with peripheral vascular disease. The nurse should include which information in the discussion with this client? Select all that apply.
☐ **1.** Avoid prolonged standing and sitting.
☐ **2.** Limit walking so as not to activate the "muscle pump."
☐ **3.** Keep extremities elevated on pillows.
☐ **4.** Keep the legs in a dependent position.
☐ **5.** Use a heating pad to promote vasodilation.

49. A father tells the nurse that his adolescent son spends lots of time in his room, his grades are falling, and he has given away a few of his favorite video games. What is the **most** appropriate action for the nurse?
☐ **1.** Give the father the telephone number for the local crisis hotline.
☐ **2.** Have the father take the adolescent to the nearest mental health outpatient facility now.
☐ **3.** Make a same-day appointment for the adolescent with his usual healthcare provider (HCP).
☐ **4.** Obtain more history information from the distraught father before making a decision.

50. A 7-year-old child is admitted to the hospital with acute rheumatic fever with chorea-like movements. Which eating utensil should the nurse remove from the meal tray?
☐ **1.** fork
☐ **2.** spoon
☐ **3.** plastic cup
☐ **4.** drinking straw

51. A client's catheter is removed 4 days after a transurethral resection of the prostate (TURP). He is experiencing urinary dribbling. What should the nurse do?
☐ **1.** Teach the client Kegel exercises.
☐ **2.** Obtain a urine culture and sensitivity analysis to screen for a urinary infection.
☐ **3.** Encourage voiding every hour to prevent dribbling.
☐ **4.** Inform him that the dribbling will stop after a few days.

52. The parent of a 2-month-old infant with colic states, "I do not know what to do anymore. She is up in the middle of the night crying all the time." What should the nurse tell the parent to do?
☐ **1.** Walk the floor with the baby at night.
☐ **2.** Take the infant for a short drive in the car.
☐ **3.** Allow the infant to cry it out in her crib.
☐ **4.** Offer cereal to fill the baby's stomach.

53. After the application of an arm cast, the client has pain on passive stretching of the fingers, finger swelling and tightness, and loss of function. Based on these data, the nurse anticipates that the client may be developing:
☐ **1.** delayed bone union.
☐ **2.** compartment syndrome.
☐ **3.** fat embolism.
☐ **4.** osteomyelitis.

54. Which is a **priority** for exercising for a client who has just had a myocardial infarction?
☐ **1.** low-back training program
☐ **2.** risk modification education
☐ **3.** strength training program
☐ **4.** jogging exercise program

55. While assessing a 4-day-old neonate born at 28 weeks' gestation, the nurse cannot elicit the neonate's Moro reflex, which was present 1 hour after birth. The nurse notifies the healthcare provider (HCP) because this may indicate which complication?
☐ 1. postnatal asphyxia
☐ 2. skull fracture
☐ 3. intracranial hemorrhage
☐ 4. facial nerve paralysis

56. The nurse is teaching the client about the appropriate use of lorazepam to manage anxiety. Which statement indicates that the client understands the nurse's teaching?
☐ 1. "I can take my medicine whenever I feel anxious."
☐ 2. "It is okay to double my dose if I need to."
☐ 3. "My medicine is not for the everyday stress of life."
☐ 4. "It is safe to have a glass of wine while taking this medicine."

57. The healthcare provider (HCP) prescribes a maternal blood test for alpha fetoprotein for a nulligravid client at 16 weeks' gestation. When developing the teaching plan, the nurse bases the explanations on the understanding that this test is used to detect which condition?
☐ 1. neural tube defects
☐ 2. Rh incompatibilities
☐ 3. inborn errors of metabolism
☐ 4. lecithin-sphingomyelin ratio

58. An unlicensed assistive personnel (UAP) recorded a client's 0600 blood glucose level as 126 mg/dL (7 mmol/L) instead of 216 mg/dL (12 mmol/L). The UAP did not recognize the error until 0900 but reported it to the nurse right away. What should the nurse do **first**?
☐ 1. Complete an incident report.
☐ 2. Wait and observe the client for symptoms of hyperglycemia.
☐ 3. Reprimand the UAP for the error.
☐ 4. Call the healthcare provider (HCP) and complete an incident report.

59. A client recovering from an abdominal hysterectomy has pain in her right calf. The nurse should:
☐ 1. palpate the calf to note pain.
☐ 2. measure the circumference of both calves and note the difference.
☐ 3. have the client flex and extend her leg and note the presence of pain.
☐ 4. raise the right leg and lower it to detect changes in skin color.

60. A client recently diagnosed with lung cancer tells the nurse that she has been having difficulty sleeping and is often preoccupied with thoughts about how her life has changed. She says, "I wish my life could just go on the way it was." Which issue should the nurse discuss with the client **first**?
☐ 1. preparing a will
☐ 2. managing insomnia
☐ 3. understanding grief
☐ 4. relieving anxiety

61. A 12-year-old has a fractured femur and is immobilized in traction as shown in the figure. What should the nurse do?

☐ 1. Add additional weight until the foot is only 2 inches (5 cm) from the bed.
☐ 2. Only offer foods that are easy to eat.
☐ 3. Place a pillow under the fractured leg to provide support.
☐ 4. Provide opportunities for age-appropriate activities.

62. The nurse is participating in a blood pressure screening event. After three separate readings taken at least 2 minutes apart, the nurse determines that a client has a blood pressure of 160/90 mm Hg. The nurse should advise the client to:
☐ 1. have blood pressure evaluated again within 1 month.
☐ 2. begin an exercise program.
☐ 3. examine lifestyle to decrease stress.
☐ 4. schedule a complete physical immediately.

63. A client's wife arrives on the nursing unit 6 hours after her husband's car accident, explaining that she has been out of town. She is distraught because she was not with her husband when he was admitted. The nurse should **first**:
☐ 1. allow her to verbalize her feelings and concerns.
☐ 2. describe her husband's medical treatment since admission.
☐ 3. explain the nature of the injury and reassure her that her husband's condition is stable.
☐ 4. reassure her that the important fact is that she is here now.

64. A client is scheduled to have a graded exercise test. The nurse explains to the client that the test will determine how:
- ☐ 1. to set the incline gradient on a treadmill.
- ☐ 2. well the body reacts to controlled exercise stress.
- ☐ 3. far he or she can walk.
- ☐ 4. long he or she can walk.

65. The mother of an infant with hemophilia tells the nurse that she is planning to do home schooling when the child reaches school age. She does not want her child in school because the teacher will not watch the child as well as she would. The mother's comments represent what common parental reaction to a child's chronic illness?
- ☐ 1. overprotection
- ☐ 2. devotion
- ☐ 3. mistrust
- ☐ 4. insecurity

66. A client with acute psychosis has been taking haloperidol for 3 days. When evaluating the client's response to the medication, which comment reflects the **greatest** improvement?
- ☐ 1. "I know these voices are not real, but I am still scared of them."
- ☐ 2. "I am feeling so restless, and I cannot sit still."
- ☐ 3. "Boy, do I need a shower. I think it has been days since I have had one."
- ☐ 4. "I am ready to talk about my discharge medications."

67. The nurse is administering an IV potassium chloride supplement to a client who has heart failure. When developing a plan of care for this client, the nurse should consider that:
- ☐ 1. hyperkalemia will intensify the action of the client's digoxin preparation.
- ☐ 2. the client's potassium levels will be unaffected by a potassium-sparing diuretic.
- ☐ 3. the administration of the IV potassium chloride should not exceed 10 mEq/h or a concentration of 40 mEq/L.
- ☐ 4. metabolic alkalosis will increase the client's serum potassium levels.

68. When assessing a client who is incontinent for risk for developing a pressure ulcer, the nurse should note which factor that can **most** alter tissue tolerance and lead to the development of a pressure ulcer?
- ☐ 1. the client's gender
- ☐ 2. exposure to moisture
- ☐ 3. presence of hypertension
- ☐ 4. smoking

69. A nurse is teaching a parenting class about how to prevent thrush (oral candidiasis). Which statement by a parent indicates more teaching is required?
- ☐ 1. "I will sterilize pacifiers."
- ☐ 2. "I should rinse my child's mouth after using a corticosteroid."
- ☐ 3. "If my child uses a spacer with asthma medications, I need to rinse it after each use."
- ☐ 4. "I should rinse my child's glass after each use."

70. A 10-year-old with a history of recent respiratory infection has swelling around the eyes in the morning and dark urine. What question should the nurse ask **first**?
- ☐ 1. "Has the child had a rash and fever?"
- ☐ 2. "Has the child had a sore throat?"
- ☐ 3. "Does the child have any allergies?"
- ☐ 4. "Does the child drink lots of liquids?"

71. Which nursing intervention is the **highest priority** during the first 24 hours postoperatively for the client who had a total laryngectomy due to cancer of the larynx?
- ☐ 1. Provide adequate nourishment.
- ☐ 2. Prevent skin breakdown around the stoma.
- ☐ 3. Maintain proper bowel elimination.
- ☐ 4. Maintain a patent airway.

72. It has been 5 months since a client lost his wife and child in a car-train accident. The nurse should determine that the client needs continuing counseling if he makes which statement?
- ☐ 1. "I am sleeping, eating, and working pretty well, but I still get so sad at times."
- ☐ 2. "I miss them so much, but I can tell I am getting better day by day."
- ☐ 3. "I wish I did not have to sleep. I hate the nightmares about what the car looked like."
- ☐ 4. "I never thought I would get over this, but I am working with my legislator for train crossing safety."

73. A client is hearing voices that are telling her to kill herself. She is demanding a knife to use on her wrists. Which is **most** appropriate intervention at this time?
- ☐ 1. Put the client in restraints after giving an IM dose of PRN medication.
- ☐ 2. Ask the client to talk about her anger and what is causing it.
- ☐ 3. Give oral PRN doses of haloperidol and lorazepam as prescribed.
- ☐ 4. Search the client's room for potential weapons after locking the unit kitchen.

74. Which measure is contraindicated when the nurse assists a child who has leukemia with oral hygiene?
- ☐ 1. applying petroleum jelly to the lips
- ☐ 2. cleaning the teeth with a toothbrush
- ☐ 3. swabbing the mouth with moistened cotton swabs
- ☐ 4. rinsing the mouth with a nonirritating mouthwash

75. The nurse realizes that a medication error has been made and a client has received the wrong medication. What should the nurse do **first**?
- ☐ 1. Assess the client's condition.
- ☐ 2. Notify the healthcare provider (HCP) of the error.
- ☐ 3. Complete an incident report.
- ☐ 4. Report the error to the unit manager.

76. The nurse is assessing a client who is 2 years of age and in the emergency department for burns on both feet, both lower legs, and the buttocks. The only area not burned from the waist down is the inside of the back of the knee. The parents inform the nurse that the child stepped into the bathtub and then sat down in the water when the water was too hot. What should the nurse do in order of priority from first to last? All options must be used.

| 1. Provide fluid resuscitation and pain medications. |
| 2. Assess burn depth in the different areas. |
| 3. Document parent-child interactions. |
| 4. Report incident to the authorities. |

| |
| |
| |
| |

77. When planning a health promotion class with a group of women, the nurse should include which information about reducing the risk of developing osteoarthritis?
- ☐ 1. Follow a high-protein diet.
- ☐ 2. Exercise for 20 minutes at least twice a week.
- ☐ 3. Prevent obesity.
- ☐ 4. Take a multivitamin supplement daily.

78. A neonate circumcised with a Plastibell 1 hour ago is brought to his mother for feeding. What should the nurse instruct the mother to do?
- ☐ 1. Read a pamphlet about circumcision care.
- ☐ 2. Remove the petroleum jelly gauze in 24 hours.
- ☐ 3. Tell the nurse when the neonate voids.
- ☐ 4. Place petroleum jelly over the site every 2 hours.

79. The nurse is assessing a client who has benign prostatic hypertrophy (BPH). The nurse should ask the client if he has:
- ☐ 1. impotence.
- ☐ 2. flank pain.
- ☐ 3. difficulty starting the urinary stream.
- ☐ 4. hematuria.

80. Which intervention should the nurse anticipate using when caring for a term neonate diagnosed with transient tachypnea at 2 hours after birth?
- ☐ 1. Monitor the neonate's color and cry every 4 hours.
- ☐ 2. Feed the neonate with a bottle every 3 hours.
- ☐ 3. Obtain extracorporeal membrane oxygenation equipment.
- ☐ 4. Provide warm, humidified oxygen in a warm environment.

81. The skin tone of a client of Vietnamese descent with dark skin who has early signs of iron deficiency anemia appears:
- ☐ 1. reddish-brown.
- ☐ 2. yellowish-brown.
- ☐ 3. black-brown.
- ☐ 4. whitish-brown.

82. Which laboratory finding is present in nephrotic syndrome?
- ☐ 1. decreased total serum protein
- ☐ 2. hypercalcemia
- ☐ 3. hyperglycemia
- ☐ 4. decreased hematocrit

83. While caring for several preterm infants in the special care nursery, which action is **most** important for preventing nosocomial infections in these neonates?
- ☐ 1. using sterile supplies for all treatments
- ☐ 2. performing thorough handwashing before giving infant care
- ☐ 3. donning cover gowns for nurses and visitors to the unit
- ☐ 4. wearing a mask, and changing it frequently when giving care

84. Which type of restraints is **best** for the nurse to use for a child in the immediate postoperative period after cleft palate repair?
- ☐ 1. safety jacket
- ☐ 2. elbow restraints
- ☐ 3. wrist restraints
- ☐ 4. body restraints

85. A nulliparous client tells the nurse that during her last pelvic examination, the healthcare provider (HCP) said that her uterus was in a severe retroverted position. The nurse determines that the client may experience:
☐ 1. frequent vaginal infections.
☐ 2. pain from endometriosis.
☐ 3. severe menstrual cramping.
☐ 4. difficulty conceiving a child.

86. A client in severe respiratory distress is admitted to the hospital. When assessing the client, the nurse should:
☐ 1. conduct a complete health history.
☐ 2. complete a comprehensive physical examination.
☐ 3. delay assessment until client's respiratory distress is resolved.
☐ 4. focus assessment on the respiratory system and distress.

87. A client has had a total hip replacement. Which sign **most** likely indicates that the hip has dislocated?
☐ 1. abduction of the affected leg
☐ 2. loosening of the prosthesis
☐ 3. external rotation of the affected leg
☐ 4. shortening of the affected leg

88. A client with schizophrenia is withdrawn, is suspicious of others, and projects blame. The client's behavior reflects problems in which stage of development as identified by Erikson?
☐ 1. trust versus mistrust
☐ 2. autonomy versus shame and doubt
☐ 3. initiative versus guilt
☐ 4. intimacy versus isolation

89. The nurse is assessing a client who has just experienced a crisis. The nurse should **first** assess the client for which behavior?
☐ 1. capability of effective problem solving
☐ 2. increased level of anxiety
☐ 3. shortened attention span
☐ 4. seeks help from others

90. A client with a new ileal conduit asks the nurse when to wear the appliance. What should the nurse tell the client?
☐ 1. "You need to wear your appliance all the time."
☐ 2. "You need to wear your appliance after you irrigate."
☐ 3. "It is only necessary to wear your appliance at night."
☐ 4. "The appliance must be worn after your meals."

91. A child has been exposed to varicella. Which precaution should the nurse institute for infection control?
☐ 1. airborne precautions
☐ 2. droplet precautions
☐ 3. contact precautions
☐ 4. indirect contact precautions

92. Which nursing goal is appropriate for a client with multiple myeloma?
☐ 1. Achieve effective management of bone pain.
☐ 2. Recover from the disease with minimal disabilities.
☐ 3. Decrease episodes of nausea and vomiting.
☐ 4. Avoid hyperkalemia.

93. After an episode of severe pain, a client says to the nurse, "The pain really frightened me. I thought I was going to die." Which statement is the **most** appropriate response from the nurse?
☐ 1. "I understand that pain can be a frightening experience."
☐ 2. "Why were you frightened? You have had pain before."
☐ 3. "There is no need to be frightened of pain."
☐ 4. "Pain cannot cause you to die. Try to relax."

94. A child returns to the pediatric unit after a bowel resection. Which action has the **highest priority**?
☐ 1. Administer IV fluids.
☐ 2. Keep the child on nothing-by-mouth status.
☐ 3. Monitor vital signs frequently.
☐ 4. Assess the child's pain level.

95. When obtaining a health history, the nurse understands that which client statement indicates the need for further follow-up?
☐ 1. "I have some shortness of breath when I exercise."
☐ 2. "No matter how much I drink, I am still thirsty all the time."
☐ 3. "I wake up early in the morning and cannot return to sleep."
☐ 4. "In the past couple of weeks, I have been having a lot of trouble urinating."

96. A young adult has been diagnosed with hypertrophic cardiomyopathy. The nurse should further assess the client for:
☐ 1. angina.
☐ 2. fatigue and shortness of breath.
☐ 3. abdominal pain.
☐ 4. hypertension.

97. The nurse should advise the mother of a toddler suspected of having pinworms to do the cellophane tape test at which time?
☐ 1. before bathing
☐ 2. after a bowel movement
☐ 3. while the child is asleep
☐ 4. after a meal

98. Which finding provides the **most** evidence that a fetus might have a gastrointestinal tract anomaly?
☐ 1. meconium in the amniotic fluid
☐ 2. low implantation of the placenta
☐ 3. increased amount of amniotic fluid
☐ 4. pre-eclampsia in the last trimester

99. Using the Morse Fall Risk Scale (see exhibit), the nurse should initiate **highest** fall risk precautions for which client?

Morse Fall Risk/Scale

Item	Scale		Scoring
1. History of falling, immediate or within 3 months	No	0	
	Yes	25	
2. Secondary diagnosis	No	0	
	Yes	15	
3. Ambulatory aid			
Bed rest/nurse assist		0	
Crutches/cane/walker		15	
Furniture		30	
4. IV/heparin lock	No	0	
	Yes	20	
5. Gait/transferring			
Normal/bed rest/ immobile		0	
Weak		10	
Impaired		20	
6. Mental status			
Oriented to own ability		0	
Forgets limitations		15	

☐ 1. an 84-year-old client with diabetes admitted with new-onset confusion who reportedly fell at home last week, is currently on bed rest, and has normal saline infusing per saline lock

☐ 2. a 48-year-old alert and oriented client with quadriplegia admitted for wound care of a stage IV pressure ulcer, receiving IV antibiotics per a peripherally inserted central catheter

☐ 3. a 62-year-old client with a history of Parkinson's disease, admitted for pneumonia and receiving IV antibiotics, who has fallen at home but is able to ambulate with a cane and who during his hospitalization has gotten out of bed without calling for assistance

☐ 4. a 27-year-old client with acute pancreatitis receiving morphine sulfate IV every 2 hours as needed for pain, no significant medical history, smokes two packs of cigarettes per day, may be up independently, and has steady gait

100. A 17-year-old gang member, who is living on the streets, is hospitalized after an overdose. When medically stable, the teen is admitted to the adolescent psychiatric unit of the same hospital. In what order of priority from first to last should the nurse explore the issues? All options must be used.

1. the reason the teen is not living with parents

2. the desire to leave or remain in the gang

3. the current level of suicidal risk

4. the desire to return home or go elsewhere after discharge

101. How does the nurse on the obstetrics unit assure client safety? Select all that apply.
☐ 1. reconciliation of medication prescriptions
☐ 2. communication among staff
☐ 3. placing culturally similar clients together
☐ 4. use of two unique identifiers
☐ 5. staff training

102. A nurse is planning care with a family of a 4-year-old in preschool who is often disruptive in class, is difficult to engage, and rarely speaks. The child flaps his arms and screeches when he is upset. What would be the **most** appropriate responses for the nurse to make to the parents? Select all that apply.
☐ 1. "Has your child received all his childhood immunizations? You know there is evidence that childhood immunizations play a role in the development of autism."
☐ 2. "Has your child been evaluated by a pediatrician? He seems to have some behaviors that are abnormal for a child of his age."
☐ 3. "How does your child behave at home? If you do not see acting out behavior at home, part of his problem may be dealing with new situations such as school."
☐ 4. "How do you respond if he disobeys or acts out at home? If your techniques help stop or prevent negative behavior, perhaps the teachers can try similar measures at school."
☐ 5. "Have you considered private school? This environment does not seem right for your child."

103. A client is anxious following a robbery. The client is worried about identity theft and states, "I could lose everything. I cannot stand the fears I have. I reported everything, but I still cannot eat or sleep." Which intervention should the nurse implement **first**?
- ☐ 1. Request a prescription for an antianxiety medication.
- ☐ 2. Provide a list of free legal resources.
- ☐ 3. Refer the client to a support group.
- ☐ 4. Listen empathetically while the client discusses the fears.

104. When a client wants to read the medical record, the nurse should:
- ☐ 1. call the healthcare provider (HCP) to obtain permission.
- ☐ 2. give the client the medical record and answer the client's questions.
- ☐ 3. tell the client to read the medical record when the HCP makes rounds.
- ☐ 4. answer any questions the client has without giving the client the medical record.

105. A nurse is relieving the triage nurse in the labor and birth unit who is going to lunch. The report indicates that there are three clients having their vital signs assessed and a fourth client is on her way to the unit from the emergency department. In which order of priority from first to last should the nurse manage these clients? All options must be used.

1. the client with clear vesicles and brown vaginal discharge at 16 weeks' gestation

2. the client with right lower quadrant pain at 10 weeks' gestation

3. the client who is at term and has had no fetal movement for 2 days

4. the client from the emergency department at term and screaming loudly because of labor contractions

106. The nurse is beginning the shift and is planning care for six clients on the postpartum unit. Three of the clients have immediate needs, and three of the clients are listed as "stable." For the **best** utilization of time and client safety, the nurse should make rounds on which client **first**?
- ☐ 1. the three clients who are reported to be stable
- ☐ 2. the mother with a 4-hour-old infant with initial blood glucose of 33 mg/dL (1.8 mmol/L) and now at 45 mg/dL (2.5 mmol/L) breast-feeding her infant
- ☐ 3. a mother who had a spontaneous vaginal birth (SVB) and received carboprost 1 hour ago for increased bleeding
- ☐ 4. a mother with a 3-day-old who had a bilirubin level of 13 mg/dL (220 µmol/L) 30 minutes ago and is now in a biliblanket at the mother's bedside

107. The nurse on the postpartum unit is caring for four couplets. There will be a new admission in 30 minutes. The new client is a G4 P4, Spanish-speaking only client with an infant who is in the special care nursery (SCN) for respiratory distress. The nurse should place the new client in a room with which client?
- ☐ 1. a G4 P4 who is 2 days postpartum with infant, Spanish speaking only
- ☐ 2. a G1 P1 who is 1 day postpartum with an infant in the SCN
- ☐ 3. a G6 P6 who gave birth 4 hours ago by cesarean section for fetal distress, infant at bedside
- ☐ 4. a G1 P1 who is a non–English-speaking client with infant in SCN for fetal distress

108. The nurse is developing a community health education program about sexually transmitted infections. Which information about women who acquire gonorrhea should be included?
- ☐ 1. Women are more reluctant than men to seek medical treatment.
- ☐ 2. Gonorrhea is not easily transmitted to women who are menopausal.
- ☐ 3. Women with gonorrhea are usually asymptomatic.
- ☐ 4. Gonorrhea is usually a mild disease for women.

109. Which client is at **greatest** risk for falling?
- ☐ 1. a 22-year-old man with three fractured ribs and a fractured left arm
- ☐ 2. a 70-year-old woman with episodes of syncope
- ☐ 3. a 50-year-old man with angina
- ☐ 4. a 30-year-old woman with a fractured ankle

110. A child with meningococcal meningitis is being admitted to the pediatric unit. In preparation for the child's arrival, the nurse should **first**:
- ☐ 1. institute droplet precautions.
- ☐ 2. obtain the child's vital signs.
- ☐ 3. ask the parent about medication allergies.
- ☐ 4. inquire about the health of siblings at home.

Answers, Rationales, and Test-Taking Strategies

*The answers and rationales for each question follow below, along with keys (🔑) to the client need (CN) and cognitive level (CL) for each question. In addition, you will also see a glossary icon (📖) highlighting specific terminology used on the licensing exam. As you check your answers, use the **Content Mastery and Test-Taking Skill Self-Analysis** worksheet (tear-out worksheet in back of book) to identify the reason(s) for not answering the questions correctly. For additional information about test-taking skills and strategies for answering questions, refer to pages 12–23 and pages 35–36 in Part 1 of this book.*

1. 3. Illegible writing is one of the most common reasons for medication errors. The **HCP** 📖 should be called to clarify the prescription. The previous medication record should not be used as a substitute for the exact prescription written by the HCP. The pharmacist or the client's family cannot interpret a prescription written by an HCP.

🔑 CN: Management of care; CL: Synthesize

2. 2. Propantheline bromide is an anticholinergic used to decrease biliary spasm. Decreasing biliary spasm helps to reduce pain in cholecystitis. Propantheline does not increase bile production or have an antiemetic effect, and it is not effective in treating infection.

🔑 CN: Pharmacological and parenteral therapies; CL: Apply

3. 3. An important function of support organizations for any health problem is to put parents of children with the condition in touch with each other. Other parents can commonly offer support and help. In some instances, organizations can offer assistance, such as providing equipment required for home care of their child with cystic fibrosis. These organizations do not obtain tutors for children, nor do they provide medications, financial assistance, or genetic counseling for parents.

🔑 CN: Management of care; CL: Apply

4. 3. Strategies for meeting client satisfaction include involving hospital department personnel to improve service. Saying, "The staff is doing the best it can," or, "I will report this to the **healthcare provider (HCP)** 📖," does not offer a practical resolution to the client's problem. Expressing a personal dislike for the food negates the client's problem and does not offer a solution.

🔑 CN: Management of care; CL: Synthesize

5. 2. Rehabilitation for a client who has sustained a cerebrovascular accident begins at the time the client is admitted to the hospital. The first goal of rehabilitation should be to help prevent deformities. This goal is achieved through such techniques as positioning the client properly in bed, changing the client's position frequently, and supporting all parts of the body in proper alignment. Passive range-of-motion exercises may also be started, unless contraindicated.

🔑 CN: Management of care; CL: Synthesize

6. 4. An involuntarily admitted client loses the right to leave the hospital until the condition is stable enough that the client no longer poses a danger to self or others. While hospitalized, the client retains all civil rights such as receiving mail, making phone calls, refusing treatment, and also receiving the least restrictive treatment. Should the involuntarily admitted client refuse treatment once admitted, he will be evaluated for the need to receive treatment against wishes in order to decrease the risk for self-harm or harm to others.

🔑 CN: Management of care; CL: Analyze

7. 2. Chewing the pill or capsule form of valproic acid can cause mouth and throat irritation and is contraindicated. Taking the pills at the same time each day is important to maintain therapeutic effectiveness of the drug. Taking the pills with food is appropriate if the client is experiencing gastrointestinal upset. Valproic acid may cause clotting problems; therefore, bruising should be reported.

🔑 CN: Pharmacological and parenteral therapies; CL: Evaluate

8. 3. The client is positioned correctly in the sidelying position. The pillows support the client's joints and do not cause unnecessary pressure on the joints or skin. It is not necessary to add another pillow under the arm or to elevate the head of the bed. The nurse should assess the client's skin for signs of breakdown, particularly at the elbows, back, hips, and heels where there were pressure points from the position in which the client was previously lying.

🔑 CN: Reduction of risk potential; CL: Evaluate

9. 2. It is the role of the surgeon or the person performing the procedure to obtain the **informed consent** 📖. This consists of informing the client about the procedure, the risks of treatment, the side effects, other types of treatments available, and the effects without the procedure. Nurses, anesthesiologists, and social workers do not obtain informed consent.

🔑 CN: Management of care; CL: Apply

10. 4. Hospice care focuses on supportive care for the client and family. Care for the family may continue throughout the bereavement period. Hospice care involves care of the client at home as well as in an inpatient setting. Although professional care is provided in hospice, family members, volunteers, and unlicensed assistive personnel (UAP) also participate in the care of the client.

CN: Basic care and comfort; CL: Apply

11. 3. One of the side effects of steroid therapy is fat deposition on the trunk and face, producing classic Cushingoid signs. Therefore, the nurse should expect to find truncal obesity. Steroids also can cause altered moods or mood swings. Typically, long-term steroid use results in weight gain. Steroids may inhibit the action of growth hormone. Therefore, a growth spurt is not likely.

CN: Pharmacological and parenteral therapies; CL: Analyze

12. 3. The nurse should not be required to participate in an abortion if it contradicts the nurse's religious beliefs. The behavior should not be reflected negatively on the nurse's evaluation. Preparing equipment and supplies for the case may be viewed as the same as circulating for the case. The nurse has a right not to participate in an abortion unless it is an absolute emergency and no one else is available to care for the client.

CN: Management of care; CL: Synthesize

13. 3. Phenytoin causes hyperplasia of the gums, and the client needs frequent dental examinations and meticulous oral hygiene. Phenytoin therapy may contribute to a folic acid deficiency, but it is not related to iron or calcium metabolism. A need for frequent eye examinations is not related to the side effects of phenytoin.

CN: Pharmacological and parenteral therapies; CL: Synthesize

14. 1. The chest is compressed with the heel of one hand positioned on the lower sternum, two fingerbreadths above the sternal notch (at the nipple line). Fingertips are used to compress the sternum in infants, and the heels of both hands are used in adult cardiopulmonary resuscitation.

CN: Safety and infection control; CL: Apply

15. 1. Nitroglycerin tablets should be taken 5 minutes apart for three doses; if this is ineffective, 911 should be called to obtain an ambulance to take the client to the emergency department. The client should not drive or have a family member drive the client to the hospital.

CN: Pharmacological and parenteral therapies; CL: Synthesize

16. 3. The client will obtain the most health benefits from aerobic exercises such as walking, biking, jogging, or swimming. Because the client has been sedentary, the nurse instructs the client to start the exercise program with walking slowly 10 minutes

four times a day and increasing to 30 to 60 minutes three to five times per week. Jogging is not a realistic exercise at this time. Playing golf is not considered an aerobic activity; therefore, it is not beneficial in lowering serum lipids. To illicit cardiovascular changes, the client would need to swim more than once a week.

CN: Health promotion and maintenance; CL: Synthesize

17. 4. The client who voices death wishes must be asked directly about thoughts of suicide and specific suicide plans. The other questions are important history questions but are not crucial to address the follow-up needed when the client verbalizes a death wish.

CN: Psychosocial integrity; CL: Synthesize

18. 3. This client should be monitored for blood dyscrasias, evidenced by decreased platelet count and white blood cell count with changes in the CBC differential. Elevated serum electrolytes, serum glucose, and sedimentation rates are not side effects of this drug.

CN: Pharmacological and parenteral therapies; CL: Apply

19. 4. The new onset of constipation may be a sign of a tumor or other health problems. Constipation is not an expected change of aging. Increased fiber and fluid intake is helpful with constipation, but in this case, the client needs to be seen by a **HCP** to rule out a health problem.

CN: Reduction of risk potential; CL: Synthesize

20. 4. Saying, "We will help you be successful so that you can stay alcohol-free," conveys interest in the client as a worthwhile individual who needs help and treatment. This statement also helps to build trust and enhances self-esteem. The other statements confront the client and may result in the client's feeling belittled, judged, and rejected.

CN: Psychosocial integrity; CL: Synthesize

21. 3. Research has shown that at least two injections daily provide improved blood glucose control and decreased incidence of target end-organ damage. Type 1 diabetes requires insulin replacement and cannot be managed with oral medications alone. It would be inappropriate to ask the **HCP** to change the insulin schedule.

CN: Pharmacological and parenteral therapies; CL: Synthesize

22. 1. Peak and trough serum levels are used to adjust the dosage within a therapeutic range. Monitoring drug levels does not prevent allergic reactions. Preventing toxicity helps decrease the risk of some side effects, but will not but not totally prevented them. Peaks and trough levels are monitored only after a drug has been given long enough to achieve therapeutic levels.

CN: Pharmacological and parenteral therapies; CL: Apply

23. 4. A glycosylated hemoglobin level gives the nurse data about the average blood glucose concentration over 2 to 3 months, providing a picture of the client's overall glucose control. A fasting serum glucose level gives a picture of the client's recent glucose level, not the overall effectiveness of the therapeutic regimen. A 1-week diet recall is not always accurate. Although a home log would provide some information about overall control and compliance, the log may not have all of the glucose levels recorded.

CN: Reduction of risk potential; CL: Evaluate

24. 3. When making rounds, nurses can note a variety of risks in the clients' rooms, in the hallways, and other areas where clients might be at risk. Using signs and color-coded armbands and keeping the bed in a low position are also useful, but making rounds offers the opportunity for nurses to intervene immediately and teach the client, family, and staff when risks are noted.

CN: Safety and infection control; CL: Synthesize

25. 1. The nurse's first action should be to clamp off the transfusion because the client is having a transfusion reaction. It is most important that the client not receive any more blood. Other measures may be appropriate after the blood has been stopped. The nurse should raise the head of the bed if the client becomes short of breath. There is no need for antibiotic therapy for a blood transfusion related to a temperature spike. The nurse can provide a cool washcloth for a headache or fever; however, this is not a priority.

CN: Pharmacological and parenteral therapies; CL: Synthesize

26. 1, 3, 4. A drop in blood pressure to 80/40 mm Hg is significant and should be reported to the **HCP** 📖. Hypotension and vasodilation may occur as a result of sympathetic nerve blockage along with the pain nerve blockage. A report of a crushing headache suggests that the epidural catheter may be dislodged in the subarachnoid space rather than the epidural space. The HCP also should be notified any time if more than 1 mL of fluid or blood is aspirated from the catheter before a bolus injection. A respiratory rate of 14 breaths/min, although somewhat decreased from baseline, is within acceptable parameters. However, if the rate drops to 10 breaths/min or less, the HCP should be notified. A pain rating of 3 out of 10 suggests that pain is being relieved with the epidural analgesia.

CN: Pharmacological and parenteral therapies; CL: Synthesize

27. 3. A client with AIDS is immunocompromised, and food safety is an important concern. Food-borne illnesses and infections can be devastating to the client with AIDS. Large, frequent meals are not necessary. Megadoses of vitamins can result in toxicities that may aggravate the client's clinical condition. Leaving food out encourages growth of microorganisms.

CN: Safety and infection control; CL: Synthesize

28. 4. This finding describes Mongolian spots, which are common in newborns of African, Asian, or Latin descent. Telangiectatic nevi, or "stork bites," are pink lesions commonly found on the back of the neck. Milia are small white papules over the nose and cheek that indicate blocked sebaceous glands.

CN: Health promotion and maintenance; CL: Analyze

29. 1. Blurred vision is a serious adverse effect of oral contraceptives, possibly because of severe hypertension as a result of the medication. If the client experiences blurred vision, she needs to contact her **HCP** 📖 immediately. Nausea, weight gain, and mild headache are common and possibly bothersome side effects and should be noted. However, they do not need to be reported immediately unless they are severe, prolonged, or accompanied by other symptoms.

CN: Pharmacological and parenteral therapies; CL: Analyze

30. 3. Nausea and vomiting, along with hypokalemia, are likely indicators of digoxin toxicity. Hypokalemia is a common cause of digoxin toxicity; therefore, serum potassium levels should be carefully monitored if the client is taking digoxin. The earliest clinical signs of digoxin toxicity are anorexia, nausea, and vomiting. Bradycardia, other dysrhythmias, and visual disturbances are also common signs. Chronic renal failure usually causes hyperkalemia. With persistent vomiting, the client is more likely to develop metabolic alkalosis than metabolic acidosis.

CN: Pharmacological and parenteral therapies; CL: Analyze

31. 2. Food sources high in calcium include steamed broccoli, dairy products, and fortified cereals. Rice, apples, and meat are not calcium-rich sources. Menopausal women need 1,500 mg of calcium daily.

CN: Reduction of risk potential; CL: Apply

32. 2. At the time a client receives a Depo-Provera injection, a follow-up appointment should be made for 3 months later. The nurse should emphasize the need to adhere to the medication schedule to prevent an unplanned pregnancy. One of the most common reasons for failure of this contraceptive is lack of adherence to the appointment schedule for injections every 3 months.

🔑 CN: Pharmacological and parenteral therapies; CL: Apply

33. 3. Panting will alleviate the client's urge to push. The client risks edema or tearing of the cervix if pushing begins before complete cervical dilation (10 cm) is achieved. Although turning the client to her left side improves uteroplacental blood flow, it will have no effect on diminishing the client's urge to push. Although focusing on an object in the room may help the client to relax, it will have no effect on diminishing the client's urge to push due to the pressure of a fetus at +1 station.

🔑 CN: Health promotion and maintenance; CL: Synthesize

34. 2, 3, 4. The client who is taking potentially nephrotoxic antibiotics should notify the **healthcare provider (HCP)** 📖 if the urine is cloudy, smoky, or pink; early signs of nephrotoxicity are manifested by changes in urine color. Straw-colored urine is normal.

🔑 CN: Pharmacological and parenteral therapies; CL: Analyze

35. 1. In clients with fluid retention, sodium restriction may be necessary to promote fluid loss. Increasing exercise will not reduce fluid retention. Exercise will promote circulation, but will not manage the fluid retention. Restricting fluid intake will not reduce retained fluids; increased fluids will increase urine output and promote improved fluid balance. Elevating the client's feet helps promote venous return and fluid reabsorption but in itself will not reduce the volume of excess fluid.

🔑 CN: Reduction of risk potential; CL: Synthesize

36. 1. The client might wear objects as a protection against specific medical disorders. Typically, these practices bring no harm to the client and should not be discouraged. The client should continue to be encouraged to follow the medical guidance of her **healthcare provider (HCP)** 📖. If the practice is not harming the client, it is inappropriate to label it quackery and demand that the client discontinue it. There is no medical evidence to support the wearing of a copper bracelet.

🔑 CN: Health promotion and maintenance; CL: Synthesize

37. 4. Normally, a neonate's heart rate should be between 120 and 160 bpm shortly after birth. The nurse should document this as a normal neonatal finding. The **HCP** 📖 does not need to be notified. Assessing for cyanosis is a routine assessment at birth, but with the neonate's heart rate at 142 bpm, cyanosis should be minimal and typically located in the hands and feet. Heart rate assessments are performed routinely according to facility protocol. For example, the heart rate is assessed soon after birth, every 15 minutes for 1 hour, every 30 minutes for 1 hour, and then every 4 hours.

🔑 CN: Health promotion and maintenance; CL: Synthesize

38. 1. The therapeutic effects of desmopressin nasal spray are relief from polydipsia and control of polyuria and nocturia in the client with diabetes insipidus. Side effects include nasal congestion and headache. Blurred vision is not related to desmopressin.

🔑 CN: Pharmacological and parenteral therapies; CL: Evaluate

39. 1. Protein and vitamin C are particularly important in promoting wound healing and recovery from infection. A diet high in carbohydrates is also essential. Because the client with an infection commonly does not feel like eating, it is important that what the client eats should be nutritious. Chicken and orange slices would help meet the client's protein and vitamin needs. A meal of a cheeseburger and fries or a cheese omelet and bacon are high in fat and low do not contain as much vitamin C as the chicken and orange slices. Gelatin salad and tea contain minimal nutrients.

🔑 CN: Basic care and comfort; CL: Apply

40. 4. Beef, liver, iron-fortified cereals, and spinach are iron-rich foods. Cheese, squash, and apples do not have significant sources of iron.

🔑 CN: Reduction of risk potential; CL: Apply

41. 2, 4. Children in respiratory distress need to be kept as quiet as possible to decrease respiratory and heart rates. Toddlers need a parent with them for security. The best way to quiet toddlers is to read or to hold them. Restraints increase heart and respiratory rates. A sedative will mask the signs of further respiratory distress. Although you could tell toddlers that a mask will help with breathing, they cannot understand the rationale and thus fully comprehend its importance. Asking the parents to leave the bedside will most likely result in greater upset, further contributing to respiratory distress.

🔑 CN: Basic care and comfort; CL: Synthesize

42. 1. Warm showers, baths, or hand soaks can help relieve joint stiffness and allow the client to more comfortably perform activities of daily living. Aspirin or other anti-inflammatory drugs should be taken before activity to help decrease inflammation

18. Which response is **most** helpful for a client who is euphoric, intrusive, and interrupts other clients engaged in conversations to the point where they get up and leave or walk away?
- ☐ **1.** "When you interrupt others, they leave the area."
- ☐ **2.** "You are being rude and uncaring."
- ☐ **3.** "You should remember to use your manners."
- ☐ **4.** "You know better than to interrupt someone."

19. The nurse is transferring a multigravid client who is at 25 weeks' gestation with preeclampsia from the obstetrical intensive care unit to the antenatal unit. To safely manage this preeclamptic client, what should be included in the transfer report about this client? Select all that apply.
- ☐ **1.** record of blood pressure trends
- ☐ **2.** record of urine protein
- ☐ **3.** edema observed by healthcare provider (HCP)
- ☐ **4.** client use of dietary sodium
- ☐ **5.** fetal position
- ☐ **6.** fetal heart rate pattern

20. The nurse is assessing fetal presentation in a multiparous client. The figure below indicates which presentation?

- ☐ **1.** frank breech
- ☐ **2.** complete breech
- ☐ **3.** footling breech
- ☐ **4.** vertex

21. A client believes she is experiencing premenstrual syndrome (PMS). The nurse should **next** ask the client about what symptom?
- ☐ **1.** menstrual cycle irregularity with increased menstrual flow
- ☐ **2.** mood swings immediately after menses
- ☐ **3.** tension and fatigue before menses and through the second day of the menstrual cycle
- ☐ **4.** midcycle spotting and abdominal pain at the time of ovulation

22. Which should the nurse closely assess in a client who is reversing from general anesthesia and receiving clindamycin?
- ☐ **1.** tachycardia
- ☐ **2.** respiratory depression
- ☐ **3.** hypotension
- ☐ **4.** renal failure

23. A client with delirium becomes very anxious and says, "I cannot stop what is happening to me. Make it stop, please!" What is the nurse's **most** appropriate response?
- ☐ **1.** "I will get you some medicine to help you relax. The more you worry, the worse it will get."
- ☐ **2.** "As soon as we know what is causing this, we can try to stop it. I will get you some medicine to help you relax."
- ☐ **3.** "I wish I could do something to make it stop, but unfortunately I cannot."
- ☐ **4.** "I will sit with you until you calm down a little."

24. A 16-year-old client is in the emergency department for treatment of minor injuries from a car accident. A crisis nurse is with the client because the client became hysterical and was saying, "It is my fault. My Mom is going to kill me. I do not even have a way home." What should be the nurse's **initial** intervention?
- ☐ **1.** Hold her hands and say, "Slow down. Take a deep breath."
- ☐ **2.** Say, "Calm down. The police can take you home."
- ☐ **3.** Put a hand on her shoulder and say, "It was not your fault."
- ☐ **4.** Say, "Your mother is not going to kill you. Stop worrying."

25. A hospitalized adolescent with type 1 diabetes mellitus is weak and nauseated with poor skin turgor. The nurse notes a fruity odor to the client's breath. The client uses insulin lispro. The last meal was lunch, 2 hours ago. Place the nursing actions in the order in which the nurse should perform them. All options must be used.

1. Obtain a fingerstick test for blood glucose.

2. Start an IV infusion with normal saline solution.

3. Administer insulin lispro.

4. Notify the healthcare provider (HCP).

26. A nurse is planning care for a hospitalized child who is 10 years of age and is delegating care to a pediatric care assistant. When a nurse delegates a task to an unlicensed assistive personnel (UAP), which factor is **most** important?
- [ ] 1. The nurse has observed the UAP perform the task.
- [ ] 2. The child and UAP have established a positive relationship.
- [ ] 3. The task is appropriate for that individual's preparation.
- [ ] 4. The UAP has previously performed the task.

27. The nurse is assessing a client with superficial thrombophlebitis in the greater saphenous vein of the left leg. The client has "aching" in the leg. Which finding indicates the nurse should contact the healthcare provider (HCP) to request a prescription to improve the client's comfort?
- [ ] 1. brown discoloration of the skin with edema in the lower left leg
- [ ] 2. dark, protruding veins of both legs that are uncomfortable when standing
- [ ] 3. absence of pain or swelling when the client dorsiflexes the left foot
- [ ] 4. red, warm, palpable linear cord along the vein that is painful on palpation

28. A client who has been recently diagnosed with acquired immunodeficiency syndrome (AIDS) inquires about hospice services. The nurse explains that hospice care is appropriate:
- [ ] 1. for clients with an inevitable death within weeks to months.
- [ ] 2. for all clients with AIDS at any stage.
- [ ] 3. only when the client has written advance directives.
- [ ] 4. when the client is ready to discuss the prognosis.

29. While assessing a neonate at age 24 hours, the nurse observes several irregularly shaped, red, flat patches on the back of the neonate's neck. The nurse interprets this as which finding?
- [ ] 1. stork bite
- [ ] 2. port-wine stain
- [ ] 3. newborn rash
- [ ] 4. café au lait spot

30. A mother who is Mexican brings her 2-month-old son to the emergency department with a high fever and possible sepsis. A lumbar puncture is prescribed, but the mother will not sign the consent until the father arrives to give permission. What should the nurse do?
- [ ] 1. Report this to the social worker.
- [ ] 2. Call the regional protective services for children.
- [ ] 3. Wait until the father arrives.
- [ ] 4. Inform the healthcare provider (HCP) that the mother has refused to have the procedure.

31. What action is **most** appropriate when dealing with a client who is expressing anger verbally, is pacing, and is irritable?
- [ ] 1. Convey empathy and encouraging ventilation.
- [ ] 2. Use calm, firm directions to get the client to a quiet room.
- [ ] 3. Put the client in restraints.
- [ ] 4. Discuss alternative strategies for when the client is angry in the future.

32. A client with Alzheimer's disease is started on a low dose of lorazepam because of agitation and a sleep disturbance. The nurse should assess the client for which complication?
- [ ] 1. nighttime agitation
- [ ] 2. extrapyramidal side effects
- [ ] 3. vomiting
- [ ] 4. anticholinergic side effects

33. The nurse is conducting a counseling session with a client experiencing posttraumatic stress disorder (PSTD) using a 2-way video telehealth system from the hospital to the client's home, which is 2 hours away from the nearest mental health facility. What are expected outcomes of using telehealth as a venue to provide health care to this client? Select all that apply. The client will:
- [ ] 1. save travel time from the house to the healthcare facility.
- [ ] 2. avoid reliving a traumatic event that might be precipitated by visiting a healthcare facility.
- [ ] 3. experience a shorter recovery time than being treated on-site at a healthcare facility.
- [ ] 4. receive health care for this mental health problem.
- [ ] 5. obtain group support from others with a similar health problem.

34. A client who is postmenopausal with an intact uterus asks the nurse why her hormone medicine has two drugs, estrogen and progesterone. Which statement by the nurse provides the client with accurate information?
- [ ] 1. "The progesterone will help prevent cervical cancer."
- [ ] 2. "The progesterone will help prevent breast cancer."
- [ ] 3. "The progesterone will help prevent liver disease."
- [ ] 4. "The progesterone will help prevent endometrial cancer."

35. A child who is of preschool age is diagnosed as having severe autism. The **most** effective therapy involves which intervention?
- [ ] 1. antipsychotic medications
- [ ] 2. group psychotherapy
- [ ] 3. 1:1 play therapy
- [ ] 4. social skills group

36. The nurse on the antenatal unit is planning care for four clients. The nurse should assess which client **first**?
- ☐ **1.** a 29-year-old client carrying twins, being treated for preterm labor at 29 weeks' gestation and receiving magnesium sulfate at 2 g/h, who has had no contractions for the past 2 hours; both twins appear stable, according to the nurse's shift report
- ☐ **2.** a 19-year-old 18 weeks intrauterine pregnancy (IUP) who is now 12 hours postmotor vehicle accident with bright red vaginal bleeding
- ☐ **3.** a client at 38 weeks' gestation hospitalized frequently during this pregnancy for placenta previa and who 2 days ago was admitted with severe bright red vaginal bleeding that has tapered off now
- ☐ **4.** a 9-week IUP hospitalized for hyperemesis gravidarum who has not vomited for the last 12 hours

37. The nurse should turn the client on bed rest every 2 hours to prevent the development of pressure ulcers. In addition, the nurse should:
- ☐ **1.** have the client walk at least twice a day.
- ☐ **2.** insert an indwelling urinary catheter.
- ☐ **3.** monitor serum albumin.
- ☐ **4.** monitor the white blood cell count.

38. A client, hospitalized with heart failure, is receiving digoxin and furosemide intravenously and now has continuous ringing in the ears. What is the appropriate action for the nurse to take at this time?
- ☐ **1.** Obtain a digoxin level to check for toxicity.
- ☐ **2.** Note the observation in the medical record, and plan to reassess in 2 hours.
- ☐ **3.** Ask the client about taking aspirin in addition to other medications.
- ☐ **4.** Discontinue the furosemide, and notify the healthcare provider (HCP).

39. A woman who speaks Spanish only and is very upset brings her child to the clinic with bleeding from the mouth. Which is the appropriate **first** action by the nurse who does not speak Spanish?
- ☐ **1.** Call for the Spanish interpreter.
- ☐ **2.** Grab the child, and take the child to the treatment room.
- ☐ **3.** Immediately apply ice to the child's mouth.
- ☐ **4.** Give the ice to the mother, and demonstrate what to do.

40. The nurse should give which discharge instructions about thermal injury to a client with peripheral vascular disease? Select all that apply.
- ☐ **1.** "Warm the fingers or toes by using an electric heating pad."
- ☐ **2.** "Avoid sunburn during the summer."
- ☐ **3.** "Wear extra socks in the winter."
- ☐ **4.** "Choose loose, soft, cotton socks."
- ☐ **5.** "Use an electric blanket when you are sleeping."

41. A client receives an IV dose of gentamicin sulfate. How long after the completion of the dose should the peak serum concentration level be measured?
- ☐ **1.** 10 minutes
- ☐ **2.** 20 minutes
- ☐ **3.** 30 minutes
- ☐ **4.** 40 minutes

42. An 86-year-old has few health problems, performs self-care, plays cards, and talks about "the good old days." The client wants to make "final" arrangements, such as completing an advance directive and planning and paying for a funeral and burial. The nurse determines that the client:
- ☐ **1.** is depressed and should be watched for further signs of depression.
- ☐ **2.** is responding in an age-appropriate manner.
- ☐ **3.** is potentially suicidal and should be placed on suicide precautions and seen by a psychiatrist.
- ☐ **4.** has a premonition about dying soon.

43. A client with hydrocephalus reports having had a headache in the morning on arising for the last 3 days, but it disappears later in the day. The nurse should:
- ☐ **1.** notify the healthcare provider (HCP).
- ☐ **2.** tell the client that this is normal because intracranial pressure (ICP) fluctuates throughout the day.
- ☐ **3.** instruct the client to increase fluid intake prior to going to bed to prevent headache in the morning.
- ☐ **4.** advise the client to request pain medication from the HCP.

44. A primigravid client visits the clinic for a routine examination at 35 weeks' gestation. The client's blood pressure is near the baseline of 120/74 mm Hg with no proteinuria or evidence of facial edema. The client asks the nurse, "What should I take if I get an occasional headache after looking at my computer at work all day?" The nurse instructs the client that she can occasionally take which over-the-counter medication?
- ☐ **1.** acetaminophen
- ☐ **2.** aspirin
- ☐ **3.** ibuprofen
- ☐ **4.** naproxen

45. A client is experiencing a flashback from the use of lysergic acid diethylamide (LSD). What should the nurse do?
- ☐ **1.** Confront the client's misperceptions.
- ☐ **2.** Reassure the client while presenting reality.
- ☐ **3.** Seclude the client until the flashback ends.
- ☐ **4.** Challenge the client's unrealistic statements.

46. A 19-year-old client has undergone an examination and had evidence collected after being raped. Her father is overheard yelling at his daughter, "You are going to tell me who did this to you. What is his name?" Which is the nurse's **best** response?
- ☐ **1.** "Please come with me, sir. I need some important information."
- ☐ **2.** "Stop yelling. You are being inappropriate."
- ☐ **3.** "Please be quiet. You are not helping your daughter this way."
- ☐ **4.** "If you do not stop yelling, I will have to call Security."

47. Which ethnic group is more likely to develop severe hypertension?
- ☐ **1.** Asian
- ☐ **2.** African
- ☐ **3.** European
- ☐ **4.** Native American/First Nations

48. A nurse is establishing priorities for home visits to a group of clients. Which client can be seen later on in the week?
- ☐ **1.** a client recently diagnosed with terminal cancer with metastasis to the brain
- ☐ **2.** a female client recently diagnosed with human immunodeficiency virus (HIV)
- ☐ **3.** a client who is to demonstrate the ability to perform an insulin injection
- ☐ **4.** a client with acquired immune deficiency syndrome (AIDS) with CD4 <200 cells/mm^2

49. During a neonate's assessment shortly after birth, the nurse observes a large pad of fat at the back of the neck, widely set eyes, simian hand creases, and epicanthal folds. Which action is **most** appropriate?
- ☐ **1.** Notify the healthcare provider (HCP) immediately.
- ☐ **2.** Ask the mother to consent to genetic studies.
- ☐ **3.** Explain these deviations to the newborn's mother.
- ☐ **4.** Document these findings as minor deviations.

50. To help prevent hip flexion deformities associated with rheumatoid arthritis, the nurse should help the client assume which position in bed several times a day?
- ☐ **1.** prone
- ☐ **2.** very low Fowler's
- ☐ **3.** modified Trendelenburg
- ☐ **4.** side lying

51. A client with severe arthritis has been receiving maintenance therapy of prednisone 10 mg/day for the past 6 weeks. The nurse should instruct the client to immediately report symptoms of:
- ☐ **1.** respiratory infection.
- ☐ **2.** joint pain.
- ☐ **3.** constipation.
- ☐ **4.** joint swelling.

52. A nurse hears a client state, "I have had it with this marriage. It would be so much easier to just hire someone to kill my husband!" What action should the nurse take?
- ☐ **1.** Since the client is still admitted to the hospital, the nurse must hold the statement in confidence.
- ☐ **2.** The nurse must start the process to warn the client's husband.
- ☐ **3.** An assessment of the client's response to treatment must be performed.
- ☐ **4.** The comment must be held in confidence because the client did not report the statement directly to the nurse.

53. When teaching unlicensed assistive personnel (UAP) about the importance of handwashing in preventing disease, the nurse should instruct the UAP that:
- ☐ **1.** "It is not necessary to wash your hands as long as you use gloves."
- ☐ **2.** "Handwashing is the best method for preventing cross-contamination."
- ☐ **3.** "Waterless commercial products are not effective for killing organisms."
- ☐ **4.** "The hands do not serve as a source of infection."

54. A 7-year-old child is admitted to the hospital with acute rheumatic fever. During the acute phase of the illness, which diversional activity would the nurse **most** discourage?
- ☐ **1.** reading a book with the father
- ☐ **2.** playing with a doll with the nurse
- ☐ **3.** watching the television with a sibling
- ☐ **4.** playing checkers with a roommate

55. Before discharge from the hospital after a myocardial infarction, a client is taught to exercise by gradually increasing the distance walked. Which vital sign should the nurse teach the client to monitor to determine whether to increase or decrease the exercise level?
- ☐ **1.** pulse rate
- ☐ **2.** blood pressure
- ☐ **3.** body temperature
- ☐ **4.** respiratory rate

56. A woman is taking oral contraceptives. The nurse teaches the client to report which complication?
- ☐ **1.** breakthrough bleeding
- ☐ **2.** severe calf pain
- ☐ **3.** mild headache
- ☐ **4.** weight gain of 3 lb (1.4 kg)

57. Which nursing action is essential for the hospitalized client with a new tracheostomy?
- ☐ **1.** Decrease secretions.
- ☐ **2.** Provide client teaching regarding tracheostomy care.
- ☐ **3.** Relieve anxiety related to the tracheostomy.
- ☐ **4.** Maintain a patent airway.

58. The nurse walks into the room of a client who has a "do-not-resuscitate" prescription and finds the client without a pulse, respirations, or blood pressure. What should the nurse do **first**?
☐ 1. Stay in the room, and call the nursing team for assistance.
☐ 2. Push the emergency alarm to call a code.
☐ 3. Page the client's healthcare provider (HCP).
☐ 4. Pull the curtain and leave the room.

59. When developing a nutritional plan for a child who needs to increase protein intake, the nurse should suggest which foods? Select all that apply.
☐ 1. whole wheat bread
☐ 2. cooked dry beans
☐ 3. peanut butter
☐ 4. yogurt
☐ 5. apple

60. Immediately after receiving an injection of bupivacaine, the client becomes restless and nervous and reports a feeling of impending doom. The nurse should:
☐ 1. ask the client to explain these feelings.
☐ 2. reassure the client that it is normal to feel restless before a procedure.
☐ 3. assess the client's vital signs.
☐ 4. administer epinephrine.

61. The nurse is conducting walking rounds and observes the client (see figure). What should the nurse do?

☐ 1. Loosen the bed restraints so the client can sit up.
☐ 2. Raise the side rails to full upright position.
☐ 3. Assess the client to determine why she wants to sit up.
☐ 4. Elevate the head of the bed.

62. A menopausal woman is taking hormone replacement therapy. The nurse teaches the client that a warning sign for endometrial cancer that needs to be reported is:
☐ 1. hot flashes.
☐ 2. irregular vaginal bleeding.
☐ 3. urinary urgency.
☐ 4. dyspareunia.

63. A client tells the nurse that she has had sexual contact with someone whom she suspects has genital herpes. The nurse should instruct the client to:
☐ 1. anticipate lesions within 25 to 30 days.
☐ 2. continue sexual activity unless lesions are present.
☐ 3. report any difficulty urinating.
☐ 4. drink extra fluids to prevent lesions from forming.

64. When explaining the risk for having a child with cystic fibrosis to a husband and wife, the nurse should tell them:
☐ 1. the risk is greatest when both clients have the recessive gene.
☐ 2. the gene is carried on the X chromosome and there is little risk.
☐ 3. the disease will only occur if the child is a male.
☐ 4. the disease does not have a genetic basis.

65. The nurse is assessing a client with peripheral arterial disease who had a femoral-popliteal bypass. Which finding indicates improved arterial blood supply to the lower extremity?
☐ 1. decrease in muscle pain when walking
☐ 2. dependent rubor
☐ 3. absence of pulse using a Doppler ultrasound
☐ 4. reduction in pitting edema

66. The nurse is caring for a client who had an open cholecystectomy 24 hours ago. The client's vital signs have been stable for the last 24 hours, but the client now has a temperature of 38.4°C (101.1°F), a heart rate of 116 bpm, and a respiratory rate of 26 breaths/min. The client has an IV infusion running at a keep-open rate. The nurse contacts healthcare provider (HCP) and receives several prescriptions (see chart).

Which prescription should the nurse implement **first**?

Prescriptions
1. Continue to check vital signs every 2 hours.
2. Draw stat blood cultures × 2.
3. CT of abdomen.
4. Start broad-spectrum IV antibiotic 4 hours after blood cultures are drawn.
5. Draw CBC, CRP, ESR, and UA with culture and sensitivity if indicated.
6. Ensure patent IV access for fluid bolus

☐ 1. Obtain blood cultures.
☐ 2. Increase the rate of the intravenous infusion.
☐ 3. Obtain CT of the abdomen.
☐ 4. Chart vital signs.

67. A client was talking with her husband by telephone, and then she began swearing at him. The nurse interrupts the call and offers to talk with the client. She says, "I cannot talk about that bastard right now. I just need to destroy something." What should the nurse do **next**?
- ☐ **1.** Tell her to write her feelings in her journal.
- ☐ **2.** Urge her to talk with the nurse now.
- ☐ **3.** Ask her to calm down or she will be restrained.
- ☐ **4.** Offer her a phone book to "destroy" while staying with her.

68. A man of Chinese descent is admitted to the hospital with multiple injuries after a motor vehicle accident. His pain is not under control. The client states, "If I could be with my people, I could receive acupuncture for this pain." The nurse should understand that acupuncture in the Asian culture is based on the theory that it:
- ☐ **1.** purges evil spirits.
- ☐ **2.** promotes tranquility.
- ☐ **3.** restores the balance of energy.
- ☐ **4.** blocks nerve pathways to the brain.

69. The nurse is caring for a multigravid client in active labor when the nurse detects variable fetal heart rate decelerations on the electronic monitor. The nurse interprets this as the compression of which structure?
- ☐ **1.** head
- ☐ **2.** chest
- ☐ **3.** umbilical cord
- ☐ **4.** placenta

70. A neonate is experiencing respiratory distress and is using a neonatal oxygen mask. An unlicensed assistive personnel (UAP) has positioned the oxygen mask as shown. The nurse is assessing the neonate and determines that the mask:

- ☐ **1.** is appropriate for the neonate.
- ☐ **2.** is too large because it covers the neonate's eyes.
- ☐ **3.** is too small because it is obstructing the nose.
- ☐ **4.** should be covered with a soft cloth before being placed against the skin.

71. Which findings should lead the nurse to suspect that a client who had a cesarean birth 8 hours earlier is developing disseminated intravascular coagulation (DIC) and report to the healthcare provider (HCP)? Select all that apply.
- ☐ **1.** petechiae on the arm where the blood pressure was taken
- ☐ **2.** heart rate of 126 bpm
- ☐ **3.** abdominal incision dressing with bright red drainage
- ☐ **4.** platelet count of 80,000/mm³ (80 × 10⁹/L)
- ☐ **5.** urine output of 350 mL in the past 8 hours
- ☐ **6.** temperature of 98.4°F (36.9°C)

72. Two days after placement of a pleural chest tube, the tube is accidentally pulled out of the chest wall. The nurse should **first**:
- ☐ **1.** immerse the tube in sterile water.
- ☐ **2.** apply an occlusive dressing such as petroleum jelly gauze.
- ☐ **3.** instruct the client to cough to expand the lung.
- ☐ **4.** auscultate the lung to determine whether it collapsed.

73. Three victims with gunshot wounds are brought to the emergency department. The nurse should take which action to preserve forensic evidence?
- ☐ **1.** Cut around blood stains to remove clothing.
- ☐ **2.** Place each item of clothing in a separate paper bag.
- ☐ **3.** Place all wet clothing in a plastic bag.
- ☐ **4.** Refrain from documenting client statements.

74. An 18-year-old female client who is sexually active with her boyfriend has a purulent vaginal discharge that is sometimes frothy. The nurse interprets this as suggesting a:
- ☐ **1.** sexually transmitted infection.
- ☐ **2.** normal variation in vaginal discharge.
- ☐ **3.** need for vaginal douching.
- ☐ **4.** side effect of a birth control method.

75. A client is admitted to the hospital with a diagnosis of a pulmonary embolism. Which problem should the nurse address **first**?
- ☐ **1.** productive cough
- ☐ **2.** activity intolerance
- ☐ **3.** difficulty breathing
- ☐ **4.** impaired gas exchange

76. A client is receiving morphine sulfate by a patient-controlled analgesia (PCA) system after a left lower lobectomy 4 hours ago. The client reports moderately severe pain in the left thorax that worsens when coughing. The nurse's **first** course of action is to:
- [ ] 1. reassure the client that the PCA system is working and will relieve pain.
- [ ] 2. encourage the client to rest; no further assessment is needed.
- [ ] 3. assess the pain systematically with the hospital-approved pain scale.
- [ ] 4. encourage the client to take deep breathes and expectorate the mucous that is stimulating the cough.

77. Which is characteristic of cardiogenic shock?
- [ ] 1. hypovolemia
- [ ] 2. increased cardiac output
- [ ] 3. decreased myocardial contractility
- [ ] 4. infarction

78. A loading dose of digoxin is given to a client newly diagnosed with atrial fibrillation. The nurse instructs the client about the medication and the importance of monitoring his heart rate. An expected outcome of this instruction is:
- [ ] 1. a return demonstration of palpating the radial pulse.
- [ ] 2. a return demonstration of how to take the medication.
- [ ] 3. verbalization of why the client has atrial fibrillation.
- [ ] 4. verbalization of the need for the medication.

79. The nurse is reviewing the laboratory results of a client with hypothyroidism. An expected finding is:
- [ ] 1. decreased thyroxine (T_4) and increased thyroid-stimulating hormone (TSH) levels.
- [ ] 2. decreased TSH and increased T_4 levels.
- [ ] 3. decreased creatine phosphokinase levels.
- [ ] 4. absence of antithyroid antibodies.

80. The nurse administers a tap water enema to a client. While the solution is being infused, the client has abdominal cramping. What should the nurse do **first**?
- [ ] 1. Clamp the tubing, and carefully withdraw the tube.
- [ ] 2. Temporarily stop the infusion, and have the client take deep breaths.
- [ ] 3. Raise the height of the enema container.
- [ ] 4. Rub the client's abdomen gently until the cramps subside.

81. The mother of a 7-month-old child born 6 weeks early asks the nurse what play activities and toys is appropriate for her child. What should the nurse suggest?
- [ ] 1. picture books
- [ ] 2. peekaboo
- [ ] 3. rattle
- [ ] 4. colored blocks

82. Which is the **most** accurate method of determining the extent of a client's fluid loss?
- [ ] 1. measuring intake and output
- [ ] 2. assessing vital signs
- [ ] 3. weighing the client
- [ ] 4. assessing skin turgor

83. The nurse uses Montgomery straps **primarily** so the client is free from:
- [ ] 1. falls.
- [ ] 2. bruises.
- [ ] 3. skin breakdown.
- [ ] 4. wandering.

84. The nurse is counseling a client regarding treatment of the client's newly diagnosed depression. The nurse emphasizes that full benefit from antidepressant therapy usually takes how long?
- [ ] 1. 1 week
- [ ] 2. 2 to 4 weeks
- [ ] 3. 5 to 7 weeks
- [ ] 4. 8 weeks

85. A multigravid client is scheduled for a percutaneous umbilical blood sampling procedure. The nurse instructs the client that this procedure is useful for diagnosing which condition?
- [ ] 1. twin pregnancies
- [ ] 2. fetal lung maturation
- [ ] 3. Rh disease
- [ ] 4. alpha fetoprotein level

86. A 70-year-old, previously well client asks the nurse, "I notice I have tremors. Is this just normal for my age?" What should the nurse tell the client?
- [ ] 1. "I would not be worried because this is common with aging."
- [ ] 2. "You should report this to the healthcare provider (HCP) because it may indicate a problem."
- [ ] 3. "You should drink orange juice when this occurs."
- [ ] 4. "You should have your blood pressure checked when this occurs."

87. A client is prescribed atropine 0.4 mg intramuscularly. The atropine vial is labeled 0.5 mg/mL. How many milliliters should the nurse plan to administer? Record your answer using one decimal place.

_____ mL.

88. A school-age child diagnosed with attention deficit hyperactivity disorder is prescribed methylphenidate. What finding should alert the school nurse to the possibility that the child is experiencing a common side effect of the drug?
- [ ] 1. loss of appetite
- [ ] 2. vomiting
- [ ] 3. photosensitivity
- [ ] 4. weight gain

89. A client has a dull headache, is dizzy, and has an increased pulse rate. The results of arterial blood gas analysis are as follows: pH, 7.26; partial pressure of carbon dioxide, 50 mm Hg (6.7 kPa); and bicarbonate, 24 mEq/L (24 mmol/L). These findings indicate which acid-base imbalance?
☐ **1.** respiratory alkalosis
☐ **2.** respiratory acidosis
☐ **3.** metabolic acidosis
☐ **4.** metabolic alkalosis

90. Which meal would be appropriate for the child with osteomyelitis to choose?
☐ **1.** beef and bean burrito with cheese, carrot and celery sticks, and a glass of milk
☐ **2.** fries, beef hot dog, and an apple
☐ **3.** potato soup, jelly sandwich, and a peach
☐ **4.** tomato soup made with water, grilled cheese sandwich, and a banana

91. The nurse is planning a continuous quality improvement (CQI) process to decrease the infection rate on the nursing unit. The nurse should consider which factors when planning the process? Select all that apply.
☐ **1.** CQI processes are required by accrediting agencies.
☐ **2.** The approach to CQI can be retrospective or concurrent.
☐ **3.** Institutional review board (IRB) approval is required.
☐ **4.** CQI is conducted by people who are not part of the process.
☐ **5.** The CQI process has a fixed end point.

92. The nurse is conducting a health assessment of an older adult. The client tells the nurse about cramping leg pain that occurs when walking for 15 minutes; the pain is relieved with rest. The lower extremities are slightly cool to touch, and pedal pulses are palpable +1. The nurse should instruct the client to:
☐ **1.** increase the length of time for walking.
☐ **2.** include more potassium in the diet.
☐ **3.** perform leg circles and ankle pumps.
☐ **4.** seek consultation from the healthcare provider (HCP).

93. A client has a newly placed tracheostomy tube. The nurse should assess the client for which possible complication?
☐ **1.** decreased cardiac output
☐ **2.** damage to the laryngeal nerve
☐ **3.** pneumothorax
☐ **4.** acute respiratory distress syndrome

94. Which comment from a client indicates a need for further instruction after being taught about taking ciprofloxacin?
☐ **1.** "I must drink 500 to 1,500 mL of water a day."
☐ **2.** "I should not take an antacid before taking the ciprofloxacin."
☐ **3.** "I should let the healthcare provider (HCP) know if I start vomiting from the ciprofloxacin."
☐ **4.** "I may get light-headed from the ciprofloxacin."

95. A multiparous client tells the nurse that she is using medroxyprogesterone for contraception. The nurse should instruct the client to increase her intake of which nutrient?
☐ **1.** folic acid
☐ **2.** vitamin C
☐ **3.** magnesium
☐ **4.** calcium

96. When reviewing the plan of care for a client with Alzheimer's disease, which intervention would the nurse question?
☐ **1.** reminiscence group
☐ **2.** walking
☐ **3.** pet therapy
☐ **4.** stress management

97. Before an incisional cholecystectomy is performed, the nurse instructs the client in the correct use of an incentive spirometer. Why is incentive spirometry essential after surgery in the upper abdominal area?
☐ **1.** The client will be maintained on bed rest for several days.
☐ **2.** Ambulation is restricted by the presence of drainage tubes.
☐ **3.** The operative incision is near the diaphragm.
☐ **4.** The presence of a nasogastric tube inhibits deep breathing.

98. The nurse should instruct the parents of a school-age child with hemophilia to implement which interventions when the child develops bleeding into a joint? Select all that apply.
☐ **1.** Have the child rest.
☐ **2.** Apply heat to the joint area.
☐ **3.** Begin factor VIII therapy.
☐ **4.** Start physical therapy.
☐ **5.** Apply a topical antifibrinolytic.

99. When cleaning the skin around an incision and drain site, what should the nurse do?
☐ **1.** Clean the incision and drain site separately.
☐ **2.** Clean from the incision to the drain site.
☐ **3.** Clean from the drain site to the incision.
☐ **4.** Clean the incision and drain site simultaneously.

100. The nurse is teaching a client about using topical gentamicin sulfate. Which comment by the client indicates the need for additional teaching?
- ☐ 1. "I will avoid being out in the sun for long periods."
- ☐ 2. "I should stop applying when the redness is gone."
- ☐ 3. "I will call the healthcare provider (HCP) if the condition worsens."
- ☐ 4. "I should apply it to large open areas."

101. Which goal is **most** important when developing a long-term care plan for a child with hemophilia?
- ☐ 1. Increase the parent's and child's knowledge about hemophilia.
- ☐ 2. Prevent injury during each stage of development.
- ☐ 3. Improve the child's self-esteem during bleeding episodes.
- ☐ 4. Manage acute pain when there is bleeding into joints.

102. When preparing a 3-year-old child to have blood specimens drawn for laboratory testing, the nurse should:
- ☐ 1. explain the procedure in advance.
- ☐ 2. explain why the blood needs to be drawn.
- ☐ 3. use distraction techniques during the procedure.
- ☐ 4. provide verbal explanations about what will occur.

103. The client has been prescribed lisinopril to treat hypertension. The nurse should assess the client for which electrolyte imbalance?
- ☐ 1. hyponatremia
- ☐ 2. hypocalcemia
- ☐ 3. hyperkalemia
- ☐ 4. hypermagnesemia

104. A usually reliable interpreter called by the nurse to help communicate with a mother of a child who does not speak English and has brought her child in for a routine visit has yet to arrive in the clinic. The nurse has paged the interpreter several times. What should the nurse do **next**?
- ☐ 1. Continue with the examination.
- ☐ 2. Reschedule the infant's appointment for later in the week.
- ☐ 3. Ask the mother to stay longer in the hope that the interpreter arrives.
- ☐ 4. Page the interpreter one more time.

105. A client with angina shows the nurse the nitroglycerin that the client carries in a plastic bag in a pocket. The nurse instructs the client that nitroglycerin should be kept in:
- ☐ 1. the refrigerator.
- ☐ 2. a cool, moist place.
- ☐ 3. a dark container to shield from light.
- ☐ 4. a plastic pill container where it is readily available.

106. A client with a chronic mental illness who does not always take her medications is separated from her husband and receives public assistance funds. She lives with her mother and older sister and manages her own medication. The client's mother is in poor health and also receives public assistance benefits. The client's sister works outside the home, and the client's father is dead. Which issue should the nurse address **first**?
- ☐ 1. family support
- ☐ 2. marital communication
- ☐ 3. financial concerns
- ☐ 4. medication compliance

107. A client is receiving total parenteral nutrition (TPN). The nurse notices that the bag of TPN solution has been infusing for 24 hours but has 300 mL of solution left. The nurse should:
- ☐ 1. continue the infusion until the remaining 300 mL is infused.
- ☐ 2. change the filter on the tubing and continue with the infusion.
- ☐ 3. notify the healthcare provider (HCP) and obtain prescriptions to alter the flow rate of the solution.
- ☐ 4. discontinue the current solution, change the tubing, and hang a new bag of TPN solution.

108. The nurse should suspect that the client taking disulfiram has ingested alcohol when the client exhibits which symptom?
- ☐ 1. sore throat and muscle aches
- ☐ 2. nausea and flushing of the face and neck
- ☐ 3. fever and muscle soreness
- ☐ 4. bradycardia and vertigo

109. A client with a history of cardiac problems is having severe chest pain. What should be the nurse's **first** response?
- ☐ 1. Notify the healthcare provider (HCP).
- ☐ 2. Administer an analgesic to control the pain.
- ☐ 3. Assess the client's pain.
- ☐ 4. Start oxygen at 2 L/min via nasal cannula.

110. Which characteristic should the nurse include in the teaching plan for a multiparous client after giving birth to a neonate diagnosed with trisomy 13?
- ☐ 1. webbed neck
- ☐ 2. small testes
- ☐ 3. congenital heart defects
- ☐ 4. polydactyly

111. A nulligravid client calls the clinic and tells the nurse that she forgot to take her oral contraceptive this morning. The nurse should tell the client to:
- ☐ 1. take the medication immediately.
- ☐ 2. restart the medication in the morning.
- ☐ 3. use another form of contraception for 2 weeks.
- ☐ 4. take two pills tonight before bedtime.

112. A client is being treated for acute low back pain. The nurse should report which of these clinical manifestations to the healthcare provider (HCP) **immediately**?
- ☐ 1. diffuse, aching sensation in the L4 to L5 area
- ☐ 2. new onset of footdrop
- ☐ 3. pain in the lower back when the leg is lifted
- ☐ 4. pain in the lower back that radiates to the hip

113. A client with type 1 diabetes mellitus asks the nurse about taking ginseng at home. The nurse should tell the client:
- ☐ 1. "No, there are no therapeutic benefits of ginseng."
- ☐ 2. "Taking ginseng will increase the risk of hypoglycemia."
- ☐ 3. "You can take the ginseng to help improve your memory."
- ☐ 4. "You can take ginseng if you take it with a carbohydrate."

114. A client has had a central venous pressure line inserted. The nurse should **immediately** report which sign to the healthcare provider (HCP)?
- ☐ 1. sharp pain on the affected side
- ☐ 2. urinary output of 50 mL/h
- ☐ 3. heart rate of 88 bpm
- ☐ 4. discomfort at the insertion site

115. The nurse teaches the client with cirrhosis that the expected outcome of taking lactulose is:
- ☐ 1. one regular bowel movement a day.
- ☐ 2. two to three soft stools per day.
- ☐ 3. four to five loose stools per day.
- ☐ 4. five to six loose stools per day.

116. The nurse is evaluating the laboratory results of a client who was recently admitted to the hospital. Which result indicates the presence of inflammation?
- ☐ 1. decreased sedimentation rate
- ☐ 2. thrombocytopenia
- ☐ 3. leukocytosis
- ☐ 4. erythrocytosis

117. The client sustained an open fracture of the femur from an automobile accident. The nurse should assess the client for which type of shock?
- ☐ 1. cardiogenic
- ☐ 2. hypovolemic
- ☐ 3. neurogenic
- ☐ 4. anaphylactic

118. The nurse is assessing a teenage girl (see figure). The nurse should describe the girl shown in the figure as having:

- ☐ 1. normal posture.
- ☐ 2. kyphosis.
- ☐ 3. scoliosis.
- ☐ 4. lordosis.

119. A client reports having pain in the casted left arm that is unrelieved by pain medication. The nurse assesses the arm and notes that the fingers are swollen and difficult to separate. What should the nurse do **first**?
- ☐ 1. Administer morphine 2 mg intravenously.
- ☐ 2. Apply an ice bag to the fingers to relieve pain.
- ☐ 3. Elevate the arm on two pillows and reassess in 30 minutes.
- ☐ 4. Call the healthcare provider (HCP) to report swelling and pain.

120. A primiparous client develops uterine atony and postpartum hemorrhage 1 hour after a vaginal birth. The healthcare provider (HCP) has prescribed IM prostaglandin F_{2a}. After administration of the medication, the nurse should observe the client for which complication?
- ☐ 1. tachycardia
- ☐ 2. hypotension
- ☐ 3. constipation
- ☐ 4. abdominal distention

121. A client receives morphine for postoperative pain. The nurse should:
- ☐ 1. take apical heart rate after each dose of morphine.
- ☐ 2. assess urinary output every 8 hours.
- ☐ 3. assess mental status every shift.
- ☐ 4. check for pedal edema every 4 hours.

122. While caring for a mother and her 1-day-old neonate born vaginally at 30 weeks' gestation, the nurse explains about the neonate's need for gavage feeding at this time instead of the mother's plan for bottle-feeding. What should the nurse include as the rationale for this feeding plan?
- ☐ **1.** The neonate has difficulty coordinating sucking, swallowing, and breathing.
- ☐ **2.** A high-calorie formula, presently needed at this time, is more easily delivered via gavage.
- ☐ **3.** Gavage feedings can minimize the neonate's increased risk of developing hypoglycemia.
- ☐ **4.** This type of feeding, easily given in the isolette, decreases the neonate's risk of cold stress.

123. The nurse is giving preoperative instructions to a client who will have a reversal of a colostomy. The nurse should prepare the client to expect which nursing actions during the immediate postoperative period? Select all that apply.
- ☐ **1.** nasogastric (NG) tube attached to low intermittent suction
- ☐ **2.** administration of IV fluids
- ☐ **3.** daily measurement of abdominal girth
- ☐ **4.** calculation of intake and output every 8 hours
- ☐ **5.** assessment of vital signs every 6 hours

124. The nurse is teaching a client with rheumatoid arthritis about how to manage the fatigue associated with this disease. Which statement indicates the client understands how to manage the fatigue?
- ☐ **1.** "I sleep for 8 to 10 hours every night so that I will have the energy to care for my children during the day."
- ☐ **2.** "I schedule afternoon rest periods for myself in addition to sleeping 10 hours every night."
- ☐ **3.** "I spend one weekend day a week resting in bed while my husband cares for the children."
- ☐ **4.** "I get up early in the morning and get all my household chores completed before my children wake up."

125. The nurse is caring for a child with hemophilia who is actively bleeding from the leg. The nurse should apply:
- ☐ **1.** direct pressure, checking every few minutes to see if the bleeding has stopped.
- ☐ **2.** ice to the injured leg area several times a day.
- ☐ **3.** direct pressure to the injured area continuously for 10 minutes.
- ☐ **4.** ice bag with elevation of the leg twice a day.

126. When assessing for signs of a blood transfusion reaction in a client with dark skin, the nurse should assess the client for:
- ☐ **1.** hypertension.
- ☐ **2.** diaphoresis.
- ☐ **3.** polyuria.
- ☐ **4.** warm skin.

127. Which is **least** likely a danger associated with pancytopenia?
- ☐ **1.** anemia
- ☐ **2.** bleeding
- ☐ **3.** infection
- ☐ **4.** hypothyroidism

128. A client suspected of being a victim of abuse returns to the emergency department and, sobbing, tells the nurse, "I guess you really know that my husband beats me and that is why I have bruises all over my body. I do not know what to do. I am afraid he will kill me one of these times." Which response **best** demonstrates that the nurse recognizes the client's needs at this time?
- ☐ **1.** "The fear that your husband will kill you is unfounded."
- ☐ **2.** "We can begin by discussing various options open to you."
- ☐ **3.** "You can legally leave your husband because he has no right to hurt you."
- ☐ **4.** "We can begin by listing ways to avoid making your husband angry with you."

129. The infusion rate of total parenteral nutrition (TPN) is tapered before being discontinued. This is done to prevent which complication?
- ☐ **1.** essential fatty acid deficiency
- ☐ **2.** dehydration
- ☐ **3.** rebound hypoglycemia
- ☐ **4.** malnutrition

130. A client has just returned from surgery for a gastrectomy. The nurse should position the client in which position?
- ☐ **1.** prone
- ☐ **2.** supine
- ☐ **3.** low Fowler's
- ☐ **4.** right or left Sims'

131. A child with heart disease starts on oral digoxin. When preparing to administer the medication, what should the nurse do **first**?
- ☐ **1.** Check the last serum electrolyte results for the child.
- ☐ **2.** Verify the dosage with a licensed practical/vocational nurse (LPN/VN) who is working that day.
- ☐ **3.** Ask the mother if she is willing to administer the medication.
- ☐ **4.** Teach the mother how to measure the child's heart rate.

132. A client with diabetes has been diagnosed with hypertension, and the healthcare provider (HCP) has prescribed atenolol, a beta-blocker. When performing discharge teaching, it is important for the nurse to emphasize that the addition of atenolol can cause:
- ☐ 1. a decrease in the hypoglycemic effects of insulin.
- ☐ 2. an increase in the hypoglycemic effects of insulin.
- ☐ 3. an increase in the incidence of ketoacidosis.
- ☐ 4. a decrease in the incidence of ketoacidosis.

133. The nurse is caring for a client who has deep partial-thickness and full-thickness burns. During the emergent (resuscitative) phase of burn management, the nurse should assess the client for a fluid shift from the:
- ☐ 1. intracellular to extracellular compartment.
- ☐ 2. extracellular to intravascular compartment.
- ☐ 3. interstitial to the intracellular compartment.
- ☐ 4. intravascular to the interstitial compartment.

134. The nurse is caring for an elderly client who has experienced a sensorineural hearing loss. The nurse anticipates that the client will exhibit which symptom?
- ☐ 1. difficulty hearing high-pitched sounds
- ☐ 2. problems with speaking clearly
- ☐ 3. inability to assign meaning to sound
- ☐ 4. vertigo when changing positions

135. The nurse is evaluating the effectiveness of fluid resuscitation during the emergency period of burn management. Which finding indicates that adequate fluid replacement has been achieved in the client?
- ☐ 1. an increase in body weight
- ☐ 2. fluid intake less than urinary output
- ☐ 3. urine output greater than 35 mL/h
- ☐ 4. blood pressure of 90/60 mm Hg

136. The parent of a child who is taking an antibiotic for bilateral otitis media tells the nurse that they have stopped the medicine since the child is better and are saving the rest of the medication to use the next time the child gets sick. What should the nurse tell the parent?
- ☐ 1. "It is important to give the medicine as prescribed."
- ☐ 2. "How do you know your child's ears are cured?"
- ☐ 3. "Your child needs all of the medicine so that the infection clears."
- ☐ 4. "Stopping the medicine is not what is best for your child!"

137. A client who comes to the emergency department with multiple bruises on her face and arms, a black eye, and a broken nose says that these injuries occurred when she fell down the stairs. The nurse suspects that the client may have been physically assaulted. What should the nurse do next?
- ☐ 1. Ask the client directly about the possibility of physical abuse.
- ☐ 2. Tell the client that it is difficult to believe that such injuries resulted from a fall.
- ☐ 3. Ask the client what she did to make someone beat her so badly.
- ☐ 4. Discuss with the client what she can do to de-escalate the situation next time.

138. What is the primary goal for the care of a client who is in shock?
- ☐ 1. Achieve adequate tissue perfusion.
- ☐ 2. Preserve renal function.
- ☐ 3. Prevent hypostatic pneumonia.
- ☐ 4. Maintain adequate vascular tone.

139. A client with emphysema has been admitted to the hospital. The nurse should assess the client further for:
- ☐ 1. frequent coughing.
- ☐ 2. bronchospasms.
- ☐ 3. underweight appearance.
- ☐ 4. copious sputum.

140. The parent of a young child diagnosed with low-dose lead exposure asks about long-term effects. Which conditions should the nurse mention as possible long-term effects to this parent? Select all that apply.
- ☐ 1. seizures
- ☐ 2. depression
- ☐ 3. hyperactivity
- ☐ 4. aggression
- ☐ 5. impulsiveness

141. Which information is appropriate to include in an incident report?
- ☐ 1. an interpretation of the likely cause of the incident
- ☐ 2. what the nurse saw and did
- ☐ 3. the client's statement about the incident that occurred
- ☐ 4. the extenuating circumstances involved in the situation

142. The nurse is preparing a teaching plan for a client who is being discharged after being admitted for chest pain. The client has had one previous myocardial infarction 2 years ago and has been taking simvastatin 40 mg for the last 2 years. After reviewing the lab results for the client's cholesterol levels (see chart), the nurse should:

Lab Report

Test	Result	Units	Reference Range
Cholesterol total	195 (5.05)	mg/dL (mmol/L)	<200 (<5.18)
Triglycerides	106 (1.20)	mg/dL (mmol/L)	<150 (<1.69)
HDL-cholesterol	69 (1.79)	mg/dL (mmol/L)	>39 (<1.03)

☐ 1. ask if the client is taking the simvastatin regularly.
☐ 2. tell the client that the cholesterol levels are within normal limits.
☐ 3. instruct the client to lower the saturated fat in the diet.
☐ 4. review the chart for lab reports of hemoglobin and hematocrit.

143. The client is to have a gastrectomy. The surgeon will use a transverse incision. Prior to surgery, the nurse is checking to be sure the correct site has been marked. Identify the site the client should have marked.

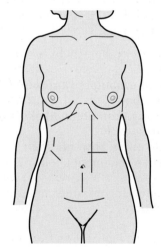

144. A 58-year-old homeless person is brought to the emergency department by the police after being found unconscious on the street. Following examination and evaluation of laboratory test results, a diagnosis of diabetic ketoacidosis is confirmed. Which information is **most** crucial to document on the client's medical record? Select all that apply.
☐ 1. size of pupils and reaction of pupils to light
☐ 2. response to verbal and painful stimuli
☐ 3. skin condition and presence of any rashes, lesions, or ulcers
☐ 4. blood pressure
☐ 5. length of time the client has had diabetes
☐ 6. hourly urine output

145. The nurse is reconciling the medications with a client who is being discharged. Which information indicates there is a "discrepancy"?
☐ 1. There is agreement between the client's home medication list and current medication prescriptions.
☐ 2. There is justification for a difference in the medication prescriptions.
☐ 3. There is lack of congruence between a client's home medication list and current medication prescriptions.
☐ 4. Sample medications have been included in the medication list.

146. The healthcare provider (HCP) has determined that a primigravid client in active labor requires a cesarean birth because of cephalopelvic disproportion. After the birth of a healthy neonate, which assessment should the nurse make **first**?
☐ 1. nasopharyngeal secretions
☐ 2. high-pitched cry
☐ 3. skull fracture
☐ 4. decreased muscle tone

147. An older adult's daughter is asking about the follow-up evaluation for her father after his pneumonectomy for primary lung cancer. The nurse should tell the daughter:
☐ 1. "The usual follow-up is chest x-ray and liver function tests every 3 months."
☐ 2. "The follow-up for your father will be a chest x-ray and a computed tomography scan of the abdomen every year."
☐ 3. "No follow-up is needed at this time."
☐ 4. "The follow-up for your father will be a chest x-ray every 6 months."

148. A parent of a toddler brings the child to the emergency department because the child has accidentally been scalded by hot water spilling from the stove. In order to differentiate the burn from potential abuse, the nurse should **first** assess the child:
☐ 1. on the back of the body.
☐ 2. on the front of the body.
☐ 3. for circular patterns.
☐ 4. on the buttocks.

149. A 17-year-old client visits the clinic at 36 weeks' gestation. The client's blood pressure is 130/90 mm Hg. On previous visits, her blood pressure ranged from 100 to 110 mm Hg systolic and 70 to 80 mm Hg diastolic. Further assessment reveals slight edema of her hands and 1+ proteinuria. The nurse anticipates that the healthcare provider (HCP) will **most** likely prescribe which treatment?
☐ **1.** IV magnesium sulfate
☐ **2.** labetalol
☐ **3.** bed rest with bathroom privileges
☐ **4.** hourly blood pressure checks

150. A female client who is 32 years of age has been diagnosed with stage 1 hypertension. The client's height is 5 feet 5 inches (165 cm), and her weight is recorded as 125 pounds (56.6 kg); she reports that she frequently eats at "fast-food" restaurants and enjoys a glass of wine to relax on weekends. In developing a teaching plan for this client, the nurse should address which topic?
☐ **1.** potential use of nitroprusside
☐ **2.** adverse effects of alcohol
☐ **3.** decreasing dietary caloric intake
☐ **4.** low-sodium food choices

151. The nurse observes that an area in the mouth of a child with leukemia is bleeding. Which item should the nurse use to promote homeostasis over the lesion?
☐ **1.** karaya gum
☐ **2.** a cotton ball imbedded with petroleum jelly
☐ **3.** a nonsticking gauze sponge
☐ **4.** a dry tea bag

152. A client with a fractured leg has been instructed to ambulate without weight bearing on the affected leg. The nurse evaluates that the client is ambulating correctly if the client uses which crutch-walking gait?
☐ **1.** two-point gait
☐ **2.** four-point gait
☐ **3.** three-point gait
☐ **4.** swing-to gait

153. Which is appropriate for the nurse to include in a plan for the prevention of pressure ulcers?
☐ **1.** daily skin cleaning with soap and hot water
☐ **2.** gentle massage of bony prominences every shift
☐ **3.** encouraging the client to sit up as much as possible
☐ **4.** systematic skin assessment at least once per shift

154. A client at 36 weeks' gestation tells the nurse, "I have been having a lot of backaches lately." After giving instructions about how to decrease the backaches, the nurse determines that the client needs further instruction when she makes which statement?
☐ **1.** "I should walk with my pelvis tilted backward."
☐ **2.** "I may need to put a board under my mattress."
☐ **3.** "I should squat and not bend to pick up objects."
☐ **4.** "I should wear flat or low-heeled shoes."

155. Which is an initial clinical manifestation of gonorrhea in men?
☐ **1.** impotence
☐ **2.** scrotal pain
☐ **3.** penile lesion
☐ **4.** urethral discharge

156. A client's blood pressure is elevated at 160/90 mm Hg. The healthcare provider (HCP) prescribed "clonidine 1 mg by mouth now." The nurse sent the prescription to pharmacy at 0710, but the medication still has not arrived at 0800. The nurse should do all **except**:
☐ **1.** check all appropriate places on the unit to which the drug could have been delivered.
☐ **2.** check the client's blood pressure.
☐ **3.** call the pharmacy.
☐ **4.** go to the pharmacy to obtain the drug.

157. The client with major depression states, "I am too tired to get out of bed to go to group therapy. I just want to rest." The nurse should tell the client:
☐ **1.** "Perhaps you will feel better later on."
☐ **2.** "I will let you rest for as long as you need."
☐ **3.** "Attending group therapy is an important part of your treatment plan."
☐ **4.** "You have been in bed long enough and need to get up."

158. After teaching the mother of a 7 month-old diagnosed with bronchiolitis, the nurse determines that the teaching has been effective when the mother states she will immediately report which sign or symptom?
☐ **1.** seven wet diapers a day
☐ **2.** temperature of 100°F (37.8°C) for 2 days
☐ **3.** clear nasal discharge for longer than 2 days
☐ **4.** longer periods of sleep than usual

159. A 4-year-old who weighs 40 lbs (18 kg) is brought to the emergency department with sudden onset of a temperature of 103°F (39.4°C), sore throat, and refusal to drink. The child will not lie down and prefers to lean forward while sitting up. What should the nurse do **next**?
☐ **1.** Give 600 mg of acetaminophen rectally, as prescribed.
☐ **2.** Inspect the child's throat for redness and swelling.
☐ **3.** Have an appropriate-sized tracheostomy tube readily available.
☐ **4.** Obtain a specimen for a throat culture.

160. Which client would benefit from the application of warm moist heat?
☐ **1.** a client with appendicitis
☐ **2.** a client with a recently sprained joint
☐ **3.** a client with a suspected malignancy
☐ **4.** a client with low back pain

161. A client is newly diagnosed with pernicious anemia. The nurse emphasizes to the client the need to increase vitamin B$_{12}$ intake by:
- ☐ 1. increasing dietary intake of vitamin B$_{12}$.
- ☐ 2. taking an oral vitamin B$_{12}$ replacement.
- ☐ 3. taking vitamin B$_{12}$ injections or nasal spray replacement.
- ☐ 4. chelation therapy.

162. The nurse has received a prescription to add 20 mEq of potassium chloride to a 1,000-mL bottle of IV fluid. The nurse has a 30-mL, multiple-dose vial of potassium chloride. The label reads 2 mEq/mL. How many milliliters should the nurse add to the IV fluid? Record your answer using a whole number.

_____ mL.

163. A client with major depression and suicidal ideation is suddenly calmer and more energetic. Which conclusion should the nurse reach?
- ☐ 1. The client is improving.
- ☐ 2. The client's medication dosage is too high.
- ☐ 3. The client is overstimulated.
- ☐ 4. The client is suicidal.

164. A multigravid client at 38 weeks' gestation is scheduled to undergo a contraction stress test. What should the nurse include in the explanation as the purpose of this test?
- ☐ 1. evaluation of fetal lung maturity
- ☐ 2. determination of the fetal biophysical profile
- ☐ 3. assessment of fetal ability to tolerate labor
- ☐ 4. determination of fetal response during movements

165. The nurse is caring for a client who has been diagnosed with atypical pneumonia. The nurse should assess this client carefully for:
- ☐ 1. high fever.
- ☐ 2. tachypnea.
- ☐ 3. dry cough.
- ☐ 4. severe chills.

166. The nurse is teaching a client with emphysema how to do pursed-lip breathing. What is the expected outcome of using pursed-lip breathing?
- ☐ 1. increased oxygenation
- ☐ 2. prolonged exhalation
- ☐ 3. increase exercise tolerance
- ☐ 4. relief from shortness of breath

167. What is the advantage of using automated medication dispensing equipment?
- ☐ 1. It facilitates the change-of-shift count of narcotics.
- ☐ 2. It keeps a record of narcotic usage.
- ☐ 3. It allows nurses unmonitored access to narcotics.
- ☐ 4. It cancels the charges for narcotics.

168. Immediately following an automobile accident, a 21-year-old client has severe pain in the right chest from hitting the steering wheel and a compound fracture of the right tibia and fibula and multiple lacerations and contusions. The priority for care is **first** to:
- ☐ 1. reduce the client's anxiety.
- ☐ 2. maintain adequate oxygenation.
- ☐ 3. decrease chest pain.
- ☐ 4. maintain adequate circulating volume.

169. While assessing a primiparous client 8 hours after childbirth, the nurse inspects the episiotomy site, finding it edematous and slightly reddened. Which interpretation by the nurse is **most** appropriate?
- ☐ 1. The client needs application of an ice pack.
- ☐ 2. The episiotomy site is infected.
- ☐ 3. A hematoma will likely develop.
- ☐ 4. The client has had a repair of a vaginal laceration.

170. When administering an IM injection, the nurse should use the Z-track technique when the medication:
- ☐ 1. takes a long time to absorb.
- ☐ 2. takes effect very quickly.
- ☐ 3. is irritating to tissues.
- ☐ 4. is viscous in consistency.

171. A client with bipolar disorder is monopolizing the use of the telephone by making several calls each day, interfering with the ability of other clients to use the telephone. The nurse should:
- ☐ 1. provide a separate phone for the client.
- ☐ 2. limit the amount of calls the client can make each day.
- ☐ 3. remind the client that others need to use the telephone.
- ☐ 4. take away the client's telephone privileges.

172. When preparing a 20-month-old for removal of a foreign body in the nasal passage by the healthcare provider (HCP), the nurse should use which method of restraint?
- ☐ 1. jacket restraint
- ☐ 2. elbow restraint
- ☐ 3. use of father to hold
- ☐ 4. papoose board

173. The nurse auscultates the lungs of a client who has been diagnosed with a tumor in the lung and notes wheezing over one lung. The nurse should assess the client further for:
- ☐ 1. the presence of exudate in the airways.
- ☐ 2. the client's history of smoking.
- ☐ 3. an indication of pleural effusion.
- ☐ 4. obstruction of the airway.

174. The nurse is teaching a client who is taking insulin about the signs of diabetic ketoacidosis, which include:
☐ **1.** Kussmaul's respirations.
☐ **2.** excessive hunger.
☐ **3.** dry, flaky skin.
☐ **4.** high blood pressure.

175. A nurse receives a lithium level report of 1.0 mEq/L (1.0 mmol/L) for a client who has been taking lithium for 2 months. How does the nurse interpret this information?
☐ **1.** an error in reporting
☐ **2.** too low to be therapeutic
☐ **3.** too high, indicating toxicity
☐ **4.** within the therapeutic range

176. A child with 20% second- and third-degree burns is admitted to the burn center. The child weighs 44 lbs (20 kg). The nurse has started an IV infusion of lactated Ringer solution and inserted an indwelling catheter. Which of the findings indicate that the child is going into shock? Select all that apply.
☐ **1.** Urinary output is 25 mL/h.
☐ **2.** Specific gravity is within normal limits.
☐ **3.** Pain is 7 on a pain scale of 1 to 10.
☐ **4.** Heart rate is elevated.
☐ **5.** Blood pressure is dropping.

177. A client has been receiving radiation therapy for 3 weeks to treat cancer and has fatigue. The nurse should consider which factor when planning to help the client cope with the fatigue?
☐ **1.** Fatigue is a temporary problem that requires no active intervention.
☐ **2.** The cause of the fatigue should be determined.
☐ **3.** Fatigue indicates that the client's cancer is not under control.
☐ **4.** A balance of activity and rest will help manage the fatigue.

178. When educating unlicensed nursing personnel (UAP) about how to prevent the development of pressure ulcers, the nurse should emphasize that **most** tissue injuries related to shearing can be prevented by:
☐ **1.** close adherence to a turning schedule.
☐ **2.** keeping the skin clean and dry.
☐ **3.** proper positioning and moving of the client.
☐ **4.** use of skin lubricants.

179. When using crutches, the nurse should instruct the client to bear weight primarily on the:
☐ **1.** axillae.
☐ **2.** elbows.
☐ **3.** upper arms.
☐ **4.** hands.

180. A child with aggressive and impulsive behaviors is admitted to the child psychiatric unit with a diagnosis of a conduct disorder. Which intervention is appropriate?
☐ **1.** Allow autonomy.
☐ **2.** Elicit descriptions of feelings.
☐ **3.** Set limits.
☐ **4.** Teach assertiveness.

181. What should the nurse do **first** when admitting a toddler with croup?
☐ **1.** Monitor vital signs.
☐ **2.** Assess respiratory status.
☐ **3.** Ensure adequate fluid intake.
☐ **4.** Place a tracheostomy set at the bedside.

182. Before the nurse administers IV replacement of 5% dextrose in water with potassium chloride, what nursing intervention must be completed **first**?
☐ **1.** adding potassium chloride to the bag at the bedside
☐ **2.** evaluating laboratory results for electrolytes
☐ **3.** priming tubing using sterile technique
☐ **4.** checking the rate for IV push administration

183. A 45-year-old client diagnosed with colon cancer states, "I do not want any treatment. I have not seen any family members in 25 years. I am a loner. Besides, I will decide when and how I want to die." In which order of priority from first to last should the nurse perform the actions? All options must be used.

1. Ask the client what methods for suicide are available.
2. Tell the client that the primary care provider will ask for a psychiatric consult.
3. Ask the client about thoughts of suicide.
4. Express concern for the client's feelings and safety.

184. Which sign is an early indication that a client has developed hypocalcemia?
☐ **1.** tingling in the fingers
☐ **2.** depressed reflexes
☐ **3.** ventricular dysrhythmias
☐ **4.** memory changes

185. The nurse is auscultating the lung sounds of a client with long-standing emphysema. The nurse is **most** likely to detect:
☐ 1. fine crackles.
☐ 2. diminished breath sounds.
☐ 3. stridor.
☐ 4. pleural friction rub.

186. A client with a paranoid personality disorder sees some clients laughing during a group activity and asks the nurse, "Why are they laughing at me? I bet they are making fun of me." Which response by the nurse is **most** appropriate?
☐ 1. "You should not let yourself get so upset."
☐ 2. "Do not worry about them. They do not mean any harm."
☐ 3. "Look. They seem to be having fun."
☐ 4. "They are laughing at a joke John told. They are not laughing at you."

187. Mebendazole is prescribed for an 8-year-old child with pinworms. The child has an 18-month-old brother and a 4-year-old sister. The nurse should be sure that the parents are also treating which family members with this drug?
☐ 1. both of the siblings
☐ 2. the parents and brother
☐ 3. everyone who lives in the household
☐ 4. the parents and sister

188. When planning a presentation on the topic of osteoporosis to a group of middle-aged women, the nurse should include which information in the presentation?
☐ 1. An early symptom of osteoporosis is the dowager's hump.
☐ 2. Women of African and Latin descent are at greater risk.
☐ 3. Loss of height is an early symptom of the disease.
☐ 4. Conventional radiographs are usually used to confirm the disease.

189. Which rationale **best** explains why the nurse should evaluate gastric residual before administering the client's next enteral feeding?
☐ 1. to determine how well nutrients are being absorbed
☐ 2. to determine if the client is receiving enough feeding
☐ 3. to prevent overdistention of the stomach
☐ 4. to prevent mixing undigested formula with partially digested formula

190. The results of which serologic test should the nurse have on the medical record before a client is started on tissue plasminogen activator or alteplase recombinant?
☐ 1. partial thromboplastin time
☐ 2. potassium level
☐ 3. Lee-White clotting time
☐ 4. fibrin split product

191. When planning the care for a client diagnosed with hepatitis A, the nurse should include which interventions? Select all that apply.
☐ 1. Implement an exercise program.
☐ 2. Provide relief from nausea and vomiting.
☐ 3. Administer pain medication.
☐ 4. Encourage multiple small meals daily.
☐ 5. Plan frequent rest periods.

192. The nurse is assessing a client who has had a myocardial infarction. The nurse notes the cardiac rhythm shown. The nurse identifies that this rhythm is:

☐ 1. atrial fibrillation.
☐ 2. ventricular tachycardia.
☐ 3. premature ventricular contractions.
☐ 4. third-degree heart block.

193. The client with borderline personality disorder spends much time around the nurse's station, making numerous minor requests. The nurse interprets these behaviors as indicating which factor?
☐ 1. fears of abandonment and attention seeking
☐ 2. enjoyment of bothering the staff
☐ 3. boredom suggesting the need for something to do
☐ 4. lack of desire for involvement in milieu activities

194. A client has soft wrist restraints to prevent the client from pulling out the nasogastric tube. Which nursing intervention should be implemented while the restraints are on the client?
☐ 1. Instruct the client not to move while the restraints are in place.
☐ 2. Remove the restraints every 4 hours to provide skin care.
☐ 3. Secure the restraints to side rails of the bed.
☐ 4. Check on the client every 30 minutes while the restraints are on.

195. A client with alcohol dependence states, "I feel so bad because of what I have done to my wife and kids. I am just no good." Which response by the nurse is **most** appropriate?
☐ 1. "Why do you think you are no good?"
☐ 2. "They will need to forgive your shortcomings."
☐ 3. "Alcohol dependence is a disease that can be treated."
☐ 4. "Alcoholism is painful for everyone involved."

196. Which statement by a parent indicates the **best** understanding of why raisins should be limited as a snack food in toddlers?
- ☐ 1. "Raisins are low in nutritional value."
- ☐ 2. "Raisins can increase tooth decay."
- ☐ 3. "Raisins are easy to choke on."
- ☐ 4. "Raisins are hard to digest entirely."

197. A client has been diagnosed with atrial fibrillation. The healthcare provider (HCP) prescribed warfarin to be taken on a daily basis. The nurse instructs the client to avoid using which over-the-counter medication while taking warfarin?
- ☐ 1. aspirin
- ☐ 2. diphenhydramine
- ☐ 3. digoxin
- ☐ 4. pseudoephedrine

198. The nurse should inform a client taking carbamazepine that it can affect other medications in which way?
- ☐ 1. It decreases the effects of oral anticoagulants.
- ☐ 2. It decreases the serum concentration of verapamil.
- ☐ 3. It increases the serum concentration of other anticonvulsants.
- ☐ 4. It increases the effects of oral contraceptives.

199. A client has been diagnosed with hepatitis A. Which goal is **most** appropriate for the client?
- ☐ 1. Achieve control of abdominal pains.
- ☐ 2. Increase activity levels gradually.
- ☐ 3. Be able to breathe without difficulty.
- ☐ 4. Experience relief from edema.

200. Which activity by the mother offers the **most** support to the child during the first few days after surgery to repair a cleft lip?
- ☐ 1. holding and cuddling the child
- ☐ 2. helping the child play with some toys
- ☐ 3. reading some of the child's favorite stories
- ☐ 4. staying at the bedside and holding the child's hand

201. Which strategy is the **most** effective for a nurse to use to reduce the number of children involved in automobile accidents who were not wearing seat belts?
- ☐ 1. Contact the local government representative to discuss new legislation about child seat belts.
- ☐ 2. Attend a school board meeting to advocate for classes teaching children seat belt safety.
- ☐ 3. Call the town mayor's office with this information so that the mayor can discuss it with the media.
- ☐ 4. Start a letter-writing campaign to the school superintendent about seat belt importance.

202. The nurse is developing a discharge plan for a client who has had a myocardial infarction. Planning for discharge for this client should begin:
- ☐ 1. on discharge from the hospital.
- ☐ 2. on discharge from the cardiac care unit.
- ☐ 3. on admission to the hospital.
- ☐ 4. four weeks after the onset of illness.

203. A child is admitted to the emergency department with dyspnea related to bronchospasms. The nurse should place the client in which position?
- ☐ 1. high Fowler's
- ☐ 2. side lying
- ☐ 3. prone
- ☐ 4. supine

204. A client's chest tube is to be removed by the healthcare provider (HCP). Which item should the nurse have ready to be placed directly over the wound when the chest tube is removed?
- ☐ 1. butterfly dressing
- ☐ 2. Montgomery strap
- ☐ 3. fine mesh gauze dressing
- ☐ 4. petrolatum gauze dressing

205. The nurse is preparing to administer IM morphine sulfate to a client who is in pain. On checking the healthcare provider's (HCP's) prescription, the nurse notes that the prescription states "morphine sulfate 60 mg IM every 4 hours as needed for pain." The usual dose of morphine is 10 to 15 mg. What is the **most** appropriate action for the nurse to take?
- ☐ 1. Administer the medication as prescribed.
- ☐ 2. Administer 15 mg of the drug.
- ☐ 3. Contact the HCP to verify the prescription.
- ☐ 4. Ask another nurse to review the prescription.

206. Following surgery for removal of a brain tumor, a client is coughing and short of breath and has a "bad" feeling. The nurse obtains the following vital signs: blood pressure of 80/60 mm Hg, pulse rate of 120 bpm, and respiratory rate of 30 shallow breaths/minute. What should the nurse do **first**?
- ☐ 1. Call the neurosurgeon.
- ☐ 2. Place the client in the Trendelenburg position.
- ☐ 3. Consult the neurologic clinical nurse specialist (CNS).
- ☐ 4. Activate the rapid response team (RRT).

207. The nurse is preparing a client for paracentesis. What should the nurse do?
- ☐ 1. Have the client void before the procedure.
- ☐ 2. Scrub the client's abdomen with an antiseptic skin cleanser.
- ☐ 3. Position the client supine.
- ☐ 4. Put the client on nothing-by-mouth (NPO) status 4 hours before the procedure.

208. Which behavior in a 20-month-old would lead the nurse to suspect that the child is being abused?
- ☐ 1. absence of crying during the examination
- ☐ 2. clinging to the parent during the examination
- ☐ 3. playing with toys on the examination room floor
- ☐ 4. talking easily with the nurse

209. What information should the nurse plan to include when teaching the client and family about a substance abuse problem?
☐ 1. the role of the family in perpetuating the problem
☐ 2. the family's responsibility for the client
☐ 3. the physical, physiologic, and psychological effects of substances
☐ 4. the reasons that could have led the client to use the substance

210. A client who has had a laparoscopic cholecystectomy receives discharge instructions from the nurse. Which statement indicates that the client has understood the instructions?
☐ 1. "I need to maintain a low-fat diet for the next 6 months."
☐ 2. "I can remove the dressing from my incision tomorrow and take a shower."
☐ 3. "I can anticipate some nausea for several days after surgery."
☐ 4. "I can return to work in 4 to 6 weeks."

211. The nurse is obtaining a health history from an adult from Mexico. The nurse should interpret the findings by understanding that in this client's culture, what are highly valued?
☐ 1. children
☐ 2. materialism
☐ 3. firstborn sons
☐ 4. the elderly

212. A client has extreme fatigue and is malnourished, and laboratory tests reveal a hemoglobin level of 8.5 g/dL (85 g/L). The nurse should specifically ask the client about the intake of food **high** in which nutrients?
☐ 1. vitamins A, E, and C
☐ 2. vitamins B_6 and B_{12}, folate, iron, and copper
☐ 3. thiamine, riboflavin, and niacin
☐ 4. vitamins A and B

213. The nurse is assessing a neonate born to a mother with type 1 diabetes. Which finding is expected?
☐ 1. hypertonia
☐ 2. hyperactivity
☐ 3. large size
☐ 4. scaly skin

214. A client who had transurethral resection of the prostate has dribbling urine after his Foley catheter is removed on the second postoperative day. The nurse notes that the client had 200 mL of urine output in the last 8 hours with a 1,000-mL intake. The nurse should **first**:
☐ 1. apply a condom catheter.
☐ 2. assess for bladder distention.
☐ 3. obtain a urine specimen for culture.
☐ 4. teach the client Kegel exercises.

215. A client has atrial fibrillation. The nurse should monitor the client for:
☐ 1. cardiac arrest.
☐ 2. cerebrovascular accident.
☐ 3. heart block.
☐ 4. ventricular fibrillation.

216. A child diagnosed with tinea is being treated with griseofulvin. What should the nurse tell the parents to do?
☐ 1. Give the medication before a meal.
☐ 2. Have the child avoid intense sunlight.
☐ 3. Give the medication for 10 days.
☐ 4. Encourage increased fluid intake.

217. The nurse is developing a care plan for a client with a diagnosis of a borderline personality disorder. Which interventions would be effective to help the client cope and control emotions? Select all that apply.
☐ 1. Assist client with identifying his/her emotions.
☐ 2. Decrease impulsivity.
☐ 3. Have client keep a journal of emotions and coping techniques.
☐ 4. Encourage the client to delay gratification.
☐ 5. Use confrontation techniques.

218. A client undergoes cystoscopy with bladder biopsy. After the procedure, which assessment is **most** appropriate for the nurse to make?
☐ 1. Assess the patency of the Foley catheter.
☐ 2. Assess urine for excessive bleeding.
☐ 3. Percuss the bladder for distention.
☐ 4. Obtain a urine specimen for culture.

219. The nurse is assessing an infant who is 6 months of age and has a black eye; the infant is brought by his mother to the quick-care clinic. The mother reports that the daycare provider told her the child "fell down the steps with his walker." What should the nurse do in order of priority from first to last? All options must be used.

| 1. Report the incident to the social services department. |
| 2. Document findings accurately. |
| 3. Ask the mother for details about the incident and the daycare center. |
| 4. Place an ice bag on the infant's eye. |
| |
| |
| |
| |

220. A client of Mexican descent has bacterial pneumonia and has a temperature of 102°F (39°C). The client tells the nurse that the client has treated the infection by drinking milk, and the nurse interprets the client's remark as:
☐ 1. confusion from fever.
☐ 2. use of the hot disease concept.
☐ 3. use of milk as a laxative.
☐ 4. the need for a dietitian to assist her with meal planning.

221. A female client with paranoid schizophrenia has been hearing negative voices and "getting special messages from various sources." Which intervention is **most** appropriate for the client's symptoms?
☐ 1. Ask her to make simple decisions.
☐ 2. Be matter-of-fact with her.
☐ 3. Monitor her reactions to television programs.
☐ 4. Reinforce appropriate dress and hygiene.

222. The nurse is talking with a client who was diagnosed with bulimia 3 months ago. The client needs more education about the illness if she makes which comments? Select all that apply.
☐ 1. "I know that this illness is chronic and intermittent. I will always have to control it."
☐ 2. "If I start severely restricting my eating, I may be building up to a bingeing episode."
☐ 3. "When I am not bingeing and purging, I can skip that eating disorder support group."
☐ 4. "I have made a real effort to be more social and involved in activities."
☐ 5. "My depression is gone, so I do not need my antidepressant any longer."

223. The nurse judges that the parents of a newborn with imperforate anus know what a low defect is when they say that the rectum:
☐ 1. is below the abdominal rectus muscle.
☐ 2. is above the abdominal rectus muscle.
☐ 3. has descended through the puborectalis muscle.
☐ 4. has ascended through the puborectalis muscle.

224. An elderly client is receiving meperidine after abdominal surgery. The nurse should observe the client for which **most** significant side effect of meperidine?
☐ 1. respiratory depression
☐ 2. dysrhythmias
☐ 3. constipation
☐ 4. seizures

225. The mother of a child with bronchial asthma tells the nurse that the child wants a pet. Which pet is **most** appropriate?
☐ 1. cat
☐ 2. fish
☐ 3. gerbil
☐ 4. canary

226. A client with iron deficiency anemia is taking iron supplements. The nurse emphasizes to the client that the drug will have increased absorption if taken with:
☐ 1. milk.
☐ 2. orange juice.
☐ 3. food.
☐ 4. beta-carotene.

227. When obtaining the nursing history of a client who has type 1 diabetes mellitus, the nurse should assess the client for which early symptom of renal insufficiency?
☐ 1. polyuria
☐ 2. dysuria
☐ 3. hematuria
☐ 4. oliguria

228. When an infant resumes taking oral feedings after surgery to correct intussusception, the parents comment that the child seems to suck on the pacifier more since the surgery. The nurse explains that sucking on a pacifier:
☐ 1. provides an outlet for emotional tension.
☐ 2. indicates readiness to take solid foods.
☐ 3. indicates intestinal motility.
☐ 4. is an attempt to get attention from the parents.

229. A client is planning to be treated for infertility with the zygote intrafallopian transfer (ZIFT) method. Which information should the nurse include when teaching the client about this type of treatment method?
☐ 1. Fertilization takes place outside of the body.
☐ 2. ZIFT is helpful for clients with bilateral blocked fallopian tubes.
☐ 3. Ova and sperm are needed for instillation into the fallopian tube.
☐ 4. Fertilized ova are instilled into the vagina to enter the uterus.

230. When assessing for oxygenation in a client with dark skin, the nurse should examine the client's:
☐ 1. skin.
☐ 2. buccal mucosa.
☐ 3. nape of the neck.
☐ 4. forehead.

231. To prevent shoulder ankyloses following chest surgery, the nurse should teach the client to:
☐ 1. turn from side to side.
☐ 2. raise and lower the head.
☐ 3. raise the arm on the affected side over the head.
☐ 4. flex and extend the elbow on the affected side.

232. A client with a tracheostomy tube coughs and dislodges the tracheostomy tube. The nurse's **first** action should be to:
- ☐ 1. call for emergency assistance.
- ☐ 2. attempt reinsertion of tracheostomy tube.
- ☐ 3. position the client in semi-Fowler's position with the neck hyperextended.
- ☐ 4. insert the obturator into the stoma to reestablish the airway.

233. The experienced licensed practical/vocational nurse (LPN/VN) under the supervision of the registered nurse (RN) team leader is providing nursing care for an infant with respiratory syncytial virus (RSV). Which tasks are appropriate for the RN to delegate to the LPN/VN? Select all that apply.
- ☐ 1. Auscultate breath sounds.
- ☐ 2. Administer prescribed aerosolized medications.
- ☐ 3. Initiate nursing care plan.
- ☐ 4. Check oxygen saturation using pulse oximetry.
- ☐ 5. Complete in-depth admission assessment.
- ☐ 6. Evaluate the parent's ability to administer aerosolized medications.

234. A first-time mother is concerned that her 6-month-old infant is not gaining enough weight. What should the nurse tell the mother?
- ☐ 1. "Birth weight doubles by 6 months of age."
- ☐ 2. "Birth weight doubles by 3 months of age."
- ☐ 3. "The baby will eat what he needs."
- ☐ 4. "You need to make sure the baby finishes each bottle."

235. When assessing a client who reports a back injury, it is critical for the nurse to question the client about:
- ☐ 1. family history of back problems.
- ☐ 2. previous hospitalizations.
- ☐ 3. personal history of illness.
- ☐ 4. mechanism of injury.

236. A client is taking metoprolol and hydrochlorothiazide. The medication is effective if it:
- ☐ 1. lowers the blood pressure.
- ☐ 2. increases the heart rate.
- ☐ 3. improves circulation in the extremities.
- ☐ 4. decreases dyspnea.

237. A client in cardiac rehabilitation would like to eat the right foods to ensure adequate endurance on the treadmill. Which nutrient is **most** helpful for promoting endurance during sustained activity?
- ☐ 1. protein
- ☐ 2. carbohydrate
- ☐ 3. fat
- ☐ 4. water

238. The nurse is examining an older adult woman with possible rheumatoid arthritis. The nurse should ask the client if she is having:
- ☐ 1. nausea.
- ☐ 2. dizziness.
- ☐ 3. fatigue.
- ☐ 4. limitation of movement.

239. The nurse instructs the client in mixing and administering regular and NPH insulin. Which statement indicates that the client needs additional instruction?
- ☐ 1. "I draw up the regular insulin first."
- ☐ 2. "I shake the bottle of NPH insulin before drawing it up."
- ☐ 3. "I store the insulin in a cool place."
- ☐ 4. "I insert the needle at a 90-degree angle."

240. The mother of a child with newly diagnosed Duchenne's muscular dystrophy asks how her child developed the disease. The nurse gives a response incorporating which statement about its transmission?
- ☐ 1. "It is an autosomal recessive genetic disorder."
- ☐ 2. "It is a genetic disorder carried by males and transmitted to male children."
- ☐ 3. "It is a disorder primarily transmitted by males in the family."
- ☐ 4. "It is a disorder usually carried by females and transmitted to male children."

241. What is a **priority** nursing goal for an infant with intussusception?
- ☐ 1. Restore fluids.
- ☐ 2. Control diarrhea.
- ☐ 3. Protect the skin.
- ☐ 4. Manage acute pain.

242. A client is trying to lose weight at a moderate pace. If the client eliminates 1,000 cal/day from his normal intake, how many pounds (or kilograms) would the client lose in 1 week?

_____ lb/kg.

243. The healthcare provider (HCP) prescribes IV cefazolin 1 g for a client. In preparing to administer the cefazolin, the nurse notes that the client is allergic to penicillin. Based on this information, what is an appropriate action for the nurse to take?
- ☐ 1. Continue to prepare to administer the cefazolin as prescribed.
- ☐ 2. Notify the HCP of the client's allergy to penicillin.
- ☐ 3. Administer the cefazolin, staying at the client's bedside during the infusion.
- ☐ 4. Call the pharmacist to verify that the cefazolin should be administered as prescribed.

244. A client is prescribed buspirone 5 mg two times a day. Which statements indicate that the client has understood the nurse's teaching about this drug? Select all that apply.
☐ **1.** "This medicine will make me sleepy."
☐ **2.** "Buspirone will relax my muscles."
☐ **3.** "My anxiety will be completely gone by tomorrow."
☐ **4.** "Buspirone will help me not to worry so much."
☐ **5.** "I will be able to focus better."

245. When a client has a tearing of tissue with irregular wound edges, the nurse should document this as:
☐ **1.** contusion.
☐ **2.** abrasion.
☐ **3.** laceration.
☐ **4.** colonization.

246. A client with schizophrenia is responding well to risperidone and is no longer psychotic. After teaching the client about managing the illness, which statement reflects a need for further intervention?
☐ **1.** "I just do not know if I can afford to keep taking medicines every day."
☐ **2.** "When my thoughts start racing, I know I need to relax more."
☐ **3.** "I can name the side effects of risperidone, but I am not having any."
☐ **4.** "I do not listen to my mom's religious beliefs about not using medicines."

247. While a mother is feeding her full-term neonate 1 hour after birth, she asks the nurse, "What are these white dots in my baby's mouth? I tried to wash them out, but they are still there." After assessing the neonate's mouth, the nurse explains that these spots indicate which condition?
☐ **1.** Koplik's spots
☐ **2.** Epstein's pearls
☐ **3.** precocious teeth
☐ **4.** thrush curds

248. A nurse is assessing a client with hepatitis A. The client reports that the appetite is poor and the presence of food causes nausea. The nurse should encourage the client to eat:
☐ **1.** high-fat foods at each meal.
☐ **2.** foods high in protein.
☐ **3.** the majority of the calories in the morning during small frequent snacks.
☐ **4.** a low-calorie diet with numerous snacks.

249. A client had a cast applied to the left femur to stabilize a fracture. To promote early rehabilitation, the nurse should **first**:
☐ **1.** call physical therapy to provide passive exercise of the affected limb.
☐ **2.** teach the client how to do isometric exercises of the quadriceps.
☐ **3.** show the family how to do active range-of-motion exercises of the unaffected limb.
☐ **4.** obtain weights so the client can exercise the upper extremities.

250. The client arrives in the emergency department following a bicycle accident in which the client's forehead hit the pavement. The client is diagnosed as having a hyphema. The nurse should place the client in which position?
☐ **1.** supine
☐ **2.** semi-Fowler's
☐ **3.** side lying on the affected side
☐ **4.** side lying on the unaffected side

251. The nurse has just received change-of-shift report for four clients. Based on this report, the nurse should assess which client **first**?
☐ **1.** a 38-year-old who is 2 days postmastectomy due to breast cancer, having difficulty coping with the diagnosis
☐ **2.** a 52-year-old with pneumonia and chronic back pain who is requesting pain medication
☐ **3.** a 36-year-old admitted after motor vehicle accident whose urine output has totaled 30 mL over the last 2 hours
☐ **4.** an 84-year-old with resolving left-sided weakness who is slightly confused and has been awake most of the night

252. An obese diabetic client who has bilateral leg aching is to start a cardiac rehabilitation with an exercise program. Using which exercise equipment will be **most** helpful to the client?
☐ **1.** stationary bicycle
☐ **2.** treadmill
☐ **3.** elliptical trainer
☐ **4.** stair climber

253. The nurse has received a change-of-shift report. The nurse should assess which client **first**?
☐ **1.** a 72-year-old admitted 2 days ago with a blood alcohol level of 0.08
☐ **2.** a 36-year-old with chest tube due to spontaneous pneumothorax with current respiratory rate 18 breaths/min and oxygen saturation 95% on oxygen at 2 L per nasal cannula
☐ **3.** a 28-year-old who is 2 days postappendectomy with discharge prescriptions written and whose husband is waiting to take her home
☐ **4.** a 62-year-old admitted with a recent gastrointestinal (GI) bleeding whose hemoglobin is 13.8 g/dL (138 g/L)

254. An infant is born with facial abnormalities, growth retardation, and vision abnormalities. These abnormalities are likely caused by maternal:
☐ **1.** alcohol consumption.
☐ **2.** vitamin B_6 deficiency.
☐ **3.** vitamin A deficiency.
☐ **4.** folic acid deficiency.

255. The adolescent with cystic fibrosis has been placed on ciprofloxacin for a lung infection. Which statement from the client indicates the need for more teaching?
- ☐ 1. "I will not take this drug with any dairy products."
- ☐ 2. "I will need to have drug levels drawn while I am on this medication."
- ☐ 3. "I should immediately report any muscle or joint pain."
- ☐ 4. "If I miss a dose, I should take it as soon as I remember."

256. A client whose condition remains stable after a myocardial infarction gradually increases activity. To determine whether the activity is appropriate for the client, the nurse should assess the client for:
- ☐ 1. edema.
- ☐ 2. cyanosis.
- ☐ 3. dyspnea.
- ☐ 4. weight loss.

257. The parents of a 7-year-old child with glomerulonephritis ask what they can do to ensure that their other children do not develop the disease. The nurse should respond with which statement?
- ☐ 1. "If you suspect your child has a urinary tract infection, see your primary healthcare provider (HCP) right away."
- ☐ 2. "I am afraid there is nothing you can do; glomerulonephritis is a genetic disorder."
- ☐ 3. "Glomerulonephritis is not contagious, so your other children will not get the disease."
- ☐ 4. "If your child has a streptococcal infection, complete the course of prescribed antibiotics."

258. A client admitted for alcohol detoxification is taking disulfiram. The nurse should instruct the client to avoid ingestion of which foods and/or liquids? Select all that apply.
- ☐ 1. aged cheeses
- ☐ 2. beer
- ☐ 3. communal wine at church
- ☐ 4. chocolates
- ☐ 5. cough syrup

259. The nurse is evaluating an infant for auditory ability. What is the expected response in an infant with normal hearing?
- ☐ 1. blinking and stopping body movements when sound is introduced
- ☐ 2. evidence of shy and withdrawn behaviors
- ☐ 3. saying "da-da" by age 5 months
- ☐ 4. absence of squealing by age 4 months

260. When admitting a neonate whose mother received magnesium sulfate, the nurse should assess the baby for which complication? Select all that apply.
- ☐ 1. increased Moro reflex
- ☐ 2. decreased muscle tone
- ☐ 3. increased respirations
- ☐ 4. decreased respirations
- ☐ 5. increased temperature

261. The neonate has a prescribed IV rate of 8 mL/h. Fluid totals are recorded every 2 hours on the even hours. There is a new prescription written at 1030 to decrease the IV rate to 6 mL/h. What is the fluid total to be infused and recorded at 1200?

_____ mL.

262. The nurse is auscultating S_1 and S_2 in a client. Identify the area where the nurse should hear S_1 the loudest.

263. While assessing the psychosocial aspects of a primigravid client at 30 weeks' gestation, what feelings are expected?
- ☐ 1. vulnerability
- ☐ 2. confirmation
- ☐ 3. ambivalence
- ☐ 4. body image disturbance

264. The nurse must be aware that adverse drug reactions in the elderly client may be underestimated because:
- ☐ 1. adverse reactions rarely have an atypical presentation.
- ☐ 2. cognitive impairment is an expected finding in the elderly client.
- ☐ 3. physical or psychological symptoms are attributed to the effects of aging.
- ☐ 4. excess sedation is difficult to assess in the elderly client.

265. A parent tells the nurse that their 8-month-old infant is anxious. Which suggestion by the nurse is **most** appropriate to help the parent lessen anxiety in the infant?
- ☐ 1. Limit holding the infant to feeding times.
- ☐ 2. Talk quietly to the infant while awake.
- ☐ 3. Play music in his room for most of the day and night.
- ☐ 4. Have a close friend keep the infant for a few days.

Answers, Rationales, and Test-Taking Strategies

The answers and rationales for each question follow below, along with keys (8➞) to the client need (CN) and cognitive level (CL) for each question. In addition, you will also see a glossary icon (▭) highlighting specific terminology used on the licensing exam. As you check your answers, use the **Content Mastery and Test-Taking Skill Self-Analysis** *worksheet (tear-out worksheet in back of book) to identify the reason(s) for not answering the questions correctly. For additional information about test-taking skills and strategies for answering questions, refer to pages 12–23 and pages 35–36 in Part 1 of this book.*

1. 1, 3, 4, 5. The fetus does go through sleep cycles, rendering it less likely to move while it is asleep. Blood glucose does cross the placenta and can affect fetal movement. Cigarette smoking causes carbon monoxide to cross the placenta, which reduces fetal oxygen. Pregnant women are more likely to notice fetal movement while they are sitting or lying down, and time of day often determines this. Most pregnant women notice fetal movement in the evening. Barometric pressure does not affect fetal activity in utero.

8➞ CN: Health promotion and maintenance; CL: Analyze

2. 1. The infant is exhibiting periodic breathing, which is normal in infants of this age. The infant typically alternates short periods of rapid, louder respirations with periods of slower, quieter respirations.

8➞ CN: Health promotion and maintenance; CL: Analyze

3. 2. *Respondeat superior* is Latin for "The master is responsible for the acts of his servants." The nurse, as an employee of the hospital, acted according to the established policy of the hospital. Because the nurse followed hospital policy, it is unlikely that this incident involved malpractice, negligence, or tort law.

8➞ CN: Management of care; CL: Evaluate

4. 3. The surgeon is required to give the client explanations and have questions answered. The nurse has no way of assessing the client's understanding without the interpreter. The client should sign the Spanish **consent** ▭ form only after receiving an explanation of the procedure, its risks, and alternatives. A family member cannot be relied on to translate the surgeon's instructions. The nurse is commonly asked to witness the explanation and to obtain the client's signature on the informed consent form. Informed consent is the provision of information concerning the procedure and its risks, not obtaining the client's signature on the form. The surgical charge nurse does not need to be notified.

8➞ CN: Management of care; CL: Synthesize

5. 4. Traveling is usually discouraged if preterm labor has been a problem, as it restricts normal movement. A client should be able to walk around frequently to prevent blood clots and to empty her bladder at least every 1 to 2 hours. Bladder infections often stimulate preterm labor, and preventing them is of great importance to this client. Contractions that recur indicate the return of preterm labor, and the **HCP** ▭ needs to be notified. Dehydration is known to stimulate preterm labor, and encouraging the client to drink adequate amounts of water helps to prevent this problem.

8➞ CN: Reduction of risk potential; CL: Evaluate

6. 2. Timolol can cause some eye discomfort when administered. It is important for the client to continue to take the drug. Glaucoma eyedrops should be administered as prescribed, not whenever the client desires. The client with glaucoma needs to take eye medication on an ongoing basis to control the disorder and prevent vision damage. There is no need to refrigerate the drug.

8➞ CN: Pharmacological and parenteral therapies; CL: Synthesize

7. 2. DVT causes edema; therefore, the **UAP** ▭ should elevate the extremity to promote venous return. Dependent positioning is appropriate for a client with arterial insufficiency. Placing a pillow under the knee would position the foot in a low position, and pressure behind the knee may obstruct venous flow. Massaging the extremity could dislodge the thrombus.

8➞ CN: Management of care; CL: Synthesize

8. 3. The bluish pigment on the buttocks and back of an infant of African descent is a common finding and should be documented as Mongolian spots in the child's **medical record** ▭. These spots typically fade by the time the child is 5 or 6 years. Additional assessment by the care provider is not indicated. The marks are not bruises.

8➞ CN: Health promotion and maintenance; CL: Synthesize

9. 1. This client has a barrel chest. The anterior-posterior diameter of the chest is larger than the transverse diameter, as is characteristic of the client with chronic obstructive pulmonary disease. Although the client may be muscular from lifting weights, the barrel chest is not associated with the client's age, height, or weight. Use of bronchodilators will not change the shape of the client's chest.

☞ CN: Physiological adaptation; CL: Analyze

10. 2. Fetal acoustic stimulation involves the use of an instrument that emits sound levels of approximately 80 dB at a frequency of 80 Hz. The sharp sound startles and awakens the fetus and is used with nonstress testing as a method to evaluate fetal well-being. A fetoscope or Doppler stethoscope is used to listen to the fetal heart rate. Nipple stimulation or intravenous oxytocin is used to stimulate contractions. Ultrasound testing is used to determine amniotic fluid volume.

☞ CN: Reduction of risk potential; CL: Apply

11. 1, 3, 4, 5. Child molesters prey on lonely children or those who spend a lot of time at home alone due to a working parent. They initially show interest and assist the child and family such as by providing rides, money, and homework help. Once trust is established, molesters push for a more sexual relationship, which they justify by pointing out what they have done to help the child. If the child tries to stop the sexual interaction or appears ready to tell someone, molesters will use threats to maintain the secret. Though some child molesters have had difficult childhoods in which they may have been molested, having them recognize that is not enough to keep them from offending again.

☞ CN: Safety and infection control; CL: Apply

12. 3. A client with severe depression may experience symptoms of psychosis such as hallucinations and delusions that are typically mood congruent. The statement "My heart has stopped and my blood is black ash" is a mood-congruent somatic delusion. A delusion is a firm, false, fixed belief that is resistant to reason or fact. A hallucination is a false sensory perception unrelated to external stimuli. An illusion is a misinterpretation of a real sensory stimulus. Paranoia refers to suspiciousness of others and their actions.

☞ CN: Psychosocial integrity; CL: Analyze

13. 2. Typically, iron supplements are needed for at least 1 month. By the end of this time, there should be a significant rise in the hemoglobin and hematocrit. Therefore, the mother needs to continue the iron supplements for several more weeks. Testing the child after only 2 weeks of treatment may not be beneficial. A significant rise in hemoglobin and hematocrit usually requires approximately 1 month of therapy. An iron-rich diet should have been started when the diagnosis was made and continued for at least the duration of iron supplement therapy.

☞ CN: Pharmacological and parenteral therapies; CL: Synthesize

14. 2. Cystic fibrosis is the most common inherited disease in children. It is inherited as an autosomal recessive trait, meaning that the child inherits the defective gene from both parents. The chances are one in four for each of this couple's pregnancies.

☞ CN: Reduction of risk potential; CL: Apply

15. 1. The dietary department should meet with the client to ensure that the foods are available and prepared according to religious beliefs. On admission, the client should be asked whether there are special dietary needs. The dietary department should be notified of these special needs, and a dietary representative should meet with the client and family when possible. The **HCP** 📖 should be consulted if a requested food is contrary to a prescribed diet restriction. The unit case manager does not need to be contacted regarding a dietary request. The rabbi is not involved in dietary requests.

☞ CN: Management of care; CL: Apply

16. 1, 2, 3. For the client with grandiose delusions, the nurse should accept the client but not argue with the delusion to build trust and the client's self-esteem. Focusing on the underlying feeling or meaning of the delusion helps to meet the client's needs. Focusing on events and topics based in reality distracts the client from the delusional thinking. Confronting the client's delusions or beliefs can lead to agitation in the client and the need to cling to the grandiose delusion to preserve self-esteem. Interacting with the client only when based in reality ignores the client's needs and therapeutic nursing intervention.

☞ CN: Psychosocial integrity; CL: Synthesize

17. 3. The nurse must act as an advocate for the client when the client cannot afford treatment. It may be possible to substitute a less expensive antibiotic. Correct procedure includes contacting the **HCP** 📖 to explain the mother's economic situation and request a substitution. For example, amoxicillin is more economical than azithromycin. If it is not possible to use another antibiotic, then the nurse can explore other avenues with the mother and/or social worker.

☞ CN: Management of care; CL: Synthesize

18. 1. Saying "When you interrupt others, they leave the area" is most helpful because it serves to increase the client's awareness of others' perceptions of the behavior by giving specific feedback about the behavior. The other statements are punitive and authoritative, possibly threatening to the client, and likely to increase defensiveness, decrease self-worth, and increase feelings of guilt.

☞ CN: Psychosocial integrity; CL: Synthesize

19. 1, 2, 3, 6. The important information to be given with a preeclamptic client should include blood pressure trends while being monitored and the protein that is and has been present in the urine as these are indicators of increasing eclampsia. Edema of the face, a history of headache, blurred vision, and epigastric pain are important as these also indicate worsening preeclampsia. The fetal position at 25 weeks is of minor importance as the fetus is constantly changing positions at this point in the pregnancy. The use of dietary sodium does not have an impact on preeclampsia. Glycosuria is an important consideration if this client has gestational diabetes but is not significant for the client with preeclampsia.

CN: Safety and infection control; CL: Synthesize

20. 3. Although breech presentations are rare, footling breech occurs when there is an extension of the fetal knees and one or both feet protrude through the pelvis. In frank breech, there is flexion of the fetal thighs and extension of the knees. The feet rest at the sides of the fetal head. In complete breech, there is flexion of the fetal thighs and knees; the fetus appears to be squatting. Vertex position occurs in 95% of births; in such cases, the head is engaged in the pelvis.

CN: Health promotion and maintenance; CL: Apply

21. 3. The timing of symptoms is important to the diagnosis of PMS. The client should keep a 3-month log of symptoms and menses. With PMS, the symptoms begin 3 to 7 days before menses and resolve 1 to 2 days after the menstrual cycle has started. Menstrual cycle irregularity and mood swings after menses are not related to PMS, and other causes should be investigated. Midcycle spotting and pain are related to ovulation.

CN: Health promotion and maintenance; CL: Analyze

22. 2. The client who has received general anesthesia with neuromuscular blocking agents must be carefully monitored when given clindamycin. A serious interaction could be enhanced, neuromuscular blockage, skeletal muscle weakness, or respiratory depression, if this combination is used during or immediately after surgery. Concurrent use should be avoided. The combined effect of the medications places the client at increased risk, and the nurse should assess the client closely for respiratory depression or paralysis. The nurse will be monitoring the client's heart rate, blood pressure, and urinary output but not specifically because of potential drug interactions and adverse effects of clindamycin.

CN: Pharmacological and parenteral therapies; CL: Analyze

23. 2. The client needs to know that there is a cause for the delirium, that there is hope for treatment, and that medications can help decrease anxiety. Giving medications can help the anxiety, but the client also needs an explanation about the condition. Saying that the more the client worries, the worse the delirium will get is inappropriate and most likely would add to the client's anxiety.

CN: Psychosocial integrity; CL: Synthesize

24. 1. The client is in a crisis and has a high anxiety level. Holding the client's hands and encouraging the client to slow down and take a deep breath conveys caring and helps decrease anxiety. Telling the client to calm down or stop worrying offers no concrete directions for accomplishing this task. It is unknown from the data who was at fault in the accident. Therefore, it is inappropriate for the nurse to state that it was not the client's fault.

CN: Psychosocial integrity; CL: Synthesize

25. 1, 4, 2, 3. The client is experiencing ketoacidosis. The nurse should first obtain the blood glucose level and then notify the **IICP** 📖 who will then prescribe the appropriate dose of insulin. Prior to administering the insulin, the nurse will start the IV infusion.

CN: Physiological adaptation; CL: Synthesize

26. 3. Tasks that the **UAP** 📖 can undertake vary greatly. The nurse must be aware of the scope of the UAP's preparation and the policies of the healthcare agency. The important consideration is that the task is appropriate for that individual and is within the guidelines for practice at the healthcare agency. The UAP can perform complicated tasks within the scope of the preparation. Although the nurse observes the UAP and evaluates the UAP on his or her ability to perform the task, the most important aspect of delegation is to delegate within the UAP's educational preparation. A positive relationship with clients, while desirable, is not essential to delegation. Delegation involves giving clear directions and following up after the task has been delegated.

CN: Management of care; CL: Analyze

27. 4. Superficial thrombophlebitis is associated with pain, warmth, and erythema. The nurse can request a prescription for warm packs to relieve the pain. Venous insufficiency causes edema and a brown discoloration of the lower leg. Varicose veins are dark, protruding veins, and symptoms of discomfort increase with standing. Pain on dorsiflexion of the foot indicates deep vein thrombosis; the client does not indicate having this pain.

🔑 CN: Physiological adaptation; CL: Synthesize

28. 1. Hospice programs are appropriate programs for clients with any type of terminal illness when death is imminent within weeks up to 6 months. Clients may discuss their prognosis of a terminal illness before it progresses to the terminal stage when a referral to hospice care is indicated. Clients are not required to have advance directives to be admitted to hospice services, but will be asked to complete them upon admission.

🔑 CN: Management of care; CL: Apply

29. 1. Several irregularly shaped red patches, common skin variations in neonates, are termed stork bites. They eventually fade away as the neonate grows older. Port-wine stains are disfiguring darkish red or purplish skin discolorations on the scalp and face that may need laser therapy for removal. Newborn rash is typically generalized over the body, not localized to one body area, and is commonly raised. Café au lait spots are brown and typically found anywhere on the body. More than six spots or spots larger than 1.5 cm are associated with neurofibromatosis, a genetic condition of neural tissue.

🔑 CN: Health promotion and maintenance; CL: Analyze

30. 3. In the traditional Mexican household, the man is the head of the family and makes the major decisions. Efforts should be made to reach the father as soon as possible to acquire his permission. It is not necessary to contact the social worker at this point. The client has not refused the procedure, so it is premature to contact the **HCP** 📖. This is not a situation of suspected child abuse.

🔑 CN: Management of care; CL: Synthesize

31. 1. At this time, the client's anger is not out of control, so empathy and talking are appropriate to diffuse the anger. Using time-out is appropriate when the client's anger is escalating and the client can no longer talk about the anger rationally. Restraints are appropriate only when there is imminent risk of harm to the client or others. Future strategies are discussed after the initial incident is resolved.

🔑 CN: Psychosocial integrity; CL: Synthesize

32. 1. In the cognitively impaired client, benzodiazepines, such as lorazepam, can increase confusion and nighttime agitation. Extrapyramidal side effects are more common with antipsychotics. Vomiting and sweating are signs of benzodiazepine withdrawal. Anticholinergic side effects are more likely with antipsychotics and tricyclic antidepressants.

🔑 CN: Pharmacological and parenteral therapies; CL: Analyze

33. 1, 2, 4. Telehealth is becoming an increasingly available way for nurses to conduct counseling sessions with clients who are at a distance from a **healthcare provider (HCP)** 📖 or healthcare facility. The client saves travel time and can avoid precipitating symptoms associated with the stress disorder that might occur as a result of a visit to a healthcare facility. The client also can access care that might not otherwise be easily available. Treatment for PSTD is long term, and there is no evidence to suggest that telehealth versus face-to-face counseling shortens recovery time. Counseling sessions using telehealth technology are conducted on an individual basis between one client and an HCP, but group support may be available if required as a part of a treatment plan.

🔑 CN: Management of care; CL: Evaluate

34. 4. A woman with a uterus who takes unopposed estrogen has an increased risk of endometrial cancer. The addition of progesterone prevents the formation of endometrial hyperplasia. Progesterone does not prevent breast, liver, or cervical cancer.

🔑 CN: Pharmacological and parenteral therapies; CL: Apply

35. 3. The pre–school-age child with severe autism will benefit from one-on-one play therapy. The therapist can develop a rapport with this child with nonverbal play. Antipsychotic medications are not indicated for the autism client. The child has difficulty with interpersonal relationships; therefore, group psychotherapy and social skills groups would not be effective.

🔑 CN: Psychosocial integrity; CL: Analyze

36. 2. The client who is 18 weeks with an intrauterine pregnancy (IUP) is not stable with bright red vaginal bleeding. Even with a nonviable fetus, the mother is in jeopardy with continued bleeding. The client who is 9 weeks IUP and has not vomited for 12 hours appears stable at this point with a nonviable fetus. The G8 also appears stable as her bleeding has tapered off since admission. The 29-week gestation client carrying twins has no information indicating that she is in jeopardy, with no contractions in the past 2 hours, and is becoming more stable.

🔑 CN: Health promotion and maintenance; CL: Synthesize

37. 3. The nurse should monitor the client's serum albumin. A decreased serum albumin indicates malnutrition and is considered a risk factor in the development of pressure ulcers. Other risk factors include immobility, incontinence, and decreased sensation. Having the client walk and inserting an indwelling catheter require a **healthcare provider's (HCP's)** 📖 prescription. The white blood cell count is monitored if an infection is present.

🔑 CN: Physiological adaptation; CL: Synthesize

38. 4. The nurse should recognize the ringing in the ears, or tinnitus, as a sign of ototoxicity probably caused by the furosemide. The appropriate action is for the nurse to stop the furosemide and notify the **HCP** 📖. If the drug is stopped soon enough, permanent hearing loss can be avoided, and the tinnitus should subside. The nurse should note the observation in the **medical record** 📖 but should not delay action. Tinnitus is not a symptom of digoxin toxicity. Aspirin can cause tinnitus, but the nurse should first investigate the obvious cause of tinnitus, which in this case is the furosemide.

🔑 CN: Pharmacological and parenteral therapies; CL: Synthesize

39. 4. Any injury to the mouth results in copious amounts of blood because the mouth is a highly vascular area. Because the nurse does not know the mother and does not speak Spanish, the most appropriate action is to give the mother the ice and demonstrate what she is to do. The child will be less fearful if the ice is applied by the mother. Calling for an interpreter is appropriate after caring for the immediate need of the child. Grabbing the child away will probably upset the mother more, further adding to the stress experienced by the child.

🔑 CN: Psychosocial integrity; CL: Synthesize

40. 2, 3, 4. The client should recognize the signs of potential thermal dangers to prevent skin breakdown and wear clean, loose, soft cotton socks so that the feet are comfortable, air can circulate, and moisture is absorbed. In the winter or if the client has cold feet, the client should be encouraged to wear an extra pair of socks and a larger shoe size. Getting a sunburn during the summer puts the client at risk for tissue injury and skin breakdown. Using a heating pad to warm the feet or using an electric blanket places the client at risk for injury and should be avoided.

🔑 CN: Reduction of risk potential; CL: Create

41. 3. The peak serum dose of an antibiotic is drawn 30 minutes after the completion of the IV dose of the antibiotic.

🔑 CN: Pharmacological and parenteral therapies; CL: Apply

42. 2. Given the client's age, making final plans is age appropriate. The absence of any signs of ill health, depression, or suicidal ideation makes the other options inappropriate.

🔑 CN: Psychosocial integrity; CL: Analyze

43. 1. ICP is highest in the early morning, and the client with hydrocephalus may be experiencing signs of increased ICP that need to be treated. The increased ICP is not related to fluid levels, and the nurse should not advise the client to increase fluid intake. While ICP does fluctuate during the day, it is highest in the morning, and the nurse should notify the **HCP** 📖. Pain medication will not treat the potentially increasing ICP and may mask important signs of increasing ICP.

🔑 CN: Physiological adaptation; CL: Synthesize

44. 1. The nurse should instruct the client that symptoms from an occasional headache due to eye strain or continuous work at a computer can be relieved by acetaminophen. Although this drug causes prostaglandin inhibition, this effect is rapidly reversed and cleared with no apparent harmful effects in pregnancy. If the headaches become more frequent or severe, the client should be instructed to contact her **healthcare provider (HCP)** 📖 immediately. Aspirin should be avoided during pregnancy because it inhibits prostaglandin synthesis. It also decreases uterine contractility and may delay the onset of labor or prolong pregnancy and labor. Aspirin decreases platelet aggregation, possibly increasing the risk of bleeding. Ibuprofen and naproxen can lead to premature closure of the fetal ductus arteriosus and decreased amniotic fluid with prolonged use. They may also prolong pregnancy or labor because of their antiprostaglandin effects.

🔑 CN: Pharmacological and parenteral therapies; CL: Synthesize

45. 2. When a client is experiencing a flashback, the nurse should stay with the client, offer reassurance, and present reality in a nonthreatening manner to minimize the client's anxiety and agitation. The client needs to be told that he or she is experiencing an effect from lysergic acid diethylamide and that he or she is safe and the flashback will end. Confronting the client's misperceptions or challenging unrealistic statements could increase anxiety and agitation, possibly leading to aggressive behavior. Secluding the client until the flashback ends usually is not necessary or appropriate unless the client threatens or demonstrates aggression toward self or others.

🔑 CN: Psychosocial integrity; CL: Apply

69. 3. Variable decelerations are associated with compression of the umbilical cord. The nurse should alter the client's position and increase the IV fluid rate. Fetal head compression is associated with early decelerations. Severe compression of the fetal chest, such as during the process of vaginal birth, may result in transient bradycardia. Compression or damage to the placenta, typically from abruptio placentae, results in severe, late decelerations.

CN: Reduction of risk potential; CL: Analyze

70. 1. The mask is appropriate because it covers the nose and mouth and fits snugly against the cheeks and chin. Masks that are too large may cover the eyes. Masks that are too small obstruct the nose. The mask does not need to be covered with a cloth.

CN: Management of care; CL: Evaluate

71. 1, 2, 3, 4. DIC is diagnosed based on clinical symptoms and laboratory findings. Findings such as excessive and unusual bruising or bleeding over areas of tissue trauma, such as IV insertion or incision sites, or application of a blood pressure cuff should be reported to the **HCP** 📖. Tachycardia and diaphoresis also may be noted. Laboratory results reveal low platelet, fibrinogen, proaccelerin, antihemophilic factor, and prothrombin levels. Bleeding time is normal, and partial thromboplastin time is increased. A urine output of 350 mL in 8 hours indicates adequate renal function. Temperature is not an indication of DIC.

CN: Physiological adaptation; CL: Analyze

72. 2. If the chest tube is accidentally pulled out (a rare occurrence), a petroleum jelly gauze and sterile 4- × 4-inch dressing should be applied over the chest wall insertion site immediately. The dressing should be covered with adhesive tape and be occlusive, and the surgeon should be notified. The lungs can be auscultated, and vital signs can be taken after the dressing is in place and the surgeon has been called. Placing the tube in sterile water will not reestablish a seal to prevent air entering the insertion site of the chest tube.

CN: Reduction of risk potential; CL: Synthesize

73. 2. Preserving forensic evidence is essential for investigative purposes following injuries that may be suspected as having criminal intent. The nurse places each item of clothing in a separate paper bag and labels it; wet clothing is hung to dry. The nurse does not cut or otherwise unnecessarily handle clothing, particularly clothing with evidence such as blood or body fluids. The nurse documents carefully the clients' description of the incident and uses quotes around the clients' exact words where possible; documentation will become a part of the clients' **medical records** 📖 and can be subpoenaed for subsequent investigation.

CN: Management of care; CL: Synthesize

74. 1. A frothy, purulent vaginal discharge in a sexually active female client is typically caused by a sexually transmitted infection such as trichomonas. Other diseases, such as chlamydia, may also be present. Both the client and the boyfriend need treatment after the disease is determined. Normal variations in female vaginal discharge should be clear to white, not frothy or purulent. The client should be instructed to wear cotton underwear and avoid pantyhose, wet gym clothes, and tight-fitting garments, such as jeans, so that air can circulate.

CN: Management of care; CL: Analyze

75. 4. Emboli obstruct blood flow, leading to a decreased perfusion of the lung tissue. Because of the decreased perfusion, a ventilation-perfusion mismatch occurs, causing hypoxemia to develop. Arterial blood gas analysis typically will indicate hypoxemia and hypocapnia. A priority objective in the treatment of pulmonary emboli is maintaining adequate oxygenation. A productive cough and activity intolerance do not indicate impaired gas exchange. The client does not demonstrate an ineffective breathing pattern; rather, the problem of impaired gas exchange is caused by the inability of blood to flow through the lung tissue.

CN: Physiological adaptation; CL: Synthesize

76. 3. Systematic pain assessment is necessary for adequate pain management in the postoperative client. Even though the client is receiving morphine sulfate by PCA, assessment is needed if the client is experiencing pain. Encouraging the client to rest or to ignore pain without further assessment is not a sufficient intervention.

CN: Basic care and comfort; CL: Synthesize

77. 3. Cardiogenic shock occurs when myocardial contractility decreases and cardiac output greatly decreases. The circulating blood volume is within normal limits or increased. Infarction is not always the cause of cardiogenic shock.

CN: Physiological adaptation; CL: Analyze

78. 1. The goal of the education program is to instruct the client to take the pulse; therefore, the expected outcome would be the ability to give a return demonstration of how to palpate the heart rate.

CN: Reduction of risk potential; CL: Evaluate

79. **1.** The nurse should expect to find decreased levels of thyroxine and triiodothyronine and increased TSH. Other indicators of hypothyroidism are the presence of antithyroid antibodies and elevation of the creatine phosphokinase (CPK-MM) level. Hypothyroidism has a metabolic effect on skeletal muscle. Muscle injury results, causing the CPK-MM to spill out of the damaged cells and into the bloodstream.

🔑 CN: Physiological adaptation;
CL: Analyze

80. **2.** If the client begins to experience abdominal cramping during administration of the enema fluid, the nurse's first action is to temporarily stop the infusion and have the client take a few deep breaths. After the cramping subsides, the nurse can continue with the enema solution. If the cramping does not subside, the nurse should clamp the tubing and remove it. Raising the height of the container will increase the flow of fluid and cause the cramping to increase. Rubbing the abdomen while infusing the enema fluid will not stop the cramping.

🔑 CN: Basic care and comfort;
CL: Synthesize

81. **3.** Although chronologically the infant is 7 months old, because of being born 6 weeks early, the child is only 5½ months old developmentally. Appropriate activities for a 5- to 5½-month-old infant include placing a rattle or ball in the infant's hand. Picture books are an appropriate choice for an infant older than 9 months. Playing peekaboo is appropriate for a 9- to 12-month-old infant. Colored blocks are appropriate for a toddler approximately age 15 to 18 months.

🔑 CN: Health promotion and maintenance;
CL: Synthesize

82. **3.** Accurate daily weight measurement provides the best measure of a client's fluid status: 1 kg (2.2 lb) is equal to 1,000 mL of fluid. To be accurate, weight should be obtained at the same time every day, with the same scale, and with minimal clothing on.

🔑 CN: Physiological adaptation;
CL: Analyze

83. **3.** The nurse uses Montgomery straps primarily to avoid the removal of long-term abdominal dressing tape and ultimate skin breakdown.

🔑 CN: Basic care and comfort; CL: Apply

84. **2.** Full benefit from an antidepressant medication usually takes about 2 to 4 weeks on an adequate dose.

🔑 CN: Pharmacological and parenteral therapies; CL: Apply

85. **3.** Percutaneous umbilical blood sampling is a useful procedure for diagnosing Rh disease, obtaining fetal complete blood count, and karyotyping chromosomes to evaluate for genetic disorders. Ultrasound commonly is used to detect twins. A lecithin-sphingomyelin ratio is the procedure of choice to diagnose fetal lung maturation. A maternal blood test is used to determine the alpha fetoprotein level.

🔑 CN: Reduction of risk potential;
CL: Apply

86. **2.** Fine tremors are the first symptom reported in 70% of clients with Parkinson's disease. A new onset of tremors needs to be investigated by the **HCP** 📖. Tremors are not an expected change with aging.

🔑 CN: Reduction of risk potential;
CL: Synthesize

87. **0.8 mL**

$$\frac{0.4 \text{ mg}}{X} = \frac{0.5 \text{ mg}}{1 \text{ mL}}$$

$$0.4 = 0.5X$$

$$\frac{0.4}{0.5} = X$$

$$0.8 \text{ mL} = X.$$

🔑 CN: Pharmacological and parenteral therapies; CL: Apply

88. **1.** Loss of appetite is one of the more common adverse effects associated with methylphenidate. Although nausea is associated with this drug, vomiting is not. Photosensitivity is not associated with this drug. Because of decreased appetite, the client will not gain more weight.

🔑 CN: Pharmacological and parenteral therapies; CL: Evaluate

89. **2.** The pH of 7.26 indicates that the body is in a state of acidosis. The elevated partial pressure of carbon dioxide value accompanied by a normal bicarbonate value indicates that the acid-base imbalance is respiratory acidosis. The additional clinical findings of headache, dizziness, and increased pulse rate, resulting from the elevated partial pressure of carbon dioxide, further support this diagnosis.

🔑 CN: Physiological adaptation;
CL: Analyze

90. **1.** Children with osteomyelitis need a diet that is high in protein and calories. Milk, eggs, cheese, meat, fish, and beans are the best sources of these nutrients.

🔑 CN: Physiological adaptation;
CL: Synthesize

91. 1, 2. The purpose of CQI is to improve a local process to benefit clients and providers; it is required by the institution, regulatory, or accrediting agencies. The approach to the problem can be retrospective or concurrent; institutional review board (IRB approval) is not required unless the results will be made available to external parties, and specific clients could be identified. CQI is performed by clinicians and managers who are part of the process being studied; the timeframe is continuous or cyclical.

CN: Management of care; CL: Synthesize

92. 4. This client has indications of peripheral artery disease (PAD) and needs additional follow-up. Increasing walking or exercising the legs and feet likely will not be sufficient to improve peripheral circulation. Muscle cramping is a result of inadequate arterial circulation. Increasing potassium will not decrease the cramping.

CN: Physiological adaptation;
CL: Synthesize

93. 2. Tracheostomy tubes are associated with several potential complications, including laryngeal nerve damage, bleeding, and infection. Tracheostomy tubes do not cause decreased cardiac output, pneumothorax, or acute respiratory distress syndrome.

CN: Physiological adaptation;
CL: Analyze

94. 1. To reduce the risk of crystalluria, the client should drink 2,000 to 3,000 mL of water a day, not 1,000 to 1,500 mL. The client should not take an antacid before taking ciprofloxacin. An antacid decreases the absorption of the drug. The client should let the **HCP** 📖 know if vomiting occurs from the medication. The client may get light-headed from the ciprofloxacin. If so, the client should not drive a motor vehicle and should contact the HCP.

CN: Pharmacological and parenteral therapies; CL: Evaluate

95. 4. The nurse should instruct the client to increase her intake of calcium because there is a slight increase in the risk of osteoporosis with this medication. Weight-bearing exercises are also advised. The drug may also impair glucose tolerance in women who are at risk for diabetes.

CN: Pharmacological and parenteral therapies; CL: Synthesize

96. 4. Stress management is not beneficial to the client with Alzheimer's disease because of cognitive impairment, confusion, and short-term memory loss. Reminiscence group, walking, and pet therapy are beneficial.

CN: Psychosocial integrity;
CL: Synthesize

97. 3. The incisions made for upper abdominal surgeries, such as cholecystectomies, are near the diaphragm and make deep breathing painful. Incentive spirometry, which encourages deep breathing, is essential to prevent atelectasis after surgery. The client is not maintained on bed rest for several days. The client is encouraged to ambulate by the first postoperative day, even with drainage tubes in place. Nasogastric tubes do not inhibit deep breathing and coughing.

CN: Physiological adaptation; CL: Apply

98. 1, 3. When a child with hemophilia develops bleeding into a joint, the parents should have the child rest and begin factor VIII therapy. If therapy is started immediately, usually other interventions such as ice are not necessary. Heat causes vasodilation and promotes bleeding. Starting factor VIII immediately helps prevent chronic joint disease. Starting physical therapy further traumatizes the joint, possibly increasing the bleeding. Applying a topical agent does not control internal bleeding.

CN: Reduction of risk potential;
CL: Create

99. 1. When cleaning the skin around an incision and drain, the nurse should clean the incision and drain separately to avoid contaminating either wound. This is applying the principle of working from the least contaminated area to the most contaminated area. In this case, both areas are fresh wounds and should be kept separate.

CN: Management of care; CL: Apply

100. 4. The aminoglycoside antibiotic gentamicin sulfate should not be applied to large denuded areas because toxicity and systemic absorption are possible. The nurse should instruct the client to avoid excessive sun exposure because gentamicin sulfate can cause photosensitivity. The client should be instructed to apply the cream or ointment for only the length of time prescribed because a superinfection can occur from overuse. The client should contact the **HCP** 📖 if the condition worsens after use.

CN: Pharmacological and parenteral therapies; CL: Evaluate

101. 2. The priority for ongoing care for this child is to prevent injury while maintaining normal growth and interests. As with all chronic illnesses, there is a potential for self-esteem problems, but no data are presented to support this as a priority for care planning. The parents should have a good understanding of the disease process and realize the importance of obtaining regular health care for their child. The client may have episodes of acute pain, for the child who has bleeding into a joint, but this is a transient situation.

CN: Reduction of risk potential;
CL: Synthesize

102. **3.** A 3-year-old child responds best to distraction during a procedure because of the typical level of cognitive development of a 3-year-old and the fear of painful events. Preparation for the procedure should be done immediately beforehand, so that the child will not become too frightened. A 3-year-old is not concerned about the why of the procedure but about whether the procedure will hurt. This child is too young for verbal explanations alone because of the limited verbal abilities at this age and the fear of a painful event.

🔑 CN: Health promotion and maintenance; CL: Synthesize

103. **3.** Lisinopril is an angiotensin-converting enzyme (ACE) inhibitor. Hyperkalemia can be a side effect of ACE inhibitors. Because of this side effect, ACE inhibitors should not be administered with potassium-sparing diuretics.

🔑 CN: Pharmacological and parenteral therapies; CL: Analyze

104. **2.** The interpreter may have been delayed. Therefore, the nurse's best action would be to reschedule the child's appointment when the interpreter can be scheduled as well. Because the mother does not speak English, there is no point in examining the infant because history information is needed and most likely would be too difficult to obtain. Asking the mother to stay longer is rude to her. Also, doing so would probably be difficult because of the communication gap. If the interpreter is delayed, paging one more time will not help.

🔑 CN: Management of care; CL: Synthesize

105. **3.** Nitroglycerin in all dosage forms (sublingual, transdermal, or intravenous) should be shielded from light to prevent deterioration. The client should be instructed to keep the nitroglycerin in the dark container that is supplied by the pharmacy, and it should not be removed or placed in another container.

🔑 CN: Pharmacological and parenteral therapies; CL: Apply

106. **4.** Medication noncompliance is a primary cause of exacerbation in chronic mental illnesses. Of the issues listed, medications should be addressed first. Other issues, such as family, marriage, and finances, can be addressed as client stabilization is maintained.

🔑 CN: Psychosocial integrity; CL: Synthesize

107. **4.** IV fluids should not be infused for longer than 24 hours because of the risk of bacterial growth in the solution. The appropriate action for the nurse to take is to discontinue the current TPN solution, change the tubing, and hang a new bag of solution. Changing the filter does not decrease the risk of contamination. Notifying the HCP 📖 for a change in flow rate is not an acceptable solution.

🔑 CN: Pharmacological and parenteral therapies; CL: Synthesize

108. **2.** The client who drinks alcohol while taking disulfiram experiences sweating, flushing of the neck and face, tachycardia, hypotension, a throbbing headache, nausea and vomiting, palpitations, dyspnea, tremor, and weakness.

🔑 CN: Pharmacological and parenteral therapies; CL: Analyze

109. **3.** The nurse's first response is to further assess the client's pain. After a thorough assessment, additional appropriate actions may be to notify the HCP 📖, administer an analgesic, and administer oxygen.

🔑 CN: Basic care and comfort; CL: Synthesize

110. **4.** Trisomy 13 (Patau's syndrome) is an autosomal disorder. Characteristics include cleft lip and palate, polydactyly, malformed ears, and mental retardation. These neonates typically die during infancy. A webbed neck is associated with Turner's syndrome (45 total chromosomes). Small testes and absence of sperm are associated with Klinefelter's syndrome (47 chromosomes). Congenital heart defects are associated with trisomy 21 (Down syndrome) and trisomy 18 (Edwards' syndrome).

🔑 CN: Physiological adaptation; CL: Synthesize

111. **1.** The nurse should instruct the client to take the medication immediately or as soon as she remembers that she missed the medication. There is only a slight risk that the client will become pregnant when only one pill has been missed, so there is no need to use another form of contraception. However, if the client wishes to increase the chances of not getting pregnant, a condom can be used by the male partner. The client should not omit the missed pill and then restart the medication in the morning because there is a possibility that ovulation can occur, after which intercourse could result in pregnancy. Taking two pills is not necessary and also will result in putting the client off her schedule.

🔑 CN: Pharmacological and parenteral therapies; CL: Synthesize

112. 2. Neurologic symptoms, such as footdrop, or bowel or bladder changes, should be reported to the **HCP** 📖 immediately. When musculoskeletal strain causes back pain, these symptoms may take 4 to 6 weeks to resolve. As an accompanying symptom of acute low back pain, the client may have a diffuse, aching sensation in the L4 to L5 area, pain in the lower back when the leg is lifted, or pain that radiates to the hip.

🔑 CN: Reduction of risk potential;
CL: Analyze

113. 2. Taking ginseng when on insulin is not encouraged because ginseng increases the risk of hypoglycemia. Ginseng can be therapeutic in certain situations but is potentially harmful for clients taking insulin. Taking ginseng with a carbohydrate will not offset the effect of the ginseng.

🔑 CN: Pharmacological and parenteral therapies; CL: Synthesize

114. 1. Sudden, sharp pain with breathing or coughing on the affected side, tachypnea, dyspnea, diminished or absent breath sounds on the affected side, tachycardia, anxiety, and restlessness indicate a pneumothorax, which can be a complication of inserting a central venous pressure line. The other findings are within normal limits.

🔑 CN: Physiological adaptation;
CL: Analyze

115. 2. The expected effect of lactulose is for the client to have two to three soft stools a day to help reduce the pH and serum ammonia levels, which will prevent hepatic encephalopathy.

🔑 CN: Pharmacological and parenteral therapies; CL: Evaluate

116. 3. Leukocytosis, an increased white blood cell count, indicates the presence of inflammation, infection, or a leukemia process. In inflammation and infection, the client's sedimentation rate is increased. Thrombocytopenia, a platelet deficiency, occurs in the client with leukemia, immunocompromised client, client with aplastic anemia, or client with other conditions. Erythrocytosis, an elevation of the red blood cell count, occurs in polycythemia vera.

🔑 CN: Physiological adaptation; CL: Analyze

117. 2. A fractured femur, especially an open fracture, can cause much soft tissue damage and lead to significant blood loss. Hypovolemic shock can develop. Cardiogenic shock occurs when cardiac output is decreased as a result of ineffective pumping. Neurogenic shock occurs as a result of an impaired autonomic nervous system function. Anaphylactic shock is the result of an allergic reaction.

🔑 CN: Physiological adaptation;
CL: Analyze

118. 4. This girl has an exaggeration of the lumbar spine, swayback, or lordosis. Kyphosis is an increased convexity or roundness of the curve of the thoracic spine. Scoliosis is a lateral curvature of the spine.

🔑 CN: Health promotion and maintenance;
CL: Analyze

119. 4. The most appropriate action is to report the swelling, loss of mobility, and unrelieved pain to the **HCP** 📖. These symptoms are indicators of neurovascular impairment. Administering opioids will not eliminate the cause of the problem, which is unrelieved pressure on nerves and blood supply. If prompt action (cutting the cast) is not taken to relieve the pressure, permanent muscular and neurologic injury may result. Applying the ice bag would have been appropriate earlier to decrease or prevent swelling, but applying it at this time could actually lead to further decreased circulation. The arm should be elevated, but the nurse cannot wait 30 minutes to reassess the client without risking permanent damage.

🔑 CN: Reduction of risk potential;
CL: Synthesize

120. 1. Prostaglandin F_{2a} promotes uterine contractions, thereby minimizing uterine atony and subsequent hemorrhage. Possible side effects include nausea, tachycardia, hypertension, and diarrhea. Abdominal distention is not associated with the use of prostaglandin F_{2a}.

🔑 CN: Pharmacological and parenteral therapies; CL: Analyze

121. 2. Morphine can cause urinary retention. The nurse should assess the client for urinary hesitancy or retention and note the urinary output. It is not necessary to take the apical heart rate after each dose of morphine. Mental status should be assessed after each dose because morphine can cause such effects as sedation, delirium, and disorientation. Assessing for pedal edema is not necessary.

🔑 CN: Pharmacological and parenteral therapies; CL: Analyze

122. 1. Before 32 weeks' gestation, most neonates have difficulty coordinating sucking and swallowing reflexes along with breathing. Increased respiratory distress may occur with bottle-feeding. Bottle-feedings can be given after the neonate shows sucking and swallowing behaviors. High-calorie formulas can be given by bottle or by gavage feeding. Although frequent feeding prevents hypoglycemia, the feeding does not have to be given via a gavage tube. Although these neonates can be stressed by cold, they can be kept warm with blankets while being bottle-fed or fed while in the warm isolette environment.

🔑 CN: Health promotion and maintenance;
CL: Apply

123. **1, 2, 4.** After bowel surgery, an NG tube attached to low intermittent suction is used to remove gastric fluids. The amount of fluid from the NG tube suction is important because it contributes to the client's overall fluid and electrolyte balance. IV fluids are used to maintain hydration, and intake and output is measured to determine hydration status. Postoperative vital signs are assessed more frequently than every 6 hours. Bowel sounds will be auscultated to determine when they return. Measuring abdominal girth is not necessary following colostomy reversal.

⁦ CN: Physiological adaptation; CL: Synthesize

124. **2.** Regularly scheduled rest periods during the day along with 8 to 10 hours of sleep at night helps relieve the fatigue, pain, and stiffness associated with rheumatoid arthritis. Even with mild rheumatoid arthritis, the client may find it difficult to perform activities of daily living without some rest periods. Spending 1 day a week in bed to relieve fatigue does not adequately manage the disease. The client must recognize the need for rest before feeling exhausted because overexertion can cause exacerbations. In addition, prolonged periods of inactivity can increase joint stiffness and pain. Getting up early to do household chores before the children are awake does not allow for adequate rest.

⁦ CN: Basic care and comfort; CL: Evaluate

125. **3.** For the child with hemophilia who is actively bleeding, the nurse should apply direct pressure to the injured area for 10 minutes continuously along with elevating the leg. The continuous application of direct pressure aids in stopping the bleeding. Elevating the leg reduces blood flow to the area, thereby minimizing the extent of blood loss. Although ice will cause local vasoconstriction and slow the bleeding, applying continuous direct pressure is essential.

⁦ CN: Physiological adaptation; CL: Synthesize

126. **2.** The nurse should assess for signs of impending shock such as diaphoresis. The client would have hypotension, dysuria, and cool skin.

⁦ CN: Pharmacological and parenteral therapies; CL: Analyze

127. **4.** Hypothyroidism is not associated with pancytopenia. Various anemias are associated with pancytopenia owing to the reduction in all cellular elements of the blood. Bleeding and clotting difficulties can be associated with pancytopenia. Infection is a common danger associated with pancytopenia.

⁦ CN: Physiological adaptation; CL: Analyze

128. **2.** The client's return to the emergency department and her statement about not knowing what to do about being abused by her husband indicate that the client is asking for help. The nurse's best course of action is to explain the various options available to her. This helps the client make decisions based on appropriate knowledge. Research reveals that women are more likely to be killed by partners than by strangers. Although the client can legally leave her husband, this answer provides the client with no safety options. Listing ways to avoid making the husband angry ignores the dynamics of abuse and blames the victim.

⁦ CN: Psychosocial integrity; CL: Synthesize

129. **3.** When dextrose is abruptly discontinued, rebound hypoglycemia can occur. The nurse should assess the client for symptoms of hypoglycemia. Essential fatty acid deficiency is very unlikely to occur because some of these fatty acids are stored. Preventing dehydration or malnutrition is not the reason for tapering the infusion rate; the client's hydration and nutritional status and ability to maintain adequate intake must be established before TPN is discontinued.

⁦ CN: Pharmacological and parenteral therapies; CL: Apply

130. **3.** The nurse places a postoperative client who has had abdominal surgery in low Fowler's position. This position relaxes abdominal muscles and promotes maximum respiratory and cardiovascular function.

⁦ CN: Reduction of risk potential; CL: Synthesize

131. **1.** It is most important to know the child's serum potassium level when administering digoxin. Digoxin increases contractility of the heart and increases renal perfusion, resulting in a diuretic effect with increased loss of potassium and sodium. Hypokalemia increases the risk of digoxin toxicity. Verifying the dosage is specified by facility policy and varies among facilities. Although the child may take the medication better from the mother than from the nurse, asking the mother to give the medication is not necessary. In addition, this would be done after the nurse has checked the electrolyte levels. Teaching the parent how to measure the child's heart rate can be done at any time, not necessarily when preparing to give digoxin.

⁦ CN: Pharmacological and parenteral therapies; CL: Synthesize

132. **2.** There is a direct interaction between the effects of insulin and those of beta-blockers. The nurse must be aware that there is a potential for increased hypoglycemic effects of insulin when a beta-blocker is added to the client's medication regimen. The client's blood sugar should be monitored. Ketoacidosis occurs in hyperglycemia. Although a decrease in the incidence of ketoacidosis could occur when a beta-blocker is added, the direct result is an increase in the hypoglycemic effect of insulin.

☛ CN: Pharmacological and parenteral therapies; CL: Apply

133. 4. During the emergent phase of burn management, there is a massive shift of fluid from the blood vessels (intravascular compartment) into the tissues (interstitial compartment). The result of this shift is hypovolemic shock and edema formation. The fluid shift is caused by increased capillary permeability that allows water, sodium, and protein to shift to the tissues. As the emergent period ends and capillary permeability returns to normal, the fluid in the interstitial compartment will return to the intravascular compartment.

☛ CN: Physiological adaptation; CL: Analyze

134. 1. The client with sensorineural hearing loss has difficulty hearing high-pitched sounds. Aging and ototoxicity are two causes of sensorineural hearing loss. The client's ability to speak is not affected. The client who cannot assign meaning to sound has central hearing loss. Vertigo is commonly an indication of an inner ear problem.

☛ CN: Physiological adaptation; CL: Analyze

135. 3. A urine output of 30 to 50 mL/h indicates adequate fluid replacement in the client with burns. An increase in body weight may indicate fluid retention. A urine output greater than fluid intake does not represent a fluid balance. Depending on the client, blood pressure of 90/60 mm Hg could indicate the presence of a hypovolemic state; by itself, it does not indicate adequate fluid replacement.

☛ CN: Physiological adaptation; CL: Evaluate

136. 3. Commonly, when a child appears better, the parents stop the medication. Unfortunately, the infection remains. Therefore, the nurse needs to explain that all of the medication must be administered to clear up the infection. Explaining why the medicine should be continued is more helpful to parents than saying it needs to be given. Telling the parent that stopping the medication is not what is best for the child implies blame and is condescending.

☛ CN: Pharmacological and parenteral therapies; CL: Synthesize

137. 1. Many clients who experience abuse are hesitant to talk about it and need help to do so. The nurse should ask the client directly about abuse when it is suspected, using a sensitive, empathetic, and compassionate approach. In this way, the client can feel comfortable revealing information about the abuse. Telling the client that it is difficult to believe her injuries resulted from a fall is not helpful because it is blameful and puts the client on the defensive. Asking the client what she did to make someone hit her or discussing what she can do the next time blames and alienates the client.

☛ CN: Psychosocial integrity; CL: Synthesize

138. 1. A primary outcome for the care of the client in shock is to achieve adequate tissue perfusion, thus avoiding multiple organ dysfunction. The lungs are susceptible to injury, especially acute respiratory distress syndrome. Vasoconstriction occurs as a compensatory mechanism until the client enters the irreversible stage of shock.

☛ CN: Reduction of risk potential; CL: Evaluate

139. 3. The client with emphysema is commonly underweight in appearance. The weight loss may be caused by the increased energy required to support the work of breathing. Frequent coughing, bronchospasms, and copious sputum are clinical manifestations of chronic bronchitis.

☛ CN: Physiological adaptation; CL: Analyze

140. 3, 4, 5. The neurologic system can be affected and cause long-term consequences in a young child exposed to lead. Common behavioral effects include hyperactivity, impulsivity, and aggression. Seizures may occur in a child with high-dose lead exposure. Depression is not usually associated with lead exposure.

☛ CN: Physiological adaptation; CL: Apply

141. 2. The incident report includes only what the nurse saw and did—the objective data. The nurse does not try to interpret the likely cause of the incident, include statements from the client about the incident, or comment on extenuating circumstances.

☛ CN: Management of care; CL: Apply

142. 2. The serum cholesterol is within normal range for this client indicating the medication is effective. Since the cholesterol levels are within normal limits, it is likely that the client is taking the medication and asking may indicate the nurse has doubts or mistrusts that the client is taking the medication. The client does not need to change the diet at this point. Hemoglobin and hematocrit are not affected by simvastatin; since liver damage is a side effect of simvastatin, the nurse could review the liver function studies.

☛ CN: Pharmacologic and parenteral therapies; CL: Synthesize

143. 3. The area on the abdomen where the transverse incision will be made should be marked by the surgeon.

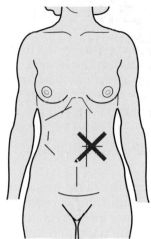

🔑 CN: Reduction of risk potential;
CL: Evaluate

144. 1, 2, 3, 4, 6. Diabetic ketoacidosis is a potentially life-threatening problem. The state of unconsciousness requires very astute monitoring of the neurologic condition. Frequent assessments of neurologic status (including the client's ability to respond to stimuli), blood pressure, and urinary output need to be documented. Assessment of skin condition for the presence of lesions, bruises, ulcers, or bumps is documented to assess for possible injuries, such as falls associated with head injury or internal injuries. Although it would be helpful to know how long the client has had diabetes, this information is not essential to document.

🔑 CN: Physiological adaptation;
CL: Analyze

145. 3. The medications prescribed for, administered to, or dispensed to the client while under the care of a healthcare organization are compared to those on the list, and any discrepancies (e.g., omissions, duplications, potential interactions) are resolved. A complete list of the client's medications is communicated to the next provider of service when a client is referred or transferred to another setting, service, practitioner, or level of care within or outside the organization. The complete, accurate list of medications is also provided to the client on discharge from the organization. The next provider of service checks the Medication Reconciliation List again to make sure it is accurate and in concert with any new medications to be prescribed.

🔑 CN: Safety and infection control;
CL: Analyze

146. 1. A neonate born by cesarean section has not had the benefit of the chest-squeezing action of a vaginal birth, which helps remove some of the nasopharyngeal secretions. The nurse should place the neonate under the radiant warmer and suction the mouth and nares with a bulb syringe to remove nasopharyngeal secretions. A high-pitched cry is associated with neurologic involvement or neonatal drug withdrawal and is unrelated to cesarean birth. Skull fractures may occur with difficult vaginal births and are not typically seen with cesarean births. Decreased muscle tone is associated with oversedation, neurologic impairment, or use of general anesthesia.

🔑 CN: Health promotion and maintenance;
CL: Analyze

147. 4. Follow-up generally involves semiannual chest radiographs. Recurrence usually occurs locally in the lungs and may be identified on chest radiographs. Follow-up after cancer treatment is an important component of the treatment plan. Serum markers (liver function tests) have not been shown to detect recurrence of lung cancer. There are no data to support the need for an abdominal computed tomography scan.

🔑 CN: Reduction of risk potential;
CL: Synthesize

148. 2. Accidental scaldings are usually splash related and occur on the front of the body. Any burns on the back of the body or in a well-defined circular or glove pattern may indicate physical abuse. Immersion burns on the buttocks are also suspicious injuries.

🔑 CN: Health promotion and maintenance;
CL: Analyze

149. 3. A client exhibiting mild preeclampsia is initially treated with activity restriction. Bed rest, or lying on the left side, decreases pressure on the vena cava and improves circulatory blood flow. Restriction of visitors and a quiet environment are also necessary. IV magnesium sulfate, a central nervous system depressant, is usually prescribed for the client with severe preeclampsia. Labetalol is used for the client with severe preeclampsia. Frequent monitoring of the client's blood pressure is important. However, hourly blood pressure checks are more routinely prescribed for the client with severe preeclampsia. Additionally, the client needs to rest, and checking her blood pressure hourly could interfere with her ability to rest.

🔑 CN: Reduction of risk potential;
CL: Synthesize

150. 4. Lifestyle modification to lower blood pressure includes weight reduction in clients who are overweight, reducing the intake of dietary sodium, and an increase in physical activity. Client teaching involves instruction on low-sodium diet and foods because of the propensity for high-sodium foods at fast-food restaurants. The client is of a normal weight, and alcohol intake is in moderation. Nitroprusside is a treatment for hypertensive crisis.

CN: Physiological adaptation;
CL: Synthesize

151. 4. A dry tea bag placed on the bleeding area can be effective to control bleeding from lesions on the oral mucosa. The tannic acid in the tea apparently helps control bleeding.

CN: Reduction of risk potential;
CL: Synthesize

152. 3. The three-point gait, in which the client advances the crutches and the affected leg at the same time while weight is supported on the unaffected extremity, is the appropriate gait of choice. This allows for non-weight bearing on the affected extremity. The two-point, four-point, and swing-to gaits require some weight bearing on both legs, which is contraindicated for this client.

CN: Reduction of risk potential;
CL: Evaluate

153. 4. The best treatment for a pressure ulcer is prevention. If a client has been determined to be at risk for developing a pressure ulcer, a systematic skin assessment should be conducted at least once per shift. Other preventive measures include daily gentle cleaning of the skin and avoiding harsh soaps and hot water, which are damaging to the skin. Massage of bony prominences is not done because it can increase damage to the underlying tissue. The client should be encouraged to change position at least every 2 hours to avoid pressure on any one area for a prolonged period.

CN: Reduction of risk potential;
CL: Synthesize

154. 1. The client needs further instructions when she says "I should walk with my pelvis tilted backward." Walking in this position puts greater strain on the back. The client should walk with her pelvis tilted forward. Pelvic tilt exercises can also help the client with backaches. Putting a board under the mattress makes the mattress firmer and provides more support. Squatting and not bending to pick up objects helps decrease back strain. Squatting involves the use of the large thigh muscles rather

than those of the back. Flat or low-heeled shoes provide better balance and greater support and can help decrease backaches.

CN: Reduction of risk potential;
CL: Evaluate

155. 4. Urethritis is usually the initial clinical manifestation of gonorrhea in men. The symptoms include a profuse, purulent discharge and dysuria. Complications are uncommon, but they include prostatitis and sterility. Impotence, scrotal pain, and penile lesions are not associated with gonorrhea.

CN: Safety and infection control;
CL: Analyze

156. 4. Although the nurse needs to obtain and administer the medication as soon as possible, it is inappropriate for the nurse to go to the pharmacy and request the drug without first calling the pharmacy and checking to see whether the medication was delivered. The drug may have been delivered to several appropriate spots on the unit, such as the client's drug bin, the transport system, or the delivery box. The nurse should assess the client's blood pressure to determine the immediacy of the condition for which the medication was prescribed.

CN: Safety and infection control;
CL: Synthesize

157. 3. The client with major depression suffers from lack of energy and withdrawal. The nurse should emphasize the importance of group involvement for the client to gain support from others and to see that others have similar problems and concerns. Attendance at group sessions and activities decreases social isolation and destructive rumination. The other statements are not therapeutic and interfere with increasing the client's involvement with others.

CN: Psychosocial integrity;
CL: Synthesize

158. 4. An infant's sleeping longer than usual can indicate that the child is expending too much energy to breathe and is tiring, suggesting that the child's condition is getting worse. This should be reported to the **healthcare provider (HCP)** 📖. Fewer than seven wet diapers a day indicates that the child is not drinking enough. A temperature of 100°F (37.8°C) for longer than 2 days should be reported. Clear nasal drainage is expected. However, yellow nasal drainage lasting longer than 24 hours should be reported.

CN: Reduction of risk potential;
CL: Evaluate

159. 3. The child is exhibiting signs and symptoms of possible epiglottitis. As a result, the child is at high risk for laryngospasm and airway occlusion. Therefore, the nurse should have a tracheostomy tube and setup readily available should the child experience an airway occlusion. Although acetaminophen is an antipyretic, the dosage of 600 mg to be administered rectally is too high. A typical 4-year-old weighs approximately 40 lb (18 kg). The recommended dose is 125 mg. When any type of respiratory illness, and especially epiglottitis, is suspected, putting any object, including a tongue depressor for inspection or a cotton-tipped applicator to obtain a throat culture, in the back of the mouth or throat or having the child open the mouth is inappropriate because doing so may predispose the child to laryngospasm or occlusion of the airway by a swollen epiglottis.

⚷ CN: Reduction of risk potential;
CL: Synthesize

160. 4. Direct application of warm moist heat would benefit a client with low back pain because the heat relaxes muscle spasms. Heat should not be applied to a client who has appendicitis because it can lead to rupture of the appendix and peritonitis. Ice is applied to recently sprained joints to help decrease edema. Applying heat to the area of a suspected malignancy can increase blood flow to the tumor and promote nourishment of the cancer cells.

⚷ CN: Basic care and comfort; CL: Analyze

161. 3. The client with pernicious anemia will require lifelong supplementation of vitamin B$_{12}$, available through injection or nasal spray administration. It must be given in these forms to ensure absorption. Oral vitamin B$_{12}$ would not be absorbed because the client lacks the intrinsic factor in the stomach necessary for absorption. Chelation therapy is used to extract metals at toxic levels such as in lead poisoning.

⚷ CN: Pharmacological and parenteral therapies; CL: Apply

162. 10 mL. To administer 20 mEq of potassium chloride, the nurse needs to administer 10 mL. The following formula is used to calculate the correct dosage:

$$20\,\text{mEq} / X\,\text{mL} = 2\,\text{mEq} / 1\,\text{mL}$$

$$X = 10\,\text{mL}$$

⚷ CN: Pharmacological and parenteral therapies; CL: Apply

163. 4. When a client with major depression and suicidal ideation displays a sudden elevation in mood, seems calmer, has more energy, and is more peaceful, the nurse should judge these behaviors as an indication that a suicide attempt is imminent. These symptoms may indicate relief from ambivalent thoughts about suicide and that the client has an immediate plan for killing himself.

⚷ CN: Psychosocial integrity;
CL: Analyze

164. 3. The purpose of a contraction stress test is to determine fetal response during labor. If late decelerations are noted with the contractions, the test is considered positive or abnormal. Fetal lung maturity is evaluated through amniocentesis to obtain the lecithin-sphingomyelin ratio. The nonstress test is part of the biophysical profile. Determining fetal response during movements is evaluated as part of the nonstress test.

⚷ CN: Reduction of risk potential;
CL: Apply

165. 3. Atypical pneumonia is characterized by a gradual onset of symptoms, such as dry cough, headache, sore throat, fatigue, nausea, and vomiting. Typical pneumonia is characterized by tachypnea, fever, chills, and productive cough with purulent sputum.

⚷ CN: Physiological adaptation;
CL: Analyze

166. 2. The primary reason for instructing the client with emphysema about how to pursed-lip breathe is to prolong exhalation. Prolonging exhalation helps to prevent bronchiolar collapse and the trapping of air. It does not directly prevent respiratory infection. Because pursed-lip breathing affects the expiratory phase of the respiratory cycle, it does not affect oxygenation. It may decrease shortness of breath, but this is not the primary reason for the technique.

⚷ CN: Reduction of risk potential;
CL: Apply

167. 2. The primary purpose of the automated dispensing machine for nurses is to keep an up-to-date record of the narcotic usage and count. The automated dispensing machine has eliminated the need for change-of-shift counts for narcotics. It does not include unmonitored access by nurses to narcotics, which would not be considered an advantage. The pharmacy has direct information about the narcotics being used on the client at what intervals and by whom, and it automatically records the charges of narcotics used. Not recording the charges would not be an advantage.

⚷ CN: Management of care; CL: Apply

168. 2. Blunt chest trauma can lead to respiratory failure. Maintenance of adequate oxygenation is the priority for the client. Decreasing the client's anxiety is related to maintaining effective respirations and oxygenation. Although pain is distressing to the client and can increase anxiety and decrease respiratory effectiveness, pain control is secondary to maintaining oxygenation, as is maintaining adequate circulatory volume.

🔑 CN: Physiological adaptation;
CL: Synthesize

169. 1. An episiotomy that is edematous and slightly reddened 8 hours after childbirth is normal. Therefore, the nurse should offer the client an ice pack to provide some relief from the perineal pain for the first 24 hours. An infection is present if greenish, purulent drainage is observed from the site. The edema and discoloration of the episiotomy at this time after childbirth are normal and do not indicate that a hematoma is likely to develop. A laceration when repaired should appear intact with edges well approximated, clean, and dry.

🔑 CN: Health promotion and maintenance;
CL: Analyze

170. 3. The Z-track technique is used with medications that are irritating to tissues. It allows the medication to be trapped in the muscle and prevents it from leaking back through the tissues.

🔑 CN: Basic care and comfort; CL: Apply

171. 2. The nurse should limit the amount of telephone calls the client can make. Setting limits for a client with bipolar disorder, mania, helps to control the hyperactive client who has excessive goal-directed activity, especially when it interferes with the rights of other clients. Giving the client access to a separate phone rewards the behavior. Reminding the client that others need to use the telephone will probably be futile because the client with mania is experiencing cognitive impairment and needs to be active. Taking away the client's telephone privileges is not the best action because the client has a right to use the telephone. The nurse is responsible for helping the client manage behavior by setting constructive limits.

🔑 CN: Psychosocial integrity;
CL: Synthesize

172. 4. Because a toddler is strong and moves frequently, the child needs to be restrained during the removal procedure by a total body restraint. To protect the child, the papoose board is best because the arms, legs, chest, and head can be fully restrained. A jacket restraint would immobilize only the child's upper body. Elbow restraints would immobilize only the child's arms. The father should be available to provide comfort before and after the procedure but not to hold the child down during the procedure.

🔑 CN: Safety and infection control;
CL: Synthesize

173. 4. Wheezing over one lung in the presence of a lung tumor is most likely caused by obstruction of the airway by a tumor. Exudate would be more likely to cause crackles. The client's history of smoking would not cause unilateral wheezing. Pleural effusion would produce diminished or absent breath sounds.

🔑 CN: Physiological adaptation; CL: Apply

174. 1. The client with diabetic ketoacidosis exhibits Kussmaul's respiration as well as flushed skin, dry mouth, urinary frequency, hyperglycemia, and ketonuria. Excessive hunger and high blood pressure are not associated with diabetic ketoacidosis.

🔑 CN: Reduction of risk potential;
CL: Apply

175. 4. For the client who has been receiving lithium therapy for the past 2 months, a maintenance serum lithium level of 0.6 to 1.2 mEq/L (0.6 to 1.2 mmol/L) is considered therapeutic. A lithium level >1.2 mEq/L (1.2 mmol/L) suggests toxicity.

🔑 CN: Pharmacological and parenteral therapies; CL: Analyze

176. 4, 5. The child is observed for shock that can occur following a severe burn. Shock is noted by the increasing heart rate and dropping blood pressure. This child has an adequate urine output (more than 1 mL/kg body weight), and the specific gravity is within normal range. Pain is expected and is not an indicator of shock.

🔑 CN: Physiological adaptation;
CL: Analyze

177. 4. The plan of care to treat fatigue associated with radiation therapy should include encouraging the client to remain active and to plan scheduled rest periods as necessary before activity. Engaging in activities, such as walking, has been shown to decrease the cycle of fatigue, anxiety, and depression that can occur during treatment. Fatigue is a very common side effect of radiation therapy that typically begins during the 3rd or 4th week of treatment and persists until after treatment ends. The presence of fatigue does not mean that the cancer is not responding to treatment or that the client has developed another health problem.

🔑 CN: Reduction of risk potential;
CL: Synthesize

178. 3. Shearing forces occur because of improper movement and positioning, which causes the underlying tissues and capillary blood supply to be pulled and disrupted. This leads to tissue trauma and the potential beginning of skin breakdown. To prevent shearing, clients should be moved with the use of lift sheets and other devices, thus preventing dragging of the skin across the mattress and linens. Clients should also be positioned and supported to prevent pulling or tension of the skin across bony prominences. Turning clients, if not done properly, can cause shearing injuries. Keeping the skin clean, dry, and moisturized is an important aspect of care, but care must be used to decrease the amount of pulling forces exerted on the tissues.

♞— CN: Reduction of risk potential;
CL: Apply

179. 4. The proper use of crutches requires supporting the body weight primarily on the hands. Improper use of crutches can cause nerve damage from excess pressure on the axillary nerve.

♞— CN: Reduction of risk potential;
CL: Apply

180. 3. The nurse promotes consistent limit setting for the client with the aggressive and impulsive behaviors of a conduct disorder. It is not appropriate for the nurse to allow autonomy or elicit a description of feelings; assertiveness classes are also inappropriate.

♞— CN: Psychosocial integrity; CL: Apply

181. 2. For the child with croup, assessing the child's respiratory status is the priority. It is especially important to assess airway patency because laryngeal spasms can occur suddenly. After the nurse has assessed the toddler's respiratory status, having a tracheostomy set at the bedside would be the next priority. Monitoring vital signs is important, as is ensuring adequate fluid intake to keep secretions loose, but assessing respiratory status is key.

♞— CN: Physiological adaptation;
CL: Synthesize

182. 2. IV solutions are prescribed based upon the fluid and electrolyte status of the client, so laboratory results should be monitored first. Safety recommendations are for standard premixed solutions. If solutions are not premixed, additives are completed by the pharmacy, not at the bedside. Potassium chloride is never given by IV push because this could be fatal. Administration guidelines require no more than 10 mEq (10 mmol/L) of potassium chloride be infused per hour on a general medical-surgical unit. An infusion device or pump is required for safe administration.

♞— CN: Pharmacological and parenteral therapies; CL: Synthesize

183. 3, 1, 4, 2. Even with such a blatant suicide clue, it is still important to confirm that he is truly suicidal. Then, it is crucial to know what methods of suicide are available to him. Before asking for a psychiatric consult, the client needs to understand that the nurse cares, is empathetic, and will take actions to protect him from harm.

♞— CN: Safety and infection control;
CL: Analyze

184. 1. Neuromuscular irritability is usually the first indication that a client has developed a low serum calcium level. Numbness and tingling around the mouth as well as in the extremities is an early sign of neuromuscular irritability. Depressed reflexes, decreased memory, and ventricular dysrhythmias are indications of hypercalcemia.

♞— CN: Physiological adaptation; CL: Analyze

185. 2. In emphysema, the anteroposterior diameter of the chest wall is increased. As a result, the client's breath sounds may be diminished. Fine crackles are present when there is fluid in the lungs. Stridor occurs as a result of a partially obstructed larynx or trachea; stridor can be heard without auscultation. A pleural friction rub is present when pleural surfaces are inflamed and rub together.

♞— CN: Physiological adaptation; CL: Analyze

186. 4. The client with paranoid personality disorder interprets the actions of others as personal threats, feels vulnerable, and is overly sensitive to others' motives. Saying "They are laughing at a joke John told. They are not laughing at you" is a simple explanation of others' behavior, which helps to decrease the client's suspiciousness and promote trust. The other statements do not help the client to realistically interpret situations and the behavior of others and are not helpful in reducing the client's suspicions or mistrust.

♞— CN: Psychosocial integrity;
CL: Synthesize

187. 4. Mebendazole is prescribed for household members older than 2 years. Although the child's 18-month-old brother would not receive the drug, the 4-year-old sister and parents would.

♞— CN: Pharmacological and parenteral therapies; CL: Synthesize

188. 3. Loss of height and back pain are early indications of the disease that are caused by collapse of the vertebrae. Later signs include the dowager's hump and loss of the waistline. The dowager's hump is a later sign of osteoporosis that occurs when the vertebrae can no longer support the upper body in an upright position. Fair-skinned, small-boned, White, and Asian women are at greater risk for osteoporosis. Conventional radiographs are little help because more than 30% of the bone mass must be lost before the disease is detected. High-density bone scans can detect the disease earlier.

⚿ CN: Reduction of risk potential;
CL: Synthesize

189. 3. The primary reason for evaluating gastric residual is to determine whether gastric emptying has been delayed and the stomach is becoming over-distended from the feeding. With delayed gastric emptying, the possibility of aspiration of the feeding into the lungs is increased. It is not possible to determine how well the client's body is absorbing nutrients or whether the client is receiving enough feeding by checking the gastric residual. It is not necessary to keep partially digested formula separate from undigested formula.

⚿ CN: Reduction of risk potential;
CL: Apply

190. 1. The baseline values of the client's partial thromboplastin time, bleeding time, and prothrombin time should be obtained. Potassium levels do not indicate a client's coagulation time. The Lee-White clotting time or baseline fibrin split product does not need to be established before starting tissue plasminogen activator or alteplase.

⚿ CN: Reduction of risk potential;
CL: Apply

191. 2, 4, 5. Clients with hepatitis A commonly experience fatigue and altered nutrition due to anorexia and nausea. Because of the severe fatigue associated with hepatitis, clients are encouraged to rest and restrict activity during the active phase of the disease. It is important that frequent rest periods be planned throughout the day. Clients may experience nausea and vomiting; thus, providing relief is important. Small, frequent meals help clients manage the anorexia associated with hepatitis. An exercise program is not appropriate due to the need for rest. Clients with hepatitis do not experience pain. All medications administered to clients with hepatitis need to be evaluated for their potential for hepatotoxicity.

⚿ CN: Physiological adaptation;
CL: Synthesize

192. 4. Third-degree heart block occurs when atrial stimuli are blocked at the atrioventricular junction. Impulses from the atria and ventricles are conducted independently of each other. The atrial rate is 60 to 100 bpm; the ventricular rate is usually 10 to 60 bpm.

⚿ CN: Reduction of risk potential;
CL: Analyze

193. 1. Clients with borderline personality disorder have fears of abandonment and seek attention. Clients are dependent and fear being alone; this stems from disapproval, feelings of being abandoned, and not having needs met earlier in their life. The nurse intervenes by reducing attention-seeking behaviors and abandonment fears to help with intense feelings and emotions.

⚿ CN: Psychosocial integrity; CL: Analyze

194. 4. The application of restraints places the client in a vulnerable, confined position. The nurse should check on the client every 30 minutes while restrained to make sure that the client is safe. The client should be able to move while the restraints are in place. The restraints should be removed every 2 hours to provide skin care and exercise the extremities. Restraints should not be secured to the side rails; they should be secured to the movable bed frame so that when the bed is adjusted, the restraints will not be pulled too tightly.

⚿ CN: Safety and infection control;
CL: Synthesize

195. 3. The most appropriate response is "Alcohol dependence is a disease that can be treated" because it conveys hope. It also emphasizes that the client has a treatable illness, which is helpful in reducing denial and guilt and encouraging the client to seek and comply with treatment. Clients often cannot answer "why" questions. The other statements are judgmental and guilt producing, possibly leading to denial and furthering the need for alcohol.

⚿ CN: Psychosocial integrity;
CL: Synthesize

196. 2. Raisins are high in nutritional value but are sticky and have a high sugar content. The raisin can stick to the teeth and act like high-sugar foods in promoting tooth decay. Although anything can be aspirated, round, hard, smooth foods are more easily aspirated than raisins, which are soft and chewy. Raisins need to be chewed thoroughly for maximum nutritional value.

⚿ CN: Health promotion and maintenance;
CL: Evaluate

197. 1. Aspirin is an antiplatelet medication. The use of aspirin is contraindicated while taking warfarin because it will potentiate the drug's effects. Diphenhydramine and pseudoephedrine do not affect blood coagulation. Digoxin is not an over-the-counter medication; it requires a prescription.

🔑 CN: Pharmacological and parenteral therapies; CL: Synthesize

198. 1. The nurse should inform the client that carbamazepine can decrease the effects of oral anticoagulants. Carbamazepine can increase the serum concentration of verapamil and can decrease the serum concentration of other anticonvulsants and the effects of oral contraceptives.

🔑 CN: Pharmacological and parenteral therapies; CL: Apply

199. 2. Viral hepatitis causes fatigue. It is important for the client to rest to allow the liver to recover. Activity levels are resumed gradually as the client begins to recover. Abdominal pain is not a common manifestation of hepatitis. The client typically does not have difficulty breathing or experience edema.

🔑 CN: Physiological adaptation; CL: Synthesize

200. 1. The mother should be encouraged to hold and cuddle her child to provide needed emotional support. Such activities as helping the child play with toys, reading stories, and staying with the child would not be contraindicated but do not offer as much emotional support as holding and cuddling.

🔑 CN: Psychosocial integrity; CL: Synthesize

201. 2. The best strategy to affect child seat belt safety is to attend the school board meeting and advocate for educational programming. The programming could be simple and done quickly. This action also targets the best audience.

🔑 CN: Health promotion and maintenance; CL: Synthesize

202. 3. A basic principle of rehabilitation, including cardiac rehabilitation, is that rehabilitation begins on hospital admission. Early rehabilitation is essential to promote maximum functional ability as the client recovers from an illness. Delaying rehabilitation activities is associated with poorer client outcomes.

🔑 CN: Basic care and comfort; CL: Apply

203. 1. The goal of the intervention is to decrease the child's work of breathing by decreasing pressure on the diaphragm and increase chest expansion by increasing the pull of gravity on the diaphragm.

Placing the client in high Fowler's position accomplishes this. Side-lying positions make it more difficult to expand the side of the lung closest to the bed. The prone or supine position does not decrease the work of breathing unless the head of the bed is raised.

🔑 CN: Physiological adaptation; CL: Synthesize

204. 4. Immediately after chest tube removal, a petrolatum gauze is placed over the wound and covered with a dry sterile dressing. This serves as an airtight seal to prevent air leakage or air movement in either direction. Bandages or straps are not applied directly over wounds. Mesh gauze allows air movement.

🔑 CN: Management of care; CL: Apply

205. 3. The most appropriate action is to contact the **HCP** 📖 to verify that the prescription is correct. Although 60 mg of morphine is a significant dose, the amount of morphine administered to a client can vary widely, especially if a client has been taking morphine for an extended period and has developed a tolerance to the medication. The safest approach is for the nurse to verify prescriptions that do not appear to fall within the norm. Administering the medication without verification is unsafe. The nurse cannot decide to reduce the amount of a prescribed medication without a prescription. Asking another nurse to review the prescription is not inappropriate; however, checking with the HCP to verify the prescription should be done.

🔑 CN: Pharmacological and parenteral therapies; CL: Synthesize

206. 4. **RRTs** 📖, or medical emergency teams, provide a team approach to evaluate and treat immediately clients with alterations in vital signs or neurological deterioration. Calling the neurosurgeon or consulting the CNS may not result in a rapid response. The Trendelenburg position is usually used in treating shock, but because the client has had brain surgery, the head should not be lower than the trunk.

🔑 CN: Physiological adaptation; CL: Synthesize

207. 1. Before paracentesis, the client is asked to void. This is done to collapse the bladder and decrease the risk of accidental bladder perforation. The abdomen is not prepared with an antiseptic cleansing solution. The client is placed in a Fowler's position. The client does not need to be put on NPO status before the procedure.

🔑 CN: Reduction of risk potential; CL: Apply

208. 1. Children who are being abused may demonstrate behaviors such as withdrawal, apparent fear of parents, and lack of an appropriate reaction, such as crying and attempting to get away when faced with a frightening event (an examination or procedure).

⚿ CN: Psychosocial integrity; CL: Analyze

209. 3. The nurse should include teaching the client and family about the physical, physiologic, and psychological effects of substances to educate them about the potential injury, illness, and disability that can result from substance use. Teaching about the role of the family in perpetuating the problem, the family's responsibility for the client, or the reasons that could have led the client to use the substance is inappropriate and based on an erroneous assumption. Including these topics blames the family for the problem and attempts to rationalize the use of the substance.

⚿ CN: Psychosocial integrity; CL: Synthesize

210. 2. Postoperative care after a laparoscopic cholecystectomy includes removal of the dressing from the incisional site the day after surgery and allowing the client to bathe or shower. The client can resume a normal diet but may wish to follow a low-fat diet for a few weeks after surgery. Nausea is not expected to last for several days after surgery. The client usually can return to work within 1 week.

⚿ CN: Reduction of risk potential; CL: Evaluate

211. 1. In Mexican culture, children are highly valued and are closely protected by godparents. The tradition of the family is all-encompassing, and the **healthcare provider (HCP)** 📖 gains trust and improved compliance rates by including the family in teaching and healthcare matters. Typically, older adults are highly regarded and respected in Asian cultures.

⚿ CN: Psychosocial integrity; CL: Apply

212. 2. Many vitamin and mineral deficiencies can result in anemia. All of these vitamins and minerals need to be assessed, preferably through a nutrition assessment. Deficiencies of vitamins A, B_6, and C result in a small cell, microcytic anemia. Folate and vitamin B_{12} deficiencies result in a large cell, macrocytic anemia. Iron, copper, and vitamin E deficiencies can also result in anemia.

⚿ CN: Physiological adaptation; CL: Analyze

213. 3. Women with diabetes mellitus generally have neonates who are large but physically immature. Other common findings in these infants are hypoglycemia, hypocalcemia, hyperbilirubinemia, polycythemia, renal thrombosis, and congestive anomalies. The neonates do not exhibit hypertonia, hyperactivity, or scaly skin.

⚿ CN: Health promotion and maintenance; CL: Analyze

214. 2. The imbalance between the client's intake and output indicates that the client may be retaining urine since the removal of his Foley catheter. The nurse's first action is to validate this assumption by assessing for bladder distention. Applying a condom catheter will not relieve urinary retention; condom catheters are meant to be used for incontinence. A urine specimen for a culture is obtained if a urinary infection is suspected, but this is not a priority at this point. Kegel exercises are helpful in controlling urinary dribbling but do not treat retention.

⚿ CN: Reduction of risk potential; CL: Synthesize

215. 2. Because of the poor emptying of blood from the atrial chambers, there is an increased risk for clot formation around the valves. The clots become dislodged and travel through the circulatory system. As a result, cerebrovascular accident is a common complication of atrial fibrillation.

⚿ CN: Physiological adaptation; CL: Analyze

216. 2. Griseofulvin is associated with photosensitivity reactions. Therefore, the nurse should instruct the parents to have the child avoid intense sunlight. Griseofulvin is best absorbed when administered after a high-fat meal. Treatment with griseofulvin typically lasts for at least 1 month. There are no indications that increased fluid intake affects absorption.

⚿ CN: Pharmacological and parenteral therapies; CL: Synthesize

217. 1, 2, 3, 4. To help the client with a borderline personality cope with and control emotions, the nurse assists the client to identify which emotions he or she is experiencing, plans to decrease the number of impulsive acts the client completes, and promotes client use of a journal in which emotions and coping techniques can be recorded. The nurse also encourages the client to delay immediate gratification of impulses. The nurse may use confrontation, but this is a component of the development of a therapeutic relationship and does not help the client cope and control emotions.

⚿ CN: Psychosocial integrity; CL: Synthesize

218. 2. After cystoscopy with biopsy, the nurse would assess for excessive hematuria, which might indicate hemorrhage caused by the biopsy. Catheters are not routinely inserted after cystoscopy. The nurse would not assess for bladder distention unless the client was having difficulty voiding. Urine cultures are not routinely prescribed after cystoscopy.

🔑 CN: Reduction of risk potential; CL: Analyze

219. 4, 3, 2, 1. The nurse first assesses and manages the physical effects of the eye injury by placing an ice pack on the eye to reduce swelling. Next, the nurse obtains as much information about the situation and the daycare center as possible. The nurse documents all physical assessment findings and information provided by the mother. Because an infant who is 6 months of age should not be in a walker unattended, and black eyes do not occur from falls with walkers, this is a potential child abuse incident; therefore, the nurse reports the incident as such using the agency's reporting structure (usually, social services department reports the incidents to the authorities).

🔑 CN: Management of care; CL: Synthesize

220. 2. The nurse interprets the client's statement as use of the hot disease concept in the Mexican culture, where the belief of a hot and cold balance of the body exists. A hot disease such as an infection is treated with the opposite, a cold food such as milk. The nurse should focus on the cultural differences and be sensitive to the cultural diversity.

🔑 CN: Health promotion and maintenance; CL: Analyze

221. 3. A client who is "getting special messages" (ideas of reference) commonly misinterprets content presented on television as containing messages for the client. Therefore, it is important for the nurse to monitor the client's reactions to television programs.

🔑 CN: Psychosocial integrity; CL: Synthesize

222. 3, 5. Not attending the support group consistently and not taking the antidepressant may lead to a relapse, and the client needs this information. Bulimia is chronic and intermittent and involves cycles of bingeing, purging, and restrictive eating. Increased socialization and activities promote healthy relationships.

🔑 CN: Psychosocial integrity; CL: Evaluate

223. 3. In a low anorectal anomaly, the rectum has descended normally through the puborectalis muscle. In an intermediate anomaly, the rectum is at or below the level of the puborectalis muscle; in a high anomaly, the rectum ends above the puborectalis muscle.

🔑 CN: Physiological adaptation; CL: Evaluate

224. 1. It is especially important for the nurse to carefully assess the elderly client for respiratory depression after administering a dose of meperidine. It may be necessary to reduce the dosage to prevent respiratory depression. Dysrhythmias, constipation, and seizures are all potential adverse effects of meperidine, but respiratory depression is most significant in the elderly.

🔑 CN: Pharmacological and parenteral therapies; CL: Analyze

225. 2. Pets are discouraged when parents are trying to allergy proof a home for a child with bronchial asthma, unless the pets are kept outside. Pets with hair or feathers are especially likely to trigger asthma attacks. A fish is a satisfactory pet for this child, but the parents should be taught to keep the fish tank clean to prevent it from harboring mold.

🔑 CN: Health promotion and maintenance; CL: Synthesize

226. 2. Ascorbic acid (vitamin C) increases iron absorption. Taking iron with a food rich in ascorbic acid, such as orange juice, increases absorption. Milk delays iron absorption. It is best to give iron on an empty stomach to increase absorption. Beta-carotene does not affect iron absorption.

🔑 CN: Pharmacological and parenteral therapies; CL: Apply

227. 1. In early renal insufficiency, the kidneys lose the ability to concentrate urine, resulting in polyuria. Oliguria occurs later. Dysuria and hematuria are not associated with renal insufficiency.

🔑 CN: Physiological adaptation; CL: Analyze

228. 1. Sucking provides the infant with a sense of security and comfort. It also is an outlet for releasing tension. The infant should not be discouraged from sucking on the pacifier. Fussiness after feeding may indicate that the infant's appetite is not satisfied. Sucking is not manipulative in the sense of seeking parental attention.

🔑 CN: Health promotion and maintenance; CL: Analyze

229. 1. The ZIFT method requires that fertilization take place outside the body. After fertilization has occurred, the fertilized eggs are transferred by laparoscopy to the open end of the fallopian tube. At least one tube must be patent for this procedure to succeed, so it is not beneficial if the client has bilateral blocked fallopian tubes. Ova and sperm are instilled in the fallopian tube for fertilization when the gamete intrafallopian transfer method is used. With in vitro fertilization, a fertilized ovum is instilled into the vagina to enter the uterus for implantation.

CN: Health promotion and maintenance; CL: Synthesize

230. 2. The nurse should examine the buccal mucosa, along with the conjunctiva and sclera, nail beds, palms, soles, lips, and tongue to assess for oxygenation in a client with dark skin.

CN: Reduction of risk potential; CL: Apply

231. 3. The nurse should teach a client who has undergone chest surgery to raise the arm on the affected side over the head to help prevent shoulder ankylosis. This exercise helps restore normal shoulder movement, prevents stiffening of the shoulder joint, and improves muscle tone and power.

CN: Reduction of risk potential; CL: Synthesize

232. 2. The nurse's first action should be to attempt to replace the tracheostomy tube immediately so that the client's airway is reestablished. Although the nurse may also call for assistance, there should be no delay before attempting reinsertion of the tube. The client is placed in a supine position with the neck hyperextended to facilitate reentry of the tube. The obturator is inserted into the replacement tracheostomy tube to guide insertion and is then removed to allow passage of air through the tube.

CN: Reduction of risk potential; CL: Synthesize

233. 1, 2, 4. LPN/VNs ▢ work collaboratively with colleagues in health care to assess, plan, and deliver quality nursing services. The experienced LPN/VN is capable of gathering data and observations including breath sounds and pulse oximetry. Administering medications, such as aerosolized medications, is within the scope of practice for the LPN/LVN. The actions that are within the scope of practice for the professional **RN** ▢ include independently completing the admission assessment, initiating the nursing care plan, and evaluating a parent's abilities, as these activities require additional education and skills.

CN: Management of care; CL: Analyze

234. 1. A general growth parameter is that the birth weight doubles in 6 months and triples in a year. Telling the mother that the baby will eat what he needs is not appropriate. The nurse needs to investigate whether the baby's weight is within the normal parameters of infant weight gain. A bottle-fed baby should not be forced to complete the bottle because this may contribute to obesity.

CN: Health promotion and maintenance; CL: Synthesize

235. 4. The mechanism of injury is always the most critical information to obtain from a client with a musculoskeletal injury. In the event of a back injury, the mechanism of injury provides the greatest clue as to the extent of injury and the proper treatment plan. The other questions are important but will not give the critical information needed related to this specific problem and injury.

CN: Physiological adaptation; CL: Analyze

236. 1. Antihypertensive medications such as metoprolol and hydrochlorothiazide work to lower the blood pressure by reducing peripheral resistance or decreasing cardiac output; the effectiveness of these drugs is noted by a lowering of the blood pressure. Vasodilators are used to improve peripheral circulation. Cardiac stimulants and antiarrhythmic drugs are used to increase heart rate. Although cardiac problems can cause dyspnea, the use of drugs to manage dyspnea depends on the underlying cause.

CN: Pharmacological and parenteral therapies; CL: Evaluate

237. 2. The stored glucose of muscle glycogen is the major fuel during sustained activity. Glucose production slows as the body begins to depend on fat stores for glucose and fatty acids. Protein is not the body's preferred energy source. Fat is a secondary source of energy. Water is not an energy source, although sufficient water is required to engage in aerobic activity without causing dehydration.

CN: Health promotion and maintenance; CL: Apply

238. 3. Typical early signs of rheumatoid arthritis are nonspecific and not necessarily related to specific joint pain. Common early symptoms include fatigue, anorexia, weight loss, and generalized feelings of stiffness. Joint swelling and limitation of movement usually occur later as joint involvement becomes more specific. Dizziness is not a sign of rheumatoid arthritis. Nausea is not typically associated with the disease process but can be related to medications prescribed to treat rheumatoid arthritis.

CN: Physiological adaptation; CL: Analyze

239. 2. NPH insulin should be rolled between the palms to mix it before drawing it up; shaking it will introduce air bubbles into the solution, which can cause inaccurate dosing. The client should draw up the insulin first, store the insulin in a cool place, and inject the insulin at a 90-degree angle.

🔑 CN: Pharmacological and parenteral therapies; CL: Evaluate

240. 4. The gene for Duchenne's muscular dystrophy is carried by women and transmitted to their male children. It involves an X-linked inheritance pattern. About one-third of new cases involve mutations.

🔑 CN: Physiological adaptation; CL: Apply

241. 4. Infants with intussusception have colic-like abdominal pain caused by the telescoping of the bowel. The nursing priority is to relieve this pain. There are no data to indicate a skin problem or dehydration. Diarrhea or constipation may precede the appearance of currant jelly stools.

🔑 CN: Physiological adaptation; CL: Analyze

242. 2 lb or 0.9 kg. One pound or 0.45 kilograms of weight is approximately equivalent to 3,500 cal. Removing 1,000 cal/day results in a 2-lb (0.9 kg) weight loss per week (7,000 cal divided by 7 days). A client who wanted to lose 1 lb (0.45 kg) in a 7-day period would need to cut out 500 cal/day (3,500 cal divided by 7 days). It is unsafe to try to lose more than 2 lb (0.9 kg)/wk.

🔑 CN: Health promotion and maintenance; CL: Apply

243. 2. The nurse should notify the **HCP** 📖 that the client is allergic to penicillin before giving the cefazolin. Cephalosporins are contraindicated in clients who are allergic to penicillin. Clients who are allergic to penicillin may have a cross-allergy to cephalosporins.

🔑 CN: Pharmacological and parenteral therapies; CL: Synthesize

244. 4, 5. Buspirone is not a benzodiazepine but acts as a serotonin agonist. Serotonin is the neurotransmitter implicated in depression. Buspirone reduces symptoms of worry, apprehension, difficulty with concentration, and irritability. It is not sedating, does not cause a high, takes 1 to 6 weeks to be effective, does not cause muscle relaxation, and does not produce dependence, withdrawal, or tolerance. Full therapeutic benefit takes 3 to 6 weeks.

🔑 CN: Pharmacological and parenteral therapies; CL: Evaluate

245. 3. The nurse should document a tearing of tissue with irregular wound edges as a laceration. A contusion or a bruise is a closed wound caused by a blunt object resulting in bleeding in underlying tissue. An abrasion is a superficial wound from a rubbing or a scraping of the surface of the skin such as from a fall. Colonization is a wound containing microorganisms.

🔑 CN: Safety and infection control; CL: Apply

246. 1. The major cause of relapse is noncompliance. If the client cannot afford to keep taking the medicines, it is a warning sign to the nurse that the client may be at risk for noncompliance. Therefore, the nurse needs to stress the need for compliance to prevent relapse. If money is a problem, a referral to a social worker may be necessary.

🔑 CN: Psychosocial integrity; CL: Evaluate

247. 2. Epstein's pearls are tiny, hard, white nodules found in the mouth of some neonates. They are considered normal and usually disappear without treatment. Koplik's spots, associated with measles in children, are patchy and bright red with a bluish-white speck in the middle. Precocious teeth are actual teeth that some neonates have at birth. Usually, only one or two teeth are present. *Candida albicans*, or thrush, is not apparent in the mouth immediately after birth but may appear a day or 2 later. This infection is manifested by yellowish-white spots or lesions that resemble milk curds and bleed when attempts are made to wipe them away.

🔑 CN: Health promotion and maintenance; CL: Analyze

248. 3. It is important to explain to the client who is having nausea that the majority of calories should be eaten in the morning because nausea most often occurs in the afternoon and evening. Small, frequent portions are best. Clients with viral hepatitis should select a diet high in calories because energy is required for healing. An intake of adequate carbohydrates can spare the protein because protein places an increased workload on the liver. Changes in bilirubin interfere with fat absorption, so low-fat diets are better tolerated.

🔑 CN: Health promotion; CL: Synthesize

249. 2. The nurse should teach the client how to do isometric exercise, contraction of the quadriceps muscle without movement of joint, to maintain muscle strength. Physical therapy may assist the client later and will then teach the client how to do active exercises and crutch walking if prescribed. The client will be able to move the unaffected limb; the family will not need to assist. If the client will be using crutches, building upper extremity strength will be helpful, but the immediate need is to maintain and develop strength in the quadriceps.

🔑 CN: Health promotion; CL: Synthesize

250. **2.** A hyphema is the presence of blood in the anterior chamber of the brain. Hyphema is produced when a force is sufficient to break the integrity of the blood vessels in the eye and can be caused by direct injury, such as penetrating injury from a small bullet or pellet, or indirectly, such as from striking the forehead on the pavement during an accident. The client is treated by bed rest in a semi-Fowler's position to assist gravity in keeping the hyphema away from the optical center of the cornea.

☞ CN: Basic care and comfort; CL: Apply

251. **3.** Urine output should be at least 500 mL in 24 hours (20 mL/h); this client's output has been just 15 mL/h for the past 2 hours requiring further assessment by the nurse. The nurse should first assess all clients and address physiological needs including pain control and safety measures; the nurse should then take time with the client having difficulty coping in order to listen and further determine her needs.

☞ CN: Reduction of risk potential;
CL: Synthesize

252. **1.** The stationary bicycle is the most appropriate training modality because it is a non–weight-bearing exercise. The time that the individual exercises on the stationary bicycle is increased with improved functional capacity. The other exercise equipment requires exercising while standing.

☞ CN: Health promotion and maintenance;
CL: Synthesize

253. **1.** The nurse should closely monitor the client admitted with an elevated blood alcohol level for several hours for signs and symptoms of withdrawal, administering sedation as needed; delirium tremens, the most severe form of withdrawal, usually peaks at 48 to 72 hours following the last drink. The client with the chest tube is not in any distress and has no pressing needs. For an older client who has had GI bleeding, a hemoglobin of 13.8 g/dL (138 g/L) is within normal limits. After assessing all clients' needs, the nurse will prepare the client who had an appendectomy for discharge as soon as possible.

☞ CN: Reduction of risk potential;
CL: Synthesize

254. **1.** Fetal alcohol syndrome is characterized by central nervous system damage, poor growth, and specific facial stigmata. As many as 90% of children with fetal alcohol syndrome have eye abnormalities. Vitamin B$_6$ and vitamin A deficiencies can affect growth and development but not with these specific effects. Folic acid deficiency contributes to neural tube defects.

☞ CN: Reduction of risk potential;
CL: Analyze

255. **2.** Therapeutic serum drug monitoring is not routinely done with ciprofloxacin. This medicine should not be taken with dairy products or other significant sources of calcium such as collard greens, calcium supplements, calcium carbonate antacids, or calcium-fortified juice. Clients may take a missed dose as soon as they remember. If it is very close to the time of the next dose, the missed dose should be omitted. The client should not take a double dose.

☞ CN: Pharmacology and parental
therapies; CL: Evaluate

256. **3.** Physical activity is gradually increased after a myocardial infarction while the client is still hospitalized and through a period of rehabilitation. The client is progressing too rapidly if activity significantly changes respirations, causing dyspnea, chest pain, a rapid heartbeat, or fatigue. When any of these symptoms appears, the client should reduce activity and progress more slowly. Edema suggests a circulatory problem that must be addressed but does not necessarily indicate overexertion. Cyanosis indicates reduced oxygen-carrying capacity of red blood cells and indicates a severe pathology. It is not appropriate to use cyanosis as an indicator for overexertion. Weight loss indicates several factors but not overexertion.

☞ CN: Reduction of risk potential;
CL: Analyze

257. **4.** The most common noninfectious renal disease in children is acute poststreptococcal glomerulonephritis. Ensuring that children diagnosed with streptococcal infections complete a full course of antibiotics will decrease their risk of developing acute glomerulonephritis. Parents should contact the primary **HCP** 📖 if they suspect a UTI; however, glomerulonephritis is not caused by a UTI. Glomerulonephritis is not a genetic disease and is not contagious, which makes answers 2 and 3 incorrect information.

☞ CN: Reduction of risk potential; CL: Apply

258. **2, 3, 5.** The client who is taking disulfiram is advised to avoid all forms of alcohol including beer, communal wine at church, and cough syrup; these can trigger a serious physical reaction. Aged cheeses and chocolate are to be avoided by the client taking monoamine oxidase inhibitors.

☞ CN: Pharmacologic and parenteral
therapies; CL: Apply

259. **1.** In response to hearing a noise, normally hearing infants blink or startle and stop body movements. Shy and withdrawn behaviors are characteristics of older children with hearing impairment. Squealing occurs in 90% of infants by age 4 months. Most infants can say "da-da" by age 9 months.

☞ CN: Health promotion and maintenance;
CL: Evaluate

260. **2, 4.** Magnesium sulfate decreases muscle contractility and crosses the placenta. Because of this, a neonate who has been exposed to this drug may have decreased muscle tone and decreased respirations. The Moro reflex will be decreased because of the decreased muscle tone. There are no findings that show magnesium sulfate has a direct effect on temperature.

🔑 CN: Pharmacological and parenteral therapies; CL: Analyze

261. **13 mL.** 1000 to 1030 = 4 mL (hourly rate 8), 1030 to 1100 = 3 mL (hourly rate 6 mL), 1100 to 1200 = 6 mL (hourly rate 6 mL). 4 + 3 + 6 = 13.

🔑 CN: Pharmacological and parenteral therapies; CL: Apply

262. S_1 is loudest at the mitral area.

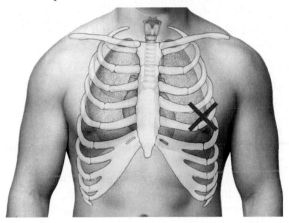

🔑 CN: Health promotion and maintenance; CL: Apply

263. **1.** During the third trimester, particularly in the 9th month of pregnancy, the client typically exhibits feelings of vulnerability and fear that the baby will be lost. Confirmation that the fetus is real occurs during the second trimester. Ambivalence is typically seen and resolved during the first trimester. Body image disturbance commonly occurs during the second trimester because of the profound changes that occur to the body during this time.

🔑 CN: Health promotion and maintenance; CL: Analyze

264. **3.** The elderly client commonly has vague or atypical responses to medications and diseases that are erroneously attributed to aging. A new cognitive change needs to be investigated and is not an expected change with aging. Changes in a client's behavior should be investigated to see whether there is a relation to excessive sedation. The nurse can interview the family members to obtain information.

🔑 CN: Health promotion and maintenance; CL: Apply

265. **2.** Infants are sensitive to stress in their caretakers. The best way to handle an anxious infant is to talk quietly, thereby soothing the infant. Limiting holding of the infant to feeding periods interferes with meeting the infant's needs for close contact, possibly compromising his ability to develop trust. Playing music in the room for most of the day and night will make it difficult for the infant to differentiate days from nights. Having a friend take the infant for several days will not necessarily take care of the problem because when the infant returns to the parents, the same behaviors will recur unless the parents makes some changes.

🔑 CN: Psychosocial integrity; CL: Synthesize

This test has 190 questions. Time yourself as you take the test so you can determine the approximate amount of time it takes to complete this many questions.

1. A primigravid client at 26 weeks' gestation asks the nurse what causes heartburn during pregnancy. The nurse should explain to the client that heartburn during pregnancy is usually caused by which factor?
- ☐ **1.** increased peristaltic action during pregnancy
- ☐ **2.** displacement of the stomach by the diaphragm
- ☐ **3.** decreased secretion of hydrochloric acid
- ☐ **4.** backflow of stomach contents into the esophagus

2. A client at a follow-up appointment after having a miscarriage 2 weeks previously yells at the nurse, "How could God do this to me? I have never done anything wrong." Which response by the nurse would be **most** appropriate at this time?
- ☐ **1.** "God can handle your anger. It is okay."
- ☐ **2.** "I know you are angry. It is so hard to lose your baby."
- ☐ **3.** "It is not God's fault. It was an accident."
- ☐ **4.** "You are a strong person. You will get through this."

3. A client who has been prescribed chemotherapy is worried and wants to take herbal treatments instead. The nurse's **best** response to the client is:
- ☐ **1.** "You are making a mistake and placing your life in jeopardy."
- ☐ **2.** "Herbal treatments are not approved by the government's regulatory agency."
- ☐ **3.** "Herbal treatments have not been researched with cancer."
- ☐ **4.** "Tell me about your concerns with chemotherapy."

4. A 4-year-old child is admitted for a cardiac catheterization. Which is **most** important to include as the nurse teaches this child about the cardiac catheterization?
- ☐ **1.** a plastic model of the heart
- ☐ **2.** a catheter that will be inserted into the artery
- ☐ **3.** the parents
- ☐ **4.** other children undergoing a catheterization

5. A client has a reddened area over a bony prominence. The nurse finds an unlicensed nursing personnel (UAP) massaging this area. The nurse should:
- ☐ **1.** reinforce the UAP's use of this intervention over the bony prominence.
- ☐ **2.** explain to the UAP that massage is effective because it improves blood flow to the area.
- ☐ **3.** inform the UAP that massage is even more effective when combined with the use of lotion.
- ☐ **4.** instruct the UAP that massage is contraindicated because it decreases blood flow to the area.

6. A worried mother confides in the nurse that she wants to change healthcare providers (HCPs) because her infant is not getting better. What is the nurse's **best** response?
- ☐ **1.** "This primary care provider has been on our staff for 20 years."
- ☐ **2.** "I know you are worried, but the primary care provider has an excellent reputation."
- ☐ **3.** "You always have an option to change. Tell me about your concerns."
- ☐ **4.** "Your infant's condition takes time to heal."

7. A mother who is breast-feeding and has known food sensitivities is asking the nurse what foods she should avoid in her diet. Which foods should the nurse advise the client to avoid? Select all that apply.
- ☐ **1.** shellfish
- ☐ **2.** eggs
- ☐ **3.** peanuts
- ☐ **4.** beef
- ☐ **5.** lamb

8. A widowed client who is receiving chemotherapy tells the nurse that he does not like to cook for himself. A community resource for this client is:
- ☐ **1.** a hospice/palliative care association.
- ☐ **2.** a home care/visiting nurses group.
- ☐ **3.** a meal delivery service.
- ☐ **4.** an association for retirees.

9. After the client has a temporary pacemaker inserted, the nurse should verify documentation on the medical record of:
☐ 1. the client's cardiovascular status.
☐ 2. the client's emotional state.
☐ 3. the type of sedation used.
☐ 4. pacemaker rate, type, and settings.

10. The nurse judges that the parent of a 9-month-old infant in a hip spica cast understands how to feed the child when the parent makes which statement?
☐ 1. "I can lay my child flat and feed that way."
☐ 2. "I will raise my child's head up and leave the hips and legs on a pillow."
☐ 3. "I can borrow a special feeding table to use."
☐ 4. "It will take two of us, one to hold and one to feed."

11. The nurse is assessing home care needs for a group of clients. Which clients qualify for home care services? The client who: (Select all that apply.)
☐ 1. requires monitoring of prothrombin time due to (warfarin) therapy.
☐ 2. needs additional instruction regarding preparation of food on a low-sodium diet.
☐ 3. has episodes of vertigo that result in falls.
☐ 4. has multiple sclerosis with an open, draining lesion on a foot.
☐ 5. needs stronger lenses for glasses.

12. Which type of mouth care is **most** appropriate when the nurse is caring for a client with dentures who has severe stomatitis?
☐ 1. using a soft toothbrush or gauze pad to provide oral hygiene
☐ 2. rinsing the mouth with a commercial mouthwash before and after each meal
☐ 3. cleansing the gums and oral mucosa with an oral swab with an astringent every shift
☐ 4. keeping dentures in place to decrease development of edema

13. The nursing staff has finished restraining a client. In addition to determining whether anyone was injured, the staff is mandated to evaluate the incident to obtain which outcome?
☐ 1. Coordinate documentation of the incident.
☐ 2. Resolve negative feelings and attitudes.
☐ 3. Improve the use of restraint procedures.
☐ 4. Calm down before returning to the other clients.

14. Two parents who are arguing in their infant's room, with voices raised and getting louder, start to hit each other. The infant is crying. Which action should the staff nurse take **next**?
☐ 1. Try to reason with both of the parents.
☐ 2. Ask one of the parents to leave the room.
☐ 3. Call security to come and break up the fight.
☐ 4. Remove the infant from the room.

15. A client asks the nurse why it is necessary to complete an advance directive on admission to the hospital. The nurse's **best** response is:
☐ 1. "This will provide a substitute for informed discussion with your healthcare provider (HCP)."
☐ 2. "It is your chance to make your wishes known if you ever become incapable of making your own decisions."
☐ 3. "Your healthcare provider will make the best decisions for you in an emergency."
☐ 4. "Are you worried that extraordinary means will be taken if you are dying?"

16. When witnessing an adult client's signature on a consent form for a procedure, the nurse verifies that the consent was obtained in an appropriate manner. What information should the nurse verify? Select all that apply.
☐ 1. that there was adequate disclosure of information
☐ 2. that the client understood the information
☐ 3. that there was voluntary consent on the client's part
☐ 4. that the client has full awareness of the potential complications
☐ 5. that the client's relative, spouse, or legal guardian was present

17. A pregnant woman at 22 weeks' gestation is diagnosed with gonorrhea. The healthcare provider (HCP) prescribes doxycycline. What should the nurse do **first**?
☐ 1. Instruct the client about the effects of the drug.
☐ 2. Make sure the record notes that the baby must receive eyedrops when born.
☐ 3. Have the HCP add a single dose of ceftriaxone.
☐ 4. Discuss with the HCP the need to change the prescription.

18. After a client undergoes a contraction stress test that is negative, what should the nurse assess **next**?
☐ 1. evidence of ruptured membranes
☐ 2. viability status of the fetus
☐ 3. indications that contractions have ceased
☐ 4. fetal heart rate patterns

19. A 2-month-old infant is at risk for an ileus after surgery to correct intussusception. What should be included in a focused assessment for this complication? Select all that apply.
☐ 1. measurement of urine specific gravity
☐ 2. assessment of bowel sounds
☐ 3. characteristics of the first stool
☐ 4. measurement of gastric output
☐ 5. bilirubin levels

20. A client with asthma who has wheezing and shortness of breath asks the nurse if it is all right to use the salmeterol inhaler during exercise. What is the nurse's **best** response?
- [ ] 1. "Yes, use the inhaler immediately for these symptoms."
- [ ] 2. "No, this drug is a maintenance drug, not a rescue inhaler."
- [ ] 3. "Use the inhaler 5 minutes before you exercise to prevent the wheezing."
- [ ] 4. "This inhaler is for allergic rhinitis, not asthma."

21. The nurse should assess the child with nephrotic syndrome for which factors? Select all that apply.
- [ ] 1. normal blood pressure
- [ ] 2. generalized edema
- [ ] 3. normal serum lipid levels
- [ ] 4. no red blood cells in the urine
- [ ] 5. elevated streptococcal antibody titers

22. A client is receiving spironolactone for treatment of bilateral lower extremity edema. The nurse should instruct the client to make which nutritional modification to prevent an electrolyte imbalance?
- [ ] 1. Increase intake of milk and milk products.
- [ ] 2. Restrict fluid intake to 1,000 mL/day.
- [ ] 3. Decrease foods high in potassium.
- [ ] 4. Increase foods high in sodium.

23. The nurse establishes the goal of preventing the development of a stress ulcer in a burn client. Which would **most** likely contribute to the achievement of this goal?
- [ ] 1. implementing relaxation exercises
- [ ] 2. administering a sedative as needed
- [ ] 3. providing a soft, bland diet
- [ ] 4. administering famotidine as prescribed

24. A nurse is assessing a client with a history of myocardial infarction who is in the surgical unit following a gastric resection. The client has chest pains. The nurse obtains the electrocardiogram (ECG) shown (see figure). What should the nurse do **first**?

- [ ] 1. Administer oxygen.
- [ ] 2. Inspect the client's incision.
- [ ] 3. Call the rapid response team.
- [ ] 4. Reposition the ECG electrodes.

25. The nurse is watching two siblings, ages 7 and 9 years, verbally arguing over a toy. The nurse has counseled the parent before about how to handle this situation. The nurse should judge that the teaching has been effective when the parent takes what action?
- [ ] 1. tells the siblings to stop arguing and shake hands
- [ ] 2. ignores the arguing and continues what she is doing
- [ ] 3. tells the children they will be punished when they go home
- [ ] 4. says they will not go out to lunch now since they have argued

26. A client is diagnosed with genital herpes (herpes simplex virus type 2, or HSV-2). The nurse should instruct the client that:
- [ ] 1. using occlusive ointments may decrease the pain from the lesions.
- [ ] 2. reducing stressful life events may decrease the incidence of herpetic outbreaks.
- [ ] 3. there are no effective drug therapies to manage herpes symptoms.
- [ ] 4. herpes is transmitted to partners only when lesions are weeping.

27. Following an infection, the client is having ototoxic effects of the vestibular branch of the acoustic nerve. The nurse should assess the client for: (Select all that apply.)
- [ ] 1. vertigo.
- [ ] 2. tinnitus.
- [ ] 3. nausea.
- [ ] 4. ataxia.
- [ ] 5. hearing loss.

28. A young adult has been bitten by a human, and the skin on the forearm is broken. The client's last tetanus shot was about 8 years ago. The nurse should prepare the client for:
- [ ] 1. an injection of tetanus toxoid.
- [ ] 2. an application of a corticosteroid cream.
- [ ] 3. closure of the wound with sutures.
- [ ] 4. testing for tuberculosis.

29. A client 6 weeks postpartum is asking the nurse about taking progesterone for birth control. Prior to discussing options, what should the nurse determine? Select all that apply.
- [ ] 1. if the client has a sexually transmitted disease
- [ ] 2. how willing her husband is to have her take the drug
- [ ] 3. if the woman is experiencing postpartum depression
- [ ] 4. that the woman is not currently pregnant
- [ ] 5. if the woman is breast-feeding

30. A mother who is visibly upset tells the nurse she wants to take her child home because the child is dying. What would be the nurse's **best** response?

☐ **1.** "I know how you feel, but the medication will make your child feel better."

☐ **2.** "I cannot let you do this without calling your healthcare provider (HCP) first."

☐ **3.** "Can you tell me why you want to take your child home now?"

☐ **4.** "I can imagine how hard this is for you, but it is not what is best for the child."

31. Several clients have been admitted to the emergency department. The nurse should assess these clients in which order from first to last? All options must be used.

1. the client who is 12 years of age with a fractured tibia

2. the client who is 8 years of age with small lacerations to legs and arms

3. the client who is 16 years of age with a "sore throat"

4. the client who is 6 months of age with diarrhea and dehydration

32. Which urine output indicates that a 5-month-old weighing 15 lb (6.8 kg) and being treated for dehydration has a normal urine output?

☐ **1.** 1 to 2 mL/kg/h

☐ **2.** 4 to 5 mL/kg/h

☐ **3.** 6 to 8 mL/kg/h

☐ **4.** 10 to 12 mL/kg/h

33. The nurses in the neonatal intensive care unit are not identifying important clinical changes in the clients that need to be documented. What should the unit director do? Select all that apply.

☐ **1.** Identify the problem at a staff meeting without placing blame on any individual or group.

☐ **2.** Ask the unit staff to develop a plan that they think will work for the unit members.

☐ **3.** Ask an experienced nurse to spend time reorienting newer staff members.

☐ **4.** Collaborate with the staff development educator to develop a plan.

☐ **5.** Ask the neonatologist to give a presentation about assessing newborns.

34. A 24-year-old client, diagnosed with acute osteomyelitis in the left leg, has acute pain in the leg that intensifies on movement. The client has a temperature of 101°F (38.3°C) and a reddened, warm area in the midcalf region over the shaft of the tibia. Based on this information, what should the nurse do?

☐ **1.** Prepare the client for possible left lower leg amputation.

☐ **2.** Instruct the client to keep the leg immobile.

☐ **3.** Develop a plan for pain management.

☐ **4.** Obtain a prescription for fluid replacement.

35. A client has undergone a vasectomy. The nurse instructs the client that he can begin having unprotected intercourse:

☐ **1.** when desired because sterilization is immediate.

☐ **2.** as soon as scrotal edema and tenderness resolve.

☐ **3.** when the sperm count reflects sterilization.

☐ **4.** after 6 to 10 ejaculations.

36. The nurse is evaluating the outcome of therapy for a client with osteoarthritis. Which indicates goals of therapy have been met?

☐ **1.** The client's joint degeneration has been arrested.

☐ **2.** The client is able to self-administer gold compound safely.

☐ **3.** The client feels better than on hospital admission.

☐ **4.** The client's joint range of motion has improved.

37. The nurse is assessing an infant diagnosed with bacterial meningitis. The nurse should ask the parent if the infant has which symptoms? Select all that apply.

☐ **1.** fever

☐ **2.** vomiting

☐ **3.** diarrhea

☐ **4.** poor feeding

☐ **5.** abdominal pain

38. To help a client prevent atelectasis and pneumonia after surgery, what should the nurse do?

☐ **1.** Administer oxygen therapy as needed to maintain adequate oxygenation.

☐ **2.** Offer pain medication before having the client deep-breathe and use incentive spirometry.

☐ **3.** Instruct the client to cough, deep-breathe, and turn in bed once every 8 hours.

☐ **4.** Encourage the client to drink 1,000 mL of fluids in 24 hours.

39. A 7-year-old child is admitted to the hospital with acute rheumatic fever. When discussing long-term care for the child with the parents, the nurse should teach them that a necessary part of this care is:

☐ **1.** physical therapy.

☐ **2.** antibiotic therapy.

☐ **3.** psychological therapy.

☐ **4.** anti-inflammatory therapy.

81. The nurse is instructing the parents of a child with acquired immunodeficiency syndrome (AIDS) how to look for signs and symptoms of infection when the child has a cut or open wound. The nurse should tell the parents to report:
☐ **1.** erythema around the area.
☐ **2.** rectal temperature higher than 100.5°F (38°C).
☐ **3.** tenderness around the area.
☐ **4.** increased warmth of the skin in the involved area.

82. The nurse is teaching a group of unlicensed assistive personnel (UAP) about providing care to clients with depression. Which approach by one of the UAPs indicates an understanding of the **most** effective approach to a depressed client?
☐ **1.** cheerful
☐ **2.** empathetic
☐ **3.** serious
☐ **4.** humorous

83. When fluids by mouth are appropriate for the infant after surgery to correct intussusception, the nurse **most** likely would initiate feeding with:
☐ **1.** cereal-thickened formula.
☐ **2.** full-strength formula.
☐ **3.** half-strength formula.
☐ **4.** oral electrolyte solution.

84. A client is taking paroxetine 20 mg PO every morning. The nurse should monitor the client for which adverse effect?
☐ **1.** hypertensive crisis
☐ **2.** sexual problems
☐ **3.** sleep disturbance
☐ **4.** orthostatic hypotension

85. The nurse is assessing a client who is in shock. Which neurologic change indicates that the client is in the progressive stage of shock?
☐ **1.** restlessness
☐ **2.** confusion
☐ **3.** incoherent speech
☐ **4.** unconsciousness

86. A child diagnosed with osteomyelitis will be discharged on IV nafcillin. After teaching the parents about adverse effects that are important to report, which effects as stated by the parents indicate that they understand the teaching? Select all that apply.
☐ **1.** sore mouth
☐ **2.** pain with urination
☐ **3.** headache
☐ **4.** stomach upset
☐ **5.** fever

87. The rapid response team arrives in the room of a client who has had a cardiac arrest. The nurse should **first** apply which piece of monitoring equipment?
☐ **1.** electrocardiogram (ECG) electrodes
☐ **2.** pulse oximeter
☐ **3.** blood pressure cuff
☐ **4.** Doppler for pulse check

88. A nurse is counseling a client who is depressed. What nursing actions promote trust between the client and the nurse? Select all that apply.
☐ **1.** Indicate an understanding for the client's feelings as well as for their cause.
☐ **2.** Listen and encourage the client to say more.
☐ **3.** Acknowledge hearing what the client said.
☐ **4.** Maintain eye contact with the client at all times.
☐ **5.** Stand very close to the client.

89. The nurse is assessing a client for heroin addiction. Which finding indicates the client has used heroin?
☐ **1.** sclera red and bloodshot
☐ **2.** pupils small and constricted
☐ **3.** pupils large and dilated
☐ **4.** drooping eyelids

90. When performing routine health evaluations in school-age children, which finding would alert the school nurse to pediculosis capitis (head lice)?
☐ **1.** spotty baldness
☐ **2.** wheals with scalp blistering
☐ **3.** frequent scalp scratching
☐ **4.** dry, scaly patches on the skin

91. When the nurse is assessing the client's abdomen, which finding **best** indicates that a client's peristaltic activity is returning to normal after surgery?
☐ **1.** The client passes flatus.
☐ **2.** The client says that she is hungry.
☐ **3.** Bowel sounds are hypoactive on auscultation.
☐ **4.** Peristalsis can be felt on abdominal palpation.

92. A client appears flushed and has shallow respirations. The arterial blood gas report shows the following: pH, 7.24; partial pressure of arterial carbon dioxide ($Paco_2$), 49 mm Hg (6.5 kPa); and bicarbonate (HCO_3), 24 mEq/L (24 mmol/L). These findings are indicative of which acid-base imbalance?
☐ **1.** metabolic acidosis
☐ **2.** metabolic alkalosis
☐ **3.** respiratory acidosis
☐ **4.** respiratory alkalosis

93. Which action is **most** important when the nurse is planning pain management for a client after a lobectomy for lung cancer?
☐ 1. repositioning the client immediately after administering pain medication
☐ 2. reassessing the client after administering pain medication
☐ 3. reassuring the client after administering pain medication
☐ 4. readjusting the pain medication dosage as needed

94. The nurse is evaluating a female client's understanding of how to prevent sexually transmitted infections (STIs). Which statement indicates that the client understands how to protect herself?
☐ 1. "I will be sure my partner uses a condom."
☐ 2. "I need to be sure to take my birth control pills."
☐ 3. "I will always douche after sexual intercourse."
☐ 4. "I will be sure to take antibiotics to prevent an STI."

95. While assessing a multigravid client at 10 weeks' gestation, the nurse notes a purplish color to the vagina and cervix. The nurse documents this as what finding?
☐ 1. Goodell's sign
☐ 2. Chadwick's sign
☐ 3. Hegar's sign
☐ 4. melasma

96. A client with bipolar disorder, mania, has flight of ideas and grandiosity and becomes easily agitated. To prevent harmful behaviors, what should the nurse do **initially**?
☐ 1. Encourage the client to stay in his room.
☐ 2. Seclude the client at the first sign of agitation.
☐ 3. Tell the client to seek out staff when feeling agitated.
☐ 4. Instruct the client to ask for medication when agitated.

97. The nurse is preparing written information for an older adult who is to manage intermittent self-catheterization. Which strategy will be **most** effective?
☐ 1. Use charts to help convey information.
☐ 2. Prepare information at a tenth-grade reading level.
☐ 3. Use short words.
☐ 4. Print the material in a condensed font.

98. The nurse should assess a child with newly diagnosed hyperthyroidism for which signs or symptoms? Select all that apply.
☐ 1. weight gain
☐ 2. dry skin
☐ 3. constipation
☐ 4. rapid pulse
☐ 5. heat intolerance

99. The nurse is planning care for four mothers and their newborns. After reviewing the clients' medical records, the nurse should make rounds on which client **first**?
☐ 1. an 18-year-old with an uncomplicated spontaneous vaginal birth 12 hours ago who has abdominal cramps
☐ 2. a 35-year-old with an uncomplicated vaginal birth 4 hours ago; the nurse's notes indicated she soaked two peripads over the last 2 hours; fundus is firm
☐ 3. a 16-year-old with a caesarean section 4 hours ago, diagnosed with preeclampsia and receiving magnesium sulfate at 2 g/h; reflexes are 2+, and the nurse's notes indicate she has a headache; vital signs are T 99.4°F (37.4°C), P 88, R 20, and BP 128/86 mm Hg
☐ 4. an 18-year-old who had a caesarian birth 2 days ago and now has severe breast pain; vital signs are T 99.8°F (37.7°C), P 96, and R 22

100. A nurse is evaluating the proper use of crutches by a client who has fractured the right leg. Which statement indicates the client is using the correct technique?
☐ 1. "I move my left leg forward first as I swing forward on my crutches."
☐ 2. "I need to increase my arm strength because my arms tingle after I use my crutches."
☐ 3. "I padded the tops of my crutches so that I can lean more comfortably on my crutches."
☐ 4. "I feel pressure on the palms of my hands when I am walking with my crutches."

101. Which factor is a **priority** when evaluating discharge plans for an older adult after a lower left lobectomy for lung cancer?
☐ 1. the distance the client lives from the hospital
☐ 2. support available for assisting the client at home
☐ 3. the client's ability to do home blood pressure monitoring
☐ 4. the client's knowledge of the causes of lung cancer

102. A primiparous client planning to breast-feed her term neonate born vaginally asks, "When will my 'real' milk come in?" The nurse explains to the client that after childbirth, breasts begin to produce milk within what time period?
☐ 1. 12 hours
☐ 2. 24 hours
☐ 3. 2 to 4 days
☐ 4. 7 days

103. The nurse is caring for an elderly, debilitated client who has been bedridden for an extended period. Which sign or symptom indicates that the client has hypoxia?
☐ 1. chills
☐ 2. productive cough
☐ 3. confusion
☐ 4. pleuritic chest pain

104. A child with rheumatic fever has polyarthritis and chorea. An echocardiogram shows swelling of the cardiac tissue. Which intervention should the nurse include in the child's plan of care?
- ☐ 1. Explain that the chorea will disappear over time.
- ☐ 2. Perform neurologic checks every 4 hours until the chorea subsides.
- ☐ 3. Promote ambulation by administering aspirin every 4 hours.
- ☐ 4. Keep the child in a slightly cool environment.

105. A 19-year-old unmarried college student who is approximately 8 weeks pregnant asks the nurse, "If I have an abortion in the next 2 or 3 weeks, how will it be done?" The nurse instructs the client that at this gestational age, an abortion is usually performed by which technique?
- ☐ 1. dilatation and curettage
- ☐ 2. menstrual extraction
- ☐ 3. dilatation and vacuum extraction
- ☐ 4. saline induction

106. The nurse is performing a respiratory assessment on a client who has a pleural effusion. The nurse would expect that the client has:
- ☐ 1. decreased breath sounds on the affected side.
- ☐ 2. normal bronchial breath sounds.
- ☐ 3. hyperresonance on percussion.
- ☐ 4. wheezing on auscultation.

107. A nurse is caring for a child with intussusception. What is an expected outcome for a goal to relieve acute pain from abdominal cramping?
- ☐ 1. The child exhibits no manifestations of discomfort.
- ☐ 2. The child is very still.
- ☐ 3. The child has a normal bowel movement.
- ☐ 4. The child has not vomited in 3 hours.

108. Gentamicin sulfate 25 mg IM has been prescribed every 6 hours. Gentamicin sulfate 40 mg/mL is available. How many milliliters (to the nearest tenth of an mL) should the nurse administer in each dose? Round to the nearest mL.

_____ mL.

109. Assessment of a 36-year-old woman who has malaise and dysuria reveals a temperature of 100°F (37.8°C) and painful blisters on the outside of her vagina. The client tells the nurse she had intercourse with a new partner 5 days ago. What should the nurse do?
- ☐ 1. Advise the client to ask her partner to use a condom.
- ☐ 2. Encourage the client to increase fluid to 3,000 mL/day.
- ☐ 3. Tell the client to use a lubricant jelly on the blisters.
- ☐ 4. Refer the client to a healthcare provider (HCP).

110. A child with leukemia fails to respond to therapy. Which statement offers the nurse the **best** guide in making plans to assist the parents in dealing with their child's imminent death?
- ☐ 1. Knowing that the prognosis is poor helps prepare relatives for the death of children.
- ☐ 2. Relatives are especially grieved when a child does well at first but then declines rapidly.
- ☐ 3. Trust in health personnel is most often destroyed by a death that is considered untimely.
- ☐ 4. It is more difficult for relatives to accept the death of a 10-year-old than the death of a younger child whose family membership has been short.

111. The nurse is caring for a child receiving a blood transfusion. The child becomes flushed and is wheezing. What should the nurse do **first**?
- ☐ 1. Notify the healthcare provider (HCP).
- ☐ 2. Administer oxygen.
- ☐ 3. Switch the transfusion to normal saline solution.
- ☐ 4. Take the child's vital signs.

112. A client who is allergic to penicillin has a prescription to receive cefazolin. The nurse should **first**:
- ☐ 1. ask if the client has taken cefazolin before without an adverse response.
- ☐ 2. verify the prescription with the healthcare provider (HCP).
- ☐ 3. administer the cefazolin as prescribed.
- ☐ 4. observe the client closely for urticaria.

113. Which nursing intervention will promote successful achievement of Erikson's stage of development for the 3-year-old toddler?
- ☐ 1. Allow the toddler to choose what time to take her antibiotic.
- ☐ 2. Encourage the toddler to assist in removing the dressing on her leg.
- ☐ 3. Allow the toddler to work on an art project that she can complete.
- ☐ 4. Encourage friends to visit the toddler in the hospital.

114. When preparing the teaching plan for a client about lithium therapy, the nurse should teach the client about:
- ☐ 1. maintaining an adequate sodium intake.
- ☐ 2. discontinuing sodium in the diet.
- ☐ 3. buying foods labeled "low in sodium."
- ☐ 4. increasing sodium in the diet.

115. A client who is undergoing radiation therapy develops mucositis. Which action should be included in the client's plan of care?
- ☐ 1. increasing mouth care to twice per shift
- ☐ 2. providing the client with hot tea to drink
- ☐ 3. promoting regular flossing of teeth
- ☐ 4. using half-strength hydrogen peroxide on mouth ulcers

116. A parent calls the Poison Control Center because her 3-year-old has eaten 10 to 12 chewable acetaminophen tablets. What should the nurse instruct the parent to do?
- ☐ **1.** Give the child a large glass of milk.
- ☐ **2.** Induce vomiting.
- ☐ **3.** Take the child to the emergency department.
- ☐ **4.** Monitor the child's respirations for 24 hours.

117. The parent of a preschool-age child tells the nurse that the child is hyperactive and something needs to be done. Which response by the nurse would be **most** appropriate initially?
- ☐ **1.** "What makes you think your child is hyperactive?"
- ☐ **2.** "What do you think needs to be done?"
- ☐ **3.** "How does your child behave normally?"
- ☐ **4.** "Does the preschool teacher think your child is hyperactive?"

118. When preparing for the discharge of a newborn after surgery to correct tracheoesophageal fistula (TEF), the nurse teaches the parents about the need for long-term health care because their child has a high probability of developing which complication?
- ☐ **1.** recurrent mild diarrhea with dehydration
- ☐ **2.** esophageal stricture
- ☐ **3.** speech problems
- ☐ **4.** gastric ulcers

119. A young adult with Hodgkin's disease has been readmitted to the hospital because of aggressive disease that is unresponsive to multiple therapies. Death appears imminent. A **priority** nursing goal for this client is to:
- ☐ **1.** reduce feelings of isolation.
- ☐ **2.** reduce fear of pain.
- ☐ **3.** reduce fear of more aggressive therapies.
- ☐ **4.** reduce feelings of social inadequacy.

120. A client is admitted in early active labor at 39 weeks' gestation with intact membranes. When assessing the fetal heart rate, the nurse locates the heart sounds above the client's umbilicus at midline. The nurse should further confirm that the fetus is lying in which position?
- ☐ **1.** cephalic
- ☐ **2.** frank breech
- ☐ **3.** face
- ☐ **4.** transverse

121. The nurse is caring for a client who has been diagnosed with pernicious anemia. Which statement by the client indicates an understanding of the treatment of pernicious anemia?
- ☐ **1.** "I will need to increase my dietary intake of foods that are high in vitamin B_{12}."
- ☐ **2.** "I will receive my first injection of vitamin B_{12} tomorrow, and I will return for a follow-up injection in 1 month."
- ☐ **3.** "I understand that the oral form of vitamin B_{12} is preferred because it is safer and less expensive than the injection form."
- ☐ **4.** "I will need to take vitamin B_{12} replacements for the rest of my life."

122. A client's 1200 blood glucose was inaccurately documented as 310 mg/dL (17.2 mmol/L) instead of 130 mg/dL (7.2 mmol/L). This error was not noticed until 1300. The nurse administered the sliding scale insulin for a blood glucose of 310 mg/dL (17.2 mmol/L). What should the nurse do **first**?
- ☐ **1.** Notify the healthcare provider (HCP).
- ☐ **2.** Assess for hypoglycemia.
- ☐ **3.** Consult with the clinical pharmacist.
- ☐ **4.** Call the charge nurse.

123. An older infant who has been injured in an automobile accident is to wear a splint on the injured leg. The mother reports that the infant has become mobile even while wearing the splint. What should the nurse advise the mother to do?
- ☐ **1.** Notify the healthcare provider (HCP) immediately to adjust the treatment plan.
- ☐ **2.** Confine the infant to one room in the apartment.
- ☐ **3.** Keep the infant in the splint at night, removing it during the day.
- ☐ **4.** Remove any unsafe items from the area in which the infant is mobile.

124. While preparing a client for surgery, the nurse assesses for psychosocial problems that may cause preoperative anxiety. Which is believed to be the **most** distressing fear a preoperative client is likely to experience?
- ☐ **1.** fear of the unknown
- ☐ **2.** fear of changes in body image
- ☐ **3.** fear of the effects of anesthesia
- ☐ **4.** fear of being in pain

125. A 56-year-old woman is admitted for a modified radical mastectomy. The client appears anxious and asks many questions. The nurse's **best** course of action is to:
- ☐ **1.** tell the client as much as she wants to know and is able to understand.
- ☐ **2.** delay discussing the client's questions with her until the convalescent phase of her care.
- ☐ **3.** delay discussing the client's questions with her until her apprehension subsides.
- ☐ **4.** explain to the client that she should discuss her questions with her healthcare provider (HCP).

126. One hour before surgery, the client asks the nurse about the risks of the surgical procedure. Which statement by the nurse is **most** appropriate?
- ☐ **1.** "What are your concerns? I can answer any questions that you have."
- ☐ **2.** "There are several risks. Did the surgeon tell you about them?"
- ☐ **3.** "It is important that your questions are answered and you understand the risks before you have surgery. I will contact the surgeon."
- ☐ **4.** "Actually, the risks associated with this procedure are minimal. The surgeon has performed this surgery many times."

127. The nurse is assessing fetal position in a 32-year-old woman in her 8th month of pregnancy. From the figure, the fetal position can be described as:

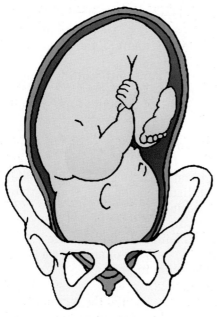

- ☐ **1.** left occipital transverse.
- ☐ **2.** left occipital anterior.
- ☐ **3.** right occipital transverse.
- ☐ **4.** right occipital anterior.

128. A child has a urinary tract infection and is being treated with antibiotics. The nurse should instruct the parents to report which symptom?
- ☐ **1.** increased urine output
- ☐ **2.** loss of appetite
- ☐ **3.** jaundice
- ☐ **4.** fever

129. After teaching a mother about the neonate's positive Babinski's reflex, the nurse determines that the mother understands the instructions when she says that a positive Babinski's reflex indicates:
- ☐ **1.** possible partial paralysis.
- ☐ **2.** possible lower limb defect.
- ☐ **3.** immature central nervous system.
- ☐ **4.** possible injury to nerves that innervate the legs.

130. The nurse should instruct a client who is taking dexamethasone and furosemide to report:
- ☐ **1.** excitability.
- ☐ **2.** muscle weakness.
- ☐ **3.** diarrhea.
- ☐ **4.** increased thirst.

131. A client with a suspected diagnosis of lung cancer has a bronchoscopy with biopsy. Following the procedure, the nurse should:
- ☐ **1.** encourage the client to gargle with oral lidocaine to decrease throat irritation.
- ☐ **2.** monitor the client for signs of pneumothorax.
- ☐ **3.** administer pain medication as needed to relieve mediastinal discomfort.
- ☐ **4.** advise the client not to talk until the gag reflex returns.

132. A nurse is preparing to administer 500 mL of an IV solution to a child over 12 hours via tubing that delivers microdrips at 60 gtt/mL. At what rate should the nurse infuse the solution?

_____ gtt/min.

133. Which technique is correct when the nurse administers a subcutaneous injection?
- ☐ **1.** Use a 1-inch (2.5-cm) needle for injection.
- ☐ **2.** Insert the needle at a 45-degree angle to the skin.
- ☐ **3.** Spread the skin tightly at the injection site.
- ☐ **4.** Draw 0.2 mL of air into the syringe before administration.

134. An elderly client hospitalized 4 days ago for treatment of acute respiratory distress has become confused and disoriented. The client has been picking invisible items off blankets and has been yelling at the daughter who is not in the room. The family tells the nurse that the client has been treated for anxiety with alprazolam for years, but alprazolam is not on the current medication list. Which safety measures should be implemented? Select all that apply.
☐ 1. The client should be placed on withdrawal precautions and treatment started immediately.
☐ 2. The client should be placed in soft restraints.
☐ 3. A prescription should be obtained to help with the hallucinations.
☐ 4. The daughter should not visit until the client is better.
☐ 5. The client's medical and mental status should be evaluated frequently and treated as needed.

135. The mother of a 3-year-old child tells the nurse her child is "fussy" and not as "easygoing" as her other children. She is having difficulty feeding the child because he fusses and cries when she serves a meal. The nurse should instruct the mother to:
☐ 1. allow the child to determine when feeding should occur.
☐ 2. not feed the child if he cries.
☐ 3. provide structured feeding times and routines.
☐ 4. give the child finger foods and let him eat when he wants.

136. When giving a client a tube feeding, the nurse should:
☐ 1. warm the feeding solution before administration.
☐ 2. place the client in a left side-lying position.
☐ 3. aspirate residual gastric contents before the feeding and discard.
☐ 4. verify position of the tube before beginning feeding.

137. A multiparous client 48 hours postpartum who is breast-feeding tells the nurse, "I am having a lot of cramping. This did not happen when I nursed my first baby." Which would be the nurse's **best** response?
☐ 1. "I will notify your healthcare provider (HCP). It is possible there are some placental fragments remaining."
☐ 2. "I need to check your lochial flow. You may have a clot that is being dislodged."
☐ 3. "You must have gotten a heavy dose of oxytocin. It should wear off soon."
☐ 4. "The cramping is normal and is caused by your baby's sucking, which stimulates the release of oxytocin."

138. The mother of a child with moderate diarrhea asks how to manage her child's illness. What should the nurse suggest?
☐ 1. Begin clear liquids for 24 hours.
☐ 2. Feed the child bananas, rice, applesauce, and toast.
☐ 3. Offer foods that are low in fat.
☐ 4. Continue the child's regular diet.

139. The nurse is performing routine tracheostomy care. Which step would be appropriate for the nurse to include in the performance of the procedure?
☐ 1. Remove the inner cannula every 2 hours for cleaning.
☐ 2. Secure the tracheostomy ties with a square knot.
☐ 3. Use cut gauze under the neck plate to protect the skin.
☐ 4. Suction the inner cannula on completion of the procedure.

140. The nurse finds a sealed container of IV 50% dextrose in a sink on the nursing unit. The nurse should:
☐ 1. leave it where found and notify the charge nurse.
☐ 2. send it to the pharmacy.
☐ 3. file an incident report.
☐ 4. discard it in a sharps container.

141. To reduce the risk of pressure ulcer formation, which activity should the nurse teach the client who is wheelchair-bound as a result of a spinal cord injury?
☐ 1. Bathe daily.
☐ 2. Eat a high-carbohydrate diet.
☐ 3. Shift your weight every 15 minutes.
☐ 4. Move from the bed to the wheelchair every 2 hours.

142. A client in the second stage of labor has had no anesthesia or analgesia. The nurse should assist the client into which position so the client can begin pushing?
☐ 1. squatting with the body curved in a C shape
☐ 2. side-lying while keeping the head elevated
☐ 3. in the knee-chest position while keeping the head down
☐ 4. squatting with the back arched

143. A client with antisocial personality disorder tells the nurse, "I punched the guy out because he deserved it, and then the cops arrested me." Which response would be **most** helpful to the client?
☐ 1. "It is wrong to punch others."
☐ 2. "If you punch people out, you will get into trouble."
☐ 3. "I would not do that again if I were you."
☐ 4. "Do not ever do that again; you are an adult."

144. The nurse is teaching an unlicensed assistive personnel (UAP) about the care of clients with self-mutilation. Which statement by the UAP would indicate teaching about self-mutilation has been effective?
- ☐ **1.** "It is a means of getting what the person wants."
- ☐ **2.** "It is a nonserious event that can be ignored."
- ☐ **3.** "It is a way to express anger and rage."
- ☐ **4.** "It is a form of manipulation."

145. The nurse is obtaining a nursing history of a client suspected of having hepatitis C. The nurse should ask the client if the client has:
- ☐ **1.** drunk contaminated water.
- ☐ **2.** traveled to India.
- ☐ **3.** had a tattoo.
- ☐ **4.** eaten shellfish.

146. A client is experiencing symptoms of early alcohol withdrawal. The client's blood pressure is 150/85 mm Hg, and the pulse is 98 bpm. The nurse should:
- ☐ **1.** administer lorazepam.
- ☐ **2.** administer an antihypertensive.
- ☐ **3.** assign an unlicensed assistive personnel (UAP) to sit with the client.
- ☐ **4.** notify the healthcare provider (HCP).

147. Which diet instructions are appropriate when teaching a client in the early stages of cirrhosis about nutritional needs? Select all that apply.
- ☐ **1.** "Limit your caloric intake so that you do not become overweight."
- ☐ **2.** "An adequate intake of protein is important to your health."
- ☐ **3.** "I encourage you to eat small, frequent meals."
- ☐ **4.** "Restrict your fluid intake to 1,000 mL/day."
- ☐ **5.** "Limit your alcohol intake to one glass of wine daily."

148. After a child returns from the postanesthesia care unit after surgery, what should the nurse assess **first**?
- ☐ **1.** the IV fluid access site
- ☐ **2.** the child's level of pain
- ☐ **3.** the surgical site dressing
- ☐ **4.** the functioning of the nasogastric tube

149. To protect a client who has received tissue plasminogen activator (t-PA) or alteplase recombinant therapy, the nurse should:
- ☐ **1.** use the radial artery to obtain blood gas samples.
- ☐ **2.** maintain arterial pressure for 10 seconds.
- ☐ **3.** administer IM injections.
- ☐ **4.** encourage physical activity.

150. A client is admitted with acute pancreatitis. The nurse should monitor which laboratory values?
- ☐ **1.** decreased urine amylase level
- ☐ **2.** increased calcium level
- ☐ **3.** decreased glucose level
- ☐ **4.** increased serum amylase and lipase levels

151. For the client with a substance abuse problem, which intervention would be **most** helpful to aid the client in dealing with feelings and concerns related to alcohol and drugs?
- ☐ **1.** individual therapy
- ☐ **2.** group sessions
- ☐ **3.** solitary activities
- ☐ **4.** recreation

152. A client has cystitis. The nurse should further assess the client for:
- ☐ **1.** flank pain.
- ☐ **2.** oliguria.
- ☐ **3.** nausea and vomiting.
- ☐ **4.** foul-smelling urine.

153. A client with acute stress disorder is telling the nurse about the tornado that leveled his house and killed his wife and baby while he was out of town on business. He states, "If only I had been at home, I could have saved them." Which response would be **most** appropriate?
- ☐ **1.** "Do not blame yourself; you will only feel worse."
- ☐ **2.** "It is not your fault, so stop feeling so guilty."
- ☐ **3.** "You might not have been at home."
- ☐ **4.** "You could not have prevented the tornado; it just happened."

154. On the first postpartum day, the nurse is caring for a primiparous client who has recently emigrated from Japan to North America and speaks only a little English. The nurse observes that the client has been bottle-feeding her neonate on occasion, but most of the neonatal care is being performed by the client's mother-in-law. Which action would be **most** appropriate?
- ☐ **1.** Notify the social worker because bonding may be affected.
- ☐ **2.** Document the unusual maternal behavior in the client's medical record.
- ☐ **3.** Determine whether this is a cultural practice for the client and her family.
- ☐ **4.** Obtain a prescription to make a home visit after the client's discharge.

155. A client is scheduled for a creatinine clearance test. What should the nurse do?
- ☐ **1.** Instruct the client about the need to collect urine for 24 hours.
- ☐ **2.** Prepare to insert an indwelling urethral catheter.
- ☐ **3.** Provide the client with a sterile urine collection container.
- ☐ **4.** Instruct the client to force fluids to 3,000 mL/day.

156. When the nurse is assessing a client's cultural adaptation, which statement is **least** sensitive to the client's needs?
- ☐ 1. "What are some of your favorite foods?"
- ☐ 2. "Describe any health problems in your past."
- ☐ 3. "Please tell me how you would like to be addressed."
- ☐ 4. "Your eyes look dark; is this normal for you?"

157. After several months of taking olanzapine, the client reports that he is no longer hearing voices of any kind. Which statement would confirm that the client is developing insight into his illness?
- ☐ 1. "That olanzapine is the best medicine I have ever had."
- ☐ 2. "I did not realize how sick I could get from a chemical brain imbalance."
- ☐ 3. "My mom is proud of me for staying on my medicines."
- ☐ 4. "I think I may be able to get a little part-time job soon."

158. A client whose job requires extensive use of a computer has developed carpal tunnel syndrome. The nurse can instruct the client to relieve the pain by managing:
- ☐ 1. decreased circulation to the brachial nerve.
- ☐ 2. muscle atrophy resulting from disuse.
- ☐ 3. median nerve compression.
- ☐ 4. progressive flexion contracture of the wrist.

159. A client is admitted to the emergency department following an overdose of barbiturates. What should the nurse do **first**?
- ☐ 1. Assess ventilation and assist ventilation as needed.
- ☐ 2. Monitor the blood pressure.
- ☐ 3. Prepare to administer blood products.
- ☐ 4. Place the client in the Trendelenburg position.

160. A client who is recovering from transurethral resection of the prostate (TURP) experiences urinary incontinence and has decreased the fluid intake because of the incontinence. What would be the nurse's **best** response to the client?
- ☐ 1. "Yes, limiting your fluids can decrease your incontinence."
- ☐ 2. "Limiting your fluids will cause kidney stones."
- ☐ 3. "Drink eight glasses of water a day and urinate every 2 hours."
- ☐ 4. "If your incontinence continues, we will reinsert your catheter."

161. The nurse is teaching a client about preventing toxic shock syndrome (TSS). Which action is a risk factor for toxic shock syndrome?
- ☐ 1. changing tampons every 3 hours
- ☐ 2. avoiding use of deodorized tampons
- ☐ 3. alternating tampons with sanitary pads
- ☐ 4. using only tampons at night

162. A client with a history of cystitis is admitted to the hospital with a diagnosis of pyelonephritis. The nurse should assess the client for:
- ☐ 1. suprapubic pain.
- ☐ 2. dysuria.
- ☐ 3. urine retention.
- ☐ 4. costovertebral tenderness.

163. A woman is taking oral contraceptives. The nurse teaches the client that medications that may interfere with oral contraceptive efficacy include:
- ☐ 1. antihypertensives.
- ☐ 2. antibiotics.
- ☐ 3. diuretics.
- ☐ 4. antihistamines.

164. A 28-year-old female client is prescribed danazol for endometriosis. The nurse should instruct the client to report:
- ☐ 1. headaches.
- ☐ 2. weight loss.
- ☐ 3. increased libido.
- ☐ 4. hair loss.

165. To which unlicensed assistive personnel (UAP) should the nurse assign a male orthodox Muslim client who needs complete morning care?
- ☐ 1. Mary, who has two other clients requiring complete morning care
- ☐ 2. Joe, who has one client requiring complete morning care
- ☐ 3. Jill, who has four clients requiring partial morning care
- ☐ 4. Jim, who has five clients requiring partial morning care

166. A client with chronic renal failure is experiencing central nervous system (CNS) changes caused by uremic toxins. Which nursing approach would be **most** appropriate for addressing these CNS changes?
- ☐ 1. Allow the client to grieve for body image changes.
- ☐ 2. Restrict foods that are high in potassium.
- ☐ 3. Restrict fluid intake to 1,000 mL/day.
- ☐ 4. Assess the client's mental status regularly.

167. The nurse is preparing to give a subcutaneous injection to an elderly, emaciated client. Which needle length and angle should the nurse plan to use to administer the injection safely?
- ☐ 1. a ½-inch (1.3-cm) needle at a 90-degree angle
- ☐ 2. a ⅝-inch (1.6-cm) needle at a 45-degree angle
- ☐ 3. a ⅜-inch (0.95-cm) needle at a 15-degree angle
- ☐ 4. a ⅝-inch (1.6-cm) needle at a 90-degree angle

168. A female client is treated for trichomoniasis with metronidazole. The nurse instructs the client that:
- ☐ 1. the medication should not alter the color of the urine.
- ☐ 2. she should discontinue oral contraceptive use during this treatment.
- ☐ 3. she should avoid alcohol during treatment and for 24 hours after completion of the drug.
- ☐ 4. her partner does not need treatment.

169. A client is in the advanced stages of osteoarthritis. Which statement **best** describes the pain that occurs in the advanced stage of the disease?
- ☐ 1. Pain occurs with minimal activity.
- ☐ 2. Crepitation develops and intensifies pain.
- ☐ 3. Joints are symmetrically affected by pain.
- ☐ 4. Fatigue accompanies pain.

170. A family may request to have a client who is Vietnamese transferred to die at home because it is traditionally believed that:
- ☐ 1. it is disloyal to leave their loved one in the hospital.
- ☐ 2. the hospital cannot be trusted.
- ☐ 3. the family can provide more comfort at home.
- ☐ 4. reincarnation will not occur in the hospital.

171. A client has just been admitted with acute delirium of unknown etiology. The client's daughter states that she is worried about her mom because she has never been this sick before. Which would be the **most** helpful statement to make to the daughter?
- ☐ 1. "Please do not worry. We will take good care of your mother."
- ☐ 2. "The healthcare provider (HCP) will prescribe tests to find out what is causing her condition."
- ☐ 3. "We can help you learn how to take care of her after she is discharged."
- ☐ 4. "It helps if you avoid arguing when she talks about seeing people who are not there."

172. A client with Alzheimer's disease is going to live with his daughter who does not work outside of the home. The nurse determines that the daughter needs further education when she makes which statement?
- ☐ 1. "I have put special locks on all the doors that Dad will not be able to unlock."
- ☐ 2. "Dad said that what he missed most while he was here was using his aftershave."
- ☐ 3. "Dad will be in a bedroom that has nothing for him to trip over getting to the bathroom."
- ☐ 4. "I have taken the knobs off of the stove so he will not be able to turn it on."

173. Allopurinol is prescribed for a client who has chronic gout. Which comment indicates that the client understands how to take the allopurinol?
- ☐ 1. "I will take the medication whenever my joints hurt."
- ☐ 2. "I must take this drug on an empty stomach."
- ☐ 3. "I should drink plenty of fluids when taking allopurinol."
- ☐ 4. "I should not take aspirin when taking allopurinol."

174. The mother calls the nurse to report that her toddler has just been burned on the arm. The nurse should advise the mother to **first**:
- ☐ 1. pack the arm in ice, and then take the child to the closest emergency department.
- ☐ 2. rub the burned area with an antibacterial ointment, and then call the child's healthcare provider (HCP).
- ☐ 3. run cool water over the burned area, and then wrap it in a clean cloth.
- ☐ 4. call the child's HCP immediately, and then wrap the arm in a clean cloth.

175. The nursing assessment of a client with osteomyelitis of the left great toe reveals pain with partial weight bearing, unsteady gait, and general weakness. Based on these data, the nurse should institute which safety measures?
- ☐ 1. bed rest
- ☐ 2. airborne precautions
- ☐ 3. referral to physical therapy
- ☐ 4. falls precautions

176. A client receiving a blood transfusion begins to have chills and headache within the first 15 minutes of the transfusion. The nurse should **first**:
- ☐ 1. administer acetaminophen.
- ☐ 2. take the client's blood pressure.
- ☐ 3. discontinue the transfusion.
- ☐ 4. check the infusion rate of the blood.

177. The family of an older adult wants their mother to have counseling for depression. During the initial nursing assessment, the client denies the need for counseling. Which statement by the client supports the fact that the client may **not** need counseling?
- ☐ 1. "My primary care provider just put me on an antidepressant, and I will be fine in a week or so."
- ☐ 2. "My daughter sent me here. She is mad because I do not have the energy to take care of my grandkids."
- ☐ 3. "Since I have gotten over the death of my husband, I have had more energy and been more active than before he died."
- ☐ 4. "My son got worried because I made this silly comment about wanting to be with my husband in heaven."

178. A client takes isosorbide dinitrate as an antianginal medication. Which statement indicates that the client understands the adverse effects of the drug?
- ☐ 1. "I should take my pulse before taking the medication."
- ☐ 2. "I should take isosorbide dinitrate with food."
- ☐ 3. "I will need to change positions slowly so I will not get dizzy."
- ☐ 4. "It is important that I report any swelling in my ankles."

179. The nurse is working on discharge plans with a client who is diagnosed with intermittent explosive disorder, characterized by sudden angry outbursts. The nurse determines that the client is ready for discharge when the client makes which comment?
- ☐ **1.** "I am just not going to let myself get angry anymore."
- ☐ **2.** "Drinking does not help, but I like being with my buddies at the bar."
- ☐ **3.** "I will be taking valproic acid and propranolol to help stay in control."
- ☐ **4.** "It would help if my mom would stop getting on my case all the time."

180. The nurse walks into a client's room to administer the 0900 medications and notices that the client is in an awkward position in bed. What is the nurse's **first** action?
- ☐ **1.** Ask the client to state his or her name.
- ☐ **2.** Check the client's name band.
- ☐ **3.** Straighten the client's pillow behind the back.
- ☐ **4.** Give the client his medications.

181. The nurse is performing the initial assessment on a middle-aged woman recently diagnosed with Cushing's syndrome. The nurse reviews the history and physical (see chart). The nurse should develop a plan with the client to manage which effect? Select all that apply.

History and Physical

A recent ground-level fall resulting in multiple bruises on both arms and left shoulder
A slow-healing laceration on the right hand from a fall 2 weeks prior.
Muscle weakness
Unable to sleep more than 2 to 3 hours at a time
Moon-faced appearance
Oily skin
Recent 20-lb (9.1-kg) weight gain

Vital signs	BP:	148/94
	Heart rate:	96/strong/regular
	Respirations:	20/regular/unlabored
	Pain:	Denies

- ☐ **1.** low blood volume
- ☐ **2.** risk for injury
- ☐ **3.** slow healing
- ☐ **4.** changes in physical appearance
- ☐ **5.** risk for infection

182. A "read-back" procedure has been implemented on a nursing unit to prevent discrepancies in telephone prescriptions and reports. This procedure should be implemented when the:
- ☐ **1.** float nurse gives a written report to the oncoming nurse.
- ☐ **2.** nurse receives a critical lab value via phone or in person from the lab.
- ☐ **3.** lab report shows up on the computerized medical record.
- ☐ **4.** unit clerk takes a telephone prescription for a stat lab test.

183. Four clients in a critical care unit have been diagnosed with *Pseudomonas aeruginosa*. The Infection Prevention and Control Department has determined that this is probably a nosocomial infection. Select the **most** appropriate intervention by the nurse. The nurse should:
- ☐ **1.** wear an N-95 mask when caring for these clients.
- ☐ **2.** initiate transmission-based precautions.
- ☐ **3.** initiate contact precautions.
- ☐ **4.** ensure that staff does not have artificial fingernails.

184. The nurse is instructing the spouse of a client who had an incision and drainage procedure for an abscess how to care for the wound at home. The nurse should instruct the spouse to:
- ☐ **1.** clean the incision and drainage sites simultaneously.
- ☐ **2.** clean from the incision site to the drainage site.
- ☐ **3.** clean from the drainage site to the incision site.
- ☐ **4.** clean each site independently.

185. After completing initial assessment rounds, which client should the nurse discuss with the healthcare provider (HCP) **first**?
- ☐ **1.** a client who was admitted from the emergency department last evening after a blow to the head who is now vomiting and confused as to time and place
- ☐ **2.** a client who returned from abdominal surgery last evening and now has a dime-sized bright red spot on the dressing
- ☐ **3.** a client who had a right total knee replacement 2 days ago and now is reporting constipation and abdominal discomfort
- ☐ **4.** a client admitted for lower extremity vasculitis and wound care who is requesting more pain medication before the next dressing change in 2 hours

186. Which is the correct knot used to secure a restraint correctly to the bedframe?

☐ **1.**

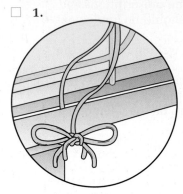

☐ **2.**

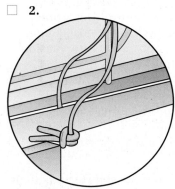

☐ **3.**

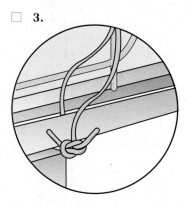

☐ **4.**

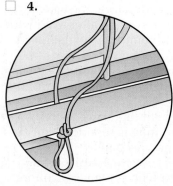

187. The obstetrical triage nurse is assessing a client with a term pregnancy. There has not been any change in the cervix for the past 2 hours despite irregular contractions. When discharging the client to her home, the nurse should tell the client to return to the hospital when which conditions occur? Select all that apply.

☐ **1.** She feels more than three contractions an hour.
☐ **2.** Contractions become more intense and closer together.
☐ **3.** She notices vaginal bleeding.
☐ **4.** She thinks the membranes have ruptured.
☐ **5.** She notices an absence of fetal movement.
☐ **6.** She feels the urge to push.

188. The parents of a newborn with Down syndrome are tearful when they tell the nurse that the diagnosis was a surprise to them. Which statement by the parents indicates that they have some understanding of Down syndrome?

☐ **1.** "Children with Down syndrome are often fearful of strangers and have difficulty making friends."
☐ **2.** "At some point during their life span, children with Down syndrome will need to be institutionalized."
☐ **3.** "Children with Down syndrome often become violent when they experience hormonal changes during puberty."
☐ **4.** "There is a broad spectrum of mental capabilities and physical characteristics of children with Down syndrome."

189. A 2-year-old is brought to the emergency department after experiencing a seizure. The child currently has the flu and has had fevers for the last 3 days. The father asks what caused the seizure to occur. The nurse's **best** response is:

☐ **1.** "Your child's seizure was likely caused by the rapid elevation of her temperature."
☐ **2.** "The seizure likely occurred because your child's temperature rose beyond a personal threshold."
☐ **3.** "Your child's seizure was likely caused by the prolonged duration of her fevers."
☐ **4.** "The seizure likely occurred because your child's immune system is not developed."

190. Thirty minutes ago, a term multigravida was 5 cm dilated, 100% effaced, and −1 station. She is now visibly uncomfortable and states that she needs to get up for a bowel movement. The **best** nursing intervention is:

☐ **1.** assist the client up to the bathroom.
☐ **2.** reassure the client that the sensation she is feeling is due to pressure from the fetal head.
☐ **3.** perform another sterile vaginal exam on the client.
☐ **4.** notify the healthcare provider (HCP) of the client's pain.

Answers, Rationales, and Test-Taking Strategies

The answers and rationales for each question follow below, along with keys ( ) to the client need (CN) and cognitive level (CL) for each question. In addition, you will also see a glossary icon ( ) highlighting specific terminology used on the licensing exam. As you check your answers, use the **Content Mastery and Test-Taking Skill Self-Analysis** *worksheet (tear-out worksheet in back of book) to identify the reason(s) for not answering the questions correctly. For additional information about test-taking skills and strategies for answering questions, refer to pages 12–23 and pages 35–36 in Part 1 of this book.*

1. 4. Heartburn is caused when stomach contents enter the distal end of the esophagus, producing a burning sensation. To avoid heartburn during pregnancy, the client should avoid spicy foods, eat smaller, more frequent meals, and avoid lying down after eating. Peristalsis usually decreases during the latter half of pregnancy. Displacement of the stomach by the uterus, not the diaphragm, may contribute to heartburn. Increased, not decreased, secretion of hydrochloric acid also contributes to heartburn during pregnancy.

CN: Basic care and comfort; CL: Apply

2. 2. Acknowledging the anger and its source encourages communication about the client's feelings. Although anger at God is common after a loss, the client is displacing the anger that she needs to deal with more directly. Telling the client that the miscarriage was an accident or that she is a strong person and will get through this ignores the client's feelings of anger and loss, thereby cutting off communication.

CN: Psychosocial integrity; CL: Synthesize

3. 4. Asking the client to speak about his concerns encourages open discussion. Telling the client that he is making a mistake is judgmental of the client's wishes and eliminates opportunities for the client to explore the situation and discuss various treatment options. Saying that herbal treatments have not been approved by the FDA or that they have not been researched is irrelevant, places a value judgment on the client's wishes, and provides no opportunity for discussion.

CN: Management of care; CL: Synthesize

4. 3. The most important aspect of teaching a preschooler is to have the family members there for support. Preschoolers are able to understand information that is individualized to their level. Including a plastic model of the heart and a catheter as part of the preoperative preparation may be helpful. The other family members will understand the heart model and catheter better than the preschooler will.

CN: Reduction of risk potential; CL: Synthesize

5. 4. Massaging an area that is reddened due to pressure is contraindicated because it further reduces blood flow to the area. In the past, massaging reddened areas was thought to improve blood flow to the area, and some nursing personnel may still believe that massaging the area is effective in preventing pressure ulcer formation. Since massaging a reddened area is contraindicated, the nurse should not encourage the UAP to continue massage or explain that it is effective. The UAP should not massage the area, nor add lotion.

CN: Management of care; CL: Synthesize

6. 3. Asking the mother to talk about her concerns acknowledges the mother's rights and encourages open discussion. The other responses negate the parent's concerns.

CN: Management of care; CL: Synthesize

7. 1, 2, 3. Some providers recommend that breast-feeding mothers avoid consuming potentially allergic foods. The top 6 foods known to cause allergies in children are shellfish, peanuts, eggs, milk, soy, and tree nuts.

CN: Health promotion and maintenance; CL: Apply

8. 3. A meal delivery service would be the most helpful to this client. There are a variety of services, some of them at no cost to the client in which a volunteer brings the meal and visits with the client and is a means to check on elderly persons who live alone. Hospice care involves daily needs for the terminally ill at home, and this client does not need this type of service. Home nursing services typically provide skilled nursing care to clients at home, and this client does not need this level of care. Associations for retired persons advocate for care and services for retirees, but do not provide services or care.

CN: Management of care; CL: Apply

9. 1. The cardiovascular status of the client is the first information documented and will validate the effectiveness of the temporary pacemaker. The client's emotional state and the type of sedation are important but not a high priority. The nurse will need to document the pacemaker information (settings of the pacemaker); this will be considered part of the cardiovascular information.

CN: Management of care; CL: Apply

10. 3. Using a special feeding table or modified high chair is the best method for an infant who is used to sitting up for feedings. The child should not be flat because of the danger of aspiration. Raising the child's head will not work as well as using a feeding table because the child is not used to lying down to eat. Two people are not necessary.

🔑 CN: Health promotion and maintenance; CL: Evaluate

11. 3, 4. The National Association for Home Care (NAHC) defines "home care" as services for people who are recovering, disabled, or chronically ill and who are in need of treatment or support to function effectively in the home environment. The client with multiple sclerosis and an open lesion is at risk for infection and will require assistance with managing the lesion. Prothrombin monitoring is usually done at the clinic or **healthcare provider's (HCP's)** 📖 office. Diet instruction can be accomplished at a healthcare facility or dietitian office. The client with vertigo should be monitored for safety in the home. Clients receiving home care services are usually under the care of a HCP with the focus of care being treatment or rehabilitation. Lenses for glasses can be evaluated at an eye clinic or an ophthalmologist's office; a prescription for stronger lenses could be written.

🔑 CN: Management of care; CL: Evaluate

12. 1. A soft toothbrush or gauze pad should be used to provide oral hygiene at least every 2 hours to promote client comfort and prevent superinfection. Commercial mouthwash is contraindicated because of high alcohol content that is irritating to inflamed mucosa. Oral swabs with an astringent should be avoided because they are drying and also can promote bacterial growth. Leaving dentures in place will have no effect on the development of edema. Additionally, further irritation of the oral mucosa may occur if dentures are left in place. Dentures should be removed to aid in relieving the client's discomfort or pain.

🔑 CN: Basic care and comfort; CL: Synthesize

13. 3. Although coordinating documentation, resolving negative feelings, and calming down are goals of debriefing after a restraint, the ultimate outcome is to improve restraint procedures.

🔑 CN: Safety and infection control; CL: Synthesize

14. 4. The situation is escalating, and the nurse's priority is to protect the infant from harm. Therefore, removal of the infant from this situation should be the first action by the nurse. Reasoning at this point or asking one of the parents to leave the room would be ineffective and may serve to further

escalate the situation. Calling security is necessary, but only after the nurse has removed the infant from the room.

🔑 CN: Management of care; CL: Synthesize

15. 2. By federal law, all clients entering a hospital or hospice program are offered the chance to make an advance directive, so that their wishes will be known and followed in an emergency. The directive is not a substitute for informed discussion with the **HCP** 📖. Worry about extraordinary means being taken can be discussed with the client later, but the client needs to be informed that the directive is a federal requirement to protect the client's autonomy.

🔑 CN: Management of care; CL: Synthesize

16. 1, 2, 3, 4. The role of the nurse in witnessing the signing of the **consent** 📖 is to witness that the client is informed of the procedure, understands the information, is aware of potential complications, and is signing of his or her own free will. It is not necessary for a spouse, relative, or guardian to be present.

🔑 CN: Management of care; CL: Apply

17. 4. Doxycycline is contraindicated in pregnancy because it can stain the teeth of the developing fetus when given during the last half of pregnancy. The nurse should withhold the drug and notify the **HCP** 📖 to change the prescription. All neonates are given prophylactic ophthalmic ointment for the prevention of ophthalmia neonatorum, conjunctivitis caused by gonorrhea.

🔑 CN: Pharmacological and parenteral therapies; CL: Synthesize

18. 3. The contraction stress test simulates labor and determines the fetal response to the labor process and the mother's contractions. Therefore, determining that contractions have ceased after the test is important. Although spontaneous rupture of membranes is a possibility after a contraction stress test, it is not a typical occurrence. The test should not affect the viability of the fetus. Fetal viability is related to gestational age. A fetus of at least 23 weeks' gestation is considered viable or capable of extrauterine life. Stating that stress test is negative means the fetal heart rate has already been interpreted and has not been found to fall during contractions.

🔑 CN: Reduction of risk potential; CL: Synthesize

19. 2, 3, 4. A postoperative ileus is a functional obstruction of the bowel. Assessment of bowel sounds, the first stool, and the amount of gastric output provide information about the return of gastric function. Measurement of urine specific gravity provides information about fluid and electrolyte status; bilirubin levels provide information about liver function, and neither of these tests needs to be included in a focused assessment for ileus.

⚷ CN: Reduction of risk potential; CL: Analyze

20. 2. Salmeterol is a beta$_2$-agonist, a maintenance drug that the asthmatic client uses twice daily, every 12 hours. Albuterol is used as the "rescue inhaler" for bronchospasms. Salmeterol can be used to prevent exercise-induced bronchospasms, but it should be taken 30 to 60 minutes before exercise. If the client is taking salmeterol twice daily, it should not be used in additional doses before exercise; twice daily is the maximum dosage. Indications for salmeterol include only asthma and bronchospasm induced by chronic obstructive pulmonary disease.

⚷ CN: Pharmacological and parenteral therapies; CL: Synthesize

21. 1, 2, 4. Nephrotic syndrome is characterized by massive proteinuria, hypoalbuminemia, edema, and hyperlipidemia and normal or lower than normal blood pressure. Elevated streptococcal antibody titers are associated with poststreptococcal glomerulonephritis, an immune complex disease.

⚷ CN: Physiological adaptation; CL: Analyze

22. 3. Aldactone is a potassium-sparing diuretic often used to counteract potassium loss caused by other diuretics. If foods or fluids are ingested that are high in potassium, hyperkalemia may result and lead to cardiac arrhythmias. Increasing the intake of milk or milk products does not affect the potassium level. Restricting fluid may elevate all electrolytes due to extracellular fluid volume depletion. By increasing foods high in sodium, water would tend to be retained and so would dilute all electrolytes in the extracellular fluid compartment.

⚷ CN: Health promotion and maintenance; CL: Synthesize

23. 4. Clients with burns are susceptible to the development of Curling's ulcer, a gastroduodenal ulcer that is caused by a generalized stress response. The stress response results in increased gastric acid secretion and a decreased production of mucus. Prevention is the best treatment, and clients are frequently treated prophylactically with antacids and H$_2$ histamine blockers such as famotidine.

⚷ CN: Reduction of risk potential; CL: Synthesize

24. 3. The client has ventricular fibrillation, an arrhythmia that can lead to cardiac arrest. Given the client's history, the nurse should call the **rapid response team** 📖 to initiate interventions to avoid cardiac arrest. After calling the team, the nurse can administer oxygen. Taking time to inspect the

incision delays the necessary intervention. This ECG strip does not show loose electrodes.

⚷ CN: Management of care; CL: Synthesize

25. 2. The best approach by the mother is not to interfere. The children need to learn how to solve disagreements on their own. If the parent always intervenes, then the children do not learn how to do this. Siblings will disagree and argue as part of normal development. Punishment, including telling the children that they will not go out to lunch, is not warranted.

⚷ CN: Health promotion and maintenance; CL: Evaluate

26. 2. Managing stressful life events can decrease the incidence of outbreaks of HSV-2. Occlusive ointments should not be applied. Antiviral therapies will not cure herpes, but they can manage symptoms and decrease the incidence of outbreaks. Clients with HSV-2 should use condoms to prevent HSV transmission. Cells can be shed at other times, not only when the vesicles are weeping.

⚷ CN: Physiological adaptation; CL: Synthesize

27. 1, 3, 4. The nurse should assess the client for adverse effects affecting the vestibular branch of the acoustic nerve, such as vertigo, nausea and vomiting with motion, and ataxia. Tinnitus, or a ringing in the ears, is a clinical manifestation of altered function of the auditory branch of the eighth cranial nerve, not the vestibular branch. The client will not have hearing loss.

⚷ CN: Physiological adaptation; CL: Analyze

28. 1. Tetanus toxoid is indicated, since there has been no booster in the last 5 years. With a human bite, there is a risk of severe infection; application of a steroid cream does not prevent infection. The closure of the wound should be delayed until it is determined that there is no infection, in approximately 24 to 48 hours. Tuberculosis is not transmitted through human bites.

⚷ CN: Reduction of risk potential; CL: Apply

29. 3, 4, 5. Before discussing the use of medroxyprogesterone acetate as a birth control option, the nurse should determine if the woman is or has been depressed because medroxyprogesterone acetate can increase depression in a client with depression. The drug can be transmitted in breast milk, and the long-term effects on the baby are not known. Women who are pregnant should not take medroxyprogesterone acetate. Medroxyprogesterone acetate does not treat or prevent sexually transmitted diseases, so this information is not essential when considering its use. Although the husband should be a part of birth control decisions, the final decision is made by the client.

🔑 CN: Pharmacological and parenteral therapies; CL: Analyze

30. 3. With a parent who is visibly upset, it is best to try to determine the cause. Therefore, asking the mother about why she wants to take the child home can provide insight into the problem. The nurse cannot stop the mother from taking her child home. However, the **HCP** 📖 should be notified about the mother's decision, and efforts are needed to explain the ramifications of taking the child home. It is inappropriate for the nurse to say "I know how you feel" or "I can imagine how hard this is" unless the nurse has had the same experience.

🔑 CN: Psychosocial integrity; CL: Synthesize

31. 4, 1, 2, 3. The infant who is 6 months of age with diarrhea is seen first because of risk for further dehydration; the nurse immediately starts an IV infusion. The client who is 12 years of age is seen next; this child is considered to require urgent care but can wait several hours. The client who is 8 years of age can be seen next; he is considered to require nonurgent care and will respond to assessment and first aid. The last client to receive care is the client who is 16 years of age; this client is considered nonurgent and likely will not require the services of the emergency department.

🔑 CN: Management of care; CL: Synthesize

32. 1. Normal urine output for an infant is 1 to 2 mL/kg/h.

🔑 CN: Physiological adaptation; CL: Evaluate

33. 1, 2, 4. All areas concerned with the safety and quality of care need to participate in the decision-making process and arrive at a plan that will meet the needs of the clients on the neonatal care unit. Identifying the problem at a staff meeting is an ideal forum to bring up the need for improvement and education. The staff is an integral part of the development team. The staff educator is an important member of the team and is responsible for orienting new nurses to the unit. Asking an experienced staff member to spend time in reorienting staff members is difficult to do as the nurses have their own clients to care for. Although the unit director can obtain additional information from the **healthcare providers (HCPs)** 📖 about the problem, the nursing staff has responsibility for assuring that they are providing safe and high-quality care.

🔑 CN: Safety and infection control; CL: Synthesize

34. 3. Based on the data given, the nurse should develop a plan with the client to manage the pain.

It is not necessary for the client to be completely immobile. There is no clinical indication that the leg will need to be amputated. A temperature of 101°F (38.3°C) would be unlikely to produce a fluid volume deficit in this client.

🔑 CN: Physiological adaptation; CL: Analyze

35. 3. After vasectomy, a sperm analysis will be performed every 4 to 6 weeks. A sperm-free analysis is necessary before the man can be considered sterile. Sperms gradually disappear from the ejaculate. Clients must be informed that conception is possible in the immediate postvasectomy period.

🔑 CN: Physiological adaptation; CL: Apply

36. 4. One outcome criterion for the client with osteoarthritis is improved joint mobility. It is probably not possible to arrest the disease. Gold compound is administered to clients with rheumatoid arthritis, not osteoarthritis. Outcome criteria should be specific; feeling better is too general to be useful.

🔑 CN: Basic care and comfort; CL: Evaluate

37. 1, 2, 4. Classic signs of meningitis in an infant include fever, poor feeding, vomiting, and irritability. Abdominal pain and diarrhea are not usual signs of meningitis; they are more commonly associated with gastroenteritis.

🔑 CN: Physiological adaptation; CL: Analyze

38. 2. Deep-breathing exercises and use of incentive spirometry are more effective when pain is minimal. A client in severe pain tends to limit movement and to breathe shallowly to decrease the pain. Enough pain medication should be given to decrease pain without depressing respirations. Administration of oxygen or increasing fluids will not prevent atelectasis or pneumonia. Deep-breathing exercises and use of incentive spirometry should be done 10 times every hour while awake. The client's position should be changed every 1 to 2 hours to allow for full chest expansion. Ambulation, not just sitting in the chair, should be implemented as soon as **healthcare provider (HCP)** 📖 approval is obtained.

🔑 CN: Reduction of risk potential; CL: Synthesize

39. 2. A child who has had rheumatic fever is likely to develop the illness again after a future streptococcal infection. Therefore, it is advised that the child receive antibiotic prophylaxis for at least 5 years and sometimes even longer after the acute attack to prevent recurrence.

🔑 CN: Physiological adaptation; CL: Synthesize

40. 4. Crowning occurs when the fetal head is visible. Anterior-posterior slit occurs as the perineum flattens and is followed by an oval opening. As labor progresses, the perineum takes on a circular shape, followed by crowning.

🔑 CN: Physiological adaptation; CL: Apply

41. 1. The first action is to increase the oxygen flow rate from 2 to 4 L/min to help ensure adequate oxygenation for the client. Although it is important to notify the **HCP** 📖 for additional prescriptions and to obtain further assessment data, such as arterial blood gas measurements, it is a priority to support the client's cardiopulmonary system. It would be appropriate to reassure the client while these other interventions are occurring.

🔑 CN: Reduction of risk potential; CL: Synthesize

42. 2. Although a cool air vaporizer may be recommended to humidify the environment, using saline nose drops and then a bulb syringe before meals and at nap and bed times will allow the child to breathe more easily. Saline helps to loosen secretions and keep the mucous membranes moist. The bulb syringe then gently aids in removing the loosened secretions. Blowing into the child's mouth to clear the nose introduces more organisms to the child. A nonprescription vasoconstrictive nasal spray is not recommended for infants because if the spray is used for longer than 3 days, a rebound effect with increased inflammation occurs.

🔑 CN: Reduction of risk potential; CL: Synthesize

43. 3. Hoarseness may indicate metastatic disease to the recurrent laryngeal nerve and is commonly noted with left upper lobe lung tumors. Diarrhea and constipation are not associated with lung cancer. Weight loss, not weight gain, can be a symptom of extensive disease.

🔑 CN: Physiological adaptation; CL: Analyze

44. 1. The nurse should determine if the **HCP** 📖 is the HCP of record and should have access to the information in the **medical record** 📖. The medical record is not for public access. The nurse would not give client information to any HCP or refuse to give information without first determining the HCP of record and/or a legitimate need to know. As an employee, the nurse should have access to medical records, but it is not acceptable to enter a medical record without justification.

🔑 CN: Management of care; CL: Synthesize

45. 1. A client with metabolic alkalosis may exhibit irritability or nervousness. Hyperventilation is a clinical manifestation of respiratory alkalosis.

Diarrhea is a possible clinical finding in metabolic acidosis. Edema is not specifically associated with an acid-base imbalance.

🔑 CN: Physiological adaptation; CL: Analyze

46. 2. An initial sign of hemorrhaging after a tonsillectomy is swallowing frequently as mucus and blood combine to increase secretions. Mouth breathing is expected after surgery because the child's mouth is very dry and the throat is sore. Because the child has been without fluids for some time, the child usually is thirsty and asks for a drink. Increased pulse rate is a later sign of hemorrhage.

🔑 CN: Reduction of risk potential; CL: Analyze

47. 1, 3, 4, 2. The nurse should first stop the transfusion. The nurse should next keep the IV open at the original blood transfusion site with normal saline at a keep-vein-open rate. Then, the nurse should administer an antihistamine. Last, the nurse should return the blood bag and blood slip to the blood bank for testing.

🔑 CN: Pharmacological and parenteral therapies; CL: Synthesize

48. 33 gtt/min
The flow rate is determined by the rate of infusion and the number of drops per milliliter of the fluid being administered: gtt/mL × mL/min = IV flow rate (gtt/min).
    Therefore:
    10 gtt/mL × 100 mL/30 min = 33 gtt/min.

🔑 CN: Pharmacological and parenteral therapies; CL: Apply

49. 4. Delusions of grandeur provide the client with an exaggerated sense of self-esteem that is unrelated to the client's actual achievements. Other, less grandiose, religious delusions may provide comfort or meaning for the client. Delusions of persecution are frequently related to safety issues. Delusions of grandeur are not about survival needs.

🔑 CN: Psychosocial integrity; CL: Analyze

50. 3. Loss of electrolytes from the gastrointestinal tract through vomiting, diarrhea, or nasogastric suction is a common cause of potassium loss, resulting in hypokalemia. Hypermagnesemia does not result from excessive loss of gastrointestinal fluids. Common causes of hypernatremia are water loss (as in diabetes insipidus or osmotic diuresis) and excessive sodium intake. Common causes of hypocalcemia include chronic renal failure, elevated phosphorus concentration, and primary hypoparathyroidism.

🔑 CN: Physiological adaptation; CL: Analyze

51. 3. It is a normal variation for women to have long-term, bilateral nipple inversion. A woman who has a unilateral nipple inversion that is a new change is at risk for a tumor; the weight of the tumor causes pulling on the nipple. A pronounced unilateral venous pattern, peau d'orange breast tissue, and breast tissue darker than the areolae are definite warning signals for breast cancer that must be reported to the **healthcare provider (HCP)** 📖 immediately.

CN: Health promotion and maintenance; CL: Analyze

52. 1. It is important for children with sickle cell disease to drink lots of fluids to help prevent a crisis. Dehydration precipitates sickling and a crisis. Although taking the child's temperature may provide information about the child's status, it will do nothing to prevent a crisis, nor will weighing the child daily. Offering the child a high-protein diet will not prevent a crisis, nor is it recommended.

CN: Reduction of risk potential; CL: Synthesize

53. 1. The nurse notifies the pediatrician because a short, webbed neck is associated with genetic deviations or chromosomal disorders such as Turner's syndrome. Cleft palate is associated with embryonic developmental failures and an abnormal opening in the palate. Potter's syndrome (renal agenesis) is characterized by an atypical facial appearance consisting of a flat nose, recessed chin, epicanthal folds, low-set abnormal ears, limb abnormalities, and pulmonary hypoplasia. Neural tube defects are associated with spina bifida or myelomeningocele.

CN: Physiological adaptation; CL: Analyze

54. 3. Diarrhea results in electrolyte loss and the nurse should assess the client for signs of hypokalemia. Clinical manifestations of hypokalemia include an irregular pulse, fatigue, muscle weakness, flabby muscles, decreased reflexes, nausea, vomiting, and ileus. Muscle spasms are not seen in hypokalemia. Thirst is a symptom of hypernatremia. Confusion can be seen in hyponatremia and hypocalcemia.

CN: Physiological adaptation; CL: Analyze

55. 1, 3, 5. Notifying the pharmacy of the nursing concerns is an appropriate first action. The nursing staff should work cooperatively with the pharmacy to develop a system that works well for both nursing and pharmacy. Constant communication with all nursing staff during the quality improvement process is integral to the final approval process of both groups. Moving the drugs to a new position within the medication system during an off shift may create errors, as medications are inserted into the system in a certain position. Leaving the decisions to the pharmacy staff eliminates the input provided by nursing, a vital link between medication and the client.

CN: Management of care; CL: Synthesize

56. 2. The client's self-report of pain is the most reliable indicator of the existence and intensity of the pain. Client response to pain is highly individualized and subjective. The nurse must respect the client's self-report.

CN: Basic care and comfort; CL: Evaluate

57. 2. Excessive milk consumption can lead to the displacement of iron-rich foods in the diet. This can result in iron deficiency anemia. Drinking excess milk will not cause vitamin C, biotin, or folate deficiencies.

CN: Health promotion and maintenance; CL: Apply

58. 2. Although all the symptoms listed can occur in cases of fat embolism syndrome, confusion is the earliest symptom noted. The confusion is caused by a low arterial oxygen level.

CN: Physiological adaptation; CL: Analyze

59. 1. An idea of reference is a person's view that other people recognize that she has an important characteristic or power. Thought insertion refers to a person's belief that others, or a specific other, can put thoughts into her mind. Visual hallucinations involve seeing objects or persons not based on reality. A neologism is a word or phrase that has meaning only to the person using it.

CN: Psychosocial integrity; CL: Analyze

60. 3. The American Academy of Pediatrics and the American College of Obstetrics and Gynecology recommend hearing screening for all newborns. Currently, more than 30 states mandate screening, which is done by otoacoustic emissions or auditory brainstem response. Newborns can hear as soon as the amniotic fluid drains from the ear canal. Even though hearing problems are not common in newborns, the mother's concerns should be addressed. Clapping to elicit a response is crude and unreliable. If done for minimal screening, the distance should be no more than 12 inches.

CN: Health promotion and maintenance; CL: Apply

61. 4. The equianalgesic dose of oral meperidine hydrochloride is up to four times the IM dose. Meperidine hydrochloride can be given orally, but it is much more effective when given IM.

CN: Pharmacological and parenteral therapies; CL: Apply

62. **1, 2, 3.** Children tend to be impulsive, which contributes to head injuries. Also, the larger size of the heads of infants and toddlers causes them to fall more easily than do older children. Falls account for one-third of all head injuries. Motor vehicle accidents account for about 80% of all severe head injuries in children. Children aged 5 to 15 are most likely to be involved in bicycle accidents as a result of only about 50% wearing helmets. Child abuse and tumors involve a much smaller number of children.

⌐☞ CN: Health promotion and maintenance; CL: Apply

63. **1.** In order to prevent disuse osteoporosis, it is important to implement weight-bearing activities as soon as medically allowed. Increasing the client's calcium intake will not prevent the development of osteoporosis without the inclusion of weight-bearing activity. Passive ROM exercises and isometric exercises do not provide the bone stress necessary to reduce the risk of osteoporosis.

⌐☞ CN: Reduction of risk potential; CL: Synthesize

64. **3.** Toddlers have temper tantrums in their attempt to develop autonomy. Toddlers should be left alone as long as they are safe during a tantrum. Moving the child to a time-out chair or punishing the child reinforces the behavior and is to be avoided. Attempting to talk to the toddler also reinforces the behavior. Additionally, at this cognitive level, toddlers do not understand as well as older children do.

⌐☞ CN: Health promotion and maintenance; CL: Synthesize

65. **1.** Because the client's temperature continues to rise in spite of recently administering ibuprofen, the nurse notifies the HCP. After notifying the HCP 📖, the nurse can bathe the client with tepid water. If the temperature cannot be lowered shortly, the client is also at risk for seizures; the nurse pads the side rails and observes for seizure activity. The nurse cannot administer another dose of ibuprofen without the HCP's orders.

⌐☞ CN: Physiological adaptation; CL: Apply

66. **3.** The Joint Commission and Health Council of Canada both mandate interactive handoff communication that allows the opportunity for questioning between the giver and receiver of client information, including up-to-date information regarding the client's care, treatment and services, current condition, and any recent or anticipated changes. Nurses have primary responsibility and accountability for utilization of all nursing care provided to clients. The nurse retains the right and has the responsibility to refrain from delegating specific activities based on individual client care needs, caregiver expertise, and/or client care program requirements.

⌐☞ CN: Management of care; CL: Apply

67. **2.** Daily skin inspection is essential in preventing pressure ulcers. Hot water is irritating to the skin and should be avoided. Massaging bony prominences is contraindicated and may actually promote skin breakdown. Prolonged, uninterrupted chair sitting should be avoided; the client's position should be adjusted at least every hour.

⌐☞ CN: Reduction of risk potential; CL: Synthesize

68. **3.** Skeletal pins should not be loose and able to move. Any pin loosening should be reported immediately. Slight serous drainage is normal and may crust around the insertion site or be present on the dressing. The pin insertion site should be cleaned with aseptic technique according to facility policy. Pin insertion sites are typically not painful; pain may be indicative of an infection and should be reported.

⌐☞ CN: Physiological adaptation; CL: Analyze

69. **4.** Acknowledging the basic feeling that the client expressed and asking an open-ended question allow the client to explain her fears. Saying, "It is normal to be scared. We will help you through it," does not focus on the client's feelings; rather, it gives reassurance. Asking if the client feels guilty for having smoked assumes guilt, which might be present, but additional information is needed to confirm. Telling the client not to be so hard on herself does not acknowledge the client's feelings at all.

⌐☞ CN: Psychosocial integrity; CL: Synthesize

70. **3.** It is important that clients with rheumatoid arthritis maintain proper posture and body alignment to support joints and decrease pain and stiffness. Clients with hip pain will be most comfortable when sitting in a straight-back chair with an elevated seat. Elevated seats avoid excessive hip flexion and place less stress on the hip joints. A recliner chair will not provide sufficient support and likely does not have an elevated seat. A couch typically has a low seat and will cause hip flexion. A rocking chair may not provide the correct joint support and is not sufficiently stable.

⌐☞ CN: Basic care and comfort; CL: Evaluate

71. **3.** Giving away personal items has consistently been shown to be an indicator of suicidal plans in the depressed and suicidal individual. The other behaviors indicate a return of interest in normal adolescent activities.

⌐☞ CN: Psychosocial integrity; CL: Synthesize

72. 3. When a neonate dies, the mother should be allowed to stay with the baby as long as she wants and say anything she wants. She is grieving and needs time with the neonate. A photograph should be taken in case the mother wants a photograph at a later time. Telling the mother that this is for the best is inappropriate because such a statement discounts the mother's feelings. Advising the mother to get pregnant again to get over the loss is not helpful because the mother needs time to grieve and be with the neonate. The nurse should remain near the mother and not delegate this responsibility to the hospital's chaplain. A chaplain or other religious member can be contacted if the mother desires.

CN: Psychosocial integrity; CL: Synthesize

73. 1. Clients typically have considerable pain for the first few days after surgery and require frequent administration of pain medication, preferably the use of opioids administered intravenously on a regular schedule or patient-controlled analgesia (PCA). The other problems are all possible complications following this type of surgery, but the priority, until noted otherwise, is to provide adequate pain control.

CL: Apply; CN: Pharmacological and parenteral therapies

74. 4. Serum albumin levels help determine whether protein intake is sufficient. Proteins are broken down into amino acids during digestion. Amino acids are absorbed in the small intestine, and albumin is built from amino acids. The red blood cell count, bilirubin levels, and reticulocyte count do not indicate protein intake.

CN: Physiological adaptation; CL: Analyze

75. 2. The client who is taking desmopressin nasal spray should not use the same naris for administration each time. The client should alternate nares every dose. The client should observe for and report promptly signs and symptoms of nasal ulceration, congestion, or respiratory infection.

CN: Pharmacological and parenteral therapies; CL: Evaluate

76. 0.5 mL

$$500 \text{ mg} / \text{mL} = 250 \text{ mg} / X \text{ mL}$$
$$X = 0.5 \text{ mL}.$$

CN: Pharmacological and parenteral therapies; CL: Apply

77. 1, 5, 6. Down syndrome is the most common trisomal abnormality. It can occur at any maternal age with the average being 27 years. The risk of bearing a Down syndrome infant increases with advanced maternal age. The syndrome is caused by nondisjunction during the first meiotic cell division, rather than autosomal dominant or recessive traits. There is no association with timing or quality of prenatal care.

CN: Health promotion and maintenance; CL: Apply

78. 1, 3, 4. The pregnant woman is not in imminent danger or likely to have a precipitous birth. The child who is 10 years of age is not at risk of infection and can be treated in an outpatient facility. First-degree burns are considered less urgent. The male with respiratory distress and coughing is transported first as he is likely experiencing smoke inhalation. The 75-year-old male with second-degree burns should also be also transported to a burn center or emergency department.

CN: Management of care; CL: Synthesize

79. 3. As with other contraceptives that are progestin based, heavy menstrual bleeding may occur. Other adverse effects include rash, acne, alopecia, fluid retention, edema, and sudden loss of vision. Depression and weight gain have been reported. For clients taking this drug, the risk of endometrial or ovarian cancer is decreased. Amenorrhea has been reported in clients after receiving four injections 3 months apart for 1 year. Depression and loss of energy have been reported.

CN: Pharmacological and parenteral therapies; CL: Create

80. 4. Because clozapine can cause tachycardia, the nurse should withhold the medication if the pulse rate is greater than 140 bpm and notify the **HCP** 📖. Giving the drug or telling the client to exercise could be detrimental to the client.

CN: Pharmacological and parenteral therapies; CL: Synthesize

81. 2. Fever is a cardinal manifestation of infection in people with AIDS. Because the major physiologic alteration in AIDS is generalized immune system dysfunction, typical indicators of the body's response to infection (e.g., erythema, warmth, tenderness) may be absent.

CN: Physiological adaptation; CL: Synthesize

82. 2. To care effectively for clients with depression, the nurse should teach the importance of demonstrating empathetic concern. Caregivers must accept clients as they are even though many will be angry and negative, acknowledge their emotional pain, and offer to help them work through their pain. For the client who is depressed, using a cheerful demeanor or a humorous, light-hearted approach may be overwhelming because the client will be unable to meet the caregiver's expectations, subsequently leading to decreased self-worth. A serious, business-like affect may threaten the client and inhibit the development of trust.

☞ CN: Management of care; CL: Evaluate

83. **4.** When a child is ready to take fluids by mouth postoperatively, clear liquids are given initially. If clear liquids are tolerated, the concentration and amount of oral feedings are gradually increased. This means advancing to half-strength and then to full-strength formula while increasing the amount given with each feeding.

☞ CN: Basic care and comfort; CL: Synthesize

84. **2.** The nurse should monitor the client taking paroxetine, a selective serotonin reuptake inhibitor, for sexual problems, such as decreased libido, impotence, and ejaculatory disturbances, because these adverse effects can occur frequently and lead to medication noncompliance. Sleep disturbances can occur with an SSRI such as paroxetine. However, this client is taking the drug every morning, which would not affect nighttime sleep. Hypertensive crisis is associated with the ingestion of foods rich in tyramine when a client is taking a monoamine oxidase inhibitor. Orthostatic hypotension is a potential adverse effect of tricyclic antidepressants.

☞ CN: Pharmacological and parenteral therapies; CL: Analyze

85. **2.** In the progressive stage of shock, the client can display listlessness or agitation, confusion, and slowed speech. Restlessness occurs in the compensatory stage. Incoherent speech and unconsciousness are clinical manifestations of the irreversible stage.

☞ CN: Physiological adaptation; CL: Analyze

86. **1, 4, 5.** Common adverse effects of nafcillin include vomiting, diarrhea, sore mouth, fever, and gastritis (stomach upset). Pain with urination and headache are not associated with this drug.

☞ CN: Pharmacological and parenteral therapies; CL: Evaluate

87. **1.** The nurse should first apply the ECG electrodes to the client's chest. If the client is found to be in ventricular fibrillation, the immediate priority is to defibrillate the client. Pulse oximetry is not an immediate priority. The client's oxygenation is evaluated in a code situation using arterial blood gas analysis. The client's blood pressure is evaluated after the ECG rhythm has been established. A

portable Doppler ultrasound unit may be needed to check for the presence of a pulse or to check the blood pressure in a code situation.

☞ CN: Safety and infection control; CL: Synthesize

88. **1, 2, 3.** Active listening facilitates trust. It means that the nurse acknowledges that he or she has heard the client and indicates in his or her own words an understanding of what the client says and the emotions underlying what is said. It also involves encouraging the client to say more. Constant eye contact and standing very close to a client can be unnerving and can hamper trust building.

☞ CN: Psychosocial integrity; CL: Synthesize

89. **2.** Heroin causes pinpoint pupils. Marijuana causes the eyes to appear red and bloodshot. Cocaine use causes pupils to dilate. Drooping of the eyelids is not typically associated with the use of any substance.

☞ CN: Pharmacological and parenteral therapies; CL: Analyze

90. **3.** A typical sign of pediculosis capitis (head lice) is frequent scratching of the scalp because the condition causes severe itching. Scratch marks are usually easily visible. Because head lice are easily transmitted to others, the child's family members and peers also should be examined for infestation. Spotty baldness, wheals, and scaly lesions are often allergic in nature.

☞ CN: Physiological adaptation; CL: Analyze

91. **1.** Passing flatus indicates the return of peristalsis, as does active bowel sounds. Hunger is not the best indicator of peristaltic return. Hypoactive bowel sounds indicate that there is some peristaltic activity, but it is limited and not yet normal. Palpation is not an appropriate method of assessing bowel activity.

☞ CN: Physiological adaptation; CL: Evaluate

92. **3.** The pH of 7.24 indicates that the client is acidotic. The Paco$_2$ value of 49 mm Hg is elevated. The HCO$_3$ value of 24 mEq/L is normal. The client is in uncompensated respiratory acidosis. Hypoventilation and a flushed appearance are additional clinical manifestations of respiratory acidosis.

☞ CN: Physiological adaptation; CL: Analyze

93. **2.** It is essential for the nurse to evaluate the effects of pain medication after it has had time to act. Although other interventions may be appropriate, continual reassessment is most important to determine the effectiveness and need for additional intervention, if any. Repositioning could provide some comfort, but assessment of the client's pain level is essential. Reassuring the client is important, but it will be of no value unless the nurse evaluates the client's pain level. To readjust the pain dosage is appropriate only if titration is prescribed by the **healthcare provider (HCP)** 📖.

🔑 CN: Basic care of comfort; CL: Synthesize

94. 1. Barrier contraceptives must be used to protect against STIs. Birth control pills and douching are not effective for prevention of STIs. Prophylactic antibiotics are not used to prevent the acquisition of STIs.

🔑 CN: Safety and infection control; CL: Evaluate

95. 2. A purplish blue discoloration of the vagina and cervix is termed Chadwick's sign; it is caused by increased vascularity of the vagina during pregnancy and is considered a probable sign of pregnancy. Goodell's sign, also considered a probable sign of pregnancy, refers to a softening of the cervix during pregnancy. Hegar's sign, also a probable sign of pregnancy, refers to a softening of the lower uterine segment. Melasma, the mask of pregnancy, refers to the pigmentation of the skin on the face during pregnancy. Melasma is considered a presumptive sign of pregnancy.

🔑 CN: Health promotion and maintenance; CL: Apply

96. 3. Initially, the nurse would tell the client to seek out staff when feeling agitated or upset to prevent violent episodes. Doing so helps the client to redirect negative feelings in an appropriate manner, such as talking. Encouraging the client to stay in his room is inappropriate because it does not help the client to deal with his feelings. Secluding the client at the first sign of agitation is not indicated and may be perceived by the client as punishment. Instructing the client to ask for medication when agitated would not be the initial course of action. The nurse would interact with the client and direct the client to an activity to decrease his anxiety before intervening with any required medication.

🔑 CN: Psychosocial integrity; CL: Synthesize

97. 3. The nurse should use short words, sentences, and paragraphs and avoid medical jargon. Correct terminology should be used when appropriate (e.g., type 1 diabetes, not "sugar diabetes"). The format should be as simple as possible; charts are not necessary and may be confusing to some clients. Information should be prepared at a fifth-grade reading level. The information should be presented in large-sized type.

🔑 CN: Psychosocial integrity; CL: Synthesize

98. 4, 5. Rapid pulse, heat intolerance, diarrhea, exophthalmos, and accelerated linear growth are more characteristic of hyperthyroidism, which is caused by an autoimmune response to thyroid-stimulating hormone receptors. Weight gain, dry skin, and constipation are characteristic of hypothyroidism, which results from a deficiency in secretion of thyroid hormone.

🔑 CN: Physiological adaptation; CL: Analyze

99. 2. The criterion for hemorrhage is saturating one pad per hour. The 35-year-old who delivered 4 hours ago had saturated a peripad per hour. Even though her fundus is firm, she may have experienced a cervical laceration, which would be the source of the bleeding. She needs to be evaluated first, based on the bleeding. The 18-year-old who has abdominal cramps is within normal limits for a G2 P2 and is experiencing afterbirth pains normally seen in a multiparous client; she will need pain medication. The 16-year-old status post cesarean section on magnesium sulfate is stable with adequate urinary output and normal reflexes. Her vital signs are within normal limits for a postpartum client. The headache is the one area of concern for this client. The 18-year-old who is 2 days postpartum with breast pain may be experiencing her milk coming in, although it does not indicate whether she is breast- or bottle-feeding; either situation may find a mother with milk developing within her system. The vital signs for this client are slightly elevated, but this may be from the milk coming in and would require nursing evaluation but is not emergent.

🔑 CN: Management of care; CL: Synthesize

100. 4. It is normal for the client to feel pressure on the palms of the hands when walking with crutches. The client should move her affected (right) leg forward first as she swings forward with the crutches. Leaning on the crutches can apply pressure to the axillae, leading to neurovascular impairment. If the client's arms are tingling after she uses her crutches, she is probably applying pressure on her axillae when walking.

🔑 CN: Reduction of risk potential; CL: Evaluate

101. 2. Because clients are discharged as soon as possible from the hospital, it is essential to evaluate the support for assistance and self-care at home. If the client has support at home, the distance from the hospital may be irrelevant. The client or support team will monitor vital signs as needed, but blood pressure monitoring is not specifically indicated. It is more important at this point for the client to understand how to manage his care at home, rather than knowing the causes of lung cancer.

CN: Management of care; CL: Analyze

102. 3. If the client begins breast-feeding early and often after childbirth, the breasts begin to fill with milk within 48 to 96 hours, or 2 to 4 days. The breasts secrete colostrum for the first 24 to 48 hours, which is beneficial to the neonate because of the immunoglobulins contained in colostrum.

CN: Health promotion and maintenance; CL: Apply

103. 3. The predominant clinical finding in elderly or debilitated clients indicating that they have hypoxia is confusion. Fever and chills, productive cough, and pleuritic chest pain could be indicative of a respiratory tract infection.

CN: Physiological adaptation; CL: Analyze

104. 1. It is important for the child and family to understand that chorea associated with rheumatic fever is not permanent. Therefore, the nurse should explain that the chorea will disappear over time. It is not necessary to assess the child's neurologic status because the chorea is self-limited and nonprogressive. Because the child has cardiac involvement, ambulation is contraindicated. Aspirin is used primarily as an anti-inflammatory drug and secondarily for pain relief. A slightly cool environment is unnecessary. Environmental temperature does not affect the child's polyarthritis and chorea.

CN: Physiological adaptation; CL: Synthesize

105. 1. When the gestation is less than 13 weeks, an elective abortion is usually performed by the dilatation and curettage method. Menstrual extraction, or suction evacuation, is the easiest method, but it is used only when the client is between 5 and 7 weeks' gestation. Dilatation and vacuum extraction is used when clients are between 12 and 16 weeks' gestation. Saline induction, used for clients between 16 and 24 weeks' gestation, involves instillation of a hypertonic saline solution into the amniotic sac to initiate expulsion. Oxytocin infusion may also be used with saline induction.

CN: Health promotion and maintenance; CL: Apply

106. 1. A pleural effusion is a collection of fluid between the pleural layers of the lung. The effusion decreases chest wall movement on the affected side. The nurse should expect the breath sounds to be decreased or diminished over the affected area. Because of the presence of fluid, percussion would elicit dullness, not hyperresonance. The nurse should not expect to hear wheezing on auscultation.

CN: Basic care and comfort; CL: Analyze

107. 1. An expected client outcome for a goal to reduce acute pain related to cramping is that the client exhibits no manifestations of discomfort, such as crying or drawing the legs to the abdomen. Being very still may indicate either a pain state or a state of relaxation, and the nurse would need to assess the client further. Having normal bowel movements and not vomiting are desired outcomes, but the goal here is to relieve the pain.

CN: Physiological adaptation; CL: Synthesize

108. 0.6 mL

$$40 \, \text{mg} / \text{mL} = 25 \, \text{mg} / X \, \text{mL}$$
$$X = 0.6 \, \text{mL}.$$

CN: Pharmacological and parenteral therapies; CL: Apply

109. 4. The client is likely exhibiting symptoms of herpes genitalis, which include painful blisters or vesicles that appear 2 to 20 days after transmission of the disease. The client was most likely exposed from her new partner. The client should be referred to an **HCP** 📖 for treatment. Having her partner wear a condom, increasing fluids, or using lubricant jelly will not treat the infection. While having her partner wear a condom will not cure the infection, having future partners wear condoms will help prevent its transmission.

CN: Management of care; CL: Synthesize

110. 2. It has been found that parents are more aggrieved when optimism is followed by defeat. The nurse should recognize this when planning various ways to help the parents of a dying child. It is not necessarily true that knowing about a poor prognosis for years helps prepare parents for a child's death, that trust in health personnel is destroyed when a death is untimely, or that it is more difficult for parents to accept the death of an older child than that of a younger child.

CN: Psychosocial integrity; CL: Synthesize

111. 3. The child is having a reaction to the blood transfusion. The priority is to stop the blood transfusion but maintain an open venous access for medication or high fluid volume delivery. Thus, switching the transfusion to normal saline solution would be done first. Since the child is having difficulty breathing, applying oxygen would be the next action. Additionally, vital signs are taken to determine the extent of circulatory involvement. Then the **HCP** 📖 would be notified and, if necessary, the crash cart would be obtained.

🗝 CN: Pharmacological and parenteral therapies; CL: Synthesize

112. 1. A client who has an allergy to penicillin may have a cross-sensitivity to cefazolin, a first-generation cephalosporin, and the drug should be given with caution. The nurse should ask the client whether the client has taken cefazolin before. The nurse should inform the pharmacy of the client's allergy after asking the client about prior use of cefazolin. The medication should not be administered until the nurse first inquires about the client's exposure to cefazolin and then consults the pharmacist or **HCP** 📖. Observing the client for urticaria is appropriate but is not an initial response.

🗝 CN: Safety and infection control; CL: Synthesize

113. 2. Toddlers are in Erikson's stage of autonomy versus shame and doubt. They want to do things on their own and experience despair when they are not allowed to be independent in areas that they are capable. Allowing the toddler to participate in the dressing change promotes the toddler's independence. Medications must be administered on a schedule to maintain therapeutic levels. Toddlers have short attention spans and would not likely complete an art project. Toddlers commonly engage in parallel play. Having another toddler visit will not aid in the achievement of Erikson's stage of development.

🗝 CN: Psychosocial integrity; CL: Analyze

114. 1. The nurse would teach the client taking lithium and his family about the importance of maintaining adequate sodium intake to prevent lithium toxicity. Because lithium is a salt, reduced sodium intake could result in lithium retention with subsequent toxicity. Increasing sodium in the diet is not recommended and may be harmful. Increased sodium levels result in lower lithium levels. Therefore, the drug may not reach therapeutic effectiveness.

🗝 CN: Pharmacological and parenteral therapies; CL: Synthesize

115. 3. Mucositis is an inflammation of the oral mucosa caused by radiation therapy. It is important that the client with mucositis receive meticulous mouth care, including flossing, to prevent the development of an infection. Mouth care should be provided before and after each meal, at bedtime, and more frequently as needed. Extremes of temperature should be avoided in food and drink. Half-strength

hydrogen peroxide is too harsh to use on irritated tissues.

🗝 CN: Reduction of risk potential; CL: Synthesize

116. 3. Acetaminophen ingestion can cause severe liver disease. The child should be evaluated in the emergency department. The child should not be offered any fluids, and the parents should not attempt to induce vomiting. Assessing the child's respirations for 24 hours will delay needed emergency treatment.

🗝 CN: Management of care; CL: Synthesize

117. 1. The best approach by the nurse is to determine why the parent thinks the child is hyperactive. Some children are very active but do not have the necessary defining characteristics of hyperactivity. Asking what the parent thinks needs to be done, how the child behaves normally, and if the preschool teacher thinks the child is hyperactive would be an appropriate follow-up question once more information is gathered from the parent to determine whether the child indeed is hyperactive.

🗝 CN: Physiological adaptation; CL: Synthesize

118. 2. Dilatation at the anastomosis site is needed during the first years of childhood in about 50% of children who have had corrective surgery for TEF. Recurrent mild diarrhea with dehydration is not likely to develop with this surgery. Speech problems can occur if other abnormalities are present to produce them; the larynx and structures of speech are not affected by TEF. Dysphagia and strictures may decrease food intake, and poor weight gain may be noted, but gastric ulcers should not develop from surgery to repair TEF.

🗝 CN: Reduction of risk potential; CL: Analyze

119. 1. Terminally ill clients most often describe feelings of isolation because they feel ignored. The terminally ill client may sense any discomfort that family and friends feel in the client's presence. Nursing interventions include spending time with the client, encouraging discussion about feelings, and answering questions openly and honestly. Reducing fear of pain or fear of more aggressive therapies is secondary to lessening the client's feelings of isolation. Reducing feelings of social inadequacy is not relevant to the terminally ill client.

🗝 CN: Psychosocial integrity; CL: Synthesize

120. 2. When the fetus is in a breech position, the fetal heart rate most often is located above the umbilicus because the fetal heart is near the top of the mother's uterus. The heart of a fetus in the cephalic position is typically located on either the left or the right side of the client's uterus. Also, because the fetal heart typically is located in the lower portion of the mother's uterus, the sounds would be heard below the umbilicus. With a face presentation, fetal heart sounds are typically located on either the left or the right side of the client's uterus; in addition, because the fetal heart typically is located in the lower portion of the mother's uterus, the sounds would be heard below the umbilicus. When the fetus is in a transverse position, the fetal heart sounds typically would be located below the umbilicus and in the midline.

　　⚷ CN: Health promotion and maintenance; CL: Analyze

121. 4. Clients who have been diagnosed with pernicious anemia are lacking adequate amounts of the intrinsic factor (IF) that is secreted by the gastric mucosa. IF is necessary for the absorption of cobalamin (vitamin B_{12}) in the distal ileum. Without the presence of IF, dietary intake of vitamin B_{12} is useless because it cannot be absorbed. Treatment of pernicious anemia includes IM injections of cobalamin, at first daily for 2 weeks, then weekly until the anemia is corrected. A maintenance schedule of monthly injections is then implemented. The injections will need to be continued for the rest of the client's life.

　　⚷ CN: Physiological adaptation; CL: Evaluate

122. 2. The nurse should first assess the client because a hypoglycemic reaction is likely to occur. At this time, the nurse also should give the client a fast-acting simple carbohydrate. Then the nurse should notify the **HCP** 📖 for prescriptions to prevent or treat severe hypoglycemia. The nurse could consult the clinical pharmacist until able to contact the HCP, but the first action is to assess the client in order to have accurate information to report. When the situation has been resolved, the nurse should document the incident and report the incident to the charge nurse.

　　⚷ CN: Reduction of risk potential; CL: Synthesize

123. 4. Safety is the priority in caring for this infant. Infants adapt easily, increasing mobility even with a splint in place. Therefore, the mother needs to ensure that the area in which the infant is mobile is safe. There is no need to contact the **HCP** 📖 to alter the treatment plan. Confining the infant to one room may not allow the child to achieve normal development. The child needs different environments for maximum development. The infant needs to wear the splint as prescribed by the HCP to ensure optimal healing.

　　⚷ CN: Safety and infection control; CL: Synthesize

124. 1. Anxiety in a preoperative client may be caused by many different fears, such as fear of the effects of anesthesia, the effects of surgery on body image, separation from family and friends, job loss, disability, pain, or death. However, fear of the unknown is most likely to be the greatest fear because the client feels helpless. Therefore, an important part of preoperative nursing care is to assess the client for anxieties and explore possible causes. Emotional support can then be offered so that the client is in the best possible psychological condition for surgery.

　　⚷ CN: Psychosocial integrity; CL: Analyze

125. 1. An important nursing responsibility is preoperative teaching. The recommended guide for teaching is to tell the client as much as she wants to know and is able to understand. Delaying discussion of issues or concerns will most likely increase the client's anxiety. Telling the client to discuss questions with the **HCP** 📖 avoids acknowledging the client's concerns.

　　⚷ CN: Psychosocial integrity; CL: Synthesize

126. 3. The client must have adequate disclosure of the risks associated with the surgery before signing the **consent** 📖 form. It is the **healthcare provider's (HCP's)** 📖 responsibility to explain the risks of any procedures and to obtain the client's informed consent. If the nurse suspects that the client has not been truly informed, it is the responsibility of the nurse to act as a client advocate and contact the surgeon to provide additional information to the client. It is not appropriate to have the client go to surgery without understanding the risks. The nurse should not minimize the procedure or dismiss the client's concerns.

　　⚷ CN: Management of care; CL: Synthesize

127. 4. In right occipital anterior lie, the occiput faces the right anterior segment of the woman's pelvis. In left occipital transverse lie, the occiput faces the woman's left hip. In left occipital anterior lie, the occiput faces the left anterior segment of the woman's pelvis. In right occipital transverse lie, the occiput faces the woman's right hip.

　　⚷ CN: Physiological adaptation; CL: Analyze

128. 4. The nurse should advise the parents to report an increasing fever, which would indicate the infection is not resolving. Increased urine output may occur, but it would be very difficult for the parent to actually determine this and it is not a cardinal sign of increasing infection. The child may have a loss of appetite related to the infection or the medication, but is not indicative of an infection that is becoming worse. The child should not have

An antihypertensive will not treat the underlying CNS irritability. If the lorazepam is effective, it will not be necessary to have someone sit with the client. At this point, it is not necessary to notify the **healthcare provider (HCP)** 📖.

🔑 CN: Management of care; CL: Synthesize

147. 2, 3. Appropriate diet instructions for the client in the early stages of cirrhosis include ensuring an adequate intake of protein and eating small, frequent meals. There is no need to limit protein intake unless the client has evidence of hepatic encephalopathy. Additionally, fluid intake is not restricted unless the client has significant ascites or edema (these typically occur later in the disease). Because of gastrointestinal dysfunction, small, frequent meals are frequently better tolerated than three regular meals. Clients with cirrhosis should be encouraged to increase their caloric intake instead of restricting it. Alcohol intake in any amount is discouraged.

🔑 CN: Physiological adaptation; CL: Synthesize

148. 3. After surgery, the nurse's initial assessment is the surgical site dressing to determine whether there is any bleeding or drainage. Once this assessment is completed, then the nurse would assess the other areas such as the IV access site, pain, and nasogastric tube function.

🔑 CN: Physiological adaptation; CL: Analyze

149. 1. The nurse should use the radial artery to obtain blood gas samples because it is easier to maintain firm pressure there than on the femoral artery. Nursing interventions to protect the client who has received t-PA or alteplase recombinant therapy include maintaining arterial pressure for 30 seconds because it takes longer for coagulation to occur with the thrombolytic agent on board. IM injections are contraindicated during thrombolytic therapy. The nurse should prevent physical manipulation of the client, which can cause bruising.

🔑 CN: Reduction of risk potential; CL: Synthesize

150. 4. Serum amylase and lipase are increased in pancreatitis, as is urine amylase. Other abnormal laboratory values include decreased calcium level and increased glucose and lipid levels.

🔑 CN: Reduction of risk potential; CL: Analyze

151. 2. For the client with an alcohol or drug problem, group sessions are helpful in dealing with emotions and concerns about alcohol and drugs. Clients with substance abuse problems identify with each other's similar experiences and can best help

each other deal with these feelings and emotions. Additionally, the members of the group are able to support and confront each other. Individual therapy is not as helpful as group sessions because group members offer peer support and confrontation when needed. Solitary activities and recreation lead to increased avoidance of the issues that must be faced and dealt with by the client. These are often areas that the client must learn to develop and manage while in recovery.

🔑 CN: Psychosocial integrity; CL: Synthesize

152. 4. Foul-smelling urine is indicative of cystitis. Other symptoms include dysuria and urinary frequency and urgency. Flank pain, nausea, and vomiting indicate pyelonephritis.

🔑 CN: Physiological adaptation; CL: Analyze

153. 4. By saying "You could not have prevented the tornado; it just happened" the nurse helps the client to develop an objective perspective and promotes a better understanding of the event. The other statements tell the client how to feel, possibly causing resistance, and thus delay therapeutic healing. Guilt and self-blame will not be decreased.

🔑 CN: Psychosocial integrity; CL: Synthesize

154. 3. In many Asian cultures, the 30 days after the birth of the neonate is a time for the mother to heal from the birth. The appropriate action by the nurse is to determine whether this is a cultural practice for this client and her family. If so, the client is behaving within her cultural practices. Teaching should be provided to both the mother and her mother-in-law. There is no indication that bonding is not taking place. Lack of bonding might be indicated if the client did not show any interest in the neonate. Documenting the client's maternal behavior in her **medical record** 📖 is a routine task. However, the nurse should not assume that this behavior is unusual because it may be reflective of the client's cultural framework. A home visit is not warranted unless there is evidence of infant neglect or the family needs additional follow-up or teaching.

🔑 CN: Health promotion and maintenance; CL: Synthesize

155. 1. A creatinine clearance test is a 24-hour urine test that measures the degree of protein breakdown in the body. The collection is not maintained in a sterile container. There is no need to insert an indwelling urinary catheter as long as the client is able to control urination. It is not necessary to force fluids.

🔑 CN: Reduction of risk potential; CL: Synthesize

156. 4. The statement, "Your eyes look dark," is the least sensitive statement because it points out an obvious difference for no real purpose. The nurse has a reason to ask the client about favorite foods and needs to know about past health problems. Also, it is appropriate for the nurse to ask the client how he or she wishes to be addressed.

CN: Psychosocial integrity; CL: Analyze

157. 2. Insight into the illness is demonstrated when the client recognizes the relationship between the chemical imbalance and his illness and symptoms. Stating that the olanzapine is the best medicine or that the client's mother is proud of him for staying on his medicines reflects awareness about the effect of medications and the need for compliance. Stating that he may be able to get a part-time job indicates an awareness of his increased capacity for work.

CN: Psychosocial integrity; CL: Evaluate

158. 3. Carpal tunnel syndrome is a condition in which the median nerve becomes compressed in the wrist. The brachial nerve is not affected. Carpal tunnel syndrome may be the result of a systemic disease, such as rheumatoid arthritis or diabetes mellitus, or it may be an occupational hazard for people whose jobs require repetitive hand movements such as someone who works long hours on a computer. It is not a condition resulting from disuse. The wrists do not develop flexion contractures with carpal tunnel syndrome.

CN: Physiological adaptation; CL: Synthesize

159. 1. Barbiturates can cause significant respiratory depression. The nurse's first action is to immediately assess the respiratory status and assist in bag-mask-valve ventilation as needed. Monitoring the vital signs is important, but respiratory care takes precedence over the blood pressure. Without other injury, blood products are not necessary. Placing the client in the Trendelenburg position will put pressure from the abdominal contents onto the diaphragm and further impair breathing.

CN: Pharmacologic and parenteral therapies; CL: Synthesize

160. 3. Clients who have undergone TURP need to be instructed to maintain an adequate fluid intake despite urinary dribbling or incontinence. The client should be advised to drink at least eight glasses of water a day to dilute the urine and help prevent urinary tract infections. Maintaining a voiding schedule of every 2 hours can help decrease incidents of incontinence. Teaching the client Kegel exercises is also beneficial for strengthening sphincter tone. The nurse should not encourage the client to decrease fluids. It is not necessarily true that a decreased intake will cause renal calculi. Threatening the client with a catheter is not beneficial, and it is not the treatment of choice for a client who is experiencing incontinence from TURP.

CN: Reduction of risk potential; CL: Synthesize

161. 4. Risk factors for TSS include the use of tampons at night, when the tampon would be in place for 7 to 9 hours. TSS can occur in other situations, but it is commonly associated with women during menses, particularly women who use tampons. The longer the tampon is left in place, the greater the risk for TSS. Changing tampons every 3 hours or more frequently, avoiding use of deodorized tampons, and alternating tampons with sanitary pads are actions that decrease the risk of TSS.

CN: Reduction of risk potential; CL: Analyze

162. 4. Costovertebral tenderness occurs on the side of the affected kidney in pyelonephritis. Dysuria, suprapubic pain, and urine retention may occur in pyelonephritis but do not specifically support a diagnosis of pyelonephritis. Dysuria, suprapubic pain, and urine retention are symptoms of cystitis, which can lead to pyelonephritis if not treated.

CN: Physiological adaptation; CL: Analyze

163. 2. Broad-spectrum antibiotics can cause decreased efficacy of oral contraceptives, placing the client at risk for an unplanned pregnancy. When a client is prescribed a course of antibiotics, a backup method of contraception should be used. Antihypertensives, diuretics, and antihistamines do not interfere with oral contraceptive efficacy.

CN: Pharmacological and parenteral therapies; CL: Apply

164. 1. Adverse effects of danazol include headaches, dizziness, irritability, and decreased libido. Masculinization effects, such as deepened voice, facial hair, and weight gain, also may occur.

CN: Pharmacological and parenteral therapies; CL: Synthesize

165. 2. The nurse should assign the Muslim male client who needs complete morning care to Joe. Muslim men cannot be cared for by female nurses. The nurse must also consider workload, and Joe has the lightest assignment.

CN: Management of care; CL: Synthesize

166. 4. Central nervous system changes include such symptoms as apathy, lethargy, and decreased concentration. Seizures and coma can also occur. The nurse should assess the client's level of consciousness at regular intervals and maintain client safety. Allowing the client to express feelings related to body image changes and restricting foods high in potassium and fluid intake are all appropriate activities, but they are not related to the central nervous system changes.

CN: Physiological adaptation; CL: Synthesize

167. 3. Elderly individuals have less subcutaneous tissue. An elderly, emaciated client will require a short needle and a shallow angle to avoid hitting an underlying bone. The nurse should choose the shortest subcutaneous needle available and use the least angle.

CN: Pharmacological and parenteral therapies; CL: Apply

168. 3. Metronidazole can cause a disulfiram-like reaction if it is taken with alcohol. Tachycardia, nausea, vomiting, and other serious interaction effects can occur. Flagyl will make the urine a darker color. Oral contraceptives should never be discontinued with trichomoniasis. The partner also requires treatment to prevent retransmission of infection.

CN: Pharmacological and parenteral therapies; CL: Synthesize

169. 1. In the advanced stages of osteoarthritis, pain can occur with minimal activity or even when the client is at rest. Crepitation can be present at any stage of the disease and does not exacerbate pain. Joints are not symmetrically affected by the disease. Symmetric joint involvement and fatigue are characteristics of rheumatoid arthritis.

CN: Physiological adaptation; CL: Analyze

170. 3. The traditional belief of Vietnamese Americans is that the family can provide more comfort for their loved one at home. It is not seen as being disloyal if their loved one dies in the hospital. The request is not based on a feeling that the hospital cannot be trusted. Vietnamese Americans accept death as a part of life and do not think that reincarnation is prevented in the hospital.

CN: Psychosocial integrity; CL: Apply

171. 2. It is important for the daughter to know that there is an underlying cause for what her mother is experiencing and that it is treatable. Telling her not to worry is a useless cliché and does nothing to inform the daughter. Talking about care after discharge implies that the delirium is irreversible. Delirium is a reversible condition.

Although not arguing with hallucinations is valid, this response ignores the daughter's concern.

CN: Psychosocial integrity; CL: Synthesize

172. 2. The client with Alzheimer's dementia should not have access to toiletries that could be swallowed (such as aftershave) unless closely supervised. Putting special locks on all the doors is appropriate to prevent wandering, thus maintaining the client's safety. Placing the client in a room that has nothing to trip over is appropriate to reduce the client's risk of falling. Taking the knobs off of the stove is appropriate to prevent possible burns.

CN: Safety and infection control; CL: Evaluate

173. 3. It is important that the client force fluids to 3,000 mL/day to avoid the development of renal calculi when taking allopurinol. Allopurinol must be taken consistently to be effective in the treatment of gout. The drug should be taken after meals to avoid gastrointestinal distress. Although the client can take aspirin when taking allopurinol, both drugs can cause gastrointestinal irritation, and the practice is not recommended if the client is sensitive to the medications.

CN: Pharmacological and parenteral therapies; CL: Evaluate

174. 3. The best advice for the nurse to give the child's mother is to run cool water over the burned area to stop the burning process. Then the area should be wrapped in a clean cloth. Once these initial actions are completed, the mother can call the child's **HCP** 📖. Packing the arm in ice may cause more damage to the burned area because cold can cause burns just as heat can. For most burns, it is not advised to apply ointment until the area has been evaluated.

CN: Reduction of risk potential; CL: Synthesize

175. 4. The client is at risk for falling, and the nurse should initiate falls precaution. The client does not require airborne precautions. There is no indication the client needs a referral to physical therapy. The client should be encouraged to maintain mobility.

CN: Reduction of risk potential; CL: Analyze

176. 3. Chills and headache are signs of a febrile, nonhemolytic blood transfusion reaction, and the nurse's first action should be to discontinue the transfusion as soon as possible and then notify the **healthcare provider (HCP)** 📖. Antipyretics and antihistamines may be prescribed. The nurse would not administer acetaminophen without a prescription from the HCP. The client's blood pressure should be taken after the transfusion is stopped. Checking the infusion rate of the blood is not a pertinent action; the infusion needs to be stopped regardless of the rate.

🔑 CN: Pharmacological and parenteral therapies; CL: Synthesize

177. 3. Resolving grief and having increased energy and activity convey good mental health, indicating that counseling is not necessary at this time. Taking an antidepressant or having less energy and involvement with grandchildren reflects possible depression and the need for counseling. Wanting to be with her dead husband suggests possible suicidal ideation that warrants serious further assessment and counseling.

🔑 CN: Psychosocial integrity; CL: Evaluate

178. 3. Common adverse effects of isosorbide are light-headedness, dizziness, and orthostatic hypotension. Clients should be instructed to change positions slowly to prevent these adverse effects and to avoid fainting. Ankle swelling is not related to isosorbide administration. The client does not need to take his pulse before taking the medication. The client does not need to take the medication with food.

🔑 CN: Pharmacological and parenteral therapies; CL: Evaluate

179. 3. Valproic acid and propranolol are often prescribed to help manage explosive anger. Recognizing the need for medications indicates readiness for discharge. Not ever getting angry is difficult, impractical, and unrealistic without specific anger management strategies. Drinking does not address anger control and suggests a risk of continued drinking. Blaming others, such as the client's mother, does not address anger control and indicates a lack of responsibility for the client's own behavior.

🔑 CN: Pharmacological and parenteral therapies; CL: Evaluate

180. 3. The nurse should first help the client into a position of comfort even though the primary purpose for entering the room was to administer medication. After attending to the client's basic care needs, the nurse can proceed with the proper identification of the client, such as asking the client his name and checking his armband, so that the medication can be administered.

🔑 CN: Basic care and comfort; CL: Synthesize

181. 2, 3, 4, 5. Cushing's syndrome results from excessive levels of cortisol. Some effects of excessive adrenocortical activity include musculoskeletal changes, and the client may be at risk for injury and falls. There is excessive protein catabolism causing muscle wasting, decreased inflammatory response, and potential for delayed healing and infection. The increased cortisol levels cause a moon-faced appearance to which clients must adjust. The skin becomes thin and fragile, and the client is also at risk for infection. Increased cortisol levels do not cause deficient fluid volume.

🔑 CN: Management of care; CL: Analyze

182. 2. For any verbal or telephone prescription or result, it is important to read back the information to assure its accuracy. It is also important to document that it was read back according to facility policy. It is not necessary to use "read-back" procedures when data are entered on the computerized medical record 📱. The unit clerk is not a licensed healthcare worker and should not take telephone prescriptions. When giving a written report, it is not necessary to "read back," but the nurse should always clarify if there is any question.

🔑 CN: Safety and Infection Control; CL: Apply

183. 4. It is well documented that the subungual areas of the hand harbor bacteria that can be transmitted to others despite aggressive handwashing procedures, and therefore, it is important that the staff on this unit do not have artificial fingernails that could be the source of the infection on this unit. The Joint Commission (TJC), in the 2011 National Patient Safety Goals (NPSG.07.01.01), includes using "the hand cleaning guidelines from the Centers for Disease Control and Prevention or the World Health Organization" to prevent infection. There is no need to institute transmission-based or contact precautions. It is not necessary to wear a mask when caring for these clients.

🔑 CN: Safety and infection control; CL: Synthesize

184. 4. The sites should be treated as separate sites to avoid cross-contamination. This adheres to the principle of cleaning from the least contaminated area to the most contaminated area. Each site is considered a separate area for wound care.

🔑 CN: Safety and infection control; CL: Apply

185. 1. Any change in level of consciousness (vomiting, severe headache that is not improving or is getting worse, memory changes, confusion, irritability, change in pupils) should be immediately reported to the HCP 📱 and further evaluated, especially in a client with head trauma. The nurse should mark a circle around the amount of drainage on a dressing after surgery so it can be monitored and reported to the HCP if it grows in size, but a dime-sized spot is not an immediate priority. Constipation and abdominal discomfort after surgery require attention but are not priority. Obtaining proper pain medication in order to promote wound care and healing must be addressed with the HCP, but it is not the first priority.

CN: Reduction of risk potential; CL: Synthesize

186. 2. In order to prevent injury to a client, restraints must be secured to the bed frame using a slipknot in order to ensure quick release if necessary. A square knot would be secure but would not be easily released in an emergency. A restraint tied in a bow at the client's side would not be easily released in an emergency. A hitch, although secure, is not easily released in an emergency.

CN: Safety and infection control; CL: Evaluate

187. 2, 3, 4, 5, 6. Because there have been no cervical changes, the client is not in labor. The client should understand to return to the hospital if the contractions become more intense and regular, if she has vaginal bleeding, if she thinks her membranes rupture, if the baby is not moving, or if she has an urge to push. Three contractions an hour would be too infrequent to indicate active labor.

CN: Management of care; CL: Apply

188. 4. The mental abilities of Down syndrome children range from severe intellectual disabilities to low average intelligence. They also exhibit a wide range of physical features including almond-shaped eyes, a small, flat nose, a small mouth with a protruding tongue, and small ears. Many also have a single crease across the palms of their hands, short stubby fingers, and straight hair that is fine and thin. Children with Down syndrome are socially 2 to 3 years behind their peers. Many children with Down syndrome will be capable of living in group homes. They may also continue living with their parents or other family members. Children with Down syndrome are well tempered and very friendly.

CN: Psychosocial integrity; CL: Evaluate

189. 2. Febrile seizures usually occur during the rise in temperature and are related to the peak of the temperature rather than the rapidity or duration of elevation. When children experience febrile seizures, fevers usually exceed 38.0°C (100.4°F). Febrile seizures are not related to the rapidity or duration of elevation. Febrile seizures are most common among children 18 months to 3 years but are not related to the maturity of their immune system.

CN: Physiological adaptation; CL: Analyze

190. 3. This client could have progressed rapidly and is now ready to deliver her infant. A sterile vaginal exam is indicated prior to getting her up to the bathroom to determine if she is fully dilated. If she is ready to deliver, she could be reassured that the sensation she is feeling is due to pressure from the fetal head. If her cervix exam is unchanged, she may need pain control interventions. The nurses' assessment findings then should be discussed with the client and the **HCP** 📖.

CN: Reduction of risk potential; CL: Apply

COMPREHENSIVE
TEST
5

This test has 236 questions. Time yourself as you take the test so you can determine the approximate amount of time it takes to complete this many questions.

1. The nurse has just received the change-of-shift report on clients in the labor, birth, recovery, and postpartum unit. Which of these clients should the nurse assess **first**?
- [ ] **1.** an 18-year-old single primigravid client, in labor for 9 hours, with cervical dilation at 6 cm, 0 station, contractions occurring every 5 minutes, and receiving epidural anesthesia
- [ ] **2.** a 24-year-old primiparous client who gave vaginal birth to a 7-lb, 3-oz (3,260-g) boy 1 hour ago, has a firm fundus and scant lochia rubra, and is attempting to breast-feed
- [ ] **3.** a 26-year-old multigravid client, in labor for 8 hours, with cervical dilation at 8 cm, 1+ station, contractions every 3 to 4 minutes, and receiving no anesthesia
- [ ] **4.** a 30-year-old multipara who gave birth to a 6-lb, 5-oz (2,863-g) girl by cesarean owing to fetal distress 3 hours ago, has a firm fundus and scant lochia rubra, and is receiving morphine by patient-controlled analgesia

2. A nurse has been working with a battered woman who is being discharged and returning home with her husband. The nurse says, "All this work with her has been useless. She is just going back to him as usual." Which statement by a nursing colleague would be **most** helpful to this nurse?
- [ ] **1.** "Her reasons for staying are complex. She can leave only when she is ready and can be safe."
- [ ] **2.** "I know it is frustrating to work with clients who do not follow our advice."
- [ ] **3.** "You did your best. You will see her again and have another chance."
- [ ] **4.** "These women almost never leave for good because of their emotional and financial dependency."

3. The nurse is to administer ergonovine maleate 200 mcg IM. The ampule label reads 0.2 mg/mL. The nurse should administer how many milliliters? Record your answer using a whole number.

_____ mL.

4. An infant is being admitted to the hospital with dehydration secondary to viral gastroenteritis. Which room assignment is the **most** appropriate for this infant?
- [ ] **1.** a semiprivate room with an 8-year-old child who has had an appendectomy
- [ ] **2.** a semiprivate room with a 10-year-old child with a closed head injury
- [ ] **3.** a private room
- [ ] **4.** a semiprivate room with a 4-year-old child with leukemia

5. An older adult is being admitted to the hospital after falling from a 6-foot ladder. Which information is **essential** for the nurse to obtain at this time? Select all that apply.
- [ ] **1.** symptoms at the time of the fall
- [ ] **2.** history of a previous fall
- [ ] **3.** location of the fall
- [ ] **4.** activity at the time of the fall
- [ ] **5.** time of the fall
- [ ] **6.** trauma after the fall
- [ ] **7.** who was present at the time of the fall

6. The nurse is caring for a client with influenza. The single most effective way to decrease the spread of microorganisms is:
- [ ] **1.** washing the hands frequently.
- [ ] **2.** having separate personal care items for the client.
- [ ] **3.** using disposable equipment.
- [ ] **4.** placing the client in isolation.

7. The nurse should be especially alert for what problem when caring for a term neonate, who weighed 10 lb (4,500 g) at birth, 1 hour after a vaginal birth?
- [ ] **1.** hypoglycemia
- [ ] **2.** hypercalcemia
- [ ] **3.** hypermagnesemia
- [ ] **4.** hyperbilirubinemia

8. A female client with infertility related to anovulatory cycles is prescribed menotropins. The nurse should assess the client for which possible adverse effect of this medication?
- [ ] **1.** pulmonary edema
- [ ] **2.** ovarian enlargement
- [ ] **3.** visual disturbances
- [ ] **4.** breast tenderness

9. An older adult is admitted to the hospital with sudden onset of severe pain in the back, flank, and abdomen. The client reports feeling weak; the blood pressure is 68/31 mm Hg. There has been no urine output. Bilateral leg pulses are weak, although bruit and pulsation are noted at the umbilicus. The nurse should **first**:
- ☐ **1.** obtain consent for emergency surgery.
- ☐ **2.** assess leg pulses with a Doppler test.
- ☐ **3.** palpate the abdomen for presence of a mass.
- ☐ **4.** start an IV infusion.

10. The nurse is teaching a client who will be undergoing a lung resection. The client is told that two chest tubes will be placed during surgery. The nurse explains that the purpose of the lower chest tube is to:
- ☐ **1.** prevent clots.
- ☐ **2.** remove air.
- ☐ **3.** remove fluid.
- ☐ **4.** facilitate "milking" of the tubes.

11. The nurse is giving care to an infant in an oxygen hood (see figure). Which interventions are indicated? Select all that apply.

- ☐ **1.** Assure that the oxygen is not blowing directly on the infant's face.
- ☐ **2.** Place the butterfly mobile on the outside of the hood.
- ☐ **3.** Immobilize the infant with restraints.
- ☐ **4.** Remove the hood for 10 minutes every hour.
- ☐ **5.** Encourage the parents to visit the child.

12. A nurse is assessing an 82-year-old for depression. Because of the client's age, the nurse's assessment should be guided by the fact that:
- ☐ **1.** sadness of mood is usually present, but it is masked by other symptoms.
- ☐ **2.** impairment of cognition usually is not present.
- ☐ **3.** psychosomatic tendencies do not tend to dominate.
- ☐ **4.** antidepressant therapies are less effective in older adults.

13. A **primary** concern of the hospitalized adolescent is:
- ☐ **1.** respect for the need for privacy.
- ☐ **2.** allowing parents to visit after hours.
- ☐ **3.** wearing a hospital gown.
- ☐ **4.** the fear of loss of control when in pain.

14. A 20-year-old single parent brings her 3-year-old son into the emergency department because he "fell." The child has bruises on his face, arms, and legs; his mother says that she did not witness the fall. The nurse suspects child abuse. While examining the child, the mother says, "Sometimes I guess I am pretty rough with him. I am alone, and I just do not know how to manage him." The nurse should ask the mother if she would find it helpful to have a referral to:
- ☐ **1.** a support group for single parents.
- ☐ **2.** a parenting education program.
- ☐ **3.** a women's support group.
- ☐ **4.** a support group for abusive parents.

15. The nurse is planning to complete assessments during the last half hour of the shift. Which assessment should be accomplished **first?**
- ☐ **1.** a postpartum couplet with the infant who has had transient tachypnea of the newborn (TTN) at birth and now has a respiratory rate of 60 breaths/minute
- ☐ **2.** a newly admitted postpartum client who is receiving magnesium sulfate at 3 g an hour initiated 10 hours ago for preeclampsia; her infant ate poorly previously and has not eaten for 4 hours
- ☐ **3.** a mother who had a cesarean section and is 6 hours after birth with the baby in special care nursery; the mother has not yet seen her baby
- ☐ **4.** a couplet with baby born at 36 weeks' gestation; the 5-lb (2,268-g) infant had initial blood glucose of 35 mg/dL (1.9 mmol/L) and when taken to the room had a glucose of 46 mg/dL (2.6 mmol/L)

16. An abused child is admitted to the hospital, and the nurse is aware that a court appearance may be necessary. To plan for this eventuality, what should be the **priority**?
- ☐ **1.** Remember the parents' and child's behavior when the child was admitted.
- ☐ **2.** Document physical findings and behaviors observed during the child's admission.
- ☐ **3.** Formulate subjective opinions about the cause of any injuries.
- ☐ **4.** Prepare answers to questions that may be asked by the attorneys.

17. A nurse who fails to check a client's armband before administering medications is:
- ☐ **1.** res judicata.
- ☐ **2.** negligent.
- ☐ **3.** stare decisis.
- ☐ **4.** vicariously liable.

18. A female client is experiencing bladder control problems. Which finding indicates the success of nursing interventions to promote urinary continence for this client?
- ☐ **1.** continence for 24 hours a day
- ☐ **2.** improvement in bladder control
- ☐ **3.** self-monitoring for urine retention
- ☐ **4.** compliance with drinking and voiding schedule

19. Before administering morphine to a client, the nurse should assess the client's: (Select all that apply.)
☐ **1.** blood pressure.
☐ **2.** respiration rate.
☐ **3.** pulse.
☐ **4.** temperature.
☐ **5.** level of consciousness.

20. A client is to receive 1 unit of packed red blood cells over 2 hours. There is 250 mL in the infusion bag. The IV administration infusion set delivers 10 gtts/mL. At what flow rate (in drops per minute) should the nurse run the infusion? Record your answer using a whole number.

_____ gtt/min.

21. A mother states that she is very angry with the healthcare provider (HCP) who diagnosed her child with leukemia. Which statement helps the nurse understand this mother's reaction?
☐ **1.** Anger is a natural result of a sense of loss and helplessness.
☐ **2.** Parents of sick children are usually unable to control their anger.
☐ **3.** Anger is rarely demonstrated by parents when coping with a sick child.
☐ **4.** The mother cannot overcome her anger in an acceptable manner.

22. Which nursing strategy would be effective in managing a client who has Alzheimer's disease and wanders?
☐ **1.** Encourage participation in activities such as board games.
☐ **2.** Discourage wandering by allowing the behavior at selected intervals.
☐ **3.** Involve the client in activities that promote walking.
☐ **4.** Promote safety by restraining the client in a geriatric chair.

23. A child who had a cast applied to his arm earlier this morning tells the nurse that his fingers are numb. The nurse should:
☐ **1.** notify the healthcare provider (HCP) who applied the cast.
☐ **2.** cut the cast to loosen it.
☐ **3.** assess the circulation to the fingers.
☐ **4.** ensure that the arm is positioned correctly.

24. A nurse is planning staffing for a nursing unit in which the primary need of the clients is learning how to manage their health problems. Which combination is the ideal mix of staff for this unit?
☐ **1.** three registered nurses (RNs)
☐ **2.** one RN and two licensed practical/vocational nurses (LPNs/VNs)
☐ **3.** one LPN/VN and two unlicensed assistive personnel (UAPs)
☐ **4.** one RN, one LPN/VN, and one UAP

25. An unlicensed assistive personnel (UAP) is taking care of a child in the arm restraint shown in the figure. To provide care for this child, the nurse should instruct the UAP to:

☐ **1.** unpin the restraint and perform range-of-motion exercises.
☐ **2.** unwrap the restraint and bathe the arm using warm water.
☐ **3.** leave the restraint in its current position.
☐ **4.** remove one tape at a time while bathing the child's arm.

26. While helping clients brought to a crisis center during a severe flood, the nurse interviews a client whose pregnant wife is missing and whose home has been destroyed. The client keeps talking rapidly about his experience and says, "I cannot see how I can ever rebuild my life." Which response by the nurse would be **most** appropriate?
☐ **1.** "If you start organizing your life now, I am sure all will be fine."
☐ **2.** "This has been a terrible experience. Tell me more about how you feel."
☐ **3.** "Let me note a few of the things you said before you continue with your story."
☐ **4.** "Spend some time thinking about this so that we can continue this conversation tomorrow."

27. A deficiency of which vitamin is thought to be the **first** step in the formation of plaque and oxidative changes in the arteries?
☐ **1.** vitamin C
☐ **2.** vitamin A
☐ **3.** vitamin E
☐ **4.** vitamin B_6

28. Which action should the nurse include in the plan of care for a child with leukemia who has an absolute neutrophil count of 400/mm^3 (0.4 × 10^9/L)?
☐ **1.** Restrict staff and visitors with active infections.
☐ **2.** Place the child in strict isolation.
☐ **3.** Consult with the primary care provider to administer an antiemetic.
☐ **4.** Increase the child's oral fluid intake.

29. A client with asthma has been prescribed beclomethasone via metered-dose inhaler. To determine if the client has been rinsing the mouth after each use of the inhaler, the nurse should inspect the client's mouth for:
- ☐ **1.** gingival hyperplasia.
- ☐ **2.** oral candidiasis.
- ☐ **3.** ulceration.
- ☐ **4.** dental caries.

30. The nurse finds a client lying on the floor next to the bed. After returning the client to bed, assessing for injury, and notifying the healthcare provider (HCP), the nurse fills out an incident report. What should the nurse do **next**?
- ☐ **1.** Give the incident report to the nurse-manager.
- ☐ **2.** Place the incident report on the medical record.
- ☐ **3.** Call the family to inform them.
- ☐ **4.** Omit mentioning the fall in the medical record documentation.

31. The nurse is caring for four clients in labor. Which client is at **most** risk for a postpartum hemorrhage?
- ☐ **1.** a client who is a gravida 4 para 3 with a history of polyhydramnios with this pregnancy
- ☐ **2.** a client who is a gravida 1 para 0 at 34 weeks' gestation with mild pregnancy-induced hypertension
- ☐ **3.** a client who is a gravida 4 para 0 with diet-controlled gestational diabetes being induced at term
- ☐ **4.** a client who is a gravida 2 para 1 term pregnancy with a history of genital herpes

32. The mother of a 2-year-old who has been bitten by the family dog asks the nurse what to do about the bite, which appears to be a minor injury. What should the nurse tell the mother?
- ☐ **1.** "You need to take the child to the local urgent care center immediately."
- ☐ **2.** "Wash the bite area with lots of running water, and then call your healthcare provider (HCP)."
- ☐ **3.** "Determine when the child's latest tetanus vaccine was administered."
- ☐ **4.** "Make an appointment to see the child's healthcare provider (HCP) now to start rabies shots."

33. The nurse is discharging a client who has been hospitalized for preterm labor. The client needs further instruction when she says:
- ☐ **1.** "If I think I have a bladder infection, I need to see my obstetrician."
- ☐ **2.** "If I have contractions, I should contact my healthcare provider (HCP)."
- ☐ **3.** "Drinking water may help prevent early labor for me."
- ☐ **4.** "If I travel on long trips, I need to get out of the car every 4 hours."

34. The nurse is conducting a routine risk assessment at a prenatal visit. Which question would be the **best** to screen for intimate partner violence?
- ☐ **1.** "Is your partner excited about your pregnancy?"
- ☐ **2.** "How safe do you feel in your home?"
- ☐ **3.** "Does your partner have an arrest record?"
- ☐ **4.** "Does your partner own a gun?"

35. A nurse is obtaining the history of an infant with suspected acute otitis media. What should the nurse ask the parent about?
- ☐ **1.** position of the infant when taking a bottle
- ☐ **2.** covering of the infant's ears when out in the cold
- ☐ **3.** thorough drying of the infant's ears after a bath
- ☐ **4.** immunization status of the infant

36. A 7-year-old has been diagnosed with bacterial meningitis. Who should receive chemoprophylaxis?
- ☐ **1.** all children at the school
- ☐ **2.** all household contacts and close contacts
- ☐ **3.** the entire community
- ☐ **4.** household contacts only

37. The mother of a newborn is concerned about the number of persons with heart disease in her family. She asks the nurse when she should start her baby on a low-fat, low-cholesterol diet to lower the risk of heart disease. The nurse should tell her to start diet modifications:
- ☐ **1.** at birth.
- ☐ **2.** at age 2.
- ☐ **3.** at age 5.
- ☐ **4.** at age 10.

38. The nurse is preparing to suction a tracheostomy for a client with methicillin-resistant *Staphylococcus aureus* (MRSA) (see figure). The nurse should:

- ☐ **1.** wear a powered air purifying respirator (PAPR) face shield.
- ☐ **2.** use goggles that include the hairline.
- ☐ **3.** change to a surgical mask.
- ☐ **4.** proceed to suction the client's tracheostomy.

39. A client is being treated for severe pediculosis. The nurse should instruct the client to treat the problem in the eyebrows and eyelashes by:
- [ ] 1. applying petroleum jelly to lashes and brows three to four times a day.
- [ ] 2. applying a pediculicide with a cotton-tipped swab to the eyebrows three times a day.
- [ ] 3. applying lindane ointment to the lashes and eyelashes three times a day.
- [ ] 4. applying bacitracin ointment to the lashes and brows three times a day.

40. The nurse is discussing safety and accident prevention with the parent of a 9-month-old. The teaching has been effective when the parent makes which statement?
- [ ] 1. "I make sure that I keep my cleaning supplies locked up."
- [ ] 2. "Sometimes she plays in the bathroom when I am cleaning in there."
- [ ] 3. "Occasionally, she gets under the chair and plays with the telephone cord."
- [ ] 4. "I have found that those child-protective cabinet locks do not work very well."

41. When assessing a child receiving tobramycin sulfate, which findings would indicate that the child is experiencing adverse effects? Select all that apply.
- [ ] 1. increased blood pressure
- [ ] 2. weight gain
- [ ] 3. rash
- [ ] 4. fever
- [ ] 5. ringing in the ears
- [ ] 6. decreased heart rate

42. The nurse instructs the client who is taking gentamicin to monitor renal function. The nurse determines that the client needs additional instruction when the client makes which statement?
- [ ] 1. "I should call you if I notice that I am not urinating as much."
- [ ] 2. "I should call you if my urine looks dark or unusual."
- [ ] 3. "I should call you if my legs swell or I notice my skin looks puffy around my eyes."
- [ ] 4. "I should call you if I have a fever."

43. A school-age child is admitted to the hospital with a vasoocclusive sickle cell crisis. How should the nurse prioritize the client's care? Place interventions in order of highest priority to lowest priority. All options must be used.

1. Administer morphine for the pain.

2. Start oxygen per nasal cannula.

3. Start an IV infusion.

4. Draw blood for electrolyte and pH balance.

44. When teaching a group of parents about the potential for febrile seizures in children, which fact should the nurse include?
- [ ] 1. The exact cause is known.
- [ ] 2. The seizures occur as the fever rises.
- [ ] 3. Children older than age 3 are most at risk.
- [ ] 4. These seizures commonly occur after immunization administration.

45. A 19-year-old primigravid client is being discharged home after hospitalization for hyperemesis gravidarum and is being referred to home health care. The nurse should develop a discharge plan that includes which interventions? Select all that apply.
- [ ] 1. Refer the client to a nutritionist for the following day.
- [ ] 2. Ensure that the client has a prescription for an antiemetic.
- [ ] 3. Ask the healthcare provider (HCP) for an anxiolytic prescription.
- [ ] 4. Encourage return to normal routine when the client feels ready.
- [ ] 5. Coordinate follow-up appointment with provider in 6 weeks.
- [ ] 6. Discuss plan of care and discharge instructions with client.

46. The nurse should instruct a woman taking folic acid supplements for folic acid deficiency anemia that:
- [ ] 1. it will take several months to notice an improvement.
- [ ] 2. folic acid should be taken on an empty stomach.
- [ ] 3. iron supplements are contraindicated with folic acid supplementation.
- [ ] 4. oral contraceptive use, pregnancy, and lactation increase daily requirements.

47. The nurse makes a home visit to a primiparous client and her neonate at 1 week after a vaginal birth. Which finding should be reported to the healthcare provider (HCP)?
☐ 1. a scant amount of maternal lochia serosa
☐ 2. the presence of a neonatal tonic neck reflex
☐ 3. a nonpalpable maternal fundus
☐ 4. neonatal central cyanosis

48. The nurse is obtaining a health history for a client with osteoporosis. What should the nurse ask the client about? Select all that apply.
☐ 1. amount of alcohol consumed daily
☐ 2. use of antacids
☐ 3. dietary intake of fiber
☐ 4. use of vitamin K supplements
☐ 5. intake of fruit juices

49. The nurse tells a rape victim that even if she was protected against pregnancy by a contraceptive and has no intention of taking any legal action against her assailant, she should still be checked by a healthcare provider (HCP) for early detection of:
☐ 1. sexually transmitted disease.
☐ 2. anxiety reaction.
☐ 3. periurethral tears.
☐ 4. menstrual difficulties.

50. A hospitalized client fell on the floor and sustained a small laceration on the hand that required stitches. The intern will suture the client's hand at the client's bedside and asks for bupivacaine with epinephrine and a suture kit in order to suture the laceration. The nurse should question:
☐ 1. the intern's ability to suture.
☐ 2. the client's room as an aseptic environment.
☐ 3. bupivacaine with epinephrine as the local anesthetic.
☐ 4. the cosmetic effect from not having a plastic surgeon do the suturing.

51. A 5-lb 8-oz (2.5 kg) baby was born 1 hour ago to a 19-year-old primigravida. The **priority** nursing assessments include monitoring the infant for:
☐ 1. jaundice and physical assessment.
☐ 2. vital signs and gestational age assessments.
☐ 3. feedings and vital signs.
☐ 4. Apgar and gestational age assessments.

52. When assessing a dark-skinned client for cyanosis, what should the nurse examine?
☐ 1. the client's retinas
☐ 2. the client's nail beds
☐ 3. the client's oral mucous membranes
☐ 4. the inner aspects of the client's wrists

53. Betamethasone syrup 0.9 mg has been prescribed. It is available in a 0.6 mg/5 mL solution. How many milliliters should the nurse administer? Record your answer using one decimal place.

_____ mL.

54. A client at 37 weeks' gestation is scheduled for a biophysical profile. What should the nurse instruct the client to do **before** the test?
☐ 1. Drink 1 to 2 L of fluid.
☐ 2. Take nothing by mouth after midnight before the test.
☐ 3. Plan to remain in the clinic for 4 hours after the test.
☐ 4. Eat a high-fiber meal after the test.

55. A 12-year-old boy has depression and post-trauma response. The boy's father is now in jail for molesting him from ages 6 to 9. Given the typical reactions of incest victims, the nurse should assess the child for which behavior? Select all that apply.
☐ 1. sexualized play
☐ 2. aggression
☐ 3. isolation at home
☐ 4. running away
☐ 5. truancy

56. The nurse has provided an in-service presentation to ancillary staff about standard precautions on the birthing unit. The nurse determines that one of the staff members needs further instructions when the nurse observes which action?
☐ 1. use of protective goggles during a cesarean birth
☐ 2. placement of bloody sheets in a container designated for contaminated linens
☐ 3. wearing of sterile gloves to bathe a neonate at 2 hours of age
☐ 4. disposal of used scalpel blades in a puncture-resistant container

57. Which is true regarding delegation of client care responsibilities? Select all that apply.
☐ 1. The nurse must know the nursing model that underlies care at the institution.
☐ 2. The nurse delegates in accordance with demands on his/her time.
☐ 3. The nurse confirms that the unlicensed assistive personnel (UAP) has experience with the delegated activity.
☐ 4. The nurse retains the right to determine which tasks are delegated.
☐ 5. The nurse must document that the task has been delegated and to whom.

58. A child with leukemia had been in remission for several years, but death is now imminent. The nurse is assisting the parents as they prepare for the child's death. Which approach will be **most** helpful?
☐ 1. Reflect to the parents that the death of a child is more difficult than that of an adult.
☐ 2. Help parents understand that grief is stronger when preceded by hope.
☐ 3. Recognize that the parents have been prepared for this death since the time of diagnosis.
☐ 4. Understand the parent's trust in the health-care system will be undermined by the death of their child.

59. The client has sore nares while a nasogastric (NG) tube is in place. Which nursing measure would be **most** appropriate to help alleviate the client's discomfort?
- ☐ **1.** Reposition the tube in the nares.
- ☐ **2.** Irrigate the tube with a cool solution.
- ☐ **3.** Apply a water-soluble lubricant to the nares.
- ☐ **4.** Have the client change position more frequently.

60. The nurse is instructing a Hindu client to increase protein in the diet. Which foods are appropriate to include in this client's diet? Select all that apply.
- ☐ **1.** lentil soup
- ☐ **2.** hamburger
- ☐ **3.** steak
- ☐ **4.** veal cutlet
- ☐ **5.** broiled fish sandwich

61. The nurse is evaluating the outcome of therapy for a client with osteoarthritis. Which finding indicates goals of therapy have been met?
- ☐ **1.** Joint degeneration has been arrested.
- ☐ **2.** The client is able to self-administer gold compound safely.
- ☐ **3.** The client feels better than on hospital admission.
- ☐ **4.** Joint range of motion has improved.

62. A child with partial- and full-thickness burns is admitted to the pediatric unit. What should be the **priority** at this time?
- ☐ **1.** preventing wound infection
- ☐ **2.** evaluating vital signs frequently
- ☐ **3.** maintaining fluid and electrolyte balance
- ☐ **4.** managing the child's pain

63. A normal, healthy infant is brought to the clinic for the first diphtheria, tetanus, and acellular pertussis (DTaP) immunization. Which route is appropriate to administer this vaccine?
- ☐ **1.** oral
- ☐ **2.** intramuscular
- ☐ **3.** subcutaneous
- ☐ **4.** intradermal

64. A child has been prescribed diphenhydramine hydrochloride to help control the itching from atopic dermatitis. The nurse should instruct the parents to report which conditions? Select all that apply.
- ☐ **1.** weight loss
- ☐ **2.** drowsiness
- ☐ **3.** thickened bronchial secretions
- ☐ **4.** upset stomach
- ☐ **5.** bradycardia

65. Assessment of a nulligravid client in active labor reveals the following: moderate discomfort; cervix dilated 3 cm, 0 station, and completely effaced; and fetal heart rate of 136 bpm. What should the nurse plan to do **next**?
- ☐ **1.** Assist the client with comfort measures and breathing techniques.
- ☐ **2.** Turn the client from the left side-lying position to the right side-lying position.
- ☐ **3.** Prepare the client for epidural anesthesia to relieve pain.
- ☐ **4.** Instruct the client that internal fetal monitoring is necessary.

66. The nurse observes that a client who has received midazolam for conscious sedation is having shallow respirations. The nurse should do all **except**:
- ☐ **1.** encourage the client to deep-breathe.
- ☐ **2.** have respiratory resuscitation equipment in the room.
- ☐ **3.** administer oxygen as prescribed.
- ☐ **4.** administer naloxone.

67. The nurse is planning to assist the healthcare provider (HCP) with a thoracentesis for a client who has a pleural effusion. Which position would be appropriate for the client to assume?
- ☐ **1.** lying supine with the arms extended
- ☐ **2.** lying prone with the head supported by the arms
- ☐ **3.** sitting upright and leaning on an overbed table
- ☐ **4.** side lying with the knees drawn up to the abdomen

68. A child who is 3 years of age has been admitted with diarrhea. He has mild dehydration (<5%). The nurse is reviewing the laboratory report of the stool specimen (see report). Based on the review of the laboratory report from the stool specimen, the nurse should do which action **first**?

Laboratory Results	
Test	**Result**
WBC	Mildly elevated
RBC	Few
Bacteria	Positive for *E. coli*
Ova and Parasites	Negative

- ☐ **1.** Start an IV infusion.
- ☐ **2.** Institute enteric precautions.
- ☐ **3.** Instruct the family to wash all family bed linens in hot water.
- ☐ **4.** Cleanse and protect the anal area.

69. A client has a coxsackie B (viral) or trypano-somal (parasite) infection. The nurse should further assess the client for:
- ☐ **1.** myocarditis.
- ☐ **2.** myocardial infarction.
- ☐ **3.** renal failure.
- ☐ **4.** liver failure.

70. The nurse observes which principles when conducting a medication reconciliation? Select all that apply.
- ☐ **1.** Medication reconciliation is an important client safety goal.
- ☐ **2.** Medication reconciliation is designed to obtain and communicate an accurate list of a client's home medications across the continuum of care.
- ☐ **3.** Only nurses or healthcare providers (HCPs) can be involved in medication reconciliation.
- ☐ **4.** Medications are considered reconciled if a medication prescription exists that is therapeutically equivalent to the one prior to admission.
- ☐ **5.** A medication is considered to be any medication prescribed by a healthcare provider (HCP).

71. A charge nurse asks a newly graduated registered nurse (RN) who normally works on a medical-surgical nursing unit to take care of two clients in the coronary care unit. The nurse has not had experience with taking care of clients on monitors or using the medications that these clients are taking. The new nurse should:
- ☐ **1.** accept the assignment and then plan to ask the nurses in the coronary care unit to administer the medications for these clients.
- ☐ **2.** explain to the charge nurse about his or her level of experience and express concerns about this assignment.
- ☐ **3.** tell the charge nurse that the assignment was to the medical-surgical unit and refuse to go to the coronary care unit.
- ☐ **4.** ask the charge nurse if the assignment can be reduced to taking care of one client.

72. The nurse is working in a newborn nursery and caring for several neonates. What precaution should be taken to prevent an infant abduction?
- ☐ **1.** Notify the hospital's security staff about anyone who appears unusual.
- ☐ **2.** Take several neonates to their mothers at the same time.
- ☐ **3.** Place the infant near the doorway of the mother's room.
- ☐ **4.** Contact the hospital's security staff if an exit alarm is triggered.

73. A client has started taking amiodarone. The nurse should inform the client that periodic laboratory tests will be done to monitor the client's:
- ☐ **1.** hemoglobin.
- ☐ **2.** liver enzymes.
- ☐ **3.** creatine kinase (CK) concentration.
- ☐ **4.** renal function.

74. The nurse is assessing a teenage girl. According to the figure, the nurse should note that the girl has:

- ☐ **1.** kyphosis.
- ☐ **2.** lordosis.
- ☐ **3.** developmental dysplasia of the hip.
- ☐ **4.** scoliosis.

75. A child with type 1 diabetes is admitted to the emergency department with hot and dry skin, rapid and deep respirations, and a fruity odor to her breath. Which task, when performed by a new graduate registered nurse (RN), requires the RN preceptor to intervene?
- ☐ **1.** assessment of the child's vital signs every 15 minutes
- ☐ **2.** verification of the child's prescription for IV insulin infusion
- ☐ **3.** providing encouragement to the child to drink some orange juice
- ☐ **4.** verification of child's glucose by finger stick

76. The unlicensed assistive personnel (UAP) approaches the nurse and states, "The client does not know what caused him to be so depressed. He must not want to tell me because he does not trust me yet." In responding to this staff member, which statement by the nurse will help the UAP understand the client's illness?
- ☐ **1.** "Endogenous depression is biochemical and is not caused by an outside stressor or problem. The client cannot tell you why he is depressed because he really does not know."
- ☐ **2.** "Endogenous depression can be caused by various stressors. Perhaps the client is not willing to tell you at this time."
- ☐ **3.** "Endogenous depression comes from within the person. It is a reaction to a loss. You need to give the client more time to identify the cause or loss."
- ☐ **4.** "Endogenous depression usually derives from past childhood conflicts. It really is not important for the client to remember what happened years ago."

77. A child's plan of care lists increasing protein intake as a goal. Which food should the nurse encourage the child to eat?
- ☐ **1.** a bacon, lettuce, and tomato sandwich
- ☐ **2.** fruit-flavored yogurt
- ☐ **3.** nacho chips and cheese sauce
- ☐ **4.** crackers with jelly

78. Thirty minutes after a Sengstaken-Blakemore tube is inserted, the client appears to be having difficulty breathing. What should the nurse do **first**?
- ☐ **1.** Remove the tube.
- ☐ **2.** Deflate the esophageal portion of the tube.
- ☐ **3.** Determine whether the tube is obstructing the airway.
- ☐ **4.** Increase the oxygen flow rate.

79. A client is admitted to the emergency department with myasthenia crisis. Place interventions in order of highest priority to lowest priority. All options must be used.

1. Check if the client missed a dose of medication.

2. Assess the client for signs of infection.

3. Check the gag reflex.

4. Prepare for intubation.

80. A 10-year-old child is diagnosed with pediculosis. The mother is concerned about the spread of the lice to children who have been in contact with her child. The nurse should instruct the mother to have her child avoid:
- ☐ **1.** sharing craft supplies.
- ☐ **2.** having contact during a swimming class.
- ☐ **3.** sharing batting helmets.
- ☐ **4.** showering after football practice.

81. A 24-year-old nulligravid client with a history of irregular menstrual cycles visits the clinic because she suspects that she is "about 6 weeks pregnant." An ultrasound is scheduled in 2 weeks. The nurse should instruct the client that this test will be done to:
- ☐ **1.** assess gestational age.
- ☐ **2.** determine a multifetal pregnancy.
- ☐ **3.** identify the gender of the fetus.
- ☐ **4.** assess of maternal pelvic adequacy.

82. The nurse is beginning the shift and is assessing the oxygen exchange on a neonate. The nurse reviews the medical record for pulse oximetry reading for the last 8 hours.

Flow Sheets

Pulse Oximetry

Time	0700	0900	1100	1300	1500
Reading	95%	90%	90%	90%	86%

The pulse oximetry reading at 1530 is 75%. What should the nurse do **first**?
- ☐ **1.** Administer oxygen via mask.
- ☐ **2.** Swaddle the neonate in heated blankets.
- ☐ **3.** Reassess the oximetry reading in 30 minutes.
- ☐ **4.** Draw blood gases for oxygen and carbon dioxide levels.

83. A client with a history of peptic ulcer disease is admitted to the hospital. Initial assessment reveals that his blood pressure is 96/60 mm Hg, his pulse rate is 120 bpm, and he has vomited coffee-ground–like material. Based on this assessment, what is the nurse's **priority** action?
- ☐ **1.** Administer an antiemetic.
- ☐ **2.** Prepare to insert a nasogastric (NG) tube.
- ☐ **3.** Collect data regarding recent client stressors.
- ☐ **4.** Place the client in a modified Trendelenburg position.

84. As a nurse begins the shift on the obstetrical unit, there are several new admissions. When anticipating priorities for the shift, the client with which condition would be a candidate for induction?
- ☐ **1.** preeclampsia
- ☐ **2.** active herpes
- ☐ **3.** face presentation
- ☐ **4.** fetus with late decelerations

85. In the early postoperative period, the nurse notes a bright red, 3″ × 5″ (7.6 × 12.7 cm) area of drainage on the client's abdominal laparotomy dressing. What should be the nurse's **first** action in response to this observation?
- ☐ **1.** Ignore it because drainage is normal.
- ☐ **2.** Increase the IV flow rate.
- ☐ **3.** Take the client's vital signs.
- ☐ **4.** Change the dressing.

86. A 6-year-old client is diagnosed with attention deficit hyperactivity disorder (ADHD). When asking this client to complete a task, what techniques should the nurse use to communicate **most** effectively with him?

☐ 1. Obtain eye contact before speaking, use simple language, and have him repeat what was said. Praise him if he completes the task.

☐ 2. Fully explain to the client the actions required of him, and offer verbal praise and a food reward for task completion.

☐ 3. Explain to the client what he is to do, the consequences if he does not comply, and follow through with praise or consequences as appropriate.

☐ 4. Demonstrate to the client what he is to do, have him imitate the nurse's actions, and give a food reward if he completes the task.

87. A 10-year-old child has blood glucose readings during a 24-hour period. Which reading requires the **most** immediate intervention?

☐ 1. 50 mg/dL (2.8 mmol/L)
☐ 2. 100 mg/dL (5.6 mmol/L)
☐ 3. 150 mg/dL (8.4 mmol/L)
☐ 4. 200 mg/dL (11.2 mmol/L)

88. A client has massive bleeding from esophageal varices. In what order from **first** to last should the nurse and care team provide care for this client? All options must be used.

1. Control hemorrhaging.

2. Replace fluids.

3. Relieve the client's anxiety.

4. Maintain a patent airway.

89. Which instruction is **most** important for the nurse to include in the teaching plan for a client who is taking phenelzine?

☐ 1. Eat a normal amount of salt in the diet.
☐ 2. Drink 10 to 12 glasses of water each day.
☐ 3. Allow 10 days to achieve therapeutic effects.
☐ 4. Avoid foods high in tyramine.

90. The nurse should closely monitor the client with an open fracture for which complication?

☐ 1. avascular necrosis
☐ 2. compartment syndrome
☐ 3. osteomyelitis
☐ 4. fat embolism syndrome

91. The nurse develops a health education program about preventing the transmission of hepatitis B. The nurse evaluates that the teaching has been effective when the participants identify which activity to be high risk for acquiring hepatitis B?

☐ 1. frequent use of marijuana
☐ 2. ingestion of large amounts of acetaminophen
☐ 3. sharing needles for drug use
☐ 4. ingestion of contaminated seafood

92. An adult client who has been treated with antidepressants for a year has had antianxiety medication added to the treatment regimen. The client says to the nurse, "I have reached the bottom of the barrel now. I have to take both fluoxetine and clonazepam to control my symptoms." What would be the **best** nurse reply to the client?

☐ 1. "If the medications work, why worry? Just take them, and be happy they are effective."

☐ 2. "I can understand your concern. Those psychiatric medications are pretty potent."

☐ 3. "It seems you are concerned your illness may be worsening. Tell me more about that."

☐ 4. "You seem to feel guilty about taking psychiatric medication for your illness. There is nothing to feel guilty about."

93. The nurse is assessing a client who has a long history of uncontrolled hypertension. The nurse should assess the client for damage in which area of the eye?

☐ 1. iris
☐ 2. cornea
☐ 3. retina
☐ 4. sclera

94. While preparing to provide neonatal care instructions to a primiparous client who gave birth to a term neonate 24 hours ago, what should the nurse include in the client's teaching plan?

☐ 1. Term neonates generally have few creases on the soles of their feet.

☐ 2. Strawberry hemangiomas—deep, dark red discolorations—require laser therapy for removal.

☐ 3. Milia are white papules from plugged sebaceous ducts that disappear by age 2 to 4 weeks.

☐ 4. If erythema toxicum is present, it will be treated with antibiotic therapy.

95. Two days after being placed in a cast for a fractured femur, the client suddenly has chest pain and dyspnea. The client is confused and has an elevated temperature. The nurse should assess the client for:

☐ 1. osteomyelitis.
☐ 2. compartment syndrome.
☐ 3. venous thrombosis.
☐ 4. fat embolism syndrome.

96. Which outcome is appropriate for the client with hepatitis B? The client will:
- ☐ 1. adhere to measures to prevent the spread of infection to others.
- ☐ 2. adhere to a low-sodium, low-protein diet.
- ☐ 3. verbalize the importance of using sedatives to provide adequate rest.
- ☐ 4. avoid social activities with friends after discharge from the hospital.

97. A 15-year-old male client on the psychiatric unit shows signs of mild intoxication. When questioned, he states that another client gave him beer, and he refuses to name the client. What should the nurse do **next**?
- ☐ 1. Telephone the client's parents.
- ☐ 2. Call a community meeting.
- ☐ 3. Urge the client to tell who gave him the beer.
- ☐ 4. Call the primary care provider.

98. The client with benign prostatic hypertrophy is being transferred from the emergency department to a surgery unit. Which information should be included in the report from the nurse in the emergency department to the nurse responsible for admitting the client?
- ☐ 1. "A urine specimen was obtained from the client and sent to the laboratory for analysis."
- ☐ 2. "The client was catheterized, and 1,100 mL of urine was obtained. The urine appeared cloudy, and a specimen was sent to the laboratory."
- ☐ 3. "The client is very cooperative. He is comfortable now that his bladder has been emptied. He had no ill effects from catheterization."
- ☐ 4. "The client was in the emergency department for 3 hours because of bladder distention. He is fine now but is being admitted as a possible candidate for surgery."

99. A client has received an overdose of sympathomimetic agents. The nurse should assess the client for which **late** signs of an overdose? Select all that apply.
- ☐ 1. hypotension
- ☐ 2. bradycardia
- ☐ 3. seizures
- ☐ 4. profound pyrexia
- ☐ 5. hypertension

100. While assessing a neonate at 4 hours after birth, the nurse observes an indentation with a small tuft of hair at the base of the neonate's spine. The nurse should document this as what finding?
- ☐ 1. spina bifida cystica
- ☐ 2. spina bifida occulta
- ☐ 3. meningocele
- ☐ 4. myelomeningocele

101. Which client is at **highest** risk for developing a urinary tract infection?
- ☐ 1. a woman who has given vaginal birth to two children
- ☐ 2. a man with an indwelling urinary catheter
- ☐ 3. a man with a past medical history of renal calculi
- ☐ 4. a woman with well-controlled diabetes mellitus

102. A nurse is administering indomethacin to a neonate. What should the nurse do to ensure that the nurse has identified the neonate correctly? Select all that apply.
- ☐ 1. Ask the parents to confirm that this is their baby.
- ☐ 2. Ask another nurse to confirm that this is the neonate for whom the medication has been prescribed.
- ☐ 3. Check the neonate's identification band against the medical record number.
- ☐ 4. Verify the date of birth from the medical record with the date of birth on the neonate's identification band.
- ☐ 5. Compare the number on the crib with the number on the neonate's identification band.

103. Which statement indicates that the client with a peptic ulcer understands the dietary modifications to follow at home?
- ☐ 1. "I should eat a bland, soft diet."
- ☐ 2. "It is important to eat six small meals a day."
- ☐ 3. "I should drink several glasses of milk a day."
- ☐ 4. "I should avoid alcohol and caffeine."

104. The client with a nasogastric (NG) tube has abdominal distention. What should the nurse do **first**?
- ☐ 1. Call the healthcare provider (HCP).
- ☐ 2. Irrigate the NG tube.
- ☐ 3. Check the function of the suction equipment.
- ☐ 4. Reposition the NG tube.

105. A male client has been diagnosed as having a low sperm count during infertility studies. After instructions by the nurse about some causes of low sperm counts, the nurse determines that the client needs further instructions when he says low sperm counts may be caused by:
- ☐ 1. varicocele.
- ☐ 2. frequent use of saunas.
- ☐ 3. endocrine imbalances.
- ☐ 4. decreased body temperature.

106. The nurse instills 5 mL of normal saline before suctioning a client's tracheostomy tube. The instillation is effective when:
- ☐ 1. the secretions are thinned.
- ☐ 2. the client coughs.
- ☐ 3. there is minimal friction when the catheter is passed into the tracheostomy tube.
- ☐ 4. there is humidification for the respiratory tract.

107. A client with emphysema is receiving continuous oxygen therapy. Depressed ventilation is likely to occur unless the nurse ensures that the oxygen is administered in which way?
- ☐ **1.** cooled
- ☐ **2.** humidified
- ☐ **3.** at a low flow rate
- ☐ **4.** through nasal cannula

108. Before cataract surgery, the nurse is to instill several types of eye drops. The surgeon writes prescriptions for 5 gtts of antibiotic in OD and 3 gtts of topical steroid drops in OD. The nurse should:
- ☐ **1.** contact the surgeon to rewrite the prescription.
- ☐ **2.** administer the antibiotic in the left eye and the steroid in the right eye.
- ☐ **3.** administer both types of drops in the right eye.
- ☐ **4.** contact the pharmacist for clarification of the prescription.

109. Which instructions about breast-feeding should the nurse include when counseling the client?
- ☐ **1.** Apply ice packs to breasts while nursing.
- ☐ **2.** Wrap breasts with ace bandages.
- ☐ **3.** Avoid fruit juices with acid.
- ☐ **4.** Use a water-based lubricant when having intercourse.

110. A client with rheumatoid arthritis tells the nurse that she feels "quite alone" in adjusting to changes in her lifestyle. The nurse should respond by:
- ☐ **1.** referring the client and her husband for counseling to decrease her sense of isolation.
- ☐ **2.** suggesting that the client develop a hobby to occupy her time.
- ☐ **3.** telling the client about her community's arthritis support group.
- ☐ **4.** recommending that the client discuss her feelings with her minister.

111. Which intervention should the nurse include in the plan of care to ensure adequate nutrition for a very active, talkative, and easily distractible client who is unable to sit through meals?
- ☐ **1.** Direct the client to the room to eat.
- ☐ **2.** Offer the client nutritious finger foods.
- ☐ **3.** Ask the client's family to bring the client's favorite foods from home.
- ☐ **4.** Ask the client about food preferences.

112. A client in a group home is very dependent on the staff but is able to make simple decisions. The client asks, "Would you do my laundry? I do not know how the machine works." Which response would be **best**?
- ☐ **1.** "Sure, I have time; I can do it for you."
- ☐ **2.** "You will have to wait; I do not have time now."
- ☐ **3.** "Can your family do it for you?"
- ☐ **4.** "Get your laundry; I will show you how the machine works."

113. The nurse is caring for a client with chronic renal failure. The nurse should monitor the client for which adverse effects of hypermagnesemia?
- ☐ **1.** flushed skin
- ☐ **2.** lethargy
- ☐ **3.** severe thirst
- ☐ **4.** tremors

114. When determining the parents' compliance with treatment for their infant who has otitis media, the nurse should ask the parents if they are:
- ☐ **1.** cleaning the child's ear canals with hydrogen peroxide.
- ☐ **2.** administering continuous, low-dose antibiotic therapy.
- ☐ **3.** instilling ear drops regularly to prevent cerumen accumulation.
- ☐ **4.** holding the child upright when feeding with a bottle.

115. When giving a change-of-shift report, which statement by the nurse is **not** appropriate?
- ☐ **1.** "Randi Smith is a 38-year-old female client of Dr. Born with cholecystitis and cholelithiasis."
- ☐ **2.** "Mrs. Jones' pain is best relieved in the left lateral Sims' position."
- ☐ **3.** "Mr. Levi is just contrary today, and nothing is going to please him."
- ☐ **4.** "Mr. Emmert was able to walk around the unit twice today with no dizziness."

116. The nurse is teaching unlicensed assistive personnel (UAP) about caring for a client who is withdrawing from alcohol and street drugs. Which communication technique when observed by the nurse indicates the UAP has understood the instructions? The UAP talks to the client using:
- ☐ **1.** matter-of-fact manner and short sentences.
- ☐ **2.** cheerful tone of voice, using humor when appropriate.
- ☐ **3.** loud voice and giving general comments.
- ☐ **4.** clear explanations in a quiet voice.

117. A couple has completed testing and is a candidate for in vitro fertilization. The nurse is reviewing the procedure with them and realizes that further instruction is needed when the woman states:
- ☐ **1.** "One of the greatest risks is multiple pregnancies."
- ☐ **2.** "I will need to redefine how I view my job if I do become pregnant."
- ☐ **3.** "The fertilization procedure can be done anytime during my cycle."
- ☐ **4.** "We can use our own eggs and sperm or someone else's."

118. When obtaining the diet history from a client with anemia, the nurse should include questions specifically about which vitamins or minerals that are **most** likely missing in this client's diet? Select all that apply.
☐ 1. vitamin B$_6$
☐ 2. vitamin K
☐ 3. vitamin B$_{12}$
☐ 4. iron
☐ 5. vitamin C

119. What is the **primary** goal of nursing care during the emergent phase after a burn injury?
☐ 1. Replace lost fluids.
☐ 2. Prevent infection.
☐ 3. Control pain.
☐ 4. Promote wound healing.

120. The nurse assesses for euphoria in a client with multiple sclerosis, looking for what characteristic clinical manifestations?
☐ 1. inappropriate laughter
☐ 2. an exaggerated sense of well-being
☐ 3. slurring of words when excited
☐ 4. visual hallucinations

121. The nurse is assessing a client with a burn injury using the "rule of nines" to determine:
☐ 1. amount of body surface area burned.
☐ 2. rehabilitation needs.
☐ 3. respiratory needs.
☐ 4. type of intravenous fluids required.

122. When assessing a 2-month-old infant, the nurse feels a "click" when abducting the infant's left hip. What should the nurse do **next**?
☐ 1. Document the finding as normal for a 2-month-old.
☐ 2. Check the lengths of the femurs to determine if they are equal.
☐ 3. Instruct the mother to keep the leg in an adducted position.
☐ 4. Reschedule the child for a follow-up assessment in 3 weeks.

123. Which laboratory tests should the nurse monitor when the client is receiving warfarin sodium therapy?
☐ 1. partial thromboplastin time (PTT)
☐ 2. serum potassium
☐ 3. arterial blood gas (ABG) values
☐ 4. prothrombin time (PT)

124. A client who had transurethral resection of the prostate (TURP) 2 days earlier has lower abdominal pain. The nurse should **first**:
☐ 1. auscultate the abdomen for bowel sounds.
☐ 2. administer an oral analgesic.
☐ 3. have the client use a sitz bath for 15 minutes.
☐ 4. assess the patency of the urethral catheter.

125. The nurse is ready to administer a partial fill of imipenem-cilastatin in the IV pump when a full partial fill bag of imipenem-cilastatin is found hanging at the client's bedside. The nurse should **first**:
☐ 1. discard the full partial fill of imipenem-cilastatin found hanging at the client's bedside.
☐ 2. check the identifying information of the full partial fill of imipenem-cilastatin found hanging at the client's bedside.
☐ 3. determine when the client received the last dose of the imipenem-cilastatin.
☐ 4. administer the new partial fill of imipenem-cilastatin.

126. A client with a moderate level of anxiety is pacing quickly in the hall and tells the nurse, "Help me. I cannot take it anymore." What would be the **best** initial response?
☐ 1. "It would be best if you would lie down until you are calmer."
☐ 2. "Let us go to a quieter area where we can talk if you want."
☐ 3. "Try doing your relaxation exercises to calm down."
☐ 4. "I will get some medicine to help you relax."

127. The nurse should plan to teach a client who is taking warfarin sodium to:
☐ 1. consult the healthcare provider (HCP) before undergoing a tooth extraction.
☐ 2. avoid the use of a toothbrush during oral hygiene.
☐ 3. use rectal suppositories to treat constipation.
☐ 4. eat green leafy vegetables.

128. A 30-year-old client hospitalized with a fractured femur, which is being treated with skeletal traction, has not had a bowel movement for 2 days. The nurse should:
☐ 1. administer a tap water enema.
☐ 2. place the client on the bedpan every 2 to 3 hours.
☐ 3. increase the client's fluid intake to 3,000 mL/day.
☐ 4. perform range-of-motion movements to all extremities.

129. A client is receiving a tube feeding and has developed diarrhea, cramps, and abdominal distention. What should the nurse do? Select all that apply.
☐ 1. Change the feeding apparatus every 24 hours.
☐ 2. Use a higher volume of formula because the formula may be too hypotonic.
☐ 3. Slow the administration rate.
☐ 4. Use a diluted formula, gradually increasing the volume and concentration.
☐ 5. Anticipate changing to a lactose-free formula.

130. A 62-year-old client who has smoked two packs of cigarettes for the last 10 years is admitted with a diagnosis of lung cancer. She reports having "no appetite" and exhibits symptoms of anorexia. The client is 5 feet, 8 inches (173 cm) tall and weighs 112 lb (50.8 kg). The client is now scheduled for a left lung lobectomy. The nurse should include which factor when planning to prevent postoperative pulmonary complications?
☐ 1. The client tends to keep her real feelings to herself.
☐ 2. The client ambulates and can climb one flight of stairs without dyspnea.
☐ 3. The client is aged 62.
☐ 4. The client's weight relative to her height is low.

131. When developing the plan of care for a 12-year-old child who is to receive chemotherapy that is associated with nausea and vomiting, the nurse should plan to administer an antiemetic at which time?
☐ 1. thirty minutes after the chemotherapy has started, then as needed
☐ 2. thirty minutes before the chemotherapy starts, then routinely
☐ 3. when the 12-year-old requests medication for nausea, then as needed
☐ 4. on starting the chemotherapy infusion, then routinely

132. The membranes of a multigravid client in active labor rupture spontaneously, revealing greenish-colored amniotic fluid. How does the nurse interpret this finding?
☐ 1. passage of meconium by the fetus
☐ 2. maternal intrauterine infection
☐ 3. Rh incompatibility between mother and fetus
☐ 4. maternal sexually transmitted disease

133. A client's arterial blood gas values are as follows:

Laboratory Results

Test	Result
pH	7.24
Paco$_2$	35 mmHg (6.7 kPa)
HCO$_3^-$	15 mEq/L (15 mmol/L)

The nurse should monitor the client for:
☐ 1. metabolic acidosis.
☐ 2. metabolic alkalosis.
☐ 3. respiratory acidosis.
☐ 4. respiratory alkalosis.

134. A client is suspected of having a slow gastrointestinal bleed. The nurse should evaluate the client for which sign?
☐ 1. increased pulse
☐ 2. nausea
☐ 3. tarry stools
☐ 4. abdominal cramps

135. The nurse is assessing a client's knowledge about coronary syndrome that was diagnosed 4 years ago. When assessing the client's learning needs, the nurse should take which information into consideration?
☐ 1. The client has had the heart condition for 4 years and is probably very knowledgeable about this disease.
☐ 2. The client's learning needs may have changed over the course of the illness.
☐ 3. The client's condition is presently stable, so there will be fewer learning needs.
☐ 4. Clients are usually more motivated to learn about their condition when they are hospitalized.

136. Which suggestion should the nurse give to an adolescent football player with Osgood-Schlatter disease of the left knee?
☐ 1. Apply ice on the knee after playing.
☐ 2. Use crutches until healing has occurred.
☐ 3. Stop playing until healing has occurred.
☐ 4. Make an appointment with a physical therapist.

137. The nurse instructs a client who is taking iron supplements that:
☐ 1. iron supplements should be taken on an empty stomach.
☐ 2. a daily bulk laxative such as psyllium hydrophilic mucilloid should be avoided.
☐ 3. the stools will become darker.
☐ 4. liquid iron supplements will not discolor teeth.

138. What should the nurse teach a client with generalized anxiety disorder to help the client cope with anxiety?
☐ 1. cognitive and behavioral strategies
☐ 2. issue avoidance and denial of problems
☐ 3. rest and sleep
☐ 4. withdrawal from role expectations and role relationships

139. After a lobectomy for lung cancer, the nurse instructs the client to perform deep breathing exercises to:
☐ 1. decrease blood flow to the lungs for rest and increased surface alveoli ventilation.
☐ 2. elevate the diaphragm to enlarge the thorax so that the lung surface area available for gas exchange is increased.
☐ 3. control the rate of air flow to the remaining lobe to decrease the risk of hyperinflation.
☐ 4. expand the alveoli and increase lung surface available for ventilation.

140. Which is the correct technique when the nurse is applying an elastic bandage to a leg?
- [ ] 1. Increase tension with each successive turn of the bandage.
- [ ] 2. Start at the distal end of the extremity and move toward the trunk.
- [ ] 3. Secure the bandage with clips over the area of the inner thigh.
- [ ] 4. Overlap each layer twice when wrapping.

141. A nulliparous client says that she and her husband plan to use a diaphragm with spermicide to prevent conception. Which should the nurse include as the action of spermicides when teaching the client?
- [ ] 1. destruction of spermatozoa before they enter the cervix
- [ ] 2. prevention of spermatozoa from entering the uterus
- [ ] 3. a change in vaginal pH from acidic to alkaline
- [ ] 4. slowing of the movement of the migrating spermatozoa

142. A client with acquired immunodeficiency syndrome (AIDS) is admitted because of paranoia and visual hallucinations probably related to progressive dementia. The client continues to be restless and have hallucinations. The nurse calls the healthcare provider (HCP) and, after explaining the situation, background, and assessment, recommends that the HCP consider writing a prescription for the client to have:
- [ ] 1. methylphenidate.
- [ ] 2. lorazepam.
- [ ] 3. trazodone.
- [ ] 4. sertraline.

143. The nurse is auscultating the lungs of a client with bacterial pneumonia. Which finding is expected?
- [ ] 1. increased fremitus
- [ ] 2. bilateral expiratory wheezing
- [ ] 3. resonance on percussion
- [ ] 4. vesicular breath sounds

144. A client is admitted with severe abdominal pains and the diagnosis of acute pancreatitis. The nurse should develop a plan of care during the acute phase of pancreatitis that will involve interventions to manage:
- [ ] 1. drug and alcohol abuse.
- [ ] 2. risk for injury.
- [ ] 3. severe pain.
- [ ] 4. ineffective airway clearance.

145. A nurse notices that a newborn has a swelling in the scrotal area. The nurse interprets this swelling as indicative of hydrocele if what else occurs?
- [ ] 1. The swollen bulge can be reduced.
- [ ] 2. The increase in scrotal size is bilateral.
- [ ] 3. The scrotal sac can be transilluminated.
- [ ] 4. The bulge appears during crying.

146. The nurse is screening clients for cancer prevention. Which is the recommended screening protocol for colon cancer in asymptomatic clients who have a low-risk profile?
- [ ] 1. Fecal occult blood testing should be performed annually after age 50 and up to age 75.
- [ ] 2. Digital rectal examinations are recommended every 5 years after age 40.
- [ ] 3. Sigmoidoscopy is recommended if symptoms of colon problems are present.
- [ ] 4. A diet low in saturated fat should be implemented after age 50.

147. A client with diabetes who takes insulin has a blood glucose level of 40. What should the nurse offer the client to begin to raise the blood glucose level? Select all that apply.
- [ ] 1. one-half cup (120 mL) of orange juice
- [ ] 2. one cup (240 mL) of milk
- [ ] 3. one-quarter cup (60 mL) of tuna
- [ ] 4. one tablespoon (15 mL) of peanut butter
- [ ] 5. one slice of bread
- [ ] 6. one-half cup (120 mL) of regular soda

148. An infant with increased intracranial pressure (ICP) on a regular diet vomits while eating dinner. What should the nurse do **next**?
- [ ] 1. Put the child on nothing-by-mouth (NPO) status for 4 hours.
- [ ] 2. Call to report this event to the healthcare provider (HCP).
- [ ] 3. Wait a few minutes, and then refeed the child.
- [ ] 4. Administer the prescribed antiemetic.

149. When preparing to draw up 8 units of a short-acting insulin and 20 units of a long-acting insulin in the same syringe, the nurse should:
- [ ] 1. inject air in the vial with the long-acting insulin first.
- [ ] 2. draw up the long-acting insulin first.
- [ ] 3. draw up either insulin first.
- [ ] 4. use a high-dose insulin syringe.

150. The mother of an infant with iron deficiency anemia asks the nurse what she could have done to prevent the anemia. The nurse should teach the mother that it is helpful to introduce solid foods into the infant's diet at age:
- [ ] 1. 3 months.
- [ ] 2. 6 months.
- [ ] 3. 8 months.
- [ ] 4. 10 months.

151. Following surgery, to evaluate the effectiveness of the client's use of an incentive spirometer, the nurse should determine if the client:
- [ ] 1. has increased circulation in the extremities.
- [ ] 2. is ready to ambulate without pain.
- [ ] 3. has stronger abdominal muscles.
- [ ] 4. can breathe more easily.

152. The nurse is caring for a client who is having an acute asthma attack. The nurse should notify the healthcare provider (HCP) when the client has:
☐ **1.** loud wheezing.
☐ **2.** tenacious, thick sputum.
☐ **3.** decreased breath sounds.
☐ **4.** persistent cough.

153. The nurse should teach the client who is receiving radiation therapy to:
☐ **1.** avoid shaving with straight-edge razors.
☐ **2.** clean the skin daily with antibacterial soap.
☐ **3.** apply moisturizing lotion before and after each treatment.
☐ **4.** keep the radiated area covered with a sterile gauze dressing.

154. A client has had a cardiac catheterization. The femoral dressing has a bright bloody drainage. What should the nurse do **first**?
☐ **1.** Assess the airway.
☐ **2.** Administer oxygen.
☐ **3.** Apply pressure to the site.
☐ **4.** Assess the pulse in the left extremity.

155. The nurse should instruct the parent of a child who is taking valproic acid that the child will need to have what routine blood analyses?
☐ **1.** complete blood count (CBC) and alkaline phosphate level
☐ **2.** cholesterol and platelet levels
☐ **3.** electrolytes and CBC
☐ **4.** platelet and fibrinogen levels

156. Bacterial conjunctivitis has affected several children at a local day care center. A nurse should advise which measure to minimize the risk of infection?
☐ **1.** Close the day care center for 1 week to control the outbreak.
☐ **2.** Restrict the infected children from returning for 48 hours after treatment.
☐ **3.** Perform thorough handwashing before and after touching any child in the day care center.
☐ **4.** Set up a conference with the parents of each child to explain the situation carefully.

157. The nurse is evaluating the client's risk for having a pressure sore. Which is the **best** indicator of risk for the client's developing a pressure sore?
☐ **1.** nutritional status
☐ **2.** circulatory status
☐ **3.** mobility status
☐ **4.** orientation status

158. A client with acute pancreatitis is put on nothing-by-mouth status, with the intent of not stimulating the pancreas. The client is prescribed an IV infusion of dextrose 5% in half-normal saline solution at 120 mL/h. After 3 days of this regimen, the nurse should observe the client for which adverse metabolic condition?
☐ **1.** ketosis
☐ **2.** hyperglycemia
☐ **3.** metabolic syndrome
☐ **4.** lactic acidosis

159. While the nurse is assisting a client to ambulate as part of a cardiac rehabilitation program, the client has midsternal burning. The nurse should:
☐ **1.** stop and assess the client further.
☐ **2.** obtain the client's blood pressure and heart rate.
☐ **3.** call for help and place the client in a wheelchair.
☐ **4.** administer nitroglycerin.

160. The nurse is counseling a client about the prevention of coronary heart disease. Which vitamins should the nurse recommend the client include in the diet to reduce homocysteine levels? Select all that apply.
☐ **1.** vitamin K
☐ **2.** vitamin B_6
☐ **3.** folate
☐ **4.** vitamin B_{12}
☐ **5.** vitamin D

161. A client has been taking dexamethasone for 2 weeks. The nurse evaluates a client's knowledge as deficient when the client says:
☐ **1.** "I cannot stop the medication all at one time."
☐ **2.** "If I forget a dose, it is no big deal; I will just take it when I remember it."
☐ **3.** "When I get a cold, I need to let my health-care provider (HCP) know."
☐ **4.** "I need to watch for an allergic reaction when I first start taking this pill."

162. A 3-month-old has moderate dehydration. The nurse should assess the client for:
☐ **1.** oliguria.
☐ **2.** bulging eyes.
☐ **3.** sunken posterior fontanelle.
☐ **4.** pale skin color.

163. The nurse is assessing a client who is suspected of being in the early symptomatic stages of human immunodeficiency virus (HIV) infection. Which indications of infection should the nurse detect during this stage?
☐ **1.** whitish yellow patches in the mouth
☐ **2.** dyspnea
☐ **3.** bloody diarrhea
☐ **4.** raised, hyperpigmented lesions on the legs

164. A primiparous client who is breast-feeding develops endometritis on the third postpartum day. What instructions should the nurse give to the mother?
- ☐ 1. The neonate will need to be bottle-fed for the next few days.
- ☐ 2. The condition typically is treated with IV antibiotic therapy.
- ☐ 3. The client's uterus may become "boggy," requiring frequent massage and oxytocics.
- ☐ 4. The client needs to remain in bed in a side-lying position as much as possible.

165. After instructing a primiparous client who is breast-feeding on how to prevent nipple soreness during feedings, the nurse determines that the client needs further instruction when she makes which statement?
- ☐ 1. "I should position the baby the same way for each feeding."
- ☐ 2. "I should make sure the baby grasps the entire areola and nipple."
- ☐ 3. "I should air-dry my breasts and nipples for 10 to 15 minutes after the feeding."
- ☐ 4. "I should not use a hand breast pump if my nipples get sore."

166. A client who has Ménière's disease is experiencing an acute attack of vertigo. The nurse should:
- ☐ 1. darken the client's room and provide a quiet environment.
- ☐ 2. provide a low-sodium, bland diet.
- ☐ 3. administer an opioid to relieve headache.
- ☐ 4. encourage fluid intake to prevent dehydration.

167. During a home visit to a primiparous client 1 week postpartum who is bottle-feeding her neonate, the client tells the nurse that her mother has suggested that she feed the neonate cereal so he will sleep through the night. What would be the nurse's **best** response?
- ☐ 1. "It is permissible to give the baby cereal if it is thinned with formula."
- ☐ 2. "The time for starting cereal varies, so check with your pediatrician."
- ☐ 3. "Formula is the food best digested by the baby until about 4 to 6 months of age."
- ☐ 4. "If cereal is given too early in life, the undigested food can lead to a need for surgery."

168. When a client reports being allergic to amoxicillin even though the medication administration record and armband do not indicate medication allergies, the nurse should:
- ☐ 1. administer the prescribed medication.
- ☐ 2. withhold the amoxicillin.
- ☐ 3. administer another, similarly acting antibiotic.
- ☐ 4. call the family to verify the client's statement.

169. While assessing a term neonate on a home visit to a primiparous client 2 weeks after a vaginal birth, the nurse observes that the neonate is slightly jaundiced and the stool is a pale, light color. The nurse notifies the healthcare provider (HCP) because these findings indicate which problem?
- ☐ 1. biliary atresia
- ☐ 2. Rh isoimmunization
- ☐ 3. ABO incompatibility
- ☐ 4. esophageal varices

170. To reduce urethral irritation, where should the nurse tape the female client's Foley catheter?
- ☐ 1. inner thigh
- ☐ 2. groin area
- ☐ 3. lower abdomen
- ☐ 4. lower thigh

171. A 6-year-old child has had heart surgery to repair tetralogy of Fallot. When developing the discharge plan, the nurse should include information about:
- ☐ 1. allowing the child to lead a normal, active life.
- ☐ 2. persuading the child to get enough rest.
- ☐ 3. treating tet spells.
- ☐ 4. having the child out of school for a month.

172. A client is recovering from abdominal surgery and has a nasogastric (NG) tube inserted. The expected outcome of using the NG tube is gastrointestinal tract:
- ☐ 1. compression.
- ☐ 2. lavage.
- ☐ 3. decompression.
- ☐ 4. gavage.

173. The nurse teaches the mother of a toddler who has had a cleft palate repair that her child is at risk for developing which problem in the future?
- ☐ 1. hearing problems
- ☐ 2. poor self-concept
- ☐ 3. a speech defect
- ☐ 4. chronic sinus infections

174. The nurse assesses a client who is receiving a tube feeding. Which situation would require prompt intervention from the nurse?
- ☐ 1. The client is sitting upright in bed while the feeding is infusing.
- ☐ 2. The feeding that is infusing has been hanging for 8 hours.
- ☐ 3. The client has a gastric residual of 25 mL.
- ☐ 4. The feeding solution is at room temperature.

175. A client has been taking furosemide for 2 days. The nurse should assess the client for:
- ☐ 1. an elevated blood urea nitrogen (BUN) level.
- ☐ 2. an elevated potassium level.
- ☐ 3. a decreased potassium level.
- ☐ 4. an elevated sodium level.

176. When suctioning the respiratory tract of a client, it is recommended that the suctioning period not exceed how many seconds?
- ☐ **1.** 5 seconds
- ☐ **2.** 10 seconds
- ☐ **3.** 15 seconds
- ☐ **4.** 20 seconds

177. An 80-year-old client with severe kidney damage is placed on life support and dialysis. Care decisions are being made by his wife, who is showing signs of early Alzheimer's disease. The client's daughter arrives from out of town with a copy of the client's living will, which states that the client did not want to be on life support. The nurse should:
- ☐ **1.** immediately inform the healthcare provider (HCP) about the living will.
- ☐ **2.** suggest to the daughter that she discuss her father's wishes with her mother.
- ☐ **3.** prepare to remove the client from life support.
- ☐ **4.** make a copy of the living will and give it to the client's wife.

178. Prior to administering plasminogen activator (t-PA) to a client admitted with a stroke, the nurse should verify that the client: (Select all that apply.)
- ☐ **1.** is older than 65 years.
- ☐ **2.** has had symptoms of the stroke <3 hours.
- ☐ **3.** has a blood pressure within normal limits.
- ☐ **4.** does not have active internal bleeding.
- ☐ **5.** has not had an alcoholic beverage within the last 8 hours.

179. A client with peripheral arterial disease has had surgery for placement of an aortobifemoral bypass graft. Immediately following surgery, what should the nurse do **first**?
- ☐ **1.** Elevate the lower extremities.
- ☐ **2.** Assist the client to use incentive spirometry.
- ☐ **3.** Start the client on a liquid diet.
- ☐ **4.** Assess peripheral pulses every 4 hours.

180. How does the nurse identify the type of presentation shown in the figure?

- ☐ **1.** frank breech
- ☐ **2.** compound breech
- ☐ **3.** complete breech
- ☐ **4.** incomplete breech

181. Following cardiac bypass surgery, the client has been referred to a cardiac rehabilitation exercise program. The client has type 1 diabetes and has bilateral leg discomfort with walking. The nurse should advise the client to exercise using a stationary bicycle and intermittent training because of the client's:
- ☐ **1.** diabetic neuropathy.
- ☐ **2.** muscle atrophy.
- ☐ **3.** Raynaud's disease.
- ☐ **4.** transient ischemic attacks.

182. Which statement indicates that the client with hepatitis B has understood the nurse's discharge teaching?
- ☐ **1.** "I will not drink alcohol for at least 1 year."
- ☐ **2.** "I must avoid sexual intercourse."
- ☐ **3.** "I should be able to resume normal activity in a week or two."
- ☐ **4.** "Because hepatitis B is a chronic disease, I know I will always be jaundiced."

183. A client who is taking olanzapine states he is being poisoned and refuses to take his scheduled medication. The nurse states, "If you do not take your medication, you will be put into seclusion." The nurse's statement is an example of which legal concept?
- ☐ **1.** assault
- ☐ **2.** battery
- ☐ **3.** malpractice
- ☐ **4.** invasion of privacy

184. A client who has been taking diazepam for 3 months for skeletal muscle spasms and lower back pain has stopped taking the medication 2 days ago because it was no longer helping. Now the pain has increased. The nurse should assess the client for: (Select all that apply.)
- ☐ **1.** insomnia.
- ☐ **2.** euphoria.
- ☐ **3.** bradycardia.
- ☐ **4.** diaphoresis.
- ☐ **5.** tremor.
- ☐ **6.** vomiting.

185. An IV infusion is to be administered through a scalp vein on an infant's head. What should the nurse tell the parents to prepare them for the procedure?
- ☐ **1.** It may be necessary to remove a small amount of hair from the infant's scalp.
- ☐ **2.** A sedative will be given to help keep the infant quiet.
- ☐ **3.** Visiting the infant will be delayed until the infusion has been completed.
- ☐ **4.** Holding the infant will be contraindicated while the infusion is being administered.

186. Which nursing goal is **most** important for a client with acute pancreatitis?
- ☐ 1. The client reports minimal abdominal pain.
- ☐ 2. The client regains a normal pattern for bowel movements.
- ☐ 3. The client limits alcohol intake to two to three drinks per week.
- ☐ 4. The client maintains normal liver function.

187. A nurse is caring for a child with type 1 diabetes mellitus at camp. The child is irritable and has a headache. What should the nurse do **first**?
- ☐ 1. Administer 2 oz (60 mL) of orange juice.
- ☐ 2. Notify the healthcare provider (HCP) about the child's status.
- ☐ 3. Check the child's blood glucose level.
- ☐ 4. Send the child back to the planned activities.

188. A client tells the nurse that her bra fits more snugly at certain times of the month and she is concerned this may be a sign of breast cancer. The best response for the nurse is to explain that:
- ☐ 1. a change in breast size should be checked by her healthcare provider (HCP).
- ☐ 2. benign cysts tend to cause the breast to vary in size.
- ☐ 3. it is normal for the breast to increase in size before menstruation begins.
- ☐ 4. a difference in the size of her breasts is related to normal growth and development.

189. Which beliefs of traditional Chinese medicine found in Asian culture should the nurse consider when planning care for a follower of traditional Chinese medicine?
- ☐ 1. Health is described as harmony between family members.
- ☐ 2. Illness is caused by an imbalance of the yin and yang.
- ☐ 3. Exercise to the point of overexertion can improve health.
- ☐ 4. Illness is caused by a change in eating habits.

190. A client is scheduled for an intravenous pyelogram (IVP). In preparation for the procedure, what should the nurse ask the client?
- ☐ 1. "Have you ever had an IVP before?"
- ☐ 2. "Do you have any allergies?"
- ☐ 3. "When was your last bowel movement?"
- ☐ 4. "Have you ever experienced urinary incontinence?"

191. Which oral contraceptive is considered safe for use while breast-feeding because it will not affect the breast milk supply once breast-feeding has been well established?
- ☐ 1. estrogen
- ☐ 2. estrogen and progestin
- ☐ 3. progestin
- ☐ 4. testosterone

192. The nurse is teaching the client to self-administer insulin. Learning goals most likely will be attained when they are established by the:
- ☐ 1. nurse and client because both need to be responsible for teaching.
- ☐ 2. healthcare provider (HCP) and client because the HCP is the manager of care and the client is the main participant.
- ☐ 3. client because the client is best able to identify his or her own needs and how to meet those needs.
- ☐ 4. client, nurse, pharmacist, and HCP so the client can participate in planning care with the entire team.

193. A multigravid client at 36 weeks' gestation who is visiting the clinic for a routine visit begins to sob and tells the nurse, "My boyfriend has been beating me up once in a while since I became pregnant, but I cannot bring myself to leave him because I do not have a job and I do not know how I would take care of my other children." What is the **priority** action by the nurse at this time?
- ☐ 1. Contact a social worker for assistance and family counseling.
- ☐ 2. Help the client make concrete plans for the safety of herself and her children.
- ☐ 3. Tell the client that she should not allow anyone to hit her or her children.
- ☐ 4. Provide the client with brochures on the statistics about violence against women.

194. Several children were admitted yesterday. In which order of priority from first to last would the nurse assess these children? All options must be used.

| 1. a 3-month-old infant with respiratory syncytial virus and stable vital signs |

| 2. a 10-month-old infant with pneumonia and respiratory rate of 50 breaths/minute |

| 3. a 3-year-old child with acute pyelonephritis and a temperature of 104.5°F (40.3°C) |

| 4. a 6-year-old child with a recent concussion and little change in vital signs |

| 5. a 12-year-old child with a fractured femur and lacerated liver |

| |

| |

| |

| |

| |

195. Sulfamethoxazole/trimethoprim has been prescribed for a client who has a urinary tract infection. When administering sulfonamides, the nurse should:
- ☐ 1. encourage the client to take the medication with meals.
- ☐ 2. instruct the client to drink at least eight glasses of water a day.
- ☐ 3. measure the client's urine output.
- ☐ 4. instruct the client that the urine may turn reddish orange.

196. A client is admitted with a diagnosis of dementia becomes agitated and violent and has bizarre thoughts. The nurse is reviewing the client's medication record. Which ordered medication would be expected to reduce agitation?
- ☐ 1. tacrine
- ☐ 2. ergoloid
- ☐ 3. diazepam
- ☐ 4. risperidone

197. A client has been diagnosed with multi-infarct (or vascular) dementia (MID). When preparing a teaching plan for the client and family, which action should the nurse indicate as the **most** critical for slowing MID?
- ☐ 1. administering anticoagulants such as warfarin
- ☐ 2. administering benzodiazepines such as lorazepam to decrease choreiform movements
- ☐ 3. managing related symptoms such as depression
- ☐ 4. managing the symptoms by increasing dopamine availability

198. While performing cardiopulmonary resuscitation (CPR) on a 5-year-old child, the nurse palpates for a pulse. Which site is **best** for checking the pulse during CPR in a 5-year-old child?
- ☐ 1. femoral artery
- ☐ 2. carotid artery
- ☐ 3. radial artery
- ☐ 4. brachial artery

199. A nurse is assessing a client with nephrotic syndrome. The nurse should assess the client for which condition?
- ☐ 1. hematuria
- ☐ 2. massive proteinuria
- ☐ 3. increased serum albumin level
- ☐ 4. weight loss

200. A child with tetralogy of Fallot and a history of severe hypoxic episodes is to be admitted to the pediatric unit. What would be **most** important for the nurse to have at the bedside?
- ☐ 1. morphine sulfate in a syringe ready to administer
- ☐ 2. oxygen tubing and flow meter plugged in
- ☐ 3. blood pressure cuff and stethoscope
- ☐ 4. suction tubing and equipment

201. When assessing pain in a client from Mexico, the nurse should understand the implications of which statement from the client about the pain experience?
- ☐ 1. "Enduring pain is a part of God's will."
- ☐ 2. "This pain is killing me."
- ☐ 3. "I have got to see a healthcare provider (HCP) right away."
- ☐ 4. "I cannot go on in pain like this any longer."

202. A client is voiding small amounts of urine every 30 to 60 minutes. What should the nurse do **first**?
- ☐ 1. Palpate for a distended bladder.
- ☐ 2. Catheterize the client for residual urine.
- ☐ 3. Obtain a urine specimen for culture.
- ☐ 4. Encourage an increased fluid intake.

203. When making rounds, which client should the nurse assess **first**?
- ☐ 1. a 16-month-old child with periorbital cellulitis who is to be discharged today
- ☐ 2. a 7-year-old child who had an appendectomy yesterday and developed peritonitis
- ☐ 3. a 10-year-old child who has just been admitted in sickle cell crisis
- ☐ 4. a 16-year-old adolescent receiving a 3rd day of chemotherapy

204. Which has the **highest priority** for the care of a client with chronic renal failure?
- ☐ 1. Apply corticosteroid creams to relieve itching.
- ☐ 2. Achieve pain control with analgesics.
- ☐ 3. Maintain a low-sodium diet.
- ☐ 4. Measure abdominal girth daily.

205. The father of an 18-month-old with no previous illness, who has been admitted to a surgery center for repair of an inguinal hernia, tells the nurse that his child is having trouble breathing. The father does not think the child choked. After telling the clerk to call the rapid response team, the nurse should take which actions? Place in order from **first** to last. All options must be used.

1. Notify the surgeon.
2. Start an intravenous infusion.
3. Assess the effectiveness of the abdominal thrusts.
4. Perform the abdominal thrust maneuver.
5. Listen for breath sounds.

206. The nurse is assessing a child's skeletal traction and notices that the weights are on the floor. What should the nurse do **next**?
- ☐ 1. Raise the weights so that the child can move up in bed.
- ☐ 2. Notify the healthcare provider (HCP) immediately.
- ☐ 3. Put the foot of the bed on blocks.
- ☐ 4. Move the child up in bed.

207. Compared to the food requirements of pre-schoolers and adolescents, the food requirements of school-age children are not as great because these children have a lower:
- ☐ 1. growth rate.
- ☐ 2. metabolic rate.
- ☐ 3. level of activity.
- ☐ 4. hormonal secretion rate.

208. When assessing a 17-year-old client with depression for suicide risk, which question would be **best**?
- ☐ 1. "What movies about death have you watched lately?"
- ☐ 2. "Can you tell me what you think about suicide?"
- ☐ 3. "Has anyone in your family ever committed suicide?"
- ☐ 4. "Are you thinking about killing yourself?"

209. Which intervention should the nurse suggest to a parent to relieve itching in a child with chickenpox?
- ☐ 1. generous amounts of fine baby powder
- ☐ 2. oatmeal preparation baths
- ☐ 3. soft towels moistened with hydrogen peroxide
- ☐ 4. cool compresses moistened with a weak salt solution

210. A woman who has preeclampsia is receiving magnesium sulfate 20 g per 500 mL of lactated Ringers via infusion pump. The prescribed rate of infusion is 2 g/h. How many mL/h should the nurse set the infusion pump for? Record your answer using a whole number.

_____ mL/h.

211. Which technique is **best** for the nurse to use in evaluating the parents' ability to administer ear-drops correctly?
- ☐ 1. Observe the parents instilling the drops in the child's ear.
- ☐ 2. Listen to the parents as they describe the procedure.
- ☐ 3. Ask the parents to list the steps in the procedure.
- ☐ 4. Ask the parents whether they have read the handout on the procedure.

212. Ibuprofen is prescribed for a client with osteoarthritis. Which instruction about ibuprofen should the nurse include in the client's teaching plan?
- ☐ 1. Report the development of tinnitus.
- ☐ 2. Increase vitamin B_{12} intake.
- ☐ 3. Take with food or antacids.
- ☐ 4. Have the complete blood count (CBC) monitored monthly.

213. A staff member states, "I do not know why Mary is so depressed. She lives in an exclusive part of town and has gorgeous clothes. Her husband seems to care about her very much. She really has it all." What should the nurse conclude from the staff member's statement?
- ☐ 1. An accurate assessment of the client has been made.
- ☐ 2. The staff member is jealous of the client.
- ☐ 3. There is no reason for the client to be depressed.
- ☐ 4. The staff member needs teaching about major depression.

214. The nurse is instructing the mother of a child with asthma about noting food triggers for asthma attacks. Which food would **most** likely be responsible for causing an allergic reaction?
- ☐ 1. fish
- ☐ 2. tossed salad
- ☐ 3. pork chop
- ☐ 4. oranges

215. Which family should the nurse determine as **most** in need of follow-up?
- ☐ 1. a single mother with a 7-month-old child whose immunizations are delayed
- ☐ 2. a two-parent family whose 3-year-old has a fractured leg from an automobile accident
- ☐ 3. a single parent with a toddler who has third-degree burns over 20% of the body
- ☐ 4. a two-parent family with a foster child who has a history of caustic liquid ingestion

216. After several hours of induction with intravenous oxytocin administered along with a primary intravenous solution of lactated Ringer's solution, assessment of a primigravida at 42 weeks' gestation reveals a fetal heart rate near the baseline at 120 bpm and strong contractions occurring every 2 to 2.5 minutes and lasting 90 to 100 seconds. In what order should the nurse perform the required actions? All options must be used.

1. Position the client in a lateral position.

2. Contact the primary care provider for further prescriptions.

3. Stop the intravenous flow of oxytocin.

4. Administer oxygen at a rate of 8 to 10 L/min.

| |

| |

| |

217. When preparing to administer a tap water enema, in which position should the nurse place the client?
- ☐ **1.** supine
- ☐ **2.** semi-Fowler's
- ☐ **3.** right lateral
- ☐ **4.** left Sims'

218. When planning care for a group of clients, the nurse should identify which client as having the **greatest** risk for the development of pressure ulcers?
- ☐ **1.** a client who ambulates four times a day
- ☐ **2.** a client with an indwelling urinary catheter
- ☐ **3.** a client who has a decreased serum albumin level
- ☐ **4.** a client with an elevated white blood cell count

219. A 16-year-old primigravida at 36 weeks' gestation who has had no prenatal care experienced a seizure at work and is being transported to the hospital by ambulance. What should the nurse do upon the client's arrival?
- ☐ **1.** Position the client in a supine position.
- ☐ **2.** Auscultate breath sounds every 4 hours.
- ☐ **3.** Monitor the vital signs every 4 hours.
- ☐ **4.** Admit the client to a quiet, darkened room.

220. An adult admitted to the hospital with a hemoglobin of 6.5 g/dL (65 g/L) is experiencing cerebral tissue hypoxia. The nurse should:
- ☐ **1.** plan frequent rest periods throughout the day.
- ☐ **2.** assist the client in ambulating to the bathroom.
- ☐ **3.** check the temperature of the water before the client showers.
- ☐ **4.** refer the client to occupational therapy for energy conservation interventions.

221. A nurse is assessing an older adult with pneumonia. Where should the nurse place the stethoscope to listen for breath sounds that will indicate the client is fully oxygenating the lung on the right side?

222. During care, the client suddenly blurts out, "My doctor just told me that I am going to have to have chemotherapy after all; I was hoping to avoid it." Which is the nurse's **most** therapeutic response?
- ☐ **1.** "Well, you are under the care of our best oncologist; I am certain the oncologist knows what is best."
- ☐ **2.** "What concerns you most about possible chemotherapy?"
- ☐ **3.** "You know, you can get a second opinion before you agree to any of that."
- ☐ **4.** "I understand how you feel. I would feel the same way."

223. Two parents who are arguing in their infant's room, with voices raised and getting louder, start to hit each other. The infant is crying. Which action should the staff nurse take **next**?
- ☐ **1.** Try to reason with both of the parents.
- ☐ **2.** Ask one of the parents to leave the room.
- ☐ **3.** Call security to come and break up the fight.
- ☐ **4.** Remove the infant from the room.

224. A hospitalized client is experiencing "fight versus flight," a stress-mediated physiologic response. As a result, the nurse should assess the client for:
- ☐ **1.** increased urinary output.
- ☐ **2.** decreased arterial blood pressure.
- ☐ **3.** increased blood glucose.
- ☐ **4.** decreased mental acuity.

225. The nurse observes an unlicensed assistive personnel (UAP) sharing extensive stories of her own mother's death with a dying client's husband. Which statement demonstrates appropriate feedback for the nurse to offer to the UAP?
- ☐ **1.** "I thought that was really great how you talked with him; he seemed really scared."
- ☐ **2.** "You provided excellent client education by sharing your stories."
- ☐ **3.** "I think it helps clients to see us as real people, and friends too, when you share your own stories."
- ☐ **4.** "It is probably best to avoid talking about your personal experience very much; keep communication client centered."

226. Assessment of a primigravida in active labor reveals cervical dilation at 9 cm with complete effacement and the fetus at +1 station. What should the nurse do when the primary care provider prescribes meperidine 50 mg intramuscular (IM) for the client?
- ☐ **1.** Administer the medication in the left ventrogluteal muscle.
- ☐ **2.** Be certain that naloxone is at the client's bedside.
- ☐ **3.** Ask the primary care provider to validate the dosage of the drug.
- ☐ **4.** Refuse to administer the medication to the client.

227. Which nursing action is appropriate when planning care for a client who is being battered? Select all that apply.
☐ **1.** Give information about a safe home.
☐ **2.** Provide a cell phone and the crisis help line telephone number.
☐ **3.** Help the client displace her feelings.
☐ **4.** Teach the client about the cycle of violence.
☐ **5.** Discuss the client's legal and personal rights.

228. Which client is at greatest risk for obtaining inadequate nutrition?
☐ **1.** the client with diabetic peripheral neuropathy
☐ **2.** the client recovering from a femur fracture
☐ **3.** the client who is breast-feeding
☐ **4.** the client with burns to 45% of the body

229. The use of a patient-controlled analgesia (PCA) pump is effective in which situation?
☐ **1.** The client achieves a therapeutic level of analgesia.
☐ **2.** The client does not become dependent on opioids postoperatively.
☐ **3.** There is decreased cost by decreasing use of intramuscular (IM) injections.
☐ **4.** The family can assist the client in managing the pain.

230. A client's chest tube is connected to a drainage system with a water seal. The nurse notes that the fluid in the water seal column is fluctuating with each breath that the client takes. The fluctuation means that:
☐ **1.** there is an obstruction in the chest tube.
☐ **2.** the client is developing subcutaneous emphysema.
☐ **3.** the chest tube system is functioning properly.
☐ **4.** there is a leak in the chest tube system.

231. A client is taking metformin. To prevent lactic acidosis when taking this drug, the nurse should instruct the client to report which symptoms? Select all that apply.
☐ **1.** hyperventilation
☐ **2.** muscle discomfort
☐ **3.** dizziness
☐ **4.** headache
☐ **5.** increased hunger
☐ **6.** tingling in the fingertips

232. The nurse is serving on a task force to update the electronic health record. The task force should ensure that the revisions of the medical record will: (Select all that apply.)
☐ **1.** aid in client care.
☐ **2.** serve as a legal document.
☐ **3.** have sufficient room for charting nurses' notes.
☐ **4.** facilitate data collection for clinical research.
☐ **5.** guide performance improvement.
☐ **6.** be written so the client can understand what is written.

233. The nurse discovers that a hospitalized client with stage 4 esophageal cancer and major depression has a gun in the home. What is the **best** nursing intervention to help the client remain safe after discharge?
☐ **1.** Give the client the number of a 24-hour crisis phone line for use, if needed.
☐ **2.** Tell the healthcare provider (HCP) the client is too high risk for discharge at this time.
☐ **3.** Have the client promise to use the gun only for home protection.
☐ **4.** Talk with the HCP about requiring gun removal as a condition of discharge.

234. A client with severe osteoarthritis and decreased mobility is moved to an assisted living facility. The nurse notices that the client smells of alcohol, is slurring words, and has six wine bottles in the trash. The client tells the nurse, "Those are my other pain medicines." Which statements by the nurse are **most** appropriate at this point? Select all that apply.
☐ **1.** "I did not realize you that your pain was not being managed with your current medication."
☐ **2.** "It is important for me to know how many bottles of wine you drank this week."
☐ **3.** "I am worried about the amount of wine you are drinking and its effects on your balance."
☐ **4.** "How are you getting all this wine?"
☐ **5.** "I am calling your healthcare provider (HCP) to have all of us to talk about better pain control without the wine."

235. Which child **most** needs a referral for developmental language delay?
☐ **1.** the 1-year-old who does not have three words
☐ **2.** the 18-month-old who only points to one body part
☐ **3.** the 2-year-old who only combines two words
☐ **4.** the 4-year-old who is difficult to understand

236. A client is being admitted with nursing home–acquired pneumonia. The unit has four empty beds in semiprivate rooms. The room that would be **most** suitable for this client is the one with a:
☐ **1.** 60-year-old client admitted for investigation of transient ischemic attacks.
☐ **2.** 45-year-old client with an abdominal hysterectomy.
☐ **3.** 24-year-old client with non-Hodgkin's lymphoma.
☐ **4.** 55-year-old client with alcoholic cirrhosis.

38. 4. The nurse is wearing protective personnel equipment appropriate for suctioning the client: goggles, gown, and respirator mask. It is not necessary to wear a PAPR face shield to suction a tracheostomy. A surgical mask does not provide maximum protection.

🗝 **CN:** Safety and infection control; **CL:** Apply

39. 1. Petroleum jelly is thought to smother the lice. Lindaine and other pediculicides should not be applied to the face or close to the eyes. Bacitracin ointment will not kill the lice.

🗝 **CN:** Pharmacological and parenteral therapies; **CL:** Apply

40. 1. A major goal of safety and accident prevention focuses on having all cleaning supplies and medications locked up as infants become mobile. The child should not play in the bathroom even if the parent is present because the child will think that it is okay to play with these items when the parent is not present. Playing with cords could lead to possible strangulation. The child-protective cabinet locks should work unless they were installed incorrectly or are defective.

🗝 **CN:** Safety and infection control; **CL:** Evaluate

41. 3, 4, 5. Common adverse effects of tobramycin include nephrotoxicity, ototoxicity, fever, and rash. Hypertension, weight gain, and decreased heart rate are not associated with this drug.

🗝 **CN:** Pharmacological and parenteral therapies; **CL:** Analyze

42. 4. Fever is generally not thought to be a sign of impaired renal function related to long-term use of gentamicin. The client should report signs of decreasing urinary function, such as decreased output, unusual appearance of the urine, or edema.

🗝 **CN:** Pharmacological and parenteral therapies; **CL:** Evaluate

43. 3, 2, 1, 4. The nurse first starts an IV as dehydration increases sickling of cells; maintaining fluid balance is a priority. The nurse next starts oxygen and then administers morphine for pain; these actions are followed by obtaining a blood sample for laboratory studies.

🗝 **CN:** Physiological adaptation; **CL:** Synthesize

44. 2. Febrile seizures commonly occur as the fever rises. The exact cause of febrile convulsions is not known. Infants and young toddlers are the age-groups primarily affected. Febrile seizures typically do not follow immunization administration.

🗝 **CN:** Health promotion and maintenance; **CL:** Apply

45. 1, 2, 4, 6. The nurse case manager should refer the client to a nutritionist so the client is aware of and can be monitored regarding her food intake to assure transition to a normal pregnancy diet with intake of adequate nutrients to support growth and development of the fetus. A PRN (as needed) prescription for an antiemetic is useful to overcome occasional episodes of nausea and vomiting. Encouraging a return to normal activities when the client feels ready gives the client a goal to look forward to, and activity is not contraindicated in hyperemesis when the client feels ready to initiate activity. Discussion of the plan of care and discharge instructions is a standard of care when discharging a client from a healthcare facility. There is no indication for an anxiolytic, and hyperemesis gravidarum typically is not associated with anxiety. Six weeks is too long to wait for a follow-up appointment post-hospitalization.

🗝 **CN:** Management of care; **CL:** Create

46. 4. Oral contraceptive use, pregnancy, and lactation are situations that increase demand for folic acid. With supplementation, a response should cause the reticulocyte count to increase within 2 to 3 days after therapy has begun. It is not necessary to take folic acid on an empty stomach. A client may safely take both iron and folic acid supplementation.

🗝 **CN:** Pharmacological and parenteral therapies; **CL:** Synthesize

47. 4. Although acrocyanosis may be present for 24 to 48 hours after birth, central cyanosis of the trunk indicates decreased oxygenation from respiratory distress or another disease state (e.g., cardiac anomalies). This should be reported to the **HCP** 📖 and evaluated further. Maternal lochia serosa in scant amount is a normal finding 1 week postpartum, as is a nonpalpable maternal fundus. Presence of a neonatal tonic neck reflex is a normal finding in a 1-week-old neonate.

🗝 **CN:** Physiological adaptation; **CL:** Analyze

48. 1, 2, 3, 4. The nurse should ask the client about alcohol use because heavy alcohol use causes fluid excretion resulting in heavy losses of calcium in urine. If the client uses antacids containing aluminum or magnesium, a net loss of calcium can occur. If the client has a high-fiber diet, the fiber can bind up some of the dietary calcium. People with hip fractures have been found to have low vitamin K intakes; vitamin K plays an important role in production of at least one bone protein. Fruit juices do not affect calcium absorption.

🗝 **CN:** Health promotion and maintenance; **CL:** Analyze

49. 1. The postrape examination is important for detecting the possibility of sexually transmitted disease, which can be spread through rape. The client should also be examined for infection that can result from trauma. Additionally, if the victim or the rapist was not using a contraceptive, postcoital contraceptive methods should be discussed. The information provided does not indicate anxiety or physical injury, such as periurethral tears, and these are not the primary reason for the examination. Menstrual difficulties are not a common result of rape.

CN: Safety and infection control; CL: Synthesize

50. 3. The nurse should question the use of a local anesthetic agent with epinephrine on the hands or feet because the epinephrine is a vasoconstrictor and can cause ischemia and gangrene of extremities. The nurse should suggest that the intern use bupivacaine without epinephrine as the local anesthetic agent. An intern should be trained in suturing small superficial incisions, and the cosmetic effect should be acceptable. The client's room should be a sufficiently aseptic environment because there is no other client in the room.

CN: Management of care; CL: Synthesize

51. 3. Infants should be monitored for hypoglycemia, temperature stability, and respiratory distress. The answer that best includes these components is monitoring the infant feedings and vital signs. Apgar assessments are done at 1 and 5 minutes of age, not at 1 hour of age. The gestational age assessment is important for this infant, but, after completion, does not require additional monitoring. The infant should be regularly assessed for jaundice as part of the physical assessment, but this is not the priority assessment at this time.

CN: Basic care and comfort; CL: Analyze

52. 3. In dark-skinned clients, cyanosis can best be detected by examining the conjunctiva, lips, and oral mucous membranes. Examining the retinas, nail beds, or inner aspects of the wrists is not an appropriate assessment for determining cyanosis in any client.

CN: Health promotion and maintenance; CL: Analyze

53. 7.5 mL

$$0.9\,mg\,/\,X\,mL \times 0.6\,mg\,/\,5\,mL$$
$$X = 7.5\,mL$$

CN: Pharmacological and parenteral therapies; CL: Apply

54. 1. A biophysical profile includes a nonstress test; evaluation of fetal breathing movements, gross body movements, and fetal tone; and amniotic fluid volume measurement. Because an ultrasound analysis is used during the test, the client should plan to drink 1 to 2 L of fluid before the test to ensure a full bladder, which provides better visualization of the fetus. The client does not need to be on nothing-by-mouth status before the test. The client does not need to remain in the clinic for 4 hours after the test. However, if the client were scheduled for a contraction stress test, she would be observed as an outpatient for 1 to 4 hours after the test to make certain that the contractions had stopped. The client does not need to eat a high-fiber meal after the test. A high-fiber meal typically is indicated after certain radiographic procedures, such as an upper gastrointestinal series.

CN: Reduction of risk potential; CL: Apply

55. 1, 2, 4, 5. Children typically act out their feelings (such as depression and anger) in response to incest. Sexualized play, aggression, running away, and truancy are typical acting-out behaviors. Isolation at home is not common for incest victims who are preadolescents.

CN: Psychosocial integrity; CL: Analyze

56. 3. One of the staff members needs further instructions when the nurse observes the staff member wearing sterile gloves to bathe a neonate at 2 hours of age. Clean gloves should be worn, not sterile gloves. Sterile gloves are more expensive than clean gloves and are not necessary when bathing a neonate. Wearing protective goggles during a cesarean birth is a standard blood precaution. Bloody sheets should be placed in a designated container. Scalpel blades, needles, syringes, and other equipment used during birthing should be disposed of safely in appropriate, labeled containers.

CN: Safety and infection control; CL: Evaluate

57. 1, 3, 4. Delegation involves the reassignment or transfer of selected aspects of a job to selected persons in selected situations. Although responsibility for completion of a task or activity can be delegated, accountability for that task remains with the RN. In delegating nursing acts, functions, or tasks, the **RN** must consider the nursing model to determine the appropriate delegation of assignment. Prior to delegation, the RN validates that the non-RN caregiver has orientation and experience in completion of the activity. The amount of time the nurse has does not direct the delegation procedure; the focus is on the task and capability of the staff to whom the task is delegated. It is not necessary to document that the task has been delegated and to whom; however, the outcome of the task should be documented by the nurse.

CN: Management of care; CL: Apply

58. 2. Parents often experience greater grief when they have experienced the hope provided by the remission of their child's disease. The nurse allows the parents to express this grief. Reactions to death of a family member are not based on the age of the dying family member. No matter how well prepared the parents may be for the death of their child, it will not make coping with death easier. Family members may displace anger and frustration on the healthcare system and **healthcare providers (HCPs)** 📖, but death does not necessarily undermine trust.

    🔑 CL: Analyze; CN: Psychosocial integrity

59. 3. Applying a water-soluble lubricant to the nares helps alleviate sore nares when an NG tube is in place. Repositioning the tube does not eliminate the possibility of irritating the nares. Irrigating the tube with a cool solution or changing positions will not relieve the local irritation from the NG tube.

    🔑 CN: Basic care and comfort;
CL: Synthesize

60. 1, 5. Hindus do not eat beef. Sufficient protein can be obtained from lentils and fish.

    🔑 CN: Health promotion and maintenance;
CL: Synthesize

61. 4. One outcome criterion for the client with osteoarthritis is improved joint mobility. It is probably not possible to arrest the disease. Gold compound is administered to clients with rheumatoid arthritis, not osteoarthritis. Outcome criteria should be specific; feeling better is too general to be useful.

    🔑 CN: Basic care and comfort; CL: Evaluate

62. 3. Although monitoring vital signs frequently is important, for the first few days the primary concern in burn care is fluid and electrolyte balance, with the goal being to replace fluid and electrolytes lost. With burns, fluid and electrolytes move from the interstitial spaces to the burn injury and are lost. These must be replaced. Once the child's fluid and electrolyte status has been addressed and fluid resuscitation has begun, preventing wound infection is a priority and efforts to control the child's pain can be initiated.

    🔑 CN: Reduction of risk potential;
CL: Synthesize

63. 2. DTaP vaccine is given intramuscularly, usually with other vaccines. As a killed virus, it can be given to immunocompromised children.

    🔑 CN: Pharmacological and parenteral therapies; CL: Apply

64. 2, 3, 4. Diphenhydramine hydrochloride is an antihistamine that blocks the effects of histamine at receptor sites and has atropine-like effects, such as dry mouth, nausea, drowsiness, tachycardia, and thickened bronchial secretions. Weight loss and bradycardia are not adverse effects of this medication.

    🔑 CN: Pharmacological and parenteral therapies; CL: Apply

65. 1. The client's assessment findings indicate that the client is in the latent phase of the first stage of labor. Therefore, the nurse should plan to assist the client with comfort measures and breathing techniques to relieve discomfort. The client can move around, walk, or ambulate at this phase of labor. If the client chooses to remain in bed, a left side-lying position provides the greatest perfusion. It is too early for the client to have an epidural anesthetic. Epidural anesthesia is usually administered when the cervix is dilated 4 to 5 cm. The fetal heart rate is normal, so internal fetal monitoring is not warranted at this time.

    🔑 CN: Health promotion and maintenance;
CL: Synthesize

66. 4. The nurse does not administer naloxone because naloxone is the antidote for morphine, not midazolam. The benzodiazepine receptor antagonist for midazolam is flumazenil. The nurse can promote oxygenation by encouraging deep breathing and administering oxygen. Resuscitation equipment should be accessible if needed.

    🔑 CN: Reduction of risk; CL: Synthesize

67. 3. The client should be seated upright with the arms raised and crossed in front and supported by the overbed table. The client's head should rest on the arms. This position allows for outward expansion of the chest wall and promotes collection of the pleural fluid at the base of the thorax. Supine, prone, and side-lying positions will not allow for sufficient chest expansion.

    🔑 CN: Reduction of risk potential;
CL: Synthesize

68. 2. The stool specimen indicates the client has *E. coli* in his stool. The nurse institutes enteric precautions and ensures that those who come in contact with the child perform good hand hygiene and wear a gown to prevent spread of infection. Restoring fluid balance is a goal of therapy, but because the dehydration is mild, oral rehydration is the first choice for replacing fluids. The nurse also cleanses and protects the anal area from irritation from the diarrhea, but on an ongoing basis and not as the priority for care. It is not necessary for the family to wash all of their bed linens, as only those in contact with the client are contaminated.

    🔑 CN: Safety and infection control;
CL: Synthesize

69. 1. Intracellular microorganisms, such as viruses and parasites, invade the myocardium to survive. These microorganisms damage the vital organelles and cause cell death in the myocardium. The myocardium becomes weak, leading to heart failure; then T lymphocytes invade the myocardium in response to the viral infection. The T lymphocytes respond to the viral infection by secreting cytokines to kill the virus, but they also kill the virus-infected myocardium. Myocardial infarction, renal failure, and liver failure are not direct consequences of a viral or parasitic infection.

🔑 CN: Safety and infection control; CL: Analyze

70. 1, 2, 4. A National Patient Safety Goal of the Joint Commission is to accurately and completely reconcile medications across the continuum of care. The requirement is that there is a process for comparing the client's current medications with those prescribed for the client while under the care of the healthcare organization. Clients are most at risk during transitions in care (hand-offs) across settings, services, providers, or levels of care. The development, reconciliation, and communication of an accurate medication list throughout the continuum of care are essential in the reduction of transition-related adverse drug events. The client or client's family is an integral component of medication reconciliation, particularly at the point of admission to, and discharge from, a healthcare facility. Any medications that the client uses, for example, over-the-counter medications, must be included in the reconciliation process.

🔑 CN: Safety and infection control; CL: Apply

71. 2. The nurse should not accept an assignment to "float" to another nursing unit for which the nurse does not have experience or adequate preparation. The first step is to discuss the situation with the person making the assignment; if the situation is not resolved, the newly graduated nurse should ask to speak with the supervisor.

🔑 CN: Management of care; CL: Synthesize

72. 1. The nurse should notify the hospital's security staff about anyone who appears unusual. Typically, the abductor is an older woman who wishes to have a baby. The nurse should take only one baby at a time to a mother to prevent the neonate being taken to the wrong mother. Infants should never be left in the hallway. When in the mother's room, the infant should be placed away from the doorway to prevent or minimize the risk of abduction of the neonate. If an exit alarm is triggered, it is possible that an abductor is running away with an infant. Staff members should investigate the alarm immediately and stop the potential abductor. Hospital security can be alerted if someone is seen exiting the unit carrying a large bag or an infant.

🔑 CN: Management of care; CL: Synthesize

73. 2. Amiodarone is metabolized in the liver and excreted in the bile and feces. Liver toxicity has been reported with the use of this drug, so the nurse will want to monitor the client's liver enzymes. Amiodarone does not affect hemoglobin, CK, or renal function.

🔑 CN: Pharmacological and parenteral therapies; CL: Apply

74. 4. The teenage girl has scoliosis, the lateral deviation of the spine. Kyphosis is noted by a forward curvature of the shoulders. Lordosis is an inward curvature of the lower back. Hip dysplasia is noted in older children by pain, but it is usually diagnosed before the child walks by noting excessive gluteal folds and limited hip abduction.

🔑 CN: Health promotion and maintenance; CL: Analyze

75. 3. The client is exhibiting symptoms that are consistent with hyperglycemia. The **RN** 📖 does not give any additional glucose. All of the other interventions are appropriate for this client. The new graduate RN notifies the **healthcare provider (HCP)** 📖 about the assessment findings.

🔑 CN: Management of care; CL: Analyze

76. 1. The cause of endogenous depression is believed to be biochemical and not a reaction to a loss. It is caused by an imbalance or decreased availability of norepinephrine, serotonin, and possibly dopamine, so the client cannot identify a specific outside cause or a loss. Reactive depression is a reaction to a loss or a stressor. It is wrong to consider that lack of trust and slow thinking are reasons why the client will not identify the cause of his depression. Problems and stressors from past childhood conflicts may be present; however, the client can discuss them with the staff when he is willing or able.

🔑 CN: Management of care; CL: Synthesize

77. 2. Yogurt is high in protein because it is made from milk. The other choices are much higher in carbohydrates than protein except for bacon, which is higher in fat.

🔑 CN: Reduction of risk potential; CL: Apply

78. 3. If the gastric balloon should rupture or deflate, the esophageal balloon can move and partially or totally obstruct the airway, causing respiratory distress. The client must be observed closely. No direct action should be taken until the condition is accurately diagnosed.

🔑 CN: Reduction of risk potential; CL: Synthesize

79. 4, 3, 2, 1. Clients with myasthenia crisis have severe muscle weakness that may result in respiratory failure requiring mechanical ventilation. The nurse's first action is to focus on assuring an adequate airway by preparing for intubation. The nurse can then assess for a gag reflex for risk of aspiration. Once the airway and risk for aspiration are assured, the nurse can assess the client for infection and medication schedule.

🔑 CN: Physiological adaptation; CL: Synthesize

80. 3. Pediculosis capitis, or head lice, can be spread by close contact or sharing of headgear or combs and brushes with other children. Sharing craft supplies, swimming, and showering usually do not provide close enough contact to permit transmission.

CN: Safety and infection control; CL: Synthesize

81. 1. In the first trimester, ultrasound scanning typically is prescribed to determine the gestational age. This is especially important for a client with a history of irregular menstrual cycles to establish an accurate birth date. There is no reason at this point in pregnancy to determine whether twins are present. This might be indicated if the fundal height were larger than the gestational age may indicate. Identifying the gender of the fetus is not a reason for an ultrasound examination unless there is a history of sex-linked genetic disorders. Pelvic adequacy can be determined by physical examination. If the client has a borderline pelvis, an ultrasound scan cannot confirm this. Pelvimetry can be done, but it is not performed as frequently as it once was.

CN: Health promotion and maintenance; CL: Apply

82. 1. The oxygen levels for this neonate have dropped during the last 8 hours; the nurse should administer oxygen, as the neonate is not obtaining adequate oxygenation on room air. The recommended pulse oximetry reading in a term neonate is 95% to 100%. Keeping the neonate warm may improve the oxygen saturation if that is the cause of the poor gas exchange, but overheating with warm blankets may increase oxygen demand. Waiting to reassess the neonate could cause the neonate to have inadequate oxygen levels unnecessarily. While blood gases may be drawn, the first action is to administer the oxygen.

CN: Management of care; CL: Synthesize

83. 2. The nurse should prepare to insert an NG tube. The data collected provide evidence that the client is experiencing an upper gastrointestinal bleed secondary to a peptic ulcer. The client will be placed on nothing-by-mouth status, and an NG tube will be inserted to provide gastric decompression and alleviate vomiting. Administering antiemetics is not a priority action for a client who is hypotensive and vomiting coffee-ground emesis. Assessment of client stressors is appropriate after emergency care has been provided and the client stabilized. A modified Trendelenburg position is inappropriate for clients who are vomiting.

CN: Reduction of risk potential; CL: Synthesize

84. 1. The client with preeclampsia would be a candidate for the induction process because ending the pregnancy is the only way to cure preeclampsia.

A client with active herpes would be a candidate for a cesarean section to prevent the fetus from contracting the virus while passing through the birth canal. The woman with a face presentation will not be able to give birth vaginally due to the extended position of the neck. The client whose fetus exhibits late decelerations without oxytocin would be at greater risk for fetal distress with use of this drug. Late decelerations indicate the fetus does not have enough placental reserves to remain oxygenated during the entire contraction. This client may require a cesarean section.

CN: Management of care; CL: Synthesize

85. 3. The sudden onset of bright red drainage of this magnitude needs to be further assessed. Assessing vital signs is an important nursing action to determine whether there have been any changes in the client's status. Additional steps would include reinforcing the dressing and notifying the **healthcare provider (HCP)** 🔲. Increasing the IV flow rate does not address the bleeding. Changing the dressing would be done only if the HCP prescribed it.

CN: Reduction of risk potential; CL: Synthesize

86. 1. Because the client with ADHD is easily distractible, it is important to obtain eye contact before explaining the task. Simple language and having him repeat what he is told are necessary because of his age. Praise encourages the client to repeat the task in the future as well as building the client's self-esteem. A full explanation with verbal praise and a food reward is inappropriate because a food reward increases the chance that he will expect a physical reward for completing tasks. In addition, a full explanation might be too confusing for someone his age. Explaining consequences focuses on punishment, rather than praise. Although demonstration and imitation is an effective teaching method, rewarding with food fosters dependence on food reward for task completion.

CN: Psychosocial integrity; CL: Synthesize

87. 1. A normal blood is 70 to 110 mg/dL. Hypoglycemia is an immediate concern. When the brain does not have enough glucose, the client will become rapidly unconscious, and, if uncorrected, seizures and death can result. A reading of 100 mg/dL is normal, and no intervention is necessary. Readings of 150 and 200 mg/dL are elevated and could cause complications, but complications from the elevation would not occur as rapidly.

CN: Reduction of risk potential; CL: Analyze

88. 4, 1, 2, 3. The goal that has the highest priority when a client has a massive bleed from esophageal varices is to maintain a patent airway.

The nurse should position the client to prevent aspiration and assess respirations and oxygen saturation. The nurse should then assist the **healthcare provider (HCP)** 📖 in controlling the hemorrhage by using esophageal balloon tamponade. Octreotide may be administered to reduce portal pressure. The third priority is to restore circulating blood volume with blood and IV fluids. Esophageal bleeding is an anxiety-provoking event for the client, and although lifesaving measures are the priority, the nurse and healthcare team should explain procedures to the client and provide reassurance as needed.

🔑 CN: Physiological adaptation;
CL: Synthesize

89. 4. A client who is taking phenelzine, a monoamine oxidase inhibitor, needs to avoid foods that are rich in tyramine because this food-drug combination can cause hypertensive crisis. The client should be given a list of foods to avoid and should report headaches, palpitations, and a stiff neck to the **healthcare provider (HCP)** 📖 immediately. The client does not need to restrict or add salt to the diet. Drinking 10 to 12 glasses of water each day is important to teach the client who is receiving lithium therapy. Antidepressant drugs take 2 to 4 weeks to achieve therapeutic effects.

🔑 CN: Pharmacological and parenteral therapies; CL: Synthesize

90. 3. Clients with open fractures are particularly susceptible to infections. If not treated promptly, these infections can lead to the development of osteomyelitis. Localized symptoms of osteomyelitis include tenderness, swelling, and warmth at the site of infection, as well as unrelieved severe bone pain. Systemic symptoms include fever, chills, night sweats, and malaise. Avascular necrosis occurs when the blood supply to a bone is interrupted, most commonly in intracapsular hip fractures. Compartment syndrome is most commonly associated with fractures of the distal humerus and proximal tibia; it results from an increase in pressure on the nerves and blood supply within a closed tissue compartment. Fat embolism syndrome is associated most frequently with fractures of the long bones, ribs, and pelvis, which may or may not be open fractures.

🔑 CN: Reduction of risk potential;
CL: Analyze

91. 3. Sharing needles is associated with increased incidence of blood-borne diseases such as hepatitis B. Hepatitis B is not spread through marijuana use. Acetaminophen taken in large amounts can cause severe hepatic necrosis but does not cause hepatitis B. Contaminated seafood is responsible for transmission of hepatitis A.

🔑 CN: Safety and infection control;
CL: Evaluate

92. 3. The nurse should confirm the client's concern about taking psychiatric medications. Suggesting that he feels guilty is probably too direct, may not be accurate, and may cut off further discussion. Expressing concern is likely to promote further discussion about the reasons for his concern. Telling the client he is correct feeds any fear or guilt he may feel, and telling him not to worry demeans his concerns.

🔑 CN: Psychosocial integrity; CL: Apply

93. 3. The retina is especially susceptible to damage in a client with chronic hypertension. The arterioles supplying the retina are damaged. Such damage can lead to vision loss. The iris, cornea, and sclera are not affected by hypertension.

🔑 CN: Physiological adaptation;
CL: Analyze

94. 3. Milia are white papules resulting from plugged sebaceous ducts that disappear by age 2 to 4 weeks. Parents should be instructed to avoid scratching them to prevent secondary infection. Term neonates generally have many creases on the soles of their feet. Preterm neonates may have only a few creases due to their immaturity. Strawberry hemangiomas are elevated areas formed by immature capillaries that will disappear over time. Port-wine stains are deep, dark red discolorations that require laser therapy for removal. Erythema toxicum is a newborn rash or "flea bite" rash that requires no treatment and disappears over time.

🔑 CN: Health promotion and maintenance;
CL: Synthesize

95. 4. Clients with fractures of the long bones such as the femur are particularly susceptible to fat embolism syndrome (FES). Signs and symptoms include chest pain, dyspnea, tachycardia, and cyanosis. Changes in mental status are caused by hypoxemia and can be the first symptoms noted in FES. The client can also be restless and febrile and can develop petechiae. Osteomyelitis is infection of the bone; signs and symptoms of osteomyelitis do not include respiratory symptoms. Compartment syndrome causes signs of localized neurovascular impairment, not systemic symptoms. Venous thrombosis occurs in the lower extremities and is caused by venous stasis.

🔑 CN: Reduction of risk potential;
CL: Analyze

96. 1. The client should be taught how to prevent the spread of hepatitis B to others. The client should eat a well-balanced, nutritional diet. There is no need to restrict sodium or protein. Sedatives should be avoided because these are usually detoxified by the liver. It is not necessary for the client to be isolated from family and friends.

🔑 CN: Safety and infection control;
CL: Evaluate

97. 2. In this situation, the nurse should call a community meeting. The community meeting serves as a forum for clients to voice their opinions about the environment, receive feedback from staff and other clients, and discuss community concerns, including exploring the problems of daily living. The community meeting can be used to increase peer support and handle confrontation when necessary. For adolescents, peer pressure is generally more effective in changing behavior than the staff's influence. Telephoning the client's parents or urging the client to tell on his friends is authoritative and may lead to increased mistrust of the staff. Calling a primary care provider is not necessary at this time. Rather, a community meeting would be helpful to discuss the problem.

🗝 CN: Management of care; CL: Synthesize

98. 2. A report about the client's condition should be as clear, pertinent, and concise as possible. It should be free of subjective information that could be interpreted differently by different caregivers. The report mentioning that a specimen was sent to the laboratory does not indicate how much urine had been drained from the client's bladder and how the urine appeared. The report describing the client as cooperative is subjective and provides only limited client data. The report that mentions that the client was in the ED for 3 hours does not mention the treatment provided.

🗝 CN: Management of care; CL: Create

99. 1, 3, 4. As the homeostatic responses begin to decompensate, late clinical manifestations from a large overdose of sympathomimetic agents include loss of function of the hypothalamus such as temperature regulation, leading to profound pyrexia, and ectopic brain activity leading to seizures. Hypotension is a late sign that occurs as the vascular system collapses. Hypertension, an earlier sign, precedes hypotension. Tachycardia occurs as a reflex to hypotension, a late sign.

🗝 CN: Pharmacological and parenteral therapies; CL: Analyze

100. 2. A small tuft of hair and an indentation at the base of the neonate's spine is termed spina bifida occulta. This condition usually occurs between the L5 and S1 vertebrae with failure of the vertebrae to completely fuse. There are usually no sensory or motor deficits with this condition. Spina bifida cystica includes meningocele, myelomeningocele, and lipomeningocele. Meningocele is characterized by a saclike protrusion filled with spinal fluid and meninges. Usually, this condition is associated with sensory and motor deficits. Myelomeningocele is characterized by a saclike protrusion filled with spinal fluid, meninges, nerve roots, and spinal cord. With myelomeningocele, there are usually sensory and motor deficits.

🗝 CN: Health promotion and maintenance; CL: Analyze

101. 2. Indwelling catheters are considered to be a major contributor to nosocomial infections. Any client with an indwelling catheter is at high risk for developing a urinary tract infection. A history of previous childbirths does not necessarily predispose a client to urinary tract infections. Clients with a history of renal calculi are not necessarily at risk for developing urinary tract infections unless the renal calculi recur. Clients with diabetes mellitus are at a higher risk for developing urinary tract infections, but this risk can be decreased by maintaining good control over blood glucose levels.

🗝 CN: Management of care; CL: Analyze

102. 3, 4. The nurse should use at least two sources of identification prior to administering medication to any client, such as the **medical record** 📖 number and the client's date of birth. It is not safe practice to ask the parent or a nurse to verify the correct neonate. It is also not safe to use the room number or crib number as a source of identification because neonates' locations in the hospital change frequently.

🗝 CN: Safety and infection control; CL: Apply

103. 4. Caffeinated beverages and alcohol should be avoided because they stimulate gastric acid production and irritate gastric mucosa. The client should avoid foods that cause discomfort; however, there is no need to follow a soft, bland diet. Eating six small meals daily is no longer a common treatment for peptic ulcer disease. Milk in large quantities is not recommended because it actually stimulates further production of gastric acid.

🗝 CN: Reduction of risk potential; CL: Evaluate

104. 3. When a client with a NG tube exhibits abdominal distention, the nurse should first check the suction machine. If the suction equipment is functioning properly, then the nurse should take other steps, such as repositioning the tube or checking tube patency by irrigating it. If these steps are not effective, then the **HCP** 📖 should be called.

🗝 CN: Reduction of risk potential; CL: Synthesize

105. 4. Increased, not decreased, body temperature resulting from occupations or infections can contribute to low sperm counts caused by decreased sperm production. Heat can destroy sperm. Varicocele, an abnormal dilation of the veins in the spermatic cord, is an associated cause of a low sperm count. The varicosity increases the temperature within the testes, inhibiting sperm production. Frequent use of saunas or hot tubs may lead to a low sperm count. The temperature of the scrotum becomes elevated, possibly inhibiting sperm production. Endocrine imbalances (thyroid problems) are associated with low sperm counts in men because of possible interference with spermatogenesis.

CN: Reduction of risk potential; CL: Evaluate

106. 1. The primary purpose of instilling 5 mL of normal saline solution before suctioning a tracheostomy tube is to thin the secretions to be suctioned. The saline may stimulate a cough; however, this is not the reason for using saline. The tracheostomy tube is larger than the suction catheter, so the catheter will easily pass into the tube without lubrication. Humidification is provided by a nebulizer if needed.

CN: Reduction of risk potential; CL: Evaluate

107. 3. The client with emphysema has a chronically elevated carbon dioxide level. As a result, the normal stimulus for breathing in the medulla becomes ineffective. Instead, peripheral pressoreceptors in the aortic arch and carotid arteries, which are sensitive to oxygen blood levels, stimulate respirations. This is in response to low oxygen levels that have developed over time. If the client receives high concentrations of oxygen, the blood level of oxygen will rise excessively, the stimulus for respiration will decrease, and respiratory failure may result. Oxygen is not cooled. Humidification or administration of the oxygen through nasal cannula will not prevent depressed ventilation if the flow rate of the oxygen is too high.

CN: Physiological adaptation; CL: Apply

108. 1. The nurse should not administer drugs without a complete prescription. In this case, the prescription does not contain information about dosage and uses abbreviations that can cause confusion. The surgeon must write a prescription using complete dosages and without abbreviations before the nurse administers the drugs. Relying on the pharmacist for clarification is inappropriate.

CN: Management of care; CL: Synthesize

109. 4. Vaginal tissue can be atrophic while breast-feeding, so the use of a water-based lubricant can help with discomfort and lubrication during intercourse. Ice is applied to decrease breast milk supply, and ace bandages are only used to dry up breast milk. Fruit juice is a health drink while breast-feeding.

CN: Health promotion and maintenance; CL: Apply

110. 3. The client should be encouraged to join the community arthritis support group so that she can share her feelings with others who are facing

similar experiences with this chronic illness and can identify with her concerns. A hobby will not help her resolve her feelings of being alone. Seeking counseling or discussing her feelings with a minister may be helpful, but these activities will not necessarily help the client to understand that there are many individuals who must adjust their lifestyles because of arthritis and that she is not alone.

CN: Health promotion and maintenance; CL: Synthesize

111. 2. For the client who is unable to sit through meals to maintain adequate nutrition, the nurse should offer the client nutritious finger foods and fluids that he can consume while "on the run." Foods high in protein and carbohydrates, such as half of a peanut butter sandwich, will help to maintain nutritional needs. Adequate fluid intake is necessary, especially if the client has been started on lithium therapy. Directing the client to his room to eat is not helpful because the client will not stay in his room long enough to eat. Asking the client's family to bring his favorite foods or asking the client about his food preferences is not helpful in ensuring adequate nutrition for the hyperactive client who is unable to sit and eat.

CN: Basic care and comfort; CL: Synthesize

112. 4. Telling the client to get her laundry and then showing her how to use the machine helps keep the client from becoming overly dependent on the nurse, establishes boundaries between the client and the nurse, and promotes positive self-worth. The statement "Sure, I have time; I will do it for you" is not therapeutic because it increases the client's dependency. Telling the client that she will have to wait because the nurse does not have time dismisses the client and insinuates that the nurse will do the laundry later, thus fostering dependency. Asking "Can your family do it for you?" is not appropriate because the client is capable of doing her own laundry. This statement places responsibility on the family instead of the client.

CN: Psychosocial integrity; CL: Synthesize

113. 2. Early signs and symptoms of hypermagnesemia include drowsiness, lethargy, nausea, and vomiting. Flushed skin is a sign of hypernatremia. Severe thirst is associated with hyperglycemia. Tremors are associated with hypomagnesemia.

CN: Reduction of risk potential; CL: Analyze

114. 4. Sitting or holding a child upright for formula feedings helps prevent pooling of formula in the pharyngeal area. When the vacuum in the middle ear opens into the pharyngeal cavity, formula (along with bacteria) is drawn into the middle ear. Cleaning the ear canals does not reduce the incidence of otitis media because the pathogenic bacteria are in the nasopharynx, not the external area of the ears. Continuous low-dose antibiotic therapy is used only in cases of recurrent otitis media, when the child finishes a course of antibiotics but then develops another ear infection a few days later. Although accumulation of cerumen makes it difficult to visualize the tympanic membrane, it does not promote inner ear infections.

CN: Health promotion and maintenance; CL: Evaluate

115. 3. Calling a client "contrary" is critical in nature and judgmental on the nurse's part. It is inappropriate for the nurse to make a comment like this at shift report or at any time. The other statements provide important and appropriate information (diagnosis, **healthcare provider's [HCP's]** 📖 name, pain relief strategies, and evaluation of ambulation).

CN: Management of care; CL: Apply

116. 1. The nurse should teach personnel to communicate with clients who are withdrawing from alcohol and street drugs in a calm, matter-of-fact manner, using short sentences and a moderate tone of voice. This approach promotes orientation, reinforces cognitive-perceptual functions, and decreases anxiety. A cheerful tone and humor are inappropriate, possibly leading to misperceptions by the client with cognitive-perceptual impairment. Using general and abstract terms and a loud tone of voice increases anxiety and may lead to misunderstanding. Lengthy explanations delivered with a quiet voice will lead to frustration and increased anxiety.

CN: Psychosocial integrity; CL: Evaluate

117. 3. The best opportunity for a successful pregnancy is when the normal menstrual cycle is created either naturally or through hormonal augmentation. Implantation can occur only when the levels of estrogen and progesterone are at particular levels. For many women, more than one fertilized egg is placed into the uterus. This increases the risk that more than one embryo will implant and reach maturity. Couples can choose to utilize their own eggs and sperm if they have been determined to be healthy, or they can choose to use donor oocytes and sperm. For many women who utilize in vitro fertilization, a career has taken precedence over having a family, and these women will need to rebalance a career with the demands of pregnancy and parenting.

CN: Physiological adaptation; CL: Evaluate

118. 1, 3, 4, 5. Vitamins B_6, B_{12}, and iron are important in the production of red blood cells. Therefore, the nurse should question the client specifically about food intake that contains these vitamins and minerals. Vitamin C helps iron absorption and plays a small role in red blood cell production. Vitamin K has little role in the production of red blood cells.

CN: Health promotion and maintenance; CL: Analyze

119. 1. During the emergent phase of burn care, one of the most significant problems is hypovolemic shock. The development of hypovolemic shock can lead to impaired blood flow through the heart and kidneys, resulting in decreased cardiac output and renal ischemia. Efforts are directed toward replacing lost fluids and preventing hypovolemic shock. Preventing infection and controlling pain are important goals, but preventing circulatory collapse is a higher priority. It is too early in the stage of burn injury to promote wound healing.

CN: Physiological adaptation; CL: Synthesize

120. 2. A client with multiple sclerosis may have a sense of optimism and euphoria, particularly during remissions. Euphoria is characterized by mood elevation with an exaggerated sense of well-being. Inappropriate laughter, slurring of words, and visual hallucinations are uncharacteristic of euphoria.

CN: Psychosocial integrity; CL: Analyze

121. 1. The "rule of nines" is used to estimate the percentage of the client's body surface area that was burned. Medical treatment, including fluid volume replacement therapy, is based on the percentage of body surface area burned. Rehabilitation needs are identified after the extent of the burn is established and are directed toward preserving the client's functional ability. Respiratory needs are determined by the location of the burn and the potential for injury from inhalation in addition to vital signs and oxygenation levels.

CN: Reduction of risk potential; CL: Analyze

122. 2. The "click" the nurse feels when abducting the femur is made by the head of the femur as it slips into the acetabulum. This is Ortolani's sign and indicates a dislocated hip. This is not a normal finding for a 2-month-old. The nurse needs to gather additional information by checking for unequal leg lengths and asymmetry of the gluteal and thigh folds. Once the nurse has obtained additional assessment information, the nurse would notify the **healthcare provider (HCP)** 📖. Usual medical treatment involves keeping the hip joint in an abducted position in a Pavlik harness. The goal of treatment is to keep the head of the femur centered in the acetabulum. Treatment needs to begin as soon as possible. Usually, the earlier treatment is started, the better the outcome.

CN: Health promotion and maintenance; CL: Synthesize

123. 4. Warfarin sodium interferes with clotting. The nurse should monitor the PT and evaluate for the therapeutic effects of coumadin. A therapeutic PT is between 1.5 and 2.5 times the control value; the PT should be established by the **healthcare provider (HCP)** 📖. It may also be reported as an international normalized ratio, a standardized system that provides a common basis for communicating and interpreting PT results. The PTT is monitored in clients who are receiving heparin therapy. Serum potassium levels and ABG values are not affected by warfarin.

🔑 CN: Pharmacological and parenteral therapies; CL: Analyze

124. 4. The lower abdominal pain is most likely caused by bladder spasms. A common cause of bladder spasms after TURP is blood clots obstructing the catheter; therefore, the nurse's first action should be to assess the patency of the catheter. Auscultating the abdomen for bowel sounds would be appropriate after patency of the catheter has been established. The nurse should assess for bladder spasms before administering an analgesic. A sitz bath would not relieve bladder spasms that are caused by an obstructed catheter.

🔑 CN: Physiological adaptation; CL: Synthesize

125. 3. The nurse should first determine whether the client received the last dose of imipenem-cilastatin. If the client did not receive the last dose, the nurse should notify the **healthcare provider (HCP)** 📖 that the client did not receive the dose, receive prescriptions, document, implement the prescriptions, and complete an incident report. The nurse should not automatically discard the partial fill of imipenem-cilastatin found at the client's bedside until further investigation is done. The nurse should recognize the cost of medications such as imipenem-cilastatin and consult the pharmacist after identifying information on the partial fill bag that was found. After verifying all information, the nurse can administer the new partial fill of imipenem-cilastatin so that the client can receive the antibiotic on time.

🔑 CN: Safety and infection control; CL: Synthesize

126. 2. For a client with moderate anxiety, the nurse should initially lead the client to a less stimulating environment and help him discuss his feelings. Doing so helps the client to gain control over anxiety that could be overwhelming. Telling the client that it would be best to lie down until he is calmer is not appropriate because the client is too anxious to benefit from this intervention. Suggesting that the client try relaxation exercises could be helpful after the nurse takes the client to a less stimulating environment and allows the client to vent and discuss his feelings. Getting some medication to help the client relax is an intervention that the nurse would carry out later after trying to help the client decrease anxiety through ventilation and relaxation exercises.

🔑 CN: Psychosocial integrity; CL: Synthesize

127. 1. Clients who are receiving anticoagulant therapy should consult the **HCP** 📖 before undergoing any dental work that will cause bleeding such as a tooth extraction. The dentist should also be aware that the client is taking anticoagulants. A soft toothbrush is desirable for oral hygiene if the client is receiving anticoagulant therapy; it helps prevent the gums from bleeding. Rectal suppositories are contraindicated during anticoagulant therapy because their insertion may cause bleeding. Stool softeners may be used instead to prevent straining, which also may promote bleeding. Green leafy vegetables should not be eaten in excess because of their vitamin K content, which may alter the effectiveness of the anticoagulant therapy.

🔑 CN: Pharmacological and parenteral therapies; CL: Synthesize

128. 3. Increasing the client's fluid intake to 3,000 mL/day, unless contraindicated, is the most appropriate action. Typically, clients who are immobilized by skeletal traction are given stool softeners. Treating constipation with diet, increased fluids, and stool softeners is preferred to the administration of an enema. Placing the client on the bedpan will not encourage a bowel movement. Range-of-motion movements maintain joint mobility but do not stimulate peristalsis.

🔑 CN: Reduction of risk potential; CL: Synthesize

129. 1, 3, 4, 5. Although about 50% of diarrhea in clients receiving tube feedings is caused by sorbitol-containing medications, the nurse should assess for other possible causes. Diarrhea can occur as a result of bacterial contamination if fresh formula is not used or stored in a refrigerator, or if the feeding apparatus is not changed at least every 24 hours. Lactose intolerance, rapid formula administration, low serum albumin level, and hypertonic solutions may also cause diarrhea. Hypotonic solutions would not be a likely cause of diarrhea, abdominal distention, or cramping.

🔑 CN: Basic care and comfort; CL: Synthesize

130. 4. Risk factors for postoperative pulmonary complications include malnourishment, which is indicated by the low weight relative to the client's height. Although keeping feelings inside can be problematic, it would not be considered a postoperative risk for pulmonary complications. The absence of dyspnea on exertion is not indicative of postoperative complications. The client's age does not necessarily place her at increased risk.

🔑 CN: Health promotion and maintenance; CL: Analyze

131. 2. Administering an antiemetic before beginning chemotherapy and then routinely around the clock helps prevent nausea and vomiting. Waiting until the client requests it may be too late because nausea is already present.

🔑 CN: Pharmacological and parenteral therapies; CL: Synthesize

132. 1. Greenish-colored amniotic fluid is caused by the passage of meconium, usually secondary to a fetal insult during labor. Meconium passage also may be related to an intact gastrointestinal system of the neonate, especially those neonates who are full term or of postdate gestational age. Amnioinfusion may be used to treat the condition and dilute the fluid. Cloudy amniotic fluid is associated with an infection caused by bacteria or a sexually transmitted disease. Severe yellow-colored fluid is associated with Rh incompatibility or erythroblastosis fetalis.

🔑 CN: Health promotion and maintenance; CL: Analyze

133. 1. The pH of 7.24 indicates that the client is acidotic. The carbon dioxide level is normal, but the HCO_3^- level is decreased. These findings indicate that the client is in metabolic acidosis. This laboratory report does not indicate that the client is in metabolic alkalosis, respiratory alkalosis, or respiratory acidosis. This laboratory report does not indicate that the client is in metabolic alkalosis, respiratory alkalosis, or respiratory acidosis.

🔑 CN: Reduction of risk potential; CL: Analyze

134. 3. Black, tarry stools indicate the presence of a slow upper gastrointestinal bleed. The longer the blood is in the system, the darker it becomes as the hemoglobin is broken down and iron is released. Vital sign changes, such as an increased pulse, are not evident with slow gastrointestinal bleeds. Nausea and abdominal cramps can occur but are not definitive signs of gastrointestinal bleeding.

🔑 CN: Physiological adaptation; CL: Analyze

135. 2. This client has lived with the diagnosis of coronary syndrome for 4 years, and, depending on the progression of the illness, the learning needs may have changed. The client may at this time have more questions about the illness and how to manage it. The nurse does not assume that the client is stable and knowledgeable about the illness just

because the diagnosis was made 4 years ago. Clients are sometimes less likely to want to learn during hospitalization because they are not feeling well enough to learn.

🔑 CN: Health promotion and maintenance; CL: Synthesize

136. 1. Most adolescents with Osgood-Schlatter disease are able to continue to exercise and use ice afterward. Ibuprofen also may be prescribed. Because Osgood-Schlatter disease is self-limited, crutches or physical therapy is usually unnecessary, and the adolescent usually does not need to stop playing sports. Only in severe cases would the adolescent have to stop playing sports.

🔑 CN: Physiological adaptation; CL: Synthesize

137. 3. Iron supplements will darken the stools. Iron supplements should not be taken on an empty stomach because they can cause gastric irritation. Iron is constipating, and a daily bulk-forming laxative should be started prophylactically. A straw should be used when taking liquid iron to avoid discoloring the teeth.

🔑 CN: Pharmacological and parenteral therapies; CL: Apply

138. 1. A client with generalized anxiety disorder needs to learn cognitive and behavioral strategies to cope with anxiety appropriately. In doing so, the client's anxiety decreases and becomes more manageable. The client may need assertiveness training, reframing, and relaxation exercises to adaptively deal with anxiety. The nurse should not encourage the client to seek avoidance or denial, but rather be engaged using cognitive and behavioral strategies. The client should not withdraw from role responsibilities or relationships. The client does not need additional rest or sleep.

🔑 CN: Psychosocial integrity; CL: Synthesize

139. 4. Deep breathing helps prevent microatelectasis and pneumonitis and also helps force air and fluid out of the pleural space into the chest tubes. It does not decrease blood flow to the lungs or control the rate of air flow. The diaphragm is the major muscle of respiration; deep breathing causes it to descend, thereby increasing the ventilating surface.

🔑 CN: Reduction of risk potential; CL: Apply

140. 2. When applying an elastic bandage to a leg, start at the distal end and move toward the trunk in order to support venous return. Tension should be kept even and not increased with each turn to prevent circulatory impairment. Overlapping each layer twice when wrapping can also impair circulation. The clips securing the bandage should be placed on the outer aspect of the leg to avoid creating a pressure point on the other leg.

🔑 CN: Reduction of risk potential;
CL: Evaluate

141. 1. Spermicidal agents work by destroying the spermatozoa before they enter the cervix. In addition, some spermicides alter the vaginal pH to a strong acidic environment, which is not conducive to survival of spermatozoa. Spermicides do not prevent the spermatozoa from entering the uterus, but the diaphragm or condom is a barrier.

🔑 CN: Pharmacological and parenteral therapies; CL: Apply

142. 4. A low dosage of sertraline is helpful in controlling dementia-induced paranoia and hallucinations. Methylphenidate would be indicated for attention deficit hyperactivity disorder. Lorazepam would be prescribed if the client were anxious and agitated. Trazodone would be used if depression were prominent.

🔑 CN: Pharmacological and parenteral therapies; CL: Synthesize

143. 1. Increased fremitus can be present in bacterial pneumonia, indicating the presence of pulmonary consolidation. Additional findings would include crackles, bronchial breath sounds, and dullness on percussion. Bilateral expiratory wheezing and resonance on percussion are not present in bacterial pneumonia. Vesicular breath sounds are normal and would not be an expected finding in bacterial pneumonia.

🔑 CN: Physiological adaptation;
CL: Analyze

144. 3. Acute pancreatitis is very painful; management involves interventions for pain. Although alcohol abuse is often implicated in pancreatitis, drug and alcohol counseling will be an individual consideration. Risk for injury and ineffective airway clearance are not typically associated with acute pancreatitis.

🔑 CN: Basic care and comfort;
CL: Synthesize

145. 3. A hydrocele, defined as fluid in the processus vaginalis, is determined when the scrotal sac can be transilluminated. A swelling in the scrotal area that can be reduced indicates an inguinal hernia. Both hydroceles and hernias can enlarge the scrotal sac, and both can be either unilateral or bilateral. A hernia typically is more obvious during crying.

🔑 CN: Reduction of risk potential;
CL: Analyze

146. 1. The screening protocol recommended by the American and Canadian Cancer Societies for early detection of cancer in asymptomatic people includes the following: Beginning at age 50, men and women should have fecal occult blood testing, flexible sigmoidoscopy, or colonoscopy every year until age 75 unless determined otherwise by a **healthcare provider (HCP)** 📖. A diet low in saturated fat and high in fruit and fiber is not a screening protocol but is good dietary advice for all clients.

🔑 CN: Health promotion and maintenance;
CL: Apply

147. 1, 2, 5, 6. To treat a low blood glucose level, the nurse should provide the client with approximately 15 g of carbohydrate and monitor the blood glucose level within 15 minutes. The orange juice, milk, bread, or soda would provide approximately 15 g of carbohydrate. Meat or fish, such as tuna, does not contain carbohydrate. Processed peanut butter may contain small amounts of carbohydrate, but it is also high in fat and protein. Peanut butter is not a good option to raise a blood glucose level in a timely manner.

🔑 CN: Reduction of risk potential;
CL: Synthesize

148. 3. Increased ICP can cause vomiting, particularly in children whose fontanelles are closed. An infant with an open anterior fontanelle may have less vomiting because the cranium can respond, expanding with increased ICP. The best course of action is to wait a few minutes and then refeed the child. Putting the child on NPO status may not be helpful because this is not a gastrointestinal problem. Because this is an expected event, notifying the **healthcare provider (HCP)** 📖 is not necessary. Antiemetics frequently make a client sleepy, making neurologic checks difficult to interpret.

🔑 CN: Physiological adaptation;
CL: Synthesize

149. 1. The air is injected into the long-acting insulin first. Air is then injected into the short-acting insulin, and the short-acting insulin is withdrawn. Then the long-acting insulin is withdrawn. It does matter which insulin is drawn up first because the nurse does not want to contaminate the short-acting insulin with the long-acting insulin. It is not necessary to use a high-dose insulin syringe to prepare 28 units of insulin.

🔑 CN: Pharmacological and parenteral therapies; CL: Apply

150. 2. Solids should be introduced at 6 months. Full-term infants use up their prenatal iron stores within 4 to 6 months after birth. Milk contains insufficient iron.

🔑 CN: Health promotion and maintenance;
CL: Apply

151. 4. Incentive spirometry promotes lung expansion and increases respiratory function. When used properly, an incentive spirometer causes sustained maximal inspiration and increased cardiac output.

Incentive spirometry does not directly promote circulation in the extremities. Using incentive spirometry will not help relieve pain or strengthen abdominal muscles.

    CN: Reduction of risk potential; CL: Evaluate

152. 3. Diminished breath sounds during an acute asthma attack are a serious sign of airway obstruction, fatigue, and impending respiratory failure. Wheezing, coughing, and the production of sputum indicate the presence of airflow through the lungs and are less ominous symptoms.

    CN: Physiological adaptation; CL: Analyze

153. 1. Clients should use an electric razor, instead of a straight-edge razor, on any skin areas that are receiving radiation. The skin should be cleaned daily with a mild soap, not harsh antibacterials. Lotion should be removed from the skin before any treatment and then reapplied after the treatment. The radiated skin area needs to be kept clean, dry, and open to air.

    CN: Basic care and comfort; CL: Synthesize

154. 3. A moderate amount of bloody drainage could indicate active bleeding. The priority action is to apply pressure to the area and call for help. Assessing the airway or pulse or administering oxygen does not address the bleeding.

    CN: Reduction of risk potential; CL: Synthesize

155. 4. Because valproic acid is associated with thrombocytopenia and hypofibrinogenemia, routine follow-up blood work would consist of monitoring platelet and fibrinogen levels for decreases. A CBC count and serum electrolyte level are not necessary. Aspartate transaminase, not alkaline phosphatase, is routinely monitored to evaluate for hepatic toxicity, a possible but rare effect of valproic acid. Valproic acid has no effect on cholesterol levels.

    CN: Pharmacological and parenteral therapies; CL: Apply

156. 3. Bacterial conjunctivitis is very contagious. Attention should be paid to thorough handwashing, a major means of stopping the transmission of the disease. Closing the day care center for 1 week is not necessary because thorough handwashing will stop the spread of the infection. Keeping the children out for 48 hours is not necessary. A child may return to day care after being treated for 24 hours. Although the parents of each child should be told about the outbreak, doing so will not help to curtail or prevent the spread of the infection.

    CN: Safety and infection control; CL: Synthesize

157. 3. The client's mobility status is the best indicator of risk for development of a pressure sore. Nutritional and circulatory status are other factors that can contribute to pressure sore development, but immobility, even in the presence of adequate nutrition and circulation, is the leading cause of pressure sores. Disorientation can cause a client to neglect making needed position changes, but the underlying factor will be immobility.

    CN: Reduction of risk potential; CL: Analyze

158. 1. Ketosis is an adaptation to prolonged fasting or carbohydrate deprivation. The body takes partially broken-down fat fragments and combines them into ketone bodies, which the brain can then use for energy. Hypoglycemia is more likely to occur than hyperglycemia, although glucagon assists in preventing this. Metabolic syndrome refers to syndrome X, which includes an abnormal lipid profile and a tendency to gain weight in the abdomen. Lactic acidosis is a metabolic reaction that occurs when oxygen is reduced or not present.

    CN: Physiological adaptation; CL: Analyze

159. 1. The nurse should stop and assess the client further. A chair should be available for the client to sit down. Obtaining the client's blood pressure and heart rate are important when exercising. These values can be used to predict when the oxygen demand becomes greater than the oxygen supply. Calling for help is not necessary for the midsternal burning. If the **healthcare provider (HCP)** has prescribed nitroglycerin, the nurse can administer it; however, stopping the activity may restore the oxygen balance.

    CN: Physiological adaptation; CL: Synthesize

160. 2, 3, 4. Vitamin B_6, folate, and vitamin B_{12} have been shown to reduce homocysteine levels. The effects of vitamins K and D have not been established with regard to homocysteine.

    CN: Health promotion and maintenance; CL: Synthesize

161. 2. The statement "If I forget a dose, it is no big deal, I will just take it when I remember it" indicates a knowledge deficit. The nurse should reinforce that the client should take dexamethasone as prescribed and at the same time each day. The drug has to be tapered off and cannot be stopped abruptly. The **healthcare provider (HCP)** should be notified when the client is under additional stress (e.g., infection, surgery, illness). The client can have an allergic reaction to inactive ingredients contained in dexamethasone.

    CN: Pharmacological and parenteral therapies; CL: Evaluate

162. 1. A child with moderate dehydration, described as a loss of 50 to 90 mL/kg of body fluid, would have oliguria, gray skin color, increased pulse rate, and poor skin elasticity. Sunken eyes, not bulging, are a sign of dehydration. The anterior fontanelle may be sunken, but the posterior fontanelle is normally closed by 6 to 8 weeks of age. A child with mild dehydration, described as a loss of <50 mL/kg of body fluid, would have pale skin color, decreased skin elasticity, decreased urine output, and normal or increased pulse rate.

CN: Physiological adaptation;
CL: Analyze

163. 1. Oropharyngeal candidiasis, or thrush, is the most common infection associated with the early symptomatic stages of HIV infection. Thrush is characterized by whitish yellow patches in the mouth. Various other opportunistic diseases can occur in clients with HIV infection, but they tend to occur later, after the diagnosis of acquired immunodeficiency syndrome has been made. Dyspnea can be indicative of pneumonia, which is caused by a variety of infective organisms. Bloody diarrhea is indicative of cytomegalovirus infection. Hyperpigmented lesions are indicators of Kaposi's sarcoma.

CN: Physiological adaptation;
CL: Analyze

164. 2. Postpartum infection is a leading cause of maternal mortality in the United States. Typical treatment for the condition is IV antibiotic therapy with drugs such as clindamycin, gentamicin, or both. Cultures of the lochia will also be obtained. The neonate can continue to breast-feed as long as the mother desires. A switch to bottle-feeding is not necessary. The uterus tends to be firm, with increased cramping to rid the uterus of the infection. The client should be encouraged to remain in Fowler's position when in bed to allow for drainage of the lochia.

CN: Physiological adaptation;
CL: Synthesize

165. 1. The mother needs further instruction when she says "I should position the baby the same way for each feeding." This can contribute to sore nipples. The position should vary for each feeding to prevent repeated pressure on the same area each time. Grasping the entire areola and nipple will help to decrease nipple soreness. Air-drying the breasts and not using a hand pump will help to decrease nipple soreness.

CN: Health promotion and maintenance;
CL: Evaluate

166. 1. During an acute attack of vertigo, it is best for the client to lie down in a darkened, quiet room and to avoid sudden position changes. A low-sodium diet may be helpful in decreasing the number of attacks, but it is not recommended during the attack. Headaches are not a component of the vertigo attack. Because vertigo is frequently accompanied by nausea and vomiting, the client will not want to eat or drink. Fluids are usually administered parenterally to maintain hydration and administer medications.

CN: Basic care and comfort;
CL: Synthesize

167. 3. The American Academy of Pediatrics recommends that all neonates should receive only formula or breast milk for the first 4 to 6 months of life. Cereal will not help the neonate sleep through the night and may result in allergies and other digestive disorders.

CN: Health promotion and maintenance;
CL: Synthesize

168. 2. Once the client has stated that he is allergic to a substance, the nurse would be negligent to ignore the client's statement and administer the substance. The nurse should check the medical record for allergies and call the **healthcare provider (HCP)** 🔖 for an alternative antibiotic prescription.

CN: Management of care; CL: Synthesize

169. 1. Jaundice that persists past the 3rd or 4th day of life and pale, light stools are associated with biliary atresia. Alkaline phosphatase levels will also be elevated. Surgical intervention is necessary to remove the blockage. Rh isoimmunization and ABO incompatibility are associated with neonatal anemia as the red blood cells are hemolyzed by the antibodies. Esophageal varices are associated with cirrhosis of the liver and large amounts of bleeding when the vessels rupture. The child with esophageal varices will exhibit manifestations of anemia such as pallor and may experience hemorrhage and shock.

CN: Physiological adaptation;
CL: Analyze

170. 1. To reduce urethral irritation and allow drainage, the nurse should tape the Foley catheter to a female client's inner thigh. Taping the catheter also prevents excessive traction against the bladder neck. Taping the catheter to the groin or lower abdomen would not allow for proper drainage and would cause urethral discomfort. Taping the catheter to the lower thigh would pull on the catheter and cause urethral irritation.

CN: Reduction of risk potential;
CL: Apply

171. 1. Most parents find it especially difficult to allow a child who was unable to be normally active before corrective heart surgery to lead a normal and active life after surgery. These parents are less likely to be apprehensive about persuading the child of the need for rest, about postoperative complications, or having the child out of school for a month. Tet spells are no longer expected after the surgical repair.

CN: Physiological adaptation; **CL:** Synthesize

172. 3. After abdominal surgery, the reason for inserting an NG tube is to decompress the gastrointestinal tract until peristaltic action returns. Compression may be used to control bleeding esophageal varices. Lavage is used to remove substances from the stomach or control bleeding. Gavage is used to provide enteral feedings.

CN: Physiological adaptation; **CL:** Evaluate

173. 3. The most common long-term problem experienced by children with cleft palate repair is speech problems. These children frequently need speech therapy for a period of time. Hearing problems may occur as a result of chronic ear infections and the placement of myringotomy tubes. A poor self-concept may develop in any child. However, if a child with a cleft palate receives adequate parenting and support, this should not occur. Chronic sinus infections are more commonly associated with asthma, not with this defect.

CN: Physiological adaptation; **CL:** Apply

174. 2. Feeding solutions that have not been infused after hanging for 8 hours should be discarded because of the increased risk of bacterial growth. Sitting the client upright during the feeding helps prevent aspiration of the feeding. A gastric residual of 25 mL is considered acceptable. A gastric residual of 100 to 150 mL, or a residual >100% of the previous hour's intake, indicates delayed emptying. The feeding solution should be at room or body temperature.

CN: Pharmacological and parenteral therapies; **CL:** Analyze

175. 3. Furosemide is a loop diuretic and inhibits the reabsorption of sodium and chloride from the proximal and distal renal tubules and the loop of Henle. Furosemide promotes sodium diuresis, resulting in a loss of potassium and serious electrolyte imbalances. Furosemide does not affect the BUN level.

CN: Pharmacological and parenteral therapies; **CL:** Analyze

176. 3. Suctioning the respiratory tract for prolonged periods depletes the client's oxygen supply and causes hypoxia. It is recommended that each suctioning period not exceed 15 seconds.

CN: Reduction of risk potential; **CL:** Apply

177. 2. The most appropriate action is to encourage the daughter to talk to her mother about the end-of-life issues first to reach a consensus or agreement. This is a family decision. Immediately informing the **HCP** or preparing to remove the client from life support would be premature if the family is not in agreement. Although a copy of the living will should be on the client's medical record, it is up to the daughter to show it to her mother.

CN: Management of care; **CL:** Synthesize

178. 2, 3, 4. Contraindications for t-PA or alteplase recombinant therapy include current active internal bleeding, 3 hours or longer since the onset of symptoms of a stroke, and severe hypertension. Age >65 years and having had an alcoholic beverage are not contraindications for the therapy.

CN: Pharmacological and parenteral therapies; **CL:** Analyze

179. 2. The nurse should assist the client to use incentive spirometry every 1 to 2 hours postoperatively to prevent atelectasis and pneumonia. Starting a liquid diet is not the highest priority as the client will have an IV infusion and might have an NG tube; adequate fluid status can be maintained until intestinal function returns. The client's extremities are kept flat or lowered to promote circulation. Elevation of extremities is used to promote venous blood flow. The nurse assesses pulses and vital signs hourly in the early postoperative course.

CN: Physiological adaptation; **CL:** Synthesize

180. 3. For a complete breech, the buttocks present, the feet and legs are flexed on the thighs, and the thighs are flexed on the abdomen. For a frank breech, the buttocks present with the hips flexed and the legs extended against the abdomen and chest. This is the most common type of breech presentation. For a compound breech, the buttocks present together with another part, such as a hand. This is a rare occurrence. For an incomplete breech, one or both feet or the knees extend below the buttocks. This can also be termed a single footling or double footling breech.

CN: Health promotion and maintenance; **CL:** Analyze

181. 1. A common complication of diabetes is diabetic neuropathy. Diabetic neuropathy results from the metabolic and vascular factors related to hyperglycemia. Damage leads to sensory deficits and peripheral pain. Muscle atrophy can result from disuse, but it is not a direct consequence of diabetes. Raynaud's disease is associated with vasospasms in the hands and feet. Transient ischemic attacks involve the cerebrum.

CN: Reduction of risk potential; **CL:** Analyze

182. 1. It is important that the client understand that alcohol should be avoided for at least 1 year after an episode of hepatitis. Sexual intercourse does not need to be avoided, but the client should be instructed to use condoms until the hepatitis B surface antigen measurement is negative. The client will need to restrict activity until liver function test results are normal; this will not occur within 1 to 2 weeks. Jaundice will subside as the client recovers; it is not a permanent condition.

⚷ CN: Reduction of risk potential; CL: Evaluate

183. 1. The nurse's statement exemplifies assault, which is the threat of being touched in an offensive way without **consent** 📖. Battery is touching another person without consent. Malpractice is care below the standard of care that results in injury. Invasion of privacy is a violation of a person's right to be left alone.

⚷ CN: Management of care; CL: Analyze

184. 1, 4, 5, 6. Diazepam is a benzodiazepine that causes symptoms of withdrawal when stopped abruptly. The nurse should assess the client for tremors, agitation, irritability, insomnia, vomiting, sweating, tachycardia, headache, anxiety, and confusion. Euphoria or elevated mood is not a symptom of benzodiazepine withdrawal.

⚷ CN: Pharmacological and parenteral therapies; CL: Analyze

185. 1. Parents are typically quick to notice changes in their infant's physical appearance. The removal of the infant's hair may be upsetting to them if they have not been told why it is being done. Hair may be removed on the scalp at the site of needle insertion for IV therapy to provide better visualization and a smooth surface on which to attach tape to secure the needle. Sedatives are not ordinarily prescribed before IV fluid administration. In most instances, it is acceptable for parents to visit their infant while the IV solution is infusing. Holding the infant is encouraged to provide comfort.

⚷ CN: Pharmacological and parenteral therapies; CL: Synthesize

186. 1. Abdominal pain can be a significant problem in acute pancreatitis. An expected outcome is to decrease or eliminate the pain the client is experiencing. Patterns of bowel elimination and liver function are not typically affected by pancreatitis. The client should avoid alcohol.

⚷ CN: Physiological adaptation; CL: Synthesize

187. 3. The most appropriate initial response by the nurse would be to test the child's blood glucose level. The child's symptoms are consistent with hypoglycemia but could also be used by the child to avoid participation in planned activities. Administering milk or fruit juice during a mild reaction may also be appropriate if testing cannot be done. Notifying the **HCP** 📖 may be appropriate after the child's glucose level has been obtained and emergency treatment has been initiated if the child is experiencing hypoglycemia. Returning the child to previous activities is not appropriate until either testing or administering treatment has been done.

⚷ CN: Physiological adaptation; CL: Synthesize

188. 3. Normally, breasts are about the same size. They can vary in size before menstruation due to breast engorgement caused by hormonal changes. It is not necessary for an **HCP** 📖 to check this slight change in breast size. The changes in breast size this client described are most likely caused by hormonal changes, not a benign cyst or normal growth and development.

⚷ CN: Health promotion and maintenance; CL: Synthesize

189. 2. Traditional Chinese medicine describes health as the balance of yin and yang. It describes health as harmony between the mind, body, and soul.

⚷ CN: Health promotion and maintenance; CL: Apply

190. 2. Before an IVP, the client should be assessed for allergies, particularly to iodine-based dyes that may be used during an IVP. Shellfish is a source of iodine, so people who are allergic to shellfish should inform the healthcare personnel and ask what type of dye is being used. Asking the client whether he or she has ever had an IVP before can help determine the degree of teaching needed before the procedure, but that is not the most important question. Neither the client's last bowel movement nor urinary incontinence has any relationship to having an IVP.

⚷ CN: Reduction of risk potential; CL: Analyze

191. 3. Progestin alone has no effect on breast milk or breast-feeding once the milk supply is well established. Estrogen suppresses milk output. Testosterone is not given as an oral contraceptive.

⚷ CN: Pharmacological and parenteral therapies; CL: Apply

192. 4. Learning goals are most likely to be attained when they are established mutually by the client and members of the healthcare team, including the nurse, pharmacist, and the **HCP** 📖. Learning is motivated by perceived problems or goals arising from unmet needs. The perception of the unmet needs must be the client's; however, the nurse, pharmacist, and HCP help the client arrive at his or her own perception of the need or reason to learn.

⚷— CN: Management of care; CL: Evaluate

193. 2. In this situation, the client has indicated that she is not willing to leave the abusive boyfriend because of potential economic concerns and other children in the household. The nurse should explain the cycle of abuse (e.g., tension-building phase, battering incident, and honeymoon phase). The priority intervention is to assist the client to make concrete plans for the safety of herself and her children. The client should identify the safest, quickest routes out of the house and be able to identify where she will go once the cycle of violence escalates. Contacting a social worker at this time is not appropriate because the client is not ready to leave the abusive situation. The nurse can tell the client that these services are available, but it is up to the client to determine whether a referral is necessary. Telling the client that she should not allow anyone to hit her or her children does not assist the client to make plans for her safety and the children's safety should the violence escalate. The client may have a flat affect or feel extreme humiliation from the abuse. The client may also be feeling that the abuse is her fault. When the client is ready to leave the abusive situation and receive continuous counseling, efforts can be made to increase her self-esteem and prevent additional violence. The client should be made aware of the available services in the community for women who are involved in abusive relationships. The location and phone numbers for available shelters should be provided to the client. Giving her a brochure related to the statistics about violence against women is not helpful and, if found by the abuser, may lead to further violence.

⚷— CN: Safety and infection control; CL: Synthesize

194. 5, 4, 3, 2, 1. The child whose condition could change most quickly should be assessed first, and the most stable child should be assessed last. The child with a lacerated liver is at the highest risk for a rapid change in condition. Therefore, this child should be assessed first because the child is at high risk for hemorrhage. The child with a recent concussion should be assessed next because the child is at high risk for increased intracranial pressure, which would be indicated as a change in neurologic status but not necessarily vital signs. The third child to be assessed is the 3-year-old child with pyelonephritis and fever. The fever needs to be acted upon, but this assessment is not as critical as that for the child with a lacerated liver and the child with a concussion. The normal respiratory rate for a 10-month-old infant is 30 breaths/minute. Although the infant is tachypneic, this is expected with pneumonia. Additionally, the infant is not in acute respiratory distress. However, the increased respiratory rate needs evaluation, so the 10-month-old infant should be assessed before the 3-month-old infant with respiratory syncytial virus who has stable vital signs and is not in acute distress.

⚷— CN: Management of care; CL: Synthesize

195. 2. The client who is taking sulfadiazine should be instructed to drink at least eight glasses of water a day to prevent the development of crystalluria. Sulfadiazine should be taken on an empty stomach with a full glass of water. It does not require that the client's urine output be measured and does not affect the color of the urine.

⚷— CN: Pharmacological and parenteral therapies; CL: Synthesize

196. 4. Risperidone is ordered for severe agitation and has a rapid response. Ergoloid and tacrine stabilize and may improve the cognitive functioning of clients with dementia. Diazepam is an antianxiety agent that would not have the desired effect on the severe agitation, violence, and bizarre thoughts.

⚷— CN: Pharmacologic and parenteral therapies; CL: Analyze

197. 1. MID results from multiple small blood clots in the brain. Therefore, the most critical factor is using anticoagulants to reduce the risk of more infarcts. Administering benzodiazepines such as lorazepam to decrease choreiform movements is associated with Huntington's disease. Although depression is common with MID, managing depression-related symptoms will not slow the progression of MID. Managing symptoms by increasing dopamine availability is appropriate for clients with Parkinson's disease.

⚷— CN: Pharmacological and parenteral therapies; CL: Synthesize

198. 2. Checking the carotid artery pulse in a child during CPR provides information about perfusion of the brain. The brachial pulse is checked in an infant because the infant's short and typically fat neck makes it difficult to palpate the carotid pulse. The femoral and radial arteries might indicate perfusion to the peripheral body sites, but the critical need is for adequate circulation to the brain.

⚷— CN: Physiological adaptation; CL: Apply

199. 2. Nephrotic syndrome is characterized by massive proteinuria caused by increased glomerular membrane permeability. Other symptoms include peripheral edema, hyperlipidemia, and hypoalbuminemia. Because of the edema, clients retain fluid and may gain weight. Hematuria is not a symptom related to nephrotic syndrome.

⚷— CN: Physiological adaptation; CL: Analyze

200. **2.** Because the child has a history of severe hypoxic episodes, having oxygen readily available at the bedside is most important. Should the child experience another hypoxic episode, oxygen could be administered easily and quickly. Although morphine causes peripheral dilation, which causes the blood to remain in the periphery, decreasing system volume and oxygen administration is the priority. Typically, a child with tetralogy of Fallot with episodes of hypoxia does not require suctioning.

CN: Physiological adaptation; CL: Synthesize

201. **1.** Although individuals differ, the most likely attitude of a Mexican-American client is to bear pain stoically, to endure pain as a part of God's will, and to delay seeking treatment.

CN: Basic care and comfort; CL: Apply

202. **1.** When a client voids frequent, small amounts, the nurse should suspect that the client is retaining urine. Palpating for a distended bladder is the first assessment that the nurse should perform to verify this suspicion. Obtaining a prescription to catheterize for residual urine may be appropriate as a follow-up activity. Obtaining a urine specimen for culture is not a first priority. The nurse would not encourage an increased fluid intake until further assessment of the situation is completed.

CN: Physiological adaptation; CL: Synthesize

203. **3.** Of the clients listed, the newly admitted client should be assessed first. This is the client who is likely to be unstable and in pain. The child to be discharged today would be considered the most stable and therefore would be assessed last.

CN: Management of care; CL: Synthesize

204. **3.** It is appropriate for the client to be on a low-sodium diet to help decrease fluid retention. Dry skin and pruritus are common in renal failure. Lotions are used to relieve the dry skin, and antihistamines may be used to control itching; corticosteroids are not used. Pain is not a major problem in chronic renal failure, but analgesics that are excreted by the kidneys must be avoided. It is not necessary to measure abdominal girth daily because ascites is not a clinical problem in renal failure.

CN: Reduction of risk potential; CL: Synthesize

205. **5, 4, 3, 2, 1.** The most frequent cause of respiratory distress in a toddler with no previous illness is foreign body aspiration. After having the clerk call for the **rapid response team**, the nurse should assess the child for breaths, and then begin abdominal thrusts. Next, the nurse (or rapid response team if present) should assess the effectiveness of the abdominal thrusts, and then start an intravenous infusion. Finally, the nurse can notify the surgeon.

CN: Reduction of risk potential; CL: Synthesize

206. **4.** The traction weights should be hanging freely to maintain pull. The child needs to be moved up in bed with the weights left untouched to continue countertraction. Then the nurse can determine whether blocks are necessary to maintain the child in the correct position. Raising the weights is inappropriate because doing so interferes with countertraction. The **HCP** does not need to be notified. The nurse can easily correct the problem by moving the child up in bed.

CN: Safety and infection control; CL: Synthesize

207. **1.** Children ages 6 to 12 have a slower growth rate than do younger children and adolescents. As a result, their food requirements are comparatively less.

CN: Health promotion and maintenance; CL: Apply

208. **4.** Asking whether the client is thinking about killing herself is the most direct and therefore the best way to assess suicide risk. Knowing whether the client has recently watched movies on suicide and death, what the client thinks about suicide, or about previous suicides of family members will not tell the nurse whether the client herself is thinking about committing suicide right now.

CN: Psychosocial integrity; CL: Synthesize

209. **2.** Because of their colloidal properties, oatmeal preparation baths typically help relieve the itching associated with chickenpox. Calamine lotion can be also be used if there are no open lesions. Baby powder is unlikely to relieve itching because it acts primarily to absorb moisture. A soft towel moistened with hydrogen peroxide is unlikely to relieve itching. Rather, hydrogen peroxide is used to clean wounds. A cool compress moistened with a weak salt solution is unlikely to relieve itching because it does not have any antipruritic properties.

CN: Basic care and comfort; CL: Synthesize

210. **50 mL/h.**

$$X = 500 \text{ mL}/20 \text{ g} \times 2 \text{ g/h}$$

$$X = 50 \text{ mL/h}$$

CN: Pharmacological and parenteral therapies; CL: Apply

211. **1.** Return demonstrations are the best way to evaluate a person's ability to perform a skill. This technique enables the teacher to observe not only the learner's sequencing of steps of the procedure but also the learner's ability to perform the skill.

🔑 CN: Health promotion and maintenance; CL: Evaluate

212. 3. Ibuprofen should be taken with food or antacids to avoid the development of gastrointestinal distress. Tinnitus is not an adverse effect of ibuprofen; it is a sign of salicylate toxicity. There is no need to increase vitamin B_{12} intake. The CBC is not typically monitored monthly, although clients should be told to report signs of unusual bleeding because ibuprofen can prolong bleeding time.

🔑 CN: Pharmacological and parenteral therapies; CL: Synthesize

213. 4. The nurse concludes that the staff member needs teaching about depression, specifically the biological basis of major depression, when the staff member states the client has no reason to be depressed because "she really has it all." Major depression, or endogenous depression, is caused by alterations of neurotransmitters, primarily serotonin and norepinephrine. Genetics and hereditary also predispose an individual to develop depression. Therefore, there may not be an external cause or a reason for depression to develop. Depression that occurs from an external cause is known as reactive depression, and it could be caused by a loss or a life stress.

🔑 CN: Management of care; CL: Analyze

214. 1. In asthma, the airways react to certain external and internal stimuli, including allergens, infections, exercise, and emotions. Food allergens commonly associated with asthma include soy, wheat, egg whites, dairy products, nuts, shellfish, and fish.

🔑 CN: Reduction of risk potential; CL: Apply

215. 3. Toddlers receive burns usually as the result of not being closely supervised. Toddlers are very inquisitive and need constant supervision; therefore, close follow-up is necessary. In addition, the child probably will need some type of wound care requiring involvement of the parent and possibly others. The amount of support available to the single parent of the 7-month-old child is not known. Although immunization schedules need to be adhered to, it is very possible for a 7-month-old to be delayed in receiving immunizations because of illness or other conflicts. An automobile accident can happen to anyone and does not indicate a lack of safety or supervision. A history of caustic liquid ingestion in a foster child may have been from a time before the child began living with the foster parents; it does not indicate a lack of safety or supervision.

🔑 CN: Management of care; CL: Evaluate

216. 3, 1, 4, 2. The nurse first should stop the intravenous flow of oxytocin because the client is exhibiting a hypertonic uterine contraction pattern caused by the oxytocin. Once the oxytocin infusion is stopped, the nurse should place the client in a lateral position to improve placental blood flow to the fetus. The nurse should next administer oxygen and then contact the primary care provider to report the situation and obtain further prescriptions.

🔑 CN: Management of care; CL: Synthesize

217. 4. When administering an enema, the nurse should position the client in a left Sims' position. Placing the client in this position facilitates the flow of fluid into the rectum and colon. It also allows the client to flex the right leg forward, adequately exposing the rectal area.

🔑 CN: Basic care and comfort; CL: Apply

218. 3. Risk factors for the development of pressure ulcers include poor nutrition, indicated by a decreased serum albumin level. According to the *Guidelines for Pressure Ulcers* published by the Agency for Healthcare Research and Quality, other risk factors include immobility, incontinence, and decreased sensation. A client who does not ambulate often can be repositioned frequently to prevent pressure ulcers. Having an indwelling urinary catheter does not normally increase the risk of developing a pressure ulcer unless pressure from the tubing impinges on urethral or other tissue. An elevated white blood cell count does not place a client at risk for pressure ulcers.

🔑 CN: Reduction of risk potential; CL: Analyze

219. 4. Because of her age and report of a seizure, the client is probably experiencing eclampsia, a condition in which convulsions occur in the absence of any underlying cause. Although the actual cause is unknown, adolescents and women older than 35 years are at higher risk. The client's environment should be kept as free of stimuli as possible. Thus, the nurse should admit the client to a quiet, darkened room. Clients experiencing eclampsia should be kept on the left side to promote placental perfusion. In some cases, edema of the lungs develops after seizures and is a sign of cardiovascular failure. Because the client is at risk for pulmonary edema, breath sounds should be monitored every 2 hours. Vital signs should be monitored frequently, at least every hour.

🔑 CN: Management of care; CL: Synthesize

220. 2. Cerebral hypoxia is commonly associated with dizziness. The greatest risk of injury to a client with dizziness is a fall. Frequent rests and energy conservation measures should be included in the client's plan of care, but safety from falls is the greatest need. Checking the shower water temperature is not critical for this client, who will not be showering because of her fall risk.

🔑 CN: Reduction of risk potential; CL: Synthesize

221. The nurse should auscultate the right lower lobe and listen as the client inhales and exhales. The nurse should be able to hear vesicular breath sounds.

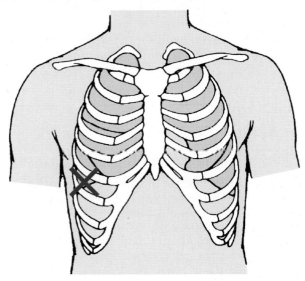

🔑 CN: Physiological adaptation; CL: Apply

222. 2. The most therapeutic nursing response is client centered and goal directed and provides an opportunity for the client to say more, for example, to express additional emotions, needs, or issues. Option 1 is nontherapeutic; it is a false reassurance. Option 3 is also nontherapeutic; the nurse offers a personal opinion of the client's situation. Option 4 is also nontherapeutic; the nurse changes the subject and appears to be uncomfortable discussing the client's concerns.

🔑 CN: Basic care and comfort; CL: Synthesize

223. 4. The situation is escalating, and the nurse's priority is to protect the infant from harm. Therefore, removal of the infant from this situation should be the first action by the nurse. Reasoning at this point or asking one of the parents to leave the room would be ineffective and may serve to further escalate the situation. Calling security is necessary, but only after the nurse has removed the infant from the room.

🔑 CN: Management of care; CL: Synthesize

224. 3. Responses to physiologic stress, such as hospitalization, surgery, or pain, are a result of catecholamine release and specifically include increased heart rate and blood pressure, increased bronchiolar dilation, water retention and decreased urinary output, increased blood glucose, and increased mental acuity.

🔑 CN: Basic care and comfort; CL: Apply

225. 4. Therapeutic communication is always purposeful, goal directed, and client centered. If self-disclosure is used by the nurse or the **UAP** 📖, it should be very focused and limited to just enough to support further communication with the client. It is not always helpful (or educational) and often inappropriate to share personal stories with clients.

🔑 CN: Management of care; CL: Synthesize

226. 4. The nurse should refuse to administer the medication to the client because of the risk of respiratory depression in the neonate. Meperidine, given IM, peaks in 30 to 60 minutes and lasts 2 to 4 hours. Based on the assessment findings, the client most likely will be giving birth within that time frame, increasing the risk for respiratory depression in the neonate, a serious consequence. Therefore, the nurse should not administer the drug. Naloxone should be readily available whenever narcotics that can result in respiratory depression are used. Asking the primary care provider to validate the dosage is not necessary. For clients in early labor, meperidine can be given IM in dosages ranging from 50 to 100 mg.

🔑 CN: Management of care; CL: Synthesize

227. 1, 2, 4, 5. When working with a battered client, the nurse should give information about a safe home and provide a cell phone and information about the crisis help line. The nurse should also help the client understand the cycle of violence as well as personal and legal rights. The nurse should help the client share and discuss her anger, frustration, guilt, shame, and other feelings. Displacing, that is, placing feelings onto another person or object, is not helpful to the client and is not a healthy way to handle feelings.

🔑 CN: Safety and infection control; CL: Synthesize

228. 4. With illness or injury, there is a need to heal or recover. To accomplish this, the client must consistently consume adequate nutrition (and protein) to maintain a positive nitrogen balance and to experience necessary growth and/or healing. The client with burns has the greatest nutritional needs, due to the extent of the injury. Clients with diabetic neuropathy can be encouraged to follow the diabetic diet plan and manage pharmacological therapy to prevent further neuropathy. The client with a fractured femur is not at risk for inadequate nutrition unless there is also a reason the client is not eating. The client who is breast-feeding needs additional calories, but if the client is eating a well-balanced diet with additional calories, the client is not at risk for obtaining inadequate nutrition.

🔑 CN: Physiological adaptation; CL: Analyze

229. 1. PCA is used to manage postoperative or persistent pain. Clients can control the administration of their own medication within predetermined safety limits; there is not a risk of dependence on opioids when using PCAs is not a concern. Family members who are not authorized agents are cautioned not to push the button for the client because this overrides some of the safety features of the PCA system. The nurse retains the responsibility for monitoring the client. Cost is not the primary factor in pain management.

⚿⛀ CN: Pharmacological and parenteral therapies; CL: Evaluate

230. 3. Fluctuation of fluid with respirations in the water seal column indicates that the system is functioning properly. If an obstruction were present in the chest tube, fluid fluctuation would be absent. Subcutaneous emphysema occurs when air pockets can be palpated beneath the client's skin around the chest tube insertion site. A leak in the system is indicated when bubbling occurs in the water seal column.

⚿⛀ CN: Reduction of risk potential; CL: Apply

231. 1, 2, 3. There is a high risk of lactic acidosis when using metformin; 50% of the cases may be fatal. A black box warning for metformin is to instruct the client to stop the drug and immediately notify the prescriber about unexplained hyperventilation, muscle pain, malaise, dizziness, light-headedness, unusual sleepiness, unexplained stomach pain, feelings of coldness, slow or irregular heart rate, or other nonspecific symptoms of early lactic acidosis. Headache, hunger, and tingling in the fingertips are not signs of lactic acidosis.

⚿⛀ CN: Pharmacological and parenteral therapies; CL: Synthesize

232. 1, 2, 4, 5. The electronic health record should contain sufficient information to identify the client, support the diagnosis, justify treatment, document the client's course and results, and facilitate continuity of care among **healthcare providers (HCPs)** 📖. The **medical record** 📖 will facilitate client care, serve as a financial and legal record, aid in clinical research, support decision analysis, and guide professional and organizational performance improvement. The medical record should be compiled concurrently and be completed at the time of discharge. Many disciplines may be authorized to make entries in the medical record. All healthcare personnel will document care on this record. The medical record is not written for clients; if clients need information, the nurse or appropriate healthcare professional can explain the information to them.

⚿⛀ CN: Management of care; CL: Synthesize

233. 4. The only action that keeps the client safe is removal of the gun. If the **HCP** 📖 is considering discharge, the client is medically stable and will not be able to remain in the medical hospital any longer. The client's lack of current suicidal ideation means he cannot be hospitalized for psychiatric reasons. While helpful, the crisis phone line number and the client's promise do not ensure safety.

⚿⛀ CN: Safety and infection control; CL: Analyze

234. 1, 2, 3, 5. Acknowledging the client's concern about pain and expressing the nurse's concern about the client's condition are important to help the client open up and gain further assessment of pain in this client. Awareness of the amount of wine consumption in a week will be helpful to guide which kind of detoxification will be needed. Expressing the nurse's concern about the client's safety is important. How the client is getting the wine is least important because there are so many possibilities, such a weekly shopping trips in the facility van or having friends or family bring it in. Notifying the primary care provider about the situation and arranging for a joint conference are important for the client's safety and recovery.

⚿⛀ CN: Safety and infection control; CL: Apply

235. 4. More than 90% of children have speech that is totally intelligible at 4 years of age. Having one word at 1 year is the expectation. Having three words is a 15-month milestone. Pointing to one body part at 18 months and combining two words at 2 years would be a normal finding.

⚿⛀ CN: Health Promotion and maintenance; CL: Analyze

236. 1. The client with a possible transient ischemic attack is the only client who has not had surgery and is not immunocompromised. The client with a recent surgery and incision should not be exposed to a client with infection. Clients with cancer or alcoholic cirrhosis are very susceptible to infection, and it would not be safe to expose them to a client with a respiratory infection.

⚿⛀ CN: Management of care; CL: Synthesize

This test has 265 questions. Time yourself as you take the test so you can determine the approximate amount of time it takes to complete this many questions. This test reflects the maximum number of questions you may receive on the actual licensing exam.

1. A client returns to the recovery room following left supratentorial surgery for treatment of a brain tumor. The nurse should place the client in which position to facilitate venous drainage?
- ☐ **1.** lying flat without a pillow with the head turned to the right
- ☐ **2.** lying flat with the head elevated on three pillows
- ☐ **3.** head of the bed elevated to 30 degrees with the head in a neutral position
- ☐ **4.** side-lying on the client's left side

2. After a bronchoscopy with biopsy, the nurse assesses the client. The nurse should report which finding to the healthcare provider (HCP)?
- ☐ **1.** green sputum
- ☐ **2.** dry cough
- ☐ **3.** hemoptysis
- ☐ **4.** laryngeal stridor

3. Which activity is **least** effective in preventing sensory deprivation during a client's stay in the cardiac care unit?
- ☐ **1.** watching television
- ☐ **2.** visiting with family
- ☐ **3.** reading the newspaper
- ☐ **4.** keeping the door closed to provide privacy

4. A 57-year-old woman with breast cancer who does not speak English is admitted for a lumpectomy. Her daughter, who speaks English, accompanies her. In order to obtain admission information from the client, what should the nurse do?
- ☐ **1.** Ask the client's daughter to serve as an interpreter.
- ☐ **2.** Ask one of the unlicensed assistive personnel (UAP) to serve as an interpreter.
- ☐ **3.** Use the limited knowledge of the client's language learned in high school along with nonverbal communication.
- ☐ **4.** Obtain a trained medical interpreter.

5. The nurse is assessing a child with suspected juvenile hypothyroidism. Which signs or symptoms should the nurse expect this child to manifest?
- ☐ **1.** short attention span and weight loss
- ☐ **2.** weight loss and flushed skin
- ☐ **3.** rapid pulse and heat intolerance
- ☐ **4.** dry skin and constipation

6. After discussing preconception needs with a nulliparous client who eats a primarily Asian diet, which client statement indicates the need for further instruction?
- ☐ **1.** "I should take folic acid supplements before I get pregnant."
- ☐ **2.** "If I become pregnant, I can continue to eat sushi twice a week."
- ☐ **3.** "I should continue to steam my vegetables rather than cooking them for a long time."
- ☐ **4.** "Eating soy products can increase my protein levels once I am pregnant."

7. A child is receiving amoxicillin for otitis media. Which action should the nurse recommend the mother do when the child develops diarrhea?
- ☐ **1.** Begin clear fluids.
- ☐ **2.** Withhold food and fluids for 2 hours.
- ☐ **3.** Offer yogurt several times a day.
- ☐ **4.** Restrict the intake of pizza.

8. A client fears chemotherapy because of the side effects. What is the nurse's **best** response to the client's concerns?
- ☐ **1.** "Your health has been excellent. It is unlikely that you will experience serious side effects."
- ☐ **2.** "We will give you medications to prevent the side effects, so you should not be too concerned."
- ☐ **3.** "Each person responds differently to chemotherapy treatments. We will monitor your responses closely."
- ☐ **4.** "You may choose not to take the chemotherapy, but you must understand that this will have an adverse effect on the course of your disease."

9. A nurse is caring for a client who has undergone a total laryngectomy for laryngeal cancer. What information is important to include in discharge teaching? Select all that apply.
☐ 1. Provide humidity at home.
☐ 2. Follow a bland diet.
☐ 3. Learn how to suction.
☐ 4. Have communication rehabilitation with a speech pathologist.
☐ 5. Attend a smoking cessation program.

10. The client received electroconvulsive therapy (ECT) an hour ago and now has a headache. Which response by the nurse is **best**?
☐ 1. "A headache is common after ECT."
☐ 2. "I will get some acetaminophen for you."
☐ 3. "A nap will help you feel better."
☐ 4. "Eat your breakfast and then let me know how you feel."

11. The nurse interprets the rhythm strip (see figure) from a client's bedside monitor as:

☐ 1. normal sinus rhythm.
☐ 2. sinus tachycardia.
☐ 3. ventricular tachycardia.
☐ 4. ventricular fibrillation.

12. The nurse is caring for a client who is 12 weeks pregnant and speaks Spanish only. Which interventions should the nurse include in the plan of care at the client's initial visit? Select all that apply.
☐ 1. Provide brochures in the client's native language.
☐ 2. Refer the client to a high-risk clinic.
☐ 3. Discuss cultural differences and emphasize the differences between cultures.
☐ 4. Arrange for an interpreter for her appointments.
☐ 5. Discuss contraception and options.
☐ 6. Review dietary intake and discuss nutrition.

13. When assessing speech development, which child should the nurse refer for further examination?
☐ 1. a 4-month-old who laughs out loud
☐ 2. a 10-month-old who says "dada" and "mama"
☐ 3. a 1-year-old who says three to five words
☐ 4. an 18-month-old who only says "no"

14. The client is started on simvastatin as a component of cholesterol management. Which laboratory test needs to be monitored while on this therapy?
☐ 1. complete blood count
☐ 2. serum glucose
☐ 3. total protein
☐ 4. liver function tests

15. A family has taken home their newborn and later received a call from the child's healthcare provider (HCP) that the phenylketonuria (PKU) levels for their newborn daughter are abnormally high. Additional testing confirmed the diagnosis of phenylketonuria. The parents refuse to believe the results as no one else in their family has the disease. The nurse explains that the disease:
☐ 1. is carried on recessive genes contributed by each parent.
☐ 2. is caused by a recessive gene contributed by either parent.
☐ 3. is cured by eliminating dietary protein for this child.
☐ 4. will not impact future childbearing for the family.

16. During a postpartum examination, the mother of a 2-week-old infant tearfully tells the nurse she feels very tired and thinks she is not a good mother to her baby. Which statement by the nurse would be **best**?
☐ 1. "The hormonal changes your body is experiencing are causing you to feel this way."
☐ 2. "Most new mothers feel the same way that you do. I hear that a lot from others."
☐ 3. "You need to have your husband and family help you so that you can get some rest."
☐ 4. "I am concerned about what you are experiencing. Tell me more about what you are thinking and feeling."

17. The nurse is caring for a client who has severe burns on the head, neck, trunk, and groin areas. Which position would be **most** appropriate for preventing contractures?
☐ 1. high Fowler's
☐ 2. semi-Fowler's
☐ 3. prone
☐ 4. supine

18. After transurethral resection of the prostate, the nurse notices that the client's urine is bright red, has numerous clots, and is viscous. Which nursing action is **most** appropriate?
☐ 1. Irrigate the catheter to remove clots.
☐ 2. Milk the catheter tube vigorously.
☐ 3. Increase the client's fluid intake.
☐ 4. Assess vital signs and notify the surgeon.

19. A client is to receive 2 g of metronidazole orally in a single dose. The medication is available in 500-mg tablets. How many tablets should the nurse administer? Record your answer using a whole number.

_____ tablets.

20. A client asks the nurse to help make out a will. The nurse should tell the client:
- [ ] 1. "I am not a lawyer, but I will do what I can for you."
- [ ] 2. "You have a long way to go before you will need to do that. Let us wait on it a while, shall we?"
- [ ] 3. "I do not believe in getting involved in legal matters, but maybe I can find another nurse who will help you."
- [ ] 4. "You need to consult an attorney because I am not trained in such matters. Is there a family lawyer you can call?"

21. After vaginal birth of a term neonate, the nurse determines that the placenta is about to separate when which occurs?
- [ ] 1. The uterus becomes oval shaped.
- [ ] 2. The uterus enlarges.
- [ ] 3. A sudden gush of dark blood occurs.
- [ ] 4. The client expends efforts pushing.

22. When preparing to present a community program about women who are victims of physical abuse, which should the nurse stress about the incidence of battering?
- [ ] 1. Death from battering is rare.
- [ ] 2. Battering is a major cause of injury to women.
- [ ] 3. Lower socioeconomic groups are primarily affected.
- [ ] 4. Physical abuse typically begins early in a relationship well before a woman gets pregnant.

23. A college student is asking the nurse about the student's grandfather, who just received a diagnosis of Huntington's disease. The student wants to know if the student will have the disease too. What should the nurse tell the student? Select all that apply.
- [ ] 1. "Huntington's disease affects men more than women."
- [ ] 2. "Huntington's disease is an autosomal dominant disease."
- [ ] 3. "Huntington's disease does not skip a generation."
- [ ] 4. "Huntington's disease is a treatable disease."
- [ ] 5. "There is a 75% chance you will have the disease."

24. The nurse notices drops of a liquid on the hallway floor of a healthcare facility. What should the nurse do **first**?
- [ ] 1. Place paper towels over the drops of liquid.
- [ ] 2. Don clean gloves and wipe up the drops of liquid.
- [ ] 3. Post "wet floor" signs around the area.
- [ ] 4. Call the Environmental Services Department.

25. A client is admitted with numbness and tingling of the feet and toes after having an upper respiratory infection and flu for the past 5 days. Within 1 hour of admission, the client's legs are numb all the way up to the hips. What should the nurse do **next**? Select all that apply.
- [ ] 1. Call the family to come in to visit.
- [ ] 2. Notify the healthcare provider (HCP) of the change.
- [ ] 3. Place respiratory resuscitation equipment in the client's room.
- [ ] 4. Check for advancing levels of paresthesia.
- [ ] 5. Have the client perform ankle pumps.

26. When assessing a client with heart failure, the nurse should report which findings to the healthcare provider (HCP)? Select all that apply.
- [ ] 1. bibasilar crackles
- [ ] 2. blood pressure 108/62 mm Hg, heart rate 88 beats/minute
- [ ] 3. O_2 saturation 94% on room air
- [ ] 4. 2-lb (0.9-kg) weight gain in 5 days
- [ ] 5. urine output of 20 mL/h
- [ ] 6. confusion

27. The nurse is caring for a client with an injury to the thalamus. The nurse should plan to:
- [ ] 1. give higher doses of pain medication.
- [ ] 2. keep patches on the client's eyes to prevent corneal abrasion.
- [ ] 3. monitor the temperature of the bathwater.
- [ ] 4. avoid turning the client.

28. A client with paranoia is having a delusion. While the client is having the delusion, what nursing intervention is **most** indicated?
- [ ] 1. Assist the client to relieve anxiety.
- [ ] 2. Ask the client what is causing the feelings of anxiety.
- [ ] 3. Present reality when the client asks about the delusion.
- [ ] 4. Allow the client to express anger and intense emotions in appropriate ways.

29. When explaining to a pregnant client about the need to take supplemental vitamins with iron during her pregnancy, the nurse should instruct the client to take the iron with which liquid to promote maximum absorption?
- [ ] 1. milk
- [ ] 2. tea
- [ ] 3. hot chocolate
- [ ] 4. orange juice

30. A client with major depression is completing his morning care independently. When the nurse approaches the client with his medication, he tells the nurse that he is a failure as a husband and a father and is worthless. His wife told the nurse previously that the client is a good provider and a wonderful father and husband. Which response by the nurse is **most** appropriate?
- [ ] 1. "You were able to shower and dress without help this morning."
- [ ] 2. "Your wife told me that you are a good husband and father."
- [ ] 3. "You do not have any reason why you should feel that way."
- [ ] 4. "This medication will help your thinking."

31. The nurse is reviewing laboratory values of a client receiving clozapine. Which laboratory value should the nurse report to the healthcare provider (HCP)?
- [ ] 1. WBC of 3,500/μL (3.5×10^9/L)
- [ ] 2. hemoglobin of 8.2 g/dL (82 g/L)
- [ ] 3. sodium level of 136 mEq/L (136 mmol/L)
- [ ] 4. hyaline casts in the urinalysis

32. Four hours after a cast has been applied for a fractured ulna, the nurse assesses that the client's fingers are pale and cool and capillary refill is delayed for 4 seconds. How should the nurse interpret these findings?
- [ ] 1. Nerve impairment is developing in the fingers.
- [ ] 2. Arterial blood supply to the fingers is decreased.
- [ ] 3. Venous stasis is occurring in the fingers.
- [ ] 4. The finding is normal for this recovery period.

33. The nurse is planning care for a client who has sustained a spinal cord injury. The nurse should assess the client for:
- [ ] 1. anesthesia below the level of the injury.
- [ ] 2. tingling in the fingers.
- [ ] 3. pain below the site of the injury.
- [ ] 4. loss of vibratory sense.

34. A client who is paraplegic cannot feel the lower extremities and has been positioned on the side. The nurse should inspect which area that is a potential pressure point when the client is in this position?
- [ ] 1. sacrum
- [ ] 2. occiput
- [ ] 3. ankles
- [ ] 4. heels

35. Which interventions are appropriate when developing a plan of care for promoting the development of a preschooler? Select all that apply.
- [ ] 1. Provide anticipatory guidance for parents.
- [ ] 2. Help the parents understand their child's behavior.
- [ ] 3. Identify deviations from normal growth and development patterns.
- [ ] 4. Determine the child's future development.
- [ ] 5. Send the child to a day care center.

36. A child who is 15 years of age is hospitalized with acute glomerulonephritis. The nurse is reviewing the client's urine chemistry laboratory reports as noted below.

Laboratory Results	
Test	**Result**
Urine specific gravity	1.035 (1.035)
Protein	12 mg/24 h (120 mg/d)
Potassium	35 mEq/24 h (35 mmol/d)
Creatinine	2 mg/24 h (17.6 mmol/d)

Which finding does the nurse draw to the attention of the healthcare provider (HCP)?
- [ ] 1. urine specific gravity
- [ ] 2. protein
- [ ] 3. potassium
- [ ] 4. creatinine

37. A client is exhibiting pressured speech, a labile affect, euphoria, and hyperactivity. The client states, "I am the savior of the city." The family states that the client has hardly slept or eaten for days. Which client need is a **priority** in the nurse's plan of care?
- [ ] 1. physical
- [ ] 2. social
- [ ] 3. spiritual
- [ ] 4. cultural

38. When assessing a neonate's temperature with a disposable digital thermometer, in which location should the nurse place the thermometer?
- [ ] 1. under the neonate's tongue
- [ ] 2. under the neonate's arm
- [ ] 3. into the neonate's rectum
- [ ] 4. into the neonate's ear

39. A neonate is receiving an IV infusion of dextrose 10% administered by an infusion pump. The nurse should verify the alarm settings on the infusion pump at which times? Select all that apply.
- [ ] 1. when the infusion is started
- [ ] 2. at the beginning of each shift
- [ ] 3. when the neonate returns from x-ray
- [ ] 4. when the neonate moves in the crib
- [ ] 5. after the parents have visited

40. A coworker confides in the nurse that she had been a lifelong friend of a client who committed suicide. The coworker states: "We just saw each other last week. I cannot believe she tried to kill herself. She told me she wanted to give me her expensive necklace because our friendship meant so much to her. She seemed really happy and content. I knew she had been feeling down the last few months. I should have known that something was wrong; I should have asked her about suicide." The nurse determines the coworker is **most** likely experiencing:
☐ **1.** secondary traumatic stress.
☐ **2.** a boundary violation.
☐ **3.** compassion fatigue.
☐ **4.** moral distress.

41. The nurse is caring for a critically ill client with the client's mother and spouse in the room. The spouse begins to shout derogatory comments to the mother, blaming her for her spouse's critical state. What should the nurse do?
☐ **1.** Try to calm both the mother and spouse by speaking in a soft voice.
☐ **2.** Step between the mother and spouse stating emphatically, "Stop!"
☐ **3.** Call the hospital Security Department.
☐ **4.** Report the details immediately to the supervisor.

42. The nurse walks into the room and finds that a client who has just had surgery is diaphoretic, appears to have no respirations, and has a barely palpable pulse. The nurse should **first**:
☐ **1.** call a code.
☐ **2.** open the airway.
☐ **3.** start rescue breathing.
☐ **4.** start cardiac compressions.

43. The nurse is planning care for a neonate to prevent neonatal heat loss immediately after birth. To conserve heat and help the infant maintain a stable temperature, the nurse should:
☐ **1.** nestle the neonate against the crib wall.
☐ **2.** place the infant skin to skin with the mother.
☐ **3.** bathe the neonate with warm water.
☐ **4.** position the neonate lying in an open crib with a diaper on.

44. The nurse observes that the client's right eye does not close completely. Based on this finding, what should the nurse do?
☐ **1.** Have the client wear eyeglasses at all times.
☐ **2.** Place an eye patch over the right eye.
☐ **3.** Instill artificial tears once a day.
☐ **4.** Cleanse the eye with a clean washcloth every shift.

45. A mother tells the nurse that she wants her 4-year-old to stop sucking her thumb. When developing the teaching plan, which intervention should the nurse suggest?
☐ **1.** Apply a special medicine that tastes terrible on the thumb.
☐ **2.** Get the child to agree to stop the thumb-sucking.
☐ **3.** Remind the child every time the mother sees the thumb in her mouth.
☐ **4.** Put the child in time-out every time the mother observes thumb-sucking.

46. The nurse is administering an intramuscular injection to an infant. Indicate the appropriate site for this injection.

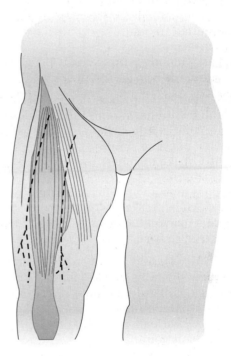

47. A 14-year-old with rheumatic fever who is on bed rest is receiving an IV infusion of dextrose 5% administered by an infusion pump. The nurse should verify the alarm settings on the infusion pump at which times? Select all that apply.
☐ **1.** when the infusion is started
☐ **2.** at the beginning of each shift
☐ **3.** when the child returns from x-ray
☐ **4.** when the child moves in the bed
☐ **5.** when the child is sleeping

48. A primigravid client at 26 weeks' gestation visits the clinic and tells the nurse that her lower back aches when she arrives home from work. The nurse should suggest that the client perform which exercise?
☐ **1.** tailor sitting
☐ **2.** leg lifting
☐ **3.** shoulder circling
☐ **4.** squatting

49. A client with diabetes is explaining to the nurse how to care for the feet at home. Which statement indicates that the client understands proper foot care?
- ☐ 1. "When I injure my toe, I will plan to put iodine on it."
- ☐ 2. "I should inspect my feet at least once a week."
- ☐ 3. "It is okay to go barefoot in the house."
- ☐ 4. "It is important to dry my feet carefully after my bath."

50. A nurse is assessing a client who has a potential diagnosis of pancreatitis. Which risk factors predispose the client to pancreatitis? Select all that apply.
- ☐ 1. excessive alcohol use
- ☐ 2. gallstones
- ☐ 3. abdominal trauma
- ☐ 4. hypertension
- ☐ 5. hyperlipidemia with excessive triglycerides
- ☐ 6. hypothyroidism

51. When performing chest percussion on a child, which technique should the nurse use?
- ☐ 1. Firmly but gently strike the chest wall to make a popping sound.
- ☐ 2. Gently strike the chest wall to make a slapping sound.
- ☐ 3. Percuss over an area from the umbilicus to the clavicle.
- ☐ 4. Place a blanket between the nurse's hand and the child's chest.

52. The nurse should assess an older adult who has diminished hearing and vision for:
- ☐ 1. feelings of disorientation.
- ☐ 2. cognitive impairment.
- ☐ 3. sensory overload.
- ☐ 4. social isolation.

53. Which child should be referred for further assessment regarding language development?
- ☐ 1. a 2-year-old who has a vocabulary of 300 words and can combine two or three words in a phrase
- ☐ 2. a 3-year-old who has a vocabulary of 900 words and can make a complete sentence of three or four words
- ☐ 3. a 4-year-old whose speech is understood 50% of the time
- ☐ 4. a 1-year-old who has a vocabulary of eight words and can say "mommy" and "daddy" with specific reference to the correct person

54. To prevent development of peripheral neuropathies associated with isoniazid administration, the nurse should teach the client to:
- ☐ 1. avoid excessive sun exposure.
- ☐ 2. follow a low-cholesterol diet.
- ☐ 3. obtain extra rest.
- ☐ 4. supplement the diet with pyridoxine (vitamin B_6).

55. The healthcare provider (HCP) has prescribed nitroglycerin to a client with angina. The client also has closed-angle glaucoma. The nurse contacts the HCP to discuss the potential for:
- ☐ 1. decreased intraocular pressure.
- ☐ 2. increased intraocular pressure.
- ☐ 3. hypotension.
- ☐ 4. hypertension.

56. A nurse is taking a medication history on a client with multiple sclerosis before administering an initial dose of baclofen. What should the nurse check **before** administering the drug? Select all that apply.
- ☐ 1. presence of muscle weakness
- ☐ 2. history of muscle spasms
- ☐ 3. serum creatinine level
- ☐ 4. serum potassium level
- ☐ 5. blood glucose

57. A client has been taking carbamazepine for 2 years. What should the nurse assess the client for? Select all that apply.
- ☐ 1. bruising
- ☐ 2. sore throat
- ☐ 3. urine retention
- ☐ 4. light-colored stool
- ☐ 5. hydration status

58. The nurse should assess the client with severe diarrhea for which acid-base imbalance?
- ☐ 1. respiratory acidosis
- ☐ 2. respiratory alkalosis
- ☐ 3. metabolic acidosis
- ☐ 4. metabolic alkalosis

59. A nurse is planning care for a client who has heart failure. Which goal is appropriate for a client with excess fluid volume?
- ☐ 1. A weight reduction of 20% will occur.
- ☐ 2. Pain will be controlled effectively.
- ☐ 3. Arterial blood gas values will be within normal limits.
- ☐ 4. Serum osmolality will be within normal limits.

60. A 7-year-old child is admitted to the hospital with the diagnosis of acute rheumatic fever. Which laboratory blood finding confirms that the child has had a streptococcal infection?
- ☐ 1. high leukocyte count
- ☐ 2. low hemoglobin count
- ☐ 3. elevated antibody concentration
- ☐ 4. low erythrocyte sedimentation rate

61. A 12-year-old client says, "Give me my pajamas. I am not putting your silly gown on." An appropriate response by the nurse should be:
- ☐ 1. "I know they are funny, but everyone here wears them."
- ☐ 2. "You do not mean that, now. A big guy like you knows how hospitals are."
- ☐ 3. "You are upset because you feel awkward and embarrassed in these gowns."
- ☐ 4. "You are upset because you think we are unreasonable."

62. After teaching the parents of a 15-month-old child who has undergone cleft palate repair how to use elbow restraints, which statement by the parents indicates effective teaching?
- ☐ **1.** "We will keep the restraints in place continuously until our healthcare provider (HCP) says it is okay to remove them."
- ☐ **2.** "We can take off the restraints while our child is playing, but we will make sure to put them back on at night."
- ☐ **3.** "The restraints should be taped directly to our child's arms so that they will stay in one place."
- ☐ **4.** "We will remove the restraints temporarily at least three times a day to check his skin, then put them right back on."

63. The nurse notes that a client is too busy investigating the unit and overseeing the activities of other clients to eat dinner. To help the client obtain sufficient nourishment, which plan would be **best**?
- ☐ **1.** Serve foods that she can carry with her.
- ☐ **2.** Allow her to send out for her favorite foods.
- ☐ **3.** Serve food in small, attractively arranged portions.
- ☐ **4.** Allow her to enter the unit kitchen for extra food as necessary.

64. The nurse should encourage women to have a "Pap test" (Papanicolaou smear) to: (Select all that apply.)
- ☐ **1.** detect precancerous and cancerous cells of the uterus.
- ☐ **2.** assess the effects of sex hormonal replacement.
- ☐ **3.** identify viral, fungal, and parasitic conditions.
- ☐ **4.** evaluate the response to chemotherapy or radiation therapy to the cervix.
- ☐ **5.** determine a diminished blood flow to the perineal mucous membrane.

65. The nurse is administering prednisone to a preschool child with nephrosis. What should the nurse do to ensure that the nurse has identified the child correctly? Select all that apply.
- ☐ **1.** Ask another nurse to confirm that this is the correct dose and correct client for whom the prednisone has been prescribed.
- ☐ **2.** Check the child's identification band against the medical record number.
- ☐ **3.** Verify the date of birth from the medical record with the date of birth on the client's identification band.
- ☐ **4.** Compare the room number on the bed with the number on the client's identification band.
- ☐ **5.** Ask the client to state the first name.

66. A client is scheduled to have surgery to relieve an intestinal obstruction. Prior to surgery, the nurse should verify that the client has:
- ☐ **1.** discontinued use of blood thinners.
- ☐ **2.** followed a low-residue diet.
- ☐ **3.** practiced abdominal muscle strengthening exercises.
- ☐ **4.** signed a last will and testament.

67. After teaching a client about collecting a stool sample for occult testing, which client statement indicates effective teaching? Select all that apply.
- ☐ **1.** "I will avoid eating meat for 1 to 3 days before getting a stool sample."
- ☐ **2.** "I need to eat foods low in fiber a few days before collecting the sample."
- ☐ **3.** "I will take the sample from different areas of the stool that I have passed."
- ☐ **4.** "I need to send the stool sample to the lab in a covered container right away."
- ☐ **5.** "I can continue to take all of my regular medications at home."

68. The nurse is preparing to administer propranolol to a client for control of migraine headaches. The client also has a prescription for sumatriptan as needed for a headache. The client's pulse rate is 56 bpm. What should the nurse do **next**?
- ☐ **1.** Contact the healthcare provider (HCP).
- ☐ **2.** Assess blood pressure.
- ☐ **3.** Administer oxygen.
- ☐ **4.** Administer sumatriptan.

69. A client with a history of type 1 diabetes mellitus and chronic obstructive pulmonary disease should have which immunization?
- ☐ **1.** influenza
- ☐ **2.** hepatitis A
- ☐ **3.** measles-mumps-rubella
- ☐ **4.** varicella

70. The mother of a toddler diagnosed with iron deficiency anemia asks what foods she should give her child. The nurse should evaluate the teaching as successful when the mother later reports that she feeds the toddler which foods?
- ☐ **1.** milk, carrots, and beef
- ☐ **2.** raisins, chicken, and spinach
- ☐ **3.** beef, lettuce, and juice
- ☐ **4.** eggs, cheese, and milk

71. When a child is able to grasp the idea that a ball continues to exist even though the child's parent placed the ball under a hat, the child is in which stage in the development of logical thinking according to Piaget?
- ☐ **1.** sensorimotor
- ☐ **2.** preoperational
- ☐ **3.** concrete operations
- ☐ **4.** formal operations

72. A nurse discusses with parents the procedures that will be performed on their neonate immediately after birth. The nurse determines that the instructions have been understood when the parent states that which procedure will be done to the neonate **first**?
- ☐ **1.** The neonate will be suctioned.
- ☐ **2.** The neonate will be dried and stimulated to cry.
- ☐ **3.** The neonate will be given oxygen.
- ☐ **4.** The neonate's umbilical cord will be cut.

73. An infusion of lidocaine hydrochloride is running at 30 mL/h. The dilution is 1,000 mg/250 mL. What dosage is the client receiving per minute? Record your answer using a whole number.

_____ mg/min.

74. A mother tells a nurse that her child has been exposed to roseola. After teaching the mother about the illness, which finding, if stated by the mother as the **most** characteristic sign of roseola, indicates successful teaching?
☐ **1.** fever and sore throat
☐ **2.** normal temperature followed by a low-grade fever
☐ **3.** high fever followed by a drop and then a rash
☐ **4.** cold-like signs and symptoms and a rash

75. A nurse is instructing a client about using nitroglycerin patches in order to prevent tolerance to the drug. The nurse should instruct the client to:
☐ **1.** remove the patch every night.
☐ **2.** use the patch only when chest pain occurs.
☐ **3.** change the site of the patch every day.
☐ **4.** apply the patch only on alternate days.

76. A client's abdominal incision eviscerates. The nurse should **first**:
☐ **1.** take the client's vital signs and call the healthcare provider (HCP).
☐ **2.** lower the client's head and elevate the feet.
☐ **3.** cover the incision with a dressing moistened with sterile normal saline solution.
☐ **4.** start an emergency infusion of IV fluids.

77. The nursing staff has safely and successfully secluded and restrained a client with acute mania who threatened the nurse and threw a chair against the wall in the community room. Which statement by the nurse is **most** helpful to the client at this time?
☐ **1.** "Threatening others and throwing furniture is not allowed."
☐ **2.** "You have been restrained until you can manage your behavior."
☐ **3.** "Since you have been here before, you know what the rules are."
☐ **4.** "We are only doing this for your own good, so calm down."

78. At what time should the blood be drawn in relation to the administration of the IV dose of gentamicin sulfate?
☐ **1.** 2 hours before the administration of the next IV dose
☐ **2.** 3 hours before the administration of the next IV dose
☐ **3.** 4 hours before the administration of the next IV dose
☐ **4.** just before the administration of the next IV dose

79. A client is taking 600 mg of valproic acid twice daily. The nurse should assess the client for which adverse effects? Select all that apply.
☐ **1.** tremors
☐ **2.** hair loss
☐ **3.** gastrointestinal upset
☐ **4.** anorexia
☐ **5.** weight gain

80. A client has a cerclage placed at 16 weeks' gestation. She has had no contractions, and her cervix is dilated 2 cm. The nurse is preparing the client for discharge. Which statement by the client should indicate to the nurse that the client needs further instruction?
☐ **1.** "I will need more frequent prenatal visits."
☐ **2.** "I should call if I am leaking fluid or have bleeding or contractions."
☐ **3.** "I can have sex again in about 2 weeks."
☐ **4.** "I can have nothing in my vagina until I am at term."

81. The nurse is admitting a 4-year-old with a possible meningococcal infection. Which type of isolation is indicated?
☐ **1.** airborne precautions
☐ **2.** contact precautions
☐ **3.** droplet precautions
☐ **4.** standard precautions

82. While preparing to administer medications to a client, the nurse compares the medication in the medication box with the healthcare provider's (HCP) prescriptions and discovers that the HCP has prescribed prednisone 15 mg PO for a client with cirrhosis and the medication in the client's medication box is prednisolone 5 mg. What should the nurse do **next**?
☐ **1.** Call the pharmacy for prednisone 15 mg.
☐ **2.** Notify the charge nurse or supervisor.
☐ **3.** Call the HCP for clarification.
☐ **4.** Contact the pharmacy about the discrepancy.

83. A parent calls the clinic after her 4-year-old choked on a peanut. The parent reports performing abdominal thrusts and the child is breathing normally now. The nurse should tell the parent to:
☐ **1.** bring the child to the emergency department to check for airway obstruction.
☐ **2.** test the child's urine for blood from internal bleeding.
☐ **3.** call the healthcare provider (HCP) if the child begins to sweat and feels dizzy.
☐ **4.** observe the child for difficulty breathing because the abdominal thrusts may have caused a pneumothorax.

84. A client is taking nonsteroidal anti-inflammatory drugs (NSAIDs) to manage pain from rheumatoid arthritis. What instruction should the nurse give the client about NSAIDs?
☐ **1.** Take the prescribed medication with food and fluids.
☐ **2.** Gradually decrease the medication dosage.
☐ **3.** Rinse the mouth with water after taking NSAIDs.
☐ **4.** Avoid driving and using machinery while taking NSAIDs.

85. The nurse is assessing a neonate at 5 minutes after birth. The nurse records the Apgar score based on the findings in the chart below.

Flow Sheets

Apgar at 5 Minutes After Birth	
Heart rate	100 bpm
Respirations	Irregular
Color	Pink
Muscle tone	Moving all four extremities
Reflexes	Cough

The nurse compares these findings to the Apgar score obtained at birth, as determined by the findings in the chart below.

Flow Sheets

Apgar at Birth	
Heart rate	120 bpm
Respirations	Slow
Color	Blue extremities
Muscle tone	Flexion of extremities
Reflexes	Grimace

What should the nurse do **next**?
☐ **1.** Notify the neonatologist on call.
☐ **2.** Continue to assess the neonate.
☐ **3.** Apply an oxygen mask.
☐ **4.** Rub the neonate's extremities.

86. It is important for nurses to communicate with clients about their health care because:
☐ **1.** consumers of health care cannot keep up with rapid advances in science.
☐ **2.** healthcare services are often specialized and fragmented.
☐ **3.** the media provides misleading information.
☐ **4.** clients are more demanding that their rights be respected.

87. The nurse should assess a newborn with esophageal atresia and tracheoesophageal fistula (TEF) for which complications? Select all that apply.
☐ **1.** copious frothy mucus
☐ **2.** episodes of cyanosis
☐ **3.** several loose stools
☐ **4.** initial weight loss
☐ **5.** poor gag reflex

88. When developing a teaching plan for a client with an infected decubitus ulcer, the nurse should tell the client that which factor is **most** important for healing?
☐ **1.** adequate circulatory status
☐ **2.** scheduled periods of rest
☐ **3.** balanced nutritional diet
☐ **4.** fluid intake of 1,500 mL/day

89. The **most** appropriate toys to give to a 5-month-old infant are:
☐ **1.** plastic toy cars.
☐ **2.** wooden puzzles.
☐ **3.** stuffed animals.
☐ **4.** soft, washable toys.

90. One staff member in a psychiatric unit says to the nurse, "Why are we carrying out suicide precautions for someone who is dying? It is pointless and a waste of time." The nurse should:
☐ **1.** assign the staff member to other clients.
☐ **2.** ask the psychiatric clinical nurse specialist to meet with the staff member.
☐ **3.** agree with the staff member and discontinue suicide precautions.
☐ **4.** call for a multidisciplinary staff meeting.

91. The nurse reviews the client's laboratory report to determine the client's blood level of valproic acid, which is 35 mcg/mL (243 µmol/L). Based on this report, what should the nurse do **first**?
☐ **1.** Withhold the next dose of valproic acid.
☐ **2.** Notify the healthcare provider (HCP).
☐ **3.** Give the next dose as prescribed.
☐ **4.** Take the client's vital signs.

92. After 2 days on a psychiatric unit, a client is still isolating himself in his room, except for meals. The client says he is uncomfortable around crowds of people. Which nursing intervention is the **most** appropriate initially?
☐ **1.** Play a game of checkers with the client in his room.
☐ **2.** Ask the client to attend a group session with the nurse.
☐ **3.** Invite the client to go for a walk with the nurse and one other client.
☐ **4.** Talk with the client in a corner of the crafts room.

93. A nurse is caring for a woman who gave birth to a term neonate at 0600. At 1600, the woman has a distended bladder and is reporting pain of 5 on a scale of 1 to 10. The nurse reviews the client's output record.

Intake and Output

Output Record

Time	0800	1000	1100	1600
	30 mL	50 mL	30 mL	60 mL

What should the nurse do **first**?
- ☐ 1. Apply a warm, moist towel over the bladder.
- ☐ 2. Ask the woman to sit on the toilet while the nurse runs water from the faucet.
- ☐ 3. Administer acetaminophen with codeine.
- ☐ 4. Use an in-and-out catheter to empty the bladder.

94. The nurse observes that a client with a history of panic attacks is hyperventilating. The nurse should:
- ☐ 1. have the client breathe into a paper bag.
- ☐ 2. instruct the client to put his head between his knees.
- ☐ 3. give the client a low concentration of oxygen by nasal cannula.
- ☐ 4. tell the client to take several deep, slow breaths and exhale normally.

95. A client at 40+ weeks' gestation visits the emergency department because she thinks she is in labor. Which is the **best** indication that the client is in true labor?
- ☐ 1. fetal descent into the pelvic inlet
- ☐ 2. cervical dilation and effacement
- ☐ 3. painful contractions every 3 to 5 minutes
- ☐ 4. leaking amniotic fluid clear in color

96. The father of a 3-week-old infant who has developed sepsis says that he feels guilty because he did not realize his infant was sick. Which response by the nurse would be **most** appropriate?
- ☐ 1. "You should have realized something was wrong; he is your son."
- ☐ 2. "Did you read the booklet on newborns that was sent home with you from the hospital?"
- ☐ 3. "What you are feeling is normal; next time, you will know what to look for."
- ☐ 4. "Babies can get sick quickly, and parents do not always realize it."

97. A mother brings a 15-month-old child to the well-baby clinic. She states the child has been taking approximately 18 to 20 oz (540 to 600 mL) of whole milk per day from a bottle with meals and at bedtime. The nurse should suggest that she begin weaning the child from the bottle to avoid risking:
- ☐ 1. malnutrition.
- ☐ 2. anemia.
- ☐ 3. dental caries.
- ☐ 4. malocclusion.

98. The registered nurse (RN) is teamed with a licensed practical/vocational nurse (LPN/VN) in caring for a group of cardiac clients on a pediatric unit. Which action by the LPN/VN indicates the nurse should intervene immediately?
- ☐ 1. The LPN/VN assists a child to the bathroom 2 hours after a cardiac catheterization.
- ☐ 2. The LPN/VN places an infant having a cyanotic episode in a knee-chest position.
- ☐ 3. The LPN/VN checks a child's apical heart rate prior to administering digoxin.
- ☐ 4. The LPN/VN brings breakfast to a child who is scheduled for an electrocardiogram.

99. A client is taking vancomycin. The nurse should report which possible side effect to the healthcare provider (HCP)?
- ☐ 1. vertigo
- ☐ 2. tinnitus
- ☐ 3. muscle stiffness
- ☐ 4. ataxia

100. The nurse hears a pregnant client yell, "Oh my! The baby is coming!" After placing the client in a supine position and trying to maintain some privacy, the nurse sees that the neonate's head is being born. What should the nurse do **first**?
- ☐ 1. Suction the mouth with two fingertips.
- ☐ 2. Check for presence of a cord around the neck.
- ☐ 3. Tell the client to bear down with force.
- ☐ 4. Advise the mother that help is on the way.

101. Which goal is a **priority** after surgical repair of a cleft lip?
- ☐ 1. Manage pain.
- ☐ 2. Prevent infection.
- ☐ 3. Increase mobility.
- ☐ 4. Develop parenting skills.

102. A client with heart failure is given a prescription for torsemide. Two days after the drug therapy is started, the nurse evaluates the torsemide as effective when the client:
- ☐ 1. has an improved appetite and is eating better.
- ☐ 2. weighs 7 lb (3 kg) less than the client did 2 days ago.
- ☐ 3. is less thirsty than before the drug therapy.
- ☐ 4. has clearer urine since starting torsemide.

103. Which technique is correct when the nurse is inserting a rectal suppository for an adult client?
- [ ] 1. Insert the suppository while the client bears down.
- [ ] 2. Place the client in a supine position.
- [ ] 3. Position the suppository along the rectal wall.
- [ ] 4. Insert the suppository 2 inches (8 to 10 cm) into the rectum.

104. In caring for the client with hepatitis B, which situation would expose the nurse to the virus?
- [ ] 1. contact with fecal material
- [ ] 2. a blood splash into the nurse's eyes
- [ ] 3. touching the client's arm with ungloved hands while taking a blood pressure
- [ ] 4. disposing of syringes and needles without recapping

105. A young woman is brought from the emergency department (ED) to the psychiatric unit. ED staff report that she is not answering questions and has been sitting in the same position in the wheelchair for 45 minutes. When her arm was extended to draw blood, she did not move her arm back to a natural position. The client's brother says he found her this way yesterday and could not get her to move on her own. Which nursing interventions have a **high priority** in this case? Select all that apply.
- [ ] 1. Ask her to describe her stressors.
- [ ] 2. Monitor her body positions to prevent injury.
- [ ] 3. Offer her nutritional shakes every 3 hours.
- [ ] 4. Encourage her to talk about her feelings.
- [ ] 5. Assist her to the bathroom every 2 hours.
- [ ] 6. Protect her from intrusions by other clients.

106. The nurse is assessing a group of children in a day care center. Which child warrants further assessment?
- [ ] 1. a child who is 12 months of age who has bruises on one side of the head
- [ ] 2. a child who is 3 years of age with a spiral fracture of the ulna whose mother does not know how the injury occurred
- [ ] 3. a child who is 4 years of age who wears the same clothes to the center every day
- [ ] 4. a child who is 2 years of age who has frequent episodes of untreated conjunctivitis

107. A client who had a total hip placement at 0900 is receiving an autologous blood transfusion that was started at 1100. At the change of shift (1500), the nurse working on the day shift reports that there is 50 mL of the unit of blood remaining to be infused. Which is a **priority** action for the nurse working on the evening shift?
- [ ] 1. Keep the blood transfusing at the same rate.
- [ ] 2. Increase the rate so it will infuse by 1600.
- [ ] 3. Discontinue the blood transfusion at the beginning of the shift.
- [ ] 4. Maintain the current rate, and discontinue the blood transfusion at 1700.

108. A client undergoes a nephrectomy. In the immediate postoperative period, which nursing intervention has the **highest priority**?
- [ ] 1. Monitor blood pressure.
- [ ] 2. Encourage the use of the incentive spirometer.
- [ ] 3. Assess urine output hourly.
- [ ] 4. Check the flank dressing for urine drainage.

109. A client is admitted with fatigue, shortness of breath, pale skin, and dried, cracked lips, tongue, and mouth. The hemoglobin is 9 g/dL (90 g/L), and red blood cell count is 3.5 million cells/mm³ (3.5×10^{12}/L). The nurse should instruct the client to:
- [ ] 1. eat foods with good sources of iron.
- [ ] 2. limit fluid intake to 1,000 mL/day.
- [ ] 3. increase the amount of carbohydrates in the diet.
- [ ] 4. eat a serving of fish with high omega 3 content two times a week.

110. When assessing a neonate 1 hour after birth, the nurse observes that the neonate exhibits slight cyanosis when quiet but becomes pink when crying. The nurse is unable to pass a catheter through the left nostril. The nurse notifies the healthcare provider (HCP) because the neonate **most** likely is exhibiting signs and symptoms of what problem?
- [ ] 1. esophageal reflux disorder
- [ ] 2. unilateral choanal atresia
- [ ] 3. respiratory distress syndrome
- [ ] 4. tracheoesophageal fistula

111. A client is receiving digoxin, and the pulse range is normally 70 to 76 bpm. After assessing the apical pulse for 1 minute and finding it to be 60 bpm, the nurse should **first**:
- [ ] 1. notify the healthcare provider (HCP).
- [ ] 2. withhold the digoxin.
- [ ] 3. administer the digoxin.
- [ ] 4. notify the charge nurse.

112. When developing a teaching plan for parents of toddlers about poisonous substances, the nurse should emphasize which safety points? Select all that apply.
- [ ] 1. Toddlers should be adequately supervised at all times.
- [ ] 2. All poisonous substances should be kept out of the reach of children and stored in a locked cabinet if necessary.
- [ ] 3. The difference between pediatric and adult dosages of medicines is significant, and adult dosages given to children can have serious, harmful effects.
- [ ] 4. Syrup of ipecac should be administered following all ingestions of poisonous substances.
- [ ] 5. Following any poisoning, the parents should call the Poison Control Center for instructions for appropriate treatment.

113. A client on a psychiatric care unit has muscle spasms in the neck and stiffness in other muscles, and the eyes are rolling upward. The client had two PRN doses of haloperidol in the last 6 hours. Of the drugs that have been prescribed for the client as needed (see chart), the nurse should administer:

> **Prescriptions**
>
> Lorazepam 1 mg IM
> Amantadine 100 mg PO
> Diphenhydramine 25 mg PO
> Benztropine 0.5 mg IM

☐ 1. lorazepam.
☐ 2. amantadine.
☐ 3. diphenhydramine.
☐ 4. benztropine.

114. After birth of a male neonate at 38 weeks' gestation, the nurse dries the neonate and places him under the radiant warmer. The nurse performs this action based on the understanding that one neonatal response to cold stress involves which factor?
☐ 1. metabolism of brown adipose tissue
☐ 2. decreased utilization of glycogen stores
☐ 3. decreased utilization of calorie stores
☐ 4. increased shivering to keep warm

115. Twenty-four hours after an appendectomy, a 16-year-old adolescent of Asian ethnicity reports no pain when asked but is frowning and has the legs drawn to the fetal position. The nurse should:
☐ 1. administer pain medication.
☐ 2. ask the adolescent what is troubling him.
☐ 3. discuss the adolescent's behavior with the parents.
☐ 4. offer a distracting activity such as a video game.

116. When developing the teaching plan for a primiparous client who is bottle-feeding her term neonate for the first feeding, what information should the nurse include?
☐ 1. Fill the entire nipple of the bottle with formula.
☐ 2. All term babies have well-developed sucking skills.
☐ 3. Bubble the baby after 2 oz (60 mL) of formula have been taken.
☐ 4. Propping of the bottle results in too much air being taken in by the baby.

117. Which topic would be **most** important to include when teaching the parents how to promote overall toddler development?
☐ 1. Language is the most important achievement.
☐ 2. Discipline is critical to appropriate development.
☐ 3. Safety is a priority concern for this age-group.
☐ 4. Eating habits that follow into adulthood begin now.

118. A client has back pain 10 minutes after a unit of packed red blood cells (RBCs) was started. The client's pulse, blood pressure, and respirations are stable, and similar to vital signs obtained before infusing the RBCs. What should the nurse do? Select all that apply.
☐ 1. Turn off the infusion of the packed RBCs.
☐ 2. Flush the Y-tubing with normal saline to clear the line.
☐ 3. Send the remaining blood to lab.
☐ 4. Prepare for cardiopulmonary resuscitation.
☐ 5. Obtain a urine specimen to send to the laboratory.

119. A primiparous client at 4 hours after a vaginal birth and manual removal of the placenta voids for the first time. The nurse palpates the fundus, noting it to be 1 cm above the umbilicus, slightly firm, and deviated to the left side, and notes a moderate amount of lochia rubra. The nurse notifies the healthcare provider (HCP) based on the interpretation that the assessment indicates which problem?
☐ 1. perineal lacerations
☐ 2. retained placental fragments
☐ 3. cervical lacerations
☐ 4. urine retention

120. While performing a gestational age assessment for a male neonate born vaginally at 37 weeks' gestation, the nurse should assess the neonate for:
☐ 1. an anterior transverse crease on the soles.
☐ 2. extensive rugae on the scrotum.
☐ 3. some cartilage in the earlobes.
☐ 4. coarse and silky scalp hair.

121. Two family members are visiting their father who is experiencing acute delirium. They are upset that their father is so disoriented. "He knows who we are, but that is about it. We do not know what to say to him." What should the nurse tell the family? Select all that apply.
☐ 1. "Answer his questions simply, honestly, slowly, and clearly."
☐ 2. "Correct him when he is hearing and seeing things that are not there."
☐ 3. "Occasionally remind him of the time, day, and place when he does not remember."
☐ 4. "Include him in your conversation, instead of talking about him while he is present."
☐ 5. "Raise your voice a bit so you are sure he hears you."

122. A 26-year-old is being treated for delirium due to acute alcohol intoxication. The client is restless, does not want to stay seated, and has a staggering gait. What should the nurse do **first**?
☐ 1. Place the client in a chair with a waist restraint.
☐ 2. Provide one-to-one supervision of the client until detoxification treatment can begin.
☐ 3. Ask the client to sit in a chair next to the nurses' station.
☐ 4. Decrease stimuli by putting the client in bed with the room door closed.

123. The nurse is monitoring a client receiving a blood transfusion when the client develops a cough with shortness of breath. The client also has a headache and a racing heart. What should the nurse do **first**?
☐ 1. Slow the infusion rate.
☐ 2. Replace the blood with saline.
☐ 3. Administer an antihistamine.
☐ 4. Place the client flat with the feet elevated.

124. The nurse should seek clarification about which prescription?
☐ 1. Give 5,000 units bolus dose of heparin IV push.
☐ 2. Give 200,000 units heparin by IV drip, and infuse over 24 hours.
☐ 3. Give 40,000 units of heparin by IV drip, and infuse over 24 hours.
☐ 4. Give 5,000 units of heparin IV piggyback every 4 to 6 hours.

125. A nurse is analyzing a client's intake and output. The client has a temperature of 102°F (38.9°C) and is receiving 2,400 mL of IV fluids per 24 hours because the client is to have nothing by mouth. Before planning nursing actions, the nurse should **first** determine:
☐ 1. the client's body mass index.
☐ 2. the amount of insensible fluid loss through the lungs and skin.
☐ 3. when the client last ate.
☐ 4. the intravenous fluid intake during the last 8 hours.

126. Two toddlers are arguing over a toy in the playroom. The nurse should say to the children:
☐ 1. "If you cannot play together, I will have to put you back in your rooms."
☐ 2. "Give the toy to me. Now neither of you will have it."
☐ 3. "Let me see if I can get both of you a similar toy."
☐ 4. "Let one of you play with it for awhile, and then give it to the other."

127. A client has been prescribed digoxin. Which symptom should the nurse tell the client to report as a potential indication of digoxin toxicity?
☐ 1. urticaria
☐ 2. shortness of breath
☐ 3. visual disturbances
☐ 4. hypertension

128. A 9-month-old infant whose parents have emigrated from Mexico presents in the clinic with severe dehydration from vomiting. The infant was seen in the clinic just 3 days ago for a well-child visit, but now the family seems very distrustful of the healthcare team. The nurse should ask the parents:
☐ 1. "Have you been speaking with a healer?"
☐ 2. "Did anything concern you about your last visit?"
☐ 3. "Has immigration been causing you problems?"
☐ 4. "Are you afraid your baby will be taken from you?"

129. A 4-year-old child continues to come to the nurses' station after being told children are not allowed there. What behavior is the child exhibiting?
☐ 1. attention-seeking behavior
☐ 2. aggressive behavior
☐ 3. resistive behavior
☐ 4. exaggerated stress behavior

130. A 5-month-old infant is brought to the emergency department with vomiting and diarrhea, which the parent states started 3 days ago. The nurse should conduct a focused assessment for which signs and symptoms? Select all that apply.
☐ 1. decreased or absent tearing
☐ 2. dry mucous membranes
☐ 3. sunken fontanelle
☐ 4. clear, pale yellow urine
☐ 5. bounding pulse

131. A client's burn wounds are being cleaned twice a day in a hydrotherapy tub. Which intervention should be included in the plan of care before a hydrotherapy treatment is initiated?
☐ 1. Limit food and fluids 45 minutes before therapy to prevent nausea and vomiting.
☐ 2. Increase the IV flow rate to offset fluids lost through the therapy.
☐ 3. Apply a topical antibiotic cream to burns to prevent infection.
☐ 4. Administer pain medication 30 minutes before therapy to help manage pain.

132. A neonate born to a primiparous client at 36 weeks' gestation in a small, rural hospital is to be transferred by ambulance to a level III nursery. To prepare the parents for the transfer, what should the nurse include in the plan of care?
☐ 1. Instruct the parents that the neonate is in critical condition.
☐ 2. Obtain the mother's consent for the neonate's transfer.
☐ 3. Allow the parents to touch the neonate before transfer.
☐ 4. Ask the father if he desires to ride in the ambulance during the transfer.

133. A multiparous client gives birth to a neonate at 24 weeks' gestation. After 12 hours, the neonate's condition deteriorates, and death appears likely within the next few minutes. The parents are Roman Catholic, and they request that the neonate be baptized. What action would be **most** appropriate?
☐ 1. Contact the hospital chaplain to perform the baptism.
☐ 2. Alert the hospital's director that a neonatal death is imminent.
☐ 3. Find a healthcare provider (HCP) who is Roman Catholic to perform the baptism.
☐ 4. Baptize the neonate, regardless of the nurse's own religious beliefs.

134. A client with bipolar disorder, manic phase, shows little interest in eating. To help the client meet recommended daily allowances of nutrients, the nurse should:
- ☐ 1. give the client half of a meat and cheese sandwich to carry with him.
- ☐ 2. inform the client that snacks are available only if he eats properly at mealtime.
- ☐ 3. tell the client to sit alone at mealtime so that he won't be distracted by others.
- ☐ 4. teach the client about proper nutrition.

135. A client has bursitis in the subacromial bursa. A nurse determines that the client understands teaching when the client says:
- ☐ 1. "I will apply moist heat to my shoulder for 20 minutes three times each day."
- ☐ 2. "I will lift 30-lb (13.5-kg) weights at least three times each day."
- ☐ 3. "I will apply dry ice to my shoulder for 20 minutes three times each day."
- ☐ 4. "I will perform 360-degree circles with my arms extended at least three times daily."

136. A client has just undergone a lumbar puncture (LP). Which finding should the nurse **immediately** report to the healthcare provider (HCP)?
- ☐ 1. The client's oral intake was 1,200 mL in the past 8 hours.
- ☐ 2. The client required analgesia for headache.
- ☐ 3. A moderate amount of serous fluid was noted on the lumbar dressing.
- ☐ 4. The client is concerned about the test results.

137. The nurse is reviewing the lab report below for a client in hospice care with breast cancer and brain metastasis. According to the information in the chart, what should the nurse do **next**?

Laboratory Results

Test	Result
Potassium	4.0 mEq/L (mmol/L)
Sodium	142 mEq/L (mmol/L)
Chloride	100 mEq/L (mmol/L)
Calcium	12.4 mg/dL (3.1 mmol/L)

- ☐ 1. Document these results on the medical record.
- ☐ 2. Report the elevated potassium level immediately.
- ☐ 3. Report the elevated calcium level immediately.
- ☐ 4. Refrain from reporting the results because the client is in hospice care.

138. A nurse is caring for a primigravid client at 40 weeks' gestation in active labor. Assessments include the following: cervix 5 cm dilated; 90% effaced; station 0; cephalic presentation and FHR baseline 135 bpm, decreases to 125 bpm shortly after onset of 5 uterine contractions and returns to baseline before the uterine contraction ends. Based on this assessment, what action should the nurse take **first**?
- ☐ 1. Position the woman on her left side, and administer oxygen via face mask.
- ☐ 2. Document findings on the woman's medical record, and continue to monitor labor progress.
- ☐ 3. Perform a vaginal exam to rule out umbilical cord prolapse.
- ☐ 4. Notify the healthcare provider (HCP) immediately, and prepare for emergency cesarean section.

139. A child with a cardiac defect assumes a squatting position. The nurse should determine that the position is effective for the child by noting:
- ☐ 1. less energy required to play with toys on the floor.
- ☐ 2. less dyspnea.
- ☐ 3. relief of abdominal pressure.
- ☐ 4. improved muscle tone.

140. A client was brought to the emergency department following a motor vehicle accident and has phrenic nerve involvement. The nurse should assess the client for:
- ☐ 1. alteration in level of consciousness.
- ☐ 2. altered cardiac functioning.
- ☐ 3. ineffective breathing pattern.
- ☐ 4. alteration in urinary elimination.

141. A primigravid client is seen for her first visit in the antenatal clinic and tells the nurse that her brother was born with cystic fibrosis (CF). When teaching the client about this disorder, the nurse should include which information? Select all that apply.
- ☐ 1. Persons of Asian descent have the highest inheritance rates.
- ☐ 2. To inherit CF, each parent must carry a recessive trait for the disease.
- ☐ 3. If both parents carry the trait, each offspring has a 25% chance of inheriting the disease.
- ☐ 4. Fetal testing can occur by checking the shape of the red blood cells.
- ☐ 5. Chorionic villi sampling (CVS) can identify prenatally if their child carries the trait or has the disease.

142. A client with a peritonsillar abscess has been hospitalized. Upon assessment, the nurse determines the following: a temperature of 103°F (39.4°C), body chills, and leukocytosis. The client begins to have difficulty breathing. In what order should the nurse perform the actions? All options must be used.

| **1.** Call the healthcare provider (HCP). |
| **2.** Open the airway. |
| **3.** Start an IV access site. |
| **4.** Explain the situation to the family. |

| |
| |
| |
| |

143. The nurse is teaching a client who has deep vein thrombosis caused by a pulmonary embolus, which has now resolved. What should the nurse tell the client?
- [ ] **1.** "Report such signs as leg swelling, discomfort, redness, or warmth."
- [ ] **2.** "Sit with your legs lower than the rest of your body."
- [ ] **3.** "Walk at least every other day."
- [ ] **4.** "Limit your fluids to 1 L each day."

144. A multiparous client and her neonate, who has been cared for in the intensive care nursery for the past 3 days because of being small for gestational age, are to be discharged. Before their release, the mother tells the nurse, "I have been living in my car for the past 2 weeks." What should the nurse do **next**?
- [ ] **1.** Notify the director of the birthing unit.
- [ ] **2.** Contact the hospital's social worker.
- [ ] **3.** Contact the client's healthcare provider (HCP).
- [ ] **4.** Notify the client's family members.

145. A client who is receiving a blood transfusion suddenly experiences chills and a temperature of 101°F (38.3°C). The client also has a headache and appears flushed. In what order from first to last should the nurse perform the actions? All options must be used.

| **1.** Obtain a blood culture from the client. |
| **2.** Send the blood bag and administration set to the blood bank. |
| **3.** Stop the blood infusion. |
| **4.** Infuse normal saline to keep the vein open. |

| |
| |
| |
| |

146. The fetus of a multigravid client at 38 weeks' gestation is determined to be in a frank breech presentation. The nurse describes this presentation to the client as which fetal part coming in contact with the cervix?
- [ ] **1.** buttocks
- [ ] **2.** head
- [ ] **3.** both feet
- [ ] **4.** shoulder

147. The nurse collects a urine specimen from a client for a culture and sensitivity analysis. What should the nurse do **next**?
- [ ] **1.** Send the specimen to the laboratory immediately.
- [ ] **2.** Send the specimen with the next pickup.
- [ ] **3.** Send the specimen the next time an unlicensed assistive personnel (UAP) is available.
- [ ] **4.** Store the specimen in the refrigerator until it can be sent to the laboratory.

148. A client in surgery has an endotracheal tube (ET) in place. The nurse should call a time-out if which requirements are not in place? Select all that apply.
- [ ] **1.** an identification band
- [ ] **2.** postoperative pain medication
- [ ] **3.** an IV line
- [ ] **4.** oxygen administration
- [ ] **5.** an anesthetist/anesthesiologist

149. A multiparous client at 16 weeks' gestation is diagnosed as having a fetus with probable anencephaly. The client is a devout Baptist and has decided to continue the pregnancy and donate the neonatal organs after the death of the neonate. Which action by the nurse would be **most** appropriate?
☐ 1. Explore his or her own feelings about the issues of anencephaly and organ donation.
☐ 2. Contact the client's minister to discuss the client's options related to the pregnancy.
☐ 3. Advise the client that the prolonged neonatal death will be very painful for her.
☐ 4. Ask the client if she has discussed this with her family.

150. A 3-month-old infant is being discharged on digoxin. The nurse should instruct the parents to report which signs and symptoms? Select all that apply.
☐ 1. signs of constipation or painful straining
☐ 2. decrease in the amount of infant formula taken or a refusal to take it
☐ 3. pulse rate >140 bpm or <100 bpm
☐ 4. signs that the infant is not following moving objects
☐ 5. sudden vomiting or sudden drowsiness

151. The nurse receives a report of a serum potassium level on an infant of 5.4 mEq/L (5.4 mmol/L). What should the nurse do **first**?
☐ 1. Notify the healthcare provider (HCP) of the abnormal level.
☐ 2. Call the laboratory to see how the specimen was obtained.
☐ 3. Connect the infant to a cardiac monitor.
☐ 4. Check the infant's last 24-hour output.

152. A client with suicidal thoughts is admitted to an adult inpatient behavioral health unit. What should the nurse do **first**?
☐ 1. Initiate suicide precautions with face-to-face observation of the client at all times.
☐ 2. Place the client on suicide watch, and have a family member remain with the client.
☐ 3. Question the client further about the suicidal thoughts and plans.
☐ 4. Confine the client to his or her room, and post a staff member at the door to observe the client's actions.

153. The nurse is caring for a client who has a history of gastric bypass surgery and is now being seen for her first prenatal visit. Which interventions should be included in the plan of care? Select all that apply.
☐ 1. Take a prenatal vitamin with 400 mcg of folic acid.
☐ 2. Refer the client to a registered dietician.
☐ 3. Draw glucose levels at each prenatal visit.
☐ 4. Counsel her she will most likely gain all of her weight back.
☐ 5. Check urine at each visit for protein and glucose.
☐ 6. Monitor with nonstress tests beginning at 20 weeks.

154. A nurse is planning care for a regressed, chronically ill client diagnosed with schizophrenia. What is the **most** appropriate milieu?
☐ 1. confrontation and peer pressure to break down the client's denial
☐ 2. reminder that all clients must participate fully in unit self-governance
☐ 3. required attendance at group activities with equal participation from all clients
☐ 4. nurturance and supportive interaction focusing on individual needs

155. The nurse is assessing a client with irreversible shock. The nurse should document which finding?
☐ 1. increased alertness
☐ 2. circulatory collapse
☐ 3. hypertension
☐ 4. diuresis

156. The nurse is caring for a client who has been diagnosed with deep vein thrombosis. When assessing the client's vital signs, the nurse notes an apical pulse of 150 bpm, a respiratory rate of 46 breaths/minute, and blood pressure of 100/60 mm Hg. The client appears anxious and restless. What should be the nurse's **first** course of action?
☐ 1. Notify the healthcare provider (HCP).
☐ 2. Administer a sedative.
☐ 3. Try to elicit a positive Homans' sign.
☐ 4. Increase the flow rate of intravenous fluids.

157. Assessment of a primigravid client in active labor reveals cervical dilation at 9 cm with complete effacement and the fetus at +1 station. What is the **most** appropriate action for the nurse to take when the healthcare provider (HCP) prescribes morphine 2 mg IM for the client?
☐ 1. Administer the medication in the left ventrogluteal muscle.
☐ 2. Be certain that naloxone is at the client's bedside.
☐ 3. Ask the HCP to validate the dosage of the drug.
☐ 4. Refuse to administer the medication to the client.

158. A client has been hospitalized with a diagnosis of myasthenia gravis. A friend is visiting the client during lunch. The nurse enters the room after the client recovered from choking on lunch. What should the nurse do **next**?
☐ 1. Instruct the client to sit at a 30-degree angle in bed when eating.
☐ 2. Tell the client to swallow when her chin is tipped down on her chest.
☐ 3. Remind the client to rest after eating.
☐ 4. Encourage the client to eat alone.

159. A nurse is assessing a client with a brain injury. What is a client's cerebral perfusion pressure (CPP) when the blood pressure (BP) is 90/50 mm Hg and the intracranial pressure (ICP) is 21? Round to the nearest whole number.

_____ mm Hg.

160. A client with a T2 to T3 spinal cord injury suddenly has a throbbing headache and blurred vision. The client is flushed and sweating on the upper trunk and face, and the hairs on the arms are raised. What should the nurse do **first**?
- ☐ 1. Raise the head of the bed.
- ☐ 2. Assess for hypotension.
- ☐ 3. Check the client for a distended bladder.
- ☐ 4. Logroll the client to see if the client is lying on a foreign object.

161. A 17-year-old unmarried primigravida client at 10 weeks' gestation tells the nurse that her family does not have much money and her dad just got laid off from his job. The nurse should **first**:
- ☐ 1. instruct the client in methods for low-cost, highly nutritious meal preparation.
- ☐ 2. determine whether the client qualifies for local assistance programs.
- ☐ 3. refer the client to a social worker for enrollment in a food assistance program.
- ☐ 4. ask the client if she has a job and the amount of income earned.

162. A client has impairments in immediate recall and short-term memory. A nurse is planning for the client's daily activities. Which action by the nurse would be **most** effective?
- ☐ 1. Write out the client's schedule in large print, and show the client where the schedule is placed.
- ☐ 2. Describe each activity and the time of the events at the beginning of the day.
- ☐ 3. Take the client to each activity if the client does not attend on time.
- ☐ 4. Tell the client about each activity 10 minutes before it begins.

163. A 17-year-old male client is being admitted to the adolescent psychiatric unit. He was brought in by the police after beating up two male peers. The client says, "They said I was gay because I had sex with an older neighbor when I was 8 years old. I am not gay!" Which nursing intervention would be appropriate? Select all that apply.
- ☐ 1. Monitor the client's level of anger and potential aggression.
- ☐ 2. Help the client express anger safely.
- ☐ 3. Assist the client in processing his feelings about the sexual abuse.
- ☐ 4. Ask the client if he would like to attend a support group.
- ☐ 5. Discuss the client's attitude about going to jail after discharge.

164. The nurse has been assigned to care for several postpartum clients and their neonates on a birthing unit. Which client should the nurse assess **first**?
- ☐ 1. a multiparous client at 48 hours postpartum who is being discharged
- ☐ 2. a primiparous client at 2 hours postpartum who gave vaginal birth to a term neonate
- ☐ 3. a multiparous client at 24 hours postpartum whose infant is in the special care nursery
- ☐ 4. a primiparous client at 48 hours postpartum after cesarean birth of a term neonate

165. A client is admitted to the hospital with malaise, headache, and cough followed by fever, chills, dyspnea, chest discomfort, myalgia, anorexia, vomiting, and diarrhea. The healthcare provider (HCP) makes the diagnosis of legionellosis (Legionnaires' disease). The client asks, "How did I get this?" Which response by the nurse is the **most** accurate?
- ☐ 1. "The bacteria thrive in warm water environments and are inhaled from contaminated water droplets."
- ☐ 2. "You inhaled the bacteria from secondary smoke."
- ☐ 3. "As ceiling fans circulate, bacteria are dispersed into the air."
- ☐ 4. "You may have swallowed contaminated water."

166. A 4-year-old child who has been ill for 4 hours is admitted to the hospital with difficulty swallowing, a sore throat, and severe substernal retractions. The child's temperature is 104°F (40°C), and the apical pulse is 140 bpm. The white blood cell count is 16,000/mm³ (16 × 10⁹/L). What is the **priority** for nursing intervention?
- ☐ 1. infection
- ☐ 2. airway obstruction
- ☐ 3. difficulty breathing
- ☐ 4. potential for aspiration

167. Which baseline laboratory data should be established before a client is started on tissue plasminogen activator or alteplase recombinant?
- ☐ 1. potassium level
- ☐ 2. Lee-White clotting time
- ☐ 3. hemoglobin level, hematocrit, and platelet count
- ☐ 4. blood glucose level

168. A client is scheduled to undergo an upper gastrointestinal (GI) series. The nurse should give the client which instructions in preparation for the test? Select all that apply.
- ☐ 1. "You will need to take a stool softener before the test to promote evacuation of the barium."
- ☐ 2. "Do not eat or drink for 8 hours before the test."
- ☐ 3. "You can expect white stools for about 48 hours after the test."
- ☐ 4. "You will experience mild stomach pain during the test."
- ☐ 5. "It is okay for you to smoke before the test."

169. Which are appropriate identifiers to use when providing care or administering medications or treatments? Select all that apply.
☐ **1.** room number
☐ **2.** bed number
☐ **3.** medical record number
☐ **4.** name band
☐ **5.** social security (social insurance) number

170. The nurse interprets the rhythm strip below from a client's bedside monitor as:

☐ **1.** normal sinus rhythm.
☐ **2.** sinus tachycardia.
☐ **3.** atrial fibrillation.
☐ **4.** ventricular tachycardia.

171. The nurse is preparing to give an IM injection to an underweight client. Which site is the safest because it has the fewest amount of blood vessels and major nerves located in the area?
☐ **1.** deltoid
☐ **2.** dorsogluteal
☐ **3.** vastus lateralis
☐ **4.** triceps

172. The nurse is planning to teach the client how to properly use a metered-dose inhaler to treat asthma. The nurse should tell the client to:
☐ **1.** rinse the mouth after each use of a steroid inhaler.
☐ **2.** inhale quickly when administering the medication.
☐ **3.** inhale the medication and then exhale through the nose.
☐ **4.** cough and deep-breathe before inhaling the medication.

173. A client is receiving a transfusion of packed red blood cells. To safely administer the blood, the nurse should:
☐ **1.** keep the blood refrigerated on the nursing unit until ready to administer.
☐ **2.** stay with the client during the first 15 minutes to detect signs or symptoms of a reaction.
☐ **3.** not infuse blood that has been hanging for more than 6 hours.
☐ **4.** administer the blood quickly to prevent wasting it if the client develops a fever.

174. A client who is receiving a blood transfusion begins to have difficulty breathing. The nurse notes an elevated blood pressure and a cough. Based on these signs, the nurse should prepare to manage which complication?
☐ **1.** anaphylactic reaction
☐ **2.** circulatory overload
☐ **3.** sepsis
☐ **4.** acute hemolytic reaction

175. The nurse is teaching a client with peptic ulcer disease how to take sucralfate. Which statement indicates that the client understands how to take the medication?
☐ **1.** "I should take the sucralfate every evening at bedtime."
☐ **2.** "It is important that I take this drug on an empty stomach."
☐ **3.** "I should avoid milk products while taking this drug."
☐ **4.** "I should have my hemoglobin checked monthly while taking sucralfate."

176. The nurse is conducting an admission interview with a client and is assessing for risk factors related to the client's safety. The nurse should include which targeted assessments? Select all that apply.
☐ **1.** suicide or self-harm ideation
☐ **2.** incentives that motivate the client
☐ **3.** recent use of substances of abuse
☐ **4.** allergic reactions or adverse drug reactions
☐ **5.** dietary preferences

177. An adult client has bacterial conjunctivitis. What should the nurse teach the client to do? Select all that apply.
☐ **1.** Use warm saline soaks four times per day to remove crusting.
☐ **2.** Apply topical antibiotic without touching the tip of the tube to the eye.
☐ **3.** Wash the hands after touching the eyes.
☐ **4.** Avoid touching the eyes.
☐ **5.** Observe isolation procedures by staying in the bedroom until the redness in the eye disappears.

178. A 31-year-old client, G3, T0, P2, Ab0, L0 at 32 weeks' gestation is being admitted to the hospital with contractions of moderate intensity occurring every 3 to 4 minutes per the client report. The client is crying on admission; the history reveals that the client has previously had two nonviable fetuses at 30 weeks' gestation. What nursing action would be the **highest priority** for this client?
☐ **1.** Assess maternal contraction and fetal heart rate pattern.
☐ **2.** Reassure the client that this baby will be healthy.
☐ **3.** Review history of prior fetal demises with client.
☐ **4.** Prepare for immediate administration of magnesium sulfate.

179. Which actions by the nurse will **most** likely ensure that the correct client receives a medication? Select all that apply.
- [ ] 1. Have the client state his or her name.
- [ ] 2. Check the name on the armband with the name on the medication.
- [ ] 3. Learn to recognize the client.
- [ ] 4. Check the client's room number.
- [ ] 5. Compare the date of birth on the client's medical record to the date of birth on the client's armband.

180. A nurse is counseling a mother with young children after the mother left her abusive husband 6 months ago. The mother says, "My 6-year-old is starting to act just like his father. I just do not know how to handle this." Which response by the nurse is **most** appropriate?
- [ ] 1. "You will have to limit your son's contact with his father."
- [ ] 2. "Counseling for your son would be helpful."
- [ ] 3. "Most boys outgrow these behaviors."
- [ ] 4. "Setting limits on his behavior is all you need to do now."

181. A 40-year-old primigravid client with AB-positive blood visits the outpatient clinic for an amniocentesis at 16 weeks' gestation. The nurse determines that the **most** likely reason for the client's amniocentesis is to determine if the fetus has which problem?
- [ ] 1. cri-du-chat syndrome
- [ ] 2. ABO incompatibility
- [ ] 3. erythroblastosis fetalis
- [ ] 4. Down syndrome

182. The nurse-manager is developing a "read-back" procedure to reduce medication administration errors. Which are purposes of the "read-back" requirement? Select all that apply.
- [ ] 1. to prohibit prescriptions and test results from being communicated verbally or by telephone
- [ ] 2. to make sure that prescriptions and test results that are communicated verbally or by telephone are clear to the receiver of the information
- [ ] 3. to make sure that prescriptions and test results that are communicated verbally or by telephone are confirmed by the individual giving the information
- [ ] 4. to minimize the risk of nonauthorized personnel from giving prescriptions that are communicated verbally or by telephone
- [ ] 5. to encourage the use of electronic medical records

183. A female client who is hospitalized for an eating disorder weighs 15 lb less than the ideal body weight. Which goal is a **priority** for this client?
- [ ] 1. The client attends all eating disorder support groups.
- [ ] 2. The client eats bigger meals at breakfast.
- [ ] 3. The client gains 1 lb per week.
- [ ] 4. The client reports an improved self-image.

184. A 16-year-old primiparous client has decided to place her baby for adoption. The adoptive parents are on their way to the hospital when the mother says, "I want to see the baby one last time." What should the nurse do?
- [ ] 1. Tell the client that it would be best if she did not see the baby.
- [ ] 2. Allow the client to see the baby through the nursery window.
- [ ] 3. Contact the healthcare provider (HCP) for advice related to the client's visitation.
- [ ] 4. Allow the client to see and hold the baby for as long as she desires.

185. A school nurse interviews the parent of a middle school student who is exhibiting behavioral problems, including substance abuse, following a sibling's suicide. The parent says, "I am a single parent who has to work hard to support my family, and now, I have lost my only son, and my daughter is acting out and making me crazy! I just cannot take all this stress!" Which concern regarding this family has **priority** at this time?
- [ ] 1. the parent's ability to emotionally support the adolescent in this crisis
- [ ] 2. potential suicidal thoughts/plans of both family members
- [ ] 3. the adolescent's anger
- [ ] 4. the parent's frustration

186. A 10-year-old child is admitted with a brain tumor. Which assessment made by the nurse is **most** critical to report to the child's healthcare provider (HCP)?
- [ ] 1. vomiting after lunch
- [ ] 2. difficulty in recalling the day of the week
- [ ] 3. blood pressure of 102/62 mm Hg
- [ ] 4. 100 mL of concentrated urine voided at one voiding

187. A client with jaundice has poor appetite, nausea, and two episodes of emesis in the past 2 hours. The client reports having spasms in the stomach area. The client does not have pruritus. The nurse should develop a care plan for which health problem **first**?
- [ ] 1. nausea
- [ ] 2. poor appetite
- [ ] 3. jaundice
- [ ] 4. abdominal spasms

188. When planning for risk management for clients who are at risk for development of pressure ulcers, the nurse should **first**:
- ☐ 1. identify at-risk clients on admission to the healthcare facility.
- ☐ 2. place at-risk clients on an every-2-hour turning schedule.
- ☐ 3. automatically place clients in specialty beds.
- ☐ 4. provide at-risk clients with a high-protein, high-carbohydrate diet.

189. The nurse is teaching a 17-year-old girl who has a severe gonorrheal infection. The nurse realizes that the girl understands the implications of her disease when she tells the nurse:
- ☐ 1. "Once I am treated, I will have immunity."
- ☐ 2. "My partner does not need treatment."
- ☐ 3. "I will not have any more problems once I learn to protect myself."
- ☐ 4. "I could have trouble getting pregnant."

190. After teaching the parent of a child with a spica cast about skin care, which parental action would indicate the need for additional teaching?
- ☐ 1. application of powder to the skin under the cast
- ☐ 2. inspection of the cast edges for smoothness
- ☐ 3. application of plastic film to cover the perineal cast area
- ☐ 4. inspection of areas inside the cast

191. The nurse-manager is teaching the staff about the medication reconciliation policy. The nurse teaches the staff that reconciliation is needed to ensure that clients are on the correct medications in which situations? Select all that apply.
- ☐ 1. admission to the hospital
- ☐ 2. transfer to the nursing home
- ☐ 3. transfer of a client from surgery to the surgical unit
- ☐ 4. admission to a home health agency from the hospital
- ☐ 5. move from a double room to a single room on the same unit

192. Sodium polystyrene sulfonate is prescribed for a client following crush injury. The drug is effective if:
- ☐ 1. the pulse is weak and irregular.
- ☐ 2. the serum potassium is 4.0 mEq/L (4.0 mmol/L).
- ☐ 3. the ECG is showing tall, peaked T waves.
- ☐ 4. there is muscle weakness on physical examination.

193. The nurse is teaching a young female about using oxcarbazepine to control seizures. The nurse determines teaching is effective when the client states:
- ☐ 1. "I will use one of the barrier methods of contraception."
- ☐ 2. "I will need a higher dose of oral contraceptive when on this drug."
- ☐ 3. "Since I am 28 years old, I should not delay starting a family."
- ☐ 4. "I must weigh myself weekly to check for sudden gain in weight."

194. A client diagnosed with chronic renal failure is undergoing hemodialysis. Postdialysis, the client weighs 59 kg. The nurse should teach the client to:
- ☐ 1. increase the amount of sodium in the diet to 4 g/day.
- ☐ 2. limit the total amount of calories consumed each day to 1,000.
- ☐ 3. increase fluid intake to 3,000 mL each day.
- ☐ 4. control the amount of protein intake to 59 to 70 g/day.

195. A client was treated for a streptococcal throat infection 2 weeks ago. The client now has been diagnosed with acute poststreptococcal glomerulonephritis. The client asks the nurse how to prevent this infection. What should the nurse tell the client?
- ☐ 1. "See your healthcare provider (HCP) for an early diagnosis and treatment of a sore throat."
- ☐ 2. "As long as you do not have a fever, it is sufficient to gargle daily with an antibacterial mouthwash."
- ☐ 3. "You may continue to utilize the previously prescribed antibiotics until they are gone."
- ☐ 4. "Unscented bar soap may be used in showers."

196. Assessment of a primigravid client in active labor reveals a cervix dilated to 5 cm and completely effaced, with the fetus at −1 station. The client has indicated that she wants a "natural childbirth" with no analgesia or anesthesia. The healthcare provider (HCP) enters the room and tells the client that it is time for an epidural anesthetic. What would be the nurse's **best** action at this time?
- ☐ 1. Ask the client if she desires an epidural anesthetic.
- ☐ 2. Tell the HCP that the client desires a "natural childbirth."
- ☐ 3. Tell the client that her labor will be more comfortable with an anesthetic.
- ☐ 4. Ask the client to discuss this with her husband and then make a decision.

197. A client is ready to be discharged following an inguinal hernia repair. Which criteria must the client meet before the nurse can discharge the client? Select all that apply.
- ☐ 1. The client has transportation home via a taxicab.
- ☐ 2. The client is able to tolerate oral fluids.
- ☐ 3. The client has pain no greater than 5 on a scale of 1 to 10.
- ☐ 4. The client can walk to the bathroom unassisted.
- ☐ 5. The client has voided.

198. The nurse is administering eyedrops to a client with glaucoma. Which is a correct technique for instilling the eyedrops? The eyedrops are placed:
- ☐ 1. in the lower conjunctival sac.
- ☐ 2. near the opening of the lacrimal ducts.
- ☐ 3. on the cornea.
- ☐ 4. on the scleral surface.

199. The nurse is teaching an older adult how to prevent falls. The nurse should tell the client to:
☐ 1. turn on bright lights in the room so the client can see items in the room.
☐ 2. instruct the client to rise slowing from a supine position.
☐ 3. encourage the client not to use assistive devices as they reduce independence.
☐ 4. instruct the client not to exercise painful joints.

200. Before inserting a nasogastric (NG) tube in an adult client, the nurse estimates the length of tubing to insert. Identify the point on the illustration where the nurse would end the measurement.

201. The nurse is designing a benchmarking study to gather information about nursing care practices for wound care. Which sources of information are used for benchmarking? Select all that apply.
☐ 1. government reports
☐ 2. literature reviews
☐ 3. standard-setting organizations
☐ 4. databases
☐ 5. clinical organization recommendations

202. A client scheduled for hip replacement surgery wishes to receive his own blood for the upcoming surgery. The nurse should:
☐ 1. document the client's request on the medical record.
☐ 2. notify the hematology laboratory.
☐ 3. notify the surgeon's office.
☐ 4. call the blood bank.

203. A client is using an over-the-counter nasal spray containing pseudoephedrine to treat allergic rhinitis. Which instruction about this medication would be **most** appropriate for the nurse to provide for the client?
☐ 1. Prolonged use of nasal spray can lead to nasal infections.
☐ 2. Pseudoephedrine is an addictive drug and must be used cautiously.
☐ 3. Overuse of pseudoephedrine can lead to increased nasal congestion.
☐ 4. A common side effect of pseudoephedrine nasal spray is thrush.

204. A 6-year-old child is admitted for an appendectomy. What is the **most** appropriate way for the nurse to prepare the child for surgery?
☐ 1. Explain how to use a patient-controlled analgesia (PCA) pump for pain control.
☐ 2. Permit the child to play with the blood pressure cuff, electrocardiogram (ECG) pads, and a face mask.
☐ 3. Show the child a video about the surgery.
☐ 4. Show the child a visual analog scale (VAS) based on a scale from 0 to 10.

205. The nurse is working on a hospital's birthing unit when a primigravid client in active labor is to receive morphine. As the nurse enters the medication room, the nurse observes a female coworker slipping a vial of morphine into the side pocket of the uniform. Which action would be **most** appropriate?
☐ 1. Contact the hospital's security chief.
☐ 2. Notify the supervisor of the unit.
☐ 3. Tell the coworker of the incident.
☐ 4. Notify the federal drug agents about the incident.

206. Which information should the nurse include when teaching the family and a client who was prescribed benztropine, 1 mg PO twice daily, about the drug therapy?
☐ 1. The drug can be used with over-the-counter cough and cold preparations.
☐ 2. The client should not discontinue taking the drug abruptly.
☐ 3. Antacids can be used freely when taking this drug.
☐ 4. Alcohol consumption with benztropine therapy need not be restricted.

207. Which information should the nurse include in a teaching plan that addresses the adverse effects of antipsychotic medication?
☐ 1. information about all potential adverse effects
☐ 2. research data about rare adverse effects
☐ 3. adverse effects that can be seen or felt
☐ 4. percentages associated with each adverse effect

208. A client has nephrotic syndrome. To aid in the resolution of the client's edema, the healthcare provider (HCP) prescribes 25% albumin. In addition to an absence of edema, the nurse should evaluate the client for which expected outcome?
- ☐ **1.** crackles in the lung bases
- ☐ **2.** blood pressure elevation
- ☐ **3.** cerebral edema
- ☐ **4.** cool skin temperature in lower extremities

209. A client has polycystic kidney disease. The client asks the nurse, "How did I get these fluid-filled bubbles on my kidneys?" How should the nurse respond to help the client understand risk factors for this disease process?
- ☐ **1.** "Secondhand smoke puts you at greater risk for developing cysts."
- ☐ **2.** "Exposure to dyes used to color fruits and vegetables increases the risk of polycystic kidney disease."
- ☐ **3.** "There is a higher incidence of polycystic kidney disease among blood relatives."
- ☐ **4.** "Drinking alcohol daily allows the kidneys to develop cysts."

210. A nurse is administering IV fluids to a dehydrated client. When administering an IV solution of 3% sodium chloride, what should the nurse do? Select all that apply.
- ☐ **1.** Measure the intake and output.
- ☐ **2.** Inspect the jugular veins for distention.
- ☐ **3.** Evaluate the client for neurologic changes.
- ☐ **4.** Encourage the client to drink more fluids.
- ☐ **5.** Insert an indwelling urinary catheter.

211. The nurse is working on a birthing unit with an unlicensed assistive personnel (UAP). The nurse determines that the UAP understands the type of information to report to the nurse when the UAP reports which information about one of the clients?
- ☐ **1.** an episode of nausea after administration of an epidural anesthetic
- ☐ **2.** contractions 3 minutes apart and lasting 40 seconds
- ☐ **3.** evidence of spontaneous rupture of the membranes
- ☐ **4.** sleeping after administration of IV nalbuphine

212. A 9-year-old child is scheduled for an electromyelogram. To prepare the child for this procedure, what should the nurse do **first**?
- ☐ **1.** Wait until just before the test to tell the child what will be done.
- ☐ **2.** Ask the child to draw a picture of the body structures involved.
- ☐ **3.** Show the child the equipment that will be used in the test.
- ☐ **4.** Verbally explain what will be done during the test.

213. The nurse is planning a program about women's health and cancer prevention for a community health fair. Which information should the nurse include? Select all that apply.
- ☐ **1.** Regular self-exams of the breast and vulva are important self-care activities.
- ☐ **2.** Cancer can be prevented by removing precancerous lesions of the vulva, cervix, or endometrium.
- ☐ **3.** Girls, age 11 to 12, should receive immunization for human papillomavirus (HPV) to prevent cervical cancer.
- ☐ **4.** Smoking cessation reduces the risk of cervical cancer.
- ☐ **5.** There is limited evidence that cancer in women is inherited.

214. A 10-year-old client with rheumatic fever is on bed rest. Which diversional activity would be appropriate for the nurse to encourage?
- ☐ **1.** watching television with the roommate
- ☐ **2.** coloring picture books with the brother
- ☐ **3.** keeping up with the school work
- ☐ **4.** building a bird house

215. Clients who are receiving total parenteral nutrition (TPN) are at risk for development of which complication?
- ☐ **1.** hypostatic pneumonia
- ☐ **2.** pulmonary hypertension
- ☐ **3.** orthostatic hypotension
- ☐ **4.** fluid imbalances

216. The nurse is to administer a bolus starting dose of heparin to a child who is taking penicillin. What should the nurse do? Select all that apply.
- ☐ **1.** Check that the dose is appropriate for the child's weight.
- ☐ **2.** Note that the onset of the medication will be immediate.
- ☐ **3.** Follow the administration of the bolus of heparin with an IV infusion of heparin 10 units/kg/h.
- ☐ **4.** Monitor partial thromboplastin time (PTT).
- ☐ **5.** Discontinue the penicillin until the PTT is at a therapeutic level.

217. The client is receiving propantheline bromide to treat cholecystitis. The nurse should evaluate the client's response to the medication by observing for which adverse effect?
- ☐ **1.** urine retention
- ☐ **2.** diarrhea
- ☐ **3.** hypertension
- ☐ **4.** diaphoresis

218. The nurse is preparing to start an IV infusion. Before inserting the needle into a vein, the nurse should apply a tourniquet to the client's arm to:
- ☐ **1.** distend the veins.
- ☐ **2.** stabilize the veins.
- ☐ **3.** immobilize the arm.
- ☐ **4.** occlude arterial circulation.

219. Prochlorperazine is prescribed postoperatively. The nurse should evaluate the drug's therapeutic effect when the client expresses relief from:
☐ **1.** nausea.
☐ **2.** dizziness.
☐ **3.** abdominal spasms.
☐ **4.** abdominal distention.

220. A 17-year-old client has been admitted to the hospital for a biopsy to confirm the diagnosis of bone cancer. The nurse should assess the client for which conditions? Select all that apply.
☐ **1.** cough
☐ **2.** dyspnea
☐ **3.** pain
☐ **4.** swelling
☐ **5.** fever
☐ **6.** anorexia

221. A nurse on the labor and birth unit transfers a primiparous client and her term neonate to the mother-baby unit 2 hours after the client gave vaginal birth to the neonate. Which information is a **priority** for the nurse to report to the nurse receiving the client on the mother-baby unit?
☐ **1.** firm fundus when gentle massage is used
☐ **2.** evidence of bonding well with the neonate
☐ **3.** labor that lasted 12 hours with a 1-hour second stage
☐ **4.** temperature of 99°F (37.4°C) and pulse rate of 80 bpm

222. A client who underwent cardiac surgery 2 days ago is recovering well. His wife, who is assisting with his care, says, "He is doing too much. I told him to let me help, but he will not let me." The nurse says to the wife, "It sounds like you need to feel you can be more helpful to him." In order to make the nonverbal behavior complement the words, the nurse should:
☐ **1.** direct the eyes at the client.
☐ **2.** direct the body and eyes at the wife and client.
☐ **3.** avoid direct eye contact with the client and wife.
☐ **4.** shift the eyes back and forth between the client and wife.

223. A nurse is having difficulty establishing a relationship with an aggressive client. What strategy will **most** likely improve the relationship?
☐ **1.** The nurse and the client agree to work to improve their involvement in the therapeutic relationship.
☐ **2.** The nurse establishes goals for having only positive interactions with the client.
☐ **3.** The nurse agrees to be submissive so the client can dominate the relationship.
☐ **4.** The nurse seeks assistance from colleagues to become more aware of the quality of the interactions and more sensitive to the dynamics of communication.

224. The charge nurse on the postpartum unit has received a report about a client who has just experienced a fetal demise and will be ready for transfer out of the labor unit in about 2 hours. The client has asked her primary nurse if she can stay on the obstetrical unit since she has found support from the nursing staff there. What action should the charge nurse on the postpartum unit take?
☐ **1.** Request a room for this client on a unit without newborns.
☐ **2.** Ask the nurse in labor and birth to discharge the mother as soon as she is physically able to leave.
☐ **3.** Talk to the mother first and decide on a location that is mutually agreeable.
☐ **4.** Admit the mother to a private room on the postpartum unit.

225. A 12-month-old child is seen in the neighborhood clinic for a regular checkup. Which statement by the child's mother about the influenza vaccine reflects the need for more teaching?
☐ **1.** "Yearly influenza vaccinations are recommended to begin as early as 6 months of age."
☐ **2.** "The *Haemophilus influenzae* vaccine my child has already received helps protect against some forms of influenza."
☐ **3.** "My child is too young to receive the live attenuated intranasal vaccine."
☐ **4.** "The first time a child receives the influenza vaccine, a second dose is recommended in 1 month."

226. A nurse is about to conduct a sexual history for a 16-year-old female who is accompanied by her mother. What is an appropriate question for the nurse to ask this client or her mother?
☐ **1.** "What do you think about having your mother leave the room now?"
☐ **2.** "Mother, do you think your daughter is sexually active?"
☐ **3.** "Mother, I am going to ask you to wait a few minutes in the waiting room now so I can complete the health history with your daughter."
☐ **4.** "The two of you seem like you share everything. I am going to ask questions about sexual history now."

227. A nurse is admitting an older female client to the gynecology surgical unit. When the nurse asks the client what medication she is taking at home, the client responds that she is taking a little red pill in the morning and a white capsule at night for her blood pressure. What action by the nurse is focused on safe, effective care of this client?

☐ 1. Consult the pharmacist regarding identification of the medications.

☐ 2. Show pictures to the client from the *Physician's Desk Reference* to identify the medications.

☐ 3. Consult the previous medical record from 2 years ago, and notify the healthcare provider (HCP) regarding medications that must be prescribed.

☐ 4. Ask a family member to bring the medications from home in the original vials for proper identification and administration times.

228. A client who had undergone an abdominal hysterectomy is in the recovery room. The surgeon has prescribed a 250-mL bolus of normal saline over 1 hour to replace blood loss. The IV solution infusing in the client was 1,000 mL normal saline with 40 mEq of potassium chloride at 100 mL/h. What should the nurse do? Select all that apply.

☐ 1. Increase the IV infusion rate to 250 mL/h for 1 hour.

☐ 2. Add 250 mL of normal saline to the current infusion bag, and continue at 100 mL/h.

☐ 3. Connect a 250-mL bag of normal saline to the Y-connector, and calculate to infuse over 1 hour.

☐ 4. Contact the healthcare provider (HCP) regarding continuation of the primary IV infusion during the bolus infusion.

☐ 5. Administer the normal saline bolus via an IV infusion pump.

229. The nurse is caring for several neonates in the newborn nursery. Precautions that should be taken to prevent an infant abduction include which measure?

☐ 1. Notify the hospital's security staff about anyone who appears unusual.

☐ 2. Take several neonates to their mothers at the same time.

☐ 3. Place the infant near the doorway of the mother's room.

☐ 4. Contact the hospital's security staff if an exit alarm is triggered.

230. Clozapine therapy has been initiated for a client with schizophrenia who has been unresponsive to other antipsychotics. The client states, "Why do I have to have a blood test every week?" Which response by the nurse would be **most** appropriate?

☐ 1. "Weekly blood tests are necessary to determine safe dosage and to monitor the effect of the medication on the blood."

☐ 2. "Weekly blood tests are done so that you can receive another week's supply of the medication."

☐ 3. "Your healthcare provider (HCP) will want to know how well you are progressing with the medication therapy."

☐ 4. "Everyone taking clozapine has to go through the same procedure because it is required by the drug company."

231. The nurse administers an intradermal injection to a client. Proper technique has been used if the injection site demonstrates:

☐ 1. minimal leaking.

☐ 2. no swelling.

☐ 3. tissue pallor.

☐ 4. evidence of a bleb.

232. The sudden onset of which sign indicates a potentially serious complication for the client receiving an IV infusion?

☐ 1. noisy respirations

☐ 2. pupillary constriction

☐ 3. halitosis

☐ 4. moist skin

233. The nurse is planning to start a blood transfusion. Which solution should the nurse select to prime the tubing when preparing to administer the blood?

☐ 1. lactated Ringer's solution

☐ 2. normal saline

☐ 3. 5% dextrose in half-normal saline

☐ 4. 5% dextrose in water

234. When preparing to insert an IV catheter to administer fluids to a client who is going to surgery, the nurse selects the median cubital vein. Identify the location of the median cubital vein on the illustration.

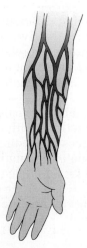

235. The mother of a 28-year-old client who is taking clozapine states, "Something is wrong. My son is drooling like a baby." What response by the nurse would be **most** helpful?
- ☐ 1. "I wonder if he is having an adverse reaction to the medicine."
- ☐ 2. "Excess saliva is common with this drug; here is a paper cup for him to spit into."
- ☐ 3. "Do not worry about it; this is only a minor inconvenience compared to its benefits."
- ☐ 4. "I have seen this happen to other clients who are taking clozapine."

236. The healthcare provider (HCP) is calling in a prescription for ampicillin for a neonate. What should the nurse do? Select all that apply.
- ☐ 1. Write down the prescription.
- ☐ 2. Ask the HCP to come to the hospital and write the prescription on the medical record.
- ☐ 3. Repeat the prescription to the HCP over the telephone.
- ☐ 4. Ask the HCP to confirm that the prescription is correct.
- ☐ 5. Ask the nursing supervisor to cosign the telephone prescription as transcribed by the nurse.

237. The nurse is planning care for a client who has been experiencing a manic episode for 6 days and is unable to sit still long enough to eat meals. Which choice will **best** meet the client's nutritional needs at this time?
- ☐ 1. Offer a green salad topped with chicken pieces.
- ☐ 2. Offer a peanut butter sandwich.
- ☐ 3. Offer a bowl of vegetable soup.
- ☐ 4. Offer to have the family bring in favorite foods.

238. Which medication should the nurse anticipate administering in the event of a heparin overdose?
- ☐ 1. warfarin sodium
- ☐ 2. protamine sulfate
- ☐ 3. vitamin K
- ☐ 4. atropine sulfate

239. The nurse has administered aminophylline to a client with emphysema. The medication is effective when there is:
- ☐ 1. relief from spasms of the diaphragm.
- ☐ 2. relaxation of smooth muscles in the bronchioles.
- ☐ 3. efficient pulmonary circulation.
- ☐ 4. stimulation of the medullary respiratory center.

240. The nurse is conducting health assessments for school-age children. A characteristic behavior of a 7-year-old girl is that she:
- ☐ 1. likes to play only with other girls.
- ☐ 2. prefers to play with her sister.
- ☐ 3. prefers to play team games.
- ☐ 4. likes to play alone.

241. A nurse is planning care for a 7-year-old who is hospitalized for a hernia repair. The nurse should assess the client for which fear common in this age-group?
- ☐ 1. separation from parents
- ☐ 2. trying something new
- ☐ 3. injury and pain
- ☐ 4. opposite-sex relationships

242. When teaching a client with bipolar disorder who has started to take valproic acid about possible side effects of this medication, the nurse should instruct the client to report which side effect?
- ☐ 1. increased urination
- ☐ 2. slowed thinking
- ☐ 3. sedation
- ☐ 4. weight loss

243. A woman who gave birth to a healthy baby 6 hours ago is having cramps in her legs. Upon further assessment, the nurse identifies leg pain on dorsiflexion. The nurse should:
- ☐ 1. tell the woman to massage the area.
- ☐ 2. apply warm compresses to the area.
- ☐ 3. instruct the woman on how to do ankle pumps.
- ☐ 4. notify the healthcare provider (HCP).

244. After instructing a 40-year-old woman about osteoporosis after menopause, the nurse determines that the client needs further instruction when the client makes which statement?
- ☐ 1. "A standard serving of yogurt is the equivalent of one glass of milk."
- ☐ 2. "Women who do not eat dairy products should consider calcium supplements."
- ☐ 3. "Women of African descent are at the greatest risk for osteoporosis."
- ☐ 4. "Estrogen therapy at menopause can reduce the risk of osteoporosis."

245. A young adult is hospitalized with a seizure disorder. The client, who is in a bed with padded side rails, has a tonic-clonic seizure. In what order from first to last should the nurse take the actions? All options must be used.

1. Loosen clothing around the client's neck.

2. Turn the client on his or her side.

3. Clear the area around the client.

4. Suction the airway.

246. A client with metastatic cancer of the liver tells the nurse about being concerned about the prognosis. The nurse should:
- ☐ 1. provide information for the client to consider a liver transplantation.
- ☐ 2. assure the client that the prescribed medications will shrink all tumor sites.
- ☐ 3. explain the effects of chemotherapy.
- ☐ 4. place emphasis on providing symptomatic and comfort measures.

247. The nurse delegates the care of a multiparous client who gave birth to a viable term neonate vaginally 30 hours ago and is preparing to be discharged to a licensed practical/vocational nurse (LPN/VN). The nurse should instruct the LPN/VN to notify the nurse if the client exhibits which sign or symptom?
- ☐ 1. pulse rate of 100 bpm
- ☐ 2. oral temperature of 99°F (37.2°C)
- ☐ 3. large amounts of perspiration
- ☐ 4. frequent voiding in large amounts

248. A client with obsessive-compulsive disorder washes the hands multiple times daily and is late for meals and milieu activities. What is **most** appropriate for the nurse to do initially?
- ☐ 1. Totally eliminate the client's ritual.
- ☐ 2. Allow the client to decide whether to attend meals and activities.
- ☐ 3. Inform the client that absence from meals and activities is not permitted.
- ☐ 4. Remind the client about meal and activity times so that the ritual can be completed on time.

249. A client with osteoarthritis purchased a copper bracelet to wear and tells the nurse that there is less pain now. Which response by the nurse is **most** appropriate?
- ☐ 1. Tell the client that copper is best applied as copper-lined gloves.
- ☐ 2. Warn the client not to spend any more money on quackery such as bracelets.
- ☐ 3. Instruct the client to remove the bracelet because the copper in it can interfere with salicylate metabolism.
- ☐ 4. Acknowledge that the client feels better, but encourage the client to continue with the prescribed therapy.

250. A woman with a history of a left radical mastectomy is being admitted for abdominal surgery. The woman has a swollen left arm. The nurse should:
- ☐ 1. take the blood pressure only in the unaffected arm.
- ☐ 2. start an IV line in the affected arm.
- ☐ 3. encourage a dependent position of the affected arm.
- ☐ 4. allow blood draws in the affected arm.

251. A 36-month-old child weighing 20 kg (44 lb) is to receive ceftriaxone 2 g IV every 12 hours. The recommended dose of ceftriaxone is 50 to 75 mg/kg/day in divided doses. The nurse should:
- ☐ 1. administer the medication as prescribed.
- ☐ 2. administer half the prescribed dose.
- ☐ 3. call the laboratory to check the therapeutic serum level of ceftriaxone.
- ☐ 4. withhold administering the ceftriaxone and notify the child's healthcare provider (HCP).

252. The nurse has provided an in-service presentation to ancillary staff about standard precautions on the birthing unit. The nurse determines that one of the staff members needs further instructions when the nurse makes which observation?
- ☐ 1. use of protective goggles during a cesarean birth
- ☐ 2. placement of bloody sheets in a container designated for contaminated linens
- ☐ 3. wearing of sterile gloves to bathe a newborn at 2 hours of age
- ☐ 4. disposal of used scalpel blades in a puncture-resistant container

253. The nurse has completed breast-feeding discharge instructions and determines the mother understands when she makes which statements? Select all that apply.
- ☐ 1. "My calorie intake will need to increase by 1,000 calories per day."
- ☐ 2. "Any drugs that I take may pass through to my breast milk."
- ☐ 3. "Babies should have six to eight wet diapers per day after the first 3 days of life."
- ☐ 4. "I have the phone number for the lactation consultant if I have questions."
- ☐ 5. "Babies should be satisfied from the feeding for 5 to 6 hours after daytime feedings."

254. The healthcare provider's (HCP's) prescription for an intravenous infusion is 3% normal saline to infuse at 125 mL/h. The client's most recent sodium level is 132 mEq/L (132 mmol/L). The nurse should:
- ☐ 1. hang 0.9% normal saline at 125 mL/h.
- ☐ 2. start the IV solution as prescribed.
- ☐ 3. consult the prescriber about the prescription.
- ☐ 4. hang the IV solution prescribed at 62 mL/h.

255. The nurse is auscultating for an aortic murmur. Indicate where the nurse should place the stethoscope to **best** evaluate the presence of this murmur.

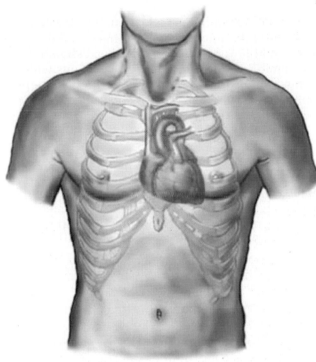

256. After a nasogastric (NG) tube has been inserted, the nurse can **most** accurately determine that the tube is in the proper place when:

☐ **1.** the client is no longer gagging or coughing.
☐ **2.** the pH of the aspirated fluid is measured.
☐ **3.** thirty milliliters of normal saline can be injected without difficulty.
☐ **4.** a whooshing sound is auscultated when 10 mL of air is inserted.

257. A client has been diagnosed with early alcoholic cirrhosis. The client should be taught that which behavior could potentially reverse the pathologic changes occurring in the liver?

☐ **1.** Do not become fatigued.
☐ **2.** Avoid drinking alcohol.
☐ **3.** Eliminate smoking.
☐ **4.** Eat a high-carbohydrate, low-fat diet.

258. A client is admitted to the emergency department with sudden onset of chest pain. Which prescriptions should the nurse implement **immediately**? Select all that apply

☐ **1.** Provide oxygen.
☐ **2.** Administer nitroglycerin.
☐ **3.** Administer aspirin.
☐ **4.** Insert a Foley catheter.
☐ **5.** Administer morphine.
☐ **6.** Administer acetaminophen.

259. Which measure should the nurse institute to help minimize joint pain in a child with rheumatic fever?

☐ **1.** massaging the affected joints
☐ **2.** applying ice to the affected joints
☐ **3.** limiting movement of the affected joints
☐ **4.** encouraging progressive weight bearing

260. To reduce the possibility of catheter-related urinary tract infections (CAUTIs), the nurse should:

☐ **1.** use sterile technique when providing catheter care.
☐ **2.** ensure that clients who are incontinent have indwelling urinary catheters.
☐ **3.** minimize urinary catheter use and duration of use in all clients.
☐ **4.** clean the periurethral area with antiseptics.

261. A client is admitted to the emergency department (ED) experiencing syncope. The nurse speaks with the family concerning the client's condition and current medications. The client's family states that the client takes several medications and has brought all the client's medications with them. To determine the correct medications required for this client, the nurse performs which step of the required process to ensure safe administration of medications?

☐ **1.** verification
☐ **2.** clarification
☐ **3.** documentation
☐ **4.** reconciliation

262. An elderly client admitted with new-onset confusion, headache, poor skin turgor, bounding pulse, and urinary incontinence has been drinking copious amounts of water. Upon reviewing the lab results, the nurse discovers a sodium level of 122 mEq/L (122 mmol/L). What actions should the nurse take? Select all that apply.

☐ **1.** Encourage fluids to 2,000 mL in 24 hours.
☐ **2.** Keep partial side rails up.
☐ **3.** Restrict fluids to 800 mL in 24 hours.
☐ **4.** Tell the family they may get the client up to walk in the halls.
☐ **5.** Prepare to insert a Foley catheter.
☐ **6.** Notify the healthcare provider (HCP).

263. Following the creation of an ileostomy, a client states, "I am really worried about how I am going to manage this thing." The **first** action of the nurse should be to:

☐ **1.** remind the client to focus energy on getting healthy.
☐ **2.** determine the client's exact concerns about the ileostomy.
☐ **3.** arrange a meeting with the client's case manager.
☐ **4.** encourage the client's spouse to talk with the client.

264. A client who is being treated for nonhealing diabetic foot ulcers tells the nurse angrily, "I am so frustrated with my doctors. The wound care doctor tells me this will not heal and I need to have my toes amputated and another doctor tells me I need to keep going with the antibiotics and dressing changes so I can save my foot. I just want to go home!" After listening to the client's concerns, the nurse should:

☐ 1. contact the client's case manager to set up a care conference.

☐ 2. assure the client that the healthcare providers (HCPs) know what they are doing.

☐ 3. remind the client of the responsibilities for health habits regarding diabetes.

☐ 4. review the healthcare providers' (HCPs') progress notes with the client.

265. While making rounds, the nurse enters a client's room and finds the client on the floor between the bed and the bathroom. In which order of priority from first to last should the nurse take the actions? All options must be used.

| 1. If no acute injury, get help, and carefully assist the client back to bed. |
| 2. Document as required by the facility. |
| 3. Assess the client's current condition and vital signs. |
| 4. Notify the client's healthcare provider (HCP) and family. |
| |
| |
| |
| |

Answers, Rationales, and Test-Taking Strategies

The answers and rationales for each question follow below, along with keys (🔑) to the client need (CN) and cognitive level (CL) for each question. As you check your answers, use the **Content Mastery and Test-Taking Skill Self-Analysis** worksheet (tear-out worksheet in back of book) to identify the

reason(s) for not answering the questions correctly. For additional information about test-taking skills and strategies for answering questions, refer to pages 12–23 and pages 35–36 in Part 1 of this book.

1. 3. The head of the bed should be elevated 30 degrees to promote venous drainage and decrease intracranial pressure. The client's head should be in a midline, or neutral, position. Clients with supratentorial surgery should be positioned on the nonoperative side to prevent displacement of the cranial contents by gravity.

🔑 CN: Reduction of risk potential; CL: Synthesize

2. 4. Laryngeal stridor is characteristic of respiratory distress from inflammation and swelling after bronchoscopy. It must be reported immediately. Green sputum indicates infection and would occur 3 to 5 days after bronchoscopy. A mild cough or hemoptysis is typical after bronchoscopy. If a tissue biopsy specimen was obtained, sputum may be blood streaked for several days.

🔑 CN: Reduction of risk potential; CL: Analyze

3. 4. Keeping the client's door closed is likely to contribute to feelings of isolation and sensory deprivation. Such activities as watching television, visiting with a relative, and reading a newspaper help prevent sensory deprivation and yet do not require physical effort.

🔑 CN: Psychosocial integrity; CL: Synthesize

4. 4. A trained medical interpreter is required to ensure safety, accuracy of history data, and client confidentiality. The medical interpreter knows the client's rights and is familiar with the client's culture. Using the family member as interpreter violates the client's confidentiality. Using the **UAP** 📖 and limited Spanish and nonverbal communication do not ensure accuracy of interpretation and back-translation into English.

🔑 CN: Management of care; CL: Synthesize

5. 4. Clinical manifestations of juvenile hypothyroidism include dry skin, constipation, sparse hair, and sleepiness. Short attention span, weight loss, moist flushed skin, rapid pulse, and heat intolerance suggest hyperthyroidism.

🔑 CN: Physiological adaptation; CL: Analyze

6. 2. The client needs further instructions when she says, "If I become pregnant, I can continue to eat sushi twice a week." Raw fish, including tuna, should be avoided while the client is pregnant because of the risk of contamination with mercury and other potential teratogens. Folic acid supplements taken before the client gets pregnant and during pregnancy can help reduce the risk of neural tube defects. Steaming vegetables reduces the risk that vitamins will be lost in the cooking water. Soy products can increase the client's protein levels.

ℎ☌ CN: Health promotion and maintenance;
CL: Evaluate

7. 3. Diarrhea is a common adverse effect of amoxicillin because the drug kills normal intestinal bacteria. Yogurt with live cultures helps restore the normal intestinal flora. Restricting the child to clear fluids will not help stop the diarrhea or recolonize the intestine. Withholding food and fluids for 2 hours is suggested when a child vomits. Pizza tends to be spicy and aggravates the diarrhea, but restricting its intake will not help the underlying problem.

ℎ☌ CN: Basic care and comfort;
CL: Synthesize

8. 3. It is normal for the client who is beginning chemotherapy to be anxious and fearful about possible side effects. It is important that the nurse listen to the client's concerns, correct any misconceptions, and explain the supportive care that will be provided during the chemotherapy treatments. The client needs to understand that individuals do respond differently to the treatments, and the experience may be very different from those of other people. A previously excellent health record does not necessarily ensure that the client will not experience side effects. Medications may lessen but not prevent the side effects, so client concerns should not be dismissed. Telling the client that he or she will die if treatment is refused does nothing to allay fears and concerns.

ℎ☌ CN: Psychosocial integrity;
CL: Synthesize

9. 1, 3, 4, 5. Home care for a client with a total laryngectomy should include a high-humidity environment, laryngectomy tube care and suctioning, speech rehabilitation, and smoking cessation. The client is not restricted to a bland diet.

ℎ☌ CN: Management of care; CL: Create

10. 2. Administering acetaminophen to the client with a post-ECT headache is the best action. Stating a headache is common after ECT and that napping will help the client feel better may be true, but it does not offer the client pain relief. Telling the client to eat breakfast and then to let the nurse know how the client feels conveys a lack of understanding to the client and dismisses the client's concern.

ℎ☌ CN: Basic care and comfort;
CL: Synthesize

11. 3. This rhythm is ventricular tachycardia, which is characterized by an absent P wave and a heart rate of 140 to 220 bpm. Ventricular tachycardia requires immediate intervention, usually with lidocaine.

ℎ☌ CN: Physiological adaptation;
CL: Analyze

12. 1, 4, 6. Providing culturally sensitive care includes providing printed material in the client's native language. There is nothing to indicate that this client is a high-risk pregnancy. Discussing cultural differences is not a priority or important at the first visit. Clients need to have an interpreter for each prenatal visit to translate and interpret questions. Contraceptive options are not a priority for the first prenatal visit. Reviewing dietary intake and discussing nutrition are important components of early prenatal care.

ℎ☌ CN: Health promotion and maintenance;
CL: Create

13. 4. An 18-month-old child should be able to say 10 or more words. Lack of speech development may indicate a lack of social stimulation, a hearing deficiency, or developmental delay. Referring the child for an evaluation may increase the child's chance of reaching the child's potential. A 4-month-old child with a healthy central nervous system and normal mental development should be able to laugh out loud if the child's environment has been caring and the child's needs are met safely and consistently. Children at age 10 months should be able to say the words "dada" and "mama" in response to the appropriate person. A 1-year-old child should have the ability to speak three to five words plus "mama" and "dada."

ℎ☌ CN: Health promotion and maintenance;
CL: Analyze

14. 4. Liver function tests, including aspartate transaminase (AST), should be monitored before therapy, 6 to 12 weeks after initiation of therapy or after dose elevation, and then every 6 months. If AST levels increase to three times normal, therapy should be discontinued. Simvastatin does not influence serum glucose, complete blood count, or total protein. Serum cholesterol and triglyceride levels should be evaluated before initiating therapy, after 4 to 6 weeks of therapy, and periodically thereafter.

ℎ☌ CN: Health promotion and maintenance;
CL: Analyze

15. 1. Phenylketonuria is a disease that is carried on the recessive genes of each parent. In order to be transmitted to a newborn, the infant inherits a recessive gene from each parent. Control of the disease is by reduction of the amino acid phenylalanine, which is present in all protein foods. The disease cannot be cured, but controlled. With each pregnancy, there is a 25% chance a child will inherit the disease.

🔑 CN: Reduction of risk potential; CL: Apply

16. 4. The nurse should convey empathy and invite the client to share more about her thoughts and feelings so that the nurse can assess the mother for possible postpartum depression, which usually occurs between 2 weeks and 3 months after the baby's birth but also can occur later. Postpartum depression is a mood disorder with symptoms of tearfulness, mood swings, despondency, feelings of inadequacy, inability to cope with the baby, and guilt about performance as a mother. Postpartum depression commonly goes undetected because of poor recognition and lack of knowledge. Hormonal changes during and after childbirth may account for some of the symptoms; however, the nurse should not assume that that is the case. Stating the client's husband and family should help her is an assumption that they are not and dismisses the client's concerns. Saying most new mothers feel the same way minimizes the client's concerns and decreases the likelihood of further disclosure by the client.

🔑 CN: Psychosocial integrity; CL: Synthesize

17. 4. Supine in extension is the position most likely to prevent contractures. Clients who have experienced burns will find a flexed position most comfortable. However, flexion promotes the development of contractures. The high Fowler's and semi-Fowler's positions create hip flexion. The prone position is contraindicated because of head and neck burns. In clients with head and neck burns, pillows should not be used under the head or neck to prevent neck flexion contractures.

🔑 CN: Reduction of risk potential; CL: Synthesize

18. 4. Blood clots are normal after transurethral resection of the prostate, but bright red urine can indicate a hemorrhage. The nurse should assess the client's vital signs and notify the surgeon. Irrigation of the catheter may help remove clots, but it does not decrease bleeding. Milking a urinary catheter or increasing fluid intake is not effective for controlling bleeding or decreasing clots.

🔑 CN: Reduction of risk potential; CL: Synthesize

19. 4 tablets

$$1{,}000 \text{ mg} = 1\text{g}$$
$$2\text{g} = 2{,}000 \text{ mg}$$
$$2{,}000 \text{ mg} \div 500 \text{ mg} = 4$$

🔑 CN: Pharmacological and parenteral therapies; CL: Apply

20. 4. A will is an important legal document. It is best to have one prepared with the help of an attorney. It would be unwise to help the client or to seek another nurse's help because a nurse is not a lawyer. Asking the client to delay preparing the will just avoids the problem.

🔑 CN: Management of care; CL: Synthesize

21. 3. A sudden gush of dark blood, a lengthening of the umbilical cord, a smaller uterus, and changing of the uterus to a round or spherical shape are impending signs of placental separation. Pushing effort from the client is not a reliable indicator for impending placental separation, nor is it necessary for placental expulsion.

🔑 CN: Health promotion and maintenance; CL: Analyze

22. 2. Battering is a major cause of injury to women. Although battering occurs in all socioeconomic groups, it may appear to be more common in members of lower socioeconomic groups because they are more likely to use emergency department services. Many women experience battery for the first time when they become pregnant. Death from battering is not rare.

🔑 CN: Psychosocial integrity; CL: Create

23. 2, 3. Huntington's disease, or *Huntington's chorea*, is an autosomal dominant genetic neurologic disease that affects descendants of an affected person at a 50% rate. Huntington's disease does not skip generations and affects men and women equally. Huntington's disease is genetically transmitted on chromosome 4, and death usually results from respiratory complications related to aspiration.

🔑 CN: Physiological adaptation; CL: Apply

24. 2. Liquids found on the floor should be removed immediately. The nurse should first put on gloves and then wipe up the liquid. Following removal, Environmental Services should be contacted to thoroughly cleanse the floor with a disinfectant solution. Placing paper towels over the drops is a safety hazard. "Wet floor" signs will be posted after the floor is cleansed by Environmental Services.

🔑 CN: Safety and infection control; CL: Synthesize

25. **2, 3, 4.** A client who has been admitted for numbness and tingling in the lower extremities that advances upward, especially after having a viral infection, has clinical manifestations characteristic of Guillain-Barré syndrome. The **HCP** ▢ must be notified of the change immediately because this disease is progressively paralytic and should be treated before paralysis of the respiratory muscles occurs. The nurse must assess the client continuously to determine how fast the paralysis is advancing. The family does not need to be called in to visit until the client is stabilized and emergency equipment is placed at the bedside. Performing ankle pumps will not relieve the numbness or change the course of the disease.

    ⚷ CN: Management of care; CL: Synthesize

26. **5, 6.** The nurse reports signs of decreased tissue perfusion to the **HCP** ▢; these include a decrease in urine output and confusion. Crackles, edema, and weight gain are monitored closely, but are not as high a priority as decreasing tissue perfusion. Vital signs and oxygen saturation are within normal limits.

    ⚷ CN: Physiological adaptation; CL: Synthesize

27. **3.** The spinal cord connects the brain to the periphery. The thalamus is located in the midbrain and integrates all sensory impulses except olfaction. The afferent impulses are received and then transmitted from the thalamus. Destruction or interruption of the neurosensory pathway results in loss of communication between the two systems. Monitoring the temperature of the bathwater is important because the client cannot feel whether the water is too hot or too cold. Damage to the thalamus does not result in loss of the corneal reflex. Loss of position and vibratory sense usually occurs with degeneration of the posterior column of the spinal cord; therefore, turning every 2 hours is critical to prevent skin breakdown related to increased capillary pressure. The nurse can give only the prescribed dosage of pain medication.

    ⚷ CN: Physiological adaptation; CL: Synthesize

28. **3.** When a client is experiencing delusion, the nurse should present reality. The nurse should tell the client that he or she does not hear the voice, see the image, or experience whatever other manifestation of the delusion that the client is experiencing. The client with paranoia is delusional, related to anxiety states, but cannot manage the anxiety at this moment. Allowing expressions of anger or other intense emotions may be harmful to the client or others. Nurses should avoid "why" questions, because such questions tend to make the client defensive.

    ⚷ CN: Management of care; CL: Synthesize

29. **4.** Absorption of supplemental iron and non-meat sources of iron is enhanced by combining them with meat or a good source of vitamin C. An acidic environment enhances iron absorption. Therefore, taking the iron on an empty stomach or with orange juice would be most effective. If gastrointestinal upset occurs, the client may take the drug with meals. However, doing so reduces iron absorption by 40% to 50%. Because milk interferes with the absorption of iron, the client should avoid taking the iron with milk. Tea has been shown to interfere with the absorption of iron. Therefore, the client should avoid taking the iron with tea. Hot chocolate, a milk product, interferes with iron absorption. Thus, the client should avoid taking the iron with hot chocolate.

    ⚷ CN: Basic care and comfort; CL: Synthesize

30. **1.** Stating "You were able to shower and dress without any help this morning" points out a visible, realistic accomplishment and strength to the client with self-deprecatory statements, thereby helping to increase the client's self-worth. The statements "Your wife told me that you are a good husband and father" and "You do not have any reason why you should feel this way" are not helpful because logical statements are ineffective in changing the thinking of a client who is depressed. The client may agree with what the nurse states but be just as depressed because intellectual understanding does not help the severely depressed client. The statement "This medication will help your thinking," although true, does not recognize the client's accomplishment and will have no positive effect on his self-esteem.

    ⚷ CN: Psychosocial integrity; CL: Synthesize

31. **1.** A low WBC may indicate the development of agranulocytosis, a serious life-threatening side effect of clozapine, and should be reported immediately. While a hemoglobin of 8.2 mg/dL is low, it is not life threatening. The sodium level of 136 mEq/L (136 mmol/L) is normal. Hyaline casts are usually caused by dehydration and indicate the need for more fluids.

    ⚷ CN: Management of care; CL: Synthesize

32. **2.** The pallor and cool temperature of the fingers and the decreased return time for capillary refill indicate decreased arterial blood supply to the fingers. These findings are not normal for any time in the recovery process. Nerve impairment includes numbness, tingling, and impaired movement of the fingers. Signs of venous stasis include edema and reddening of the fingers, not pallor and cool temperature.

    CN: Physiological adaptation; CL: Analyze

33. 1. The spinal cord connects the brain to the periphery. Destruction or interruption of the neurosensory pathway results in loss of communication between the two systems. Transection of the spinal cord renders the individual in a complete state of anesthesia below the level of injury. Tingling in the fingers may be related to spinal cord disease or to improper positioning of the extremity. Loss of position and vibratory sense usually occurs when the individual has degeneration of the posterior column of the spinal cord.

    CN: Physiological adaptation; CL: Analyze

34. 3. Common pressure points in the side-lying position include the ears, shoulders, ribs, greater trochanter, medial and lateral condyles, and ankles. The sacrum, occiput, and heel are pressure points in the supine position.

    CN: Basic care and comfort; CL: Analyze

35. 1, 2, 3. Goals for promoting healthy development in preschoolers include anticipatory guidance, helping parents understand their child's behavior, identifying deviations from the norm, and assessing parent-child interaction. No one can assess or determine the child's future development, and trying to do so can limit the potential the child may achieve. Although learning to interact with others is important, sending the child to a day care center is not essential to promote healthy development. The nurse can encourage the parents to provide opportunities for the child to play with others.

    CN: Psychosocial integrity; CL: Create

36. 1. The nurse verifies that the **HCP** has noted the elevated specific gravity. Clients with glomerulonephritis have concentrated urine from oliguria caused by the inflammation of the glomeruli. The other laboratory results are in normal range.

    CN: reduction of risk potential; CL: Analyze

37. 1. The client's physical needs are a priority in the nurse's plan of care. The lack of fluid and caloric intake can lead to dehydration and cardiac collapse. The lack of sleep and rest can lead to exhaustion and death. Social, spiritual, and cultural needs are important client needs but not as important as the physical needs during an acute manic episode.

    CN: Psychosocial integrity; CL: Synthesize

38. 2. The correct method of assessing a neonate's temperature is to place the thermometer under the neonate's arm for an axillary reading. The oral route is not appropriate for obtaining the temperature in a neonate, because the neonate is unable to close the mouth around the thermometer, thus leading to an inaccurate reading. Additionally, inserting a thermometer into a neonate's mouth may cause trauma to delicate tissues. Rectal temperatures may be indicated in some circumstances, but they are generally to be avoided in neonates because of the risk of injury to or perforation of the delicate rectal mucosa. Only a specialized tympanic membrane device should be used to obtain a temperature reading via the ear. Inserting a disposable digital thermometer into the neonate's ear may cause trauma to the delicate tissues.

    CN: Basic care and comfort; CL: Apply

39. 1, 2, 3. The alarm settings on infusion pumps should be verified at the time the infusion is started, at the beginning of each shift, and when the client is moved. The neonate can move in bed, but if the alarm is triggered, the nurse should verify the settings. Unless the neonate has moved or been taken out of the crib, it is not necessary to check alarm settings after the parents visit.

    CN: Safety and infection control; CL: Apply

40. 4. Moral distress occurs when one is unable to act because of internal or external constraints. The nurse is not able to change the way she interacted with her friend the last time she saw her and is feeling anguish. Secondary traumatic stress is distress that is a result of hearing firsthand traumatic experiences of another. A boundary violation is behavior by a professional that has violated the limits of a professional-client relationship. Compassion fatigue is disengagement on the part of the caregiving professional.

    CN: Management of care; CL: Analyze

41. 3. Contacting the Security Department is a proactive response in a situation that may become more volatile. A soft voice by the nurse may not even be heard in this situation. To state "Stop!" in this situation is not helpful and does not deal with the escalating risk. Once Security has been notified, the nurse should also report the incident to the supervisor.

    CN: Management of care; CL: Synthesize

42. **2.** The most appropriate immediate response is to open the airway. The nurse then should look, listen, and feel for respirations. Noting none, the nurse calls a code and attempts ventilations with a bag mask or mask with a one-way valve until the full code team responds. Using standard precautions with the mask protects the nurse from exposure to possible client microorganisms.

    CN: Physiological adaptation;
CL: Synthesize

43. **2.** Thermoregulation of the neonate is a critical intervention for the nurse caring for neonates. The preferred method of thermoregulation for healthy term newborns is to place them skin to skin with the mother. Wrapping and placing a hat on the newborn is another way to conserve heat and prevent heat loss. With the neonate lying against a crib wall, heat transfers away from the infant to the cooler surface (conduction). If the neonate is wet, the warmer water on the surface of the neonate evaporates to the cooler air (evaporation). If the neonate is lying in an open crib with a diaper on, the body naturally loses heat to the surrounding cooler air as it radiates from the warm body to the cooler room (radiation).

    CN: Management of care;
CL: Synthesize

44. **2.** When the blink reflex is absent or the eyes do not close completely, the cornea may become dry and irritated. Placing a patch over the eye is the most appropriate intervention to prevent eye injury. Making sure the client wears eyeglasses at all times will not help protect the eye from injury. Instilling eye drops once a day will not adequately relieve the potential for injury from a dry and irritating ocular environment. A normal saline solution should be used to moisten the eye, not tap water.

    CN: Health promotion and maintenance;
CL: Synthesize

45. **2.** A 4-year-old is old enough to be able to cooperate and stop the behavior. Therefore, the first step is to obtain the child's cooperation. When this has occurred, then the mother makes sure it is okay to remind the child when the behavior is viewed. Using a substance that does not taste good is not effective as the child may suck it off and does not promote health behavior. The mother also should be encouraged to praise the child when she sees her not engaging in the behavior; "time-out" is considered a punishment and does not promote the desired behavior.

    CN: Health promotion and maintenance;
CL: Create

46. The vastus lateralis in the thickest part of the anterolateral thigh is a safe injection site for infants. The needle should be inserted at a 90-degree angle to the long axis of the femur.

    CN: Safety and infection control;
CL: Apply

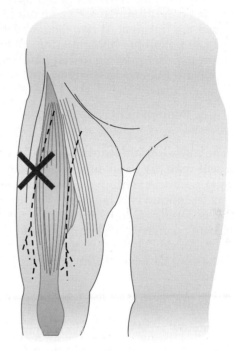

47. **1, 2, 3.** The alarm settings on infusion pumps should be verified at the time the infusion is started, at the beginning of each shift, and when the client is moved. The child can move in bed or sleep, but if the alarm is triggered, the nurse should verify the settings.

    CN: Safety and infection control;
CL: Apply

48. **1.** Tailor sitting, also referred to as cobbler's or butterfly pose, is an excellent exercise that helps to strengthen the client's back muscles and also prepares the client for the process of labor. The client should be encouraged to rest periodically during the day and avoid standing or sitting in one position for a long time. Leg lifts are helpful for leg aches. Shoulder circling exercises are helpful for neck and upper backaches. Squatting is not helpful for alleviating lower backaches.

    CN: Basic care and comfort;
CL: Synthesize

49. **4.** It is important to dry the feet carefully after a bath to prevent a fungal infection. Clients with diabetes should seek medical attention when they injure their toes or feet to prevent complications. Iodine is highly toxic to the tissues.

Clients with diabetes should inspect their feet daily and should wear shoes that support their feet while in the house.

⚷ CN: Reduction of risk potential;
CL: Evaluate

50. 1, 2, 3, 5. Pancreatitis, a chronic or acute inflammation of the pancreas, is a potentially life-threatening condition. Excessive alcohol intake and gallstones are the greatest risk factors. Abdominal trauma can potentiate inflammation. Hyperlipidemia is a risk factor for recurrent pancreatitis. Hypertension and hypothyroidism are not associated with pancreatitis.

⚷ CN: Reduction of risk potential;
CL: Analyze

51. 1. The nurse should firmly yet gently strike the chest wall with the hand cupped to make a hollow popping sound. A slapping sound indicates that an incorrect technique is being used. The area over the rib cage is percussed to loosen mucus from the underlying lung passages. The child should wear a thin piece of clothing (T-shirt) over the chest area to protect the skin without diminishing the effect of the percussion.

⚷ CN: Reduction of risk potential;
CL: Analyze

52. 4. Social isolation is a concern for an older adult who has diminished hearing and vision. Feeling disoriented may be related to cognitive problems rather than diminished hearing and vision. Diminished hearing and vision is related to the aging process and does not result in impairment of the older adult's thought processes. The client with impaired hearing and vision is unlikely to experience sensory overload.

⚷ CN: Psychosocial integrity;
CL: Synthesize

53. 3. At age 4, a child's speech should be understood most of the time even by people who do not know the child. According to the Denver Developmental Screening Examination, a child aged 2 years should have a vocabulary of 300 words, be able to combine two or three words, and ask for what he or she wants by name. By age 3, the child should have a vocabulary of 900 words and can use a complete sentence of three or four words. A 1-year-old has a vocabulary of at least eight words and can reference people and objects.

⚷ CN: Health promotion and maintenance;
CL: Analyze

54. 4. Isoniazid competes for the available vitamin B_6 in the body and leaves the client at risk for developing neuropathies related to vitamin deficiency. Supplemental vitamin B_6 is routinely prescribed to address this issue. Avoiding sun exposure is a preventive measure to lower the risk of skin cancer. Following a low-cholesterol diet lowers the individual's risk of developing atherosclerotic plaque. Rest is important in maintaining homeostasis but has no real impact on neuropathies.

⚷ CN: Pharmacological and parenteral therapies; CL: Synthesize

55. 2. Nitroglycerin causes vasodilation, which results in increased intraocular pressure. The vasodilatory effects of the medication can trigger an attack, causing pain and loss of vision. Hypotension is a common side effect of nitroglycerin, which dilates the blood vessels, but is not a concern in the client with glaucoma.

⚷ CN: Pharmacological and parenteral therapies; CL: Synthesize

56. 1, 2, 3, 5. The nurse should ask the client with multiple sclerosis about areas of muscle weakness because baclofen may increase the weakness. The nurse should ask the client about a history of muscle spasms. Baclofen is effective against involuntary spasms resistant to passive movement for clients with multiple sclerosis and paralysis. Baclofen is not effective against the spasticity of cerebral origin, such as with cerebral palsy and Parkinson's disease. The nurse should ask the client about the client's liver and renal function because baclofen is metabolized and excreted by these organs. The nurse should check the laboratory values reflecting the function of the kidneys and liver, which include serum creatinine and blood urea nitrogen levels. The nurse should also check blood glucose levels because baclofen can increase blood glucose. Clients with diabetes taking antidiabetic medication may need to adjust the dosage. Potassium is not affected by the drug, so the nurse does not need to check the serum potassium level.

⚷ CN: Pharmacological and parenteral therapies; CL: Apply

57. 1, 2, 4. The nurse should assess the client for signs of bone marrow depression, manifested by bruising or unusual bleeding, and signs of infection such as a sore throat. The nurse should also assess the client for signs of hepatic dysfunction, such as light-colored stool or dark-colored urine. Although the nurse may want to check the client's urinary function and hydration status, urine output and hydration are not specific monitoring needs related to long-term use of carbamazepine.

⚷ CN: Pharmacological and parenteral therapies; CL: Analyze

58. 3. A client with severe diarrhea loses large amounts of bicarbonate, resulting in metabolic acidosis. Metabolic alkalosis does not result in this situation. Diarrhea does not affect the respiratory system.

⚷ CN: Reduction of risk potential;
CL: Analyze

59. 4. Serum osmolality indicates the water balance of the body. A normal plasma osmolality between 275 and 295 mOsm/kg (mmol/kg) indicates that the fluid volume excess has been resolved. A weight reduction of 10% may not necessarily return the client to a state of normal serum osmolality. Clients with excess fluid volume do not necessarily have pain or abnormal arterial blood gas values.

CN: Reduction of risk potential;
CL: Synthesize

60. 3. Exactly why rheumatic fever follows a streptococcal infection is not known, but it is theorized that an antigen-antibody response occurs to an M protein present in certain strains of streptococci. The antibodies developed by the body attack certain tissues such as in the heart and joints. Antistreptolysin O titer findings show elevated or rising antibody levels. This blood finding is the most reliable evidence of a streptococcal infection.

CN: Reduction of risk potential;
CL: Analyze

61. 3. The nurse uses active listening, in which the client's feelings are reflected back to him. Telling the client that everyone wears them does not consider the client's feelings. Telling the client that what he said is not what he meant discounts the validity of his statement. Interpreting the reason for the client being upset as the rule being unreasonable does not take into account how it affects the client personally.

CN: Psychosocial integrity;
CL: Synthesize

62. 4. Elbow restraints help to keep the child from placing fingers or any other object in the mouth that would cause injury to the operative site. The restraints are worn at all times except when they are removed to check the skin. Because of the risk for skin breakdown, the restraints are removed periodically during the day to assess the child's underlying skin. It is advisable to remove only one restraint at a time while keeping hold of the child's hand on the unrestrained side. Toddlers are quick and usually want to explore the area in the mouth that the surgery has made feel different. The restraints should be in place at all times during sleep and play to prevent inadvertent injury to the operative site. Taping the restraints directly to the skin is not advised because skin breakdown can occur when tape is reapplied to the same area over several weeks. The restraints can be fastened to clothing to keep them from slipping.

CN: Safety and infection control;
CL: Evaluate

63. 2. Because the client is very active, it would be best to give her food she can carry with her and eat as she moves. Neither allowing the client to send out for her favorite foods nor serving food in small, attractively arranged portions will address her need to be active. Allowing the client in the unit kitchen is impractical, and she most likely would be too busy to eat anyway.

CN: Basic care and comfort;
CL: Synthesize

64. 1, 2, 3, 4. The purposes of the Pap (Papanicolaou) smear include to detect precancerous and cancerous cells of the cervix; to assess the effects of sex hormonal replacement; to identify viral, fungal, and parasitic conditions; and to evaluate the response to chemotherapy or radiation therapy to the cervix.

CN: Health promotion and maintenance;
CL: Apply

65. 2, 3. The nurse should use at least two sources of identification before administering medication to any client. The identification can include the **medical record** 🖵 number and the client's date of birth. It is not necessary to check the client and dose for this drug with another nurse. It is also not safe to use the room number or bed number as a source of identification as clients' locations in the hospital are frequently changed. The nurse should not assume that the child will give a correct first name.

CN: Safety and infection control;
CL: Apply

66. 1. Nurses should verify that clients having surgery discontinued use of any blood thinners to prevent postoperative bleeding. Prior to bowel resection, the client should follow a high-residue diet with increased fluids. Abdominal tightening exercises are not necessary before this surgery. Clients may write a will before surgery, but the nurse does not have to inquire about it.

CN: Reduction of risk potential;
CL: Synthesize

67. 1, 3. When a client collects stool for occult blood, the nurse should instruct the client to avoid eating meat, especially red meat, for 1 to 3 days before the sample collection because meat eliminated in the stool can lead to false-positive results. Eating foods high in fiber a few days before sample collection may be recommended because doing so improves the chances of finding occult blood if a lesion is present. The client should take stool samples from different sites of the stool for a better sample. The stool sample should be covered to protect everyone from body secretions. The specimen does not have to be sent to the laboratory immediately. Some medications, herbs, foods, and activities can lead to false results of the occult testing. For example, iron pills, turnips, and horseradish lead to false-positive results. Vitamin C leads to false-negative results. Some anti-inflammatory drugs and aspirin should be avoided due to antiplatelet properties that increase the risk of gastrointestinal bleeding.

CN: Reduction of risk potential; CL: Evaluate

68. 2. One of the actions of propranolol, a drug used in the treatment of migraine headaches, is to inhibit arterial vasodilation. The nurse should assess the client's blood pressure to evaluate overall circulatory response to the medication. Until the nurse determines the client's blood pressure, there is no immediate need to contact the **HCP** ☐. There is no immediate need to administer oxygen. The client has not indicated pain; it is not necessary to administer the sumatriptan at this time.

CN: Pharmacological and parenteral therapies; CL: Synthesize

69. 1. The client with diabetes and a chronic respiratory condition is most at risk for influenza and should receive the vaccine yearly. Diabetes and chronic respiratory conditions do not increase the risk of hepatitis A. An adult client is not as likely to need the measles-mumps-rubella or varicella immunizations, but titers can be checked if the client has not had childhood immunizations or the disease.

CN: Reduction of risk potential; CL: Apply

70. 2. Good sources of dietary iron include red meats, poultry, green leafy vegetables, and dried fruits such as raisins. Milk products are poor sources of iron. Carrots are high in vitamin A.

CN: Reduction of risk potential; CL: Evaluate

71. 1. During the tertiary circular reaction stage of the sensorimotor stage (12 to 18 months of age), the infant comes to understand causality and object permanence, recognizing that objects placed out of sight continue to exist. During the preoperational stage (ages 2 to 6), the child's perception is based on how he or she views an event. The concrete operational stage (ages 6 to 12) is the beginning of concrete, logical thinking. During the formal operational stage (ages 13 to 18), the child is able to perform abstract reasoning.

CN: Health promotion and maintenance; CL: Analyze

72. 2. The neonate will be simultaneously dried and stimulated to cry immediately upon birth. If the neonate does not cry as a result of these measures, the ABCs (airway, breathing, and circulation) of cardiopulmonary resuscitation will be followed. Positioning the neonate and suctioning or clearing the airway ensure that the airway is clear so that the first breath the neonate takes is air, rather than fluid or particulate matter. Breathing will be stimulated once the airway is clear, and then heart rate will be validated either apically or through the cord. The cord may be cut in order to hand the neonate to the mother for nursing. In many instances, the infant is placed on the mother's abdomen before the cord is cut.

CN: Health promotion and maintenance; CL: Evaluate

73. 2 mg/minute
First, calculate the concentration of mg/mL:

$$\frac{\overset{4}{\cancel{1,000}} \text{ mg}}{\underset{1}{\cancel{250}} \text{ mL}} = 4 \text{ mg / mL}.$$

Next, multiply the number of milligrams per milliliter by the pump setting in milliliters per hour:

$$\frac{4 \text{ mg}}{1 \text{ }\cancel{mL}} \times \frac{30 \text{ }\cancel{mL}}{1 \text{ h}} = 120 \text{ mg/h}.$$

Next, divide the milligrams per hour by 60 to obtain milligrams per minute:

$$120 \text{ mg/h} \div 60 \text{ minutes} = 2 \text{ mg/min}.$$

CN: Pharmacological and parenteral therapies; CL: Apply

74. 3. Children with roseola have a high fever for 3 days, which drops suddenly. Then a nonpruritic rash appears, typically lasting for 1 to 2 days. High fever followed by a rash is a characteristic sign. Associated symptoms include cold symptoms, cough, and lymphadenopathy.

CN: Physiological adaptation; CL: Evaluate

75. 1. The client may become tolerant of the antianginal effects of nitrates. Removing nitrates for 8 hours each day is usually effective in preventing tolerance. Nitrate patches should not be used on an as-needed basis. Sites should be rotated daily to prevent skin irritation, but this is not related to tolerance. Removing the patch for only 8 hours is sufficient to prevent tolerance, and skipping days could impact the drug's effectiveness.

CN: Pharmacological and parenteral therapies; CL: Apply

76. 3. When an incision eviscerates, it is a medical emergency. The nurse's first response is to apply a sterile dressing that has been moistened with sterile normal saline solution. The client should also be placed in semi-Fowler's position to release any tension on the abdominal area. Vital signs should be taken, and an IV line may be started for emergency treatment; however, the first action is to protect the wound and abdominal contents.

CN: Reduction of risk potential; CL: Synthesize

77. 2. The nurse should tell the client in a simple, matter-of-fact manner the purpose of the restraints to help the client understand why restraints are necessary. Long explanations and interactions with the acutely manic and agitated client are not appropriate or therapeutic at this time because the client with a high level of anxiety has difficulty focusing and processing. Saying "Threatening others and throwing furniture is not allowed" could lead the client to believe he is being punished. Reminding the client that the client has "been here before and knows what the rules are" and "We are only doing this for your own good, so calm down" are condescending and verbalizing the expectation that the client can control the illness.

✂— CN: Psychosocial integrity; CL: Synthesize

78. 4. To determine how low the gentamicin serum level drops between doses, the trough serum level should be drawn just before the administration of the next IV dose of gentamicin sulfate.

✂— CN: Pharmacological and parenteral therapies; CL: Apply

79. 1, 2, 3, 5. Anorexia or loss of appetite is not associated with valproic acid. Adverse effects include tremors, transient hair loss, gastrointestinal upset, and weight gain.

✂— CN: Pharmacological and parenteral therapies; CL: Analyze

80. 3. Intercourse commonly stimulates uterine contractions. The prostaglandins found in semen can also initiate contractions. After placement of a cerclage for advanced dilation and contractions, the client is considered at high risk for preterm birth and should be seen by her **healthcare provider (HCP)** 📖 more frequently. The client should call the HCP immediately if she sees signs of complications, such as leaking fluid (rupture of membranes), vaginal bleeding, and contractions (particularly with a cerclage in place). Anything in the vagina may initiate contractions and the labor process.

✂— CN: Reduction of risk potential; CL: Evaluate

81. 3. Meningococcal infections are spread through close mucous membrane or respiratory contact with large respiratory droplets. Meningococcal infections are not spread by small airborne organisms or contact with a person's skin or contaminated items. Standard precautions, used when touching body fluids, are not sufficient to prevent the spread of meningitis.

✂— CN: Safety and infection control; CL: Apply

82. 3. The nurse should contact the **HCP** 📖 for clarification of the prescription. The nurse must be vigilant when comparing medication in the medication box to the prescription; prednisolone, for example, is three to five times more potent than prednisone. The nurse cannot make a pharmacy substitution change without prescriptive authority. The prednisolone is not returned until a clarification prescription is obtained to determine the substitution drug and dosage is correct. It is not necessary to contact the charge nurse or supervisor, as the nurse must first clarify the prescription with the HCP. The nurse reports the incident according to agency policy and notifies all involved of the change in the prescription.

✂— CN: Pharmacological and parenteral therapies; CL: Synthesize

83. 1. The nurse should instruct the mother to bring the child to the emergency department. If aspirated, nuts may swell leading to an airway obstruction after the initial event; endoscopy may be required to remove remaining fragments. Bleeding from trauma to internal organs after abdominal thrusts is rare. There are no signs of shock to suggest anaphylaxis. There is no indication of the presence of a pneumothorax.

✂— CN: Physiological adaptation; CL: Synthesize

84. 1. Gastric upset is an adverse effect of NSAIDs. Taking these drugs with food and fluids minimizes this effect. The dosage of NSAIDs does not need to be tapered. Because NSAIDs do not cause drowsiness or stomatitis, the client does not need to restrict driving or rinse the mouth.

✂— CN: Pharmacological and parenteral therapies; CL: Synthesize

85. 2. The neonate's Apgar score has been improving since birth. (The birth score is 6; the current score is 9.) The nurse should continue to assess the neonate. There is no indication that oxygen is needed since the color is improving, and stimulating the baby is not necessary as the baby is now flexing the extremities.

✂— CN: Management of care; CL: Synthesize

86. 2. Managing clients' health involves many specialized areas, such as respiratory therapy, medicine, laboratory, social services, and technical monitoring. One of the significant roles of the nurse is to ensure clear communication with the client and among the healthcare team. Due to expanded media coverage of healthcare issues, clients may be more aware of healthcare issues, but may not be able to determine if the information is accurate or pertains to them. Because of increasing numbers of media sources, both digital and print, it is difficult for consumers to keep up with all of the advances in the science of health care. Clients are more aware of their rights because of media exposure and information disseminated by healthcare facilities. However, respect for the client's rights should be the nurse's concern as well, and communication should not be impacted by a client's knowledge or demand for those rights.

🔑 CN: Health promotion and maintenance; CL: Apply

87. 1, 2. The initial signs of esophageal atresia and TEF include lots of frothy mucus and unexplained episodes of cyanosis usually caused by overflow of mucus from the esophagus. Loose stools and poor gag reflex are not signs of TEF. Initial weight loss is common in newborns and not related to TEF.

🔑 CN: Reduction of risk potential; CL: Analyze

88. 1. Adequate circulatory status is the most important factor in the healing process of an infected decubitus ulcer. Blood flow to the area must be present to bring nutrients and prescribed antibiotics to the tissues. Rest and a balanced diet are essential to health maintenance but are not the priority for healing an infected decubitus ulcer. A fluid intake of 2,000 to 3,000 mL/day, if not contraindicated, is recommended to provide hydration to the client's tissues.

🔑 CN: Reduction of risk potential; CL: Synthesize

89. 4. Soft, washable toys are appropriate for infants, who tend to place everything in their mouths. These toys are not harmful. Plastic toys cannot be manipulated by a child of this age, and the child would put the car in the mouth, which may not be safe due to small parts that may be swallowed or aspirated. Games and puzzles are too advanced for a 5-month-old, and the child could put the pieces in the mouth and swallow them. Some stuffed animals have eyes that can be swallowed or aspirated.

🔑 CN: Reduction of risk potential; CL: Apply

90. 4. The nurse should call for a multidisciplinary staff meeting because there is a need for staff members to share their feelings of anger, frustration, and grief. Because nurses focus on saving human lives, any feelings of hopelessness regarding a dying client can interfere with the client's care and management. Assigning the staff member to other clients ignores the staff member's need to work through feelings. Calling the clinical nurse specialist to deal with the staff member does nothing to help other staff. The psychiatric clinical nurse specialist would

be included in the staff meeting to help the entire staff deal with their feelings. Agreeing with the staff member and discontinuing suicide precautions is highly inappropriate.

🔑 CN: Management of care; CL: Synthesize

91. 3. The nurse should give the next dose as prescribed because the blood level is 35 mcg/mL, which is lower than the normal range of 50 to 100 mcg/mL. Withholding the next dose, notifying the **HCP** 📖, and taking the client's vital signs are not indicated in this situation.

🔑 CN: Pharmacological and parenteral therapies; CL: Synthesize

92. 3. Going for a walk with the nurse and another client is a more gradual introduction to being with others. The goal is to gradually encourage interaction with others; playing games in the client's room promotes continued isolation. Going to a group session and participating in crafts are exposing the client to large groups too rapidly.

🔑 CN: Psychosocial integrity; CL: Synthesize

93. 4. The client is not emptying her bladder after repeated attempts. The nurse should now use an in-and-out catheter to empty the bladder. While the other comfort measures may be helpful, this client has not completely emptied her bladder since childbirth and will be at risk for a urinary tract infection and postpartum hemorrhage.

🔑 CN: Management of care; CL: Synthesize

94. 1. The best way to ease symptoms caused by hyperventilation is to have the client breathe into a paper bag. This helps to raise carbon dioxide level, which encourages deeper, slower breathing. The symptoms of hyperventilation will not be alleviated by having the client put his head between his knees, giving the client low concentrations of oxygen, or having the client take deep, slow breaths and exhaling normally.

🔑 CN: Basic care and comfort; CL: Synthesize

95. 2. True labor is present when cervical dilation and effacement occur. Fetal descent into the pelvic inlet is an indication that labor will begin soon. However, for a nulligravid client, this may take 1 to 2 weeks. Painful contractions every 3 to 5 minutes may be Braxton Hicks contractions. Contractions that disappear when the client lies down are a sign of false labor. Although leaking amniotic fluid should be reported, it is not a sign of true labor.

🔑 CN: Health promotion and maintenance; CL: Analyze

96. 4. The signs and symptoms of sepsis in a neonate, such as changes in appearance and behavior, are almost imperceptible. Often, the parents' only problem is that the neonate does not look "right." Fever and localized response, which are clues to infections in older children, are often absent in the neonate. Telling the father that he should have realized something was wrong is condescending and serves only to further the father's guilt feelings. Asking the father whether he read the booklet from the hospital implies that the father is at fault. One experience would not necessarily ensure that the father would be able to detect sepsis another time.

⚷ CN: Psychosocial integrity;
CL: Synthesize

97. 3. Nursing bottle caries occur when a child is routinely given a bottle of milk or juice at nap and bedtime. When teeth become coated in sugar before sleep, the lack of activity in the child's mouth for several hours during sleep allows the sugar to convert to acid, leading to decay. A child drinking 18 to 20 oz of whole milk in a day should not be malnourished, although she may lack essential vitamins and iron. Anemia may occur if she is only drinking milk because it contains no iron; however, the mother indicates she is eating meals. Regardless, children of this age should be taking no more than 16 oz of milk per day, and most children at this age should be drinking from a cup. The mother should be instructed to wean the child to a cup one feeding at a time until the child is completely weaned to a cup for all feedings. The last bottle-feeding to be replaced is usually the night bottle. Malocclusion of the teeth does not occur at 15 months. If the child were to continue to suck on a bottle until age 4 years or later, then malocclusion may occur.

⚷ CN: Health promotion and maintenance;
CL: Apply

98. 1. Because the femoral artery is usually used as the access site during a cardiac catheterization, children are required to remain on bed rest (with the head only slightly elevated) for several hours after the procedure to avoid arterial bleeding at the site. A knee-chest position is the correct position for an infant during a cyanotic episode as it will create peripheral resistance to the extremities, shunting blood to the heart. The apical heart rate is assessed prior to administering this medication; administration can be performed by an experienced **LPN/VN** 📖, although medication is checked with the **RN** 📖 prior to administration. Because echocardiography is noninvasive, there is no need to withhold meals before this procedure.

⚷ CN: Management of care; CL: Analyze

99. 2. The client should report tinnitus because vancomycin can affect the acoustic branch of the eighth cranial nerve. Vancomycin does not affect the vestibular branch of the acoustic nerve; vertigo and ataxia would occur if the vestibular branch were involved. Muscle stiffness is not associated with vancomycin.

⚷ CN: Pharmacological and parenteral therapies; CL: Analyze

100. 2. In an emergency in which the neonate's head is already being born, the first action by the nurse should be to check for the presence of a cord around the neonate's neck. If the cord is present, the nurse should gently remove it from around the neck. The mother should be told to breathe gently and avoid forceful bearing-down efforts, which could lead to lacerations. Although blood and bodily fluid precautions are always present in client care, this is an emergency. If possible, the nurse should put on gloves. Suctioning the mouth can be done after the nurse has checked that the cord is not around the neonate's neck. Telling the mother that help is on the way is not reassuring because emergency medical technicians may take some time to arrive. Birth is imminent because the neonate's head is emerging.

⚷ CN: Reduction of risk potential;
CL: Synthesize

101. 2. After surgery, the most important nursing goal is to prevent infection. Surgery involves an incision, which places the infant at risk for infection. The infant with this type of procedure does have discomfort, which can be relieved with acetaminophen, and managing pain is important but not the priority. The infant may be in arm restraints or have the cuff of the sleeve pinned to the diaper or pants. It is important that the infant not touch the incision line or disrupt the sutures, but the infant is not at risk for problems related to immobility. There is no indication that the parents need to improve their skills, but the nurse can support the family as they would be reacting normally with a first reaction of shock.

⚷ CN: Reduction of risk potential;
CL: Analyze

102. 2. The primary reason to give a diuretic to a client with heart failure is to promote sodium and water excretion through the kidneys. As a result, the excessive body water that tends to accumulate in a client with heart failure is eliminated, which causes the client to lose weight. Monitoring the client's weight daily helps evaluate the effectiveness of diuretic therapy. Clients should be advised to weigh themselves daily. An increased appetite or decreased thirst does not establish the effectiveness of the diuretic therapy, nor does having clearer urine after starting torsemide.

⚷ CN: Pharmacological and parenteral therapies; CL: Evaluate

103. 3. The client should be placed in a side-lying position and encouraged to take a deep breath during the insertion of the suppository. Placing the suppository along the rectal wall promotes absorption of the medication and helps avoid placing it into a stool mass. The nurse should insert the suppository 3 to 4 inches into the rectum of an adult client.

CN: Reduction of risk potential;
CL: Apply

104. 2. Hepatitis B virus is spread through contact with blood, body fluids contaminated with blood, and such body fluids as cerebrospinal, pleural, peritoneal, and synovial fluids; semen; and vaginal secretions. The risk of transmission of hepatitis B through feces is low. Touching the client without gloves is acceptable when there is no danger of contact with blood or body fluids. Recapping a used needle is a common source of needlestick injuries; needles should be properly disposed of uncapped.

CN: Safety and infection control;
CL: Apply

105. 2, 3, 5, 6. Safety and physiological needs are crucial initially for a client who is unable to meet her own needs. Identifying her stressors and feelings will be important later when she is responding to questions and her environment.

CN: Psychosocial integrity;
CL: Synthesize

106. 2. Signs of child abuse include injury with a history that is inconsistent with the nature of the injury, or unusual injuries for the age of the child. A spiral fracture of a child is always investigated as potential child abuse as this injury is often due to twisting of an extremity. It is not unusual for a child who is learning to walk to have bruises. Wearing the same clothes is not an indication of abuse or neglect. The child with conjunctivitis requires health care, but having frequent episodes is not an indication of abuse or neglect.

CN: Reduction of risk potential;
CL: Analyze

107. 3. In most agencies, it is a policy to discard the autologous blood after 4 hours of transfusing, due to an increased risk of infection. Increasing the infusion rate could cause fluid overload. Monitoring blood transfusions is a serious nursing responsibility, and because it is the change of shift, there is increased risk of error.

CN: Safety and infection control;
CL: Synthesize

108. 3. After a nephrectomy, a specific aspect of immediate postoperative management includes monitoring urine output at least hourly. Monitoring blood pressure and encouraging the use of incentive spirometry are other important considerations, but because of the surgical disruption of the urinary system, urine output is a priority. Measurement of urine output should also include an estimation of the amount of urine drainage on the flank dressing.

CN: Reduction of risk potential;
CL: Synthesize

109. 1. The client is demonstrating signs of anemia and should increase the iron in the diet. Foods such as red meats, beets, and cabbage are good sources of iron. The client should not limit the fluid intake to 1,000 mL/day, but should maintain an adequate fluid intake of about 3,000 mL/day. Carbohydrates will not provide the necessary dietary intake of iron. While fish is a healthy choice, beef, lamb, and iron-rich vegetables are more important in the diet at this time.

CN: Health promotion and maintenance;
CL: Synthesize

110. 2. Infants are obligatory nose breathers except when crying. The observation that the infant has slight cyanosis when quiet but becomes pink when crying and the inability to pass a catheter through the left nostril suggest that the neonate is exhibiting symptoms of unilateral choanal atresia. With this condition, one of the nasal passages is blocked by an abnormality of the septum. Surgical intervention is necessary to open the nostril. Typically, a neonate with esophageal reflux disorder exhibits episodes of apnea and vomiting after eating. Respiratory distress syndrome commonly occurs in preterm neonates who lack surfactant to maintain lung expansion. Common findings include sternal retractions, tachypnea, grunting respirations, nasal flaring, cyanosis, pallor, hypotonia, and bradycardia. A neonate with tracheoesophageal fistula commonly exhibits cyanosis during feedings and vomiting.

CN: Reduction of risk potential;
CL: Analyze

111. 2. The nurse's initial response should be to withhold the digoxin. The nurse should then notify the **HCP** 📖 if the apical pulse is 60 bpm or lower because of the risk of digoxin toxicity. The charge nurse does not need to be notified, but the nurse needs to document the notification and follow-up in the **medical record** 📖.

CN: Pharmacological and parenteral therapies; CL: Synthesize

112. 1, 2, 3, 5. Safety measures for poisonous substances include close supervision of children, safely storing toxic substances, teaching proper dosages and differences between adult and child doses, and the proper way to contact the Poison Control Center for instructions. Poison Control should be notified as soon as the poisoning has occurred and airway and circulation have been assessed. Poison Control will direct any further treatment. Syrup of ipecac is rarely used today in the treatment of ingested substances due to the potential for aspiration. It is contraindicated in cases of arsenic poisoning, seizures, and the ingestion of petroleum or corrosive substances.

☞ CN: Safety and infection control; CL: Create

113. 4. Dystonic adverse effects of haloperidol, especially oculogyric crises, are painful and frightening. IM benztropine is the fastest and most effective drug for managing dystonia. Lorazepam is an antianxiety medication and is not effective for treatment of dystonia. Although amantadine and diphenhydramine can be used for extrapyramidal symptoms, oral medications do not work as quickly, and amantadine may worsen psychotic symptoms.

☞ CN: Pharmacological and parenteral therapies; CL: Synthesize

114. 1. Neonates burn brown adipose tissue (fat) as a response to cold stress. In addition, there is increased utilization of glycogen and calorie stores. Hypoglycemia may result from becoming stressed by a cold environment. Neonates do not have the ability to shiver.

☞ CN: Health promotion and maintenance; CL: Apply

115. 1. While the adolescent is denying pain, he is displaying objective signs of pain. Adults of Asian ethnicity typically display stoic behavior, and the 16-year-old most likely would try to conform to this cultural norm. The nurse should administer an analgesic and assure the client that taking medication will speed the recovery process. The nurse must also reassess the client after administering the pain medication and document the response. The reassessment is typically done 30 minutes after a parenteral analgesic and an hour after an oral analgesic. People who identify with the Asian culture infrequently report concerns, and, therefore, asking the client about what is troubling him is unlikely to provide the nurse with additional information. The adolescent's behavior is consistent with postoperative pain. If the parents are stoic, discussing the adolescent's behavior may not be productive. At this stage of treatment, distractions can be used in conjunction with medication, but should not be substituted for them.

☞ CN: Basic care and comfort; CL: Synthesize

116. 1. Formula should fill the entire nipple of the bottle while the baby is sucking. This decreases the amount of air taken in by the baby; taking in too much air can lead to regurgitation. Not all babies at term are born with well-developed sucking skills. Some neonates are sleepy and do not suck well. For the first feeding, the baby should be bubbled after taking one-fourth to one-half ounce of formula and then again when the infant has finished the feeding. Bottle propping can lead to aspiration, decreased infant bonding, and aspiration of formula. However, it is not associated with the intake of too much air.

☞ CN: Health promotion and maintenance; CL: Synthesize

117. 3. Because of toddlers' high energy and poor impulse control, safety is a priority concern for this age-group. Language is important in toddler development, but not the most important at this time. While parents should set clear guidelines for behavior, the priority for toddlers is ensuring safety. Diet habits should be developed at this time, but the most important subject to teach parents of toddlers is safety.

☞ CN: Safety and infection control; CL: Synthesize

118. 1, 3, 4, 5. When a client begins to have back pain with administration of blood, the nurse should suspect a hemolytic reaction, and the blood transfusion should be stopped immediately. Any remaining blood and the tubing should be sent to the lab. The nurse should prepare for a reaction from mild to severe, including the need for cardiopulmonary resuscitation, because even a small amount of mismatched blood can lead to a major reaction. The nurse should obtain a urine specimen to send to the laboratory to check for hemoglobin because RBC hemolysis filters through the kidneys from the reaction. The nurse should stop the IV line with the Y-tubing for the blood and not flush the line with saline so that the client does not receive any more blood. The tubing should be changed so that a tube without blood can be used for infusions.

☞ CN: Pharmacological and parenteral therapies; CL: Synthesize

119. 2. At 4 hours postpartum, the fundus should be midline and at the level of the umbilicus. Whenever the placenta is manually removed after birth, there is a possibility that all of the placenta has not been removed. Sometimes, small pieces of the placenta are retained, a common cause of late postpartum hemorrhage. The client is exhibiting signs and symptoms associated with retained placental fragments. The client will continue to bleed until the fragments are expelled. Perineal and cervical lacerations are characterized by bright red bleeding and a firmly contracted fundus at the level that is expected. Urine retention is characterized by a full bladder, which can be observed by a bulge or fullness just above the symphysis pubis. Also, the client's fundus would be deviated to one side and boggy to the touch.

⚼ CN: Reduction of risk potential; CL: Analyze

120. 3. A neonate born at 37 weeks' gestation will have some cartilage in the earlobes, fine and fuzzy hair, scant to moderate rugae in the scrotum, and a breast nodule diameter of 4 mm. Neonates born before 36 weeks' gestation will have only an anterior transverse crease on the soles of the feet. Extensive rugae on the scrotum are a typical finding in neonates born at 39 weeks' gestation or later. Coarse and silky scalp hair typically is found in neonates that are born at 39 weeks or later.

⚼ CN: Health promotion and maintenance; CL: Analyze

121. 1, 3, 4. Clear communication is crucial for a client with delirium. The family must include the client in all conversations and keep him oriented to time and place. It is inappropriate to argue with a client's hallucinations because they are real to the client. Speaking more loudly will not help this client hear more distinctly and may increase the client's confusion.

⚼ CN: Management of care; CL: Synthesize

122. 2. One-to-one supervision provides safety until appropriate detoxification can be given. Restraints are the last intervention after less restrictive alternatives have been tried. It is unlikely that the client can cooperate with staying in a chair. Putting the client in bed in his or her room puts the client at risk for falling, and a closed door prevents close observation.

⚼ CN: Safety and infection control; CL: Synthesize

123. 1. The nurse should recognize that the client's clinical manifestations indicate fluid overload and decrease the infusion rate so the client's circulation can handle the extra fluid. Antihistamines are used for allergic reactions. The nurse should place the client in an upright position with the feet down so that blood or fluid volume can drain to the lower extremities and relieve some of the extra fluid load on the heart. The nurse does not need to replace the blood with another type of fluid because the client's response is not a blood transfusion reaction.

⚼ CN: Pharmacological and parenteral therapies; CL: Synthesize

124. 2. 200,000 units of heparin is too large of a dose. Heparin may be given in a 5,000-unit bolus dose IV; then 20,000 to 40,000 units infused over 24 hours with a dose adjusted to maintain desired APTT, or 5,000 to 10,000 units IV piggyback every 4 to 6 hours.

⚼ CN: Pharmacological and parenteral therapies; CL: Apply

125. 2. Insensible fluid loss is invisible vaporization from the lungs and skin and assists in regulating body temperature. The amount of water loss is increased by accelerated body metabolism, which occurs with increased body temperature. The client's body mass index does not directly influence calculating fluid therapy.

⚼ CN: Management of care; CL: Analyze

126. 3. A toddler has not developed the concept of sharing, so two similar toys must be provided to prevent disagreements. Playing together in harmony is not the developmental level of a toddler. They play side by side, but not together. Threatening to put the children in their rooms does not solve the problem, nor does taking away the toy.

⚼ CN: Health promotion and maintenance; CL: Synthesize

127. 3. Visual disturbances are a symptom of digoxin toxicity. These disturbances can include double, blurred, or yellow vision. Cardiovascular manifestations of digoxin toxicity include bradycardia hypotension, other dysrhythmias, and pulse deficit. Gastrointestinal symptoms include anorexia, nausea, and vomiting.

⚼ CN: Pharmacological and parenteral therapies; CL: Analyze

128. 2. In order to reestablish trust, the nurse should first try to determine if something happened at the last visit that was upsetting for the family. Dislocation of a body part can be seen as a source of illness among persons of Mexican ethnicity. At a well-child visit, the **healthcare provider (HCP)** 📖 would have palpated the fontanelle. If it is now sunken from dehydration, the parents may blame the provider for the illness. This belief is referred to as *caida de la mollera*. The family may have talked with a traditional healer, but following this line of questioning first may appear that the nurse considers the healer as an adversary. Asking about immigration makes a stereotypical assumption. Asking if the family is afraid the baby will be taken from them may be suggesting something the family has never considered and may cause unnecessary distress.

⚼ CN: Psychosocial integrity; CL: Synthesize

129. 1. The child wants attention from the nurse, even if the behavior is met by a negative response. Aggression, resistance against authority, and exaggerated stress are behaviors that can be associated with a 4-year-old. However, coming to the nurses' station after being told not to do so is not an example of these behaviors.

CN: Psychosocial integrity; CL: Analyze

130. 1, 2, 3. Clinical manifestations of dehydration include decreased tearing; dry mucous membranes; sunken fontanelles; weight loss; behavioral changes; scanty, concentrated urine; and a thready, fast pulse. Clear, pale yellow urine would indicate adequate hydration. A bounding pulse would indicate fluid volume excess.

CN: Physiological adaptation; CL: Analyze

131. 4. Hydrotherapy wound cleaning is very painful for the client. The client should be medicated for pain about 30 minutes before the treatment in anticipation of the increased pain the client will experience. Wounds are debrided, but excessive fluids are not lost during the hydrotherapy session. However, electrolyte loss can occur from open wounds during immersion, so the sessions should be limited to 20 to 30 minutes. There is no need to limit food or fluids 45 minutes before hydrotherapy unless it is an individualized need for a given client. Topical antibiotics are applied after hydrotherapy.

CN: Reduction of risk potential; CL: Create

132. 3. When a neonate is being transferred to a neonatal care center (level III nursery), the parents should be allowed to see and touch the neonate, if possible, before transfer. The parents should be given the location and telephone number of the unit to which the neonate is being transferred. This helps to keep the parents informed. The parents are already aware of the neonate's condition and should recognize that it is critical if the neonate is being transferred to a neonatal care center. The parents have signed **consent** for treatment on admission, and in most states another consent is not necessary. Asking whether the father would like to ride in the ambulance with the neonate during the transfer is inappropriate. Most ambulances or transferring vehicles (e.g., helicopters, airplanes) do not allow family members to accompany the ill client. Space in the motor vehicle, helicopter, or plane is limited. In addition, most transferring vehicles do not have insurance to cover family members should an accident occur during transfer.

CN: Management of care; CL: Synthesize

133. 4. Tenets of the Roman Catholic Church hold that it is acceptable for anyone, regardless of religious belief, to baptize a neonate. For Roman Catholic families, baptism ensures entry into heaven. Local practice may vary, and in some situations, the parents may prefer to have a Roman Catholic person perform the rites; however, this person may not be available until after the death. The parents may wish to have a priest contacted for grief support. Notification of the hospital's director is not necessary.

CN: Management of care; CL: Synthesize

134. 1. The best nursing intervention is giving the client finger foods high in protein and calories that he can eat while he paces or walks. Informing the client that snacks are available if he eats properly at mealtime is inappropriate because the client is too busy and distracted to sit and eat an entire meal. Telling the client to sit alone at mealtime to decrease distractions will not help him, because the client is in a manic state, is easily distracted, and needs to move. Teaching the client about proper nutrition ignores his need for adequate intake. The client would be unable to focus on the nurse's teaching.

CN: Basic care and comfort; CL: Synthesize

135. 1. Moist heat is a nonpharmacologic pain management strategy that may alleviate pain and reduce the dose of analgesic, if required. Heat dilates blood vessels and decreases inflammation. Lifting and circular exercises will aggravate the already-inflamed joint. Cold constricts blood vessels, and dry ice is not used on the body.

CN: Basic care and comfort; CL: Evaluate

136. 3. For an LP, a needle is inserted into the subarachnoid space to obtain a specimen of spinal fluid for diagnostic testing. Fluid on the lumbar dressing indicates cerebrospinal fluid (CSF) leakage and must be reported to the **healthcare provider (HCP)** immediately. The client should be encouraged to drink fluids after an LP to facilitate production of CSF. It is normal to have a mild headache due to the removal of CSF samples for laboratory analysis. Although the concerns of the client should be discussed with the HCP at some point, the CSF leakage is a priority and should be reported immediately.

CN: Reduction of risk potential; CL: Analyze

137. 3. The normal calcium level is 9.0 to 10.5 mg/dL. Hypercalcemia is commonly seen with malignant disease and metastases. The other laboratory values are normal. Hypercalcemia can be treated with fluids, furosemide, or administration of calcitonin. Failure to treat hypercalcemia can cause muscle weakness, changes in level of consciousness, nausea, vomiting, abdominal pain, and dehydration. Although the client is on hospice care, she will still need palliative treatment. Comfort and risk reduction are components of hospice care.

CN: Reduction of risk potential; CL: Synthesize

138. 2. The nurse would document these findings as "early" decelerations. Early decelerations are thought to be the result of vagal nerve stimulation caused by compression of the fetal head during labor. They are considered normal physiologic response to labor and do not require any intervention. Early decelerations do not require position change or oxygen, as they are not a sign of fetal distress. Variable decelerations are thought to be due to umbilical cord compression. Early decelerations are not emergent and do not require immediate reporting to the **healthcare provider (HCP)** or preparing for cesarean section.

CN: Management of care; CL: Synthesize

139. 2. A child with a cardiac defect finds that squatting decreases venous return and workload to the heart and increases comfort and blood flow to the lungs. Squatting traps blood in the lower extremities so less blood is returned to the right atrium. Squatting does not make it easier for the child to play with toys. Squatting does not relieve abdominal pressure; it may even increase it slightly. Squatting has no effect on muscle tone. When done by a child with a cardiac defect, it is not meant as an exercise but is a compensatory process used to reduce dyspnea.

CN: Physiological adaptation; CL: Evaluate

140. 3. The diaphragm is the major muscle of respiration; it is made up of two hemidiaphragms, each innervated by the right and left phrenic nerves. Injury to the phrenic nerve results in hemidiaphragm paralysis on the side of the injury and an ineffective breathing pattern. Consciousness, cardiac function, and urinary elimination are not affected by the phrenic nerve.

CN: Management of care; CL: Analyze

141. 2, 3, 5. Cystic fibrosis is most common in those of the Caucasian race. As an autosomal recessive disease, for an infant to be affected, each parent must carry a recessive trait. If both parents carry the trait, each offspring has a 25% chance of inheriting the disease, a 50% chance of being a carrier, and a 25% chance of being unaffected. The shape of red blood cells is altered with sickle cell disease rather than CF. CVS testing can identify whether a fetus is or is not affected.

CN: Health promotion and maintenance; CL: Create

142. 2, 3, 1, 4. An open airway is essential to survival. The nurse should first ensure an open airway. Next, the nurse should start an IV and then notify the **HCP**. Finally, the nurse should inform the family of the situation and, if appropriate, allow them to remain with the client.

CN: Management of care; CL: Synthesize

143. 1. Prevention of another pulmonary embolus is important; the nurse should teach the client to observe for signs of clot formation to prevent a potentially fatal episode and maintain cardiopulmonary integrity and adequate ventilation and perfusion. Elevation of the lower extremities, not lowering them, promotes venous return to the heart. Ambulation must be done several times each day. Limiting fluid intake increases blood viscosity, promoting clot formation.

CN: Health promotion and maintenance; CL: Synthesize

144. 2. When a client is being released from the hospital with her neonate and the nurse learns that the client is homeless, the nurse should contact the hospital's or unit's social worker. Social workers have access to resources to assist the client to find temporary shelter in emergencies. The director of the birthing unit does not need to be notified. The director's responsibilities are primarily administrative. The client's **HCP** can be notified once the social worker has offered assistance to the client. The HCP may cancel the release of the neonate until temporary housing is located. Notifying the client's family is inappropriate. The client may not have any immediate family members, or there may be some stress between the client and family.

CN: Management of care; CL: Synthesize

145. 3, 4, 1, 2. The client is experiencing a septic reaction to the blood transfusion. The nurse's first action is to stop the infusion and notify the **healthcare provider (HCP)** and blood bank. The nurse then uses an infusion of normal saline to keep the vein open. Next, the nurse obtains a sample of the client's blood for a blood culture, and last, the nurse sends the blood bag and the administration set to the blood bank for culture.

CN: Pharmacological and parenteral therapies; CL: Synthesize

146. 1. In a frank breech, the buttocks alone are at the cervix, while the knees are extended to rest on the chest. In a cephalic presentation, the head is the fetal body part first coming in contact with the cervix. Both feet at the cervix is termed double footling breech. In a shoulder presentation, one of the shoulders (actually the acromion process) presents to the cervix. Typically, the fetus is lying horizontally (transverse lie).

CN: Health promotion and maintenance; CL: Apply

147. 1. A specimen for culture and sensitivity should be sent to the laboratory promptly so that a smear can be taken before organisms start to grow in the specimen.

⚷ CN: Reduction of risk potential;
CL: Apply

148. **1, 3, 4, 5.** The nurse is responsible for the client's safety in the operating room. The nurse should call a **time-out** 📖 if the client is not properly identified with an identification band. In addition, an IV line and oxygen should always be established when an ET tube is placed. This practice applies whenever a client's airway is compromised enough for intubation to occur, not only in the operating room environment. An anesthetist or anesthesiologist should be present during surgery to manage the airway. Postoperative pain medication is administered in the recovery room.

⚷ CN: Safety and infection control;
CL: Synthesize

149. **1.** Anencephaly is a neural tube defect that is not compatible with life, although some infants with anencephaly live for several days before death occurs. When the client has decided to continue the pregnancy and donate the neonatal organs after the death of the neonate, the nurse should remain nonjudgmental. The nurse should explore his or her feelings about the issue of anencephaly and organ donation. The nurse should not make judgments about the client's position, nor should the nurse try to persuade the client to terminate the pregnancy. Contacting the client's minister to explore the client's options is not appropriate. As a devout Baptist, the client probably has already discussed the matter with her minister. Telling the client that the neonatal death will be prolonged and painful to her is not helpful. Death may occur very soon after birth. Contacting the client's family members is not appropriate. The client may wish not to discuss the matter with her family.

⚷ CN: Management of care; CL: Synthesize

150. **2, 3, 4, 5.** Anorexia is commonly the first indication of digoxin toxicity. Arrhythmias are also common with digoxin toxicity. Although bradycardia is the most common sign of toxicity, other tachycardic arrhythmias can occur. A normal pulse rate for a 3-month-old child at rest is about 120 bpm. Blurred vision can be associated with digoxin toxicity and may be detected in an infant if he or she stops following moving objects. Sudden vomiting or drowsiness can be associated with digoxin toxicity. Constipation is not associated with digoxin toxicity and is not an adverse effect of digoxin.

⚷ CN: Pharmacological and parenteral therapies; CL: Synthesize

151. **2.** If the specimen was from a fingerstick and not a venous sample, the potassium level can be falsely elevated. Because the finger is squeezed to obtain the sample, cells may have been broken from the pressure of squeezing. When the cells break, they release potassium, which will falsely elevate the potassium level in the result. Calling the **HCP** 📖 without first checking the source of the sample would not give the HCP accurate and complete information. A cardiac monitor would not be necessary if the potassium level is falsely elevated. The last 24-hour output would only indicate that the infant is voiding in an adequate amount. This may or may not have an influence on the infant's potassium level.

⚷ CN: Reduction of risk potential;
CL: Synthesize

152. **3.** The level of lethality of a client's suicidal thoughts depends on the presence or absence of a plan. If the client has a plan, the nurse must know what it is and whether or not the client has access to the means to complete suicide. The initiation of suicide precautions is necessary whenever a client threatens suicide, but first it is important to discover more information about what the client is thinking and planning. Unless the client has at his or her disposal the means to harm himself or herself or is constantly trying to harm himself or herself with objects on the unit, placing the client on a suicide watch or confining the client to his or her room is an overreaction to the client's disclosure of suicidal ideation.

⚷ CN: Safety and infection control;
CL: Synthesize

153. **1, 2, 5.** Prenatal care includes a general supplementation of 400 mcg of folic acid, and clients with a history of gastric bypass should be referred to a dietician to determine adequate nutrient intake. All pregnant clients have their urine routinely checked for protein and sugar. There is no indication for checking glucose levels at each prenatal visit in clients who have undergone gastric bypass. Gastric bypass clients are not at risk of gaining all of their weight back. No evidence supports implementing stress tests at 20 weeks.

⚷ CN: Health promotion and maintenance;
CL: Create

154. **4.** Due to the client's psychosis and difficulties coping, a positive, supportive environment is essential to limit further regression and help the client engage in her own treatment. Confrontation and peer pressure are the type of milieu more suited to a chemically dependent client. While involvement in self-governance can be therapeutic, forcing a psychotic client to participate in self-governance before he or she is ready could actually hinder treatment and recovery. Although group activities are commonly required in treatment programs, a client who is very disturbed or confused is not forced to attend. Also, the client must participate when and how the client feels comfortable, rather than mandating a specific amount of participation. Equal participation by clients does not ensure a therapeutic milieu or speed the client's recovery.

🔑 CN: Psychosocial integrity; CL: Synthesize

155. 2. Severe hypoperfusion to all vital organs results in failure of the vital functions and then circulatory collapse. Hypotension, anuria, respiratory distress, and acidosis are other symptoms associated with irreversible shock. The client in irreversible shock will not be alert.

🔑 CN: Reduction of risk potential; CL: Analyze

156. 1. Pulmonary embolism is a potentially life-threatening complication of deep vein thrombosis. The client's change in mental status, tachypnea, and tachycardia indicate a possible pulmonary embolism. The nurse should promptly notify the **HCP** 📖 of the client's condition. Administering a sedative without further evaluation of the client's condition is not appropriate. There is no need to elicit a positive Homans' sign; the client is already diagnosed with deep vein thrombosis. Increasing the IV flow rate may be an appropriate action but not without first notifying the HCP.

🔑 CN: Reduction of risk potential; CL: Synthesize

157. 4. The nurse should refuse to administer the medication to the client because of the risk of respiratory depression in the neonate. Morphine, given IM, peaks in 30 to 60 minutes and lasts 4 hours. Based on the assessment findings, the client most likely will be delivering within that time frame, increasing the risk of respiratory depression in the neonate, a serious consequence. Therefore, the nurse should not administer the drug. Naloxone should be readily available whenever opioids that can result in respiratory depression are used. Asking the **HCP** 📖 to validate the dosage is not necessary.

🔑 CN: Management of care; CL: Synthesize

158. 2. Bending the chin down toward the chest decreases the risk of food entering the trachea and causing aspiration into the lungs. The client should sit up at a 90-degree angle when eating. Although eating and talking increase the risk of aspiration as well as muscle fatigue, the nurse should encourage the client to have visitors but avoid talking while chewing and swallowing. The client should rest before eating because muscle fatigue can contribute to choking.

🔑 CN: Reduction of risk potential; CL: Synthesize

159. 42 mm Hg
To obtain CPP, use this formula:
    CPP = mean arterial pressure (MAP) – ICP.
    To obtain the MAP, use this formula:

$$MAP = \left[\text{systolic BP} + (2 \times \text{diastolic BP})\right] \div 3$$

$$MAP = \left[90 + (2 \times 50)\right] \div 3 = 63.3$$

$$CPP = 63.3 - 21 = 42.3\,\text{mm Hg.}$$

🔑 CN: Physiological adaptation; CL: Apply

160. 1. The client with a spinal cord injury above T6 who suddenly experiences clinical manifestations of autonomic stimulation, such as flushing, sweating, and piloerection, is demonstrating life-threatening autonomic dysreflexia. The cluster of manifestation results from noxious stimuli, such as a full bladder, or lying on a foreign object, such as a plastic cap or crinkled paper, which the client cannot feel. As soon as the noxious stimulus is removed, the manifestations begin to subside. When the client demonstrates clinical manifestations of autonomic dysreflexia, the nurse should first elevate the head of the bed immediately to decrease the intracerebral pressure caused by the hypertension that developed from autonomic stimulation. The nurse can next check for a distended bladder or foreign object. The client's blood pressure will be elevated; the nurse should assess vital signs frequently.

🔑 CN: Management of care; CL: Synthesize

161. 3. The nurse should refer the client to a social worker for assistance in enrolling in the WIC program. This program provides assistance for foods such as milk, cereal, and infant formula. Instructing the client in low-cost, highly nutritious meal preparation will not meet the client's need for additional funds for food. Determining whether the client qualifies for state assistance is part of the role of the social worker, not the nurse. Asking the client if she has a job and the amount of income earned is not within the role of the nurse. The social worker can determine whether the family income guidelines are met for state and federal assistance.

🔑 CN: Management of care; CL: Synthesize

162. 4. Telling the client about one activity at a time with 10 minutes' notice gives the client time to prepare for that activity. Writing out the schedule does not ensure that the client will remember to look at it. It is overwhelming to explain an entire day's schedule all at once to a client diagnosed with dementia. Leading a client to an activity after the fact doesn't allow the client to prepare.

🔑 CN: Psychosocial integrity; CL: Synthesize

163. 1, 2, 3, 4. Safety of others is a priority, and the nurse must monitor the client's anger and potential for aggression. The nurse should also find safe ways for the client to express the client's anger and any other feelings about the abuse. A referral to a support group is appropriate because anger management groups are one way to assist the client in learning to manage anger. Nothing about jail is mentioned in the question. Discussion of jail does not help the client address the client's issues with anger and the abuse causing the anger.

⚷— CN: Management of care; CL: Synthesize

164. 2. The primiparous client at 2 hours postpartum who delivered a term neonate vaginally should be assessed first because this client is at risk for postpartum hemorrhage. Early postpartum hemorrhage typically occurs during the first 24 hours postpartum. Once the nurse has assessed the client's fundus, lochia, and vital signs, a determination about the stability of the client can be made. After this assessment, the nurse can provide care to the other clients, who are of lesser priority than the newly delivered primiparous client.

⚷— CN: Management of care; CL: Synthesize

165. 1. Legionellosis is a pneumonia caused by the bacterium *Legionella pneumophila* that thrives in water that is 95°F to 115°F (35°F to 46°C). When a building's hot water plumbing has water at this temperature, the bacteria thrive; then they may be transmitted via inhalation from air conditioning, showers, spas, and whirlpools. The bacteria are not transmitted via smoke or ceiling fan blades or by swallowing contaminated water.

⚷— CN: Health promotion and maintenance; CL: Synthesize

166. 2. The child's signs and symptoms in conjunction with the acute onset suggest possible croup or epiglottitis. The priority diagnosis at this time is airway obstruction. The airway may become completely occluded by the epiglottis at any time. Although the child has an infection, and the client has respiratory distress, the immediate priority is to establish and maintain a patent airway. No evidence is provided to support the potential for aspiration.

⚷— CN: Reduction of risk potential; CL: Analyze

167. 3. The baseline laboratory data that are established before a client is started on tissue plasminogen activator or alteplase recombinant include hematocrit, hemoglobin level, and platelet count.

⚷— CN: Reduction of risk potential; CL: Apply

168. 2, 3. The client should be instructed not to eat or drink for 8 to 12 hours before the test. Stools will be white for up to 72 hours following the procedure as the barium is eliminated from the body. Laxatives and fluids will be encouraged after the procedure to help prevent barium impaction, but the client will not be given stool softeners or laxatives before the procedure. The client should not experience pain during the procedure. The nurse should also instruct the client to stop smoking at midnight the night before the test.

⚷— CN: Reduction of risk potential; CL: Apply

169. 3, 4. A National Patient Safety Goal of the Joint Commission is to improve the accuracy of client identification; to attain that goal, healthcare personnel must use at least two client identifiers when providing care, treatment, or services. The **medical record** ▢ number and name as printed on the client's name band are appropriate identifiers. Because the client can change rooms and beds, these are not to be used as identifiers. Social security number is not used as an identifier for healthcare or treatment purposes.

⚷— CN: Safety and infection control; CL: Apply

170. 3. This rhythm is atrial fibrillation. It is characterized by an irregular QRS interval, no definite P waves before the QRS waves, and a ventricular rate >100 bpm.

⚷— CN: Reduction of risk potential; CL: Analyze

171. 3. The vastus lateralis site is the preferred IM site for all ages because it does not have any major nerves or blood vessels located near it. The deltoid and dorsogluteal muscles have major nerves and blood vessels located nearby. The triceps is not an acceptable muscle for IM injections because it is not well developed in most clients.

⚷— CN: Pharmacological and parenteral therapies; CL: Apply

172. 1. Clients should be instructed to rinse their mouths after using a steroid inhaler to avoid developing thrush. Clients should also be instructed to inhale slowly through the mouth and then hold the breath as they count to 10 slowly. It is not necessary for the client to cough and deep-breathe before using the inhaler.

⚷— CN: Pharmacological and parenteral therapies; CL: Synthesize

173. 2. The nurse should stay with the client during the first 15 minutes of a blood transfusion because this is when reactions are most likely to occur. Blood products should never be refrigerated on the nursing unit. Blood that has not been infused after 4 hours should not be infused. The blood should be infused over the specific time prescribed by the **healthcare provider (HCP)** 📖. If a fever develops, the transfusion should be stopped immediately, and the blood reaction policy of the facility should be followed.

🔑 CN: Pharmacological and parenteral therapies; CL: Synthesize

174. 2. The symptoms of difficulty breathing, elevated blood pressure, and cough are indicative of circulatory overload. Circulatory overload occurs when blood is infused more rapidly than the circulatory system can accommodate. Anaphylactic reactions are manifested by urticaria, wheezing, and shock. Sepsis begins with a rapid onset of chills and fever. Acute hemolytic reaction is typically manifested by chills, fever, low back pain, and flushing.

🔑 CN: Pharmacological and parenteral therapies; CL: Analyze

175. 2. Sucralfate should be taken on an empty stomach 1 hour before or 2 hours after meals and at bedtime. It is usually taken four times a day. There is no need to avoid milk products while taking the drug. Sucralfate does not affect hemoglobin levels.

🔑 CN: Pharmacological and parenteral therapies; CL: Evaluate

176. 1, 3, 4. When assessing client safety, the nurse assesses suicide thoughts or plan, recent use of illicit drugs (as they may cause impaired judgment or thought processes), and previously experienced allergic reactions and adverse reactions to medications. Note that safety involves many aspects of care. Incentives and diet preferences (allergies would be previously noted) are not directly related to safety, although they may be part of an overall assessment.

🔑 CN: Reduction of risk potential; CL: Synthesize

177. 1, 2, 3, 4. The client with conjunctivitis can use warm soaks to remove crusting. The nurse should teach the client to dispose of the soaks by wrapping them in a separate bag to avoid spreading bacteria. Topical antibiotics are used to treat the infection. The client should avoid contaminating the tip of the medication dispenser. Bacterial conjunctivitis requires containing the spread of the infection. The client should avoid touching the eyes. If the client does touch the eyes, the client should wash the hands after touching the eyes. The client does not need to be isolated.

🔑 CN: Reduction of risk potential; CL: Create

178. 1. The physical aspects of care have a higher priority than do the psychosocial aspects. The client report is part of the electronic **medical record** 📖,

but the maternal contraction pattern and the fetal heart rate pattern must be completed immediately upon admission to establish a baseline. The need for a tocolytic agent cannot be determined until the maternal fetal unit has been assessed. Assessment of the circumstances and etiologies of the prior fetal demises are important but are not of the highest importance. The psychosocial aspects are very important in the care of this client and can briefly be discussed as the physical aspects of assessment are being completed, but in-depth psychosocial care will need to wait until the physical aspects have been completed.

🔑 CN: Safety and infection control; CL: Synthesize

179. 2, 5. Two sources of identification must be confirmed before administering medication to a client. A source of information can be the client's record number, name, or date of birth, as noted on the client's armband. A client may be confused or hard of hearing and may give a wrong name or answer to a wrong name; thus, having the client state his or her name or respond to his or her name is not safe practice. Client recognition is not sufficient identification for administering medication. Clients change rooms frequently, so a room number is not a source of identification for administering medication.

🔑 CN: Pharmacological and parenteral therapies; CL: Apply

180. 2. Children who witness domestic violence commonly grow up to be victims or abusers. Counseling helps interrupt the pattern of violence in families. Limiting contact between the father and child does not address the child's behavior, and outgrowing violent behaviors is not likely without other interventions. Setting limits on violent behaviors alone does not address the child's feelings and needs.

🔑 CN: Psychosocial integrity; CL: Synthesize

181. 4. Because of the client's age, the amniocentesis is most likely being done to evaluate for Down syndrome (trisomy 21). Women older than 35 years are at higher risk for having a child with Down syndrome. Cri-du-chat syndrome is a genetic disorder involving a short arm on chromosome 5. This disorder is not associated with mothers who are older than 35 years. The client is AB positive, so the amniocentesis is not being done for ABO incompatibility, in which the mother is type O and the fetus is type A, B, or AB. The amniocentesis is not being done to detect erythroblastosis fetalis because the mother is Rh positive.

🔑 CN: Reduction of risk potential; CL: Analyze

182. 2, 3. A National Patient Safety Goal of the Joint Commission is to improve the effectiveness of communication among caregivers. The requirement for verbal or telephone prescriptions, or for telephonic reporting of critical test results, is to verify the complete prescription or test result by having the person receiving the information record and "read back" the complete prescription or test result. Effective communication that is timely, accurate, complete, unambiguous, and understood by the recipient reduces error and results in improved client safety. "Read-back" procedures are not intended to discourage or prohibit telephone communications among **healthcare providers (HCPs)** 💻 or to promote use of electronic **medical records** 💻. Safety procedures, such as provider identification codes, are in place for HCPs to give verbal or telephone prescriptions.

⚷ CN: Safety and infection control;
CL: Apply

183. 3. The actual desired weight gain of 1 lb per week is the most measurable goal for the client. Attending all eating disorder support groups is a goal, but is not as important as actual weight gain. The client can eat a larger meal at breakfast and then not eat sufficient food and over exercise for the remainder of the day. The client's improved self-image is important, but actual weight gain is again a priority.

⚷ CN: Physiologic adaptation;
CL: Synthesize

184. 4. The nurse should allow the client to see and hold the baby for as long as she desires. Such activities provide memories for the mother and assist in the grieving process. There is a possibility that the client may change her mind about the adoption. In most states, there is a defined period (6 months to 1 year or longer) before an adoption becomes final. If the client changes her mind about the adoption, the nurse should accept the client's decision and notify the **HCP** 💻 and social worker. Telling the client that it would be best if she did not see the baby is imposing the nurse's value system on the client. Allowing the client to see the baby through the nursery window is inappropriate because the client should be allowed to touch and hold the baby. Contacting the HCP for advice related to the client's visitation is not necessary.

⚷ CN: Management of care; CL: Synthesize

185. 2. The parent's expression of stress and grief and the adolescent's behavior and drug use could be preludes to suicide, especially since another member of the family succeeded in suicide. Suicide attempts are more likely in families in which there has been a previous suicide attempt or suicide death, especially for young people. The parent's ability to emotionally support the adolescent in this crisis has been compromised, but the safety of both supersedes this concern. Assuring the client's and parent's safety is more important than dealing with anger or frustration at this point. Though the emotional states of both the parent and the child are important, one is not more important than the other.

⚷ CN: Safety and infection control;
CL: Analyze

186. 2. A decrease or change in the level of consciousness is an early indication of increased intracranial pressure (ICP) and should be reported to the child's **HCP** 💻 as soon as possible to try and control the pressure so that it does not increase further. Vomiting can be a sign of increased ICP that occurs with a brain tumor, but it usually occurs unrelated to food and in the morning upon arising. Blood pressure increases with a brain tumor due to pressure on the brain stem. Concentrated urine is a sign of dehydration and is not related to the signs of a brain tumor.

⚷ CN: Physiological adaptation;
CL: Analyze

187. 1. The nurse should first plan to relieve the nausea and vomiting; if these continue, the client is at risk for dehydration and electrolyte imbalance. The client's poor appetite is likely related to the underlying health problem and is not the priority; the nausea may adversely affect the appetite, and relieving the nausea may allow the client an opportunity to eat and drink. The client has jaundice but does not have uncomfortable symptoms such as pruritus. The abdominal spasms may be related to nausea and vomiting and can be assessed again when the nausea and vomiting have stopped.

⚷ CN: Reduction of risk potential;
CL: Analyze

188. 1. All clients who are at risk for pressure ulcer development should be identified on admission to healthcare facilities so that preventive actions can be implemented by the nursing staff. These preventive actions need to be individualized to the client, so automatic placement of all at-risk clients on an every-2-hour turning schedule, a specialty bed, or a high-protein, high-carbohydrate diet is not appropriate.

⚷ CN: Reduction of risk potential;
CL: Apply

189. 4. With a severe gonorrheal infection, scarring of the fallopian tubes may occur, and becoming pregnant may be difficult or impossible. If the girl's partner is not treated, she can be reinfected. There is no immunity against gonorrhea, and, if exposed again, the girl can again become infected. Although a condom may provide some protection against contracting gonorrhea, it is not an adequate protection against the condition and will not help clear up an existing infection. It is only with proper antibiotic administration that the condition can be eradicated.

CN: Safety and infection control; CL: Evaluate

190. 1. Powder should not be applied to the skin beneath the cast because powder can cause irritation and skin breakdown. The parent would need further teaching about avoiding this measure. Checking the smoothness of the cast edges, covering the cast around the perineum, and inspecting inside the cast are all appropriate actions for the child with a spica cast to help prevent skin breakdown.

CN: Basic care and comfort; CL: Evaluate

191. 1, 2, 3, 4. The goal of "medication reconciliation" is to ensure that clients are on the right medication after any transfer, admission, or discharge. It is not necessary to reconcile the medications if the client moves to a different room on the same floor. It is estimated that more than half of medication errors occur during these transitions, and medication reconciliation can reduce errors by 70% or more. The Joint Commission requirements mandate medication reconciliation programs.

CN: Pharmacological and parenteral therapies; CL: Apply

192. 2. Following crush injury, serum potassium rises to high levels. Sodium polystyrene sulfonate is a potassium binding resin. The resin combines with potassium in the colon and is then eliminated, and serum potassium levels should come back to normal. Normal serum potassium is 3.5 to 5.3. Weak, irregular pulse and tall peaked T waves on ECG are signs of hyperkalemia, and muscle weakness is a sign of hypokalemia.

CN: Pharmacological and Parenteral Therapies; CL: Evaluate

193. 1. An alternative or additional method of birth control must be used since oxcarbazepine reduces the effectiveness of oral contraceptives. Higher doses of oral contraceptives will not help in achieving this purpose, but the client needs an additional or alternative method of birth control. The client does not need advice about when to start her family. A side effect of oxcarbazepine may be weight gain, but it is typically gradual.

CN: Pharmacological and Parenteral Therapies; CL: Apply

194. 4. Hemodialysis clients have their protein requirements individually tailored according to their postdialysis weight. The protein requirement is 1.0 to 1.2 g/kg body weight per day. Hence, for a 59-kg weight, the amount of protein will be 59 to 70 g/day. Sodium should be restricted to 3 g/day.

The client should obtain sufficient calories; if calories are not supplied in adequate amount, the body will use tissue protein for energy, which will lead to a negative nitrogen balance and malnutrition. Fluid intake needs to be restricted. The fluid amount is restricted to 500 to 700 mL plus the urine output.

CN: Pharmacological and parenteral therapies; CL: Synthesize

195. 1. Acute poststreptococcal glomerulonephritis usually follows a streptococcal throat or skin infection by 1 to 2 weeks. *Streptococcus*-type infections require medical intervention with antibiotics. Antibacterial mouthwashes do not kill streptococci. Previously prescribed antibiotics may not be effective against streptococci, and may also be expired. Bar soap fragrance has no impact on its ability to kill bacteria that reside on the skin.

CN: Health promotion and maintenance; CL: Synthesize

196. 1. To be a true client advocate, the nurse should ask the client if she desires an epidural anesthetic even though the client has indicated a desire for "natural childbirth." The client has a right to change her mind and also a right to refuse treatment. The client, not the nurse, should be the one to tell the **HCP** that she does not want an epidural anesthetic; the nurse should support the client's decision. Although telling the client that her labor will be more comfortable with an anesthetic provides the client with information, a statement such as this can be viewed as an attempt to change the client's mind. The client may wish to discuss this situation with her husband, but she does not have to do so.

CN: Management of care; CL: Synthesize

197. 2, 4, 5. In order to meet the criteria for discharge from same-day surgery, the postoperative client must be able to take fluids by mouth, walk without hypotension, void, and be escorted by a responsible adult who will drive the client home. Transportation home via a taxicab is not a sufficient escort to assist a client home after surgery. The client may be discharged with severe pain as long as the client can ambulate safely. The nurse should make sure the client has a prescription for pain medication.

CN: Safety and infection control; CL: Evaluate

198. 1. Eyedrops are correctly instilled by placing them in the lower conjunctival sac. Eyedrops should not be placed near the lacrimal ducts, to decrease the chance of the medication's being systemically absorbed. Placing the drops on the cornea or sclera is uncomfortable for the client and may cause the medication to run out of the eye socket instead of being absorbed.

CN: Pharmacological and parenteral therapies; CL: Evaluate

199. 2. Normal age-related changes can predispose older adults to falling and include vision, hearing, cardiovascular, musculoskeletal, and neurological changes. One of the most common problems facing older adults is the loss of tissue elasticity that affects the arteries. This loss of elasticity results in a decrease in tissue recoil and leads to changes in blood pressure with position changes. When they rise too quickly from a supine position, they feel light-headed and dizzy and can fall. The nurse should instruct clients to change positions slowly and to dangle the legs a few minutes when arising from a supine position. When aging, the lens of the eye becomes sensitive to very bright light that can cause a glare and visual disturbances that can lead to falls. Rooms should be well lit, but not with bright lights that cause a glare. Neurological changes are seen in impaired reflexes and thus postural instability. This loss of postural stability leads to falls. The need of assistive devices (hand rails, cane, walkers) helps reduce falls and promote independence. If joint pain develops and remains untreated, it can cause older adults to become sedentary or immobile. This disuse of muscles contributes to muscle weakness and falls. Nursing interventions should be directed at encouraging regular ambulation and joint movement (range of motion).

🔑 CN: Reduction of risk potential; CL: Synthesize

200. When measuring for NG tube insertion, the nurse would end the measurement at the xiphoid process.

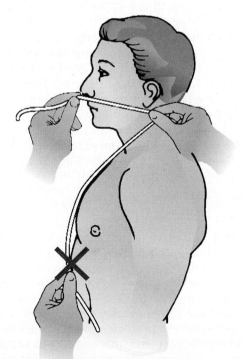

🔑 CN: Safety and infection control; CL: Apply

201. 1, 2, 3, 4. Benchmarking is a technique for learning from the success of others in an area where care improvement is desired by comparing the data from others with the data about the nursing problem for which improvement is sought. Sources of information for benchmarking include literature reviews, databases, unions, standard-setting organizations, local organizations, universities, the government, staff or customer interviews, and questionnaires. A recommendation from a clinical organization does not necessarily indicate that success has been attained.

🔑 CN: Management of care; CL: Apply

202. 3. The nurse should call the surgeon's office so that arrangements can be made for the client to donate a unit of his blood for possible future autotransfusion. This must be done in sufficient time before surgery so that the client is not at risk for being anemic at the time of the scheduled procedure. The client's request must be scheduled through the surgeon's office because the surgeon has ultimate responsibility for the client. The nurse can document that the surgeon's office was notified of the client's request. Notifying the hematology laboratory or blood bank is not an appropriate response.

🔑 CN: Pharmacological and parenteral therapies; CL: Synthesize

203. 3. Overuse of nasal spray containing pseudoephedrine can lead to rhinitis medicamentosa, which is a rebound effect causing increased swelling and congestion. Use of pseudoephedrine nasal spray does not cause infections or thrush. Pseudoephedrine is not addictive.

🔑 CN: Pharmacological and parenteral therapies; CL: Synthesize

204. 2. The best way to teach a child about surgery is through play. The nurse can let the child handle the items that will be used for monitoring, such as the blood pressure cuff and the ECG pads. The child will become more familiar with the face masks he sees the surgical team wearing in the operating room after playing with one and wearing it before surgery. A child of this age-group does not understand detailed explanations of how to use equipment, such as a PCA, a VAS, or even a video. The pain scale that should be used for children is the FACES scale.

🔑 CN: Basic care and comfort; CL: Synthesize

205. 2. When a nurse observes the theft of an opioid, it is the responsibility of the nurse to report the incident to the supervisor of the unit. The supervisor of the unit can confront the coworker and notify the hospital's chief of security about the incident. In some situations, the drug-abusing coworker may be offered drug counseling. In situations in which the drugs are being sold, the police should be notified. The nurse should not confront the coworker because this may put the nurse in danger. It is not the responsibility of the nurse to notify federal drug agents about the incident.

🔑 CN: Management of care; CL: Synthesize

206. 2. The nurse should teach the client and family the importance of not discontinuing benztropine abruptly. Rather, the drug should be tapered slowly over a 1-week period. Benztropine should not be used with over-the-counter cough and cold preparations because of the risk of an additive anticholinergic effect. Antacids delay the absorption of benztropine, and alcohol in combination with benztropine causes an increase in central nervous system depression; concomitant use should be avoided.

🔑 CN: Pharmacological and parenteral therapies; CL: Synthesize

207. 3. The nurse needs to focus on adverse effects that can be seen or felt, using a simple, brief, written description of the benefits of the medication and a list of common adverse effects and how to cope with them. The written format helps the client and family feel more in control by participating in treatment. They also can use the written information as a helpful resource for review. Information about all potential adverse effects, including percentages associated with each, will cause undue anxiety in the client and possibly overwhelm the client and family, negatively affecting compliance. The nurse should use discretion in selecting the content of educational sessions.

🔑 CN: Health promotion and maintenance; CL: Synthesize

208. 2. Albumin is a colloid that remains in the intravascular space, pulling fluid out of the intracellular and interstitial space. The client with nephrotic syndrome loses excessive amounts of protein, mainly albumin, in the urine. Because fluid is drawn into the intravascular space, blood pressure will increase. Crackles in the lung bases and cerebral edema are signs of circulatory overload or fluid volume excess. When edema is present in the lower extremities, the skin feels cool to the touch unless an infection is present.

🔑 CN: Physiological adaptation; CL: Evaluate

209. 3. Although it is not clearly understood why cysts form in polycystic kidney disease, the condition is known to be inherited. Environmental exposures such as smoking and breathing secondhand smoke promote development of bladder cancer. Although drinking alcohol requires the kidneys to excrete the alcohol, it is not thought to cause the kidneys to develop cysts. Exposure to dyes used in foods does not increase the risk for polycystic disease.

🔑 CN: Physiological adaptation; CL: Synthesize

210. 1, 2, 3. A 3% sodium chloride solution is hypertonic; it will pull fluid into the intravascular compartment and may increase renal perfusion, so intake and output should be monitored. As fluid is pulled into the vasculature, the client may demonstrate signs of fluid overload such as jugular vein distention. Hypernatremia and hyperchloremia will produce neurologic signs and symptoms. Fluids should not be forced in a client with fluid overload. There is no need for an indwelling urinary catheter.

🔑 CN: Reduction of risk potential; CL: Apply

211. 3. The nurse expects the **UAP** 📖 assigned to several clients in labor to notify the nurse if the UAP observes that one of the clients has evidence of spontaneous rupture of the membranes. When the membranes rupture spontaneously, there is danger of a prolapsed cord, a medical emergency requiring a cesarean birth. Nausea may occur after administration of an epidural anesthetic, but this is not a priority or emergency. Having contractions that are 3 minutes apart and last for 40 seconds is normal during active labor. Because nalbuphine is an analgesic, it is normal for a client to fall asleep after IV administration of this drug.

🔑 CN: Management of care; CL: Evaluate

212. 2. Before teaching a school-age child about a medical or nursing procedure, it is best to become familiar with the child's knowledge level. The nurse can then begin by explaining about the body structure involved in the procedure. Children of this age should be told about the unknown procedures far enough in advance for them to prepare for what is going to happen to them. Showing the child the equipment and explaining what is going to be done during the test should be done after the child is allowed to express what he knows about what is going to happen to him.

🔑 CN: Psychosocial integrity; CL: Synthesize

213. 1, 2, 3, 4. Educating women about risk factors for cancers of the reproductive system is important. The nurse should encourage women to do breast and vulva self-exams. Limiting sexual activity during adolescence, using condoms, having fewer sexual partners, and not smoking reduce the risk of cervical cancer. Cancer can be prevented from occurring when screening reveals precancerous conditions of the vulva, cervix, or endometrium. Also, routine screening increases the chance that a cancer will be identified in its early stage. Immunization against HPV is recommended for preteen girls to prevent cervical cancer. Many cancers in women, particularly breast cancer, have a genetic basis, and the woman's genetic history is an important tool in identifying risk.

CN: Health promotion and maintenance; CL: Create

214. 3. The client should be encouraged to keep up with the school work. The developmental task of the school-age child is industry versus inferiority. Keeping up with the peers is very important to this age-group. Watching television does provide rest, but it does not lead to a feeling of accomplishment. Coloring pictures is not an appropriate pastime for this age-group. Making crafts may be too strenuous of an activity for a client on bed rest.

CN: Health promotion and maintenance; CL: Synthesize

215. 4. Clients receiving TPN are at risk for a number of complications, including fluid imbalances such as fluid overload and hyperosmolar diuresis. Other common complications include hyperglycemia, sepsis, pneumothorax, and air embolism. Hypostatic pneumonia, pulmonary hypertension, and orthostatic hypotension are not complications of TPN.

CN: Pharmacological and parenteral therapies; CL: Analyze

216. 1, 2, 4. Heparin dosage in children is based on the child's weight. A bolus of heparin is administered by the IV route, and the onset of action is immediate. The PTT is an indicator of the effectiveness of heparin. Following the heparin with a continuous infusion of heparin would cause life-threatening anticoagulation in this child. Penicillin and cephalosporins potentiate the effects of heparin, so the heparin must be carefully titrated to obtain maximum effect without causing an overdose. However, the antibiotic should not be discontinued.

CN: Pharmacological and parenteral therapies; CL: Synthesize

217. 1. Propantheline bromide is an anticholinergic drug. Common adverse effects include urine retention and constipation; flushed, dry skin; and dry mouth, nose, and throat. Orthostatic hypotension may also occur. Diarrhea and diaphoresis are adverse effects of cholinergic drugs.

CN: Pharmacological and parenteral therapies; CL: Analyze

218. 1. Applying a tourniquet obstructs venous blood flow and, as a result, distends the veins. A tourniquet does not stabilize veins or immobilize the arm, nor is it applied to occlude arterial circulation.

CN: Pharmacological and parenteral therapies; CL: Apply

219. 1. Prochlorperazine is administered postoperatively to control nausea and vomiting. Prochlorperazine is also used in psychotherapy because of its effects on mood and behavior. It is not used to treat dizziness, abdominal spasms, or abdominal distention.

CN: Pharmacological and parenteral therapies; CL: Evaluate

220. 1, 2, 3, 4. Cough and dyspnea can be present at the time of diagnosis of bone cancer, indicating that the cancer has metastasized to the lungs. About one-quarter of all adolescents with bone cancer have lung metastasis at the time of diagnosis. Pain and swelling result from the inflammation caused by the bone tumor and the increased vascularity of the tumor. At the time of diagnosis, fever, anorexia, and decreased range of motion have not occurred. The tumor involves the bone, so there is pain when pressure is exerted on the involved bone, but range of motion is not affected. Fever and anorexia can occur if extensive metastasis has occurred.

CN: Health promotion and maintenance; CL: Analyze

221. 1. The priority assessment is that the client has a firm fundus when gentle massage is used. This indicates that the client's fundus may be soft or "boggy" when it is not massaged. The receiving nurse should assess the client's fundus soon after admission and continue to monitor the client's fundus, lochia, and pulse rate. Postpartum hemorrhage is associated with uterine atony. Maternal-infant bonding is a process that usually starts on day 2 and ends at week 1. A 12-hour labor is normal. The temperature and pulse are within normal limits.

CN: Management of care; CL: Analyze

222. 2. Assuming cultural appropriateness of eye contact with the client and his wife, this body language would make the nurse's nonverbal message congruent with the nurse's verbal message and demonstrate empathy. Directing the eyes only toward the client, rather than including the wife, ignores the wife. Avoiding eye contact with the client and wife or shifting the gaze between the client and wife conveys a lack of assurance about the nurse's focus and comments.

CN: Psychosocial integrity; CL: Apply

223. 4. Colleagues can be a source of suggestions and validation of communication strategies. The nurse has identified difficulty with the relationship and should seek assistance before discussing improved involvement with the client because improved involvement may not be the most appropriate approach. Positive and negative interactions occur in relationships. The frequency of both types of interactions determines the quality of an interpersonal relationship. In a therapeutic relationship, both parties contribute to the relationship; neither one should dominate or be submissive.

🔑 CN: Psychosocial integrity; CL: Synthesize

224. 3. The nurse on the postpartum unit should discuss with the client what her wishes are and mutually agree on a location. The charge nurse better understands the current and future needs of the client experiencing this type of loss as the client may or may not be thinking well or clearly at the moment. The postpartum unit is full of sounds of infants, and although being in a room by herself may support the need for separation, it is often in the best interest of the client to locate her away from the noise of the babies. Placing the client on another unit will remove her from the support she is seeking. On the other hand, she will not be hearing crying infants. This has often been the location for someone experiencing a loss. Discharging the mother home as soon as she is stable physically is also a possibility, but the nurse must also assess the client's emotional stability and preferences for grieving.

🔑 CN: Management of care; CL: Synthesize

225. 2. *Haemophilus influenzae* is a bacterium that can cause severe disease in children younger than 5 years, but it does not cause influenza. Yearly vaccination for influenza is recommended to begin at 6 months. The live vaccine is not recommended for children younger than 2 years or with respiratory disease. A second vaccine 4 weeks after the first is recommended the first time a child younger than 9 years receives the flu vaccine.

🔑 CN: Health promotion and maintenance; CL: Apply

226. 3. Confidentiality and privacy are critical developmental needs for the adolescent. These needs are important to enable the nurse to establish a relationship of trust with the adolescent. A sexual history should be conducted with a teen without parents. Therefore, the nurse should not ask the mother to provide information or put the daughter in a position of having to make a decision about her mother remaining in the room. Inform the adolescent that this information is confidential and will not be shared with the parent. Inform the adolescent that issues of abuse or life-threatening issues are required by law to be disclosed to the authorities, and all other information is private.

🔑 CN: Management of care; CL: Synthesize

227. 4. It is critical for medication safety to know the name, dosage, and times of administration of the medication taken at home. The family should bring the medication bottles to the hospital. The nurse should document the medication on the **medical record** 📖 from the bottles to ensure accuracy before the medication is prescribed and administered. The pharmacist is a helpful resource, but the safest way to identify the medication is in its original container. It is not safe to assume the client could correctly identify the medications from a drug book. The medication regimen may have changed since the record 2 years ago.

🔑 CN: Pharmacological and parenteral therapies; CL: Synthesize

228. 3, 4, 5. The additional fluids should run through a separate line using a Y-connector. The nurse must contact the surgeon to clarify if the client should receive the additional 100 mL/h of IV fluids containing potassium chloride during the bolus infusion. Rapid infusion of potassium chloride can cause hyperkalemia with adverse cardiac outcomes such as arrhythmias. Bolus infusions of IV fluids should be run via an infusion pump to avoid excess fluid administration. Increasing the current IV infusion rate or adding additional fluids to the existing infusion is not safe because the current infusion contains potassium.

🔑 CN: Pharmacological and parenteral therapies; CL: Synthesize

229. 1. The nurse should notify the hospital's security staff about anyone who appears unusual. Typically, the abductor is an older woman who wishes to have a baby. The nurse should take only one baby at a time to a mother to prevent the neonate being taken to the wrong mother. Infants should never be left in the hallway. When in the mother's room, the infant should be placed away from the doorway to prevent or minimize the risk of abduction of the neonate. If an exit alarm is triggered, it is possible that an abductor is running away with an infant. Staff members should investigate the alarm immediately and stop the potential abductor. Hospital security can be alerted if someone is seen exiting the unit carrying a large bag or an infant.

🔑 CN: Management of care; CL: Apply

230. 1. The client needs specific information about the effects of the drug, specifically that the drug can cause agranulocytosis. The statement about weekly blood tests to determine safe dosage and monitoring for effects on the blood gives the client specific information to ensure follow-up with the required protocol for clozapine therapy. Lack of accurate knowledge can lead to noncompliance with necessary follow-up procedures and noncompliance with medication. The supply of medication is not dependent on blood testing. Telling the client that the **HCP** 📖 wants to know the progress does not provide specific information for this client. The blood tests are not required by the drug company.

🔑 CN: Pharmacological and parenteral therapies; CL: Synthesize

231. 4. A properly administered intradermal injection shows evidence of a bleb at the injection site. There should be no leaking of medication from the bleb; it needs to be absorbed into the tissue. Lack of swelling at the injection site means that the injection was given too deeply. The presence of tissue pallor does not indicate that the injection was given correctly.

> 🔑 CN: Pharmacological and parenteral therapies; CL: Evaluate

232. 1. A serious complication of IV therapy is fluid overload. Noisy respirations can develop as a result of pulmonary congestion. Additional symptoms of fluid overload include dyspnea, crackles, hypertension, bounding pulse, and distended neck veins.

> 🔑 CN: Pharmacological and parenteral therapies; CL: Analyze

233. 2. Only isotonic (normal) saline should be used when administering a blood transfusion. The use of dextrose or lactated Ringer's solution will cause the hemolysis of red blood cells.

> 🔑 CN: Pharmacological and parenteral therapies; CL: Apply

234. 3. The median cubital vein is located in the approximate center of the antecubital space.

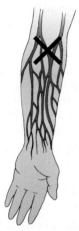

> 🔑 CN: Pharmacological and parenteral therapies; CL: Apply

235. 2. Telling the mother that excess saliva is a common adverse effect of the drug is most helpful because it gives her information about the problem, thereby helping to decrease her anxiety about what is occurring with her son. By offering the paper cup, the nurse also demonstrates concern for the client, thereby leading to increased trust. Saying "I wonder if he is having an adverse reaction to the medicine" shows the nurse's lack of knowledge about the drug, decreases confidence in the nurse, and indicates poor judgment. Saying "Do not worry about it, it is only a minor inconvenience compared to its benefits" or telling the mother that the nurse has seen this happening to other clients is insensitive and does not assuage the mother's anxiety.

> 🔑 CN: Pharmacological and parenteral therapies; CL: Synthesize

236. 1, 3, 4. The nurse should write down the prescription, read the prescription back to the **HCP** 🖥, and receive confirmation from the provider that the prescription is correct as understood by the nurse. It is not necessary for the HCP to come to the hospital to write the prescription on the **medical record** 📖 or to have the nursing supervisor cosign the telephone prescription.

> 🔑 CN: Safety and infection control; CL: Apply

237. 2. Giving the client finger foods that have protein, carbohydrates, and calories supplies energy and allows the client to eat while on the move. A salad or soup is very difficult for the client to eat while moving and may not supply the nutrients needed. Favorite foods from home may or may not be appropriate to eat while walking.

> 🔑 CN: Basic care and comfort; CL: Apply

238. 2. Protamine sulfate is a heparin antagonist. It is administered intravenously very slowly (over at least 10 minutes). Warfarin sodium and ASA have anticoagulant properties and would be contraindicated. Atropine sulfate is an anticholinergic drug and would not be effective in treating a heparin overdose.

> 🔑 CN: Pharmacological and parenteral therapies; CL: Apply

239. 2. Aminophylline, a bronchodilator that relaxes smooth muscles in the bronchioles, is used in the treatment of emphysema to improve ventilation by dilating the bronchioles. Aminophylline does not have an effect on the diaphragm or the medullary respiratory center and does not promote pulmonary circulation.

> 🔑 CN: Pharmacological and parenteral therapies; CL: Evaluate

240. 1. Seven-year-olds like to play with friends of the same sex. In early school-age years, children enjoy the company of same-sex friends. Relatives become second-choice friends to those from school. Team games can be competitive, and the ego of a 7-year-old may be too fragile to endure losing the game without losing self-confidence. Infants enjoy solitary play. The school-age child enjoys cooperative play with friends of the same sex and age.

> 🔑 CN: Health promotion and maintenance; CL: Analyze

241. 2. Trying something new is usually frightening for a 7-year-old. Separation anxiety is the most common fear between the ages of 5 months and 5 years of age. Injury and pain are a common fear of the preschool child. Fear of the opposite sex is common during adolescence.

CN: Health promotion and maintenance; CL: Analyze

242. 3. Valproic acid causes sedation as well as nausea, vomiting, and indigestion. Sedation is important because the client needs to be cautioned about driving or operating machinery that could be dangerous while feeling sedated from the medication. Valproic acid does not cause increased urination, slowed thinking, or weight loss. However, some clients may experience weight gain.

CN: Pharmacological and parenteral therapies; CL: Synthesize

243. 4. The client is experiencing signs of thrombophlebitis. The nurse should notify the **HCP** 📖 because emboli formation is a potential risk. Massaging the area may cause the thrombus to dislocate and become an embolus. Warm compresses will increase circulation to the area and may precipitate embolus formation. Ankle pump exercises are helpful in preventing thrombophlebitis but will not prevent further risk of embolus formation at this time.

CN: Reduction of risk potential; CL: Synthesize

244. 3. Small-boned, fair-skinned women of northern European descent are at the greatest risk for osteoporosis, not women of African descent. One standard serving of yogurt is the equivalent of one glass of milk. Women who do not eat dairy products, such as women who are lactose intolerant, should consider using calcium supplements. Inadequate lifetime intake of calcium is a major risk factor for osteoporosis. Estrogen therapy, or some of the newer medications that are not estrogen based, can greatly reduce the incidence of osteoporosis.

CN: Reduction of risk potential; CL: Evaluate

245. 3, 1, 2, 4. The goal of care for a client who is having a seizure is to prevent respiratory arrest and aspiration. The nurse should first clear the area around the client. Next, the nurse should loosen clothing around the client's neck and turn the client on the side. As needed, the nurse can then suction the airway and administer oxygen.

CN: Reduction of risk potential; CL: Synthesize

246. 4. There is no cure for metastatic cancer of the liver; palliative nursing care is required. Liver transplants are not recommended for the client with widespread malignant disease. Prescribed medications will not make metastatic lesions shrink. There is nothing to indicate that the client is receiving chemotherapy; therefore, explaining its effects would not be helpful.

CN: Physiological adaptation; CL: Synthesize

247. 1. During the first week postpartum, the client's pulse rate should be slow, with an average of 60 to 70 bpm. A pulse of 100 bpm warrants further investigation to rule out a possible infectious process or postpartum hemorrhage. An oral temperature of 99°F (37.2°C) is within normal limits. Excessive perspiration and frequent voiding in large amounts are caused by the normal diuresis that occurs as the body returns to its prepregnant state.

CN: Management of care; CL: Synthesize

248. 4. The nurse should remind the client about meal and activity times so that the ritual can be completed beforehand and not interfere with meals and activities. The client must be allowed to complete the ritual because it keeps anxiety in check. Totally eliminating the client's ritual will increase anxiety and the need for the handwashing. Allowing the client to decide to attend meals and activities is not appropriate or in the client's best interest because the client must perform the ritual to assuage anxiety. Informing the client that absence from meals and activities is not permitted scolds the client, increasing anxiety and the need for the ritual.

CN: Psychosocial integrity; CL: Synthesize

249. 4. The nurse should acknowledge that the client feels better but should also remind the client to continue the drug therapy and other self-care activities of rest, exercise, joint protection, and adequate nutrition. Wearing the copper-lined gloves is not harmful, and the nurse should not instruct the client to remove the gloves or label it quackery. Copper does not interfere with salicylate metabolism.

CN: Psychosocial integrity; CL: Synthesize

250. 1. Lymphedema occurs frequently after radical mastectomy when lymph nodes are removed. Aplasia, or the absence of lymph nodes, prevents proper lymph drainage. The tissue swelling is caused by obstructed lymph flow in the extremity. The blood pressure is taken in the unaffected arm to avoid further accumulation of lymphedema. An IV line should not be started in the affected arm. The nurse would encourage the client to elevate the extremity above the level of the heart. Blood draws in the affected arm should not be allowed.

CN: Physiological adaptation; CL: Synthesize

251. 4. The child's **HCP** ⌨ should be notified because the maximum daily recommended dosage for ceftriaxone for this child's weight would be 1,500 g/day, and giving this dose would administer 4 g/day. The nurse cannot administer a different dose than that prescribed. There is no therapeutic serum level of ceftriaxone.

🔑 CN: Pharmacological and parenteral therapies; CL: Synthesize

252. 3. One of the staff members needs further instructions when the nurse observes the staff member wearing sterile gloves to bathe a newly delivered neonate. Clean gloves should be worn, not sterile gloves. Sterile gloves are more expensive than clean gloves and are not necessary when bathing a newly delivered neonate. Goggles should be worn when there is a possibility of blood and body fluid spatter. Bloody sheets should be placed in labeled containers for contaminated linens. Scalpel blades are disposed of in specified containers.

🔑 CN: Safety and infection control; CL: Evaluate

253. 2, 3, 4. Maternal intake will need to increase approximately 500 cal/day while breast-feeding. It is true that many drugs taken by the mother cross through breast milk. When any medication is taken by the breast-feeding mom, the medication should be determined to be safe with the OB's or pediatrician's office. Infants who have six to eight wet diapers per day have had an adequate intake of breast milk. If there are fewer, the mother should try to increase the frequency of the infant's feedings. Within the first 24 to 72 hours of life, there will be fewer wet diapers as the mother's milk has not come in yet. Prior to discharge, clients should know how to access community resources to support breast-feeding. After a mother's breast milk is in at about the 3rd day after birth, the infant should be satisfied for approximately 1½ to 3 hours after feeding. There is a need for more frequent feedings with breast-fed infants than bottle-fed as the fat content in the breast milk is lower.

🔑 CN: Health promotion and maintenance; CL: Evaluate

254. 3. Three percent saline is a hypertonic solution, which will pull fluid from the interstitial and intracellular spaces into the bloodstream. Its use is usually reserved for severe hyponatremia (sodium <115 mEq/L). If this client were experiencing a fluid volume deficit, this IV solution could worsen the condition. The nurse should consult with the **HCP** ⌨ about this prescription. The nurse does not have prescribing rights and cannot change the prescription. The IV rate of 62 may still be dangerous for this client, and the rate was prescribed at 125 mL/h.

🔑 CN: Pharmacologic and parenteral therapy; CL: Analyze

255. Correct answer: "X" right of the sternum at the second intercostal space is the best place for listening for the aortic valve sounds.

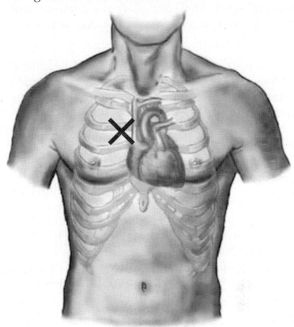

🔑 CN: Physiological adaptation; CL: Apply

256. 2. Measuring the pH of the aspirated gastric fluid is the most accurate determination of the placement of the NG tube. A pH lower than 4 indicates that the tube is in the stomach. Whether or not the client is gagging or coughing is not an accurate way to determine if the tube is placed correctly. No fluids should be inserted into the tube until the placement has been determined. Inserting air into the tube and listening for the resulting whoosh can be used, but this is not as accurate as pH measurement.

🔑 CN: Reduction of risk potential; CL: Evaluate

257. 2. Alcoholic cirrhosis is associated with excessive alcohol intake. In the early stages, the liver develops fatty changes. If alcohol intake stops, the fatty changes can be reversed. Avoiding overexertion is important in the client with cirrhosis, but it does not reverse the disease. Stopping smoking is a positive, healthy lifestyle change, but it does not have an impact on cirrhosis. A diet high in carbohydrates and low in fat is also recommended for the client with cirrhosis, but the diet does not reverse the pathologic changes that have occurred in the liver.

🔑 CN: Reduction of risk potential; CL: Synthesize

258. 1, 2, 3, 5. When emergently managing chest pain, the nurse can use the memory mnemonic MONA to plan care: morphine, oxygen, nitroglycerin, and aspirin. A Foley catheter is not included in the emergent management of chest pain and can be inserted when the pain has been relieved and the client is stable. Acetaminophen is not used to manage chest pain.

🔑 CN: Physiologic adaptation;
CL: Synthesize

259. 3. In rheumatic fever, the joints—especially the knees, ankles, elbows, and wrists—are painful, swollen, red, and hot to the touch. Limiting movement of the affected joints typically minimizes pain. Massaging the joints likely will not aid in pain relief because the pain is due to the disease process and subsequent inflammation in the joint. Applying ice to the affected joints likely will not aid in pain relief because the inflammation, edema, and effusion are too deep in the joint tissue. Exercise should be avoided because of the increased workload placed on the heart muscle. This is in contrast to usual recommendations for clients with other forms of arthritis. Despite joint involvement in rheumatic fever, permanent deformities do not occur.

🔑 CN: Basic care and comfort;
CL: Synthesize

260. 3. Minimizing urinary catheter use and duration of use in all clients, particularly those at higher risk for CAUTI or mortality from catheterization such as women, the elderly, and clients with impaired immunity, will reduce the opportunity for infection. The nurse should avoid the use of urinary catheters for clients who are incontinent; a bladder training program and frequent use of the toilet are preferred; external catheters may be used if necessary in incontinent clients. The nurse should not clean the periurethral area with antiseptics; cleansing the meatal surface during daily bathing or showering is appropriate. Using sterile technique to help reduce CAUTI is not necessary. Hand hygiene immediately before and after insertion or any manipulation of the catheter device or site is sufficient.

🔑 CN: Reduction of risk potential;
CL: Synthesize

261. 2. Clarification is the process of confirming the appropriate medication and doses for any client. Verification is the process of collecting medication history. Reconciliation is the process of documenting medication prescription changes for a client across the continuum of care. Documentation is included as a step in the three steps of a formal medication reconciliation program.

🔑 CN: Management of care; CL: Apply

262. 2, 3, 5, 6. The client is hyponatremic; the nurse should notify the **HCP** 📖, restrict fluids, and prepare to insert a Foley catheter to ensure accurate intake and output. Side rails should be up in order to maintain client safety; it is not safe for the client to be ambulating in the hallway with family at this time. Encouraging fluids would not be beneficial and could be harmful.

🔑 CN: Physiological adaptation;
CL: Synthesize

263. 2. While it is important to present options and help find solutions to the client's financial concerns, the nurse must first listen carefully to those concerns and allow the client to verbalize related emotions in order to identify the client's needs. Reminding the client to focus on getting well does not address the client's concerns or needs. Arranging a meeting with the case manager is premature as the nurse needs to first determine what the client's needs are. Until the nurse understands the client's needs, the nurse should not encourage the spouse to discuss the client's bill with the business office.

🔑 CN: Management of care; CL: Synthesize

264. 1. The nurse is ultimately responsible to coordinate the client's care while hospitalized; therefore, it is the nurse's responsibility to arrange a care conference to help get the client's questions, concerns, and frustrations addressed. Assuring the client that the **HCPs** 📖 know what they are doing does not address the client's concern or frustration with receiving conflicting information. While it is true that the client is ultimately responsible for health, asking the client to accept the consequences is a form of blaming the client. The HCPs' progress notes will not provide information that will address the client's concern or resolve the conflicting courses of action that the two HCPs are proposing.

🔑 CN: Management of care; CL: Synthesize

265. 3, 1, 4, 2. The nurse should first assess the client, and then, if there is no acute injury, help the client get back into bed. The nurse must notify the **HCP** 📖 and the family of the fall and finally, document the event on the client's health record.

🔑 CN: Safety and infection control;
CL: Synthesize

Appendices

Alabama Board of Nursing
PO Box 303900
Montgomery, AL 36130-3900
Phone: (334) 293-5200
Fax: (334) 293-5201
Web site: http://www.abn.alabama.gov

Alaska Board of Nursing
550 W. Seventh Avenue, Suite 1500
Anchorage, AK 99501-3567
Phone: (907) 269-8161
Fax: (907) 269-8196
Web site: https://www.commerce.alaska.gov/web/
cbpl/ProfessionalLicensing/BoardofNursing.aspx

College and Association of Registered Nurses of Alberta
11620 168 Street
Edmonton, AB T5M 4A6
Phone: (780) 451-0043
Fax: (780) 452-3276
Web site: http://www.nurses.ab.ca/Carna/index.aspx

Arizona State Board of Nursing
4747 N. 7th Street, Suite 200
Phoenix, AZ 85014
Phone: (602) 771-7800
Fax: (602) 771-7800
Web site: http://www.azbn.gov

Arkansas State Board of Nursing
University Tower Building
1123 S. University Avenue, Suite 800
Little Rock, AR 72204-1619
Phone: (501) 686-2700
Fax: (501) 686-2714
Web site: http://www.arsbn.arkansas.gov

College of Registered Nurses of British Columbia
2855 Arbutus Street
Vancouver, BC V6J 3Y8
Phone: (604) 736-7331
Fax: (604) 738-2272
Web site: https://www.crnbc.ca

California State Board of Registered Nursing
1747 N. Market Boulevard, Suite 150
Sacramento, CA 95834
Phone: (916) 322-3350
Fax: (916) 574-8637
Web site: http://www.rn.ca.gov

Colorado Board of Nursing
1560 Broadway Street, Suite 1370
Denver, CO 80202

Phone: (303) 894-2430
Fax: (303) 894-2430
Web site: http://www.dora.state.co.us/Nursing

Connecticut Board of Examiners for Nursing
Department of Public Health
410 Capitol Avenue, MS# 13PHO
PO Box 340308
Hartford, CT 06134-0328
Phone: (860) 509-7624
Fax: (860) 509-7553
Web site: http://www.ct.gov/dph/site/default.asp

Delaware Board of Nursing
861 Silver Lake Boulevard
Cannon Building, Suite 203
Dover, DE 19904
Phone: (302) 744-4500
Fax: (302) 739-2711
Web site: http://dpr.delaware.gov/boards/nursing/
index.shtml

District of Columbia Board of Nursing
Department of Health
Health Professional Licensing Administration
899 N. Capitol Street, NE
Washington, DC 20002
Phone: (877) 672-2174
Fax: (202) 727-8471
Web site: http://doh.dc.gov/service/board-nursing

Florida Board of Nursing
4052 Bald Cypress Way, Bin C02
Tallahassee, FL 32399-3252
Phone: (850) 245-4125
Fax: (850) 245-4172
Web site: http://floridasnursing.gov

Georgia Board of Nursing
237 Coliseum Drive
Macon, GA 31217-3858
Phone: (478) 207-2440
Fax: (877) 371-5712
Web site: http://sos.ga.gov/index.php/licensing/
plb/45

Hawaii Board of Nursing
Professional and Vocational Licensing Division
PO Box 3469
Honolulu, HI 96801
Phone: (808) 586-3000
Fax: (808) 586-2689
Web site: http://hawaii.gov/dcca/pvl/boards/
nursing

Idaho Board of Nursing
280 N. 8th Street, Suite 210
PO Box 83720
Boise, ID 83720
Phone: (208) 334-3110
Fax: (208) 334-3262
Web site: http://ibn.idaho.gov

Illinois Department of Professional Regulation
James R. Thompson Center
100 W. Randolph Street, Suite 9-300
Chicago, IL 60601
Phone: (312) 814-2715
Fax: (312) 814-3145
Web site: http://www.idfpr.com

Indiana State Board of Nursing
Professional Licensing Agency
402 W. Washington Street, Room W072
Indianapolis, IN 46204
Phone: (317) 234-2043
Fax: (317) 233-4236
Web site: http://www.in.gov/pla

Iowa Board of Nursing
River Point Business Park
400 S.W. 8th Street, Suite B
Des Moines, IA 50309-4685
Phone: (515) 281-3255
Fax: (515) 281-4825
Web site: https://nursing.iowa.gov

Kansas State Board of Nursing
Landon State Office Building
900 S.W. Jackson Street, Suite 1051
Topeka, KS 66612
Phone: (785) 296-4929
Fax: (785) 296-3929
Web site: http://www.ksbn.org

Kentucky Board of Nursing
312 Whittington Parkway, Suite 300
Louisville, KY 40222
Phone: (502) 429-3300
Fax: (502) 429-3311
Web site: http://kbn.ky.gov

Louisiana State Board of Nursing
17373 Perkins Road
Baton Rouge, LA 70810
Phone: (225) 755-7500
Fax: (225) 755-7585
Web site: http://www.lsbn.state.la.us

Maine State Board of Nursing
158 State House Station
Augusta, ME 04333
Phone: (207) 287-1133
Fax: (207) 287-1149
Web site: http://www.maine.gov/boardofnursing

College of Registered Nurses of Manitoba (CRNM)
890 Pembina Highway
Winnipeg, MB R3M 2M8

Phone: (204) 774-3477
Fax: (204) 775-6052
Web site: http://www.crnm.mb.ca

Maryland Board of Nursing
4140 Patterson Avenue
Baltimore, MD 21215
Phone: (410) 585-1900
Fax: (410) 358-3530
Web site: http://mbon.maryland.gov

Massachusetts Board of Registration in Nursing
Commonwealth of Massachusetts
239 Causeway Street, Suite 500, 5th Floor
Boston, MA 02114
Phone: (617) 973-0900
Fax: (617) 973-0984
Web site: http://www.mass.gov/eohhs/gov/
departments/dph/programs/hcq/dhpl/
nursing

Michigan Department of Licensing and Regulatory Affairs
Bureau of Health Professions
611 W. Ottawa Street
PO Box 30670
Lansing, MI 48909
Phone: (517) 335-0918
Fax: (517) 241-1431
Web site: http://www.michigan.gov/lara

Minnesota Board of Nursing
2829 University Avenue SE, Suite 200
Minneapolis, MN 55414
Phone: (612) 617-2270
Fax: (612) 617-2190
Web site: http://www.state.mn.us/portal/mn/jsp/
home.do?agency=NursingBoard

Mississippi Board of Nursing
1080 River Oaks Drive, Suite A100
Flowood, MS 39232
Phone: (601) 664-9303
Fax: (601) 664-9304
Web site: http://www.msbn.state.ms.us

Missouri State Board of Nursing
3605 Missouri Boulevard
PO Box 656
Jefferson City, MO 65102-0656
Phone: (573) 751-0681
Fax: (573) 751-0075
Web site: http://www.pr.mo.gov/nursing.asp

Montana State Board of Nursing
PO Box 200513
Helena, MT 59620-0513
Phone: (406) 841-2340
Fax: (406) 841-2305
Web site: http://bsd.dli.mt.gov/license/bsd_boards/
nur_board/board_page.asp

Nebraska Advanced Practice Registered Nurse Board
Office of Nursing and Nursing Support
DHHS, Division of Public Health, Licensure Unit
301 Centennial Mall South
Lincoln, NE 68509-4986
Phone: (402) 471-6443
Fax: (402) 471-1066
Web site: http://dhhs.ne.gov/publichealth/Pages/crl_nursing_nursingindex.aspx

Nevada State Board of Nursing
5011 Meadowood Mall Way, Suite 300
Reno, NV 89502
Phone: (775) 687-7700
Fax: (775) 687-7707
Web site: http://nevadanursingboard.org

Nurses Association of New Brunswick
165 Regent Street
Fredericton, NB E3B 7B4
Phone: (506) 458-8731
Fax: (506) 459-2838
Web site: http://www.nanb.nb.ca

Nurses Association of Registered Nurses of Newfoundland and Labrador
55 Military Road
St. John's, NL A1C 2C5
Phone: (709) 753-6040
Fax: (709) 753-4940
Web site: https://www.arnnl.ca

New Hampshire Board of Nursing
21 South Fruit Street
Concord, NH 03301-2341
Phone: (603) 271-2323
Fax: (603) 271-6605
Web site: http://www.state.nh.us/nursing

New Jersey Board of Nursing
PO Box 45010
124 Halsey Street, 6th Floor
Newark, NJ 07101
Phone: (973) 504-6430
Fax: (973) 648-3481
Web site: http://www.state.nj.us/lps/ca/medical.htm

New Mexico Board of Nursing
6301 Indian School Road, NE
Albuquerque, NM 87110
Phone: (505) 841-8340
Fax: (505) 841-8347
Web site: http://www.bon.state.nm.us

New York State Board of Nursing
Education Building
89 Washington Avenue
2nd Floor West Wing
Albany, NY 12234
Phone: (518) 474-3817 ext. 120
Fax: (518) 474-3706
Web site: http://www.op.nysed.gov/prof/nurse

North Carolina Board of Nursing
4516 Lake Boone Trail
Raleigh, NC 27607
Phone: (919) 782-3211
Fax: (919) 781-9461
Web site: http://www.ncbon.com

North Dakota Board of Nursing
919 S. 7th Street, Suite 504
Bismark, ND 58504
Phone: (701) 328-9777
Fax: (701) 328-9785
Web site: http://www.ndbon.org

Registered Nurses Association of Northwest Territories and Nunavut
#3 483 Range Lake Road
Yellowknife, NT X1A 3R9
Phone: (867) 873-2745
Fax: (867) 873-2336
Web site: http://www.rnantnu.ca

College of Registered Nurses of Nova Scotia
Suite 4005, 7071 Bayers Road
Halifax, NS B3L 2C2
Phone: (902) 491-9744
Fax: (902) 491-9510
Web site: http://www.crnns.ca

Ohio Board of Nursing
17 S. High Street, Suite 400
Columbus, OH 43215-3413
Phone: (614) 466-6940
Fax: (614) 466-0388
Web site: http://www.nursing.ohio.gov

Oklahoma Board of Nursing
2915 N. Classen Boulevard, Suite 524
Oklahoma City, OK 73106
Phone: (405) 962-1800
Fax: (405) 962-1821
Web site: http://www.ok.gov/nursing

College of Nurses of Ontario
101 Davenport Road
Toronto, ON M5R 3P1
Phone: (416) 928-0900
Fax: (416) 928-6507
Web site: http://www.cno.org

Oregon State Board of Nursing
17938 S.W. Upper Boones Ferry Road
Portland, OR 97224
Phone: (503) 673-0685
Fax: (503) 673-0684
Web site: http://www.osbn.state.or.us

Pennsylvania State Board of Nursing
PO Box 2649
Harrisburg, PA 17105-2649
Phone: (717) 783-7142
Fax: (717) 783-0822
Web site: http://www.dos.pa.gov/ProfessionalLicensing/BoardsCommissions/Nursing/Pages/default.aspx#.ViVO1X6rTcu

The Association of Registered Nurses of Prince Edward Island
53 Grafton Street
Charlottetown, PEI C1A 1K8
Phone: (902) 368-3764
Fax: (902) 628-1430
Web site: http://www.arnpei.ca

Ordre des infirmières et infirmiers de Québec
4200, boulevard Dorchester Ouest
Westmount, QB H3Z 1V4
Téléphone: (514) 935-2501
Télécopieur: (514) 935-1799
Web site: http://www.oiiq.org

Rhode Island Board of Nursing
Registration and Nursing Education
105 Cannon Building
Three Capitol Hill
Providence, RI 02908
Phone: (401) 222-5700
Fax: (401) 222-3352
Web site: http://www.health.ri.gov/for/nurses/index.php

Saskatchewan Registered Nurses' Association
2066 Retallack Street
Regina, SK S4T 7X5
Phone: (306) 359-4200
Fax: (306) 359-0257
Web site: http://www.srna.org

South Carolina State Board of Nursing
110 Centerview Drive, Suite 202
Columbia, SC 29210
Phone: (803) 896-4550
Fax: (803) 896-4515
Web site: http://www.llr.state.sc.us/pol/nursing

South Dakota Board of Nursing
4300 South Louise Avenue, Suite 201
Sioux Falls, SD 57106-3115
Phone: (605) 362-2760
Fax: (605) 362-2768
Web site: http://doh.sd.gov/boards/nursing

Tennessee State Board of Nursing
227 French Landing, Suite 300
Heritage Place, Metro Center
Nashville, TN 37243
Phone: (615) 532-5166
Fax: (615) 741-7899
Web site: http://tn.gov/health/topic/nursing-board

Texas Board of Nursing
333 Guadalupe Street, Suite 3-460
Austin, TX 78701
Phone: (512) 305-7400
Fax: (512) 305-7401
Web site: http://www.bon.state.tx.us

Utah State Board of Nursing
Heber M. Wells Building, 4th Floor
160 East 300 South

Salt Lake City, UT 84111
Phone: (801) 530-6628
Fax: (801) 530-6511
Web site: http://www.dopl.utah.gov/licensing/nursing.html

Vermont State Board of Nursing
Office of Professional Regulation
National Life Building North F1.2
Montpelier, VT 05620-3402
Phone: (802) 828-2396
Fax: (802) 828-2484
Web site: http://www.vtprofessionals.org/opr1/nurses

Virginia Board of Nursing
Department of Health Professions
Perimeter Center
9960 Mayland Drive, Suite 300
Henrico, VA 23233
Phone: (804) 367-4515
Fax: (804) 527-4455
Web site: www.dhp.virginia.gov/nursing

Washington State Nursing Care Quality Assurance Commission
Department of Health
PO Box 47864
Olympia, WA 98504-7864
Phone: (360) 236-4700
Fax: (360) 236-4738
Web site: http://www.doh.wa.gov/LicensesPermitsandCertificates/NursingCommission

West Virginia Board of Examiners for Registered Professional Nurses
101 Dee Drive
Charleston, WV 25311
Phone: (304) 558-3596
Fax: (304) 558-3666
Web site: http://www.wvrnboard.com

Wisconsin Department of Regulation and Licensing
1400 E. Washington Avenue
Madison, WI 53703
Phone: (608) 226-2112
Fax: (608) 261-7083
Web site: http:www.drl.wi.gov/board_detail.asp?boardid+42&locid=0

Wyoming State Board of Nursing
1810 Pioneer Avenue
Cheyenne, WY 82001
Phone: (307) 777-7601
Fax: (307) 777-3519
Web site: http://nursing.state.wy.us

Yukon Registered Nurses Association
Suite 204
4133-4th Avenue
Whitehorse, YT Y1A 1H8
Phone: (867) 667-4062
Fax: (867) 668-5123
Web site: http://yrna.ca

Bibliography

1. The Nursing Care of the Childbearing Family

Lippincott Williams & Wilkins. (2013). *Lippincott nursing procedures* (6th ed.). Philadelphia, PA: Author.

Pillitteri, A. (2014). *Maternal & child health nursing: Care of the childbearing and childrearing family* (7th ed.). Philadelphia, PA: Lippincott Williams & Wilkins.

Ricci, S., & Kyle, T. (2013). *Maternity and pediatric nursing* (2nd ed.). Philadelphia, PA: Lippincott Williams & Wilkins.

Simpson, K. R., & Creehan, P. A. (2014). *Association of women's health, obstetric, and neonatal nurses (AWHONN) perinatal nursing* (4th ed.). Philadelphia, PA: Lippincott Williams & Wilkins.

2. The Nursing Care of Children

Kyle, T., & Carman, S. (2013). *Essentials of pediatric nursing* (2nd ed.). Philadelphia, PA: Lippincott Williams & Wilkins.

Lippincott Williams & Wilkins. (2013). *Lippincott nursing procedures* (6th ed.). Philadelphia, PA: Author.

Pillitteri, A. (2014). *Maternal & child health nursing: Care of the childbearing and childrearing family* (7th ed.). Philadelphia, PA: Lippincott Williams & Wilkins.

Ricci, S., & Kyle, T. (2013). *Maternity and pediatric nursing* (2nd ed.). Philadelphia, PA: Lippincott Williams & Wilkins.

3. The Nursing Care of Adults with Medical and Surgical Health Problems

Ellis, J., & Hartley, C. (2011). *Managing and coordinating nursing care* (5th ed.). Philadelphia, PA: Lippincott Williams & Wilkins.

Karch, A. (2014). *Lippincott's nursing drug guide.* Philadelphia, PA: Lippincott Williams & Wilkins.

Lippincott Williams & Wilkins. (2013). *Lippincott nursing procedures* (6th ed.). Philadelphia, PA: Author.

Marquis, B., & Huston, C. (2015). *Leadership roles and management functions in nursing* (8th ed.). Philadelphia, PA: Lippincott Williams & Wilkins.

Smeltzer, B., et al. (2014). *Brunner and Suddarth's textbook of medical-surgical nursing* (13th ed.). Philadelphia, PA: Lippincott Williams & Wilkins.

Taylor, C., et al. (2015). *Fundamentals of nursing* (8th ed.). Philadelphia, PA: Lippincott Williams & Wilkins.

Weber, J. R., & Kelley, J. (2014). *Health assessment in nursing* (5th ed.). Philadelphia, PA: Lippincott Williams & Wilkins.

4. The Nursing Care of Clients with Psychiatric Disorders and Mental Health Problems

Andrews, M., & Boyle, J. (2012). *Transcultural concepts in nursing care* (6th ed.). Philadelphia, PA: Lippincott Williams & Wilkins.

Boyd, M. A. (2015). *Psychiatric nursing: Contemporary practice* (5th ed.). Philadelphia, PA: Lippincott Williams & Wilkins.

Karch, A. (2014). *Lippincott's nursing drug guide.* Philadelphia, PA: Lippincott Williams & Wilkins.

Videbeck, S. (2014). *Psychiatric mental health nursing* (6th ed.). Philadelphia, PA: Lippincott Williams & Wilkins.

Content Mastery and Test-Taking Skill Self-Analysis

Use the chart below to identify the subject matter and the reason you missed the question. Place a check mark in the columns for questions you did not answer correctly and why, and then total each column. The key ( ) to effective review is to understand your knowledge deficits and focus additional review on those subjects and reasons for not answering the question.

Review Strategies

Test Number	Subject (Care of childbearing family, care of children, care of adults, care of clients with psychiatric disorders and mental health problems)	Score

Total number of questions missed:

Use the chart below to identify the subject matter and the reason you missed the question. Use the following codes to note the client need area of the question you missed:

MC = Management of care; SI = Safety and infection control; HM = Health promotion and maintenance; PA = Physiological adaptation; PI = Psychosocial integrity; PP = Pharmacological and parenteral therapies; RR = Reduction of risk potential; BC = Basic care and comfort

Question #	Client need	Misread/ misunder-stood the question	Missed key word(s)	Did not read all options	Changed answer	Missed certain type of ques-tions (often multiple response questions)	Did not remember subject matter	Did not under-stand subject matter	Did not recognize rationale for correct answer	Made an incor-rect guess	Did not under-stand meaning of term in question	Other
1												
2												
3												
4												
5												
6												
7												
8												
9												
10												
11												
12												
13												
14												
15												
16												
17												
18												
19												
20												

(continued)

Question #	Client need	Misread/ misunder- stood the question	Missed key word(s)	Did not read all options	Changed answer	Missed certain type of ques- tions (often multiple response questions)	Did not remember subject matter	Did not under- stand subject matter	Did not recognize rationale for correct answer	Made an incor- rect guess	Did not under- stand meaning of term in question	Other
21												
22												
23												
24												
25												
26												
27												
28												
29												
30												
31												
32												
33												
34												
35												
36												
37												
38												
39												
40												
41												
42												
43												
44												
45												
46												
47												
48												
49												
50												
51												
52												
53												
54												
55												
56												
57												
58												
59												
60												
61												
62												
63												

Question #	Client need	Misread/misunderstood the question	Missed key word(s)	Did not read all options	Changed answer	Missed certain type of questions (often multiple response questions)	Did not remember subject matter	Did not understand subject matter	Did not recognize rationale for correct answer	Made an incorrect guess	Did not understand meaning of term in question	Other
64												
65												
66												
67												
68												
69												
70												
71												
72												
73												
74												
75												
76												
77												
78												
79												
80												
81												
82												
83												
84												
85												
86												
87												
88												
89												
90												
91												
92												
93												
94												
95												
96												
97												
98												
99												
100												
101												
102												
103												
104												
105												

(continued)

Question #	Client need	Misread/ misunder- stood the question	Missed key word(s)	Did not read all options	Changed answer	Missed certain type of ques- tions (often multiple response questions)	Did not remember subject matter	Did not under- stand subject matter	Did not recognize rationale for correct answer	Made an incor- rect guess	Did not under- stand meaning of term in question	Other
106												
107												
108												
109												
110												
111												
112												
113												
114												
115												
116												
117												
118												
119												
120												
121												
122												
123												
124												
125												
126												
127												
128												
129												
130												
131												
132												
133												
134												
135												
136												
137												
138												
139												
140												
141												
142												
143												
144												
145												
146												
147												
148												

Question #	Client need	Misread/ misunder- stood the question	Missed key word(s)	Did not read all options	Changed answer	Missed certain type of ques- tions (often multiple response questions)	Did not remember subject matter	Did not under- stand subject matter	Did not recognize rationale for correct answer	Made an incor- rect guess	Did not under- stand meaning of term in question	Other
149												
150												
151												
152												
153												
154												
155												
156												
157												
158												
159												
160												
161												
162												
163												
164												
165												
166												
167												
168												
169												
170												
171												
172												
173												
174												
175												
176												
177												
178												
179												
180												
181												
182												
183												
184												
185												
186												
187												
188												
189												
190												

- How many questions in each area of client needs did you miss?
- How does this compare with other exam results from this review?

Lower _____ Same _____ Higher _____ NA _____

If you missed questions because you misread questions, missed key words, or changed answers, review *Lippincott's Q&A for NCLEX-RN* Part I.

If you missed questions because you did not remember or understand the content, review that content in *Lippincott's Q&A for NCLEX-RN* Part II and your other nursing references.

If you missed questions because you did not pace yourself, practice taking timed test questions and pacing yourself to allow for sufficient time for all questions.

What is the pattern of the types of questions you are missing?

_____

_____

_____

What is your action plan for further study?

_____

_____

_____